PERIODONTICS

Sixth Edition

Commissioning Editor: Alison Taylor
Development Editor: Lulu Stader
Project Manager: Frances Affleck
Designer/Design Direction: Kirsteen Wright
Illustration Manager: Bruce Hogarth

Sixth Edition

PERIODONTICS

B. M. Eley BDS FDSRCS PhD

*Formerly Professor and Vice-Chairman, Division of Periodontology and Preventive Dentistry,
Guy's, King's and St Thomas' Dental Institute, London, UK*

M. Soory FDSRCS PhD FHEA

Periodontology, King's College London Dental Institute, London, UK

J. D. Manson MChD PhD FDSRCS

Formerly Senior Lecturer in Periodontology, Eastman Dental Institute, London, UK

SAUNDERS

ELSEVIER

Edinburgh   London   New York   Oxford   Philadelphia   St Louis   Sydney   Toronto   2010

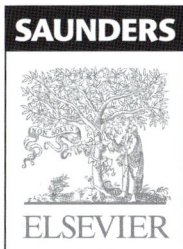

SAUNDERS
ELSEVIER

© 2000, J. D. Manson and B. M. Eley.
© 2004, 2010, Elsevier Limited. All rights reserved.

First published 1983
Second edition 1989
Third edition 1995
Fourth edition 2000
Fifth edition 2004
Sixth edition 2010
  Reprinted 2010 (twice)

ISBN: 9780702030659

British Library Cataloguing in Publication Data
A catalogue record for this book is available from the British Library

Library of Congress Cataloging in Publication Data
A catalog record for this book is available from the Library of Congress

Notice
Knowledge and best practice in this field are constantly changing. As new research and experience broaden our
knowledge, changes in practice, treatment and drug therapy may become necessary or appropriate. Readers are
advised to check the most current information provided (i) on procedures featured or (ii) by the manufacturer
of each product to be administered, to verify the recommended dose or formula, the method and duration of
administration, and contraindications. It is the responsibility of the practitioner, relying on their own experience
and knowledge of the patient, to make diagnoses, to determine dosages and the best treatment for each individual
patient, and to take all appropriate safety precautions. To the fullest extent of the law, neither the Publisher nor the
Editors assume any liability for any injury and/or damage to persons or property arising out or related to any use
of the material contained in this book.

The Publisher

ELSEVIER
your source for books,
journals and multimedia
in the health sciences
www.elsevierhealth.com

Working together to grow
libraries in developing countries

www.elsevier.com | www.bookaid.org | www.sabre.org

ELSEVIER   BOOK AID
             International   Sabre Foundation

The
publisher's
policy is to use
**paper manufactured
from sustainable forests**

Printed in China

Contents

Preface to the sixth edition

Knowledge encompassing the aetiopathogenesis of periodontal diseases and their management has advanced slowly but surely over the decades. Periodontology is a relatively small monospeciality, which represents extraordinary scope for academic development and clinical practice, bordering on boundaries of other speciality disciplines. It includes the areas of microbiology, inflammatory pathology, immunology, genetics and dental medicine in the aetiopathogeneses of periodontal diseases; and concepts of dental hygiene, restorative dentistry, dental medicine for adjunctive therapy and surgical intervention as required, for their management.

This unique presentation provides the basis of a multidisciplinary approach to the management of diseases of the periodontium with a possible outcome on systemic conditions, notably those included in the metabolic syndrome. There are several adjunctive treatment measures to combat its inflammatory pathogenesis which could impact on the inflammatory loading associated with these systemic diseases. Current thinking on the subject points to applications of the risk factors for periodontal diseases as markers of susceptibility to diseases associated with an over-exuberant inflammatory response such as rheumatoid arthritis and other auto-immune diseases; in addition to associations seen with metabolic and cardiovascular diseases. A cause and effect relationship is more difficult to prove.

Essential features of these developments and implications on treatment are covered in this edition.

Basic concepts of dental hygiene underpin the successful outcome of initial treatment and more sophisticated interventions in the management of periodontal diseases, with emphasis on a team approach incorporating the patient and operator. Health education in this context needs universal application within the profession.

Increasingly, the importance of genetic susceptibility has been underscored, in the presence of the primary aetiological agent, plaque. This often explains diversity in disease presentation and response to treatment methods in a range of age groups; also influenced by environmental factors, such as smoking.

A multifactorial basis for the aetiology and pathogenesis of periodontal diseases and diverse treatment options make it a challenging discipline that has shown progressive evolution with time.

We would like to thank Mr C.A. Waterman for his help with the chapter on mucogingival problems and their treatment and Professor R.M. Watson for his help with the section on dental implants.

J.D.M.
M.S.
B.M.E.

Preface to the first edition

There is now a considerable body of knowledge about the aetiology and pathogenesis of periodontal disease. Yet this knowledge is scarcely applied; chronic gingivitis and chronic inflammatory periodontal disease remain universal and tooth loss in the adult is still regarded by many people as an inevitable part of the ageing process. There are several reasons for this sorry state of affairs, including socio-economic factors beyond the influence of the dental profession. One factor which is wholly dependent upon the profession, is the standard of undergraduate teaching. Periodontics still occupies a minor position in the curriculum of many dental schools and is regarded by too many undergraduates and dentists as an esoteric subject peripheral to the main body of conservative dentistry.

This basic text has been written in an attempt to make our understanding of periodontal disease accessible to the undergraduate, to hygienists and to any interested reader. The main emphasis is on the plaque theory and on the prevention and early diagnosis of the disease. I have tried to avoid too great an emphasis on surgical techniques. Periodontics is not a surgical discipline; such techniques have to be resorted to only when prevention, early diagnosis and treatment techniques fail.

I am indebted to many of my colleagues, recognized in the text, for providing illustrative material, to Dr Barry Eley for his valuable comments, to Mr James Morgan of the Eastman Dental Hospital and Mr Peter Gordon for help with photography and to Mrs Jenny Halstead for her drawings without which this text would be incomplete.

J.D.M.

Dedication

To my late wife in heaven, Julie
B.M.E.

To my husband and son for their support and encouragement
M.S.

To my wife for her patience and help over all these years
J.D.M.

The periodontal tissues

The masticatory system consists of the mandible, maxilla, temporomandibular joints, muscles of mastication and teeth with associated periodontal tissues comprising gingivae, periodontal ligament, cementum and alveolar bone.

It is essential to view this system as an interdependent functional unit. Breakdown of the dentition may affect other components of the masticatory system; alterations in the functional activity of the muscles of mastication or temporomandibular joints can affect the dental tissues. Like all vital tissues, the tissues of the masticatory system are in a state of constant activity. There is constant turnover of cells and their matrices in a cyclical manner, associated with cell proliferation, synthesis of collagen and apoptosis. This activity is influenced by age, nutritional and hormonal status and by functional demand. It is also affected by disease.

Knowledge of the periodontal tissue in health is essential to an understanding of its behaviour in disease.

THE GINGIVAE

INTRODUCTION

The gingiva is that part of the oral mucosa which surrounds the tooth and covers the alveolar ridge. It is part of the tooth-supporting structure of the periodontium, and by forming a connection with the tooth via the gingival sulcus, it protects the underlying tissues of the tooth attachment from the oral environment. Being tooth dependent, when teeth are extracted, the gingivae disappear.

Like all vital tissues the gingiva can adapt itself to changes in its environment, and the mouth which is the first part of the alimentary tract and the site of the initial preparation of food in digestion may be regarded as a relatively hostile environment. The oral tissues are exposed to an enormous range of stimuli. The temperature and consistency of food and drink, its chemical composition, acidity and alkalinity vary considerably. The number of bacteria in the mouth is immense and their variety beyond exact definition. Add to this the insults and irritations of dental manipulations and one can only be impressed by the sheer resilience of the oral mucosa and the efficiency of gingival defence mechanisms, which include:

1. The salivary flow and contents of saliva, e.g. lysozyme, immunoglobulin (Ig) A
2. Cell turnover and surface desquamation
3. The activity of the immune mechanisms.

The junction between the tooth and the oral mucosa, the dentogingival junction, is unique and peculiarly vulnerable. It is the only attachment in the body between a soft tissue and a calcified tissue which is exposed to the external environment. This junction is a highly dynamic tissue with its own battery of protective mechanisms.

Healthy gingiva is pink, firm, knife-edged and scalloped to conform to the contour of the teeth (**Fig. 1.1**). Its colour may vary with the amount of melanin pigmentation in the epithelium, the degree of keratinization of the epithelium and the vascularity and fibrous nature of the underlying connective tissue (**Fig. 1.2**). In the Caucasian individual pigmentation is minimal; in patients of African or Asian origin brown or blue-black areas of pigmentation may cover a great part of the gingiva; in Mediterranean people occasional patches of pigmentation are found. It is important to distinguish physiological pigmentation from that which occurs in some diseases and with metal contamination.

The gingiva is divided into two zones: the marginal gingiva and attached gingiva (**Fig. 1.3**).

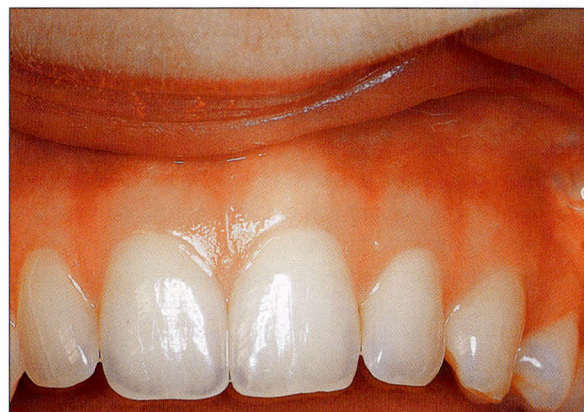

Fig. 1.1 Healthy gingivae in a girl of 19 years.

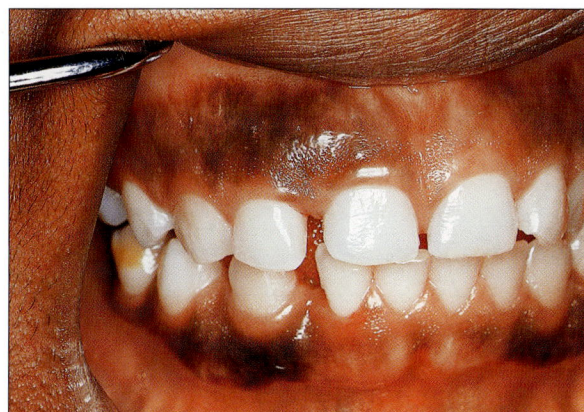

Fig. 1.2 Healthy gingivae in a black girl of 16 years showing normal melanin pigmentation.

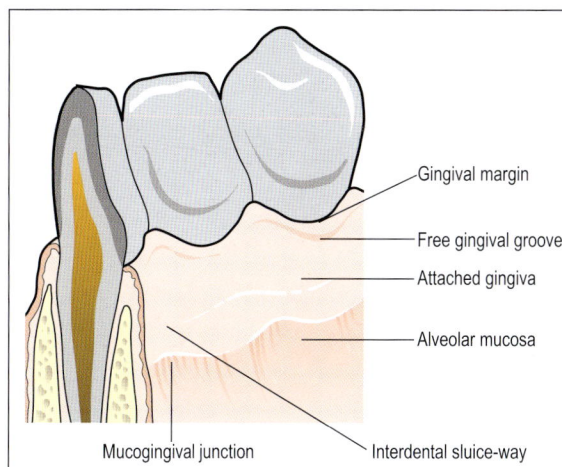

Gingival margin
Free gingival groove
Attached gingiva
Alveolar mucosa
Mucogingival junction
Interdental sluice-way

Fig. 1.3 Diagram illustrating the anatomical features of the gingiva.

THE GINGIVAL MARGIN

The marginal gingiva forms a cuff 1–2 mm wide around the neck of the tooth and is the external wall of the gingival crevice which is 0–2 mm deep. This cuff can be separated from the tooth by careful manipulation of a blunt probe. Between the teeth the margin forms a cone-shaped gingival papilla, the labial surface of which is frequently indented by a groove called a 'sluice-way'. The papilla fills the space in the interdental embrasure apical to the contact point and its facial-lingual shape conforms to the curvature of the cemento-enamel junction to form the interdental col (**Figs 1.4, 1.5**).

The surface of the gingival margin is smooth in contrast to that of the attached gingiva, from which it is demarcated by an indentation called the 'free gingival' groove (see **Fig. 1.3**).

ATTACHED GINGIVA

The attached gingiva or 'functional mucosa' extends from the free gingival groove to the mucogingival junction where it meets the alveolar mucosa (see **Figs 1.1–1.3**). The attached gingiva is a mucoperiosteum which is tightly bound to the underlying alveolar bone. At the mucogingival junction the mucoperiosteum splits so that the alveolar mucosa is separated from the periosteum by a loose, highly vascular, connective tissue. Thus the alveolar mucosa is a relatively loose and mobile tissue, deep red, in marked contrast to the pale pink attached gingiva (see **Fig. 1.1**). The surface of the attached gingiva is stippled like orange peel. This stippling varies considerably. It is most prominent on facial surfaces and often disappears in old age. There is some doubt about the cause of the stippling but it appears to coincide with epithelial rete pegs.

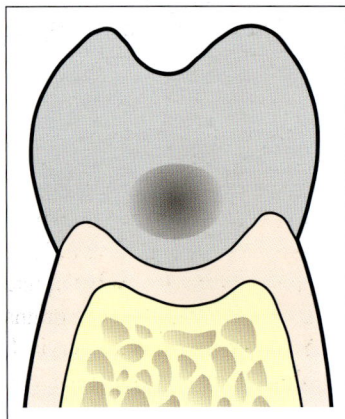

Fig. 1.4 The interdental gingiva in the shape of a 'col' reflects the contours of the tooth contact area.

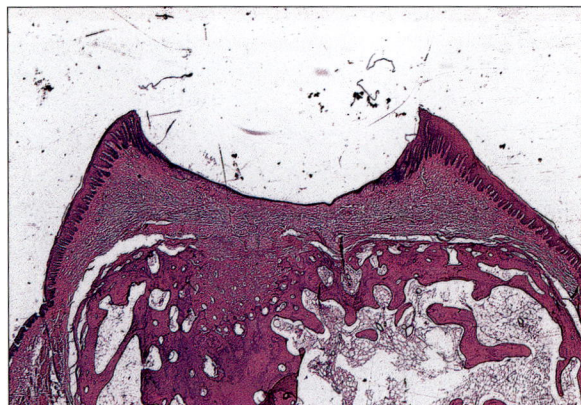

Fig. 1.5 Histological section of the interdental 'col' area showing alveolar bone, gingival connective tissue and surface epithelium which is thin in the deepest part of the 'col'.

The width of the attached gingiva can vary from about 0 to 9 mm. It is usually widest in the incisor region (3–5 mm) and narrowest over mandibular canines and premolars. In the past it has been assumed that some attached gingiva is necessary to maintain the health of the gingival margin by separating the stable margin from the mobile alveolar mucosa, but this does not appear to be the case in the clean mouth. This variation in width has given rise to controversy about what form of anatomy is compatible with health, and techniques have been devised to widen areas of attached gingiva considered to be too narrow irrespective of whether disease is present or not. Any width, even a zero width, is acceptable if the tissue is healthy.

MICROSCOPIC FEATURES OF THE GINGIVA

The gingival margin consists of a core of fibrous connective tissue covered by stratified squamous epithelium which, like all squamous epithelium, undergoes constant renewal by continuous cell reproduction in its deepest layers and shedding of the superficial layers. The two activities are held in balance so that the thickness of the epithelium remains constant. It has the characteristic layers of squamous epithelium:

1. The basal or formative cell layers of columnar or cuboidal cells
2. The prickle-cells or spinous layer (stratum spinosum) of polygonal cells
3. The granular layer (stratum granulosum), in which the cells are flatter and contain many particles of keratohyaline
4. The cornified layer (stratum corneum) in which the cells have become flat and shrunken, and keratinized or parakeratinized.

The mitotic rate of oral epithelium varies from place to place, with age and also from one animal to another. Turnover times in the experimental animal are said to be: palate, tongue and cheek 5–6 days, gingiva 10–12 days.

Like all epithelial cells, gingival epithelium cells are connected to each other and to the underlying connective tissue corium by thickenings on the periphery of the cells called hemidesmosomes. The epithelium is joined to the underlying corium by a thin basal lamina made of a protein-polysaccharide complex which is permeable to fluid. Seen by electron microscopy it can be resolved into two layers, the lamina lucida and the lamina densa.

The epithelium of the outer or oral surface of the gingival margin is keratinized or parakeratinized while the epithelium of the inner or crevicular surface is thinner and not keratinized. Contrary to popular opinion, non-keratinized oral epithelium is not necessarily always more permeable than keratinized epithelium. Intact epithelium is an effective barrier against microorganisms which can breach damaged epithelium, but intact epithelium is permeable to many smaller substances such as the molecules of skin antiseptics, topical anaesthetics and vasodilators, e.g. glyceryl trinitrate.

Pigmentation is produced by pigment-forming melanocytes. However, variation in pigmentation is not produced by variation in the number of these cells but by genetically determined variation in their pigment-producing capacity. The ratio of melanocytes to the keratin-producing epithelial cells is relatively constant at 1:36 cells.

The gingival connective tissue is made up of a mesh of collagen fibre bundles running in a ground substance which contains blood vessels and nerves plus fibroblasts, macrophages, mast cells, lymphocytes, plasma cells and other cells of the defence system, which are more numerous near the junctional epithelium, where immune activity is maintained. In common with other connective tissues, the gingival fibrous connective tissues are composed of a specialized fibroblast cell and a collagenous fibrous network embedded in an extracellular matrix composed of proteoglycans and other matrix glycoproteins. The normal connective tissue function involves constant remodelling of the matrix components and is dependent upon the interactions between the cells and the matrix molecules in their environment. This involves the production and attachment to their receptors of signal molecules such as growth and differentiation factors and cell adhesion molecules, and their interaction with components of the extracellular matrix. Various proteoglycans appear to play an important role in tissue remodelling and the maintenance of structural integrity.

THE GROUND SUBSTANCE

Connective-tissue cells and fibres, together with vessels and nerves, are embedded in an amorphous, non-fibrous and non-cellular matrix made up of glycosaminoglycans (GAGs), proteoglycans and glycoproteins. All the components of the matrix are synthesized and secreted by fibroblasts. The most common GAG is hyaluronic acid (hyaluronan), large amounts of which are found in gingiva. Proteoglycans are composed of a central protein core to which is attached a variable number of highly anionic GAG chains.

The structure of proteoglycans depends on the type of GAG chains attached to its protein core. The soft tissues such as the gingival tissue and the periodontal ligament (see below) contain small dermatan sulphate proteoglycans and a larger molecular weight chondroitin sulphate proteoglycan, versican, which is capable of interacting with hyaluronan (Embery et al 1987; Larjava et al 1992). GAGs are long unbranched polysaccharides which can bind large amounts of water. As a result of this, tissues containing large amounts of GAG resist compressive forces well. Versican, hyaluronan and link proteins in the periodontal ligament have been shown to play an important role in experimental tooth movement in the rat model (Sato et al 2002). GAG also facilitates the transport of nutrients through the extracellular spaces. The matrix also transports metabolic products, cells and chemical messengers known as cytokines which moderate cellular function. Proteoglycans are also present on cell surfaces, for example syndecan and CD44, where they function in the control of cell attachment, migration and proliferation and the binding of growth factors such as transforming growth factor beta (TGF-β) (Gallagher et al 1986).

One of the most important glycoproteins is fibronectin. This is a large protein which binds to cells, collagen and proteoglycans. It is important in promoting the adhesion of fibroblasts to the extracellular matrix, and also plays a role in the alignment of collagen fibres.

THE GINGIVAL FIBRES

The connective tissue of the gingiva (**Fig. 1.6**) is organized to keep the gingival margin tight around the neck of the tooth and to maintain the integrity of the dentogingival attachment.

The arrangement of these fibres is complicated but they have been described as being divided into several discernible groups of collagen fibre bundles:

1. Dentogingival or free gingival fibres which are attached to cementum and fan out into the gingiva and over the alveolar margin to merge with the periosteum of the attached gingiva
2. Alveolar-gingival or alveolar crest fibres which arise from the alveolar crest and run coronally into the gingiva
3. Circular fibres which encircle the tooth
4. Trans-septal fibres which run from tooth to tooth coronally to the alveolar septum.

There is a great deal of interlinking between fibre groups and special stains are needed to define the fibres.

Collagen is synthesized by fibroblasts and is secreted in an inactive form, procollagen, which is then converted into tropocollagen. In the extracellular space, tropocollagen is polymerized into collagen fibrils which are then aggregated into collagen bundles by the formation of cross-linkages. Different forms of collagen may be secreted and each is

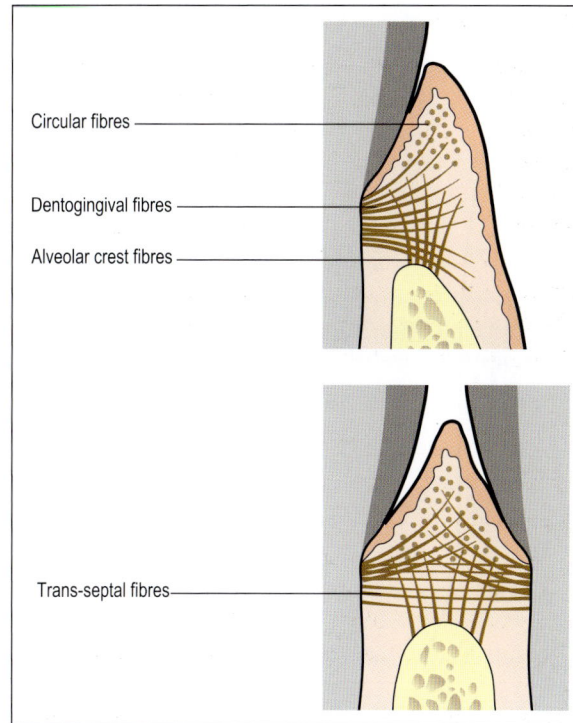

Fig. 1.6 Gingival fibre groups: dentogingival, circular, alveolar crest and trans-septal fibres.

based on variations in the composition of the basic tropocollagen molecule. The most common form found in the gingiva is Type I collagen which forms the major fibre bundles and the loose collagenous fibres. Some Type III and V collagens are also present. Type VI collagen is present in the basement membranes of blood vessels and the overlying epithelium.

GINGIVAL BLOOD, LYMPH AND NERVE SUPPLY

The gingiva has a rich blood supply derived from three sources: supraperiosteal and periodontal ligament vessels plus alveolar vessels, which emerge from the alveolar crest (**Fig. 1.7**). These link in the gingiva to form capillary loops in the connective-tissue papillae between the epithelial rete pegs. Lymphatic drainage starts in connective-tissue papillae and drains into regional lymph nodes: from the mandibular gingiva into the cervical, submandibular and submental nodes; from the maxillary gingiva into the deep cervical lymph nodes.

The nerve supply is derived from branches of the trigeminal nerve. A number of nerve endings have been identified in the gingival connective tissue as tactile corpuscles, and temperature and pain receptors.

THE INTERDENTAL GINGIVA

The gingiva between the teeth is concave and has been described as a 'col' which joins the facial and lingual papillae (see **Figs 1.4, 1.5**). Where teeth make contact, the cols conform to the shape of the teeth apical to the contact area. Where neighbouring teeth do not contact, there is no col and the interdental gingiva is flat or convex.

The epithelium of the col is very thin, not keratinized, and made up of only a few cell layers. Its structure probably reflects its sheltered position. Turnover of interdental epithelial cells is the same as that of the rest of the gingiva.

The interdental region is of special importance as it is the site of the most persistent bacterial stagnation and its structure makes it especially vulnerable. *It is the site of the initial lesion in gingivitis.*

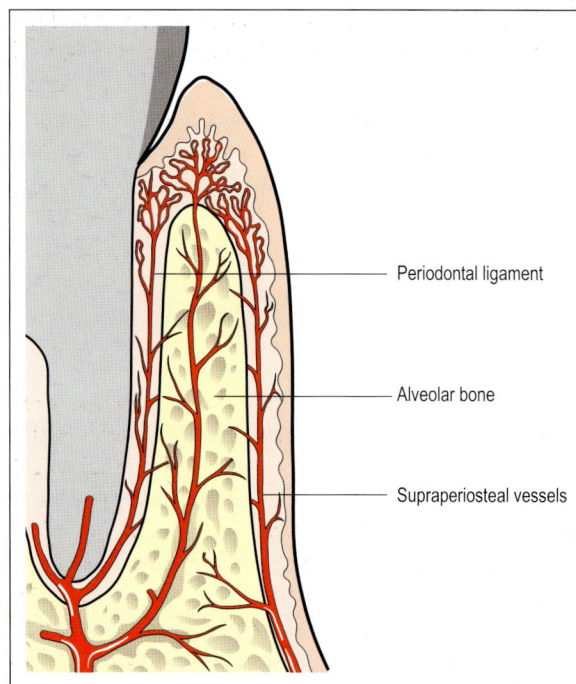

Fig. 1.7 The rich gingival blood supply derives from the: periodontal ligament, alveolar bone and supraperiosteal vessels.

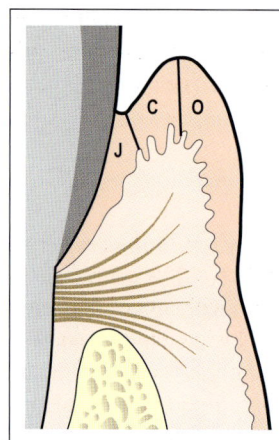

Fig. 1.8 The dentogingival junction. There are three zones of gingival epithelium: oral epithelium (O), crevicular (or sulcus) epithelium (C) and the junctional epithelium (J).

THE DENTOGINGIVAL JUNCTION

It is possible to define three zones of gingival epithelium (**Fig. 1.8**). Oral epithelium extends from the mucogingival junction to the gingival margin where crevicular (or sulcular) epithelium lines the gingival crevice (or sulcus). At the base of the crevice, the connection between the gingiva and the tooth is mediated by a special kind of epithelium called junctional epithelium.

In health, the junctional epithelium lies against enamel and extends to the cemento-enamel junction. If there is gingival recession, the junctional epithelium lies on cementum. Thus the base of the gingival crevice is the free surface of the junctional epithelium. It is said that in perfect health, the depth of the crevice is zero so that there is no crevicular epithelium and oral epithelium therefore merges directly into the junctional epithelium. This does not occur in humans.

At an ultrastructural level, a very thin basement lamina lies between the junctional epithelial cells and the connective-tissue corium, and between the junctional epithelium and the tooth surface. The latter basement lamina and related hemidesmosomes form the 'epithelial attachment', which is a product of epithelial cells. If gingivectomy is carried out and the junctional epithelium is completely removed, on healing a new gingival margin plus new junctional epithelium are formed whether the gingiva is on enamel, dentine or cementum.

The junctional epithelium is very fragile and does not form a barrier against probing. Its cells are larger than those of oral epithelium and loosely connected together, indeed the cell-to-cell connection is more fragile than the attachment to the tooth surface. Unlike keratinized epithelial cells of the crevice, the cells of the junctional epithelium can attach via hemidesmosomes to tooth surface.

The junctional epithelium in adults is about 40 cells long from apex to crevicular surface but varies from 0.25 to 1.35 mm; in the young it is a narrow sleeve as thin as 3–4 cells; in the adult it is 10–20 cells wide. Although it undergoes constant renewal, with cell division taking place throughout its structure, the junctional epithelium is relatively homogeneous and without any pattern of cell differentiation. Although the turnover time for human junctional epithelium is not known, in other primates it is said to be approximately 4–6 days, i.e. half that of oral epithelium which is roughly 10–12 days. Desquamation of the junctional epithelium takes place through the small free area at the base of the gingival crevice. Listgarten (1972) has calculated that the rate of cellular exfoliation from a unit surface of junctional epithelium is 50–100 times as fast as that from a unit of oral gingival epithelium. A small number of leucocytes (neutrophils) are often found within the junctional epithelium.

In contrast to oral gingival epithelium and crevicular epithelium, the junctional epithelium is relatively permeable and allows a two-way movement of a variety of substances:

1. From corium into the crevice: Gingival fluid exudate, polymorphonuclear leucocytes, various cells of the immune system plus immunoglobulins and complement. It is the exit point for most of the leucocytes found in saliva. In inflammation the movement of fluid and cells increases and as the population of leucocytes increases, the junctional epithelium may degenerate and become even more permeable. Some research workers believe that in perfect health, there is no passage of gingival fluid into the crevice.

2. From crevice into the corium: Foreign materials such as carbon particles, trypan blue (mol. wt 960) and many other substances inserted into the gingival crevice are found subsequently in the gingival corium and the bloodstream. *Microorganisms cannot penetrate junctional epithelium* but a large number of substances, some of them with high molecular weights, have been shown to pass through the intercellular spaces of the junctional epithelium. This is an extremely important finding as it is believed that gingival inflammation is initiated by bacterial enzymes, and metabolic products, which diffuse from the crevice through the junctional epithelium into the gingival connective tissue.

Because of the permeability of junctional epithelium it is inevitable that the tissue defence mechanisms should be in a constant state of alertness and this is manifested by an infiltration of inflammatory cells, lymphocytes and plasma cells in the underlying corium. This used to be interpreted as a sign of disease but indicates constant activity of defence mechanisms in health.

FORMATION OF THE DENTOGINGIVAL ATTACHMENT

There has been some controversy about the origin and structure of the attachment tissues but using electron microscope findings and the results of autoradiographic studies of cellular activity, a consensus seems to have been achieved.

When enamel formation is complete the reduced enamel epithelium is attached to enamel by a basal lamina and hemidesmosomes. As the tooth penetrates the oral mucosa, the reduced enamel epithelium unites with the oral epithelium and with continuing eruption this epithelium condenses along the crown. Ameloblasts gradually atrophy and are replaced by squamous epithelium, i.e. the junctional epithelium which forms a collar around the fully erupted tooth. As already described, junctional epithelium, like all squamous epithelium, is a constantly renewing structure with epithelial cells moving coronally to be shed at the free surface into the bottom of the crevice.

GINGIVAL CREVICULAR FLUID

If a filter paper strip is inserted into the gingival crevice it will absorb fluid already in the crevice and may also provoke an outward flow of fluid. This also happens in mastication, on tooth brushing and with any other stimulation of the gingivae; the flow is greatly increased when the gingivae are inflamed. Sex hormones, oestrogen and progesterone appear to increase the flow, perhaps by causing increased permeability of gingival blood vessels. Certain chemotactic factors found in plaque may also increase the flow. This fluid is an inflammatory exudate and carries polymorphonuclear leucocytes and other antimicrobial substances. It forms part of the defence mechanism of the dentogingival junction. If a patient is on systemic tetracyclines the drug finds its way via gingival blood vessels, connective tissue and junctional epithelium into the gingival crevice. In summary, the fluid performs the following functions:

1. It washes the crevice, carrying shed epithelial cells, leucocytes, bacteria and other debris
2. The plasma proteins may influence the epithelial attachment to the tooth
3. It contains antimicrobial agents, e.g. lysozyme
4. It carries polymorphonuclear leucocytes and macrophages, which are capable of phagocytosing bacteria. It also transports immunoglobulins IgG, IgA, IgM and other factors of the immune system.

The amount of gingival crevicular fluid can be measured and used as an index of gingival inflammation. Its composition may also be determined by a variety of biochemical and immunocytochemical techniques, and it may relate to the severity of the underlying periodontal pathology.

THE PERIODONTAL LIGAMENT

A ligament is a bond, usually linking two bones together. The root of the tooth is connected to its socket in alveolar bone by a dense fibrous connective tissue which can be regarded as a ligament. Above the alveolar crest it is continuous with the gingival connective tissue and at the apical foramina with the pulp. Considerable research has been carried out into the structure, function and composition of the periodontal ligament for both functional and clinical reasons. It has the following functions:

- It is the tissue of attachment between the tooth and alveolar bone. Thus, it is responsible for resisting displacing forces and protects the dental tissues from the effects of excessive occlusal loads
- It is responsible for maintaining the tooth in a functional position during tooth eruption and the changes in tooth position which follow tooth extraction, tooth attrition or excessive occlusal loading
- Its cells form, maintain and repair alveolar bone and cementum
- Its mechanoreceptors are involved in the neurological control of mastication
- It has a rich blood supply which anastomoses with that in the marrow spaces of the bone and the gingiva and facilitates these functions.

The periodontal ligament not only connects the tooth to the jaw bone but also supports the tooth in the socket and absorbs loads imposed on the tooth thus protecting the tooth especially at the root apex. The cells of the ligament maintain and repair alveolar bone and cementum. The ligament is a reservoir from which bone and cementum forming cells are derived;

precursor cells are formed from stem cells in the bone marrow, and from there migrate into the periodontal ligament (Nagatomo et al 2006). The proprioceptor nerve endings in the ligament form part of the extremely refined neurological control of mastication and the mechanoreceptors monitor changes in pressure within the ligament space. The anastomosis of the blood supply and tissue fluid between the bone marrow spaces is very important in the maintenance of an adequate supply during compression of the ligament during functional movements. All these points are more fully discussed below.

STRUCTURE AND FUNCTION

The thickness of the ligament varies from about 0.3 to 0.1 mm. It is widest at the mouth of the socket and at the apex, and narrowest at the level of the axis of rotation of the tooth, which is slightly apical to the middle of the root. In health there is a normal range of tooth mobility. Incisors are more mobile than posterior teeth; mobility is greatest on awakening and reduces through the day. As in other parts of the skeleton, functional stresses are essential to the maintenance of the periodontal ligament's tissues. When functional stresses are heavy, the ligament becomes thicker and when a tooth is functionless the ligament can become as thin as 0.06 mm. With ageing, the ligament also becomes thinner.

The ligament consists of well-organized collagen fibre bundles about 5 µm in diameter in a ground substance matrix through which vessels and nerves course. The fibre bundles, which are inserted at one end into cementum and at the other into the socket wall as Sharpey's fibres, are usually described in identifiable groups according to their predominant orientation (**Fig. 1.9**):

1. Alveolar crest fibres run from the cementum at the neck of the tooth to the alveolar crest
2. Horizontal fibres run from cementum to the alveolar crest
3. Oblique fibres form the main component of the ligament and run from the bone in a slightly apical direction to be inserted in the cementum so that they appear to be suspending the tooth in its socket
4. Apical fibres radiate from the apex to the base of the socket. One can also include the inter-radicular fibres which are found in the furcation of multirooted teeth and like trans-septal fibres run from root to root coronal to the alveolar crest.

A single fibre bundle is difficult to trace from tooth to bone. It has been claimed that an intermediate plexus is present in the midsection of the ligament during eruption, after which it disappears. However, this has been more recently questioned. It now appears that in the fully erupted tooth, fibres cross the entire width of the periodontal space but branch *en route*

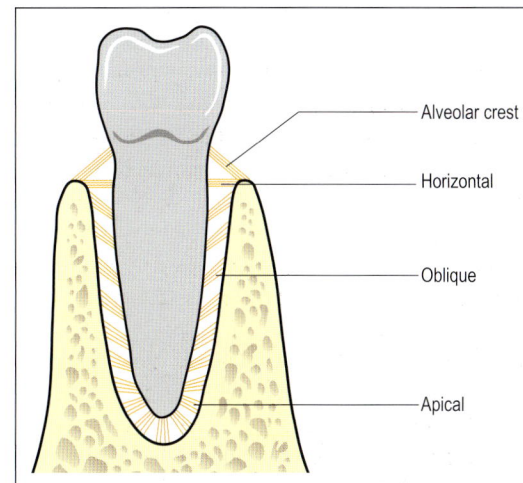

Fig. 1.9 Periodontal ligament fibre bundles.

and join neighbouring fibres to form a complex three-dimensional network. The principal fibres of the ligament do not run a straight course as they pass from bone to tooth but appear to follow a wavy pathway. Apart from these major fibre bundles, there are also less regularly orientated collagen fibre bundles.

EXTRACELLULAR MATRIX COMPONENTS OF THE PERIODONTIUM

Collagen

The periodontal ligament collagen is mostly Type I. This variety of collagen is the major protein component of most connective tissues including skin, gingiva and bone. It contains two identical α^1 chains and a chemically different α^2 chain. It is low in hydrolysine and glycosylated hydroxylysine. The periodontal ligament is also relatively rich in Type III collagen (about 20%) which consists of three α^1 III chains. It is high in hydroxyproline, low in hydroxylysine and contains cysteine. Most major periodontal ligament fibres are composed of Type I collagen. Much of the collagen is gathered together to form bundles which are approximately 5 μm in diameter and these are known as the principal fibres. The principal fibres appear to be more numerous, but smaller at their attachment to cementum than at the alveolar bone. Type III collagen is present in similar proportions to those found in embryonic tissues, and this probably reflects the high turnover rate within the ligament. Type III is more fibrillar and extensible than Type I and may be important in maintaining the integrity of the ligament during the small vertical and horizontal movements which occur during chewing.

In addition to their structural role, the extracellular matrix have also been shown to be involved either directly or indirectly in promoting cell attachment and differentiation and as a chemotactic agent for both fibroblasts and macrophages (Fulcher et al 2006).

Small amounts of other collagens are also present. Type IV is localized to basement membranes and collagen V is distributed in the matrix of the lamina propria, in close association with cells and finally type VI collagen has a microfibrillar distribution (Romanos et al 1993). Types V and XII are co-distributed with type III collagen which surrounds type I collagen in Sharpey's fibres.

The main collagen in the organic matrix of bone and cementum collagen is type I and this is virtually insoluble due to cross-links which provide the structural and mechanical stability for normal function (Bartold 2006).

Oxytalan fibres

The human periodontal ligament also contains oxytalan fibres. The ultrastructural characteristics of these fibres suggest that they are immature elastic fibres. Their function remains unknown but their fibres are thicker and more numerous in teeth which carry high loads, including abutment teeth for bridges and teeth being moved by orthodontic treatment. Thus, oxytalan fibres may have a role in tooth support. However, these fibres remain unchanged in the periodontal ligament of teeth with reduced masticatory loading. In humans, true elastic fibres are restricted to the walls of blood vessels.

Ground substance of the periodontal ligament

The ligament ground substance is an amorphous matrix of glycosaminoglycans (GAGs), proteoglycans and glycoproteins, and plays an extremely important role in the absorption of functional stresses. The GAGS are represented by several species including chondroitin sulphate, dermatan sulphate, keratin sulphate and hyaluronan (Mariotti 1993). The periodontal ligament ground substance composition is similar to that of gingival ground substance and contains hyaluronic acid (hyaluronan), small dermatan sulphate proteoglycans and a larger molecular weight chondroitin sulphate proteoglycans, versican, decorin, biglycan and syndecan, which are capable of interacting with hyaluronan (Embery et al 1987; Larjava et al 1992).

It is presumed that GAGs, proteoglycans and glycoproteins are secreted by fibroblasts. These molecules turn over at an even faster rate than collagen. They have many important functions including ion and water binding and exchange, control of collagen fibrillogenesis and fibre orientation. Their water binding functions are thought to produce a hydraulic cushion in the periodontal ligament. This cushioning effect is probably more important in resisting the forces of mastication than traction on the ligament fibres. Proteoglycans also regulate cell adhesion and growth, and have the capacity to bind and regulate growth factor activity (Bartold 2006).

The glycoproteins include the high molecular weight, insoluble, fibre-forming glycoprotein, fibronectin which is present both intra- and extracellularly (Midwood et al 2006). The structure consists of two identical disulphide-linked polypeptide chains and contains a sequence, arginine-glycine-aspartate (RGD) that binds to cells, as well as other sites that bind to collagen, heparin and fibrin (Mariotti 1993). This is thought to promote the attachment of cells to the substratum and especially to collagen. Furthermore, cells preferentially adhere to fibronectin which may be involved in cell migration and orientation (Berkowitz et al 1992). Fibronectin may have considerable biological significance within the ligament in view of its high rate of turnover. Immunochemical techniques have revealed that fibronectin is uniformly distributed throughout the periodontal ligament both during eruption and in fully erupted teeth (Steffensen et al 1992; Romanos et al 1993). However, fibronectin is expressed particularly strongly along attachment sites of the periodontal ligament collagen fibres to cementum but not to alveolar bone (Matsuura et al 1995). It is also found in the endosteal spaces, periosteum and bone lining cells at their interface with alveolar bone (Steffensen et al 1992). In the cementum its expression is weaker than in the periodontal ligament (Zhang et al 1993). Fibronectin has also been localized in the basement membrane and lamina propria (Steffensen et al 1992) with a fibrillar and diffuse distribution (Romanos et al 1993).

Ultrastructural studies (Zhang et al 1993) have localized fibronectin over collagen fibres and at certain sites at the cell-collagen interface. As loss of fibronectin has been observed during the terminal maturation of many connective tissue matrices, its continued presence within the periodontal ligament may be indicative of either the ligament retaining immature characteristics or its high turnover.

In addition to its main function as an adhesive protein, fibronectin is involved in blood coagulation, wound healing and chemotaxis (Mariotti 1993).

Another glycoprotein, termed tenascin has also been identified in the periodontal ligament and this is also characteristic of immature connective tissue. It was thought to play a prominent role in developmental processes but it has been shown that transgenic mice in which the tenascin gene is not present, nevertheless develop normally (Saga et al 1992). In contrast to other major extracellular matrix proteins, the expression of tenascin is only maintained during wound healing and in a few adult tissues including bone marrow and the periodontal tissues. In the periodontal tissues, unlike fibronectin, it is not uniformly localized throughout the periodontal ligament but rather concentrated adjacent to the alveolar bone and the cementum (Steffensen et al 1992; Becker et al 1993). It is found between less densely packed collagen fibrils of the periodontal ligament (Zhang et al 1993) and accumulated towards the alveolar bone and cementum (Steffensen et al 1992) with only weak expression throughout the alveolar bone matrix. Cementum also shows weak expression of this protein, which may have been deposited prior to mineralization (Zhang et al 1993). It is also found in the basement membrane and lamina propria (Becker et al 1993).

Some elastic fibres are present in the gingival and periodontal connective tissue and elastin, a very flexible and insoluble protein, is the major component of these (Mariotti 1993). Laminin is found exclusively in the basement membrane where it is believed to mediate the attachment of epithelium cells to type IV collagen (Mariotti 1993). In the periodontium, it has been located in the basal lamina of blood vessels and the oral, sulcus and junction epithelium (Steffensen et al 1992). Vitronectin is a protein that promotes the attachment and spreading of cells and it has been found on the cells lining the alveolar bone and cementum (Steffensen et al 1992) and also associated with the connective tissue fibres of the gingiva and periodontal ligament (Matsuura et al 1995).

CELLS OF THE PERIODONTAL LIGAMENT

The periodontal ligament tissue is developmentally derived from the inner layer of the dental follicle shortly after root development starts (Ten Cate 1994) but it is also considered that cells migrating from the dental papilla to the dental follicle also have the potential to form the periodontal ligament during odontogenesis (Palmer & Lubbock 1995). Mature periodontal ligament is a highly vascular and cellular tissue.

Fibroblasts are the most abundant cell type in the periodontal ligament and are aligned along and between the collagen fibres. It is possible that the periodontal ligament fibroblasts are motile contractile cells capable of generating a force for tooth eruption (Berkowitz et al 1992). Much of the evidence for this comes from research on the behaviour and appearance of periodontal fibroblasts in cell culture. *In vitro* periodontal fibroblasts can organize a fibrous network and can generate significant forces.

Under normal conditions *in vivo* periodontal ligament fibroblasts are primarily involved in protein synthesis. They synthesize and secrete collagen, GAGs, proteoglycans and glycoproteins. Because of the high turnover of collagen and proteoglycan within the ligament, these cells are actively engaged in protein synthesis for long periods and appear plump with abundant cytoplasm.

In addition, there is evidence that fibroblasts are also responsible for collagen degradation within the ligament (Eley & Harrison 1975). Periodontal ligament fibroblasts are also phagocytic and can take up damaged collagen fibrils. These fibrils can be seen within intracellular vacuoles in these cells at various levels of degradation (**Figs 1.10, 1.11**). The time taken for intracellular degradation of collagen may be about 30 min.

While gingival fibroblasts maintain the synthesis and integrity of the gingival connective tissue, periodontal ligament fibroblasts have specialized functions which are concerned with the formation and maintenance of the periodontal ligament including its repair or regeneration following damage (Berkowitz et al 1995). Although both gingival and periodontal ligament fibroblasts are similar in appearance when grown in culture, they have very important functional differences. Thus, in animal studies, it has been found that when tooth roots were covered with periodontal ligament cells grown in culture and then re-implanted *in vivo*, they acted as progenitor cells and gave rise to the formation of new periodontal ligament tissue (Van Dijk et al 1991; Lang et al 1995, 1998). In marked contrast, gingival fibroblasts failed to produce new tissue. Also, the total protein and extracellular matrix protein production have been shown to be higher in periodontal ligament compared with gingival fibroblasts (Somerman et al 1988; Kuru et al 1998). Moreover, the response of these two cell types to attachment factors (Somerman et al 1989), extracellular matrix proteins (Giannopoulou & Cimasoni 1996) and growth factors have been found to be different.

In addition, some of the periodontal ligament cells have been shown to possess osteoblast-like characteristics, including the production of osteonectin (Somerman et al 1990; Nohutcu et al 1996), osteocalcin (Nojima et al 1990) and high levels of alkaline phosphatase (Kawase et al 1988). These studies indicate that phenotypically distinct and functional

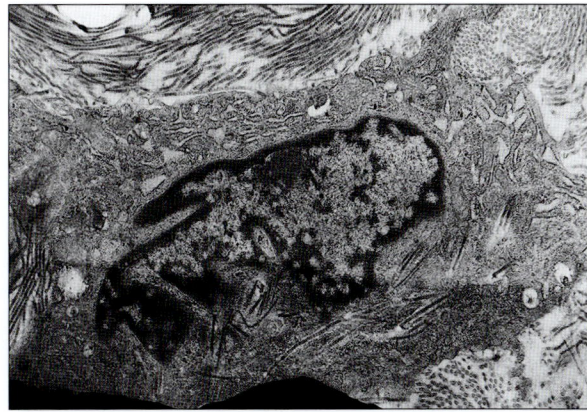

Fig. 1.10 An electron micrograph of a fibroblast containing multiple banded collagen fibrils within membrane-bound phagolysosomes.

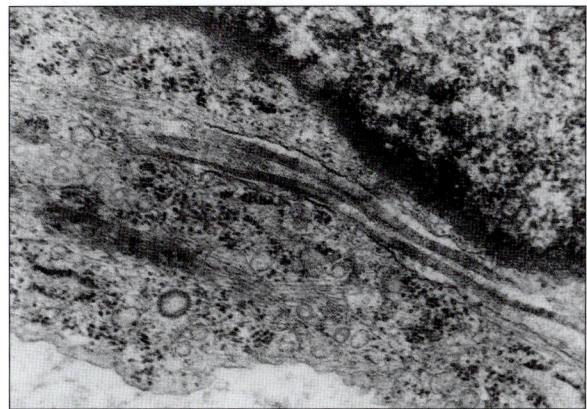

Fig. 1.11 A higher power electron micrograph of part of a fibroblast. It shows intracellular banded collagen fibrils within a membrane-bound vesicle (phagolysosome).

sub-populations of cells of both fibroblast and osteoblast/cementoblast lineage exist in the periodontal ligament and these cells probably include some stem and precursor cells important in repair and regeneration.

Osteoblasts, cementoblasts, osteoclasts and cementoclasts may also be found lining the endosteal and periosteal bone surfaces and the cementum surface. These cells are only conspicuous when active deposition of bone and cementum is taking place, at which time these cells also appear plump. Multinucleated cells (osteoclasts and cementoclasts) appear on bone and cementum surfaces when resorption is taking place, and indeed there appears to be no reason to differentiate between them since they both resorb mineralized tissue.

All of these cell types derive from stem and precursor cells in the ligament and/or alveolar bone marrow (see below). Osteoclasts and cementoclasts are derived from blood-borne precursors of marrow origin, which originate from mononuclear phagocyte cell precursors. Precursor and stem cells for all these connective cells are also present in the ligament (see below).

Groups of epithelial cells, the 'epithelial rests of Malassez', which are remnants of the Hertwig root sheath, are found close to the cementum. They may play a part in the formation of dental cysts. Histochemical and electron microscope studies reveal little activity in these cells. They may, however, proliferate to form cysts or tumours if appropriately stimulated (e.g. by chronic inflammation).

Defence cells may also be present in the periodontal ligament including macrophages, mast cells and eosinophils, as in other connective tissues.

It is important to recognize that the collagen of the periodontal ligament undergo constant remodelling, i.e. resorption of old fibres and formation of new ones, and the fibroblasts are involved in both processes.

Autoradiographic studies demonstrate a high rate of collagen turnover which is greatest at the alveolar crest and at the apex. The turnover of collagen in the periodontal ligament is said to be faster than in any other connective tissue. This probably reflects the constant functional demand placed on teeth.

Of major importance is the capacity of the periodontal ligament for repair and regeneration, which is reflected in the complex and heterogeneous sub-populations of cells of this tissue (Lekic & McCulloch 1996). The cementoblasts, osteoblasts and osteoclasts, which maintain and remodel the cementum and alveolar bone on the borders of the periodontal ligament, are also considered part of this tissue (Berkowitz et al 1995). In addition, other mesenchymal cells, which may include stem and progenitor cells are also present and are key cells in the regenerative processes.

Stem and progenitor cells

The periodontal ligament and the marrow spaces of the alveolar bone contain stem and progenitor cells which function as the precursor cells for the more specialized cells in the mesenchymal cell population that is continually renewing under physiological conditions due to cell death and terminal differentiation (Berkowitz et al 1995; Nagatomo et al 2006). Chen et al (2006) showed that the periodontal ligament of both healthy and diseased teeth contained cells with consistent identification as putative stem cells. They also showed that the presence of an inflammatory reaction associated with periodontitis enhanced the number of these cells.

A number of recent studies have investigated the origin and location of the progenitor cell populations in the periodontal ligament. It has been suggested that after the embryological development of the periodontal ligament from undifferentiated mesenchymal cells, some progenitor cells remain in the mature tissue (Hassell 1993). It is thought that this progenitor population is located perivascularly adjacent to blood vessels (Lekic & McCulloch 1996). It was suggested that these cells may give rise to periodontal ligament fibroblasts and also migrate towards the bone and cementum surfaces, where they may differentiate into osteoblasts or cementoblasts, respectively.

The cells present in the vascular channels of the alveolar bone, which migrate towards the periodontal ligament, may be another source of progenitors. This suggestion was supported by a study in which root slices were cultured in vitro with cells derived from the rat calvaria (Melcher et al 1987). It is also possible that separate precursor cells may be present for each distinct mature cell type.

Periodontal ligament stem cells show similar characteristics to bone marrow stromal stem cells and combinations of these cell types can be used on scaffolds with suitable bioactive agents to promote regeneration of matrix tissue and bone (Bartold et al 2006). These precursor cell populations undoubtedly play a major role in periodontal homeostasis and the regenerative healing process.

BLOOD SUPPLY

The rich blood supply to the periodontal ligament is mainly derived from the appropriate superior and inferior alveolar arteries, although arteries from the gingiva, such as the lingual and palatine arteries, may also be involved through anastomosis of the two supplies (**Fig. 1.7**). The arteries supplying the ligament branch off from the artery supplying the pulp before it enters the apical foramina. The ligament also receives a secondary rich supply from the vessels supplying the alveolar bone and there is massive anastomosis between vessels in the marrow spaces and the ligament via multiple foramina in the cribriform plate. This dual supply allows the ligament to survive following removal of the root apex during certain endodontic procedures.

Fenestrated capillaries are present in the periodontal ligament and this contrasts with other fibrous connective tissues which usually have continuous capillaries. The presence of fenestrated capillaries in large numbers is therefore a specialized feature of the periodontal ligament. Fenestrated capillary beds differ from continuous capillary beds in that the diffusion and filtration capabilities are greatly increased. It is possible that the capillary fenestrations are related to the high metabolic requirements of the periodontal ligament and its high rate of turnover.

The dense anastomosis of deep and superficial vessels at the gingival margin leads to a crevicular plexus of capillary loops which completely encircles each tooth within the connective tissue beneath the region of the gingival crevice. Each loop consists of one or two thin (8–10 µm in diameter) capillary ascending loops and one or two descending post-capillary venules. The crevicular capillary loops arise from a circular plexus, which is comprised of 1–4 intercommunicating vessels (6–30 µm in diameter) lying at the level of the junctional epithelium. They are separated from other more marginally situated loops just below the gingival surface.

The veins within the ligament do not usually accompany the arteries. Instead they pass through the cribriform plate to drain into intra-alveolar networks. Anastomosis with veins in the gingiva also occurs and a dense venous network is particularly prominent around the apex of the alveolus.

NERVE SUPPLY

The nerve supply to the periodontal ligament is of two types: sensory and autonomic. There are two types of sensory fibre, proprioceptive and pain, which supply the ligament's pressure and pain receptors. The pressure (proprioceptive) receptors are spindle-shaped structures and this function is central to the control of the masticatory system in chewing, swallowing and talking. Pain fibres terminate as free nerve endings. The autonomic fibres are associated mainly with the supply of the periodontal blood vessels. Compared with other dense connective tissues, the periodontal ligament is well innervated.

Nerve bundles from the trigeminal nerve follow the blood vessels. They are derived from two sources. Some nerve bundles branch off the nerve supplying the pulp before it enters the apical foramen and supply the ligament directly. Other sensory fibres enter the middle and cervical portions of the ligament from the nerve supply to the alveolar bone and enter the ligament as finer branches through the multiple foramina in the cribriform plate.

Periodontal nerve fibres are both myelinated and non-myelinated. The myelinated fibres are 5–15 µm in diameter and are all sensory fibres which respond to pressure. The non-myelinated fibres are about 0.5 µm in diameter and are both sensory pain and autonomic fibres.

About 75% of the mechanoreceptors within the periodontal ligament have their cell bodies in the trigeminal ganglion, while the remaining 25% have cell bodies in the mesencephalic nucleus.

Most research has been carried out into the mechanoreceptors and the discharge of afferent impulses from single nerve fibres dissected free from the inferior alveolar nerve in animals (Berkowitz et al 1992). The discharge appears to vary according to the direction and amplitude of the displacing force. These fibres show directional sensitivity in that they respond maximally to a force applied to the tooth crown in one particular direction. Their conduction velocities place them within the A_β group of fibres. The response characteristics of these mechanoreceptors can vary from rapidly adapting through to slowly adapting but it is not clear whether the rapidly, medium and slowly adapting mechanoreceptors are really different types of receptor. All of their sensory endings appear to be similar and are encapsulated Ruffini-like terminals. Furthermore, the response characteristics appear to be dependent upon the position of the ending within the ligament relative to the position of loading.

The proprioceptor nerve endings in the ligament form part of the extremely refined neurological control of mastication. The mechanoreceptors in the periodontal ligament monitor changes in pressure within the ligament space, and as forces increase greater numbers of mechanoreceptors are stimulated. This results in increasing numbers of impulses passing via the sensory nerves to the trigeminal nuclei. This in turn results in inhibitory impulses passing to the motor nucleus which reduces the number of motor impulses to the muscle fibres, reducing or stopping masticatory forces. A similar reflex arc passes from the muscle spindle receptors which monitor muscle stretch. The loads in mastication, swallowing and speaking vary considerably in amount, frequency, duration and direction, and in normal function, the structure of the ligament usually absorbs these effectively and transmits them to the supporting bone.

Little is known about pain fibres within the ligament, but it is presumed that they are fine non-myelinated nerves terminating in free nerve endings. There is a similar lack of information on the fine non-myelinated autonomic nerves. These fibres are 0.2–1 μm in diameter and are important in the control of the regional blood flow.

TOOTH SUPPORT MECHANISM

The proprioceptor nerve endings in the ligament form part of the extremely refined neurological control of mastication and thus protect the ligament from damage (see above). In addition, blood supply, the ground substance and collagen bundles all take part in the absorption of functional stresses and their transmission to the bones.

The periodontal ligament may be treated as a viscous hyperelastic fibre reinforced compressible system; with tremendous capacity for deformation which is essentially non-linear. It behaves differently during compression and tension forces (Zhurov et al 2007). The vascular-ground substance complex is a shock absorbing system and the fibre-bundle system is a suspensory system limiting tooth movement and transmitting strain to the supporting bone (Bartold 2006). Thus, when a force is applied to a tooth a series of events follow:

1. The initial displacement of the tooth is associated with intravascular and extravascular fluid movement through blood vessels and through bone spaces
2. As the load increases, the collagen fibre bundles take the strain and become extended. They are not elastic and they do not stretch
3. With further pressure, the alveolar process distorts
4. If the load is sufficiently powerful and prolonged, the tooth substance itself, i.e. the dentine, distorts.

This has been described as a viscoelastic system in which the vascular, tissue fluid and ground substance components provide the viscous response while the fibrous tissue and bone provide elasticity. When an axial load is applied to a tooth, there appears to be a biphasic response, the elastic phase preceding the viscous phase. It is an extremely versatile and resilient system which can cope with the variable loads imposed on the tissues by the mastication of a heterogeneous diet. However, it can break down when subject to abnormal loads or when involved in inflammation.

Axial forces are absorbed most readily. On loading, the wavy principal fibres assume their full length and the tooth is depressed in the socket. Lateral and rotational forces are absorbed less easily. On the tension side, fibres extend; on the pressure side, fibres are compressed. Further compression results in bone resorption and further tension, on bone deposition.

All teeth are slightly mobile and that mobility is influenced by:

1. The quantity and duration of the applied load
2. Length and shape of the root or roots and therefore the position of the axis of rotation. Inevitably, mobility of the lower incisor with

a relatively short and conical root is easier to elicit than that of the multirooted upper first molar with its large root base

3. The status of the supporting tissues, i.e. thickness of collagen fibre bundles and proportion of mature collagen (the erupting tooth is more mobile than the fully erupted tooth) and the state of aggregation of the ground substance. In pregnancy, some increase in tooth mobility is caused by hormone-induced disaggregation.

CEMENTUM

Cementum is the calcified connective tissue which covers the root dentine and the periodontal fibre bundles are inserted into it. It can be regarded as a 'bone of attachment' and is the only specifically dental tissue of the periodontium. It is pale yellow and softer than dentine, and in some animals is present on the crowns of the teeth as an adaptation to a herbivorous diet. In humans its relationship to the enamel margin varies, it may abut on or overlap enamel but it may be separated from the enamel by a thin band of exposed dentine. The thickness of cementum varies considerably and the coronal third may be only 16–60 μm. When exposed by gingival recession or pocketing, this very thin layer of cervical cementum can be easily removed by the toothbrush or dental instrumentation so that the very sensitive dentine is exposed. In contrast, the apical third can be 200 μm or even thicker. Cementum is formed slowly throughout life and is resistant to resorption. A layer of uncalcified matrix, the precementum, is laid down by the cementoblasts prior to calcification and a layer of this uncalcified matrix is always present on its surface within the periodontium and may be responsible for its resistance to resorption. Cementum can triple its thickness throughout life and is avascular and without innervation. It is more permeable than dentine, but this permeability decreases with age. Continual cemental formation is necessary to accommodate changes in fibre insertion within the periodontal ligament as a result of tooth movement and ligament turnover.

Like other calcified tissues, bone and dentine, it consists of collagen fibres embedded in a calcified organic matrix. It contains by weight 65% of inorganic material, mainly hydroxyapatite, 23% of organic material and 12% water. By volume, these proportions are 45%, 33% and 22%, respectively.

There are two main types of cementum: cellular and acellular. The former contains cementocytes in lacunae which, like osteocytes in bone, communicate with each other through a network of canaliculi. Acellular cementum forms a thin surface layer, often confined to cervical portions of the root. It does not contain cementocytes within its substance but as cementoblasts populate its surface, the term 'acellular' may not be wholly appropriate. The degree of mineralization varies in different parts of the tissue and some acellular zones may be as highly calcified as dentine. Cementoblasts are responsible for the synthesis and secretion of the components of organic matrix and also for its calcification and are morphologically and functionally identical to osteoblasts. As cementum formation proceeds, the cementoblasts become entrapped and are then referred to as cementocytes. It has been suggested that there may be two populations of cementoblasts, which can be distinguished by their phenotype and developmental origin (Ten Cate 1997). Thus, while cells associated with acellular cementum may be derived from the dental follicle, cells from cellular cementum may originate from the progenitor cells migrating from the alveolar bone endosteal spaces. It is probable that precursor and stems cells for cementoblasts are present in the periodontal ligament close to the cemental surface as well as the alveolar bone. Several bioactive agents such as bone morphogenic proteins (BMPs) have been shown to enhance cementogenesis by stimulating stem cell-like activity within the periodontium. In addition, phosphates are regulators of cementoblast SIBLING (small integrin-binding ligand N-linked glycoprotein) gene expression *in vitro* (Popowics et al 2005). These factors have important implications on periodontal regeneration *in vivo*.

The principal inorganic component is hydroxyapatite, although other forms of calcium phosphate are present to a higher degree than in other calcified tissues. The organic content is primarily collagen which is virtually all type I.

During calcification hydroxyapatite crystals are first deposited on the surface of collagen fibrils parallel to their surface and then within the cementoid matrix. These crystals are similar to those seen in bone and are thin and plate-like. They are on average 55 nm wide and 8 nm thick. The cementum surface is formed into conical projections about single fibrils or bundles.

The prime function of cementum is to give attachment to collagen fibres of the periodontal ligament. There are two arrangements of collagen fibrils in cementum. The principal fibrils are those of the periodontal ligament embedded as Sharpey's fibres in the calcified matrix and incorporated in the cementum as it is laid down. They are arranged at right angles to the cementum surface. The other fibrils form a dense and irregular meshwork within the matrix. In acellular cementum, the Sharpey's fibres are closely packed and largely calcified; in cellular cementum they are more widely spaced and partly calcified.

Unlike bone there is no evidence of cementum remodelling, i.e. of internal resorption and deposition; however, there is continuous, slow apposition of surface cementum as cementoblast activity continues at a low level throughout life. Cementoid or precementum is the name given to the cementum matrix prior to calcification and a layer of this is always present on its surface. Its resistance to resorption is a feature which allows orthodontic tooth movement. The precise reasons for its resistance to resorption are unknown but it may be related to differences between the physiochemical or biological properties of bone and cementum.

The greatest thickness of cementum is formed at the apex and in furcation areas. With attrition, i.e. wear of the occlusal surface of the tooth, compensatory deposition of apical cementum takes place which, together with bone deposition at the alveolar crest and at the socket fundus, maintains the vertical dimension of the face. At the tooth apex the cementum forms a constriction so that the root canal exit is very narrow.

Excessive formation of cementum, hypercementosis, may follow pulp disease or occlusal stress. A generalized hypercementosis involving all teeth may be hereditary; it also occurs in Paget's disease. Occasionally, cementicles, small spherical masses of cementum, may be found attached to the cementum surface or free in the periodontal ligament.

Cementum resorption can be a consequence of excessive occlusal stress, orthodontic movement, pressure from tumours or cysts or deficiencies of calcium or vitamins A and D. It is also found in metabolic diseases but the pathogenesis is obscure. Repair of these areas may occur if the cause is removed. Occasionally, ankylosis of the cementum and socket bone takes place. Root fracture may be followed by the formation of a cementum callus, but this repair process does not demonstrate the highly organized remodelling capacity of bone.

Resorption is carried out by multinuclear cells resembling osteoclasts, termed cementoclasts or odontoclasts. These cells undoubtedly arise from myelomonocytic cells in a similar way to osteoclasts. The resorptive lacunae resemble those seen in bone and the cementoclasts are seen at the resorptive front. If the force is large the resorption can also involve the underlying root dentine.

Areas of previous resorption can also be repaired by the laying down of further cementum by cementoblasts which probably develop from stem cells in the periodontal ligament. Repair cementum resembles cellular cementum.

ALVEOLAR BONE

That part of the maxilla and mandible which supports and protects the teeth is known as alveolar bone and an arbitrary boundary at the level of the root apices separates alveolar bone from the body of the maxilla or mandible.

Alveolar bone has its embryological origin from the initial condensation of ectomesenchyme around the early tooth germ (Ten Cate 1997). The alveolar processes are tooth dependent and are present as long as they house the teeth. It is comprised of the alveolar bone proper, in which the Sharpey's fibres are embedded, the compact bone, comprised of the oral and buccal cortical plates and the cancellous bone located between them.

Apart from supporting the teeth, the bone of the maxilla and mandible also gives attachment to muscles, provides a framework for the bone marrow and acts as a reservoir for ions, in particular calcium. The alveolar bone is dependent on the presence of teeth for its development and maintenance and thus after tooth extraction, it atrophies and in anodontia it is absent.

Bone is a mineralized connective tissue and consists by weight of about 60% inorganic material, about 25% organic material and about 15% of water. By volume, these proportions are 36%, 36% and 28%, respectively. The mineral phase consists of hydroxyapatite, in the form of needle-like crystallites or thin plates about 8 nm thick and of variable length. About 90% of the organic material is in the form of type I collagen. In addition, there are small amounts of other proteins, e.g. osteonectin, osteocalcin, osteopontin and proteoglycans. Two small molecular weight chondroitin sulphate (CS) proteoglycans have been identified in alveolar bone, namely decorin and biglycan, containing one and two CS chains, respectively (Waddington & Embery 1991).

Osteoblasts synthesize and regulate the deposition of the bone organic matrix including collagen type 1, proteoglycan, osteonectin, osteocalcin, bone sialoprotein and osteopontin. They also express and release alkaline phosphatase and this has been shown to be closely associated with new bone formation. Osteoblasts also control the process of mineralization.

Anatomically, no distinct boundary exists between the body of the maxilla or mandible and their respective alveolar processes. However, as a result of functional adaption, two parts of the alveolar process can be distinguished. The first, the alveolar bone proper, consists of a thin lamella of bone which surrounds the root of the tooth. It gives attachment to the principal fibres of the periodontal ligament. The collagen fibres of the periodontal ligament are inserted into this bone to produce what is called 'bundle bone'. The periodontal ligament fibres embedded in the bone are called Sharpey's fibres. This bone is also called the cribriform plate. As the name implies the cribriform plate is perforated like a sieve so that a large number of vascular and neural connections can be made between the periodontal ligament and the trabecular spaces. The second part, the supporting bone, is the bone which surrounds the alveolar bone proper and gives support to the socket. This has facial and lingual plates of compact bone between which is cancellous trabeculation (spongy bone). This cancellous bone is orientated around the tooth to form support for the alveolar bone proper.

The bone of the alveolar process is in no fundamental way different from bone in any other part of the body. In compact bone, the lamellae are arranged in two major patterns. At the periosteal or endosteal surfaces, they are arranged in concentric layers conforming to the bony surface contour. If the bone volume is sufficient, they may be also arranged as small concentric layers around a central vascular canal. This system is known as a haversian system and may be comprised of up to 20 concentric layers. The central haversian canals are connected by transversely running Volkmann's canals. Spongy or cancellous bone consists of widely spaced concentric or transverse lamellae enclosing the marrow spaces.

The shape of the jaws and the morphology of the alveolar processes vary between individuals and the size, shape and thickness of cortical plates and interdental septa vary in different parts of the same jaw. The margin of the alveolar crest usually runs parallel to the amelocemental junction at a remarkably constant distance of 1–2 mm, but this relationship may vary with the alignment of the tooth and the contour of the root surface. Where a tooth is displaced out of the arch, the overlying alveolar plate may be very thin or even perforated so that fenestrations (circumscribed defects) or dehiscences (splits) are formed. These defects occur more frequently in facial than in lingual bone and are more common over anterior than posterior teeth, although they are seen over the palatal root of the upper first molar if the roots are very divergent. These defects are very important clinically, because where they occur, the root of the tooth is covered only by mucoperiosteum, i.e. periosteum and the overlying gingiva, which may atrophy under irritation and thus expose the root. Where tooth roots approximate, interdental bone may be absent.

Five cell types can be identified in bone. Bone forming cells, osteoblasts, are found on the surface of the bone. They become trapped in their own secretion and subsequently become incorporated in the matrix as osteocytes. Large multinucleated cells, osteoclasts, are responsible for resorbing bone. In addition, osteoprogenitor cells are present and they appear as long, thin cells. These are a stem cell population to generate osteoblasts. They are situated close to the blood vessels of the marrow and periodontal ligament. When bone is not undergoing active deposition or resorption, then its quiescent surface is lined by relatively undifferentiated cells known as bone lining cells which may represent inactive osteoblasts. Active osteoblasts contain extensive rough endoplastic reticulum, numerous mitochondria and vesicles and an extensive Golgi apparatus. They manufacture and secrete type I collagen and proteoglycans and bring about mineralization.

Like all bone, alveolar bone undergoes constant remodelling as a response to mechanical stress and to metabolic need for calcium and phosphorus ions. In health, the remodelling process maintains the total volume of bone and its overall anatomy relatively stably. In the primate, the teeth drift mesially as interproximal tooth surface wear takes place, together with resorption on the mesial and deposition on the distal surfaces of the socket wall.

The resorbing surface of the bone shows resorption concavities, known as Howship's lacunae, in which lie osteoclasts. These vary in size and may be up to $100\,\mu m$ in diameter. The multinucleated osteoclast forms by the fusion of cells of the myelomonocyte cell line. The part of the osteoclast which lies adjacent to the bone surface has a foamy, striated appearance which is known as the brush border. Ultrastructurally, the brush border consists of many tightly packed microvilli which are coated with fine bristle-like structures. This zone may limit the diffusion of enzymes and ions to create an isolated microenvironment within which resorption can take place. These cells have less endoplastic reticulum than osteoblasts but a very prominent Golgi apparatus and are also motile. They secrete cysteine- and metalloproteinases and hydrogen ions (see Table 5.1 and **Fig. 5.3**). Bone resorption takes place in two stages. Initially, the mineral phase is removed, and later the organic matrix. The regulation of these events involves close cooperation between osteoblasts and osteoclasts (see Ch. 5).

Proteins mainly associated with bone and cementum

Mesenchymal stem cells seeded on custom made glass-ceramic scaffolds show significant differentiation demonstrating osteogenic markers such as alkaline phosphatase, osteocalcin, osteonectin and osteopontin in the absence of stimulatory agents (Dyson et al 2007). This demonstrates the osteosupportive capacity of the porous apatite-wollastonite glass-ceramic scaffold used and has applications in periodontal regenerative therapy for intrabony defects.

Osteonectin

Osteonectin is an acid phosphate containing glycoprotein rich in cysteine which is mainly secreted by osteoblasts. It is composed of a single polypeptide chain and has a strong affinity for calcium ions, due to its phosphate ions, and type I collagen (Sage & Borstein 1991). It has been suggested that the phosphate groups may be crucial for initiating the mineralization process. Osteonectin is one of the major non-collagenous proteins of bone and has also been located in basal lamina (Bilezikian et al 1996). In addition, it has been found in the periodontal ligament, particularly strongly around the Sharpey fibres, at the attachment sites between the ligament and alveolar bone and cementum (Matsuura et al 1995).

Osteocalcin

Osteocalcin is also called bone gla protein because it contains γ-carboxyglutamic acid (gla) residues and is a small protein that is mainly secreted by osteoblasts (Mariotti 1993). It becomes incorporated in the mineralized matrix of bone soon after its secretion and it has been suggested that it plays a crucial role in the mineralization process. It is probable that the gla sites on the protein act as calcium ion binding sites. The expression of osteocalcin by the cells lining the tooth root surface has been shown during tooth root development in mice (D'Errico et al 1997).

Bone sialoprotein protein

Bone sialoprotein protein (BSP), also known as BSP II, is a phosphoglycoprotein containing up to 20% of sialic acid residues that also has an RGD sequence (Bilezikian et al 1996). It has a restricted pattern of expression and is primarily found in bone (Fujisawa et al 1995). BSP expression marks a late stage of osteoblast differentiation and an early stage of matrix mineralization (Lekic et al 1996; Gordon et al 2007). There is also weak expression in the periodontal ligament at attachment sites with alveolar bone and cementum (Matsuura et al 1995). In addition, it is expressed by cells lining the root surface at early stages of cementogenesis during tooth development (MacNeil et al 1995, 1996). The cementoblasts appear to secrete this protein on to the root surface which then becomes covered by cementum. Although the precise function of this protein is not yet known, it may serve as an attachment factor since it has an affinity for collagen fibres and enhances the attachment of osteoblasts and fibroblasts to plastic surfaces.

Osteopontin

Osteopontin is also termed BSP I due to its high sialic acid content and is a glycophosphoprotein. It is found primarily in bone and in addition to an RGD cell attachment sequence it has an affinity for calcium ions (MacNeil et al 1995). Although its precise functions are unclear it is expressed prior to mineralization and appears to be involved in the attachment and movement of osteoblasts and osteoclasts. It has also been suggested (MacNeil et al 1995) that it functions as an inhibitor of mineralization during periodontal ligament development. In this regard, it has been shown to be distributed in a non-specific fashion throughout the periodontal ligament of the developing mouse molar tooth germ between 21 and 42 development days. However, in contrast, D'Errico et al (1997) reported that osteopontin was not expressed in the periodontal ligament by day 41 but was expressed by the cells lining the tooth root surface. It has also been shown to be expressed in regenerating alveolar bone adjacent to a fenestration wound in rats, prior to the expression of BSP (II) (Lekic et al 1996).

REGULATION OF TISSUE TURNOVER IN THE PERIODONTIUM

The regulation of tissue turnover depends on the recruitment and stimulation of the appropriate cells at the requisite time and often on the differentiation of appropriate stem and precursor cells in the functioning mature cells. Most of these functions are controlled by growth factors released by cells and these are described below.

GROWTH FACTORS IN PERIODONTAL TISSUE TURNOVER

Growth factors are proteins or polypeptides capable of initiating the proliferation of cells that are in a quiescent state by stimulating DNA synthesis and progression of the cell cycle. They primarily have a paracrine or autocrine action and exert their effects by binding to specific transmembrane receptors on target cells which generate a cascade of intracellular molecular signals (Ioannidou 2006). In this way, they regulate the activation and proliferation of the signalled cells and also regulate a number of other factors including cell migration and cell synthesis which are essential events in healing. Therapeutic applications include the use of stem cells which have tremendous potential for specific targeted activity, with growth factors which could favourably effect periodontal regeneration (Ioannidou 2006). The biological actions of PDGF, TGF, FGF, IGF and EGF on periodontal cells and tissues involved in regeneration have been reviewed recently (Dereka et al 2006).

Platelet-derived growth factor

Platelet-derived growth factor (PDGF) plays an important role not only in wound healing but also in normal tissue turnover. It is released primarily by platelets but is also synthesized by macrophages, fibroblasts, osteoblasts, endothelial cells and myoblasts. It consists of a dimer of two glycoprotein subunits, A and B and there are therefore three possible combinations, PDGF-AA, PDGF-BB, PDGF-AB. PDGF acts by binding to two distinct cell surface receptors, termed PDGF-receptor (PDGFR)-α and PDGFR-β on target cells. Recombinant human (rh) PDGF-BB is a potent stimulator of mitogenic activity in human periodontal ligament cells. Er: YAG laser application in combination with rh PDGF-BB showed significant fibroblast attachment on diseased root surfaces (Belal et al 2007).

A number of *in vitro* studies have demonstrated that PDGF can stimulate proliferation (Anderson et al 1998), DNA synthesis (Blom et al 1994) and collagen production by periodontal ligament cells. It is also chemotactic for these cells (Nishimura & Terranova 1996) and also for osteoblasts. PDGF-BB appears to be more effective than the other isoforms in promoting mitogenesis and chemotaxis of these cells *in vitro* and it has also been shown to act synergistically with other growth factors both *in vitro* and *in vivo* (Ioannidou 2006). The effect of rh PDGF-BB on release of ICTP (the pyridinoline cross-linked carboxy terminal telopeptide of Type 1 collagen) an established biomarker of bone synthetic activity, was investigated in periodontal bone defects (Sarment et al 2006). There was a direct effect on ICTP released from the wound in response to the growth factor, indicative of bone turnover in the osseous defect.

Transforming growth factors

Transforming growth factors (TGFs) are a family of structurally and functionally different proteins that have been isolated from normal and neoplastic tissues. The bone induction capacity of bone morphogenetic and osteogenetic proteins (BMPs/Ops) of the TGF-β superfamily have potential for periodontal bone regeneration, as demonstrated in primates and humans. They are able to stimulate de novo bone formation and act as soluble signals for tissue induction and morphogenesis of the multicellular mineralized tissues of the periodontium (Ripamonti 2007). TGF-β is encoded by five different genes yielding five isoforms TGF-β1 to TGF-β5 which display different spatial and temporal patterns of expression during healing (Frank et al 1996). TGF-β is present in high concentrations in platelets and is also produced by activated macrophages and neutrophils (Igarashi et al 1993). Three distinct receptors for these factors, type I, type II and type III are present on almost all normal cells. TGF-α stimulates epithelial and endothelial cells and acts through the receptor of another growth factor, epithelial growth factor.

The biological effects of TGF-β are highly diverse. It has been shown to be chemotactic for macrophages and gingival and periodontal ligament mesenchymal cells (Nishimura & Terranova 1996) to stimulate the proliferation of gingival and periodontal ligament mesenchymal cells (Anderson et al 1998). It has also been shown to selectively stimulate the synthesis of extracellular matrix proteins such as collagen, fibronectin, tenascin and proteoglycans (Irwin et al 1994) by these cells and to inhibit the growth of epithelial, endothelial and certain mesenchymal cells (Lu et al 1997). In addition, TGF-β1 alone or in combination with PDGF increases the proliferation of periodontal ligament mesenchymal cells more than those from gingival tissue.

Fibroblast growth factor

Fibroblast growth factors (FGFs) are a family of polypeptides which are potent mitogens and chemoattractants for endothelial and mesenchymal cells (Bilezikian et al 1996). The two most studied forms of this family are acid FGF (aFGF) and basic FGF (bFGF). Acid FGF stimulates endothelial cell proliferation. Basic FGF is widely distributed in nearly all tissues including gingiva, periodontal ligament and bone (Bilezikian et al 1996; Goa et al 1996; Murata et al 1997).

bFGF has been reported to stimulate periodontal ligament and endothelial cell migration. When applied topically to experimentally prepared periodontal tissue defects in beagle dogs and non-human primates, bFGF (FGF2) induced significant periodontal tissue regeneration with new cementum and alveolar bone formation (Murakami 2007). Devising a suitable carrier in the form of a scaffold for bFGF could enhance the potential for periodontal regeneration.

Epidermal growth factor

Epidermal growth factor (EGF) is a small polypeptide which stimulates the proliferation of epithelial, endothelial and mesenchymal cells (Bilezikian et al 1996). It is present in most human extracellular fluids including plasma, saliva, milk, amniotic fluid and urine. EGF is mitogenic for periodontal ligament cells (Blom et al 1994). It was also found to stimulate the growth of gingival cells *in vitro* (Irwin et al 1994). It also showed a slight chemotactic effect on periodontal ligament cells but suppressed their collagen synthesis.

Insulin-like growth factor

Insulin-like growth factors (IGFs) are a family of single chain proteins. IGF-I and IGF-II are anabolic peptides structurally and functionally related to insulin. They are synthesized in the liver, smooth muscle and placenta and transported via the plasma. IGFs play an important role in the biology of orofacial tissues, including the development and regeneration of the periodontium. Several IGF components have been located in cementum. Periodontal ligament fibroblasts could respond in a paracrine manner to this reservoir (Gotz et al 2006). This also has therapeutic applications for regeneration of lost tissue. They are also present in bony tissues as a result of their synthesis by osteoblasts and the release of stored peptides from the bone matrix (Bilezikian et al 1996). Both gingival and periodontal mesenchymal cells show a dose-dependent migratory response to the presence of IGF-I and II and IGF-I (Nishimura & Terranova 1996). They also increase DNA synthesis and protein production by periodontal ligament cells (Blom et al 1994).

Bone morphogenic proteins

Bone morphogenic proteins (BMPs) are part of the large TGF-β superfamily (Meikle 2007; Bilezikian et al 1996). Localization of members of the BMP family in the embryological development of the skeleton has provided strong evidence that they play an important role in mediating skeletal patterning as well as bone cell differentiation (Bilezikian et al 1996). Furthermore, the BMPs are considered to be responsible for the inductive abilities of demineralized bone allografts used in periodontal therapy (see Ch. 19). In addition, BMP-2 has been shown to stimulate osteocalcin and alkaline phosphatase expression by cultured periodontal ligament cells (Hughes 1995). BMPs also have been shown to induce bone and cartilage formation when implanted subcutaneously. They play an important role in the induction of cells responsible for regeneration of periodontal tissues (Ripamonti & Renton 2006).

The regulation of tissue turnover in the various periodontal tissues will now be separately described.

EPITHELIUM

Stratified squamous epithelium continually renews itself by division of cells in the basal layer and shedding of keratinocytes from the surface. The turnover time for skin is 12–75 days, oral epithelium 8–40 days and junctional epithelium 4–11 days. Systemic hormones influence this process, with oestrogen stimulating cell division and corticosteroids inhibiting it. Local factors appear to play a more important role in its regulation. There is a negative feedback control system on keratinocytes by substances known as chalones. The precise nature of these is unknown but their function could be due to one or more growth factors or cytokines. They act on cells in the basal layer and inhibit their division. Epithelial turnover is also affected by a number of growth factors including, epidermal growth factor (EGF), platelet-derived growth factor (PDGF) and transforming growth factors alpha (TGF-α) and beta (TGF-β). EGF and TGF-α are known to stimulate epithelial cell proliferation whilst TGF-β appears to have an inhibitory effect.

The differentiation of epithelium is also profoundly affected by the underlying connective tissue lamina propria. The nature of the connective tissue or chemical messages from it determines the nature of the overlying epithelium for instance whether it is keratinized or not. Thus, in the free gingival graft it is the nature of the underlying connective tissue which determines the type of epithelium which forms.

PERIODONTAL LIGAMENT

The periodontal ligament is constantly breaking down and renewing its constituent tissues. In health, this process is carefully controlled and is in balance. The tooth responds to functional demands and rates of turnover reflect increases or decreases in function. Recent studies have shown that periodontal diseases may pose a threat to general health. Useful inflammatory markers of systemic exposure from periodontal diseases are needed. Parameters of the host response to periodontal infections such as matrix metalol-proteinases, cytokines, chemokines, inflammatory markers and antibodies to periodontal pathogens have been used (Pussinen et al 2007). Serum markers of periodontal diseases could prove to be of value for patients with co-existing systemic diseases.

Connective tissue turnover in the periodontium is five times higher than alveolar bone and 15 times higher than the dermis of normal skin. Fibroblasts are responsible for both the synthesis (p. 87) and degradation of all components of the extracellular matrix. They secrete collagenolytic enzymes (collagenases) and these are part of a family of matrix metalloproteinases (MMPs) (Table 1.1) which require the presence of metallic cations such as magnesium and calcium for their activity (Reynolds et al

Table 1.1 *The principle members of the family of metalloproteinases (MMPs), including collagenases*

MMP	Other name	Principal source	Main substrates
MMP-1	Collagenase 1	Fibroblasts and other CT cells of mesenchyme origin including macrophages	Helical region of collagen types I, II, III, VIII, X Gelatins (limited) Proteoglycan core protein (limited)
MMP-8	Collagenase 2	Inflammatory cells, e.g. PMNs	As above
MMP-13	Collagenase 3	Human tumours and bone cells	As above
MMP-2	Gelatinase A	Fibroblasts and other CT cells of mesenchyme origin	Gelatins Specific locus of collagen IV Collagens V, VII, X, XI Elastin
MMP-9	Gelatinase B	PMNs, macrophages and osteoclasts	As above
MMP-3	Stromolysin 1	Fibroblasts and other CT cells of mesenchyme origin	Proteoglycan core protein Non-helical regions of collagen IV Collagens X, XI Procollagens I, II, III Fibronectin Laminin Gelatins (limited) Elastin (limited)
MMP-10	Stromolysin 2	Inflammatory cells, e.g. PMNs	As above
MMP-11	Stromolysin 3	Fibroblasts and human breast tumour cells	As above
MMP-7	Matrilysin	Macrophages and fibroblasts	As for stromolysins
MMP-12	Metalloelastase	Macrophages	As for stromolysins Elastin
MMP-14	Membrane type	Cell membranes	Progelatinase A

1994; Reynolds 1996). There are two distinct forms of collagenase, one originating from fibroblasts and other connective tissue cells of mesenchymal origin (MMP-1) and the other from polymorphs (MMP-8) (Table 1.2). Human tumours and bone cells also synthesize another collagenase (MMP-13 or collagenase 3). In addition, macrophages and monocytes synthesize and secrete in response to specific stimuli MMP-1 (Machein & Conca 1997; Welgus et al 1990; Campbell et al 1991). The other proteinases in the group include the gelatinases, stromolysins, matrilysins, metalloelastases and membrane associated MMPs. Gelatinases A and B (MMP-2 and MMP-9) which degrade a specific locus on collagen IV, gelatins, collagens V, VII, X and XI and elastin are also synthesized and secreted by connective tissue and inflammatory cells, respectively. Macrophages produce and secrete mainly MMP-9 but also some MMP-2 (Machein & Conca 1997; Welgus et al 1990; Campbell et al 1991). Stromolysins 1 and 2 (MMP-3 and MMP-10) degrade proteoglycan protein core, the non-helical regions of collagen IV, X, XI, laminin, fibronectin and procollagens I, II. They are also found in fibroblasts and inflammatory cells, respectively. Macrophages secrete only small amounts of MMP-3 when appropriately stimulated (Machein & Conca 1997; Welgus et al 1990; Campbell et al 1991). Another possibly related proteinase (MMP-11) with a similar substrate spectrum is secreted by human tumour cells. Matrilysin (MMP-7) is found in macrophages and has a similar action to the stromolysins. Another similar enzyme, with

Table 1.2 *The mechanisms of expression, transcription, release and activation of metalloproteinases by various cell types*

	CELL TYPE						
	PMN	**Macrophage**	**Fibroblast**	**Osteoblast**	**Osteoclast**	**Endothelial cell**	**Keratinocyte**
Enzyme expressed	MMP-8, 9	MMP-1, 2, 3, 9, 12	MMP-1, 2, 3, 7, 11	MMP-9	MMP-1, 2, 3, 9	MMP-1, 2, 3, 9	
Signals for transcription	Unknown	IL-1, TNF-α, EGF, TGF-α, PDGF	IL-1, TNF-α, EGF, TGF-α, PDGF	IL-1, TNF-α, PGE₂, Vitamin D₃	Signals from osteoblast	IL-1, TNF-α, EGF, TGF-α, PDGF	IL-1, TNF-α, EGF, TGF-α, PDGF
Release of enzyme	Granule release	Transcriptional activation	Transcriptional activation	Transcriptional activation	Transcriptional activation	Transcriptional activation	Transcriptional activation
Response time	Seconds	6–12 h	6–12 h	6–12 h	6–12 h	6–12 h	6–12 h
Duration of action	Minutes	Days	Days	Days	Days	Days	Days
Activation of pro-enzyme	Oxidative pathways in phagosome	Plasminogen activator, stromolysin and serine proteinases	Plasminogen activator, stromolysin and serine proteinases	Plasminogen activator, stromolysin and serine proteinases	Cysteine proteinases	Plasminogen activator, stromolysin and serine proteinases	Plasminogen activator, stromolysin and serine proteinases

MMP, matrix metalloproteinases; EGF, epidermal growth factor; IL, interleukin; TGF, transforming growth factor; TNF, tumour necrosis factor; PDGF, platelet-derived growth factor.

elastin as a primary substrate, is MMP-12 found in macrophages. Both of these proteinases are known as punctuated MMPs because they lack the C-terminal domain. The final proteinase in this group is a membrane bound MMP (MMP-14), which seems to be involved in a pathway leading to the activation of gelatinase-A.

During physiological turnover, the production and secretion of MMPs and other proteinases is carefully controlled by growth factors and cytokines (Table 1.2).

There are two main ways in which MMPs are generated by cells, transcriptional activation by growth factors and triggered release from PMN lysosomal granules (Ryan et al 1996). In mesenchymal cells and keratinocytes, certain growth factors, IL-1β, TNF-α, PDGF, TGF-α, EGF, appear to upregulate collagenase expression, while other factors, IFN-γ, TNF-β and glucocorticoids, downregulate this process. The genetic regulation involves signal transduction mechanisms leading to transactivation of the activator protein-1 element on the gene by transcription proto-oncogenes (Ryan et al 1996). Of relevance to bone resorption, parathyroid hormone, and prostaglandin PGE₂ can also increase collagenase secretion in bone cells. In relation to other MMPs the process is probably very similar and in this regard, it has recently been shown that interleukin-1β can upregulate MMP-3, at both the mRNA and protein level, in periodontal ligament cells (Nakaya et al 1997) and may thus have this role for this proteinase.

Neutrophil MMP regulation is mediated primarily by granule release rather than transcriptional events which results in a more immediate but less sustained response by this cell. MMPs are normally under tight regulation not only at the level of gene expression but also extracellularly after secretion, and disruption of this regulation can lead to pathological breakdown of connective tissue.

The MMPs are characterized by a five domain molecular structure: the signal peptide, the propeptide, the catalytic site, the hinge region and the pexin-like domain (Ryan et al 1996). These enzymes are not stored in cells other than PMNs but are secreted as inactive or latent pro-enzymes. In the activation process, the secreted pro-enzyme first loses its signal peptide. The function of the propeptide domain is to maintain enzyme latency until a signal is given for activation (Woessner 1994). During activation, the propeptide domain is cleaved off in several steps.

In cells of mesenchymal origin, activation can be carried out by serine proteinases such as plasmin and elastase and other MMPs such as stromolysins and only a small percentage of the enzyme may be activated to perform a designated physiological function. Neutrophil MMPs are activated within the phagosome by oxidative pathways (Sorsa et al 1994). PMN activation generates hydrogen peroxide, which in the presence of chlorine ions, is converted by myeloperoxidase to hypochlorous acid. This reactive oxygen species then activates the pro-MMP.

The collagenases (Ryan et al 1996) uniquely show specificity for the fibrillar collagens, while the gelatinases degrade denatured collagens and tissue constituents such as basement membrane type IV collagen (Table 1.1).

Inhibitors of MMPs play an important role in regulation since an imbalance between the amount of activated enzyme and their inhibitors can lead to pathological breakdown of extracellular matrix. The natural inhibitors of MMPs are the tissue inhibitors of MMPs (TIMPs) and alpha-2-macroglobulin (α²M) (Ryan et al 1996). TIMPs probably control MMP activities pericellularly, whereas α²M functions as a regulator in body fluids. During inflammation, however, this large molecular weight protein leaves blood vessels and may be found in the exudate within the extracellular matrix. α²M functions by entrapment of the susceptible proteinase followed by cleavage of a peptide bond in the bait region, a venus-fly trap-like mechanism. The TIMPs are widely distributed in tissue fluids and are expressed by fibroblasts, keratinocytes, endothelial cells, monocytes and macrophages (Ryan et al 1996). They are capable of inactivating all the MMPs, binding strongly to their catalytic domains and they may also prevent the activation of some latent MMPs. TIMP-1 is a glycoprotein, whereas TIMP-2 is its non-glycosylated counterpart. TIMP-3 has only just been isolated. TIMPs can be inactivated by reduction and alkylation and by serine proteinase proteolysis. TIMP-1 is associated with MMP-1, -9 and TIMP-2 with MMP-2. TIMP-1 is upregulated by retinoids, glucocorticoids, IL-1, EGF, TGF-β, TNF-α, whereas TIMP-2 is downregulated by TGF-β.

Other MMPs and cysteine and serine proteinases can also attack collagens, usually after primary cleavage by specific collagenases from fibroblasts and macrophages (MMP-1) or inflammatory cells (MMP-8). This type of collagen degradation takes place in the extracellular space, usually at times of major remodelling or during pathological states such as inflammation (see below). Elastase and cathepsin G (Table 1.3) are

Table 1.3 *The cellular distribution of serine and cysteine proteinases in inflammatory cells*

Proteinase	PMN	Macrophage
Serine		
Elastase	+++++	++
Cathepsin G	++	+
Cysteine		
Cathepsin B	+++	+++
Cathepsin L	+	+

mainly produced by PMNs but are also produced and secreted by monocytes and macrophages. Cathepsin B and L (Table 1.3) are synthesized and secreted mainly by monocytes and macrophages (Reddy et al 1995). All of these proteinases are produced and secreted following the appropriate stimuli.

Active collagenase cleaves collagen at a specific site and separates small segments of fibrils from the fibre bundle. These small collagen segments may be further degraded in the extracellular environment by other MMPs or other proteinases or they may be phagocytosed by fibroblasts or other phagocytic cells and degraded intracellularly by lysosomal enzymes (see below).

Under physiological conditions, the normal turnover of soft connective tissue probably does not involve specific collagenases (MMP-1 or MMP-8) since little or no collagenase can be detected in these tissues during health (Everts et al 1996). The normal turnover of soft connective tissue is likely to take place intracellularly within the lysosomal apparatus of fibroblasts after the phagocytosis of redundant collagen fibrils. This probably involves a multistep process as follows (see **Figs 1.10, 1.11** and Table 1.1):

1. The recognition of redundant collagen fibrils destined for degradation by membrane-bound receptors, probably integrins, on the surface of fibroblasts
2. Partial enclosure of the fibril by the fibroblast
3. Partial digestion of the fibril and its surrounding non-collagenous proteins by a MMP, probably gelatinase A (MMP-2)
4. Phagocytosis of the fibril and its segregation within a membrane bound body (phagolysosome)
5. Fusion of a lysosome containing destructive enzymes with this vacuole to form a digestive lysosome
6. Final digestion of the enclosed collagen fibrils by cysteine proteinases such as cathepsins B and L.

The modulation of this process is carried out under the influence of growth factors and cytokines including TGF-α and IL-1α. In this regard, TGF-α increases collagen fibril phagocytosis while IL-1α inhibits this process (Everts et al 1996).

The evidence for the precise mechanisms involved in these processes has been built up over recent years and is briefly described below.

First, membrane-bounded, intracellular collagen fibrils are frequently found in fibroblasts within two types of vacuole, one where the space between the fibril is filled with electron-dense material and the other with electron-lucent material (Everts et al 1996). The number of these collagen-containing vacuoles in fibroblasts is greater in tissues with a high connective tissue turnover than those with a low one. In addition, these vacuoles have been seen commonly in fibroblasts in the human periodontal ligament (**Figs 1.10, 1.11**) and gingival connective tissue (Eley & Harrison 1975). Although these vacuoles are most common in fibroblasts, they have also been seen in epithelial cells, macrophages, osteoblasts, cementoblasts, chondrocytes, odontoblasts and smooth muscle cells and this suggests that this process goes on in many connective tissues (Everts et al 1996).

Second, these intracellular fibres cannot be newly synthesized collagen for the following reasons (Everts et al 1996):

- Procollagen is secreted into the extracellular space and only then becomes aggregated into cross-banded fibrils
- Factors which block collagen synthesis have no influence on the number of intracellular collagen-containing vacuoles
- Factors which block phagocytosis completely inhibit the formation of intracellular collagen-containing vacuoles.

Third, the recognition and internalization of collagen fibrils probably involves integrins on the surface of the fibroblasts. Fibrils destined for degradation are surrounded by a meshwork of non-collagenous proteins including proteoglycans, glycoproteins and collagens V and VI. These may play a role in these

processes because integrin recognizable sequences are present on several collagens and glycoproteins such as fibronectin (Everts et al 1996).

Fourth, collagenase is not involved in processing these fibrils before they are internalized (Everts et al 1996) because:

- Factors which inhibit collagenase do not affect collagen fibril uptake by fibroblasts
- IL-1α, either alone or with EGF, stimulates the secretion of collagenase, while TGF-β inhibits its secretion
- TGF-β stimulates phagocytosis of collagen fibrils by fibroblasts, while IL-1α inhibits this process.

Therefore, there is an inverse relationship between collagenase secretion and phagocytosis of collagen fibrils by fibroblasts. However, selective inhibition of gelatinase A (MMP-2) does inhibit collagen fibril phagocytosis and prevents intracellular digestion. Thus, this enzyme may partially digest collagen fibrils prior to phagocytosis (Everts et al 1996).

Finally, the intracellular digestion of collagen fibrils involves cysteine proteinases such as cathepsins B and L (Everts et al 1996). This is because:

- Selective inhibition of cysteine proteinases increases the number of collagen containing vacuoles in fibroblasts and prevents their digestion
- Selective inhibition of cysteine proteinases prevents the release of collagen degradation products into the culture medium
- Selective inhibition of individual cysteine proteinases has proved that cathepsin B is involved in this process (Van Noorden & Everts 1991).

There are probably two pathways of collagen degradation:

1. The collagenase independent intracellular route (**Fig. 1.12**) of major importance in normal collagen turnover.
2. The collagenase-mediated extracellular route (**Fig. 1.13**), which is of importance in major tissue remodelling involving large amounts of collagen breakdown and during inflammation. This involves the secretion of a number of MMPs by fibroblasts and other cells including collagenases (MMP-1 and MMP-4), gelatinases A and B (MMP-2 and MMP-9) and stromolysins (MMP-3 and MMP-11).

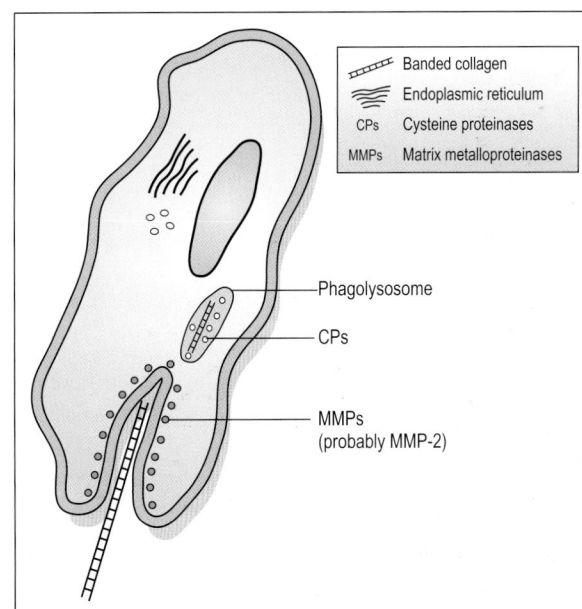

Fig. 1.12 A schematic presentation of the intracellular pathway of collagen degradation. Under physiological balanced conditions, this pathway is considered to be the major route of degradation. Collagen fibrils are engulfed by a fibroblast, and during this process the fibril is partially digested by a membrane-bound matrix metalloproteinase (MMP), probably gelatinase A (MMP-2). It is then taken up into a phagosome where it is further degraded by cysteine proteinases (CPs).

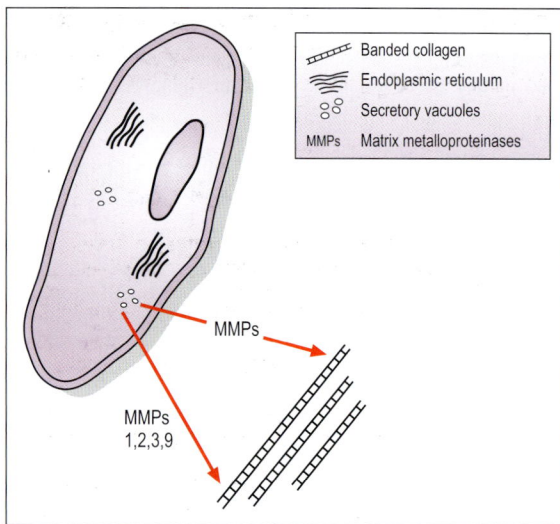

Fig. 1.13 A schematic presentation of the extracellular pathway of collagen degradation. Digestion of relatively large amounts of collagen occurs primarily in the extracellular space under the influence of a variety of enzymes secreted by the fibroblast. The most important of these are the metalloproteinases including gelatinase A (MMP-2), gelatinase B (MMP-9), collagenase (MMP-1) and stromolysin (MMP-3).

The mechanisms controlling connective tissue turnover are only partly understood (see above). Some cytokines stimulate collagen, fibronectin and proteoglycan synthesis and secretion and these include fibroblast growth factor (FGF), platelet-derived growth factor (PDGF) and transforming growth factor alpha (TGF-α) and beta (TGF-β). Other cytokines such as interleukin-1 (IL-1) and interferon gamma (IFN-γ), platelet-derived growth factor (PDGF) and transforming growth factor alpha (TGF-α) can stimulate collagenase secretion (Table 1.2). However, the control mechanisms governing the secretion of these cytokines is not fully understood.

BONE

Bone turnover takes place continually throughout life with bone deposition mediated by osteoblasts which is linked to bone resorption largely mediated by osteoclasts.

Osteoblasts are responsible for the synthesis of the bone matrix and its subsequent calcification. Initially, uncalcified matrix or osteoid is formed and this mineralized as a result of deposition of crystals of hydroxyapatite.

Osteoclasts are only formed at bone surfaces undergoing resorption. However, bone resorption cannot take place unless both osteoclasts and osteoblasts are present. Osteoblasts control the functions of osteoclasts through regulating hormones and local messengers (see Ch. 5, p. 94). Osteoblasts express at least two cytokines, receptor activator of NF kappa B ligand (RANKL) and macrophage colony stimulating factor (M-CSF), essential for osteoclast differentiation (Kobayashi & Udagawa 2007). Recent genetic studies indicate that osteoclasts also regulate the differentiation of osteoblasts *in vivo*; emphasizing the importance of communication between the two cell types during bone remodelling. Stimulated osteoblasts secrete procollagenase which when activated can remove the non-mineralized collagenous surface of bone. Osteoclasts then spread over the bone surface and beneath their ruffled borders secrete acid which dissolves the mineral phase (see **Fig. 5.4**). They also secrete lysosomal cysteine proteinases such as cathepsins B and L which are active at acid pHs and are probably responsible for removing the collagenous matrix.

This process is regulated by systemic hormones such as parathyroid hormone (PTH), vitamin D$_3$ and calcitonin and local produced factors such as prostaglandin E$_2$ (PGE$_2$), leukotrienes and cytokines such as IL-2, IL-3 and IL-6 and growth factors such as TNF-α and -β, TGF-β, PDGF (see **Fig. 5.3**).

RADIOGRAPHIC APPEARANCE OF THE PERIODONTAL TISSUES

The radiographic image represents the product of the radiodensity of the various tissues which lie in the path of the X-ray beam so that only the most radio dense tissues may be discernible. Thus, interdental bone registers while buccal and lingual plates of bone may be almost completely obscured by the image of the tooth (**Fig. 1.14**).

The discernible anatomical features on the radiograph are as follows:

The socket walls and crest of the interdental septa register as linear radio-opacities, the white line of the lamina dura outlining the socket (**Fig. 1.15**). The presence and clarity of these features reflect the contour of the alveolar crest and of the tooth socket, and variations in the thickness of these white lines, or their complete absence, do not necessarily mean that disease is present.

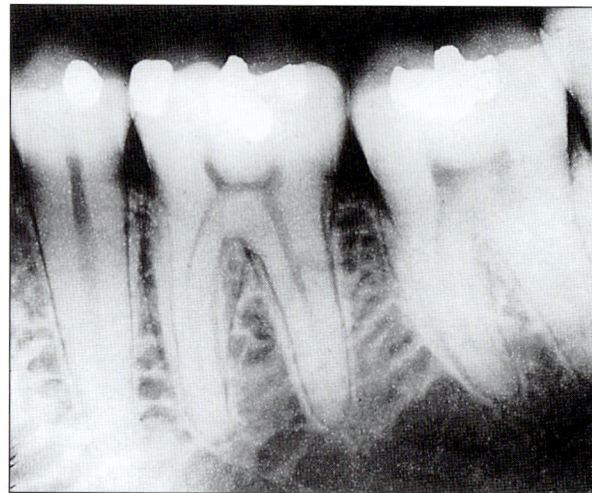

Fig. 1.14 Radiographic appearance of healthy tooth supporting tissue. The alveolar crest and sockets are delineated by a radio-opaque line. The images of the buccal and lingual plates of bone are obscured by the image of the tooth.

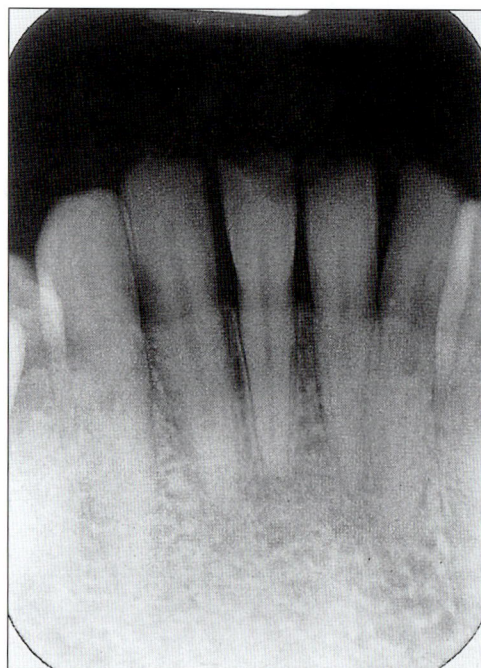

Fig. 1.15 Radiograph of the lower incisors shows that the image of the crest of the alveolar septa is less defined than between molars (Courtesy of Dr A. Sidi).

Because the facial-lingual width of the interdental septum between molars is substantial, the image of the crest is well delineated. The interdental septa between premolars and incisors are much narrower, therefore they are more radiolucent and the images of the crests tend to be less well defined (**Fig. 1.16**).

The periodontal space between the calcified structures is extremely narrow and shows as a thin dark line around the root. Where the proximal tooth surface is wide, this line is likely to be clearer than where the interproximal dimension is narrow and in some cases it may not be discernible at all. Increased functional stress produces a thickened periodontal ligament which is reflected on the radiographic film (**Fig. 1.16**). A composite image of the cancellous bone trabeculation is projected on to the radiograph and the image density reflects the density of the bone.

Cementum is discernible only when hypercementosis has taken place.

As the radiographic image can be distorted easily by alterations in beam angle and variation in exposure time and developing time, it is essential to use a completely standardized procedure. Lack of standardization makes comparison impossible and misdiagnosis possible.

AGE CHANGES IN THE PERIODONTIUM

Because destructive periodontal disease tends to manifest itself most frequently in early middle age and is more advanced in the older individual, it was regarded as part of the ageing process. This is not the case. Age changes do take place in the healthy periodontal tissues; periodontal disease is not one of them. It is important to distinguish true age changes from the effects of trauma and disease which may accompany age.

The vasculature, the gingiva, periodontal ligament, cementum and alveolar bone demonstrate age changes and it is possible that the vascular changes, e.g. thickening of vessel walls, narrowing of the lumen, even arteriosclerosis, are central to changes in the tissues generally. Briefly, these consist of loss of cellularity and increasing fibrosis. There may also be loss of ground substance and thickening of basement membranes.

In the periodontal ligament, fibre bundles are thicker and less distinct. Cementum, especially in the apical area, is thicker largely as a compensation for attrition of occlusal tooth surfaces.

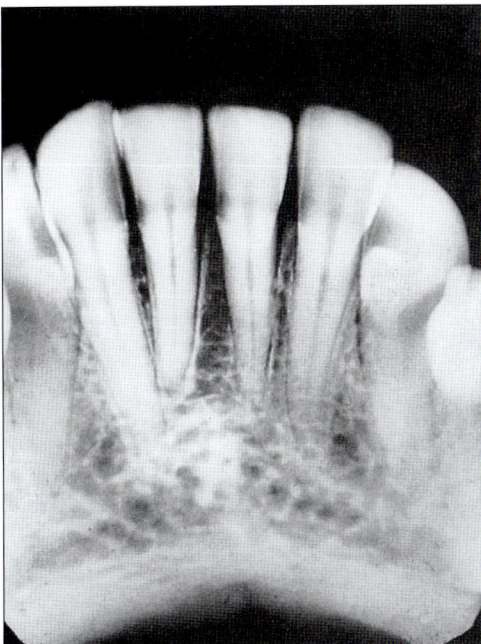

Fig. 1.16 Widening of the periodontal space at 1/1 indicating thickened ligament as response to increased occlusal stress.

The alveolar bone becomes less vascular and many haversian systems are closed. Some osteoporosis may be evident but this is not usually as severe as in the long bones. Finally, in old age, wound healing may be slower.

REFERENCES

Anderson TJ, Lapp CA, Billman MA, et al: Effects of transforming growth factor β and platelet-derived growth factor on human gingival fibroblasts grown in serum-containing and serum-free medium, *J Clin Periodontol* 25:48–55, 1998.

Bartold PM: Periodontal tissues in health and disease: introduction, *Periodontol 2000* 40:7–10, 2006.

Bartold MP, Shi S, Gronthos S: Stem cells and periodontal regeneration, *Periodontol 2000* 40:164–172, 2006.

Becker J, Schuppan D, Muller S: Immunohistochemical distribution of collagen types I, III, IV, VI, of undulin and tenascin in oral fibrous hyperplasia, *J Oral Pathol Med* 22:463–467, 1993.

Belal MH, Watanabe H, Ichinose S, et al: Effect of Er. YAG laser combined with rh PDGF-BB on attachment of cultured fibroblasts to periodontally involved root surfaces, *J Periodontol* 78:1329–1341, 2007.

Berkowitz BMB, Holland GR, Moxham BJ: *A Colour Atlas and Textbook of Oral Anatomy, Histology and Embryology*, ed 2, London, 1992, Wolfe Publishing, pp. 172–174, 182–183.

Berkowitz BMB, Moxham BJ, Newman HN: *Periodontal Ligament in Health and Disease*, ed 2, Barcelona, 1995, Mosby-Wolfe.

Bilezikian JP, Raisz LG, Rodan GA: *Principles of Bone Biology*, San Diego, 1996, Academic Press.

Blom S, Holmstrup P, Dabelsteen E: A comparison of the effect of epidermal growth factor, platelet-derived growth factor and fibroblast growth factor on rat periodontal ligament fibroblast-like cells' DNA synthesis and morphology, *J Periodontol* 65:373–378, 1994.

Campbell EJ, Cury JD, Shapiro SD, et al: Neutral metalloproteinases produced by human mononuclear phagocytes. Cellular differentiation markedly alters cell phenotype for serine proteinases, metalloproteinases, and tissue inhibitor of metalloproteinases, *J Immunol* 146:1286–1293, 1991.

Chen SC, Marino V, Gronthos S, et al: Location of putative stem cells in human periodontal ligament, *J Periodontal Res* 41:547–553, 2006.

Dereka XE, Markopoulou CE, Vrotsos IA: Role of growth factors on periodontal repair, *Growth Factors* 24:260–267, 2006.

D'Errico JA, MakNeil RL, Takata T, et al: Expression of bone associated markers by tooth root lining cells in situ and in vitro, *Bone* 20:117–126, 1997.

Dyson JA, Genever PG, Dalgarno KW, et al: Development of custom-built bone scaffolds using mesenchymal stem cells and apatite-wollastonite glass ceramics, *Tissue Eng* 13:2891–2901, 2007.

Eley BM, Harrison JD: Intracellular collagen fibrils in the periodontal ligament of man, *J Periodontal Res* 10:168–170, 1975.

Embery G, Picton D, Stanbury JB: Biochemical changes in the periodontal ligament ground substance associated with short-term intrusive loading in adult monkeys, *Arch Oral Biol* 32:545–549, 1987.

Everts V, Van der Zee E, Creemers L, et al: Phagocytosis and intracellular digestion of collagen, its role in turnover and remodelling, *Histochem J* 28:229–245, 1996.

Frank S, Madlener M, Werner S: Transforming growth factor β1, β2 and β3 and their receptors are differentially regulated during normal and impaired wound healing, *J Biol Chem* 271:10188–11019, 1996.

Fujisawa R, Nodaska Y, Kuboki Y: Further characterization of the interaction between bone sialoprotein (BSP) and collagen, *Calcifying Tissue Internation* 56:140–144, 1995.

Fulcher JA, Hashimi ST, Levroney EL, et al: Galectin-1-matured human monocyte-derived dendritic cells have enhanced migration through extracellular matrix, *J Immunol* 177:216–226, 2006.

Gallagher JT, Lyon M, Steward WP: Structure and function of heparan sulphate proteoglycans, *Biochem J* 236:313–323, 1986.

Giannopoulou C, Cimasoni G: Functional characteristics of periodontal and gingival fibroblasts, *J Dent Res* 75:895–902, 1996.

Goa J, Jordan TW, Cutress TW: Immunolocalization of basic fibroblast growth factor (bFGF) in human periodontal ligament (PDL) tissue, *J Periodontal Res* 31:260–264, 1996.

Gordon JA, Tye CE, Sampaio AV, et al: Bone sialoprotein expression enhances osteoblast differentiation and matrix mineralization in vitro, *Bone* 41:462–473, 2007.

Gotz W, Heinen M, Lossdorfer S, et al: Immunohistochemical localization of components of the insulin-like growth factor system in human permanent teeth, *Arch Oral Biol* 51:387–395, 2006.

Hassell TM: Tissues and cells of the periodontium, *Periodontol 2000* 3:9–38, 1993.

Hughes FJ: Cytokines and cell signalling in the periodontium, *Oral Dis* 1:259–265, 1995.

Igarashi A, Okochi H, Bradham DM, et al: Regulation of connective tissue growth factor gene expression in human skin fibroblasts and during wound repair, *Mol Biol Cell* 4:637–645, 1993.

Ioannidou E: Therapeutic modulation of growth factors and cytokines in regenerative medicine, *Curr Pharm Des* 12:2397–2408, 2006.

Irwin CR, Schor SL, Ferguson MWJ: Effects of cytokines on gingival fibroblasts in vitro are modulated by extracellular matrix, *J Periodontal Res* 29:309–317, 1994.

Kawase T, Sato S, Miake K, et al: Alkaline phosphatase of human periodontal ligament fibroblast-like cells, *Adv Dent Res* 2:234–239, 1988.

Kobayashi Y, Udagawa N: Mechanisms of alveolar bone remodelling, *Clin Calcium* 17:209–216, 2007.

Kuru L, Griffiths GS, Parkar MH, et al: Flow cytometry analysis of gingival and periodontal ligament cells, *J Dent Res* 77:555–564, 1998.

Lang H, Schüler N, Arnhold S, et al: Formation of differentiated tissues in vivo by periodontal cell populations cultured in vitro, *J Dent Res* 74:1219–1225, 1995.

Lang H, Schüler N, Nolden R: Attachment formation following replantation of cultured cells into periodontal defects – a study in minipigs, *J Dent Res* 77:393–405, 1998.

Larjava H, Häkkinen L, Rahemtulla F: A biochemical analysis of human periodontal tissue proteoglycans, *Biochem J* 284:267–274, 1992.

Lekic P, McCulloch CA: Periodontal ligament cell populations: the central role of fibroblasts in creating a unique tissue, *Anat Rec* 245:491–500, 1996.

Listgarten MA: Normal development, structure, physiology and repair of the gingival epithelium, *Oral Sci Rev* 1:3–67, 1972.

Lu H, Mackenzie IC, Levine AE: Transforming growth factor-β response and expression in junctional and oral gingival epithelial cells, *J Periodontal Res* 32:682–691, 1997.

Machein N, Conca W: Expression of several matrix metalloproteinase genes in human monocytic cells, *Adv Exp Med Biol* 421:247–251, 1997.

MacNeil LR, Berry J, D'Errico J, et al: Role of two mineral-associated adhesion molecules, osteopontin and bone sialoprotein, during cementogenesis, *Connect Tissue Res* 33:1–7, 1995.

MacNeil LR, Berry J, Strayhorn C, et al: Expression of bone sialoprotein mRNA by cells lining the mouse tooth rot during cementogenesis, *Arch Oral Biol* 41:827–835, 1996.

Mariotti A: The extracellular matrix of the periodontium; dynamic and interactive tissues, *Periodontol 2000* 3:39–63, 1993.

Matsuura M, Herr Y, Han KY, et al: Immunochemical expression of extracellular matrix components of normal and healing periodontal tissues in the beagle dog, *J Periodontol* 66:579–593, 1995.

Meikle MC: On the transplantation, regeneration and induction of bone: the path of bone morphogenetic proteins and other skeletal growth factors, *Surgeon* 5:232–243, 2007.

Melcher AH, McCulloch CAG, Cheong T, et al: Cells from bone synthesize cementum-like and bone-like tissue in vitro and may migrate into the periodontal ligament in vivo, *J Periodontal Res* 22:246–247, 1987.

Midwood KS, Mao Y, Hsia HC, et al: Modulation of cell-fibronectin matrix interactions during tissue repair, *J Investig Dermatol Symp Proc* 11:73–78, 2006.

Murakami S: Periodontal regeneration by FGF2, *Clin Calcium* 17:249–255, 2007.

Murata M, Hara K, Saku T: Dynamic distribution of basic fibroblast growth factor during epulis formation: an immunohistochemical study in an enhanced healing process in the gingiva, *J Oral Pathol Med* 26:224–232, 1997.

Nagatomo K, Komaki M, Sekiya I, et al: Stem cell properties of human periodontal ligament cells, *J Periodontal Res* 41:303–310, 2006.

Nakaya H, Oates TW, Hoany HM, et al: Effects of interleukin-1β on matrix metalloproteinase-3 levels in human periodontal ligament cells, *J Periodontol* 68:517–533, 1997.

Nishimura F, Terranova VP: Comparative study of the chemotactic responses of periodontal ligament cells and gingival fibroblasts to polypeptide growth factors, *J Dent Res* 75:986–992, 1996.

Nohutcu RM, McCauley LK, Shigeyama Y, et al: Expression of mineral-associated proteins by periodontal ligament cells: in vitro vs ex vivo, *J Periodontal Res* 31:369–372, 1996.

Nojima N, Kobayashi M, Shionome M, et al: Fibroblast cells derived from bovine periodontal ligaments have the phenotypes of osteoblasts, *J Periodontal Res* 25:179–185, 1990.

Palmer RM, Lubbock MJ: The soft tissues of the gingiva and periodontal ligament: are they unique? *Oral Dis* 1:230–237, 1995.

Popowics T, Foster BL, Swanson EC, et al: Defining the roots of cementum formation, *Cells Tissues Organs* 181:248–257, 2005.

Pussinen PJ, Paju S, Mantyla P, et al: Serum microbial and host derived markers of periodontal diseases: a review, *Curr Med Chem* 14:2402–2412, 2007.

Reddy VY, Zhang Q-Y, Weiss SJ: Pericellular mobilization of tissue-destructive cysteine proteinases, cathepsins B, L, and S, by human monocyte-derived macrophages, *Proc Natl Acad Sci U S A* 92:3849–3853, 1995.

Reynolds JJ: Collagenases and tissue inhibitors of metalloproteinases; a functional balance in tissue degradation, *Oral Dis* 2:70–76, 1996.

Reynolds JJ, Hembry RM, Meikle MC: Connective tissue degradation in health and periodontal disease and the role of matrix metalloproteinases and their natural inhibitors, *Adv Dent Res* 8:312–319, 1994.

Ripamonti U: Recapitulating development: a template for periodontal tissue engineering, *Tissue Eng* 13:51–71, 2007.

Ripamonti U, Renton L: Bone morphogenetic proteins and the induction of periodontal tissue regeneration, *Periodontol 2000* 41:73–87, 2006.

Romanos GE, Strub JR, Bernimoulin JP: Immunochemical distribution of extracellular proteins as a diagnostic parameter in healthy and diseased gingival tissue, *J Periodontol* 64:110–119, 1993.

Ryan ME, Ramamurthy S, Golub LM: Matrix metalloproteinases and their inhibition in periodontal treatment, *Curr Opin Periodontol* 3:85–96, 1996.

Saga Y, Yagi T, Ikawa Y, et al: Mice develop normally without tenascin, *Genes Dev* 6:1821–1831, 1992.

Sage EH, Borstein P: Extracellular proteins that modulate cell-matrix interactions. SPARC, tenascin, and thrombospondin, *J Biol Chem* 266:14831–14834, 1991.

Sarment DP, Cooke JW, Miller SE, et al: Effect of rh PDGF-BB on bone turnover during periodontal repair, *J Clin Periodontol* 33:135–140, 2006.

Sato R, Yamamoto H, Kasai K, et al: Distribution pattern of versican, link protein and hyaluronic acid in the rat periodontal ligament during experimental tooth movement, *J Periodontal Res* 37:15–22, 2002.

Somerman MJ, Archer SY, Imm GR, et al: A comparative study of periodontal ligament cells and gingival fibroblasts in vitro, *J Dent Res* 67:66–70, 1988.

Somerman MJ, Foster RA, Imm GR, et al: Periodontal ligament cells and gingival fibroblasts respond differently to attachment factors in vitro, *J Periodontol* 60:73–77, 1989.

Somerman MJ, Young MF, Foster RA, et al: Characteristics of human periodontal ligament cells in vitro, *Arch Oral Biol* 35:241–247, 1990.

Sorsa T, Ding Y, Sato T, et al: Effects of tetracyclines on neutrophil, gingival and salivary collagenases: a functional and Western blot assessment with special reference to their cellular sources in periodontal disease, *Ann N Y Acad Sci* 732:112–131, 1994.

Steffensen B, Duong AH, Milam SB, et al: Immunohistochemical localization of cell adhesion proteins and integrins in the periodontium, *J Periodontol* 63:584–592, 1992.

Ten Cate AR: *Oral Histology. Development, Structure and Function*, ed 4, St Louis, 1994, Mosby.

Ten Cate AR: The development of the periodontium – a largely ectomesenchymally derived unit, *Periodontol 2000* 13:9–19, 1997.

Van Dijk LJ, Schakenraad JM, Van der Voort HM, et al: Cell-seeding of periodontal ligament fibroblasts. A novel technique to create new attachment. A pilot study, *J Clin Periodontol* 18:196–199, 1991.

Van Noorden CJF, Everts V: The selective inhibition of cysteine proteinases by Z-Phe-AlaCH₂F suppresses digestion of collagen by fibroblasts and osteoclasts, *Biochem Biophys Res Commun* 178:178–184, 1991.

Waddington RJ, Embery G: Structural characterization of human alveolar bone proteoglycans, *Arch Oral Biol* 36:859–866, 1991.

Welgus HG, Campbell EJ, Cury JD, et al: Neutral metalloproteinases produced by human mononuclear phagocytes. Enzyme profile, regulation, and expression during cellular development, *J Clin Invest* 86:1496–1502, 1990.

Woessner J Jr: The family of matrix metalloproteinases, *Ann N Y Acad Sci* 732:11–21, 1994.

Zhang X, Schuppan D, Becker J, et al: Distribution of undulin, tenascin, and fibronectin in the human periodontal ligament and cementum: comparative immuno-electron microscopy with ultra-thin cryosections, *J Histochem Cytochem* 41:245–251, 1993.

Zhurov AI, Limbert G, Aeschlimann DP, et al: A constitutive model for the periodontal ligament as a compressible transversely isotropic visco-hyperelastic tissue, *Comput Methods Biomech Biomed Engin* 10:223–235, 2007.

FURTHER READING

Berkowitz BMB, Moxham BJ, Newman HN: *Periodontal Ligament in Health and Disease*, ed 2, Barcelona, 1995, Mosby-Wolfe.

Berkowitz BMB, Holland GR, Moxham BJ: *A Colour Atlas and Textbook of Oral Anatomy, Histology and Embryology*, ed 2, London, 1992, Wolfe Publishing Ltd.

Williams DM, Hughes FJ, Odell EW, et al: *The Normal Periodontium. Pathology of Periodontal Disease*, Oxford, 1992, Oxford Medical Press, pp. 17–31.

The oral mucosa is bathed in saliva and exposed to the passage of food, the oral flora and stimulus or injury from toothbrushes and other oral hygiene aids, as well as other objects that people put in their mouths such as cigarettes, pipes, hairgrips and so. Considering the variety of such factors, the variations in temperature, pH values, range of textures and the diversity of oral habits, the oral mucosa demonstrates remarkable adaptability and resistance.

The tooth surface which is also exposed to these factors may become covered wholly or in part by a number of deposits, pellicle, plaque, food debris, calculus, materia alba and stains.

SALIVA

Saliva plays a vital role in maintaining the integrity of the oral tissues, in food digestion and in speech. As every clinician knows, there is considerable variation in the rate of secretion from the several salivary glands. This is influenced by neurotransmission mechanisms in response to olfactory, gustatory and masticatory stimuli, and even the thought of food can increase secretion. The average unstimulated or resting flow rate is about 0.3–0.4 mL/min but in some people can reach about 2 mL/min. The stimulated flow rate can vary between 0.2–6.0 mL/min.

COMPOSITION

Saliva is 99.5% water plus 0.5% organic and inorganic substances. The organic fraction contains both large and small molecules; the former is mainly protein in the form of glycoproteins together with some gammaglobulins, serum albumin and enzymes; the latter include glucose, urea and creatinine. The inorganic fraction consists of calcium, phosphorus, sodium, potassium and magnesium as well as dissolved carbon dioxide, oxygen and nitrogen. The main salivary enzyme is amylase but in disease, many enzymes produced by bacteria and leucocytes are found. Most of the organic fraction is produced by the salivary gland cells and the remainder is transported into saliva from the blood. Among the compounds transported from the blood are the electrolytes, albumin, immunoglobulins G, A and M, and vitamins, drugs and hormones. Indeed there is a good correlation between plasma and salivary levels of hormones and medications.

FUNCTION

Saliva has a number of functions:

1. In the digestive process it helps to form the food bolus and provides amylase for the digestion of starch.
2. The flow of viscous fluid helps to remove bacterial and food debris.
3. Bicarbonates and phosphates buffer food and bacterial acids.
4. Salivary mucin and other constituents protect the oral mucosa and tooth surfaces in a variety of ways:
    (a) Salivary glycoproteins cover and lubricate the mucosa. This protective action becomes more obvious when it is removed, as in xerostomia (dry mouth) caused by pathology of the salivary glands. The oral mucosa becomes dry and red, bleeds readily and is prone to infection.
    (b) The antibacterial enzyme lysozyme acts by splitting bacterial cell walls and acting as a scavenger.
    (c) Antibacterial gammaglobulin (antibody), mostly immunoglobulin A (IgA), appears to have two forms of protective action:
        (i) It prevents the attachment of bacteria and viruses to the tooth surface and oral mucosa.
        (ii) It reacts with food antigens to neutralize their effect.
    (d) Leucocytes: Saliva contains a large number of leucocytes which migrate through the junctional epithelium and, as stated, the number of salivary leucocytes increases when there is gingival inflammation.
    (e) The enzyme sialoperoxidase has antibacterial activity, especially against lactobacilli and streptococci.
    (f) The mineral components, in particular calcium and phosphorus ions, act to maintain tooth integrity by modulating ion diffusion and preventing the loss of mineral ions from the tooth tissue. The interchange of minerals between tooth structure and saliva goes on constantly and decalcification of enamel may be remineralized.
5. The water and mucin (glycoprotein) form the lubricant essential to speech in making smooth the movements and contacts of the lips, and the tongue against the teeth and palate which enable us to form consonants.

ORAL BACTERIA

At birth the mouth is sterile but within a few hours microorganisms appear, mainly *Streptococcus salivarius*. By the time the deciduous teeth erupt, a complex flora is present. Bacteria are present in saliva, on the tongue and cheeks, on tooth surfaces, especially in fissures, and in the gingival crevice. The number of bacteria in saliva can be measured in thousands of millions/mL but the largest population of bacteria is found on the dorsum of the tongue. Even the healthy gingival crevice contains more bacteria than are free in saliva, and in periodontal disease, the crevicular population multiplies.

One can regard the various parts of the mouth, i.e. tongue, cheeks, tooth fissures, saliva, gingival crevices, as consisting of different ecosystems in which different varieties of bacteria are found in balance with one another and with the tissues. The dominant organisms are streptococci. The number and variety vary from person to person, from one part of the mouth to another, even on different surfaces of the same tooth, before and after eating or toothbrushing. Age, diet, composition of saliva and its rate of flow as well as systemic factors influence the oral flora (see pp. 34, 36, 57 and Chs 3, 4 and 5).

TOOTH DEPOSITS

DENTAL PLAQUE: A HOST-ASSOCIATED BIOFILM

Dental plaque is a bacteria biofilm which is a complex association of many different bacterial species together in a single environment. This arrangement can have major advantages to bacteria and the host. For instance the bacteria in this arrangement are more resistant to external environmental changes and have lower nutritional requirements. An example of the former property is that the susceptibility of bacteria to antimicrobial agents is significantly reduced by the biofilm structure (Costerton et al 1987).

The plaque biofilm community is initially formed through bacterial interaction with the tooth, and then through physical and physiological interactions between different species within the microbial mass. Furthermore, the bacteria within the plaque biofilm are also influenced by host-mediated environmental factors. In this regard, periodontal health can be regarded as a state of balance in which the bacterial population co-exists with the host and no irreparable damage occurs to either the bacteria or the host. However, disruption of this balance may cause alterations in both the host and biofilm bacteria and result ultimately in destruction of periodontal tissues.

Dental plaque displays properties that are typical of biofilms and microbial communities in general, a clinical consequence of which is a reduced susceptibility to antimicrobial agents as well as pathogenic synergism (Marsh 2005).

Structure and composition of dental plaque

Dental plaque can be broadly classified as supragingival or subgingival plaque. Supragingival plaque is found at or above the gingival margin and may be in direct contact with the gingival margin. Subgingival plaque is found below the gingival margin, between the tooth and the gingival sulcular tissue and is described in a separate section below.

Dental plaque is composed primarily of microorganisms and 1 g of plaque (wet weight) contains approximately 2×10^{11} bacteria (Socransky et al 1963; Gibbons et al 1963). It has been estimated that more than 325 different bacterial species may be found in plaque (Moore 1987) from the potential of more than 500 species recorded from oral samples (Whittaker et al 1996). Non-bacterial microorganisms are also occasionally found within plaque and these include *Mycoplasma* species, yeasts, protozoa and viruses. The microorganisms exist within an intracellular matrix that also contains a few host cells, such as epithelial cells and leucocytes.

Approximately 70–80% of plaque is microbial and the rest represents extracellular matrix. The intercellular matrix, which accounts for about 20% of plaque mass, consists of organic and inorganic materials derived from saliva, gingival crevicular fluid and bacterial products. Organic constituents of the matrix include polysaccharides, proteins, glycoproteins and lipids. The most common carbohydrate produced by bacteria is dextran; there is also some levan and galactose. The principal inorganic components are calcium, phosphorus, traces of magnesium, sodium, potassium and fluoride. The inorganic salt content is highest on the lingual surface of the lower incisors. Calcium ions may actually aid adhesion between bacteria and between bacteria and the pellicle. The source of both the organic and inorganic components is primarily saliva and as the mineral content increases, the plaque mass may be calcified to form calculus (see below).

Plaque formation

The main stages in supragingival plaque formation are:

- Pellicle formation
- Initial colonization
- Secondary colonization and plaque maturation.

Pellicle formation

Within seconds of tooth cleaning a thin layer of salivary protein, largely glycoprotein, is deposited on to the tooth surface (as well as on to restorations and dentures). This layer, called acquired salivary pellicle, is thin (0.5 μm), smooth, colourless and translucent. It adheres firmly to the tooth

surface and can be removed only by positive friction. There appears to be an electrostatic affinity between hydroxyapatite and certain salivary components such as glycoprotein. Initially the pellicle is bacteria free.

The specific components of pellicles on different surfaces vary in composition and studies of early (2 h) enamel pellicle show that its amino-acid composition differs from that of saliva (Scannapieco & Levine 1990) indicating that pellicle forms from selective absorption of salivary macromolecules.

The function of salivary pellicle is mainly protective. In this regard, salivary glycoproteins and salivary calcium and phosphate ions are adsorbed on to the enamel surface and this process may compensate for tooth loss from attrition and erosion. Pellicle also restricts the diffusion of acid products of sugar breakdown. It can bind other inorganic ions such as fluoride which promote remineralization. Pellicle also may contain antibacterial factors including IgG, IgA, IgM, complement and lysozyme.

As dental pellicles are formed on non-shedding surfaces, they also provide a substrate on which bacteria progressively accumulate to form plaque. The exact function of the many individual components of saliva in plaque formation is unclear and the potential number of permutations between the 80 or more salivary components and the 500 or more bacterial species in the oral cavity is immense. It is believed that some salivary components aid plaque formation by being involved in bacterial agglutination or by acting as nutritional substrates, while others may block microbial adhesion to host surfaces.

The various salivary bacterial interactions are set out below:

1. Bacteria can bind to receptors in pellicle via adhesins. However, the same components free within saliva may also bind to the bacterial adhesins and thus hinder their binding to the tooth and foster their clearance from the mouth
2. Salivary components may interact with the bacteria through multivalent binding to cause agglutinization which may increase their rate of clearance from the mouth. Alternatively, small aggregates of bacteria might adhere to the tooth
3. Some salivary components are toxic to oral bacteria and may lyse their cell membranes
4. Salivary components may serve as a nutritive source for bacteria.

Initial colonization

Very soon, indeed within minutes, after the pellicle has been deposited, it is populated by bacteria. Bacteria may deposit directly on to enamel but usually they attach to pellicle and the bacterial aggregates may be coated in salivary glycoprotein. In primitive peoples on a 'natural' diet of hard and fibrous food occlusal surfaces and contact areas are subject to considerable wear so that bacterial deposition is minimal. When a soft 'civilized' diet is used, tooth wear is slight or absent and bacterial deposition is encouraged. Accumulations are greatest in sites sheltered from functional friction and tongue movement. The interdental region below the contact area is the site of greatest plaque thickness.

Within the first few hours, species of *Streptococcus* and a little later *Actinomyces* attach to the pellicle and these are the initial colonizers (Doyle et al 1982). During the first few days this bacterial population grows along and spreads out from the tooth surface so that under an electron microscope one can see palisades of organisms rather like skyscrapers, one layer on top of another radiating from the surface (Lundquist et al 1989). These parallel columns of bacteria are separated by narrow spaces and plaque growth proceeds by the deposition of new species into these spaces. These newly deposited species attach to the pioneering bacteria using specific molecular lock and key mechanisms. In this regard, new bacteria derived from saliva or the surrounding mucous membrane appear to sense the bacteria-laden nature of the tooth surface and attach by a bonding interaction with already attached plaque bacteria. These associations are known as intergeneric co-aggregations and are mediated by specific attachment proteins that occur between the partner cells (Kolenbrander 1988).

Supragingival plaque formation is also pioneered by bacteria with an ability to form extracellular polysaccharides which allow them to adhere to the tooth and each other and these include *Streptococcus mitior*, *S. sanguis*, *Actinomyces viscosus* and *A. naeslundii*.

These two phases of initial plaque formation take about 2 days. Plaque grows by both internal multiplication and surface deposition. However, internal multiplication slows considerably as plaque matures.

Secondary colonization and plaque maturation

The secondary colonizers enter plaque on the back of the primary plaque formers and take advantage of the changes in environment that occur as the result of primary plaque growth and metabolism. First, in this process, any remaining interstitial spaces formed by the bacteria interactions described above become occupied by Gram-negative cocci such as *Neisseria* and *Veillonella* species. Second, after 4–7 days of unchecked plaque formation, gingival inflammation will develop. During this process, the environmental conditions will gradually change causing further selective changes. This includes the opening up of the gingival crevice as a site for further bacterial growth and the initiation of gingival crevicular fluid flow. This in turn produces a supply of further nutrients from the serum. This enables other bacteria with different metabolic requirements to enter plaque and these include Gram-negative rods such as *Prevotella, Porphyromonas, Capnocytophaga, Fusobacterium* and *Bacteroides* species. By 7–11 days the complexity of plaque increases still further by the appearance of motile bacteria such as spirochaetes and *Vibrios*. Further bacterial interactions occur between a number of different species (Kolenbrander et al 1989; Kolenbrander & London 1993). These secondary colonizers also form the main groups of bacteria from which subgingival plaque may subsequently form.

Thus, a complex microflora is established which represents a balanced equilibrium of organisms or microbial ecosystem on the tooth surface (**Fig. 2.1**). The mature plaque is packed full of a myriad of indigenous bacterial species and this makes it difficult for exogenous bacterial species to colonize it (Christersson et al 1985). Thus dental plaque, like other indigenous flora on the skin, oral and other mucous membranes and in the gut, is highly protective in preventing the ingress of pathogenic species. Moore et al (1982) have isolated 166 different bacterial species from supragingival plaque.

Interestingly, a recent study (Sanai et al 2002) of 150 children aged 8–11 showed that 31% of them already harboured putative periodontal pathogens including *Porphyromonas gingivalis*, *Prevotella intermedia* and *P. nigrescens* in their mouths. It was also found that two-thirds of the isolates from these subjects carried the erm (F), erythromycin resistance, and tet (Q), tetracycline resistance genes.

At a clinical level dental plaque is a soft, non-calcified layer of bacteria which accumulates on and adheres to teeth and other objects in the mouth, e.g. restorations, dentures and calculus. In thin layers it is scarcely visible and can be revealed only by the use of a disclosing agent (**Fig. 2.2**). In thick layers it can be seen as a yellowish or grey deposit which cannot be removed with mouthwash or by irrigation but can be brushed off. It is unusual to find it on the masticatory surface of the tooth unless that tooth is out of function, when gross deposits may form.

Plaque deposition and food intake

Plaque will form in patients and animals fed by a stomach tube, although in diminished amounts. There is some debate as to whether the frequency of meals or the amount of food eaten influences the amount of plaque deposited. However, plaque bacteria do use nutrients which can diffuse easily into the plaque, e.g. soluble sugars, sucrose, fructose, glucose, maltose and lactose. Starches may also serve as a bacterial substrate.

Dextran is the most important extracellular bacterial product because of its relative insolubility and adhesive properties. It can be produced from sucrose in the diet and influences plaque deposition and metabolism. Plaque forms more rapidly during sleep than following meals because the mechanical action of eating plus the stimulated salivary flow deters plaque deposition. Eating hard, coarse and fibrous food deters plaque formation and this fact is used in the experimental production of plaque. Gingivitis in the dog can be produced by feeding a soft diet for as short a time as 4 days.

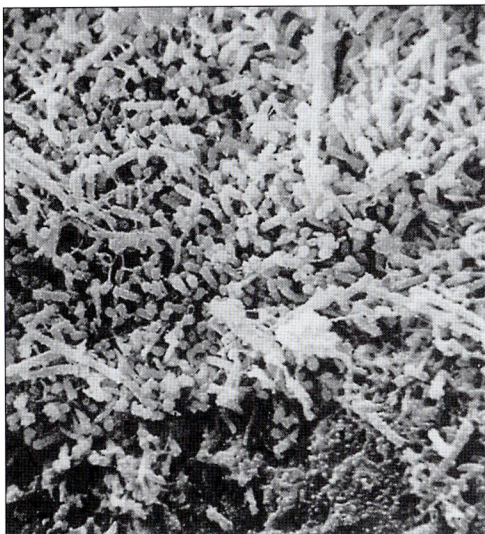

Fig. 2.1 Scanning electron micrograph of organisms in mature plaque (× 1400) (Courtesy of Dr HN Newman and the publishers of the British Dental Journal).

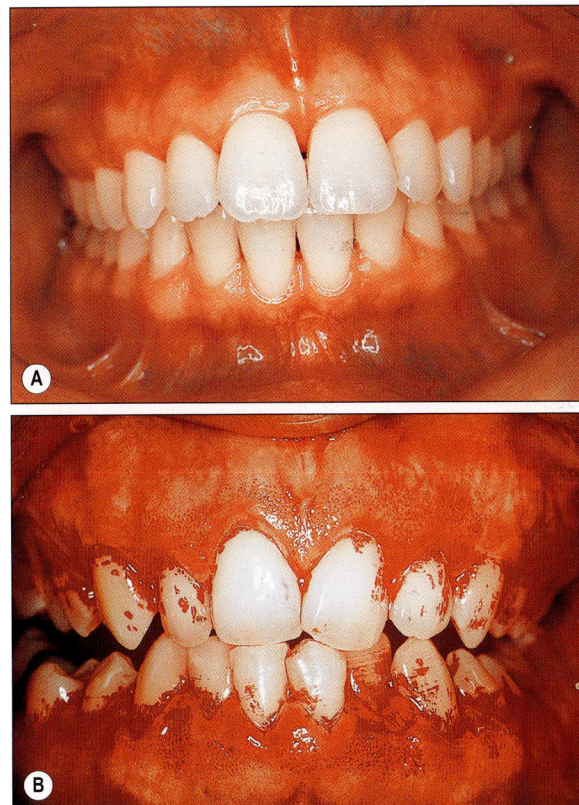

Fig. 2.2 (A) Plaque deposits seen prior to the use of a disclosing agent (B) as revealed by disclosing agent.

Although some debate still lingers about the benefits of finishing meals with apples, celery and carrots, these are preferable to the usual very sweet dessert offerings. Certainly vigorous mastication which produces natural tooth wear on both occlusal and interproximal surfaces minimizes plaque deposition.

MATERIA ALBA

This is a yellowish or whitish, soft, loose deposit found in neglected mouths (**Fig. 2.3**). It consists of a mass of microorganisms, desquamated epithelial cells, food debris, leucocytes plus salivary deposits. Its structure is amorphous and unlike plaque it can be removed easily and washed away with a water spray.

DENTAL CALCULUS (TARTAR)

Calculus, the 'stony crust' that forms on teeth, has long been associated with periodontal disease. Along with other pathological calcifications, e.g. kidney stones and gallstones, dental calculus is described in ancient medical writings. Calculus is a calcified mass which forms on and adheres to the surface of teeth and other solid objects in the mouth, e.g. restorations and dentures, which are not exposed to friction. Calculus is calcified plaque. Stages in its formation can be studied by collection on plastic veneers attached to teeth or dentures.

Calculus is rarely found on deciduous teeth and is not common on the permanent teeth of young children. However, by the age of 9 it is found frequently and it is present in virtually all adult mouths.

Deposits are classified according to their relationship to the gingival margin, i.e. they are either supragingival or subgingival.

SUPRAGINGIVAL CALCULUS

By definition this is found coronal to the gingival margin (**Fig. 2.4**). It is deposited first on tooth surfaces opposite salivary ducts, on the lingual surfaces of lower incisors and the buccal surfaces of upper molars, but it may be deposited on any tooth or denture not adequately cleaned, as for example the occlusal surface of an unopposed tooth. It is light yellow unless stained by other factors (e.g. tobacco, wine, betel nut), fairly hard, brittle and easily detached from the tooth by a suitable instrument.

SUBGINGIVAL CALCULUS

This is attached to root surface and its distribution is not related to the salivary glands but to the presence of gingival inflammation and pocketing, a fact reflected by its old name 'ceruminal calculus'. It is dark green or

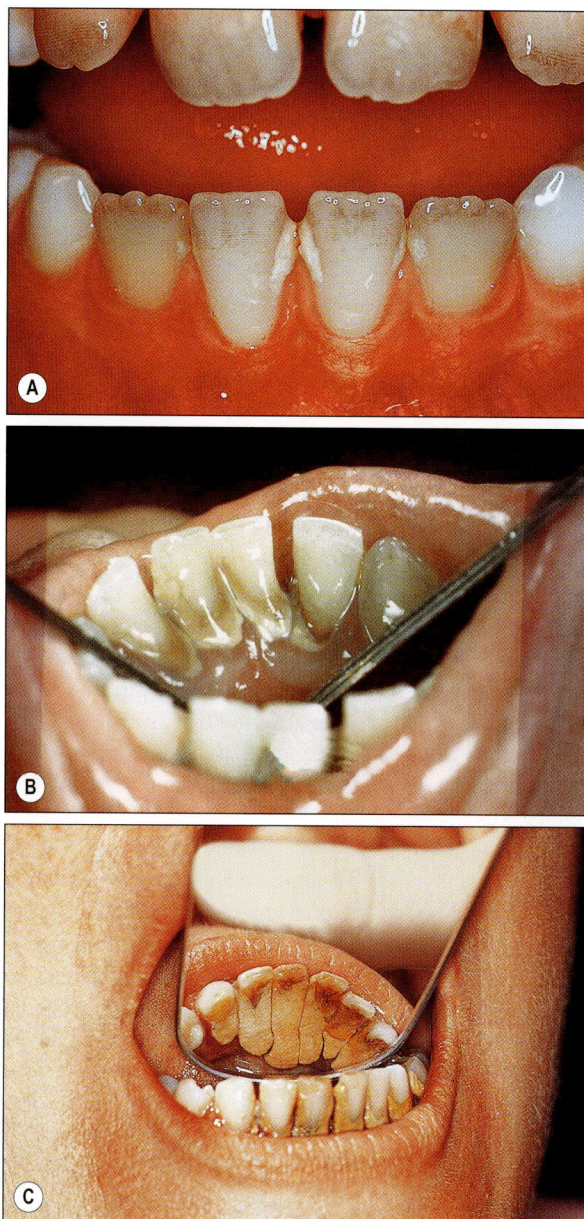

Fig. 2.4 Supragingival calculus around the lower incisors: (A) small deposits, (B) moderate deposits (C) large deposits in a high calculus forming patient.

black, much harder than supragingival calculus and more tightly adherent to the tooth surface. It may be found on roots close to the apical limit of a deep pocket, in severe cases as far down as the apex of the tooth. It can be difficult to detect on clinical examination. Sometimes its presence can be seen as a darkening of the thin overlying layer of gingiva, and its presence can be revealed directly by detaching the gingiva with a carefully directed blast of warm air. Cautious probing along the root surface with a fine probe will reveal deposits; if thick enough these may be seen on radiographs.

COMPOSITION OF CALCULUS

The composition of calculus varies slightly with the age of the deposit, its position in the mouth and even the geographical location of the individual.

It consists of 80% inorganic matter, some water and an organic matrix of protein and carbohydrate which includes desquamated epithelial cells, gram positive filamentous bacteria, cocci and leucocytes. The proportion of filamentous forms in calculus is greater than in the rest of the mouth. The inorganic fraction consists mainly of calcium phosphate as

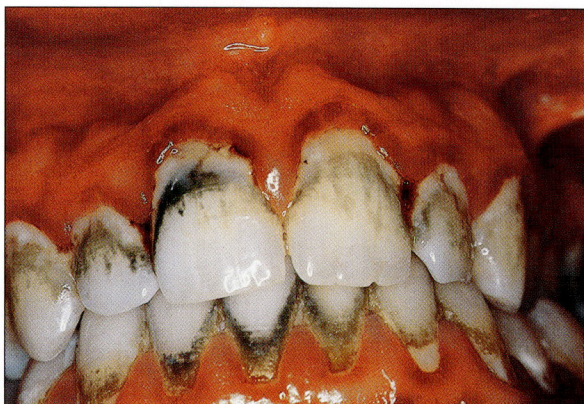

Fig. 2.3 Soft deposits of materia alba and calculus in a very dirty mouth.

hydroxyapatite, brushite, whitlockite and octacalcium phosphate. There are also small amounts of calcium carbonate, magnesium phosphate and fluoride. The fluoride content of calculus is many times higher than in plaque. The surface of calculus is covered by bacterial plaque but the centre of thick deposits may be sterile.

The obvious differences in appearance and distribution of supragingival and subgingival calculus suggest that their composition and mode of deposition may be different.

The composition of subgingival calculus is very similar to that of supragingival calculus except that its Ca/P ratio is higher and its sodium content greater. Salivary proteins are not found in subgingival calculus, indicating a non-salivary source for this deposit.

THE DEPOSITION OF CALCULUS

Calculus is mineralized bacterial plaque but not all plaque mineralizes. Supragingival calculus is rarely seen on the facial surface of lower molars but commonly on facial surfaces of upper molars which are opposite the mouth of the parotid ducts. Perhaps 90% of all supragingival calculus on a dentition is on the lower incisors which are bathed in saliva directly from the submandibular and sublingual salivary glands. Precipitation of mineral salts into plaque may be seen only hours after plaque deposition but is more usual 2–14 days after plaque is formed. Mineral in supragingival calculus derives from saliva, that in subgingival calculus from gingival fluid exudate. In early plaque, concentrations of calcium and phosphorus ions are high; indeed the concentration of calcium in plaque is about 20 times that in saliva, but no apatite crystals are present. Furthermore, there is no evidence that hydroxyapatite crystals form spontaneously in saliva. Some trigger appears to be necessary and it is generally believed that some element in plaque acts as a seeding or nucleation site where crystallization can start. Electron microscope studies suggest that apatite crystals are formed either in or on filamentous microorganisms but as calculus can be formed in germ-free animals it is likely that other factors can act as a seed. Once calcification is started it can continue by crystal growth.

Various theories have been put forward for the mechanism of initial mineralization:

1. Saliva can be regarded as an unstable supersaturated solution of calcium phosphate. As CO_2 tension is relatively low in the mouth, CO_2 can be lost from saliva with deposition of insoluble calcium phosphate
2. During sleep salivary flow is reduced and ammonia is formed from salivary urea, producing a rise of pH which favours precipitation of calcium phosphate
3. Protein may hold calcium in high concentrations but when saliva contacts the teeth the protein comes out of solution leading to precipitation of calcium and phosphate ions.

Hidaka and Oishi (2007) studied the effects of food components on the *in vitro* formation of calcium phosphate precipitates. They found that carbohydrate and oil enhanced dental calculus formation or re-mineralization of tooth enamel, while protein food decreased it.

Whichever of these mechanisms operates, the calcified deposit fixes the plaque in position against the tooth and gingiva. Calculus is attached to the pellicle, to irregularities in the tooth surface or via filamentous organisms which penetrate the surface of cementum.

BACTERIAL VIABILITY WITHIN CALCULUS

Supragingival calculus contains unmineralized channels and lacunae (Tan et al 2004) and the viability of bacteria within these areas has been investigated using a bacterial viability stain on cryostat sections viewed under a fluorescent microscope. Control sections were heat treated prior to staining. Calculus samples were obtained from patients with moderate to severe chronic periodontitis. Four additional whole calculus samples were also viewed under a confocal laser scanning microscope. Nine further samples were aerobically and anaerobically cultured after UV irradiation to kill surface bacteria.

Viable bacteria, identified using the bacterial viability stain, were found in the cavities and lacunae in the calculus cryosections. Similar findings were found in samples viewed under the confocal laser scanning microscope. Of the nine cultured samples, five showed positive growth of bacteria under both aerobic and anaerobic conditions, one showed only aerobic growth and one showed no growth. The three controls showed no growth. Thus, both viable aerobic and anaerobic bacteria are present within these cavities in calculus and these could provide a reservoir of bacteria for subgingival growth unless this calculus is completely removed in treatment.

TOOTH STAINS

Many substances form stains which are tenaciously fixed to the tooth surface and require professional cleaning for removal. Tobacco, wine, metal salts, chlorhexidine mouthwash, etc. produce characteristic stains. A green stain is found on children's teeth which may be the pigmentation of salivary pellicle by chromogenic bacteria.

Stains are unsightly but there is no evidence that they cause gingival irritation or act as a focus for plaque deposition.

THE SUBGINGIVAL FLORA

Subgingival bacterial colonization only occurs if supragingival plaque and gingivitis are present. It does not occur as a simple apical downgrowth of plaque but rather by the slow apical movement of pioneer bacteria which may be attracted by nutrient and oxygen tension gradients (Newman 1977). This initial pioneering growth is followed by progressive colonization by other indigenous bacteria and multiplication of those species that are particularly well adapted to the subgingival conditions, such as Gram-negative rods and spirochaetes. This is partly due to the environment but also to symbiotic relationships between different bacterial species and selective inhibition of some species by others.

Morphological studies of subgingival plaque (Mousques et al 1980) show a differentiation of tooth associated and tissue associated regions. Tooth associated plaque is associated with calculus formation and root caries, whereas tissue associated plaque is potentially important in soft tissue destruction. Anaerobic *Actinomyces* species are associated with the root surface, forming discrete colonies or continuous layers. Other bacteria remain unattached and free within the protected environment of the pocket, which provides them with many of the trace substances that they require. The subgingival flora is a very complex community of many different species.

METHODS OF INVESTIGATING SUBGINGIVAL FLORA

The composition of dental plaque and the identification of individual bacterial species can be partially or fully determined in a number of ways. These are dark ground or phase contrast microscopy (Listgarten 1986), culture techniques, immunological techniques including immunofluorescence (Zambon et al 1985; Zambon et al 1986) or enzyme linked immunosorbent assay (ELISA) (Ebersole et al 1984), DNA probes (French et al 1986) and other molecular biological techniques and enzyme-based assays (Loesche 1986). (These are more fully described in Ch. 14, p. 181). Precise speciation of bacteria in culture can be carried out with a variety of laboratory-based methods including selective sub-cultures, biochemical tests, SDS PAGE, gene probes, ribotyping, DNA fingerprinting and cell wall long chain fatty acid analysis (Genco et al 1986; Greenstein 1988).

However, it must be realized that whatever methods are used to determine the bacteria present in the subgingival flora, the picture will always be incomplete and sometimes can be very misleading. It will also depend on the methods used for collection. The flora contains either facultative or strict anaerobic bacteria and many bacteria will only be preserved if strict anaerobic conditions are adhered to during both collection and culture. Furthermore, it is estimated that less than 50% of the bacteria in the subgingival flora are culturable even with special selective culture conditions. The best examples of this are the spirochaetes which may account for between 40% and 60% of the total flora. In addition, a considerable number of both Gram-positive and -negative bacterial species can only be cultured with difficulty using very selective techniques. Also, some Gram-positive bacteria may appear as Gram-negative when grown in poor cultural conditions.

The latest molecular techniques which detect bacteria on the basis of their genetic composition have yielded very different compositions to cultural techniques using the same sample. Thus, the composition of the subgingival flora is still incomplete and may appear different as these new techniques yield information.

Finally, DNA and RNA probes and monoclonal antibodies are available for some subgingival bacteria and can detect these species when they are present. They are very specific and can only detect the species to which they are directed and will thus only detect bacteria already suspected to be present.

NOMENCLATURE OF ANAEROBIC RODS IN THE SUBGINGIVAL FLORA

The nomenclature of oral black-pigmented Gram-negative anaerobic rods has recently changed as a result of extensive investigations of these bacteria. The principal changes have been reviewed by van Steenbergen et al (1991) and are shown in Table 2.1.

In addition, *Wolinella recta* has been re-named *Campylobacter recta* and more recently *Bacteroides forsythus* been re-named *Tannerella forsythensis* (Klein & Gonçalves 2003). Subdivision of some current species will probably occur soon, as our knowledge increases and the next likely division will probably affect *Fusobacterium nucleatum*.

Several new species with very fastidious growth requirements making them difficult to cultivate routinely are beginning to be reported from subgingival plaque samples (Tanner 1991). These include Gram-positive bacteria such as *Eubacterium* species including *E. timidum*, *E. brachy* and *E. nodatum* (Holdeman et al 1980), *S. oralis* and *S. gordonii* (Kilian et al 1989) and *A. georgiae*, *A. gerencseriae* (Johnson et al 1990). Fastidious Gram-negative bacteria reported include *F. alocis* and *F. sulci* (Cato et al 1985), *Mitsuokella dentalis*, a motile Selenomonas (Moore et al 1987), *Treponema socranskii* sub-species (Smibert et al 1984) and *B. forsythus* (Tanner et al 1986).

SUBGINGIVAL FLORA IN HEALTH AND DISEASE

Dark ground and phase contrast microscopy studies have shown that in periodontal health there is a very scant subgingival flora consisting of non-motile rods and cocci (Listgarten & Hellden 1978; Listgarten 1992). In gingivitis there is a marked decrease in the proportion of cocci and a parallel increase in motile rods and spirochaetes. In chronic adult periodontitis the number of motile rods and spirochaetes show further increases. There is also evidence that the numbers of spirochaetes and motile rods are greater in pockets with recurrent periodontitis than those that remain inactive (Listgarten 1984; Listgarten et al 1984).

Cultural studies have identified about 300 bacterial species in the periodontal pocket, some of which occur infrequently and in low numbers (Slots & Listgarten 1988). The healthy gingival sulcus contains a scant microflora dominated by Gram-positive facultative species of *Streptococcus* and *Actinomyces* and a similar flora is found in successfully treated periodontal pockets. In chronic gingivitis Gram-negative anaerobic bacteria make up about 45% of the culturable flora (Slots 1979). The predominating bacteria are *Actinomyces* species, *Streptococcus* species, *F. nucleatum*, *P. intermedia* and various non-pigmenting *Bacteroides* species. In advancing adult periodontitis, the proportions of these bacteria continue to increase until Gram-negative bacteria form about 75% and anaerobic and facultative bacteria about 90% of the cultural flora. Common Gram-negative bacteria in chronic adult periodontitis include *Porphyromonas gingivalis*, *Prevotella intermedia*, *F. nucleatum*, *Capnocytophaga* species, *Campylobacter* (formerly *Wolinella*) *recta*, *Eikenella corrodens* and *Actinobacillus actinomycetemcomitans* (now *Aggregatibacter actinomycetemcomitans*), seen in cultural studies (Slots 1979; Slots & Genco 1984), and spirochaetes seen by dark ground microscopy.

The description of the precise bacterial species present in the subgingival flora associated with health, gingivitis and progressive periodontitis has been refined as the speciation of the flora has developed in recent years. These bacterial species have recently been reviewed and described by Tanner (1991) and are listed in Tables 2.2, 2.3 and 2.4. Various combinations of the bacteria shown in Table 2.4 have been reported as increasing at sites with progressive periodontitis in many studies on patients in different parts of the world. In this regard, a recent study of 148 Chinese adult patients aged 30–59, with chronic periodontitis found an increase in a number of these species, notably *Porphyromonas gingivalis*, *T. denticola*, *Tannerella forsythensis* (*B. forsythus*) and *C. recta*, at sites with progressive periodontitis (Papapanou et al 1997).

The composition of the pocket flora may vary from one individual to another and from one tooth site to another. The predominance of certain bacteria in the pocket does not necessarily indicate that these bacteria are exclusive pathogens since all the different bacterial species which predominate the pocket flora in various proportions and frequencies originate from the normal oral flora (Theilade 1986).

Table 2.1 *The nomenclature of black pigmented anaerobes*

Former name	New name
Black-pigmented *Bacteroides*	Black-pigmented anaerobic rods
Bacteroides gingivalis	*Porphyromonas gingivalis*
Bacteroides endodontalis	*Porphyromonas endodontalis*
Bacteroides corporis	*Porphyromonas corporis*
Bacteroides melaninogenicus	*Porphyromonas melaninogenicus*
Bacteroides denticola	*Porphyromonas denticola*
Bacteroides loescheii	*Porphyromonas loescheii*

Table 2.2 *Bacterial species associated with health*

Gram-positive rods	
Actinomyces israelli	Rothia dentocariosa
Actinomyces naeslundii	Actinomyces gerencseriae
Actinomyces odontolyticus	
Gram-positive cocci	
Streptococcus mitis	Streptococcus sanguis
Streptococcus oralis	Streptococcus gordonii
Peptostreptococcus micros	
Gram-negative rods	
Selenomonas sputigena	Prevotella intermedia
Capnocytophaga gingivalis	Fusobacterium nucleatum subsp. *vincentii*

Table 2.3 *Bacterial species associated with gingivitis*

Similar proportions in health, gingivitis and periodontitis	Elevated in gingivitis	Elevated in gingivitis and periodontitis
Actinomyces gerencseriae Actinomyces naeslundii Bacteroides gracilis Capnocytophaga ochracea Haemophilus aphrophilus Propionibacter acnes Gamella (Streptococcus) morbillorula Veillonella parvula	Actinomyces naeslundii III Campylobacter concisus Streptococcus anginosis Streptococcus sanguis	Prevotella intermedia Eubacterium timidum Fusobacterium nucleatum Campylobacter recta

Table 2.4 *Bacterial species associated with progression periodontitis*

Gram-positive rods	Gram-positive cocci
Eubacterium brachy Eubacterium nodatum Eubacterium timidum Propionibacter acnes Lactobacillus minutus	Peptostreptococcus micros Peptostreptococcus anaerobius Peptostreptococcus acnes

Gram-negative rods	Gram-negative spirochaetes
Porphyromonas gingivalis Prevotella intermedia Prevotella denticola Prevotella oralis Bacteroides forsythus Actinobacillus actinomycetemcomitans Eikenella corrodens Campylobacter recta Fusobacterium nucleatum subsp. nucleatum Fusobacterium alocis Selenomonas sputigena Selenomonas flueggei	Borrelia vincentii Treponema denticola Treponema macrodentium Treponema oralis Treponema socranskii

Yoshida et al (2003) used PCR to divide *A. actinomycetemcomitans* (now *Aggregatibacter actinomycetemcomitans*) into five serotypes (*a–e*) and investigated their distribution and that of *P. gingivalis* in the subgingival flora of 328 systemically healthy Japanese adults. *A. actinomycetemcomitans* was found in 19.8% and *P. gingivalis* in 27.1% of these subjects. In terms of *A. actinomycetemcomitans* serotypes, one serotype was found in 52%, two in 25% and three in 9.3% of the *A. actinomycetemcomitans*-positive sites. *A. actinomycetemcomitans* serotype *c* was detected in a very high proportion (76.39%) of the sites also positive for *P. gingivalis*. Thus, it may be possible that this serotype prefers a different environment to the others.

Klein and Gonçalves (2003) investigated the prevalence of *T. forsythensis* and *P. gingivalis* in subgingival plaque samples from patients with different periodontal status. *T. forsythensis* was not detected in any sample from healthy sites in any group but was detected in 70% of diseased sites from early to moderate chronic periodontitis patients and 100% of sites from advanced chronic periodontitis patients. In addition, both *T. forsythensis* and *P. gingivalis* were detected in 30% of sites with early to moderate

chronic periodontitis and 90% of those with advanced chronic periodontitis. This indicates a possible association between chronic periodontitis severity and the presence of *T. forsythensis* and/or *T. forsythensis* and *P. gingivalis*.

Huang et al (2003) separated *T. forsythensis* (*B. forsythus*) into 11 genotypes using arbitrarily primed (AR)-PCR and investigated their distribution in 64 Japanese periodontitis subjects related to their periodontal status. The majority (80.9%) of these genotypes were types I, II, III and IV (accounting for 39.7%, 20.6%, 10.3% and 10.3%, respectively). Types I and III were most commonly found in chronic periodontitis subjects (80.8% and 85.7%, respectively). Types II and IV were most commonly found in aggressive (juvenile) periodontitis subjects. Except for three subjects, who harboured two different genotypes, all subjects were infected with one genotype only. These results suggest that different genotypes may be associated with different types of periodontal disease.

Yang et al (2004) compared the prevalence and level of *P. gingivalis* and *T. forsythensis* in subgingival plaque samples from both healthy individuals and periodontal patients in different age groups. *P. gingivalis* was found in 85.7% ($p = 0.0001$) and *T. forsythensis* in 60.7% ($p = 0.0002$) of diseased subjects compared to 23.1% and 39.6%, respectively, in healthy subjects. *P. gingivalis*, but not *T. forsythensis*, was detected more frequently in any diseased group than in the healthy group in every age group ($p = 0.0001$). No significant difference was found in the prevalence of *P. gingivalis* and *T. forsythensis* among age groups. The mean level of *P. gingivalis* and *T. forsythensis* was significantly higher in diseased groups than in the healthy group ($p = 0.0001$). Thus, both these bacteria appear to be closely associated with chronic periodontitis.

Most clinical studies assume that the subgingival microbiota is similar from one geographic location to another (Haffajee et al 2004). This group investigated the composition of the subgingival microbiota in chronic periodontitis subjects from four countries (Brazil, Chile, Sweden and USA). They found that the microbial profiles of subgingival plaque samples from chronic periodontitis subjects in four countries showed surprisingly marked differences and that these differences persisted after adjusting for age, mean pocket depth, gender and smoking status.

Tanner et al (2006) felt that the association of bacterial species with early disease might be useful in determining which microbes initiate periodontitis and they hypothesized that the microbiota of subgingival and tongue samples might differ between early periodontitis and health. They carried out a cross-sectional evaluation of 141 healthy and early periodontitis adults with the use of oligonucleotide probes and PCR. They found that most species differed in associations with sample sites and most subgingival species were associated with subgingival samples. Few species were detected more frequently in early periodontitis by DNA probes. *P. gingivalis* and *T. forsythia* (*T. forsythensis*) were associated with early periodontitis by direct PCR. They also found that the microbiota of tongue samples were less sensitive than those of subgingival samples in detecting periodontal species, and there was overlap in species detected in health and early periodontitis. Thus, the bacteria associated with early periodontitis seem to be similar to those found in more advanced disease.

REFERENCES

Cato EP, Moore LVH, Moore WEC: Fusobacterium alocis sp. nov., Fusobacterium sulci sp. nov. from the human gingival sulcus, *Int J Syst Bacteriol* 35:475–477, 1985.

Christersson LA, Slots J, Zambon JJ, et al: Transmission and colonization of Actinobacillus actinomycetemcomitans in localized juvenile periodontitis, *J Periodontol* 56:127–131, 1985.

Costerton JW, Cheng KJ, Geesey CG, et al: Bacterial biofilms in nature and disease, *Ann Rev Microbiol* 41:435–464, 1987.

Doyle RJ, Nesbitt WE, Taylor KJ: On the mechanism of adherence of streptococcus sanguis to hydroxyapapatite, *FEMS Microbiol Lett* 57:1194–1201, 1982.

Ebersole JL, Frey DE, Taubman MA, et al: Serological identification of oral Bacteroides sp. by enzyme-linked immunosorbent assay, *J Clin Microbiol* 19:639–644, 1984.

French CK, Savitt ED, Simon SL, et al: DNA probe detection of periodontal pathogens, *Oral Microbiol Immunol* 1:58–62, 1986.

Genco RJ, Zambon JJ, Christersson LA: Use and interpretation of microbiological assays in periodontal disease, *Oral Microbiol Immunol* 1:73–79, 1986.

Gibbons RS, Socransky SS, Sawer B, et al: The microbiota of the gingival crevice of man. II. Predominant cultivable organisms, *Arch Oral Biol* 8:281–289, 1963.

Greenstein G: Microbiological assessments to enhance periodontal disease diagnosis, *J Periodontol* 59:508–515, 1988.

Haffajee AD, Bogren A, Hasturk H, et al: Subgingival microbiota of chronic periodontitis subjects from different geographic locations, *J Clin Periodontol* 31:996–1002, 2004.

Hidaka S, Oishi A: An in vitro study of the effect of some dietary components on calculus formation: regulation of calcium phosphate precipitation, *Oral Dis* 13:296–302, 2007.

Holdeman LV, Cato EP, Burnmeister JA, et al: Description of Eubacterium timidum sp. nov., Eubacterium brachy sp. nov., Eubacterium nodatum sp. nov. isolated from human periodontitis, *Int J Syst Bacteriol* 30:163–169, 1980.

Huang Y, Umeda M, Takeuchi Y, et al: Distribution of Bacteroides forsythus genotypes in a Japanese periodontitis population, *Oral Microbiol Immunol* 18:208–214, 2003.

Johnson JL, Moore LVH, Kaneko B, et al: Actinomyces georgiae sp. nov., Actinomyces gerencseriae sp. nov., designation of two genospecies of Actinomyces naeslundii, and inclusion of A. naeslundii serotypes II and III and Actinomyces viscosus serotype II in A. naeslundii genospecies 2, *Int J Syst Bacteriol* 40:273–286, 1990.

Kilian M, Mikkelson L, Henrichsen J: Taxonomic study of viridans streptococci: description of Streptococcus gordonii sp. nov., and amended descriptions of Streptococcus sanguis (White & Niven 1946), Streptococcus oralis (Bridge & Sneath 1982) and Streptococcus mitis (Andrewes & Horder 1906), *Int J Syst Bacteriol* 39:471–484, 1989.

Klein MI, Gonçalves RB: Detection of Tannerella forsythensis (Bacteroides forsythus) and Porphyromonas gingivalis by polymerase chain reaction in subjects with different periodontal status, *J Periodontol* 74:798–802, 2003.

Kolenbrander PE: Intergenic coaggregation among human oral bacteria and ecology of dental plaque, *Ann Rev Microbiol* 42:627–656, 1988.

Kolenbrander PE, Anderson RN, Moore LV: Coaggregation of Fusobacterium nucleatum, Selenomonas flueggei, Selenomonas infelix, Selenomonas sputigena with strains from 11 genera of oral bacteria, *Infect Immun* 57:3194–3203, 1989.

Kolenbrander PE, London J: Adhere today, here tomorrow: Oral bacterial adherence, *J Bacteriol* 175:3247–3252, 1993.

Listgarten MA: Subgingival microbiological differences between periodontally healthy sites and diseased sites prior to and after treatment, *Int J Periodontics Restorative Dent* 4:27, 1984.

Listgarten MA: Direct microscopy of periodontal pathogens, *Oral Microbiol Immunol* 1:31–36, 1986.

Listgarten MA: Microbial testing in the diagnosis of periodontal disease, *J Periodontol* 63:332–337, 1992.

Listgarten MA, Hellden L: Relative distribution of bacteria at clinically healthy and periodontally diseased sites in humans, *J Clin Periodontol* 5:115–132, 1978.

Listgarten MA, Levin S, Schifter CC, et al: Comparative differential dark-field microscopy of subgingival bacteria from tooth surfaces with recent evidence of recurring periodontitis and from non-affected sites, *J Periodontol* 55:398–401, 1984.

Loesche WJ: The identification of bacteria associated with periodontal disease and dental caries by enzymatic methods, *Oral Microbiol Immunol* 1:65–70, 1986.

Lundquist B, Emilson CG, Wennerholm K: Relationship between streptococci in saliva and their colonization to the tooth surface, *Oral Microbiol Immunol* 4:71–76, 1989.

Marsh PD: Dental plaque: biological significance of a biofilm and community life-style, *J Clin Periodontol* 32:7–15, 2005.

Moore WEC, Holdeman LV, Smibert RM, et al: Bacteriology of experimental gingivitis in young adult humans, *Infect Immun* 38:651–667, 1982.

Moore WEC: Microbiology of periodontal disease, *J Periodontal Res* 22:335–341, 1987.

Moore LVH, Johnson JL, Moore WEC: Selenomonas noxia sp. nov., Selenomonas flueggei sp. nov., Selenomonas infelix sp. nov., Selenomonas dianae sp. nov.,

Selenomonas artemidis sp. nov. from human gingival crevice, *Int J Syst Bacteriol* 36:271–280, 1987.

Mousques T, Listgarten MA, Phillips RW: The effect of scaling and root planing on the composition of human microbial flora, *J Periodontal Res* 15:144–151, 1980.

Newman HN: Ultrastructure of the apical border of dental plaque. In Lehner T, editor: *The Borderland between Caries and Periodontal Disease*, London, 1977, Academic Press, pp 79–103.

Papapanou PN, Baelam V, Luan WM, et al: Subgingival microbiota in adult Chinese: prevalence and relation to periodontal disease progression, *J Periodontol* 68:651–666, 1997.

Sanai Y, Persson GR, Starr JR, et al: Presence and antibiotic resistance of Porphyromonas gingivalis, Prevotella intermedia, and Prevotella nigrescens in children, *J Clin Periodontol* 29:929–934, 2002.

Scannapieco FA, Levine MJ: Saliva and dental pellicles. In Genco RJ, Goldman HM, Cohen DW, editors: *Contemporary Periodontics*, St Louis, 1990, Mosby, Ch. 2.

Slots J: Subgingival microflora and periodontal disease, *J Clin Periodontol* 6:351–352, 1979.

Slots J, Genco RJ: Black-pigmented Bacteroides species, Capnocytophaga species and Actinobacillus actinomycetemcomitans in human periodontal disease: virulence factors, colonization, survival and tissue destruction, *J Dent Res* 63:412–421, 1984.

Slots J, Listgarten MA: Bacteroides gingivalis, Bacteroides intermedius and Actinobacillus actinomycetemcomitans in human periodontal diseases, *J Clin Periodontol* 15:85–93, 1988.

Smibert RM, Johnson JL, Ranney RR: Treponema socranskii subsp. socranskii subsp. nov., Treponema socranskii subsp. buccule subsp. nov., Treponema socranskii subsp. paerdis subsp. nov. isolated from human periodontitis, *Int J Syst Bacteriol* 34:457–462, 1984.

Socransky SS, Gibbons RS, Dale AC, et al: The microbiota of the gingival crevice of man. I. Total microscopic and viable counts of specific microorganisms, *Arch Oral Biol* 8:275–279, 1963.

Tan BTK, Mordan NJ, Embleton J, et al: Study of bacterial viability within human supragingival calculus, *J Periodontol* 75:23–29, 2004.

Tanner ACR: Microbial succession in the development of periodontal disease. In Hamada S, Holt SC, McGhee JR, editors: *Periodontal Disease: Pathogens and Host Immune Responses*, Tokyo, 1991, Quintessence, pp 13–25.

Tanner ACR, Listgarten MA, Ebersole JL, et al: Bacteroides forsythus sp. nov., a slow-growing fusiform Bacteroides sp. from the human oral cavity, *Int J Syst Bacteriol* 36:213–221, 1986.

Tanner ACR, Paster BJ, Lu SC, et al: Subgingival and tongue microbiota during early periodontitis, *J Dent Res* 85:318–323, 2006.

Theilade E: The non-specific theory in microbial etiology of inflammatory periodontal diseases, *J Clin Periodontol* 13:905–911, 1986.

van Steenbergen TJM, van Winkelhoff AJ, de Graaff J: Black-pigmented oral anaerobic rods: Classification and role in periodontal disease. In Hamada S, Holt SC, McGhee JR, editors: *Periodontal Disease: Pathogens and Host Immune Responses*, Tokyo, 1991, Quintessence, pp 41–52.

Whittaker CJ, Klier CM, Kolenbrander PE: Mechanisms of adhesion by oral bacteria, *Ann Rev Microbiol* 50:513–552, 1996.

Yang H-W, Huang Y-F, Chou M-Y: Occurrence of Porphyromonas gingivalis and Tannerella forsythensis in periodontally diseased and healthy subjects, *J Periodontol* 75:1077–1083, 2004.

Yoshida Y, Suzuki N, Nakano Y, et al: Distribution of Actinobacillus actinomycetemcomitans serotypes and Porphyromonas gingivalis in Japanese adults, *Oral Microbiol Immunol* 18:135–139, 2003.

Zambon JJ, Reynolds HS, Chen P, et al: Rapid identification of periodontal pathogens in subgingival dental plaque. Comparison of indirect immunofluorescence microscopy with bacterial culture for detection of Bacteroides gingivalis, *J Periodontol* 56(Special Issue):32–40, 1985.

Zambon JJ, Bochacki V, Genco RJ: Immunological assays for putative periodontal pathogens, *Oral Microbiol Immunol* 1:39–44, 1986.

Host–parasite interaction

3

The description of periodontal anatomy in Chapter 1 provides little idea of the continuous activity of living tissue. Health is not a static condition; it is a dynamic state in which the living and functioning organism or tissue remains in balance with a constantly changing environment. These changes in the environment provoke corresponding alterations in tissue activity so that normal function can continue. This constant process of readjustment to maintain normal tissue activity, normal function and ultimately the continuity of life is known as homeostasis. If an environmental change is so great that homeostasis cannot be maintained, the activity of the tissues becomes abnormal, normal function cannot be continued and the change in tissue activity is perceived as disease.

Bacteria constitute an important part of our environment; indeed life without bacteria would be impossible. Usually, all external surfaces in nature including those of living tissues are covered by bacteria. The skin and the gut are no exceptions and the oral mucosa as part of the gut is covered by many species of bacteria, the oral flora. Bacteria attach themselves to surfaces by a number of means: by the microscopic roughness of the surface, by hairlike extensions on the surface of the bacteria and by natural glues made of proteins and polysaccharides, as in the glycoprotein of the salivary pellicle described in Chapter 2.

Where different life forms exist together there is competition for existence, therefore mechanisms have evolved which help one form to protect itself from another. As the tissues of the body have evolved together with their microorganisms over millions of years, one would expect that these defence mechanisms would have been perfected and that a state of harmony or balance between the host and its bacteria would have been achieved. If such a balance had not been established, as explained by Darwin's theory of natural selection, at least one of the species involved would have died out. In fact we live quite happily in a state of partnership (symbiosis) with most of the bacteria on our bodies and only under certain circumstances do we suffer from their presence. For example, both dental caries and periodontal disease are caused by bacteria which are normally resident in our mouths. In primitive man and in so-called 'primitive' communities today the prevalence of dental disease is very low, and bacterial plaque occurs in much smaller quantities and only rarely apical to the tooth-contact area. By contrast in 'civilized' man, bacterial plaque may be found on almost all tooth surfaces and dental disease is rampant. The change in texture of our diet and its large component of refined and easily fermentable carbohydrates have altered the oral environment in such a way that bacterial stagnation takes place around the teeth and gum margin, with resultant imbalance in the bacteria–tissue relationship and the production of substances which have the capacity for damaging the tissues. This is amply demonstrated in animals which do not normally suffer from dental diseases and which develop periodontal disease and caries when fed on a soft, sticky diet rich in carbohydrate.

DEFENCE MECHANISMS

A number of mechanisms operate to protect the body from attack by foreign bodies and toxins, including infection by bacteria (**Fig. 3.1**). These mechanisms can be classed as:

1. Non-specific mechanisms
2. Mechanisms specific to invading foreign proteins called antigens which stimulate the immune system.

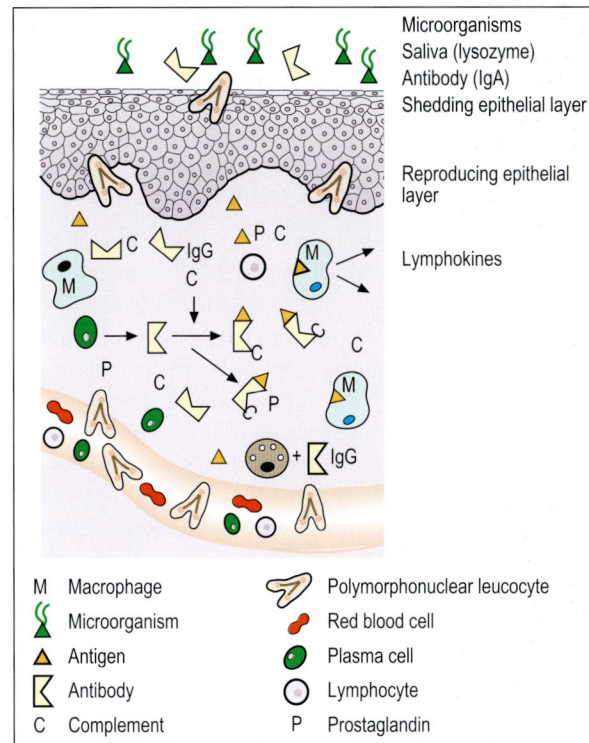

Fig. 3.1 Diagram to show the multiplicity of factors that take part in the tissue defence system.

NON-SPECIFIC PROTECTION MECHANISMS

There are five non-specific protection mechanisms:

1. Bacterial balance

The mouth as a whole and various zones in the mouth, including what has been called the 'crevicular domain', can be viewed as ecosystems in which a balance exists between the different species of microorganisms and between this flora and the tissues. Upset in this balance is most commonly seen after prolonged use of antibiotics which suppress some types of bacteria and allow others to flourish to the detriment of the tissues, e.g. the production of the fungal infection, Candida (thrush) after the use of some antibiotics.

2. Surface integrity

The surface integrity of skin and mucous membrane barriers, including the gingiva, is maintained by the continuing renewal of the epithelium from its base and desquamation of the surface layers. These two activities balance so that the thickness of the epithelium remains constant. The efficiency of the surface barrier is enhanced by keratinization and parakeratinization. The junctional epithelium, although semi-permeable, has a very high rate of cell turnover.

3. Surface fluid and enzymes

All vital surfaces are washed by fluids which are the products of surface glands and which contain substances capable of attacking foreign material, e.g. gastric acid, lysozyme in tears washing the eyeball, and sebum from

27

skin hair follicles. Saliva bathes the oral mucosa and contains antibacterial substances. The gingival fluid exudate flows through the junctional epithelium into the gingival crevice and this fluid contains phagocytic leucocytes and their enzymes.

4. Phagocytosis

Certain cells in the bloodstream and in the tissues are capable of engulfing and digesting foreign material. The two most important phagocytic cells are the polymorphonuclear leucocyte and the macrophage (Greek: big eater) (M in **Fig. 3.1**).

Polymorphonuclear leucocytes (PMNs, neutrophils)

PMNs are the most common of the white blood cells. Produced in the bone marrow they are the most important blood cell for protecting the body against acute invasion by bacteria. Because they possess an amoeba-like ability to change shape and move rapidly, they can pass through the walls of capillaries and move through the tissues, including gingival connective tissue and junctional epithelium. The direction in which they move is determined by chemical substances, mainly derived from bacteria or the complement cascade. These attract PMNs to the site of damage where foreign particles are engulfed and digested. While their role is primarily defensive, PMNs can also produce proteolytic enzymes which can destroy the surrounding tissue.

Macrophages (monocytes)

The macrophage is an indiscriminate scavenger of foreign material. It starts life as a monocyte which moves into the tissues and matures to become the extremely efficient phagocyte, the macrophage, which is capable of digesting large foreign particles. If a bacterial disease lasts more than a few days, the number of monocytes in the tissues increases until there may be as many monocytes as PMNs. Unlike PMNs, monocytes are capable of several divisions within the tissues which progressively increase the number of macrophages.

While PMNs are the main line of defence in acute infection the monocytes are more important in long-term chronic infection. The macrophages also take up antigens from the circulating fluid for processing and presentation to the lymphocytes.

Phagocytosis is aided by a battery of nine related proteins known as 'complement'. The complement cascade is initiated by the combination of immunoglobulin and the C1 component. The final product of the cascade is an esterase which damages cell membranes and leads to bacteriolysis. Two intermediary products, C3a and C5a, are produced which attach to receptor sites on mast cells and inflammatory cells. They release histamine and other substances from mast cells and prostaglandins from inflammatory cells, and these released substances increase vascular permeability. They are also chemotactic to PMNs. C3a also aids phagocytosis by attaching the antigen to the phagocyte via the C3 receptor on the surface of PMNs and macrophages (monocytes).

In addition, after detecting infection macrophages can secrete interleukin (IL)-6 (see Table 3.1) which can stimulate hepatocytes in the liver to secrete a mannose-binding protein which can bind to some bacterial capsules resistant to complement binding (Janaway 1993). After binding it can activate the complement cascade.

There are diseases in which leucocyte-forming tissues become deficient and the number of PMNs may fall to almost zero (leucopenia).

Phagocytic cells in the gingival crevice

Both PMNs and macrophages migrate from the gingival tissues through the junctional epithelium into the gingival crevice/periodontal pocket. The rate of this cellular migration increases with increasing inflammation

within the tissues. It is, however, known that the phagocytic capacity of PMNs and probably macrophages is much less within the crevice than in the tissues. The presence on the surface of the phagocytic cells of immunoglobulin type II and III receptors (Fcγ R II and III) is essential for phagocytosis to occur. In this regard it has been shown (Sugita et al 1993) that there appears to be a downregulation of Fcγ R III in PMNs harvested from gingival crevicular fluid (GCF). Furthermore, more recent studies (Miyazaki et al 1997) have compared the presence and synthesis of these receptors in both GCF and peripheral blood. They found that the synthesis and expression of both Fcγ R II and III were lower in GCF PMNs than in peripheral blood PMNs. In addition, the downregulation of these receptors in GCF PMNs significantly correlated with their reduced phagocytic capacity. Thus, it appears that GCF PMNs are characterized by reduced surface expression and synthesis of Fcγ receptors and this appears to be responsible for their lack of phagocytic capacity.

5. The inflammatory reaction

The inflammatory reaction is stimulated by tissue injury and infection, and leads to changes in the local microcirculation. This produces hyperaemia, increased vascular permeability and the formation of a fluid and cellular exudate. In this way serum proteins and phagocytic cells accumulate around the irritant.

Innate immunity cannot protect against all infections as microbes evolve rapidly enabling them to devise means of evading these defence mechanisms. To counter these changes, vertebrates have developed a unique system of adaptive immunity which enables the body to recognize, remember and respond to any bacteria, virus or cancer cell even if it has never faced it before.

SPECIFIC PROTECTIVE MECHANISMS

The adaptive immune system

The unique surveillance and attack system developed to the full by mammals has three main characteristics:

1. It can distinguish between itself and the enemy, i.e. between 'self' and 'non-self' so that it does not attack parts of itself. This recognition system can go wrong and in certain diseases known as autoimmune diseases the defence system attacks pieces of its own body.
2. The defences contain elements specific against any given antigen. This is possible because each antigen contains specific amino acid sequences or 'flags' which the immune system uses to recognize 'non-self'. Antigens are proteins and because of their novelty the body does not resist the invasion on the first attack of bacteria or viruses containing them, but within a few days or weeks the immune system will have developed specific 'answers' to each antigen. Certain non-protein substances, known as haptens, can become antigenic by associating with proteins.
3. The system has a memory. The first contact with the antigen produces a primary response in which the uneducated or virgin lymphocytes (the main cell in the immune system) proliferate and mature, and the antigen is memorized so that further contact provokes a ready secondary response.

Overview

The adaptive immune system is brought about by the actions of an array of cells which take up, process, present and react to foreign proteins known as antigens (Nossal 1993). Antigen presenting cells such as macrophages

Table 3.1 *The origin and functions of cytokines: interleukins, colony stimulating factors (CSF), tumour necrosis factors (TNF), interferons and others*

Cytokine	Source	Effector function
Interleukin (IL)		
IL-1α, IL-1β	Monocytes, macrophages, antigen presenting cells, NK, B cells, endothelial cells	Co-stimulates T-cell activity by enhancing production of cytokines including IL-2 and its receptor; enhances B-cell proliferation and maturation; stimulates and enhances NK cytotoxicity; induces IL-1, 6, 8, TNF, GM-CSF and PAGE$_2$ by macrophages; pro-inflammation by inducing cytokines and ICAM-1 and VCAM-1 on endothelium; induces fever, APP, bone resorption by osteoclasts; induces proliferation of activated B- and T-cells; enhances cytotoxic killing of tumour cells and bacteria by monocytes/macrophages
IL-2	Th1 cells	Induces proliferation of activated T and B cells; enhances NK cytotoxicity and killing of tumour cells and bacteria by monocytes/macrophages
IL-3	T cells, NK and mast cells	Growth and differentiation of haemopoietic precursor cells. Mast cell growth
IL-4	Th1 and Th2, NK, NK-T cells, αβT, mast cells	Induces Th2 cells; stimulates proliferation of activated B and T cells, mast cells; upregulates MHC class II and B cells and hence inhibits Th1 differentiation; increases macrophagocytosis; induces switch to IgG1 and IgE
IL-5	Th2 and mast cells	Produces proliferation of eosinophils and activated B cells and induces switch to IgA
IL-6	Th2 cells, monocytes, macrophages, dendritic cells, bone marrow stroma	Differentiation of myeloid stem cells and of B cells to plasma cells; induces APP and enhances T-cell proliferation
IL-7	Bone marrow stroma	Induces differentiation of lymphoid stem cells into progenitor
IL-8	Monocytes, macrophages and endothelial cells	Mediates chemotaxis and activation of neutrophils
IL-9	Th cells	Induces proliferation of thymocytes and enhances mast cell growth. Synergizes with IL-4 in switching to IgG1 and IgE
IL-10	Th cells, T cells, B cells, monocytes, macrophages	Inhibits IL-2 secretion and Th1. Downregulates MHC class II and cytokine (including IL-12) production by monocytes, macrophages and dendritic cells, thereby inhibiting Th1 differentiation. Inhibits T-cell proliferation and enhances B-cell differentiation
IL-11	Bone marrow stroma	Promotes differentiation of pro-B cells and megakaryocytes. Induces APP production
IL-12	Monocytes, macrophages, dendritic cells, B cells	Critical cytokine to Th1 differentiation and proliferation and IFN-γ production by Th1, CD8+, γδT and NK cells. Enhances NK and CD8+ toxicity
IL-13	Th2 and mast cells	Inhibits activation and cytokine secretion by macrophages, co-activates B-cell proliferation. Upregulates MHC class II and CD23 on B-cells and monocytes. Induces switch to IgG1 and IgE. Induces VCAM-1 on endothelial cells
IL-15	T cells, NK, monocytes, dendritic cells, B cells	Induces proliferation of T, NK and activated B cells and cytokine
IL-16	Th and T cells	Chemo-attractant for CD4 T cells. Monocytes and eosinophils. Induces MHC class II presentation
IL-17	T cells	Pro-inflammatory. Stimulates production of TNF, IL-1β, -6, -8 and G-CSF
IL-18	Macrophages and dendritic cells	Induces IFN-γ production by T cells. Enhances NK cytotoxicity
IL-19	Monocytes	Modulation of Th1 activity
IL-20	Probably keratinocytes	Probably regulates inflammatory responses in the skin
IL-21	Th cells	Regulation of haemopoiesis; NK cell differentiation and B-cell activation. T-cell costimulation
IL-22	T cells	Inhibits IL-4 production by Th2
IL-23	Dendritic cells	Induces proliferation and IFN-γ production by Th1 cells. Induces proliferation of memory cells
Colony stimulating factors (CSF)		
GM-CSF	Th, macrophages, fibroblasts, mast cell and endothelial cells	Stimulates growth of progenitors of monocytes, neutrophils, eosinophils and basophils. Activates macrophages
G-CSF	Fibroblasts and endothelial cells	Stimulates growth of progenitors of neutrophils
M-CSF	Fibroblasts and endothelial cells	Stimulates growth of progenitors of monocytes
SLE	Bone marrow stroma	Stimulates stem cell division
Tumour necrosis factor (TNF)		
TNF (TNF-α)	Th, monocytes, macrophages, dendritic and mast cells. NK and B cells	Tumour cytotoxicity; cachexia (weight loss); induces cytokine secretion; induces E-selection on endothelial cells; activates macrophages; anti-viral
Lymphotoxin (TNF-β)	Th1 and T cells	Tumour cytotoxicity; enhances phagocytosis by neutrophils and macrophages; involved in lymphoid organ development; anti-viral
Interferons (IFN)		
IFN-α	Leucocytes	Inhibits viral replication; enhances MHC class I presentation
IFN-β	Fibroblasts	Inhibits viral replication; enhances MHC class I presentation
IFN-γ	Th1, T cell 1, NK	Activates macrophages and switch to IgG2a; antagonizes several IL-4 actions; inhibits proliferation of Th2
Others		
TGF-β	Th3, B cells, monocytes and macrophages	Pro-inflammatory of chemo-attraction of monocytes and macrophages but also anti-inflammatory by inhibiting lymphocyte proliferation. Induces switch to IgA; promotes tissue repair
LIF	Thymic epithelium, bone marrow stroma	Induces APP
Eta-1	T cells	Stimulates IL-12 production and inhibits IL-10 production by macrophages
Oncostatin	T cells and macrophages	Induces APP

APP, acute phase protein; B cells, B lymphocytes; GM-CSF, granulocyte-macrophage colony stimulating factor; ICAM, intercellular adhesion molecule; Ig, immunoglobulin; LIF, leukaemia inhibitory factor; MHC, major histocompatibility complex; NK, natural killer cell; PG prostaglandin; SLF, steel locus factor; T cell, T lymphocyte; Th, T helper lymphocyte; TGF, transforming growth factor; VCAM, vascular cell adhesion molecule.

roam the body ingesting the antigen they find and fragmenting it into antigenic peptides. Within the cell these species of peptide are joined to the major histocompatibility complex (MHC) molecules and displayed on the surface of the cell. Thymus-dependent (T) lymphocytes have antigenic surface receptors which recognize the specific antigenic peptide-MHC combinations. The T lymphocytes are activated by that process and divide to produce memory and effector cells. The effector cells secrete chemical signals (lymphokines) which mobilize other components of the immune system. One set of cells that respond to these signals are B lymphocytes which also have specific receptor molecules on their surface but unlike T lymphocytes can recognize parts of the whole antigen free in solution. When activated, they differentiate into plasma cells that secrete specific antibodies which are soluble forms of their receptors. By binding to antigen the antibodies can neutralize them or precipitate their destruction by activating the complement cascade or enabling phagocytic cells to destroy them. Some B lymphocytes also persist as memory cells.

Development of immune cells

It is known that the cells concerned with immunity all develop from stem cells in the bone marrow (Weissman & Cooper 1993). One group of these cells, T lymphocytes, is dependent on the thymus gland for its development and if this gland is removed in a fetal animal T-cell immunity does not develop. In birds, another group of cells is similarly dependent on a sac in the hind gut known as the bursa of Fabricius and are known as bursal dependent or B lymphocytes. In mammals B lymphocyte development takes place in the bone marrow.

Cells destined to become T lymphocytes migrate early in fetal life to the thymus where they divide and differentiate. They give rise to successive bands of cells which migrate to the lining epithelia of body orifices and later to the lymphoid organs. The first cells going to the epithelia develop T-cell receptors (TCR) with gamma-delta chains, whereas the later ones going to the lymphoid organs develop TCRs with alpha-beta chains and will develop into helper (T4) and killer (T8) lymphocytes.

B lymphocytes develop under the influence of the stromal cells which produce factors needed for their growth and development. They develop interleukin (IL)-7 receptors which are stimulated by IL-7 from the stromal cells. They then progressively develop and express specific antibody receptors. They form the heavy chain first, then add the light chain and ultimately express the complete specific immunoglobulin (Ig) receptor. They produce additional Ig alpha and beta chains which associate with the Ig molecule to produce the complete receptor. If the developing B lymphocytes react with large amounts of self antigens then they are signalled to undergo programmed death (apoptosis). The clones that survive this process migrate to the lymphoid organs.

The T lymphocyte pathway is more complex and they pass through a number of challenges in their development. As they develop, they make and express either CD4 or CD8 receptors. CD4 cells react with Class II MHC and become T4 helper cells and CD8 cells react with Class I MHC and become T8 killer cells. Following this the cells make and express the specific TCR. They are first tested to see whether they detect antigens presented by other cells, an essential feature of T cells. Cells which react with self MHC survive and those which do not undergo apoptosis. They also die if they react with large amounts of self antigen. The surviving T lymphocytes migrate to the lymphoid organs and these are the cells which can recognize both foreign peptides and self-MHC.

Development of the specific receptors

There is tremendous diversity of both the TCR and Ig receptors on T and B cells, respectively (Janaway 1993; Marrak & Kappler 1993). This is determined during their development in a unique way. Both the antibody and

TCR genes are inherited as gene fragments known as mini genes which are functional only after they join together to form complete genes. This process only occurs in individual lymphocytes as they develop. The order in which they join and the joining process itself produce immense diversity. Immunoglobulins consist of heavy and light chains joined together to form a Y shape. Each cell produces one type of heavy and one type of light chain to produce together the unique Ig receptor. Each chain consists of combinations of the products of mini genes which are shuffled to produce myriad different combinations. Diversity springs from the size of the mini gene families which are divided into variable (V) of which there are more than 100, Diversity (D) of which there are 12 and Joining (J) of which there are 4. There are also constant (C) mini genes which only vary slightly to affect the function of the antibody and not its specificity. During development the shuffling of these mini genes into different VDJC combinations produces 4800 different heavy chains and 400 VDJ combinations in the light chains making 1 920 000 antibody genes. In addition, special enzymes insert a few extra DNA coding units at VD or DJ junctions which further increases diversity.

The alpha-beta or gamma-delta chains of the TCR of T lymphocytes are constructed in a similar way producing similar levels of diversity.

Lymphoid tissues

Nearly all the T lymphocytes in the lymphoid organs and over 90% of those in the blood have alpha-beta TCRs whereas virtually all such cells associated with epithelia have gamma-delta TCRs (Lydyard & Grossi 1993). In the lymphoid organs T and B cells which have matured but are not associated with immune responses reside in separate domains. After stimulation by antigen the cells which will participate in antibody production form new structures known as germinal centres. Three types of cells, T4 helper lymphocytes, B lymphocytes and dendritic cells, which are types of antigen presenting cell, predominate in the interface between B and T cell domains.

Lymphocyte circulation

Lymphocytes constantly circulate around the body to provide each lymphoid organ a rapid sampling of all the lymphocytes that may possess receptor for foreign antigens already attracting the body's attention (Weissman & Cooper 1993). They pass into the lymphoid organs through a specialized blood vessel known as a high endothelial venule (HEV). Only lymphocytes expressing homing receptors that match the receptors on the HEV can pass through. There are two types of receptors, one which matches lymph nodes and one which matches lymphoid organs of the GI tract. When T and B cells become activated they stop producing these homing markers and produce another integrin VCAM-1 which matches receptors on blood vessels so that they pass through inflamed vessels into infected tissues.

The immune response and function (Fig. 3.2)

Antigens are first taken up by antigen presenting cells (Janaway 1993; Marrak & Kappler 1993; Paul 1993). These include macrophages throughout the body, follicular dendritic cells in lymphoid organs and dendritic and Langerhans cells present throughout the mucosal surfaces. All these cells carry the CD4 surface marker. Antigens usually in the form of infecting organisms are phagocytosed by these cells and broken down within phagolysosomes into their constituent peptides. A Class II MHC molecule made in the endoplasmic reticulum (ER) is transported to the vesicle. A covering protein chain keeps the molecule inactive until it reaches the antigenic peptide within its processing vesicle. In this vehicle, the chain falls away enabling the MHC molecule to bind to any antigenic peptides

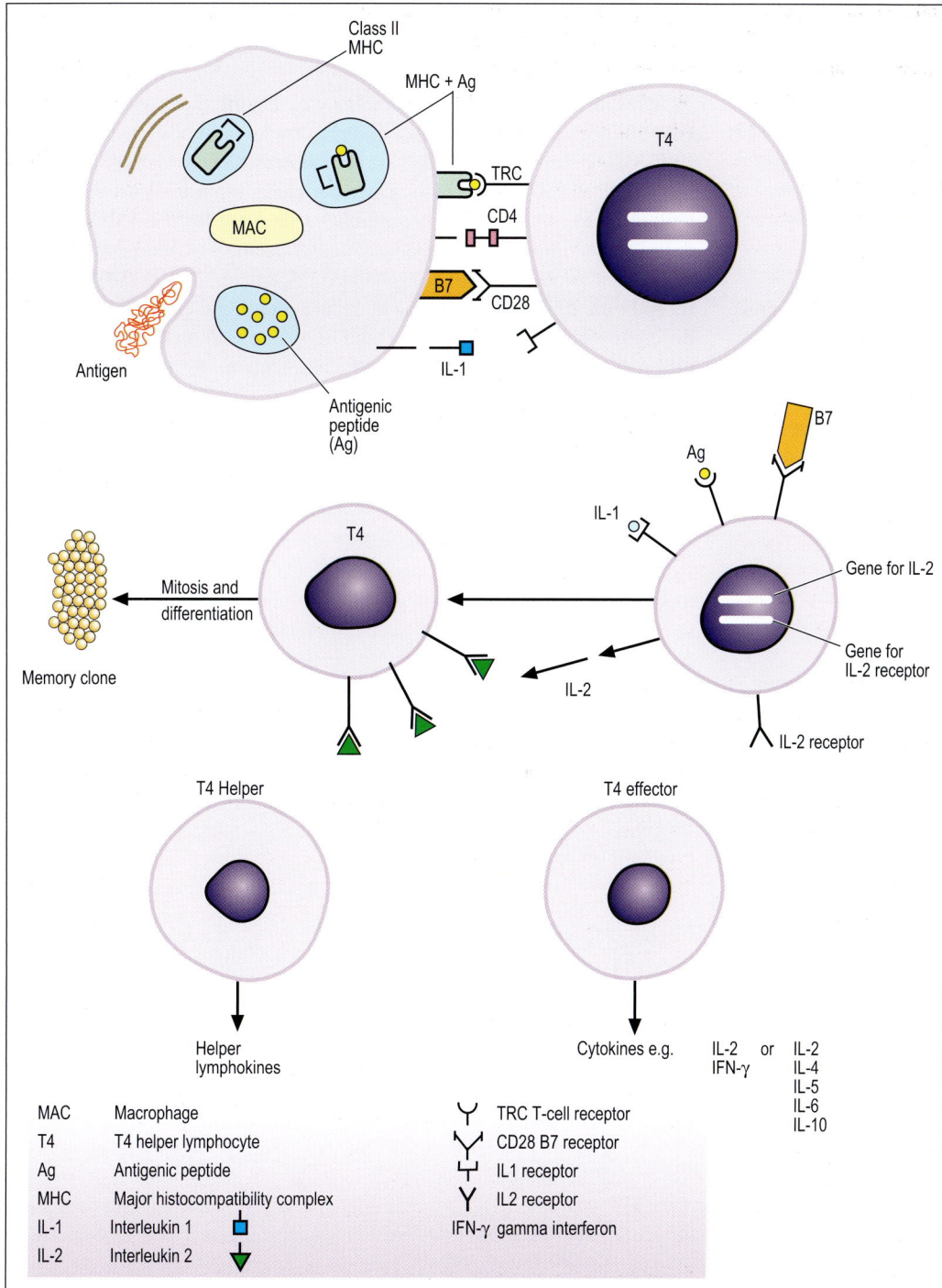

Class II
MHC

MHC + Ag

TRC

CD4

B7

CD28

IL-1

T4

Antigen

MAC

Antigenic
peptide
(Ag)

B7

Ag

IL-1

Gene for IL-2

Gene for
IL-2 receptor

IL-2 receptor

T4

Mitosis and
differentiation

Memory clone

IL-2

T4 Helper

T4 effector

Helper
lymphokines

Cytokines e.g.   IL-2   or   IL-2
IFN-γ   IL-4
IL-5
IL-6
IL-10

MAC	Macrophage		TRC	T-cell receptor
T4	T4 helper lymphocyte			CD28 B7 receptor
Ag	Antigenic peptide			IL1 receptor
MHC	Major histocompatibility complex			IL2 receptor
IL-1	Interleukin 1		IFN-γ	gamma interferon
IL-2	Interleukin 2			

Fig. 3.2 Diagram to show the primary stages in the immune reaction.

there. The complex then moves to the cell surface where it is presented so that it can be detected by T and B cells with the appropriate specific antigen receptor.

Antigenic peptides held in the groove of the Class II MHC molecule are recognized by T4 helper lymphocytes carrying CD4 marker and the appropriate TCR. The binding of the antigen to the receptor interacts with the biochemical message system in the T4 cell which will tell the cell to divide, grow, differentiate and produce its products. The lymphocyte must also receive a second message at the same time for these events to occur and if this is not received the cell will be programmed to die rather than develop. A molecule known as B7 serves this purpose and is presented at the same time by the antigen presenting cell and reacts with a CD28 receptor on the T-helper cell. B7 is only produced by infected cells and thus protects against stimulation by autoantigens.

During this process, IL-1 is also produced by the macrophage (Table 3.1) and reacts with its receptor on the T4 cell (Rook 1993). This activates the appropriate genes in the T4 cell to produce IL-2 and IL-2 receptor. Stimulation by IL-2 and other cytokines causes cell division and results in the production of a clone of memory T4 cells and effector T4 cells. The effector T4 helper lymphocytes produce helper lymphokines which stimulate T4, T8 and B lymphocytes reacting to the same antigen.

T4 immunity controlling intracellular parasites (Fig. 3.2)

Effector T4 lymphocytes produce lymphokines which activate macrophages containing the antigens to destroy the material within their vesicles (Paul 1993). This response occurs with intracellular bacterial or protozoan infections such as tuberculosis, leprosy, Leishmania etc. The

T4 cells consist of two subsets of cells and one (TH1) secretes predominantly IL-2 and gamma interferon (IFN-γ) and the other (TH2) IL-2, IL-4, IL-5, IL-6 and IL-10 (Table 3.1). The type of T4 response may affect the outcome. IFN-γ induces macrophages to produce tumour necrosis factors (TNF) and chemicals such as nitric oxide and toxic forms of oxygen which lead to microbial destruction in the phagosome. The other response activates B lymphocytes.

Humoral immunity (Fig. 3.3)

The antibody receptor on the surface of a B lymphocyte can recognize foreign antigens in the bloodstream and binds to it (Paul 1993). The antigen is taken into the cell and placed with a vesicle inside the cell. Class II MHC molecules made in the ER are delivered to the vesicle as previously described. It is then presented on the cell surface where it is detected by the appropriate clone of T4 helper lymphocytes. The TCR and CD4 bind to the antigen and MHC respectively. B cells also need a second signal from the T-helper cell. This comes from the production and presentation of CD40 by the helper cell which binds to the CD40 receptor on the B cell. The T4 cell produces helper lymphokines which then switch on the signal system

which results in division, differentiation to plasma cells and antibody production. These helper lymphokines (Table 3.1) include IL-2, IL-4, IL-5, IL-6 and IFN-γ (Feldmann 1993).

When differentiation of B lymphocytes begins they cease to display their antibody receptor molecule and prepare for antibody production. The antibodies produced by the cell are the same as those which are presented by the cell as antigen receptors. Different kinds of antibody are made each with the same specificity by a different variation of the antibody molecule during development. This is done by altering the so-called constant part of the heavy chain, again by gene rearrangement. This creates different receptor areas on this part of the molecule enabling the antibodies to go to different parts of the body. After binding to antigens on the microbe these different antibody types can activate complement, promote phagocytosis (opsonization) or activate mast cells.

All antibody molecules have the same basic structure with two specific antigen-combining sites and a single receptor-binding site. There are five types of antibody molecule each made by a separate group of plasma cells. These are: IgG, IgM, IgA, IgE and IgD. IgG and IgM are found mainly in blood and inflammatory exudates. IgG is the most abundant and is a single Ig molecule with a receptor area for the C3 and Ig gamma receptors on macrophages and polymorphs. IgM is a polymer of five Ig molecules with the same receptors as IgG. IgA is a dimer and has a secretory piece added between the two molecules by cells in secretory glands which allows it to pass through glandular epithelium into the secretion where it binds to the surface of mucous membranes. IgE binds to receptors on mast cells and basophils and causes a release of mediators.

The main function of these antibody types is as follows:

- IgG
    - Antitoxin
    - Opsonin
    - Complement activation
    - Neutralizes virus in blood
- IgM
    - Opsonin
    - Bacterial agglutination
- IgA
    - Prevents viral attachment
    - Neutralizes virus on mucous membrane
    - Prevents bacterial adherence on mucous membrane
    - Antitoxin
- IgE
    - Degranulates mast cells
    - Promotes inflammation
    - Stimulates the production of some factors which may be lethal to parasites
    - Attaches to macrophages and may bind parasites
- IgD
    - Possible role in B cell function.

In terms of humoral immune function in periodontal disease it has been shown that the serum level of anti-*Porphyromonas gingivalis* titre significantly correlated with the detection and number of *P. gingivalis* at periodontitis sites in patients with both adult periodontitis and early onset periodontitis (Kajima et al 1997). There were higher levels of *P. gingivalis* at early onset periodontitis sites compared with adult periodontitis sites but no differences in the serum IgG titres.

T8 immunity controlling viral infection (Fig. 3.4)

Class I MHC molecules are manufactured by practically all body cells in their ER and they bind to peptides that originate from proteins in the cytosolic compartment of the cell (Paul 1993). Viruses infect this area of

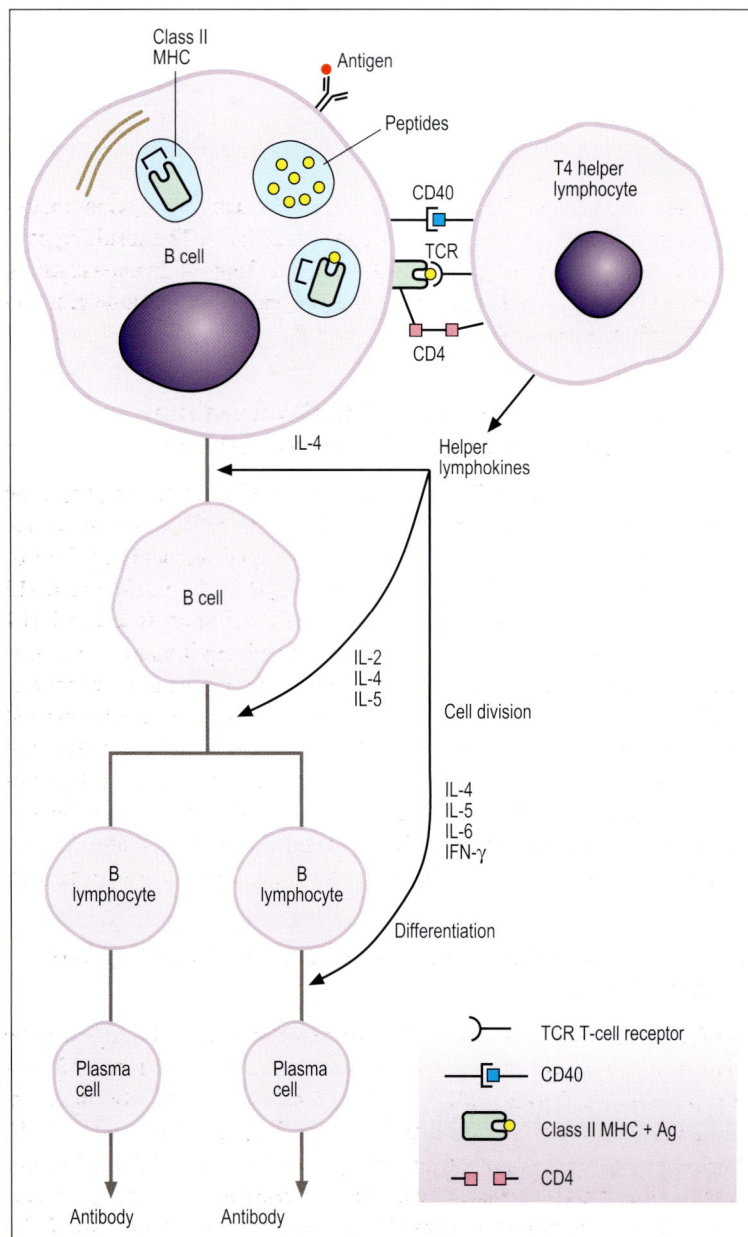

Fig. 3.3 Diagram to show the principal events in humoral immunity.

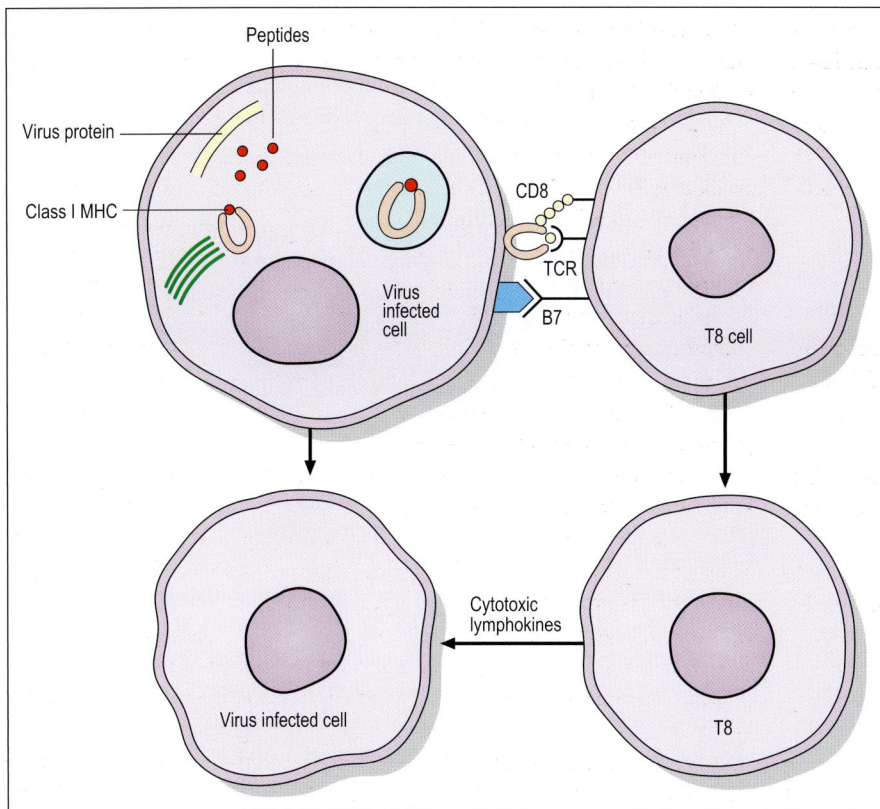

Fig. 3.4 Diagram to show the main stages in T8 immunity to control viral infections.

the cell and some of the viral proteins are broken down to peptides. They are pumped by a transport system into the ER. There the Class I MHC molecules are synthesized as long chains of amino acids which shape themselves around the antigenic peptide to form the complete molecule. This signals for it to be transported to the surface in a vesicle to be displayed on the surface of the cell. Here it can be detected by a killer T8 lymphocyte which expresses the CD8 protein. Again, two stimuli are needed to activate the cell, one from the Class I MHC and antigen and the other from B7 which is synthesized and expressed by the body cell when it presents a foreign peptide. This links to the CD28 receptor on the T8 cell.

When activated, the killer T8 lymphocyte acts directly and indirectly to kill the infected cells. They secrete perforin and other proteins that disrupt the cellular membrane and may also release molecules that promote programmed cell death or apoptosis. They also release IFN-γ and TNF (Table 3.1) which limit viral multiplication inside a cell and also attract macrophages and other phagocytes which can destroy the cell.

Hypersensitivity

Although the activity of the immune system has the primary function of defending the body, once set in motion its activity can become excessive and lead to gross tissue damage. This excessive activity is called hypersensitivity (Lichtenstein 1993). There are four main types of hypersensitivity. Types I, II and III are called immediate reactions and depend on antibody-antigen reactions. Type I is related to the production of IgE antibodies which attach to receptors on mast cells and basophils resulting in the release of the contents of their granules and membranes which mediate the allergic responses. The granular mediators are histamine and platelet activating factor and the lipid mediators are leukotrienes and prostaglandin D. These dilate and increase the permeability of blood vessels, stimulate mucus production and constrict bronchial smooth muscle. Conditions caused by these reactions include hay fever, asthma, urticaria and anaphylaxis. Type II reactions involve the production of IgG antibody which activates complement on cell surfaces harbouring the antigen

and cause cell damage. Type III (Arthus) reactions involve IgG antibody-antigen complexes reacting within blood vessel walls. The resulting activation of complement damages the vessel wall. Type IV hypersensitivity is termed delayed and is essentially the cell-mediated immune reaction described in the last section.

T-helper (CD4) cell subsets and their role in the determination of the type of immune reaction

There are four subsets of T-helper (Th) cells: the Th precursor (Thp), the Th non-determined (Th0), the Th1 and Th2 effector cells. Th1 cells secrete large amounts of IFN-γ, IL-2 and TNF-β and small amounts of TNF-α, GM-CSF and IL-3, while Th2 cells secrete IL-3, IL-4, IL-5, IL-6 and IL-13 in large amounts and TNF-α, GM-CSF in small amounts. In general Th1 cells secrete cytokines which stimulate cell-mediated immunity which is effective against intracellular pathogens which grow within macrophages, while Th2 cells produce cytokines that stimulate B-cell differentiation and humoral immunity with antibody production (Roitt & Delves 2001). The results of Th2 cytokine stimulation can be varied with different types of pathogen as IL-4 can stimulate IgE production, IL-5 can stimulate the proliferation of eosinophils and IL-3/IL-4 can stimulate mast cell proliferation and IL-4/IL-5/IL-6 stimulates the generation of an IgG antibody response.

Role of the antigen presenting cells (APC) in Th1 or Th2 determination

Antigen presenting cells (APC), in particular dendritic cells, appear to be pivotal in driving the differentiation towards either the Th1 or Th2 phenotype (Roitt & Delves 2001). IL-12 seems to be particularly important for the production of Th1 cells and IL-4 for the production of Th2 cells. Invasion of monocyte/macrophage phagocytes by intracellular pathogens such as viruses and some bacteria induces the secretion of copious amounts of IL-12 which in turn stimulates IFN-γ production by natural killer (NK) cells. These two cytokines drive the differentiation of the Th1 phenotype whilst inhibiting the development of a Th2 response. Secretion of IL-4 by APCs results in a Th2 response and is stimulated by pathogens which do not grow within body cells or monocyte/macrophage phagocytes. The effects of IL-4 are dominant over those of IL-12 and therefore the response depends on the relative amounts of IL-4 and IL-12 and secreted IFN-γ. IL-4 downregulates the expression of IL-12 receptors (IL-12Rs) on responding cells. In particular it effects the expression of the β_2 subunit which is necessary for the recognition of IL-12.

A special population of NK cells known as NK-T cells when stimulated rapidly release IL-4 and related cytokines (Roitt & Delves 2001). There is also some evidence for sub-populations of APCs which specialize in the stimulation of either Th1 or Th2 immune responses.

Gingival epithelium contains Langerhans cells (LCs) and is a site for the trafficking of these cells (Jotwani & Cutler 2003). In patients with chronic periodontitis the lamina propria also contains CD83+ mature dendritic cells (mDCs) and CD4+ T lymphocytes. In addition to LCs the gingival lamina propria contains dermal DCs and these increase in number during chronic periodontitis. Furthermore, DCs, LCs and B lymphocytes co-express CD83 in chronic periodontitis patients and contribute to the mDCs pool. Mature DCs were found to associate with clusters of CD4+ T lymphocytes in the lamina propria. This evidence (Jotwani & Cutler 2003) suggests that multiple DC subsets mature in the gingiva and that mature DCs engage in antigen presentation with CD4+ T lymphocytes during chronic periodontitis.

PERIODONTAL PATHOLOGY

The periodontal tissues are subject to two types of environmental factor:

1. A mechanical system in which the varying stresses of mastication demand constant modulation of the periodontal ligament, alveolar bone and cementum
2. Those oral factors described in Chapter 2, in particular the bacterial ecosystem of the gingival crevice.

In health the periodontal tissues metabolize and function normally in harmony with these two milieu, and because of the adaptability of vital tissues a balance can be maintained within broad environmental limits.

The periodontal tissues may undergo a variety of pathological changes, inflammatory, degenerative and neoplastic. They may also be involved in autoimmune diseases. Inflammation is by far the most common form of periodontal pathology. This may be restricted to the gingivae, that is gingivitis, or involve the deeper periodontal tissues, i.e. periodontitis. Inflammation may be acute or chronic. By definition, acute inflammation comes on suddenly, is painful and is of short duration. Chronic inflammation comes on slowly, is rarely painful and is of long duration. Acute gingivitis is usually caused by specific infection or injury. Acute periodontitis may follow a blow to a tooth or develop as a complication of chronic periodontitis. Chronic gingivitis and chronic periodontitis are successive stages in chronic inflammatory periodontal disease, and although gingival inflammation is the essential precursor to chronic periodontitis this progression is not inevitable.

Epidemiological studies indicate that this progression seems to take place in a much smaller proportion of individuals than was previously believed. Unfortunately, we cannot yet predict in which individual the progression from gingivitis to periodontitis will take place, and much current research is directed at trying to define the person who is 'at risk'. A great deal of epidemiological and clinical research in the past decade has highlighted considerable variation in clinical features and rates of disease progression, and although all cases of periodontitis involves loss of connective tissue attachment to the root surface in the presence of gingival inflammation (Papapanou 1994), it is now common practice to speak of periodontal diseases in the plural. This is not only because of the considerable variation in most features of the disease, even in the otherwise healthy individual, but also because this variation in the periodontal lesion does not appear to bear a clear and simple relationship to the causal agent, the quantity of related bacterial plaque or the types of bacteria in the plaque.

These variables are in:

1. The distribution, extent and severity of gingival inflammation
2. The presence or absence of gingival ulceration
3. The quantity of plaque and its bacterial constituents
4. The extent and distribution of areas of loss of periodontal attachment, i.e. periodontitis
5. The rapidity of loss of attachment and alveolar bone
6. The form of the bone lesion
7. The humoral and cellular component of the lesion described above.

This variation is further confused in the presence of systemic factors, genetic, hormonal, nutritional, haematological and pharmaceutical, as described in Chapter 6.

In terms of the most common form of periodontal disease, adult chronic periodontitis, this manifests itself in a least two clinical entities. In one form it remains stable over many years and then may or may not slowly progress but never endangers the dentition. In another form it may rapidly and episodically progress to producing marked tissue destruction (Seymour 1987). Adult periodontitis is primarily caused by bacteria in dental plaque, with some evidence that specific periodontal pathogens may be responsible for its progression. However, some individuals harbour these bacteria and show no signs of progression whilst others with the same bacteria show varying rates of progression from slow to rapid. Patient susceptibility to periodontal disease is of the utmost importance to its outcome and it seems likely that the host response to these bacteria is of fundamental importance (Seymour 1991; Seymour et al 1993).

Histological studies support this concept and have shown that the infiltrate of the periodontal lesion consists of macrophages and lymphocytes. T lymphocytes appear to dominate the stable lesion whereas the proportion of B lymphocytes and plasma cells increase markedly in the progressive lesion (Seymour 1991; Seymour et al 1993). A great deal of evidence has accumulated that indicates that the stable lesion, which has the same features as the early lesion of experimental gingivitis, has all the characteristics of a Th1 immune response while that of a progressive lesion, which has the same features as the established lesion of experimental gingivitis, resembles a Th2 immune response (Seymour & Gemmell 2001). It is as yet unclear what leads to the switch from Th1 to Th2 in this situation. This concept will be considered further in Chapter 5.

A clinical and laboratory study (Erciyas et al 2006) was set up to determine whether there was any change in T-lymphocyte subsets in patients with chronic periodontitis and after periodontal treatment. It showed that the local CD4+/CD8+ ratio was low in chronic periodontitis but improved following its treatment suggesting that CD4+ and CD8+ T lymphocytes could play a significant role in chronic periodontitis pathobiology.

Natural killer T (NKT) cells are a unique T lymphocyte subset that has been implicated in the regulation of immune responses associated with a broad range of diseases including autoimmunity, infectious diseases, and cancer. In contrast to conventional T cells, NKT cells are reactive to major histocompatibility complex (MHC) class I-like molecule CD1d (Amanuma et al 2006). This group carried out an immunohistochemical analysis on cryostat sections of gingival tissues from 19 patients with periodontitis and eight patients with gingivitis using antibodies to CD1a, b, c, d, NKT cells, CD83, CD3 and CD19. Their findings suggested that CD1d-expressing B cells could activate NKT cells by CD1d-restricted manner and this NKT cell activation may play roles in pathogenesis of periodontal diseases.

REFERENCES

Amanuma R, Nakajima T, Yoshie H, et al: Increased infiltration of CD1d+ and natural killer T cells in periodontal disease tissues, *J Periodontal Res* 41:73–79, 2006.

Erciyas K, Orbak R, Kavrut F, et al: The changes in T lymphocyte subsets following periodontal treatment in patients with chronic periodontitis, *J Periodontal Res* 41: 165–170, 2006.

Feldmann M: Cell cooperation in the antibody response, In Roitt I, Brostoff J, Male D, editors: *Immunology*, ed 3, St Louis, 1993, Mosby, pp 7.1–7.16.

Janaway CA: How the immune system recognizes invaders, *Sci Am* September:41–47, 1993.

Jotwani R, Cutler CW: Multiple dendritic cell (DC) subpopulations in human gingiva and association of mature DCs with CD4+ T-cells, *J Dent Res* 82:736–741, 2003.

Kajima T, Yano K, Ishikawa I: Relationship between serum antibody levels and subgingival colonisation of Porphyromonas gingivalis in patients with various types of periodontitis, *J Periodontol* 68:618–625, 1997.

Lichtenstein LM: Allergy and the immune system, *Sci Am* September:85–91, 1993.

Lydyard P, Grossi C: Cells involved in the immune response. In Roitt I, Brostoff J, Male D, editors. *Immunology*, ed 3, St Louis, 1993, Mosby, pp 2.1–2.20.

Marrak P, Kappler JW: How the immune system recognizes the body, *Sci Am* September:49–55, 1993.

Miyazaki A, Kobayashi T, Suzuki T, et al: Loss of Fcγ receptors and impaired phagocytosis of polymorphonuclear leucocytes in gingival crevicular fluid, *J Periodontal Res* 32:439–446, 1997.

Nossal GVA: Life, death and the immune system, *Sci Am* September:21–30, 1993.

Papapanou PN: Epidemiology and natural history of periodontal disease. In Lang NP, Karring T, editors. *Proceedings of the 1st European Workshop on Periodontology*, London, 1994, Quintessence Publishing, pp 23–41.

Paul W: Infectious disease and the immune system, *Sci Am* September:57–63, 1993.

Roitt IM, Delves PJ: *Essential Immunology*, ed 10, Oxford, 2001, Blackwell Science. Ch. 10, pp 177–199.

Rook R: Cell-mediated immune reactions. In Roitt I, Brostoff J, Male D, editors. *Immunology*, ed 3, St Louis, 1993, Mosby, pp 2.1–2.20.

Seymour GJ: Possible mechanisms involved in the immunoregulation of chronic inflammatory disease, *J Dent Res* 66:2–9, 1987.

Seymour GJ: Importance of the host response in the periodontium, *J Clin Periodontol* 18:421–426, 1991.

Seymour GJ, Gemmell E, Reinhardt RA, et al: Immunopathogenesis of chronic inflammatory periodontal disease: cellular and molecular mechanisms, *J Periodontal Res* 28:478–486, 1993.

Seymour GJ, Gemmell E: Cytokines in periodontal disease: where to from here? *Acta Odontol Scand* 59:167–173, 2001.

Sugita N, Suzuki T, Yoshi H, et al: Differential expression of CR3, FcεRII and FcγRIII on polymorphonuclear leukocytes, *J Periodontal Res* 28:363–372, 1993.

Weissman IL, Cooper MD: How the immune system develops, *Sci Am* September:33–39, 1993.

4

The aetiology of periodontal disease

PRIMARY FACTORS

The primary cause of periodontal disease is bacterial irritation. However, small amounts of plaque are compatible with gingival and periodontal health (Lang et al 1973) and some patients can resist larger amounts of plaque for long periods without developing destructive periodontitis although they exhibit gingivitis.

A number of other factors, local and systemic, predispose towards plaque accumulation or alter the gingival response to plaque. These may be regarded as secondary aetiological factors.

THE PLAQUE THEORY

A relationship between oral hygiene and gingival disease is described in ancient writings. Today a great deal of evidence has been amassed to support this idea.

The evidence stems from clinical observation, epidemiological studies, clinical and microbiological research and, most recently, immunological investigations. This evidence can be summarized as follows:

1. The number of bacteria in the inflamed gingival crevice or periodontal pocket is greater than in a healthy crevice.
2. In the presence of gingival inflammation or periodontal pocketing, the number of organisms in the mouth increases.
3. Injection of human oral bacteria into guinea-pigs produces abscess formation, i.e. these bacteria can be pathogenic.
4. Epidemiological studies of many population groups in different parts of the world demonstrate a direct correlation between the amount of bacterial deposit as measured by the oral hygiene indices (Ch. 10) and the severity of gingival inflammation.
5. Epidemiological data show a direct correlation between oral hygiene status and the degree of periodontal destruction as indicated by radiographic evidence of alveolar bone loss.
6. The experimental production of gingival inflammation by the withdrawal of all forms of oral hygiene. Löe et al (1965) showed that when 12 students stopped cleaning their teeth, thus allowing plaque to accumulate around the gingival margin, gingival inflammation always appeared. When tooth cleaning was resumed and the plaque removed the inflammation disappeared (**Fig. 4.1**).
7. The above experiment when repeated in Beagle dogs produced the same result. Indeed, feeding experimental animals on a soft, sticky diet is sufficient to produce periodontal disease.
8. Epidemiological studies demonstrated that oral hygiene control reduced the incidence of gingivitis.
9. Gingival inflammation produced by the withdrawal of oral hygiene measures can be prevented by the use of non-specific antiseptic mouthwashes, e.g. chlorhexidine gluconate, in both man and experimental animals (Ch. 15).
10. Topical or systemic antibiotics will reduce gingival inflammation (Ch. 16).
11. Mechanical irritants, such as rough or overhanging filling margins, do not produce persistent gingival inflammation unless the fillings are covered by bacterial plaque.
12. In germ-free animals, mechanical abuse of the gingivae by placing silk ligatures between the teeth does not appear to produce gingival

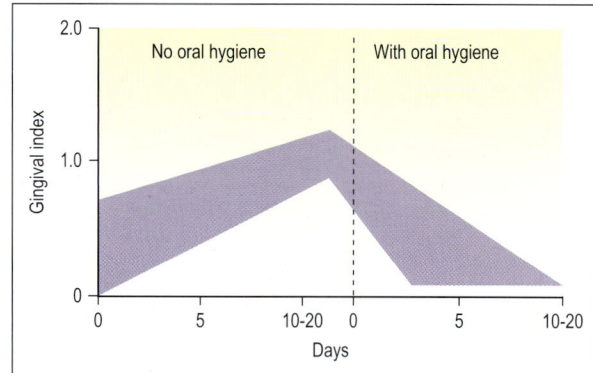

Fig. 4.1 The development of gingival inflammation with the withdrawal of oral hygiene measures, followed by resolution of inflammation as plaque control is resumed (Courtesy of Dr H. Löe).

inflammation or alveolar bone loss. When bacteria are introduced both gingival inflammation and bone loss result.
13. Cultures of bacteria from human periodontal pockets can produce enzymes which can degrade gingival and periodontal connective tissue (Ch. 5).
14. In periodontal disease there is a raised antibody titre to plaque bacteria. These antibodies can be detected in blood and crevicular fluid.
15. Lymphocytes and immunoglobulin-producing plasma cells are present in gingival connective tissue and gingival fluid, and increase in amount where there is evidence of gingival inflammation.
16. *In vitro* lymphocytes are activated by plaque deposits and there is a direct correlation between the severity of periodontal disease and lymphocyte transformation.
17. When healthy young adults abstained from oral hygiene measures for 28 days the resultant accumulation of bacterial plaque and associated gingival inflammation were correlated with an increase in lymphocyte transformation and release of migration inhibition factor. These cellular responses returned to base-line values 28 days after plaque was removed (Lehner et al 1974).

Although each piece of evidence taken by itself might be questioned, the aggregate provides powerful support for the plaque theory. A further conclusion from the evidence is that it takes a certain minimum amount of time for plaque products to produce inflammation. Lang et al (1973) showed that if teeth are cleaned at intervals of 48 h, no gingivitis results but if cleaning is delayed for 72 h gingival inflammation is produced.

SPECIFIC AND NON-SPECIFIC BACTERIAL THEORIES OF THE AETIOLOGY OF PERIODONTAL DISEASE

Recently it has become popular to speak of different periodontal diseases with possible different causes. However, only three inflammatory periodontal diseases – adult chronic periodontitis (Ch. 8), juvenile periodontitis (Ch. 23) and acute ulcerative gingivitis (Ch. 25) – can be recognized as distinctive. Chronic periodontal disease includes conditions which range from gingivitis to advanced periodontitis with varying rates of progression and a diversity of clinical forms. The condition may or may not progress and when it does it may go through periods of progression, inactivity and regression (Goodson et al 1982). The controversy between the specific and non-specific theories of the microbial aetiology of inflammatory periodontal disease has continued for nearly 100 years and is discussed below.

Specific theory

According to the pure specific theory a single specific pathogen is the cause of inflammatory periodontal disease, as in the case of the well-known exogenous bacterial infections of man, such as pneumococcal pneumonia, typhoid, tuberculosis and syphilis. If this were the case, treatment would be directed towards the elimination of the specific pathogen from the mouth with the appropriate narrow-spectrum antibiotic. Following this, plaque control would no longer be necessary since plaque without the specific pathogen would be non-pathogenic (Theilade 1986). However, no one single pathogen has been found and many suspected periodontal pathogens have been suggested, including *Actinomycetes*, spirochaetes and a number of Gram-negative anaerobic rods (Socransky et al 1982). Much recent work has centred around three bacterial species – *Porphyromonas gingivalis*, *Prevotella intermedia* and *Aggregatibacter actinomycetemcomitans* (Slots 1986) and spirochaetes (Listgarten & Levin 1981; Loesche 1988). However, none of these bacteria are foreign invaders since they are all members of the normal oral flora. Although they often make up a larger proportion of the subgingival flora in diseased sites with recent evidence of progression, they are also present in smaller numbers in non-progressive pockets and in the absence of disease (Ch. 2). Several of these organisms fulfil some of the criteria set up by Socransky (1979) to indicate pathogenicity, including quantitative association with disease, altered immune response, animal pathogenicity and the possession of virulence factors. However, none have yet been shown to fulfil Socransky's other criteria that disease should be cured by eliminating the suspected species without otherwise changing plaque. Such specific treatment is not effective and even the strongest supporters of the specific theory advocate (Goodson et al 1979) non-specific plaque control with subgingival scaling supplemented by the most broad-spectrum antibiotic, tetracycline (Ch. 17). It should also be noted that over 50% of the subgingival flora cannot be cultivated, and modern genetic methods of detecting bacteria have yielded different compositions from culture techniques (Ch. 2). Thus the bacteria detected from any given site at any given time depend on the methods used to collect and detect them.

Studies of the bacteria associated with active stages of chronic periodontitis are hampered by the fact that the disease is a dynamic condition and may have short periods of active disease progression and long periods of inactivity (Goodson et al 1982). The chances of taking a bacterial sample from the right place at the right time, coinciding with active disease, are therefore very small and probably have never been achieved.

Non-specific theory

According to pure non-specific theory the indigenous oral bacteria colonize the gingival crevice to form plaque in the absence of effective oral hygiene (Theilade 1986). Inflammatory periodontal disease develops when bacterial proliferation exceeds the threshold of host resistance and is caused by the effects of the total plaque flora. All plaque bacteria are thought to have some virulence factors causing gingival inflammation and periodontal destruction. It is implied that plaque will cause disease regardless of its composition. Total plaque control is therefore considered necessary in the prevention and treatment of inflammatory periodontal diseases. This traditional measure, combined where necessary with subgingival scaling and root planing, has proved effective. However, the pure non-specific theory does not consider that variations in the composition of the subgingival flora may have implications for its pathogenic potential. Moreover, it does not explain why some patients or tooth sites have lifelong contained

gingivitis, whereas others experience slowly or rapidly progressive periodontitis. This may, however, be due to differences in the general or local host resistance rather than changes in the bacterial flora.

It seems likely, therefore, that a modern theory of the microbial aetiology of periodontal diseases should be a compromise between the extreme versions of the specific and non-specific theories.

Unified theory of the bacterial aetiology of chronic periodontitis

The modern version of the specific theory (Socransky 1979) has abandoned the idea of a single periodontal pathogen and states that periodontal disease can be initiated by any of a number of different pathogens. It states that 6–12 bacterial species may be responsible for the majority of cases of destructive periodontitis and additional species may be responsible for a small number of other cases. On the other hand, the supporters of the non-specific theory agree that some indigenous bacteria are more commonly associated with disease than others and possess important virulence factors. The modern versions of two theories therefore appear to have much in common and a unified theory is possible (Theilade 1986).

All bacterial plaque may contribute to the pathogenic potential of the subgingival flora to a greater or lesser degree by its ability to colonize and evade host defences and provoke inflammation and tissue damage. Any composition of plaque in sufficient quantity in the gingival crevice causes gingivitis but only in some cases does it lead to destructive periodontitis.

Different combinations of bacteria may be present in individual lesions and together produce the necessary virulence factors. As over 300 species of bacteria make up the oral flora, it is not surprising that different indigenous bacteria predominate in different stages of disease and in different persons and different sites within the same mouth. The increased virulence of the subgingival flora seems to be due to the emergence of a plaque ecology unfavourable to the host but favourable to the growth of bacteria with pathogenic potential (Theilade 1986).

Over the last 25 years, a selected number of bacteria from the subgingival flora have been shown to relate positively to periodontal disease progression (Socransky 1970; van Palenstein Helderman 1981; Genco et al 1988; Loesche 1988; Socransky & Haffajee 1990; Zambon 1990). These studies showed positive correlations between their presence and numbers and signs of disease such as inflammation, increased probing depth and loss of attachment. There is also accumulated evidence that the microflora of the periodontal pocket at possible active sites, i.e. those which have shown significant attachment and bone loss within short time intervals, is characterized by the presence of *Porphyromonas gingivalis*, *Prevotella intermedia*, *Bacteroides forsythus*, *Peptostreptococcus micros*, *Campylobacter recta*, *Fusobacterium nucleatum* and *A. actinomycetemcomitans* (Tanner et al 1984; Slots et al 1985, 1986; Dzink et al 1985, 1988; Moore et al 1991). Other studies (van Winkelhoff et al 2002) have shown that *A. actinomycetemcomitans*, *Porphyromonas gingivalis*, *Prevotella intermedia*, *Bacteroides forsythus*, *F. nucleatum* and *Peptostreptococcus micros* were significantly more prevalent in the pockets of patients with chronic periodontitis than those of healthy controls. Furthermore, other retrospective studies (Slots et al 1986; Bragd et al 1987; Wennström et al 1987; Slots & Listgarten 1988) have suggested that microbiological assays for critical levels of the target bacteria *A. actinomycetemcomitans*, *Porphyromonas gingivalis* and *Prevotella intermedia* at subgingival sites might be of diagnostic value. However, it should be noted in these studies that the samples were taken after breakdown had occurred and although they showed an association between the number of these bacteria and previous attachment loss at the site they were not shown to be predictive of future attachment loss.

It should also be realized that the correlations in all these studies do not distinguish between bacteria which may be pathogenic and non-pathogens which have proliferated because of disease associated tissue change such as deepened pockets, increased serum factors from exudate and blood or bacterial shifts that may have promoted their growth (Listgarten 1992). Unfortunately, it is not possible to determine in any particular patient which of the many bacteria colonizing their pockets are pathogenic or contributing to disease at any one point in time. Furthermore, the pathogenicity of bacterial species may differ at different stages of periodontal disease and a sequence of different bacteria may succeed one another as the conditions for their optimum growth alter.

Some researchers (Slots et al 1986; Bragd et al 1987) have postulated that some bacterial species may act as markers for disease since they are often associated with clinical signs of disease (Ch. 14). In this regard some retrospective studies relating bacterial species numbers to periodontal progression have shown correlations with numbers of *Porphyromonas gingivalis*, *Prevotella intermedia* and *A. actinomycetemcomitans* and have suggested that critical levels of these bacteria might be predictive for a site at risk for periodontal breakdown. Other retrospective studies using the BANA test have shown that higher numbers of *Treponema denticola*, *Porphyromonas gingivalis* and *Bacteroides forsythus* correlate with apparent periodontal progression (Schmidt et al 1988). However, the retrospective nature of the correlations in these studies cannot be related to prospective disease activity.

In a prospective study (Listgarten & Levin 1981) of a population on maintenance following treatment for periodontitis, the percentage of spirochaetes and motile rods at baseline were shown to be predictive of future disease progression occurring during the 1 year of the study. In a further 3-year prospective study (Listgarten et al 1986), similar findings were found for patients receiving irregular widely spaced maintenance visits but not for a control group receiving regular 3-monthly maintenance. Similar lack of reliability was found in attempting to predict future episodes of periodontal breakdown using *P. gingivalis*, *Prevotella intermedia* and *A. actinomycetemcomitans* as indicators in a 3-year prospective study of patients on regular maintenance following treatment of periodontitis (Listgarten et al 1991).

DNA probes can now be used to detect specific bacteria in clinical samples. One group (Liu et al 2003) constructed and labelled a DNA probe for *Porphyromonas gingivalis* based on a fragment encoding for the fimbriae subunit protein. It was shown to be specific for *P. gingivalis* and was used to detect *P. gingivalis* in subgingival plaque samples from 100 Chinese chronic periodontitis patients and 100 healthy controls. The numbers of *P. gingivalis* were significantly higher in the diseased group and also positively correlated with probing depths and mobility.

Similar findings have been reported in different parts of the world and a recent retrospective study of 148 Chinese adult patients aged 30–59 with chronic periodontitis found an increase in certain species, notably *P. gingivalis*, *T. denticola*, *B. forsythus* and *C. recta*, at sites with progressive periodontitis (Papapanou et al 1997). This type of study, however, does not show that any of these bacteria are predictive of periodontal progression.

It should also be realized that the correlations in all these studies do not distinguish between bacteria which may be pathogenic and non-pathogens that have proliferated because of disease-associated tissue changes such as deepened pockets, increased serum factors from exudate and blood or bacterial shifts, which may have promoted their growth (Listgarten 1992). Unfortunately, it is not possible to determine in any particular patient which of the bacteria colonizing their pockets are pathogenic or contributing to disease at any one point in time. Furthermore, the pathogenicity of bacterial species may differ at different stages of periodontal disease, and a sequence of different bacteria may succeed one another as the conditions for their optimum growth alter.

Having outlined the theories of bacterial involvement it needs to be emphasized that disease is produced by the interaction of oral bacteria with the tissue defences, i.e. host factors (Ch. 6).

SECONDARY FACTORS

Secondary factors may be local or systemic. A number of local factors, in the gingival environment, predispose towards the accumulation of plaque deposits and prevent their removal. These are called plaque-retention factors. The systemic or host factors modify the response of the gingivae to local irritation.

LOCAL FACTORS

These are:

1. Faulty restorations
2. Carious cavities
3. Food impaction
4. Badly designed partial dentures
5. Orthodontic appliances
6. Malalignment of teeth
7. Lack of lip-seal or mouth-breathing
8. Developmental grooves on cervical enamel or root surface
9. Tobacco smoking. This may have both local and systemic effects.

Faulty restorations

Faulty restorations are probably the most common factor favouring plaque retention. Overhanging filling margins are extremely frequent and result from careless use of matrix bands and the failure to polish margins (**Fig. 4.2**). At one time it was assumed that rough filling margins in proximity to the gingival margin actually irritated the tissue but there is no evidence for this. If there is no plaque accumulation on the restoration margin inflammation does not occur.

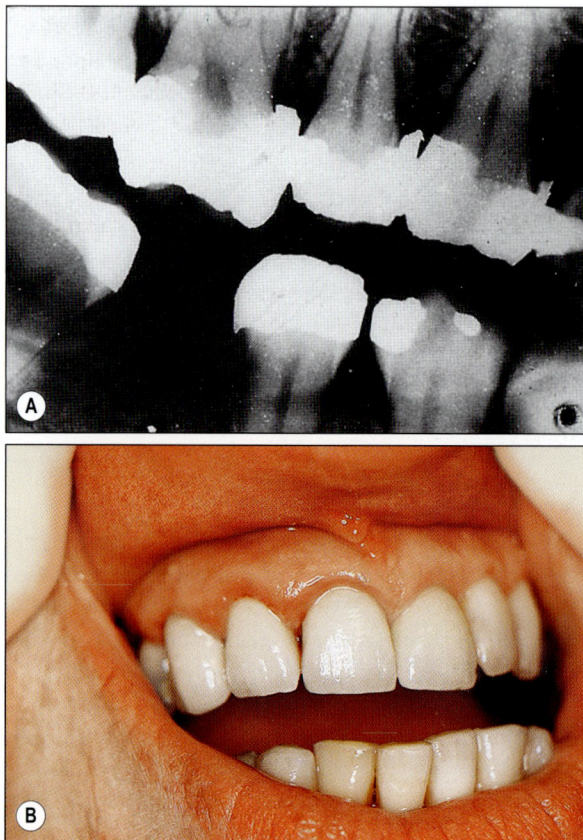

Fig. 4.2 (A) Radiograph showing overhanging restorative margins. (B) Gingival inflammation related to the subgingival placement of the margins of porcelain crowns on the upper right central and lateral incisors.

Badly contoured restorations, particularly over-contoured and bulbous crowns and fillings, may impede effective toothbrushing.

Carious cavities

Carious cavities, particularly those close to the gingival margin, encourage plaque stagnation.

Food impaction

Food impaction is the forceful wedging of food against the gingiva between teeth. Where teeth have drifted apart food wedging can take place, especially in the presence of an opposing 'plunger cusp'. It is questionable whether actual physical trauma occurs but food impaction sites are usually sites of plaque stagnation.

Badly designed partial dentures

Dentures are foreign bodies which can cause tissue irritation in a number of ways. Ill fitting or inadequately polished dentures will tend to act as foci for plaque collection. Dentures which are tissue borne frequently sink into the mucosa and compress the gingival margins causing inflammation and tissue destruction. These effects are compounded when the dentures are inadequately cleaned and worn during sleep. A further consequence of the badly designed partial denture is excessive occlusal stress on abutment teeth (**Fig. 4.3**), and this together with plaque-induced gingival inflammation is an extremely common cause of tooth loss.

Orthodontic appliances

Orthodontic appliances are worn both at night and by day and unless the patient is instructed in cleaning the appliance plaque accumulation is inevitable. As most orthodontic patients are young, a severe inflammation with gingival swelling can occur (**Fig. 4.4**).

Tooth malalignment

Tooth malalignment predisposes to plaque retention and makes plaque removal difficult (**Fig. 4.3**). Unless the patient's oral hygiene technique is very thorough tooth malalignment is frequently accompanied by gingival

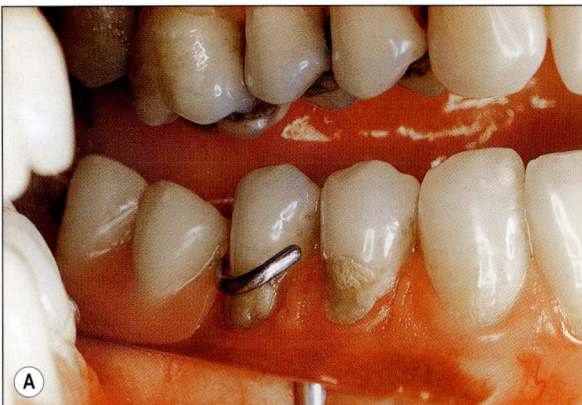

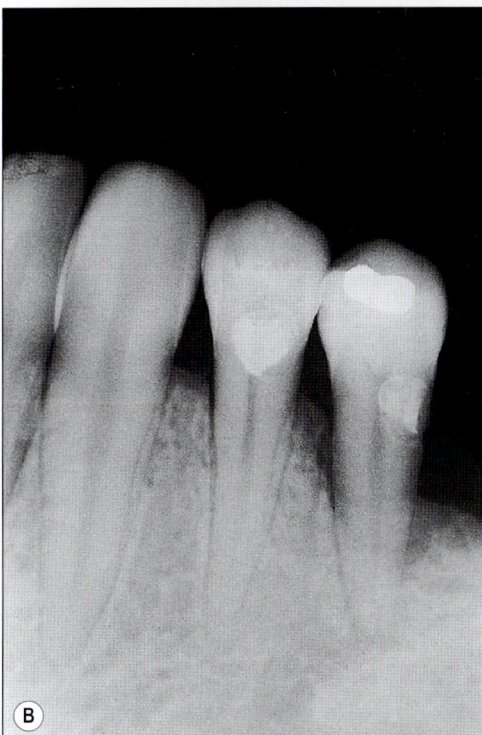

Fig. 4.3 (A) The incorrect placement of a clasp of a chrome cobalt lower partial denture so that it stress the tooth and traumatizes the interdcontoural papilla between the lower right first and second premolars. (B) Radiograph showing bone loss and widening of the periodontal ligament of lower second premolar.

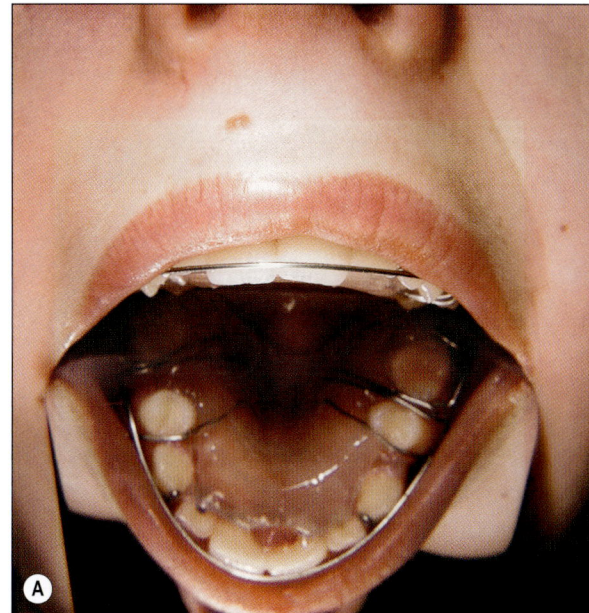

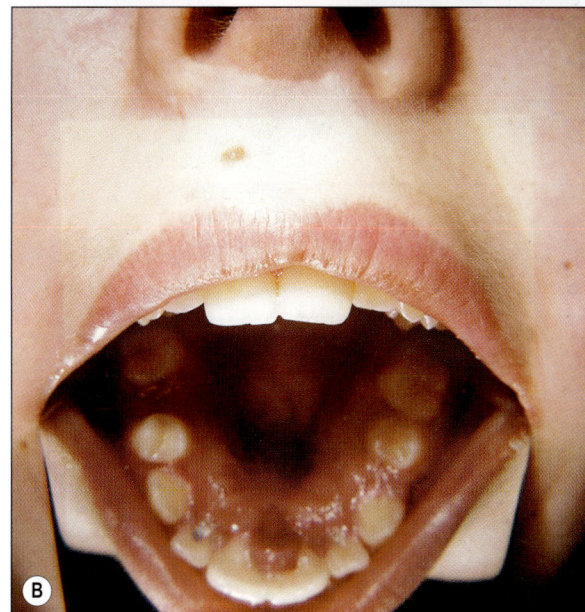

Fig. 4.4 (A) An upper removable orthodontic appliance in place in the mouth. (B) Severe gingival inflammation and enlargement palatally to the teeth covered by the appliance.

inflammation and may provide a case for orthodontic treatment (**Fig. 4.5**). However, it is important to be certain that orthodontic movement is justified. If a patient's oral hygiene is poor it may be just as bad if the teeth are straight. On the other hand, if a patient's oral hygiene overcomes the difficulties caused by malalignment no orthodontic treatment is required, at least on periodontal grounds. Orthodontic treatment is indicated where the patient's home care is effective in all areas except where there is malalignment. It is then likely that creating a good alignment will also be followed by gingival health.

Other discrepancies in tooth and jaw relationship may also produce gingival inflammation. In a very deep overbite upper incisors may impinge on lower labial gingiva or lower incisors on upper palatal gingiva, causing inflammation and tissue destruction in the presence of plaque.

Failure to replace a missing tooth may result in plaque and calculus accumulations on the non-functional opposing teeth.

Lack of lip-seal

There is some uncertainty about the influence of lip-posture on gingival health but a commonly occurring clinical phenomenon is a hyperplastic gingivitis in anterior segments (**Fig. 4.6**), usually the upper incisor regions, where there is lack of lip-seal. Indeed, in many cases the area of hyperplasia is clearly delineated by the lip-line. Although lack of lip-seal is frequently associated with mouth-breathing (**Fig. 4.7**), inadequate lip-seal may be present, even when the patient breathes through the nose. With the lips apart the gingivae in the front of the mouth are not bathed in saliva. This seems to have two effects: (1) the normal cleansing action of saliva is diminished so that plaque accumulation is encouraged; (2) dehydration of the tissues may impair their resistance.

Developmental grooves

Grooves on the root surface or the cervical crown lead to plaque accumulation and are impossible to clean. This may result in local areas of gingivitis and pocketing, most commonly seen palatal to the upper incisors (**Fig. 4.8**). The canine fossa on the mesial surface of the upper first premolar may also act in this way.

Tobacco smoking

The most obvious effect of tobacco smoking is tooth staining, but a large number of studies have shown that tobacco smoking has an influence on the prevalence and severity of periodontal diseases (Heitz-Mayfield 2005). The effect of smoking on plaque and calculus deposition, gingival inflammation and bleeding, pocket depth and bone loss, as well as the bacteriology of plaque and features of the tissue response, have been investigated.

Pindborg (1947) found that smokers had more calculus than non-smokers, and this was confirmed by many other studies such as those by Ainamo (1971) and Sheiham (1971), who also found that plaque deposits were greater in smokers. These early studies showed that the standard of oral hygiene in smokers was significantly poorer than in non-smokers, and Macgregor (1984, 1985) found that smokers spend less time brushing their teeth than non-smokers.

Young smokers appear to have the same degree of, or slightly more gingival inflammation than non-smokers, but in older age groups signs of

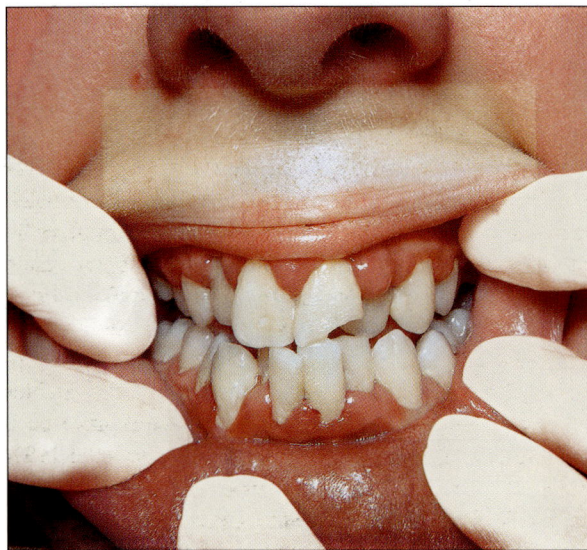

Fig. 4.5 Severe gingival inflammation and false pocketing associated with poor oral hygiene complicated by severe anterior tooth crowding.

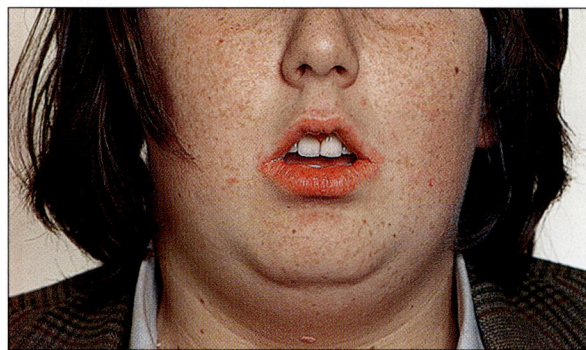

Fig. 4.7 Lack of lip-seal in a 12-year-old girl.

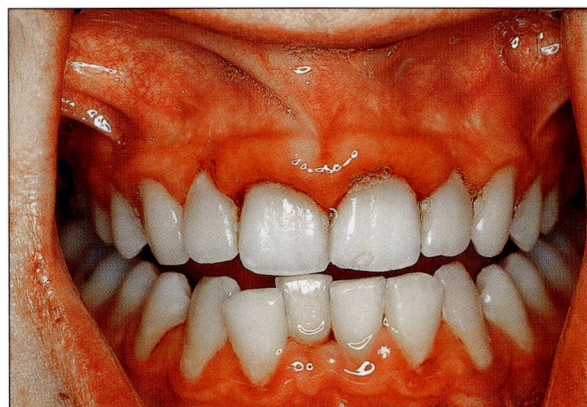

Fig. 4.6 Gingival oedematous enlargement associated with plaque deposits and lack of lip seal.

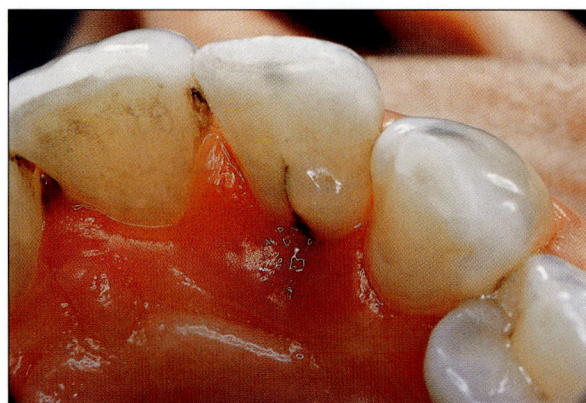

Fig. 4.8 Localized gingival inflammation and pocketing palatal to an upper left central in relation to a palatal groove which extends on to the coronal part of the root.

inflammation are less in smokers. Bergström and Floderus-Myrhed (1983) and other workers have found less gingival bleeding in smokers than non-smokers, a finding which Palmer (1987) suggests could be due to vaso-constriction of gingival vessels, but may also be attributable to the heavier keratinization of the gingivae in smokers. The gingivae of smokers contain an increased number of keratinized cells (Calonius 1962).

Pocket depth (Feldman et al 1983; Stoltenberg et al 1993) and alveolar bone loss (Arno et al 1959; Bergström et al 1991) have been found to be greater in smokers than non-smokers. A study of 70-year-old Swedes also demonstrated that toothlessness was higher in smokers and former smokers than in non-smokers (Österberg & Mellstrom 1986). Furthermore, the occurrence of refractory periodontitis, i.e. where there has been persistent failure of periodontal treatment, is found more commonly in smokers than in non-smokers (MacFarlane et al 1992).

The relationship between smoking and poor oral hygiene and its consequences is well established, but where smokers and non-smokers with comparable levels of oral hygiene are studied it is found that smoking per se has an additional significant association with periodontal disease severity. Ismail et al (1983) looked at data from epidemiological studies of 3000 individuals in the USA, adjusting the data for age, sex, race, socio-economic status, oral hygiene and frequency of toothbrushing, and found that smokers had a higher Periodontal Index score in all age groups than non-smokers. Bergström et al (1991) examined alveolar bone loss in 210 subjects aged 24–60 years, smokers, former smokers and non-smokers, and found a correlation between bone loss and smoking which was not plaque related.

Thomson et al (2007) sought to quantify the association between cigarette smoking patterns and periodontal attachment loss by age 32. Periodontal examinations were conducted at ages 26 and 32 in a long-standing prospective study of a birth cohort born in Dunedin (New Zealand) in 1972/1973. Longitudinal categorization of smoking exposure was undertaken using data collected at ages 15, 18, 21, 26 and 32. Compared with never-smokers, long-term smokers (and other age-32 smokers) had very high odds ratios for having one or more sites with at least 5 mm AL, and were more likely to be incident cases after age 26. Two-thirds of new cases after age 26 were attributable to smoking. There were no significant differences in periodontal health between never-smokers and those who had quit smoking after age 26. Thus current and long-term smoking in young adults is detrimental to periodontal health, but smoking cessation may be associated with a relatively rapid improvement in periodontitis.

Several investigations have been made into the nature of this direct effect, possibly changes in plaque and pocket flora, and various components of the tissue reaction. Bacteriological studies (Bastiaan & Waite 1978; Bardell 1981) have produced rather unclear results about differences in the make-up of plaque flora or in the rate of plaque formation in smokers and non-smokers. However, several changes in the tissue response have been noted.

Smoking appears to produce vasoconstriction of the gingival vasculature and as, Palmer (1987) points out, 'reduction in the vascular component of the inflammatory response may reduce the availability of serum-derived protective factors such as antibodies and a decrease in the passage of leucocytes into the periodontal tissues'. McLaughlin et al (1993) found that smoking produces a marked but transient increase in gingival fluid flow rate, which they felt might reflect changes in blood flow known to be produced by nicotine. Armitage and Turner (1970) showed that nicotine from cigarettes and cigars could pass through the oral mucosa and also, in the study of the toxicity of nicotine from cigarettes, they showed a 50% or more inhibition of function of oral neutrophils (Armitage et al 1975). In an earlier study, Eichel and Shahrick (1969) reported that tobacco smoke produced 50–100% inhibition of oral leucocytes due to loss of motility, which they ascribed to such substances as acrolein and cyanide in tobacco smoke.

Oral keratinocytes are the first cells to come into contact with tobacco products from smoking. A more recent study by Johnson and Organ (1997) investigated the effects of nicotine on human gingival keratinocytes (obtained from healthy gingival tissue) in culture in respect of their release of inflammatory mediators. They found that exposure to nicotine did not alter the production of prostaglandin E_2; it did, however, produce an increase in the level of interleukin (IL)-1α both in the supernatant and lysed cells. This may have significance, since IL-1α is known to play a central role in the regulation of inflammation.

In a study of refractory periodontitis by MacFarlane et al (1992), abnormal PMNs phagocytosis was found. Both the motility and chemotactic ability of PMNs can be impaired by even small amounts of tobacco smoke (Bridges et al 1977). Peacock et al (1993) have shown that, in tissue culture of human gingival fibroblasts, continuous nicotine exposure enhances attachment of fibroblasts, and at low concentrations of nicotine cell replication is stimulated

The role of smoking in the aetiology of acute ulcerative gingivitis has been much speculated upon. When this form of periodontal disease was very common many studies found a relationship between the prevalence and severity of ANUG (or ANUG, Vincent's disease, trench mouth, etc., see Ch. 25) and smoking. Stammers (1944) examined 1017 cases of ANUG and found that almost all of them were smokers, and in looking at 3880 naval recruits aged 17–21 years, Massler and Ludwick (1952) found 20 cases of ANUG, 19 of them smokers, a finding more recently confirmed in an Edinburgh study in which Kowolik and Nisbet (1983) found that 98 out of 100 individuals with ANUG were smokers. No mechanism has so far been defined to explain this relationship, but there is little doubt that smoking has multiple deleterious effects on the tissues, on vascularity and on the immune system.

A large amount of research indicates that tobacco use is directly related to the prevalence and incidence of a whole variety of medical problems including lung and possibly other cancers, pulmonary, cardiovascular and gastrointestinal disease and low birth weight (Bartecchi et al 1994). Over the last 50 years evidence has accumulated that smoking is also related to the prevalence and severity of periodontal diseases (Haber et al 1993; Ryder 1996) and subsequent tooth loss (Mohlin et al 1979; Alvesalo et al 1982; Österberg & Mellstrom 1986; Ahlquist et al 1989; Holm 1994; Ragnarsson et al 1992; Ryder 1996). Furthermore, recent studies have shown that smoking may still be a significant risk factor in the development and progression of periodontal disease when the other risk variables such as oral health behaviour and sociodemographic factors have been accounted for (Ahlberg et al 1996; Beck et al 1990; Croucher et al 1997; Dolan et al 1997; Grossi et al 1994, 1995; Horning et al 1992; Locker & Leake 1993; Norderyd & Hugoson 1998; Stoltenberg et al 1993).

In Europe and the USA more than one-quarter of the adult population smoke and in many other countries the proportions are even higher (Centers for Disease Control and Prevention 1993; Council on Scientific Affairs 1990; Bartecchi et al 1994; MacKenzie et al 1994). Thus, the association between cigarette smoking and periodontal disease represents a significant problem. Although the percentage of male adults who smoke appears to be gradually declining in developed countries the percentage of females is increasing (Bartecchi et al 1994; MacKenzie et al 1994). Furthermore, the use of tobacco products by young people appears to be increasing again (Centers for Disease Control 1989).

The relationship between tobacco products and periodontal diseases can be considered in six areas:

- Its effect on the prevalence and severity of periodontal diseases
- Its possible association with refractory periodontitis
- The role of smokeless tobacco products on the periodontal tissues
- The possible mechanisms of its effects on the periodontal tissues
- Its effects on the response to periodontal treatment
- Smoking cessation in periodontal disease prevention.

Those sections dealing with its response to treatment will also be covered in Chapters 15, 19, 20 and 21.

Its effect on the prevalence and severity of periodontal diseases

Acute necrotizing ulcerative gingivitis (ANUG)

A clear association between smoking and ANUG (see also Ch. 25) was demonstrated over 50 years ago (Stammers 1944; Pindborg 1947, 1949). Stammers (1944) examined 1017 cases of ANUG and found that nearly all of them were smokers. More recently, in a study in Edinburgh, Kowolik and Nisbet (1983) found that 98 out of 100 individuals with ANUG were smokers. This evidence has been reviewed by Macgregor (1992). More recently, a similar association has been found between smoking and the ANUG-like lesions of HIV infected individuals (Swango et al 1991).

Chronic gingivitis and periodontitis

Earlier cross-sectional studies of the relationship between smoking and the severity of periodontal disease were contradictory and inconclusive (Massler & Ludwick 1952; Arno et al 1958; Schei et al 1959; Solomon et al 1968; Sheiham 1971; Preber et al 1980; Bergström 1981; Preber & Kant 1973; Bergström and Floderus-Myrhed 1983; Macgregor et al 1985; Preber and Bergström 1986a). Some investigators reported less gingival inflammation and particularly less gingival bleeding in smokers compared with non-smokers (Massler & Ludwick 1952; Bergström and Floderus-Myrhed 1983; Preber & Bergström 1985; Bergström 1990) whilst other studies (Arno et al 1958; Preber & Kant 1973; Preber et al 1980) showed more gingival inflammation in smokers. There were also reports of an increase (Sheiham 1971; Preber & Kant 1973; Preber et al 1980; Bergström 1981; Bergström and Floderus-Myrhed 1983) or no difference (Macgregor et al 1985; Bergström & Preber 1986; Bergström 1990) in the amounts of plaque in smokers compared to non-smokers. Gingival crevicular fluid (GCF) flow was reported to increase immediately following smoking (McLaughlin et al 1993). However, it was found to be diminished in chronic smokers (Bergström & Preber 1986).

A clear correlation between probing depths and alveolar bone loss was reported by most earlier researchers (Arno et al 1959; Schei et al 1959; Solomon et al 1968; Summers & Oberman 1968; Ismail et al 1983; Bergström and Floderus-Myrhed 1983) but some others (Sheiham 1971; Preber & Kant 1973) reported no clear relationship. Some workers (Schei et al 1959; Sheiham 1971; Preber et al 1980; Ismail et al 1983) have suggested that the differences in attachment loss between smokers and non-smokers may be due to poor oral hygiene in smokers.

However, over the last 10–12 years, cross-sectional studies on much larger groups of subjects have demonstrated a much clearer relationship between smoking and periodontal disease (Ryder 1996; Molloy et al 2004). In a number of these studies the plaque accumulation levels were either balanced between the groups of smokers and non-smokers (Bergström & Elíasson 1987a, 1987b; Bergström 1989; Linden & Mullally 1994) or plaque levels were minimal in both groups (Grossi et al 1994, 1995). In both of these situations, the smoking group was found to have deeper periodontal pockets and greater probing attachment loss (Bergström & Elíasson 1987a; Bergström 1989; Linden & Mullally 1994; Grossi et al 1994; Martinez-Canut et al 1995) and/or alveolar bone loss (Bergström & Elíasson 1987a; Grossi et al 1995) than the non-smoking group. Similar findings have also been reported from other large cross-sectional studies (Feldman et al 1983; Anerud et al 1991).

The strength of the association in both case-control and prospective studies can be measured by the relative risk, which is often expressed as the odds ratio. In this process the various risk factors are assigned as categories and these are then statistically correlated with each other to produce relative risk odds. The numerous cross-sectional studies which have reported

odds ratios (Ismail et al 1983; Haber & Kent 1992; Jette et al 1993; Grossi et al 1994, 1995) have generally reported odds ratios between 2 and 6. In one of these studies (Haber & Kent 1992), current and former smokers were found to be more prevalent in a population of patients from American periodontal practices with moderate to advanced periodontitis when compared to the referring general practice or the general population.

More recently, several longitudinal studies of the relationship between smoking and periodontal disease have been reported (Bolin et al 1986; Bergström and Preber 1994; Beck et al 1997; Machtei et al 1997; Bergström et al 2000). In a 10-year longitudinal radiographical study of alveolar bone loss which began in 1970, it was shown that in those subjects which had a least 20 teeth at the start of the study, smoking was a significant predictor of future bone loss (Bolin 1986). In a 5-year study of attachment loss in 800 community dwelling adults, smokers were found to be an increased risk for attachment loss (Beck et al 1997). A further longitudinal study (Machtei et al 1997), in which a wide range of clinical, microbiological and immunological indicators were correlated with disease progression, reported that over the 1 year period of the investigation, smokers exhibited greater attachment and bone loss in comparison to non-smokers. Smokers were shown to be at significantly greater risk for further attachment loss when compared with non-smokers with an odds ratio of 5.4. Similar findings were found in a 10-year prospective study (Bergström et al 2000).

Paulande et al (2004) carried out a 10-year prospective study of 50-year-old individuals to compare the incidence of periodontal bone loss with potential risk factors. The subject sample was generated from an epidemiological survey performed in 1988 of subjects living in a district of Sweden. A randomized sample of 15% of the 50-year-old inhabitants in the county was drawn. At the 10-year follow-up in 1998, 320 (75%) of the 449 individuals examined at baseline were available for re-examination. Full-mouth clinical and radiographic examinations and questionnaire surveys were performed in 1988 and 1998. A total of 295 individuals (69%) had complete data for inclusion in the analysis of radiographic bone changes over 10 years. Non-parametric tests, correlations and stepwise multiple regression models were used for statistical analysis of the data. The mean alveolar bone level in 1988 was 2.2 mm and a further 0.4 mm was lost over the 10 years. Of the subject sample, 8% showed no loss, while 5% experienced a mean bone loss of more than 1 mm. Smoking was found to be the strongest individual risk predictor. When only those individuals who had continued with the habit during the entire 10-year follow-up period were included, the relative risk was increased but this was not the case for subjects who had quit smoking before the baseline examination. Stepwise multiple regression analysis revealed that smoking, percentage of approximal sites with probing pocket depth >4 mm, the number of teeth and systemic disease were significant explanatory factors for 10-year bone loss. For non-smokers, statistically significant predictors were number of teeth, mean alveolar bone loss, percentage of periodontally healthy approximal sites and educational level. It is possible that the inclusion of smokers in risk analysis for periodontal diseases may obstruct the detection of other risk factors.

The dose response

A relationship has also been found between the prevalence of moderate to advanced periodontitis and the number of cigarettes smoked per day (Brandtzaeg & Jamison 1964; Ismail et al 1983; Haber & Kent 1992; Haber et al 1993; Grossi et al 1994, 1995) and the number of years that the patients had smoked (Haber & Kent 1992; Martinez-Canut et al 1995; Jette et al 1993; Grossi et al 1994, 1995). The term 'pack years' (packs of cigarettes smoked per day multiplied by the number of years the subject has smoked for) is currently used to quantify this effect. One of the large studies (Grossi et al 1995) which investigated bone loss in 1361 subjects between 25 and 75, years reported odds ratios for heavy smokers of 7.28 and light smokers of 3.25. Another study (Alpagot et al 1996) reported that probing depth was significantly correlated with pack years. Furthermore, years of exposure to tobacco products have been shown to be a significant risk factor for periodontal disease in 1156 community dwelling New England elders, regardless of other social and behavioural factors (Jette et al 1993).

A Spanish study of 889 subjects (Martinez-Canut et al 1995) reported that gingival recession, probing depth and probing attachment level were significantly related to smoking status and that the attachment levels were proportionate to the cigarettes smoked per day. They found that smoking one cigarette per day, up to 10 and up to 20 increased probing attachment level by 0.5%, 5% and 10%, respectively. However, these effects were only statistically significant in the latter group and this led them to conclude that tobacco usage increases disease severity, and this effect is clinically evident above a certain level of usage.

The suggestion of greater periodontal destruction above a certain level of smoking was also made in an earlier study (Wouters et al 1993). Expressed as a percentage of tooth root length in 723 dentate adults, alveolar bone loss was shown to be significantly lower in individuals smoking more than 5 g of tobacco per day compared with subjects smoking less. Norderyd and Hugoson (1998) also found that moderate to heavy smokers (more than 10 packs per day) were associated with severe periodontitis whereas light smokers were not.

The strong association between smoking and periodontal disease severity is consistent with the hypothesis that smoking has cumulative detrimental effects (Horning et al 1992). Furthermore, the evidence above suggests that the more the patient smokes the greater the degree of periodontal disease and that this effect may worsen above a certain threshold.

However, it should be remembered that all retrospective studies have determined smoking status by interview or questionnaire and are subject to recall bias. Also some studies which have quantified lifetime exposure by pack years and current levels of smoking may not reflect past exposure. One way to overcome these problems is to measure smoking levels by serum cotinine levels and two recent studies have used this method. Cotinine is the principle metabolite of nicotine and as such provides a valuable quantitative measure of smoking status. Gonzalez et al (1996) showed that the severity of periodontal destruction, measured either by probing attachment level or radiographical crestal bone height, statistically positively correlated with serum cotinine levels and Machtei et al (1997) showed that patient cotinine levels correlated with outcomes of progressive periodontal breakdown.

Effects of cessation of smoking

There is good evidence that the severity of periodontal disease is less in former smokers than those who continue to smoke. Haber and Kent (1992) after controlling for age and sex, compared the odds ratio for the presence of moderate to advanced periodontitis in smokers, non-smokers and former smokers and found a ratio of 3.3 comparing smokers and non-smokers and one of 2.1 comparing former smokers with non-smokers. Thus there appears to be considerable benefit in stopping smoking both as regards its effects on periodontal disease and on the more serious associated medical conditions. Furthermore, a longitudinal study (Bolin et al 1993) found that the progression of bone loss was significantly retarded in those who gave up smoking during the study as compared with those who continued to smoke. Also prospective observations on tooth loss in 248 women and 977 men, with a mean follow up time of 6 years, indicated that individuals who continued to smoke cigarettes had a 2.4–3.5 risk of tooth loss compared with non-smokers (Krall et al 1997). The rates of tooth loss were significantly reduced in men after they quit smoking but remained higher than those for non-smokers. They concluded that stopping smoking significantly benefits an individual's likelihood of tooth retention, but it may take decades for the individual to return to the rate of tooth loss observed in non-smokers.

From all these more recent studies, a general pattern of effects has emerged with smokers having:

- Greater alveolar bone loss
- Increased numbers of deep pockets
- Increased rate of disease progression
- Increased calculus formation
- Less clinically apparent gingival inflammation
- Less gingival bleeding than non-smokers.

Possible association with refractory periodontitis

Tobacco smoking may play a significant role in the development of refractory periodontitis (Adams 1992; MacFarlane et al 1992) and this is shown by the fact that an unusually high percentage of refractory periodontitis patients have been found to be smokers (MacFarlane et al 1992).

The role of smokeless tobacco products on the periodontal tissues

The use of tobacco products such as snuff and chewing tobacco are popular in many countries in Asia and may often be combined with other products such as Betel nut. The relationship between these products and oral leukoplakia and carcinoma is well known and documented (Ernster et al 1990; Creath et al 1991; Wray & McGuirt 1993) and these lesions are commonly found in areas of the mouth where the tobacco product is placed. Their use has also been related to cardiovascular mortality (Bolinger et al 1994).

Although individual cases of ANUG, chronic periodontitis and gingival recession have been reported in smokeless tobacco users (Hoge & Kirkham 1983; Offenbacher & Weathers 1985; Christen et al 1979), a clear relationship to chronic periodontitis has not been demonstrated. In one study of large numbers of smokeless tobacco users (Robertson et al 1990) there was a significant increase in localized gingival recession and attachment loss, and this was found in buccal areas, adjacent to where the product was placed.

Some investigators have proposed that local exposure to high concentrations of tobacco products may play a role in local attachment loss and this could be due to their effects on local defence mechanisms (Robertson et al 1990; Ernster et al 1990; Payne et al 1994). In addition, the high concentrations of nicotine from these products could alter the local gingival blood flow (Johnson et al 1991). Finally, it has been shown that smokeless tobacco extracts affect the secretion of monocyte inflammatory mediators (Payne et al 1994).

The possible mechanisms of its effects on the periodontal tissues

Tobacco smoking has widespread systemic effects, many of which may provide mechanisms for the increased susceptibility to periodontitis and the poorer response to treatment (Palmer et al 2005) and some of these are outlined below.

Microbiology

Several investigations have been made into possible changes in plaque and pocket flora produced by smoking. However, some bacteriological studies (Bastiaan & Waite 1978; Bardell 1981) produced rather unclear results. One possible hypothesis for these effects is that smoking produces effects on plaque growth and maturation leading either to more plaque or to the presence of different or more virulent bacteria. In this regard, the earlier studies (Pindborg 1947, 1949; Ainamo 1971; Sheiham 1971) found that plaque deposits were greater in smokers than non-smokers and that their standard of oral hygiene was significantly poorer. In addition, Macgregor (1984, 1985) found that smokers spend less time brushing their teeth than non-smokers. However, later studies (Bastiaan & Waite 1978; Bergström 1989; Bergström & Elíasson 1987a; Feldman et al 1983; Bergström et al 1991) have shown little difference in the levels of plaque accumulation in smokers compared to non-smokers. This may reflect better standards of oral hygiene in the population as a whole in more recent times. Furthermore, in respect of the possible role of smoking alone, cross-sectional studies, where plaque levels were controlled to a minimum in both the smoking and non-smoking groups studied, showed that alveolar bone loss was greater in the smoking group (Bergström 1989; Bergström & Elíasson 1987a; Bergström et al 1991). Similar results were found in a retrospective study (Ismail et al 1983). They looked at data from epidemiological studies of 3000 individuals in the USA, adjusting the data for age, sex and socioeconomic status and oral hygiene and frequency of toothbrushing. They found that smokers had a higher periodontal index score in all age groups and found evidence for a direct correlation between smoking and the periodontal index score. Thus, the amount of plaque present does not seem to be responsible for the differences.

On the other hand, several studies have shown that greater accumulations of supra- and subgingival calculus appear to form in smokers compared with non-smokers (Pindborg 1947, 1949; Ainamo 1971; Feldman et al 1987; Linden & Mullally 1994). Subgingival calculus might act as a tissue irritant as a result of substances absorbed into its surface or might create a local environment which promotes the growth of pathogenic bacteria. In this regard, it has been shown that the periodontal pockets of smokers are more anaerobic than those of non-smokers (Kenny et al 1975). This profound anaerobic environment could promote the growth of periodontopathic Gram-negative anaerobic species. However, neither earlier (Kenny et al 1975; Bardell 1981) nor later studies (Preber et al 1992; Stoltenberg et al 1993) have supported this view. Cultural and microscopic studies (Kenny et al 1975) showed no differences in the bacterial composition of subgingival plaque between smokers and non-smokers. Furthermore, more recent studies (Preber et al 1992; Stoltenberg et al 1993) showed no significant differences in the recovery of *P. gingivalis*, *Prevotella intermedia*, *B. forsythus* and *A. actinomycetemcomitans* from deep pockets in the two groups. There are, however, two recent studies which suggest that smokers may have higher numbers of *B. forsythus* (Zambon et al 1996) and *T. denticola* (Umeda et al 1998) in their subgingival flora. Apart from these two reports, to date, there is no evidence to support the view that smoking adversely affects the periodontal tissues by altering the composition of plaque.

However, microorganisms and smoke products could act synergistically to produce adverse effects on the periodontal tissues. In this regard, Andreou et al (2004) have shown that smoke-derived aryl hydrocarbons and bacterial LPS may act additively to inhibit bone formation which may in part explain why periodontal bone loss is greater and bone healing is less successful in smokers than non-smokers with periodontal infections.

Effect of smoking on the periodontal tissues

It has been known for some time that both tobacco smoke and tobacco components may reduce gingival blood flow and gingival bleeding (Bergström & Floderus-Myrhed 1983). This could either be due to vasoconstriction of gingival vessels or to the heavier keratinization of the gingiva in smokers and in this last regard, the gingiva of smokers has been shown to contain an increased number of keratinized cells (Calonius 1962). Earlier studies of the effects of nicotine on gingival blood flow using a heat diffusion technique showed a decrease in flow (Clark et al 1981). However, more recent studies in the effects of cigarette smoking on gingival blood flow using laser Doppler probes has yielded contradictory results (Baab &

Oberg 1987). Inconclusive results have also been obtained in studies of possible thermal damage by cigarette smoke (Bastiaan 1979).

Smoking appears to first produce a nicotine-related transient initial increase in gingival fluid flow rate (McLaughlin et al 1993) and then a prolonged vasoconstriction of the gingival vasculature (Clarke et al 1981). This in turn tends to reduce the clinical signs of gingivitis. This effect seems to be a direct effect of absorbed nicotine on the vessels since studies which have compared the clinical response in smokers and non-smokers with identical plaque levels showed that the gingival index and gingival bleeding were significantly lower in smokers (Bergström 1990). Similar findings were seen in experimental gingivitis studies comparing smokers and non-smokers (Danielsen et al 1990).

Imirzalio et al (2005) shown that smoking may reduce the apoptotic mechanism in the oral cavity resulting in epithelial cell hyperplasia and a significant increase in thickness of the overlying orthokeratin layer.

Smokers have also been shown to have a lower level of crevicular fluid than non-smokers with either an identical healthy clinical status (Holmes 1990) or a similar diseased clinical status (Kinane & Radvar 1997) and this also appears to be related to nicotine-related vasoconstriction. With respect to these vascular changes it has been shown that nicotine from cigarettes and cigars can pass through the oral mucosa to directly affect the vasculature (Armitage & Turner 1970). The reduction in the vascular component of the inflammatory response may reduce the availability of serum-derived protective factors such as antibodies and a decrease in the passage of leucocytes into the periodontal tissues (Palmer 1987).

Effect of smoking on the local and general host response

A number of investigators have examined the role of smoking in altering the host response by:

- Impairing the response of the host against infection (Seymour 1991)
- Changing the response so that it was more destructive to the tissues (Lamster 1992).

Effects on polymorphonuclear leucocyte function

Fully functional phagocytes are key components of the defence system against infections and it has been shown that smoking can have deleterious effects on various neutrophil functions (Eichel & Shahrick 1969; Armitage et al 1975; Bridges et al 1977; Kenny et al 1977; Kraal et al 1977; Codd et al 1987; Nowak et al 1990; Kalra et al 1991; Lannan et al 1992; Selby et al 1992; Ryder et al 1994; Totti et al 1994). In this regard, it has been shown that tobacco smoke can impair the motility and chemotaxis of oral (Eichel & Shahrick 1969; Kenny et al 1977) and peripheral (Bridges et al 1977; Lannan et al 1992; Selby et al 1992) neutrophil polymorphonuclear leucocytes (PMNs). Impaired phagocytosis has also been shown in PMNs from patients with refractory periodontitis, a majority of whom are smokers (MacFarlane et al 1992). In addition, smoking has been shown to impair the oxidative burst of PMNs (Kalra et al 1991).

Eichel and Shahrick (1969) ascribed the smoking effects on oral leucocytes to acrolein and cyanide in tobacco smoke. However, the most researched tobacco component is undoubtedly nicotine. Armitage and Turner (1970) showed that nicotine from cigarettes and cigars could pass through the oral mucosa into the connective tissue. At low concentrations nicotine appears to stimulate PMN chemotaxis (Totti et al 1994) but at higher concentrations it impairs motility, chemotaxis and phagocytosis of PMNs (Armitage et al 1975; Ryder 1994). However, nicotine is only one of over 2000 potentially toxic substances in tobacco smoke (International Agency for Research on Cancer 1986) and many of these could have harmful effects on the periodontal tissues.

Güntsch et al (2006) compared the level of crevicular PMN function in 60 periodontally healthy smokers and non-smokers and found that cigarette smoking adversely affected PMN viability and function.

Alvi et al (1995) showed that tooth site GCF elastase concentrations were lower in smokers than non-smokers and the reasons for this are not clear. Elastase is produced locally by PMNs and is not found in normal serum. Therefore vasoconstriction would not account for this effect. It may be that the PMNs are less functional or are present in reduced numbers in the gingival crevices of smokers (Wolff et al 1994).

Effects on adhesion molecules

To mount a successful response to bacteria, inflammatory and immune cells must arrive at the inflammatory site in appropriate numbers and this depends on appropriate signalling and the presence of appropriate adhesion molecules at their site of entry. Nicotine increases the expression of intracellular adhesion molecule (ICAM) -1 and endothelial leucocyte adhesion molecule (ELAM)-1 on human umbilical cord vein cells (endothelial cells) and also appears to increase the amount of soluble ICAM-1 in the serum of smokers (Koundouros et al 1996). These adhesion molecule changes may affect leucocyte binding to endothelial cells lining the capillaries and post-capillary venules and, thus may impede the recruitment of defence cells to the area of microbial challenge.

Effects on cytokines

A number of recent reports have suggested that cytokine levels may be influenced by smoking. Tappia et al (1995) have shown that the plasma response of smokers following lipopolysaccharide stimulation differed from that of non-smokers in that smokers had significantly more tumour necrosis factor alpha (TNF-α), interleukin (IL) -6 and the acute phase protein, α2-macrogobulin. Boström et al (1998a,b) have also reported that the GCF levels of TNF-α were significantly higher in both untreated and treated smoking chronic periodontitis patients in comparison with corresponding non-smoking patients. In addition, Kuschner et al (1996) have reported a dose-dependent effect of smoking on IL-1, IL-6, IL-8 and monocyte chemotactic protein (MCP)-1 levels. All this research suggests that smoking is associated with the local production of greater quantities of pro-inflammatory cytokines and acute phase proteins which could in turn lead to more severe destructive inflammation in the periodontal tissues.

Oral keratinocytes are the first cells to come into contact with tobacco products from smoking. A recent study (Johnson & Organ 1997) investigated the effects of nicotine on human gingival keratinocytes, obtained from healthy gingival tissue, in culture in respect of their release of inflammatory mediators. They found that exposure to nicotine did not alter the production of prostaglandin E$_2$. However, it did produce an increase in the level of IL-1α both in the supernatant and lysed cells. This may have significance since IL-1α is known to play a central role in the regulation of inflammation and this could contribute to the effects reported in the previous paragraph.

In contrast to these studies, one investigation using nicotine levels within the normal plasma range suggested that nicotine exerts a negative immunoregulatory effect through modulation of cytokine production by mononuclear cells in particular IL-2, TNF-α. Another study (Bernzweig et al 1998) found that exposure of gingival mononuclear cells to nicotine decreased IL-1β. However, this study used 75 times the salivary nicotine concentration of smokers in this study so its relevance must be questioned.

Effects on immune response

Smoking also appears to reduce immunoglobulin production (Holt 1987; Johnson et al 1990). Macrophages play a key role as antigen presenting cells in both cell-mediated and humoral immunity utilizing the class II major histocompatibility complex (MHC) (Ch. 3). In this regard, it has been shown that alveolar macrophages from smokers have reduced expression of class II MHC (Pankow et al 1991; Mancini et al 1993). This may lead to a reduction of both the humoral and cell mediated responses to invading microbes.

Smoking has been shown to reduce the serum concentration of IgG (Ferson et al 1979; Gulsvik & Fagerhol 1979; Andersen et al 1982; Hersey et al 1983; Robertson et al 1984; McSharry et al 1985). Smokers have been also found to have decreased levels of salivary IgA antibodies (Bennet & Read 1982). Furthermore, smokers appear to have depressed numbers of T-helper lymphocytes which are key components of the immune system (Costabel et al 1986; Ginns et al 1982).

Gunsolley et al (1997) have shown that smoking may modify the concentrations of some IgG subclasses in some racial groups and blacks with adult periodontitis who smoked had lower IgG1, while those with early onset periodontitis had lower IgG2. In this latter regard, Quinn et al (1996) has also shown that smoking reduces the levels of IgG2 in early onset periodontitis cases. This may be significant since this class of antibody is associated with the response to carbohydrate haptens commonly found on oral pathogens (Ling et al 1993).

A clear picture of these changes in response has not yet appeared, however it is clear that smoking can alter both the extent and type of immune reaction. Interestingly, serum conversion following hepatitis B vaccine occurs more slowly in smokers than non-smokers, and the frequency of subjects achieving a successful response is lower for smokers (Struve et al 1992; Roome et al 1993).

In relation to putative periodontal pathogens it has been found that smokers have reduced titres of serum IgG antibodies to *P. intermedia* and *F. nucleatum* compared to non-smokers (Haber 1994). In early onset periodontitis patients, it has also been found that the level of IgG2 antibodies to *A. actinomycetemcomitans* is lower in smokers than non-smokers (Tangada et al 1997).

Graswinckel et al (2004) investigated the plasma levels of immunoglobulin (Ig) G, A and M antibodies in periodontitis patients in relation to disease severity, smoking, the presence and prevalence of periodontopathogens. A total of 29 patients with severe periodontitis, 51 with moderate periodontitis and 55 controls without periodontal destruction were enrolled; 18 were diagnosed with aggressive periodontitis and 62 with chronic periodontitis. Total IgG, IgA and IgM as well as IgG isotypes were analysed in plasma samples. Levels of total IgG, IgA and IgM did not differ between patients and controls but in periodontitis, higher levels of IgG1 and IgG2 were found. Smoking appeared to be significantly and inversely related to antibody levels in periodontitis, in particular for total IgG and IgG2. The absence of an elevated total IgG and IgG2 in smoking patients was irrespective of severity, prevalence of periodontal pathogens and diagnosis. The elevation of total IgG and IgG1 and IgG2 in non-smoker periodontitis patients was observed in patients with moderate periodontitis and to a greater extent in patients with severe periodontitis, but was independent whether patients were infected with *A. actinomycetemcomitans* or *Porphyromonas gingivalis* and independent of disease type. These findings on antibody levels may be one of several mechanisms related to the effect of smoking on the severity of periodontitis.

Effects on healing

A relationship between smoking and bone mineral content, particularly osteoporosis, has also been found (Daniell 1983; Hollenbach et al 1993). However, the possible effects of this finding on the alveolar bone is unclear.

It has been shown that low doses of nicotine can be stored in and released by periodontal fibroblasts (Hanes et al 1991) but it is not clear as to whether fibroblasts exposed to nicotine have impaired (Raulin et al 1988) or enhanced (Peacock et al 1993) function. Peacock et al (1993) have shown that in tissue cultures of human gingival fibroblasts continuous nicotine exposure enhances attachment of the fibroblasts, and at low concentrations of nicotine cell replication is stimulated. Conversely, Raulin et al (1988) showed that exposure of human fibroblasts to levels of nicotine similar to those found in the serum of smokers reduced their attachment to glass and root surfaces *in vitro*. Nicotine has also been shown to suppress the proliferation of cultured osteoblasts but to stimulate their production of alkaline phosphatase (Fang et al 1991). However, all these changes have been demonstrated *in vitro* and therefore their effects on the cells of the normal periodontium can only be surmised.

Thus, tobacco smoke may induce or exacerbate periodontal disease by direct local damage, by altering the host response or by altering the normal repair mechanisms of the periodontal tissues.

Effects on the response to periodontal treatment

It is known that smoking has a very significant adverse effect on the response to all forms of periodontal treatment (Preber and Bergström 1986b, 1990; Miller 1987; Goultschin et al 1990; Jones & Triplett 1992; Ah et al 1994; Newman et al 1994) and this will be fully described in Chs 15, 19, 20, 25.

Smoking cessation in periodontal disease prevention

Informing patients about the dangers of smoking and encouraging them to stop smoking is an important function in preventing periodontal disease initiation and progression (Bolin et al 1993; Telivuo et al 1992) and this will be described in Chapter 11.

Alcohol consumption

Tezal et al (2004) carried out a cross-sectional study of 13 198 subjects in the Third National Health and Nutrition Examination Survey (NHANES III) aged 20 and older into the relationship between alcohol consumption and periodontitis severity. Alcohol intake was represented both as a continuous variable and dichotomized using 5, 10, 15 and 20 drinks/week as cut-off points. Periodontal disease was represented by clinical attachment loss (CAL) and was assessed both as a continuous variable and dichotomized as <1.5 mm and >1.5 mm. Independent effect of alcohol on CAL was assessed by weighted multiple linear and logistic regression analyses adjusting simultaneously for the effects of age, gender, race, education, income, smoking, diet, diabetes, gingival bleeding and the number of remaining teeth. There was a significant linear relationship between number of drinks per week and log CAL ($p = 0.0001$). Thus, alcohol consumption may be associated with increased severity of periodontitis in a dose-dependent fashion. However, prospective studies and studies of the mechanisms are needed to confirm the role of alcohol as a risk factor for periodontal disease.

Trace elements

One cross-sectional epidemiological investigation involving 4290 subjects aged 20–80 years old (Meisel et al 2005) suggested an association between magnesium deficiency and severity of chronic periodontitis.

Obesity

Genco et al (2005) studied the relationship between obesity, periodontal disease and insulin resistance by using data from in the Third National Health and Nutrition Examination Survey (NHANES III). They concluded that obesity was a significant predictor of periodontal disease and this relationship appeared to be mediated by insulin resistance.

Linden et al (2007) investigated whether there was an association between obesity and periodontitis in a homogeneous group of 60–70-year-old Western European men. The study also explored whether a high body mass index (BMI) in early life could predict poor periodontal status in

later life. They found that obesity was associated with periodontitis in the homogeneous group of 60–70-year-old European men investigated, however, high BMI levels in early life did not predict periodontitis in later life in the men studied.

The same association has been also shown by (Ylöstalo et al 2008).

SYSTEMIC DISEASE

Molloy et al (2004) showed an association between some systemic diseases, including diabetes, coronary heart disease and stomach ulcers, and periodontal disease severity (see also Ch. 6).

HOST FACTORS

FACTORS AFFECTING SUSCEPTIBILITY TO PERIODONTAL DISEASE

Genetic factors

Genetic susceptibility to chronic periodontitis may greatly increase its rate of progression such that destructive disease occurs in the early adult years. Some of these cases may be termed rapidly progressive periodontitis (Ch. 23). Conversely, patients genetically resistant to periodontitis show little or no signs of attachment loss throughout their lives (**Fig. 4.9**) and may keep well supported teeth into old age with little or no periodontal treatment. In this regard, epidemiological studies have shown that the amount of periodontal attachment loss is greater in some patients than others, even when differences of oral hygiene are taken into account (Löe et al 1978). In addition, other epidemiological studies from a number of different countries have indicated that about 10% of subjects experience severe periodontal destruction with rapid progression and tooth loss, while about 10% appear to be resistant to destructive periodontitis, despite the continued presence of plaque and gingivitis (Löe et al 1978; Page & Schroeder 1986; Papapanou et al 1989). The remaining 80% of subjects appear to be susceptible to slowly progressive periodontitis which rarely results in tooth loss if they receive adequate periodontal treatment. Their rate of disease progression depends much more on their individual oral hygiene status. Thus, it is important to identify each patient's individual susceptibility to periodontitis since this will determine the type and frequency of treatment that they will require.

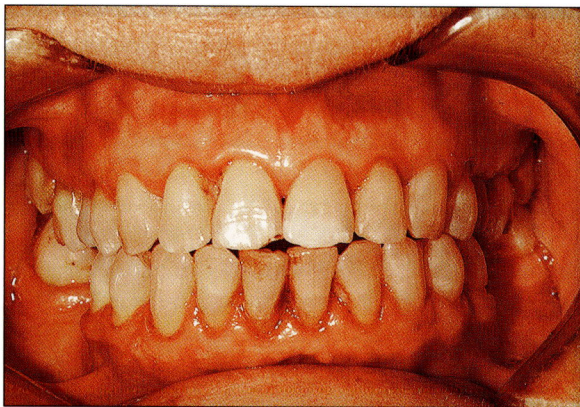

Fig. 4.9 An 85-year-old woman with minimal attachment loss. She has only attended a dentist on four occasions during her life and has lost one tooth, a lower right first molar due to caries when she was 30 years of age. She has relatively poor oral hygiene and has gingivitis and supragingival calculus deposits. However, the only attachment loss found was slight buccal gingival recession on a few teeth. All the probing depths were minimal, and there was no radiographic evidence of alveolar bone loss. Her younger sister, aged 81 years, has all her teeth and a similar periodontal condition.

Genetic factors may also play a role in the onset and severity of gingivitis in children. In this regard Dashash et al (2007) investigated the role of the polymorphism of a variable number of tandem repeats of interleukin-1 receptor antagonist gene (IL-1RN) on gingivitis in children. They found that IL-1Ra gene polymorphisms could play an active role in the pathogenesis of gingivitis in Caucasian children and that the IL-1RN*2 allele could be a protective marker against gingivitis.

Twin studies have shown that a significant variance in the susceptibility to chronic periodontitis may be attributable to genetic factors (Michalowicz et al 1991; Michalowicz 1994) but attempts to identify specific genetic markers have proved difficult (Hart & Kornman 1997).

The type of immune response mounted to any particular pathogen is genetically determined by the amino acid sequence of the major histocompatibility complex (MHC) receptor molecule (Nossal 1993). Therefore, the immune response of an individual to any particular pathogen could determine their susceptibility to the disease mediated by that pathogen. It follows from this that the type of immune response mounted against periodontal pathogens could in part determine an individual's susceptibility to periodontitis. In this regard it has been recently shown that different levels of IgG subgroups are produced against *P. gingivalis* in healthy subjects and treated and maintained chronic periodontitis patients and untreated chronic periodontitis patients (Sakai et al 2001). Furthermore, this group also showed that there was a positive statistical correlation between IgG2 levels and progressive bone loss.

One type of genetic marker tested recently has been that coding for proteins of the pro-inflammatory cytokines such as interleukin (IL)-1 and tumour necrosis factor alpha (TNF-α) which are key regulators of host responses to microbial infection (Kornman et al 1997b). IL-1 is also a major modulator of extracellular matrix degradation and bone resorption (Ch. 5). It has been shown that the specific genotype of the polymorphic IL-1 gene cluster was associated with the severity of chronic periodontitis in a group of non-smokers and statistically significantly distinguished individuals with severe periodontitis from those with mild disease. Functionally the specific periodontitis-associated IL-1 genotype comprised a variant of the IL-1β gene that is associated with high levels of IL-1 production. The specific association found in this study was with the presence of allele 2 of the IL-1α with allele 2 of the IL-1β gene and this composite genotype has been found to occur in 29.1% of Northern European subjects. No association was found for either single alleles of this gene or for alleles of the TNF genes (Kornman et al 1997b).

In this study (Kornman et al 1997a) the smokers were separated into a separate group to the non-smokers because of the known association between tobacco smoking and the severity of periodontitis (see above). They found that in smokers severe periodontitis was not associated with the genotype. It was, however, found that 86% of the severe periodontitis patients were accounted for by either smoking or the IL-1 genotype.

Some new single nucleotide polymorphisms of TNF-α have been observed in a large proportion of Japanese subjects. The frequency of Japanese subjects that carried at least one variant in these TNF-α polymorphisms was significantly higher in subjects with severe periodontitis than healthy subjects (Soga et al 2003) and thus they could play a role in chronic periodontitis susceptibility in these subjects.

In addition, in this regard, another research group (Gore et al 1988) has determined the distribution of IL-1α and β genotypes in patients with adult chronic periodontitis and their matched healthy controls. The subjects were 32 Caucasian adult periodontitis patients matched for sex and age with 32 control Caucasian subjects with no clinical signs of periodontal disease. They found that the frequency of IL-1β genotypes including allele 2 of the IL-1β +3953 restriction length bi-allelic polymorphism was significantly increased in patients with advanced adult periodontitis compared with those with early and moderate disease. Furthermore, the presence of allele 2 of this type was associated with increased production of

IL-1β by activated peripheral blood polymorphonuclear leucocytes from patients with advanced disease, although this increase did not reach statistical significance. The findings also showed a significant linkage disequilibrium between allele 2 of the IL-1β +3953 polymorphism and allele 2 of the bi-allelic IL-1α −889 polymorphism in periodontitis patients compared with healthy controls. These findings support further the possible role of IL-1α and β gene polymorphisms in the susceptibility to adult chronic periodontitis.

A number of other studies addressing this issue have also been published (Price et al 1999; Ehmke et al 1999; Engebretson et al 1999; Galbraith et al 1999; McGuire et al 1999; Armitage et al 2000; McDevitt et al 2000). However, the results of these have been varied with some supporting and some not supporting this relationship. A further case control study of this relationship (Papapanou et al 2001) showed that although the composite IL-1 genotype did correlate with the severity of chronic periodontitis in patients it failed to distinguish between periodontitis patients and healthy controls.

Tai et al (2002) compared polymorphisms of the IL-1α, IL-1β and IL-1 receptor antagonist (IL-1ra) genes in 47 generalized early onset periodontitis (G-EOP) and 97 healthy Japanese subjects. All these genes are found in the same area of the long arm of chromosome 2. IL-1ra protein attaches to the IL-1 receptor to block IL-1 attachment and thus its function. It is difficult on the basis of the clinical criteria and ages (23–35 years) of the G-EOP subjects to know whether they represented rapidly progressive periodontitis or post juvenile periodontitis cases or both. They found no differences between the groups of polymorphisms of IL-1α or IL-1β but did find a significant difference ($p = 0.005$, OR 4.12) of polymorphisms of the IL-1ra gene. However, another study of a Chilean population (Quappe et al 2004) of the role of the IL-1α and -1β genes in the progression of aggressive periodontitis supported a positive association between this condition and the presence of the IL-1β +3954 allele 2 polymorphism.

In another Chilean study, López et al (2005) carried out an investigation to determine the prevalence of the IL-1α 889 and IL-1β +3954 (previously +3953) polymorphisms and their association with periodontitis. A case-control study of 330 cases of periodontitis patients and 101 healthy controls was performed. Genomic DNA was analysed for polymorphism in the IL-1α gene at site 889 and IL-1β gene at site +3954 by polymerase chain reaction (PCR) amplification followed by restriction enzyme digestion and gel electrophoresis. Demographic and socioeconomic characteristics of subjects were similar in cases and in controls and a higher but non-significant frequency of the heterozygous IL-1α 889 locus was found in cases but not controls. The frequency of the heterozygous IL-1β +3954 locus was significantly higher in cases than in controls and was associated with periodontitis ($p = 0.001$). The homozygous status for allele 1 of the IL-1β +3954 was a protective factor for periodontitis ($p = 0.001$). The prevalence of positive genotype (at least one allele 2 present at each locus) was significantly higher in cases (26.06%) than in controls (9.9%) and was significantly associated with periodontitis ($p = 0.001$), irrespective of the smoking status and periodontitis severity. Sensitivity of positive genotype was 26%, the specificity 90%, and the positive predictive value 89%. Within the limits of this study, the results show that individuals carrying the positive genotype have significantly greater risk for developing periodontitis.

Moreira et al (2007) also found that the IL-1α (+889) gene polymorphism was associated with chronic periodontal disease in a sample of Brazilian individuals.

In this regard, Li et al (2004) also investigated whether specific interleukin (IL)-1 genotypes and/or alleles could be used to predict susceptibility to generalized AgP (GAgP) in Chinese subjects The GAgP group consisted of 122 patients, and the control group of 95 healthy subjects. Single nucleotide polymorphisms at IL-1α (+4845) and IL-1β (−511, +3954) were analysed by standard polymerase chain reaction-restriction fragment length polymorphism (PCR-RFLP) assay. The polymorphism of a variable number tandem repeat (VNTR) in intron 2 of IL-1RN was detected by PCR amplification and fragment size analysis. There was no significant association of IL-1 polymorphisms with GAgP in the unstratified subjects. However, when cases were stratified by gender, the frequencies of A2+ genotype and allele 2 at IL-1α +4845 were significantly increased in male patients compared to male controls genotype ($p = 0.039$). The frequency of IL-1β −511 A1/A2 heterozygote was significantly increased in male GAgP group compared with male controls ($p = 0.048$). In females, no significant differences were found between patients and controls in corresponding analyses at all polymorphic loci. A possible combined effect of IL-1β −511 polymorphism and smoking on the elevated risk to GAgP was observed. Thus, the polymorphisms of IL-1α +4845 and IL-1β −511 may play a role in determining GAgP susceptibility in Chinese males. Furthermore, a possible combined effect of the polymorphism of IL-1β −511 and smoking on GAgP susceptibility was suggested.

Two other studies failed to show any relationship between IL-1 polymorphisms and chronic periodontitis severity. One of these (Sakellari et al 2003) looked at the prevalence of IL-1α +4845 and IL-1β +3954 in a Greek population one group of which were healthy subjects and the other had chronic periodontitis. A high percentage of these polymorphisms were seen in this Greek population but it showed no relationship to the presence or absence of chronic periodontitis. The other study (Jepsen et al 2003) found no relationship between IL-1 polymorphisms and the severity of gingivitis in an experimental gingivitis study.

The relationship between smoking and IL-1 gene polymorphisms has been investigated (Meisel et al 2004). They found a gene-environmental interaction between these two factors. They also found that smokers bearing the genotype-positive IL-1 allele combination had an increased risk of periodontitis. However, this IL-1 genotype had no influence on non-smokers. This shows the importance of excluding smokers from genetic studies of periodontal disease susceptibility because of its strong influence.

Takeuchi-Hatanaka et al (2008) previously found that expression of interleukin IL-12RB2 molecule was a crucial regulatory factor in the T-helper type (Th) 1 differentiation of T cells. In order to elucidate the role of the cell-mediated immune (CMI) response in the pathogenesis of periodontitis, Japanese periodontal patients were subjected to single nucleotide polymorphism (SNP) analyses of the 5′ flanking region of IL-12RB2, whose variants are frequently detected in lepromatous leprosy patients, in which the very weak cellular immune response is caused by low expression of IL-12RB2. The gene polymorphisms of the 5′ flanking region of IL-12RB2 were examined in subjects with several types of periodontal disease and in healthy controls. Serum immunoglobulin (Ig) G antibody titres against periodontopathic bacteria were measured and compared in periodontal patients with and without variant alleles of IL-12RB2. They found that the frequencies of variant alleles of IL-12RB2 were significantly higher in aggressive periodontitis patients as compared with healthy controls or chronic periodontitis patients. Serum IgG titres against all periodontal bacteria examined in subjects carrying variant alleles were higher than those in subjects without variant alleles. They concluded that IL-12RB2 SNPs could be useful as genetic markers to access the susceptibility of the general population to periodontal disease. Low CMI responses or high humoral responses are associated with the pathogenesis of inflammatory periodontal diseases.

IL-2 is an immune reaction activator and pro-inflammatory cytokine from Th1 cells (Ch. 3) and this has also been investigated for its association with severe periodontitis. A total of 113 non-smoking, medically healthy, Brazilian subjects of 25 years and above were recruited and divided into periodontally healthy (44), subjects with moderate (31) and advanced (33) chronic periodontitis (Scarel-Caminaga et al 2002). DNA was extracted from buccal epithelial cell scrapings and the PCR-RFLP technique was used to detect polymorphism −300 (T-G) in the promoter region of the IL-2 gene. No significant differences in the studied polymorphism was

seen between the three groups. However, when the healthy and moderate periodontitis groups were merged and compared with the advanced periodontitis group a significant ($p = 0.027$) difference in the TT versus TG/GC genotypes was found. This indicated that individuals with the T allele were half as likely to develop advanced periodontitis than the other genotypes. Furthermore, the homozygous TT subjects were 2.5 times less likely to develop advanced periodontitis than the heterozygous or GG homozygous subjects. Since gene polymorphisms may vary between racial groups, these finding may not necessarily relate to other racial groups.

IL-4 promotes the immune response and two of its polymorphisms have been associated with asthma, atopy and more lately with aggressive periodontitis in Caucasians (Pontes et al 2004). There appear to be racial differences in the polymorphisms of this gene and the association between these IL-4 polymorphisms and chronic periodontitis have therefore been compared in a Brazilian population of African origin (Pontes et al 2004). No significant differences were found in the genotype frequencies between the periodontitis and control groups and it was concluded that IL-4 polymorphisms were not related to periodontal disease susceptibility in this population.

IL-10 is an anti-inflammatory cytokine and 3 dimorphic polymorphisms within the IL-10 promoter gene have been recently recognized which appear to effect its regulation and expression. Yamazaki et al (2001) investigated the prevalence of these haplotypes in chronic adult periodontitis, generalized early onset periodontitis and healthy subjects. Although they reported different haplotypes between Japanese and Caucasian subjects they found no differences between the periodontal patient and control groups. Another study on IL-10 polymorphisms (Gonzales et al 2002) confirmed the lack of association with adult periodontitis and also showed that they had no association with juvenile (aggressive) periodontitis. However in contrast, Berglundh et al (2003) found a positive relationship between polymorphisms of this gene at position −1087 and the severity of chronic periodontitis in a Swedish population. Interestingly, it has also been found that mice engineered to lack a functional IL-10 gene exhibit 30–40% greater and more accelerated alveolar bone loss ($p = 0.006$) than the normal control mice (Al-Rasheed et al 2003). Sasaki et al (2004) also found that the IL-10 [−]/[−] mouse was highly susceptible to bone loss induced by *P. gingivalis*, and that this was mediated via an IL-1-independent pathway (see also Ch. 5). In addition, Cullinan et al (2008) showed that either the ATA/ACC or the ACC/ACC genotype of interleukin 10 contributed to the progression of periodontal disease.

Another study (Moreira et al 2005) showed an increased susceptibility to chronic periodontitis and rapidly progressive periodontitis from a functional interleukin-1 (β)-gene polymorphism in Brazilian subjects.

Scarel-Caminaga et al (2004) investigated single-nucleotide polymorphisms (SNPs) in the IL-10 promoter gene to chronic periodontitis (CP). DNA was obtained from 67 CP patients and 43 control subjects, all non-smokers. The −1087 SNP was investigated by DNA sequencing, and the −819 and −592 SNPs by restriction fragment length polymorphism of PCR products. Frequencies of −819 and −592 SNPs showed differences between the control and CP groups. The ACC haplotype was more prevalent in the control group and the ATA haplotype more prevalent in the CP group. The ATA haplotype seemed to increase susceptibility to CP in women (odds ratio (OR) = 2.57). The heterozygous haplotype GCC/ACC was predominant in the control group (OR = 8.26; $p = 0.001$). Thus, specific haplotypes and SNPs in IL-10 promoter gene appear to be associated with susceptibility to CP in Brazilian patients.

IL-6 is a pro-inflammatory cytokine and is a key regulator of the host response to microbial infection. Polymorphisms of the gene of this cytokine have been investigated (Holla et al 2004) at positions −597(G/A), −572 (G/C) and −174(G/C). They analysed the allele, genotype, and haplotype distributions of the IL-6 promoter variants in a case control study with 148 chronic periodontitis patients and 107 healthy controls. They found significant differences in the distributions of alleles and genotypes of IL-6 (−572 G/C) polymorphism between patients and controls ($p > 0.01$). It was due to an under-representation of the −572 G/C heterozygotes in chronic periodontitis patients (6.1%) compared with controls (19.6%). Although no variant 'C/C' homozygotes were detected in the cases and controls in this study, heterozygosity appeared to protect against chronic periodontitis, representing a 73% reduction in risk compared with the wild-type homozygotes. However, there was no significant differences in the genotype or allele frequencies between both groups for IL-6 −597(G/A) and -174 (G/C) polymorphisms. This study appears to show that −572 (G/C) polymorphism of the IL-6 gene may be one of the protective factors associated with lower susceptibility to chronic periodontitis.

Another study (Nibali et al 2008) investigated the possible role of IL-6 genetic polymorphisms and haplotypes in the predisposition to aggressive periodontitis (AgP). Their study supported the hypothesis of a link between IL-6 genetic factors and AgP and highlighted the importance of two IL-6 polymorphisms (−1363 and −1480) in modulating disease phenotype and susceptibility.

Tervonen et al (2007) compared the frequencies of cytokine and receptor molecule genotypes in patients with chronic periodontitis with the corresponding frequencies in a reference population. They also studied the relationship between periodontal disease severity and polymorphisms in the related genes. CD14, IL-6, TNF-α, IL-10, IL-1α, IL-1β, and TLR-4 polymorphisms of 51 periodontitis patients were studied using polymerase chain reaction. They found no statistically significant differences between the frequencies of the cytokine genotypes in the periodontitis patients and in the reference group. However, the extent of periodontal disease was higher in subjects with the T-containing genotype of CD14−260 and the GG genotype of IL-6 174 when compared with the extent in the rest of the group. Subjects carrying the composite genotype of the above two were most severely affected by periodontal disease. Thus, possible association may exist between the carriage of the T-containing genotype of CD14−260 and the GG genotype of IL-6 174 and the extent of periodontal disease.

Wagner et al (2007) investigated the association of polymorphisms in the osteoprotegerin (OPG) and interleukin 1 (IL-1) genes with chronic periodontitis (CP) in 194 subjects, 97 patients and 97 controls. They confirmed the association between the IL-1 polymorphisms and CP but found no association between the OPG polymorphisms and CP.

A number of other studies have looked at other gene polymorphisms. Trevilatto et al (2003) showed a positive relationship between polymorphisms of the IL-6 gene at position −174 and the severity of chronic periodontitis in a Caucasian Brazilian population. However, again in a Brazilian population, polymorphisms of the IL-4 gene at position 590(C-T) were found to have no relationship to the severity of chronic periodontitis (Scarel-Caminaga et al 2003).

Interleukin (IL)-18 regulates the expression of the pro-inflammatory cytokine interferon gamma. Folwaczny et al (2005) investigated the putative involvement of six different IL-18 gene polymorphisms in predisposition to destructive periodontal disease in 129 Chronic periodontitis patents and 121 controls. However, they found that these IL-18 gene polymorphisms were not associated with destructive periodontal disease.

A single nucleotide polymorphism of the TGF-β1 gene promoter has been associated with an increased risk for asthma and other allergies (de Souza et al 2003b). Holla et al (2002) compared five polymorphisms of the TGF-β1 gene and the severity of chronic periodontitis and found also no relationship between them. A single nucleotide polymorphism of the TGF-β1 gene promoter has been found in 58% of moderate to severe chronic periodontitis Caucasian subjects compared with 38% of healthy subjects. Thus it may play a small role in chronic periodontitis susceptibility (de Souza et al 2003b).

Folwaczny et al (2004a) found no association between the −308 TNF-α gene polymorphism and periodontal disease in a study of 81 patients with generalized chronic periodontitis and 80 healthy controls.

Tumour necrosis factor receptor 2 (TNFR2) is one of the cell surface receptors for TNF-α. Recent studies have suggested that TNFR2 gene polymorphism is involved in autoimmune and other diseases (Shimada et al 2004). This group studied the relationship of TNFR2 (+587T/G) gene polymorphism with chronic periodontitis (CP). 196 unrelated subjects (age 40–65 years) with different levels of CP were identified according to established criteria, including measurements of probing pocket depth (PPD), clinical attachment level (CAL), and alveolar bone loss (BL). All subjects were of Japanese descent and non-smokers. Single nucleotide polymorphism at position +587(T/G) in the TNFR2 gene was detected by a polymerase chain reaction-restriction fragment length polymorphisms (PCR-RFLP) method. The frequency of the +587G allele was significantly higher in severe CP patients than in controls. In addition, mean values of PPD, CAL, and BL were significantly higher in the +587G allele positive than in the negative subjects. Thus, the TNFR2 (+587G) polymorphic allele could be associated with severe CP in Japanese subjects.

mRNA expression of cytokines has also been studied in this regard. Bickel et al (2001) investigated mRNA expression for IFN-γ, IL-1β, IL-2, IL-4, IL-5, IL-6 and TNF-α in six patients observed over 6 years. Their expression at biopsied sites exhibiting severe, progressive periodontitis, stable periodontitis or health were compared. However, while marked variations were seen between sites in individual patients no significant differences were observed between the sites of each disease category.

Park et al (2008) found that the haplotypes of T950C and G1181C polymorphisms in the osteoprotegerin (OPG) gene may be useful genetic markers for the prediction of periodontitis. However they suggested that further studies in a larger population would be required to determine whether these alleles directly contribute to periodontitis susceptibility.

Meuric et al (2008) demonstrated a critical role for the oxyR gene in the aerotolerance of P. gingivalis. The ahpC-F, batA, and hem genes were slightly overexpressed (between 1.65-fold and 2-fold) after exposure to atmospheric oxygen compared to anaerobic conditions. The level of transcription of dps, ftn, tpx, and rgpA genes increased >2.5-fold, and the expression of ahpC-F, dps, ftn, and tpx was partially or completely OxyR-dependent. A different transcription pattern of P. gingivalis genes was observed, depending on the stimulus of oxidative stress. These workers also presented new evidence that the expression of tpx, encoding a thiol peroxidase, is partially OxyR-dependent and is induced after atmospheric oxygen exposure.

A single-nucleotide promoter polymorphism in the CD14 gene has been associated with various inflammatory conditions. Folwaczny et al (2004b) sought to determine the frequency of the CD14−159C-to-T polymorphism among subjects with periodontitis and healthy control individuals. 70 patients with periodontal disease and 75 healthy controls were genotyped for this polymorphism. Overall, the frequency for the CD14−159T allele in patients with periodontitis was 39.3% and 48.0% for male and female controls ($p = 0.135$). However, the CD14−159C allele was significantly more prevalent ($p = 0.013$) among females with periodontitis as compared with healthy control subjects. In contrast, the distribution of the CD14−159C-to-T polymorphism showed no significant difference among males with and without periodontitis ($p = 0.816$). Thus, the C-159T promoter polymorphism of the CD14 gene was associated in female but not in male patients with periodontal disease.

Donati et al (2005) investigated the association of gene polymorphisms related to some immune regulation components (G-308A TNF-α, Q551R IL-4RA and C-159T CD14) with severe chronic periodontitis. This suggested that the -159 CD14 gene polymorphism might be associated with chronic periodontitis in Caucasian subjects of a north European origin.

Bacterial components are recognized by CD14 and toll-like receptor 4 (TLR4), resulting in a NF-B-based inflammatory response. For this reason, Laine et al (2005) investigated the occurrence of CD14−260C>T, TLR4 299Asp>Gly, and 399Thr>Ile gene polymorphisms in adult periodontitis.

DNA was collected from 100 patients with severe periodontitis and from 99 periodontally healthy controls. The gene polymorphisms were determined by the PCR technique. The CD14–260T/T genotype was found in 34.0% of periodontitis patients and in 20.2% of controls ($p<0.004$) showing that the CD14–260T/T genotype might contribute to the susceptibility to severe periodontitis in Dutch Caucasians.

The leucocyte Fc receptor for immunoglobulin G (IgG) (Fcγ R) plays a major role in handling pathogens and immune complexes and polymorphisms of the gene for this receptor could be associated with periodontitis. Kobayashi et al (2003) found a significant over-expression of the Fcγ RIIa-R131 allele in patients with both systemic lupus erythematosus (SLE) and chronic periodontitis compared to healthy subjects with no periodontal disease and SLE subjects with no periodontitis. Thus the Fcγ RIIa-R131 allele may be associated with a higher risk of progression of chronic periodontitis.

Another group (Loos et al 2003) investigated Fcγ receptor polymorphisms in 68 periodontitis patients and 61 healthy controls. Twelve of the periodontitis group were classified as aggressive periodontitis cases (AgP). The frequency of the Fcγ RIIIa-V158 allele was 53% in the patient group and 39% in controls ($p = 0.034$). The carriage rate in AgP cases was even higher (63%). The frequency of the Fcγ R IIa-H131 allele was 58% in the patient group, 79% of AgP cases and 51% in controls. For AgP versus controls this was significant ($p = 0.013$). The frequency of the Fcγ RIIa-H/H131 allele was also significantly higher in the AgP group than the controls ($p = 0.02$). Thus some of these polymorphisms may have some relationship to the severity of periodontitis particularly AgP. However, it would be wrong to draw firm conclusions from a relatively small study group particularly of AgP cases such as this one, although similar findings have been reported by Nibali et al (2006).

Functional polymorphisms of immunoglobulin G (IgG) Fc receptors IIIa and IIIb (Fcγ RIIIa and Fcγ RIIIb) have been shown as risk factors for periodontitis (Yamamoto et al 2004). This group investigated whether Fcγ RIIa polymorphism was associated with a disease risk as well. A total of 1221 Caucasian adults were used in the study of which 422 subjects had moderate to severe chronic periodontitis. They were assigned to two groups, diseased and healthy. The Fcγ RIIa genotype for three bi-allelic polymorphisms (Fcγ RIIa-R/R131, R/H131 and H/H131) was determined by means of allele-specific polymerase chain reactions. The distribution of Fcγ RIIa genotype between the patient and control groups was significantly different, with enrichment of the high ligand-binding genotype Fcγ RIIa-H/H131 in the patients ($p = 0.04$). Multivariate logistic regression model demonstrated that subject age, gender, smoking, and the Fcγ RIIa genotype were significantly associated with severity of chronic periodontitis. For smokers, there was a significant over-representation of Fcγ RIIa-H/H131 in the patient group compared with the control group ($p = 0.03$). Additionally, smokers with Fcγ RIIa-H/H131 exhibited significantly greater mean clinical attachment loss than those with Fcγ RIIa-R/H131 and R/R131 ($p = 0.04$). However, they found no association between Fcγ RIIa genotype and the disease susceptibility or severity in subjects who had never smoked. This suggests that the Fcγ RIIa-H/H131 genotype may be associated with chronic periodontitis risk in Caucasian smokers.

Another study (Sahingur et al 2003) investigated the association of -455 G/A fibrinogen gene polymorphism in chronic periodontitis by comparing 79 chronic periodontitis patients with 75 periodontally healthy controls matched for gender, age and race. They found that the frequency of the rare allele on the b-fibrinogen gene (H2H2) was 13% for the chronic periodontitis patients and 3% for the healthy controls ($p = 0.01$). The distribution of H1H1 and H1H2 genotypes were 48% and 39% in the chronic periodontitis patient group and 70% and 27% in the control group ($p = 0.01$). Serum fibrinogen levels were also significantly higher in the patient group compared to the control group. This indicates that a significantly higher proportion of chronic periodontitis patients exhibit genotypes associated with higher fibrinogen levels compared to healthy subjects and that this might increase their susceptibility to chronic periodontitis.

It has also been suggested that a protease:inhibitor imbalance could affect susceptibility to chronic periodontitis (Cox 1995; Fokkema et al 1998; see also Ch. 5). Fokkema et al (1998) compared the periodontal status of subjects with severe a1PI deficiency to that of normal controls and found a significant increase in severe periodontitis in the a1PI deficient subjects. Also, Peterson and Marsh (1979) reported a 34% prevalence of a1PI deficient phenotypes in 50 subjects with severe periodontitis. This seems to represent a dramatic increase in mild and intermediate a1PI deficiencies in this condition compared to either a periodontally healthy control group or the regional USA background level. This proportion is also higher than the reported levels of a1PI deficient phenotypes in the worldwide population (Hutchison 1998; WHO 1998). However, another investigation (Scott et al 2002) could not find an association between mutant PI* alleles and periodontitis in a small, controlled study. It is therefore likely that larger well designed studies will be necessary to resolve this issue since a small group of subjects is unlikely to contain sufficient numbers of a1PI deficient individuals.

With regards to matrix metalloproteinases (MMPs), de Souza et al (2003) found a positive relationship for polymorphisms of MMP-1 promoter gene in a Brazilian population. Also, Izakovi et al (2004) examined the association between three promoter polymorphisms of the MMP-1 gene and chronic periodontitis susceptibility and/or severity in a Czech population. They showed that these all showed significant association with chronic periodontitis ($p<0.05$). However, the level of correlation was relatively weak and other co-factors, such as smoking affected the results. Therefore, their results showed that these polymorphisms possibly had only a small effect on the pathogenesis of chronic periodontitis. Another study by Cao et al (2005) suggested that a single nucleotide polymorphism in the MMP-1 promoter region of −607 bp may be associated with generalized aggressive periodontitis in Chinese population.

The plasminogen activating system is a protease/inhibitor system central to extracellular matrix remodelling with a suggested role in periodontal disease pathology (De Carlo et al 2007). A few studies have reported polymorphisms in the genes of plasminogen activator inhibitors to be associated with periodontal disease severity and two gene polymorphisms – a BamHI restriction fragment length polymorphism in the urokinase plasminogen activator gene (uPA) and a HindIII restriction fragment length polymorphism in the plasminogen activator inhibitor type 1 gene (PAI-1) – have been associated with conditions having a vascular component. The objective of this study was to assess the association of these gene polymorphisms with alveolar bone loss in adult chronic periodontal disease. The genotype of the subjects was determined by polymerase chain reaction and amplification of whole blood. Pertinent histories were obtained by interview and alveolar bone loss was assessed from current radiographs. The subjects were 77 elderly patients with a normal distribution of alveolar bone loss. They showed a significant association between levels of alveolar bone loss and these polymorphisms in the uPA and PAI-1 genes. Controlling for the contributions of smoking or diabetes to periodontal bone loss, estimated odds ratios for predicting lower levels of alveolar bone loss, associated with a greater degree of periodontal health, were strongest when defined by the concurrent presence of a homozygous urokinase plasminogen activator genotype and the nuclease-sensitive plasminogen activator inhibitor type 1 (HindIII) allele. Thus the urokinase plasminogen activator (BamHI) and plasminogen activator inhibitor type 1 (HindIII) genotypes may serve as useful markers for severity of bone loss associated with periodontal disease.

There is little information on the association between alcohol consumption and periodontitis risk (Nishida et al 2004). Alcohol is first oxidized in the body by alcohol dehydrogenase (ADH) into aldehyde. The aldehyde is then oxidized by aldehyde dehydrogenase (ALDH) into acetate.

Asian people often have polymorphisms of the alcohol metabolizing genes such as ADH2 and ALDH2 and these play a key role in alcohol hypersensitivity in some Asians. This hypersensitivity is highest in the atypical homozygotes, ALDH2 *2/*2 followed by the heterozygotes ALDH2 *1/*2 and is lowest in the homozygotes, ALDH2 *1/*1 (Nishida et al 2004). The frequencies of the ALDH2 *2/*2, ALDH2 *1/*2, ALDH2 *1/*1 genotypes are 6%, 38% and 56% in Japanese subjects.

Nishida et al (2004) assessed whether alcohol consumption and ALDH2 genotype were associated with periodontitis in Japanese periodontitis and healthy subjects. Subjects' life styles were assessed by a self-administered questionnaire and the percentage of probing depths = 4 mm were used as the periodontal parameter. ALDH2 genotypes were determined by the use of a PCR/RFLP method. Multiple logistic analyses showed that alcohol consumption was significantly associated with periodontitis (OR 1.98). There was no significant relationship between periodontal status and the ALDH2 genotypes. However, ALDH2 *1/*2 subjects who consumed =33 g/day of alcohol had a significantly higher percentage of probing depths = 4 mm than those whose alcohol consumption was lower, while there was no significant difference in periodontal status associated with alcohol consumption in ALDH2 *1/*1 subjects. Thus these results suggest that alcohol consumption may be a risk factor for periodontitis in ALDH2 *1/*2 subjects who consume large amounts of alcohol.

It has also been shown that oestrogen receptor-α (ER-α) gene polymorphisms are associated with alterations in bone mineral density and osteoporosis in females (Zhang et al 2004) and this group has investigated the relationship between ER-α gene polymorphisms and periodontitis. They recruited 90 patients with aggressive periodontitis, 34 patients with chronic periodontitis and 91 healthy controls, all belonging to the Han Chinese race. They found that detection frequency of XX genotype was significantly higher in the chronic periodontitis patients than in the healthy controls ($p<0.05$) and that the difference between the female chronic periodontitis patients and healthy controls was more statistically significant ($p<0.01$). In contrast, there was no significant difference between the male patients and controls. Thus, in the female Han Chinese population, the XX genotype may be a risk indicator for chronic periodontitis.

Genetic polymorphisms in the vitamin D receptor (VDR) gene may be associated with bone homeostasis and diseases in which bone loss is a cardinal sign. de Brito Junior et al (2004) investigated 44 healthy individuals (control group) and 69 subjects with chronic periodontitis to determine whether chronic periodontal disease in a Brazilian population is associated with polymorphisms in the VDR gene. DNA was obtained from the subjects' epithelial cells by scraping the buccal mucosa. Two polymorphisms in the VDR gene were analysed by polymerase chain reaction, followed by TaqI and BsmI restriction endonuclease digestion. They found that TaqI and BsmI polymorphisms of the VDR gene were associated with clinical attachment loss due to periodontal disease in a Brazilian population ($p = 0.005$).

Smoking is a risk factor for the development and severity of periodontitis. Therefore, individual susceptibility to periodontitis may be influenced by the polymorphisms of genes coding for enzymes metabolizing tobacco-derived substances. Kim et al (2004) investigated three important enzymes, cytochrome P450 (CYP) 1A1, CYP2E1 and glutathione S-transferase (GST) M, involved in the metabolic activation and detoxification of tobacco-derived substances. The prevalence of the polymorphisms of these genes was examined in 115 patients with periodontitis as well as in 126 control subjects. Significantly increased risk for periodontitis was observed for subjects with the polymorphic CYP1A1 m2 allele (OR = 2.3) and the GSTM1 allele (OR = 2.1). However, no association was observed for the CYP2E1 Pst1 polymorphism. These results suggest

that the GSTM1 and CYP1A1 polymorphisms may play an important role in risk for periodontitis.

However, some tested polymorphisms of cytokine and other genes are proving either negative or playing possible minor roles in this relationship. It is likely that in the future other genes coding for other key factors that play a role in the pathogenesis of periodontal disease will be investigated for their possible association with the susceptibility to chronic periodontitis. Furthermore the relationships between periodontal disease susceptibility and gene polymorphisms are likely to be varied and complex.

Thus, there is limited evidence that some polymorphisms in the genes encoding IL-1, Fcγ receptors, IL-10 and the vitamin D receptor, may be associated with periodontitis in certain ethnic groups (Loos et al 2005). However, relatively large variations in carriage rates of the Rare (R)-alleles among studies on any polymorphism have been observed. The available studies appear to be under-powered and do not adequately take into account other pertinent risk factors for periodontitis. Future studies should include larger cohorts, should clearly define phenotypes and should adequately control for other risk factors. In addition to the candidate gene approach, alternative strategies need to be considered to elucidate the gene variations, which confer risk for periodontitis.

The current models of periodontal disease susceptibility attribute it to an imbalance between the associated microbiota and alterations in phagocyte and/or cytokine function or specific immune or other host responses (Hart & Kornman 1997; Korman et al 1997). Host responses are likely to vary as a result of genetic variation.

The possible effects of genetic factors on the presence of viable periodonto-pathogenic bacteria

Nibali et al (2007) studied whether gene polymorphisms of inflammatory markers were associated with the presence of viable periodonto-pathogenic bacteria. They found that both Fc receptor and IL-6–174 polymorphisms were associated with increased odds of detecting *A. actinomycetemcomitans*, *P. gingivalis*, and *T. forsythensis* after adjustment for age, ethnicity, smoking, and periodontitis extent. These findings support the hypothesis that complex interactions between the microbiota and host genome may be at the basis of susceptibility to aggressive periodontitis.

PSYCHOLOGICAL STRESS FACTORS

Psychological stress can play a role in many conditions and probably mediates its effects both biochemically and behaviourally, the first by affecting the immune system and the second through altered compliance and health behaviour (Andersen et al 1994). It could affect the course of periodontal disease in both these ways.

It has already been shown that negative-life-events may play a role in acute or chronic oral symptoms (Marcenes et al 1993) and it has been suggested that such factors could also play a role in the patient's susceptibility to periodontal disease progression although this has been questioned (Wilton et al 1988; Sculley et al 1991). It has, however, been suggested that the apparent lack of relationship could have been due to small sample size, unsuitable selection criteria and the recording of one rather than several life events (Marcenes & Sheiham 1992). In this regard a recent case control study has investigated the possible role of several life events on chronic periodontitis (Croucher et al 1997). 100 dental patients, matched for age and sex, were used in the study and they reported 43 life events on a positive–negative impact scale. These were then compared with the periodontal status along with oral health behaviour, tobacco use and sociodemographics. The study showed that the severity of chronic periodontitis significantly correlated with the negative impact of life events, the number of negative life events, high level of dental plaque, tobacco smoking and being unemployed. Conversely, positive life events were associated with better periodontal health. The negative life event variables remained statistically significant after adjusting for oral health behaviour and sociodemographic variables but not tobacco smoking.

Hugoson et al (2002) examined 298 older adults from a Swedish epidemiological study in respect of the relationship of negative life events to the severity of periodontal disease. They found that loss of a spouse and the personality trait of exercising extreme external control were significantly associated with severe periodontal disease.

It has been postulated by Locker (1989) that factors in the social environment which lead to stress which then impacts on psychological process and behaviour may lead to an increase in disease susceptibility. It is also possible that negative life events are important determinants of smoking which is itself a major risk factor for periodontitis (see above). The study of Croucher et al (1997) would suggest that psychological factors and oral health risk behaviours cluster together as important determinants of susceptibility to periodontitis.

It also been found that the levels of salivary cortisol were both positively associated with stress and the extent and severity of periodontitis (Hilgert et al 2006).

However, one study (Solis et al 2004) failed to show any association between anxiety and depression symptoms, and psychosocial stress factors and periodontal disease severity.

Peruzzo et al (2007) carried out a systematic review of stress and psychological factors as possible risk factors for periodontal disease. Within the limitations of the systematic review, the majority of studies showed a positive relationship between stress/psychological factors and periodontal disease.

The possible role of psychological stress in producing a poor response to treatment of chronic periodontitis has also been investigated (Axtellius et al 1988). Two groups of patients, one responding well to periodontal treatment (respondent group) and one failing to respond (non-respondent group), were compared. Somatic and psychological data were obtained by interviews and psychological tests and these variables were then statistically compared in the two groups. The results showed that the non-respondent group patients demonstrated a passive, dependent personality and indications of more psychological strain whereas those in the respondent group displayed a more rigid personality and had experienced less stressful events in the past.

Several models have been used to suggest the role of psychosocial factors in periodontal disease. None have adopted the life-course approach, which emphasizes the importance of exposures over time and at critical points of a person's life (Nicolau et al 2007). The study design was a cross-sectional survey of 330 Brazilian women randomly selected from a larger sample of mothers whose children participated in a study on chronic oral disease using a life-course framework. Each woman was clinically assessed for the presence of periodontal disease. An interview collected information on socioeconomic, behavioural and family-related factors at two periods of the participant's life (childhood and adulthood). The main outcome variable was loss of periodontal attachment. Data analysis used logistic regression. High levels of periodontal disease were predicted by <4 years of education, past and present smoking, high levels of paternal discipline in childhood and low levels of emotional support in adulthood. The influence of childhood factors was not attenuated by adulthood circumstances. Thus, psychosocial factors in childhood and adulthood were associated with high levels of periodontal disease in adulthood.

Two other studies have related susceptibility to periodontal disease to depressive mood (Saletu et al 2005) and a poor response to treatment by anxiety (Vettore et al 2005).

Stress factors have been shown to affect the immune system by a number of mechanisms. In this regard, Houri-Haddad et al (2003) have shown that mice immunized with *P. gingivalis* and exposed to isolation and restraint stress exhibited a lower IgG1/IgG2a ratio to this bacterium. This suggests an elevated Th1 response during stress.

All other host factors are described in Chapter 6.

REFERENCES

Adams DF: Diagnosis and treatment of refractory periodontitis, *Curr Opin Dent* 2:33–38, 1992.

Ah MKB, Johnson GK, Kaldahl WB, et al: The effect of smoking on the response to periodontal therapy, *J Clin Periodontol* 21:91–97, 1994.

Ahlberg J, Tuominen R, Murtomaa H: Periodontal status among male industrial workers in Southern inland with or without access to subsidized dental care, *Acta Odontol Scand* 54:166–170, 1996.

Ahlquist M, Bengtsson C, Hollender L, et al: Smoking habits and tooth loss in Swedish women, *Community Dent Oral Epidemiol* 17:144–147, 1989.

Ainamo J: The seeming effect of tobacco consumption on the occurrence of periodontal disease and caries, *Suomen Hammaslaakariseeuran Toimituksia* 67:87–94, 1971.

Alpagot AL, Wolffe LF, Smith QT, et al: Risk indicators for periodontal disease in a racially diverse urban population, *J Clin Periodontol* 23:983–988, 1996.

Al-Rasheed A, Scheerens H, Rennick DM, et al: Accelerated alveolar bone loss in mice lacking interleukin-10, *J Dent Res* 82:632–635, 2003.

Alvesalo I, Reisin S, Hay J, et al: Effects of fluoride and regular dental care on personal dental expenditures of young adults in Finland, *Community Dent Oral Epidemiol* 10:15–22, 1982.

Alvi AL, Palmer RM, Odell EW, et al: Elastase in gingival crevicular fluid from smokers and non smokers with chronic inflammatory periodontal disease, *Oral Dis* 1:110–114, 1995.

Andersen BL, Kiecolt-Glaser JK, Glaser R: A biobehavioural model of cancer stress and disease course, *American Psychologist* 49:389–404, 1994.

Andersen P, Pederson OF, Bach B, et al: Serum antibodies and immunoglobulins in smokers and non-smokers, *Clin Exp Immunol* 47:467–473, 1982.

Andreou V, D'Addario M, Zohar R, et al: Inhibition of osteogenesis in vitro by a cigarette smoke-associated hydrocarbon combined with Porphyromonas gingivalis lipopolysaccharide: reversal by Resveratrol, *J Periodontol* 75:939–948, 2004.

Anerud A, Löe H, Boysen H: The natural history and clinical course of calculus formation in man, *J Clin Periodontol* 18:160–170, 1991.

Armitage AK, Dollery CT, George CF, et al: Absorption and metabolism of nicotine from cigarettes, *Br Med J* 4:313–316, 1975.

Armitage AK, Turner DM: Absorption of nicotine in cigarette and cigar smoke through oral mucosa, *Nature* 226:1231–1232, 1970.

Armitage GC, Wu Y, Wang HY, et al: Low prevalence of periodontitis-associated interleukin-1 composite genotype in individuals of Chinese heritage, *J Periodontol* 71:164–171, 2000.

Arno A, Waerhaug J, Lovdal A, et al: Incidence of gingivitis as related to sex, occupation, tobacco consumption, toothbrushing and age, *Oral Surg Oral Med Oral Pathol* 11:587–595, 1958.

Arno A, Schei O, Lovdal A, et al: Alveolar bone loss as a function of tobacco consumption, *Acta Odontol Scand* 17:3–10, 1959.

Axtellius B, Soderfeldt B, Nilsson A, et al: Therapy-resistant periodontitis. Psychological characteristics. *J Clin Periodontol* 25:482–491, 1988.

Baab DA, Oberg PA: The effect of cigarette smoking on the gingival blood flow in humans, *J Clin Periodontol* 14:418–424, 1987.

Bardell D: Viability of six species of normal oropharyngeal bacteria to cigarette smoke in vitro, *Microbios* 32:7–13, 1981.

Bartecchi CE, MacKenzie TD, Schrier RW: The human costs of tobacco use, *N Engl J Med* 331:907–912, 1994.

Bastiaan RJ: The effects of tobacco smoking on the periodontal tissues, *J West Soc Periodontol Periodontal Abstr* 27:120–125, 1979.

Bastiaan RJ, Waite IM: Effects of tobacco smoking on plaque development and gingivitis, *J Periodontol* 49:480–482, 1978.

Beck JD, Koch GC, Rozier RG, et al: Prevalence and risk indicators for periodontal attachment loss in a population of older community-dwelling blacks and whites, *J Periodontol* 61:521–528, 1990.

Beck JD, Cusmano L, Green-Helms W, et al: A 5-year study of attachment loss in community-dwelling older adults; incidence density, *J Periodontal Res* 32:506–515, 1997.

Berglundh T, Donati M, Hahn-Zoric M, et al: Association of the -1087 IL-10 gene polymorphism with severe chronic periodontitis in Swedish Caucasians, *J Clin Periodontol* 30:249–254, 2003.

Bergström J: Short-term investigation on the influence of cigarette smoking upon plaque accumulation, *Scand J Dent Res* 89:235–238, 1981.

Bergström J: Cigarette smoking as a risk factor in chronic periodontal disease, *Community Dent Oral Epidemiol* 17:245–247, 1989.

Bergström J: Oral hygiene compliance and gingivitis expression in cigarette smokers, *Scand J Dent Res* 98:497–503, 1990.

Bergström J, Eliasson S: Noxious effect of cigarette smoking and periodontal health, *J Periodontal Res* 22:513–517, 1987a.

Bergström J, Eliasson S: Cigarette smoking and alveolar bone height in subjects with a high standard of oral hygiene, *J Clin Periodontol* 14:466–469, 1987b.

Bergström J, Preber H: Influence of cigarette smoking on the development of experimental gingivitis, *J Periodontal Res* 21:668–676, 1986.

Bergström J, Preber H: Tobacco use as a risk factor, *J Periodontol* 65:545–550, 1994.

Bergström J, Elíasson S, Preber H: Cigarette smoking and periodontal bone loss, *J Periodontol* 62:242–246, 1991.

Bergström J, Floderus-Myrhed B: Co-twin study of the relationship between smoking and some periodontal disease factors, *Community Dent Oral Epidemiol* 11:113–116, 1983.

Bergström J, Eliasson S, Dock J: 10-year prospective study of tobacco smoking and periodontal health, *J Periodontol* 71:1338–1347, 2000.

Bernzweig E, Payne JB, Reinhardt RA, et al: Nicotine and smokeless tobacco effects on gingival and peripheral blood mononuclear cells, *J Clin Periodontol* 25:246–252, 1998.

Bickel M, Axtelius B, Solioz C, Attström R: Cytokine gene expression in chronic periodontitis, *J Clin Periodontol* 28:246–252, 2001.

Bolin A, Lavsted S, Frithiof L, et al: Proximal alveolar bone loss in a longitudinal radiographic investigation. IV. Smoking and some other factors influencing the progress in individuals with at least 20 remaining teeth, *Acta Odontol Scand* 44:263–269, 1986.

Bolin A, Eklund G, Frithiof L, et al: The effects of changed smoking habits on marginal alveolar bone loss, *Swed Dent J* 17:211–216, 1993.

Bolinger G, Alfredsson L, Englund A, et al: Smokeless tobacco use and increased cardiovascular mortality amongst Swedish construction workers, *Am J Public Health* 84:399–404, 1994.

Boström L, Linder LE, Bergström J: Influence of smoking on the outcome of periodontal surgery. A 5-year follow-up, *J Clin Periodontol* 25:194–201, 1998a.

Boström L, Linder LE, Bergström J: Clinical expression of TNF-a in smoking-associated periodontal disease, *J Clin Periodontol* 25:767–773, 1998b.

Bragd L, Dahlén G, Wikström M, et al: The capability of Actinobacillus actinomycetemcomitans, Bacteroides gingivalis and Bacteroides intermedius to indicate progressive periodontitis, *J Clin Periodontol* 14:95–99, 1987.

Brandtzaeg P, Jamison HC: A study of periodontal health and oral hygiene in Norwegian army recruits, *J Periodontol* 35:302–307, 1964.

Bridges RB, Kraal JH, Huang LJT, et al: The effects of tobacco smoke on chemotaxis and glucose metabolism of polymorphonuclear leucocytes, *Infection and Immunology* 15:115–123, 1977.

Calonius PEB: A cytological study on the variation of keratinization in the normal oral mucosa of young males, *J West Soc Periodontol* 10:69–74, 1962.

Cao Z, Li C, Jin L, et al: Association of matrix metalloproteinase-1 promoter polymorphism with generalized aggressive periodontitis in a Chinese population, *J Periodontal Res* 40:427–431, 2005.

Centers for Disease Control, Tobacco use among high school students-United States, *MMWR Morb Mortal Wkly Rep* 40:617–619, 1989.

Centers for Disease Control and Prevention, *MMWR Morb Mortal Wkly Rep* 42:230–232, 1993.

Christen AG, Armstrong WR, McDaniel RK: Intraoral leukoplakia, abrasion, periodontal breakdown and tooth loss in a snuff dipper, *J Am Dent Assoc* 98:584–586, 1979.

Clarke NG, Shephard BC, Hirsch RS: The effects of intra-arterial epinephrine and nicotine on gingival circulation, *Oral Surg Oral Med Oral Pathol* 52:577–582, 1981.

Codd EE, Swim AT, Bridges RB: Tobacco smokers neutrophils are desensitised to chemotactic peptide-stimulated oxygen uptake, *J Lab Clin Med* 110:648–652, 1987.

Costabel U, Bross KJ, Reuter C, et al: Alterations in immunoregulatory T-cell subsets in cigarette smokers. A phenotypic analysis of bronchoalveolar and blood lymphocytes. *Chest* 90:39–44, 1986.

Council on Scientific Affairs, The worldwide smoking epidemic. Tobacco trade, use and control, *JAMA* 263:3312–3318, 1990.

Cox SW: Extending the scope of gingival crevicular fluid elastase research, *Oral Dis* 1:103–105, 1995.

Creath CJ, Cutter G, Bradley DH, et al: Oral leukoplakia and adolescent smokeless tobacco use, *Oral Surg Oral Med Oral Pathol* 72:35–41, 1991.

Croucher R, Marcenes WS, Torres MCMB, et al: The relationship between life-events and periodontitis. A case-control study. *J Clin Periodontol* 54:481–487, 1997.

Cullinan MP, Westerman B, Hamlet SM, et al: Progression of periodontal disease and interleukin-10 gene polymorphism, *J Periodontal Res* 43:328–333, 2008.

Daniell HW: Post menopausal tooth loss. Contribution to edentulism by osteoporosis and cigarette smoking, *Arch Intern Med* 143:1678–1682, 1983.

Danielsen B, Manji F, Nagelkerke N, et al: Effect of cigarette smoking on transition dynamics in experimental gingivitis, *J Clin Periodontol* 17:159–164, 1990.

Dashash M, Drucker DB, Hutchinson IV, et al: Interleukin-1 receptor antagonist gene polymorphism and gingivitis in children, *Oral Dis* 13:308–313, 2007.

de Brito Junior RB, Scarel-Caminaga RM, Trevilatto PC, et al: Polymorphisms in the vitamin D receptor gene are associated with periodontal disease, *J Periodontol* 75:1090–1095, 2004.

De Carlo AA, Grenett H, Park J, et al: Association of gene polymorphisms for plasminogen activators with alveolar bone loss, *J Periodontal Res* 42:305–310, 2007.

de Souza AP, Trevilatto PC, Scarel-Caminaga RM, et al: Analysis of the TGF-b1 promotor polymorphism (C-509T) in patients with chronic periodontitis, *J Clin Periodontol* 30:519–523, 2003b.

Dolan TA, Gilbert GH, Ringelberg ML, et al: Behavioural risk indicators of attachment loss in Floridians, *J Clin Periodontol* 24:223–232, 1997.

Donati M, Berglundh T, Hytönen AM, et al: Association of the -159 CD14 gene polymorphism and lack of association of the -308 TNFα, Q551R IL-4RA polymorphisms with severe chronic periodontitis in Swedish Caucasians, *J Clin Periodontol* 32:474–479, 2005.

Dzink JL, Tanner ARC, Haffajee AD, et al: Gram negative species associated with active destructive periodontal lesions, *J Clin Periodontol* 12:648–659, 1985.

Dzink JL, Haffajee AD, Socransky SS: The predominant cultivable microbiota of active and inactive lesions of destructive periodontal diseases, *J Clin Periodontol* 15:316–323, 1988.

Ehmke B, Kress W, Karch H, et al: Interleukin-1-haplotype and periodontal disease progression following therapy, *J Clin Periodontol* 26:810–813, 1999.

Eichel G, Shahrick HA: Tobacco smoke toxicity: loss of human oral leucocyte function and fluid cell metabolism, *Science* 166:1424–1428, 1969.

Engebretson SP, Lamster IB, Herrera-Abreu M, et al: Interleukin gene polymorphism on expression of interleukin-1b and tumor necrosis factor alpha in periodontal tissue and gingival crevicular fluid, *J Periodontol* 70:567–573, 1999.

Ernster V, Grady DG, Green JC, et al: Smokeless tobacco use and health effects amongst baseball players, *JAMA* 264:218–224, 1990.

Fang MA, Frost PJ, Iida-Klein A, et al: Effects of nicotine on cellular function in UMR 106–101 osteoclast-like cells, *Bone* 12:283–286, 1991.

Feldman RS, Bravacos JS, Rose CL: Association between smoking different tobacco products and periodontal disease indexes, *J Periodontol* 54:481–487, 1983.

Feldman RS, Alman JE, Chauncey HH: Periodontal disease indexes and tobacco smoking in healthy aging men, *Gerodontics* 3:43–46, 1987.

Ferson MA, Edwards A, Lind GW, et al: Low natural killer cell activity and immunoglobulin levels associated with smoking in human subjects, *Int J Cancer* 23:603–609, 1979.

Fokkema SJ, Timmerman MF, Van der Weijden FA, et al: A possible association of a1-antitrypsin deficiency with the periodontal condition in adults, *J Clin Periodontol* 25:617–623, 1998.

Folwaczny M, Glas J, Török HP, et al: Lack of association between the TNF α G -308 A promoter polymorphism and periodontal disease, *J Clin Periodontol* 31:449–453, 2004a.

Folwaczny M, Glas J, Török HP, et al: The CD14 [−] 159C-to-T promoter polymorphism in periodontal disease, *J Clin Periodontol* 31:991–995, 2004b.

Folwaczny M, Glas J, Török HP, et al: Polymorphisms of the interleukin-18 gene in periodontitis patients, *J Clin Periodontol* 32:530–534, 2005.

Galbraith GM, Hendley TM, Sanders JJ, et al: Polymorphic cytokine genotypes as markers of disease severity in adult periodontitis, *J Clin Periodontol* 26:705–709, 1999.

Genco RJ, Zambon JJ, Christersson LA: The role of specific bacteria in periodontal disease: The origin of periodontal infections, *Adv Dent Res* 2:245–259, 1988.

Genco RJ, Grossi SG, Ho A, et al: A proposed model linking inflammation to obesity, diabetes, and periodontal infections, *J Periodontol* 76:2075–2084, 2005.

Ginns LC, Goldenheim PD, Miller LG: T-lymphocyte subsets in smoking and lung cancer. Analysis of monoclonal antibodies and flow cytometry, *Am Rev Respir Dis* 126:265–269, 1982.

Gonzalez YM, De-Nardin A, Grossi SG, et al: Serum cotinine levels, smoking and periodontal attachment loss, *J Dent Res* 75:796–802, 1996.

Gonzales JR, Michel J, Diete A, et al: Analysis of genetic polymorphisms at the interleukin-10 loci in aggressive and chronic periodontitis, *J Clin Periodontol* 29:816–822, 2002.

Goodson JM, Haffajee AD, Socransky SS: Periodontal therapy by local delivery of tetracycline, *J Clin Periodontol* 6:83–92, 1979.

Goodson JM, Tanner ACR, Haffajee AD, et al: Patterns of progression and regression of advanced destructive periodontal disease, *J Clin Periodontol* 9:472–481, 1982.

Gore EA, Sanders JJ, Pandey JP, et al: Interleukin-1b+3953 allene2: association with disease status in adult periodontitis, *J Clin Periodontol* 25:781–795, 1988.

Goultschin J, Cohen HD, Donchin M, et al: Association of smoking with periodontal treatment needs, *J Periodontol* 61:364–367, 1990.

Graswinckel JEM, van der Velden U, van Winkelhoff AJ, et al: Plasma antibody levels in periodontitis patients and controls, *J Clin Periodontol* 31:562–568, 2004.

Grossi SG, Zambon JJ, Ho AW, et al: Assessment of risk for periodontal disease. I. Risk indicators for attachment loss, *J Periodontol* 65:260–267, 1994.

Grossi SG, Genco RJ, Machtei EE, et al: Assessment of risk for periodontal disease. I. Risk indicators for alveolar bone loss, *J Periodontol* 66:23–29, 1995.

Gulsvik A, Fagerhol MK: Smoking and immunoglobulin level, *Lancet* 1:449, 1979.

Gunsolley JC, Pandey GP, Quinn SM, et al: the effect of race, smoking and immunoglobulin allotypes on IgG subclass concentrations, *J Periodontal Res* 32:381–387, 1997.

Güntsch A, Erler M, Preshaw PM, et al: Effect of smoking on crevicular polymorphonuclear neutrophil function in periodontally healthy subjects, *J Periodontal Res* 41:184–188, 2006.

Haber J: Cigarette smoking: a major risk factor for periodontitis, *Compend Contin Educ Dent* 15:1002–1014, 1994.

Haber J, Kent RL: Cigarette smoking in periodontal practice, *J Periodontol* 63:100–106, 1992.

Haber J, Wattles J, Crowley M, et al: Evidence for cigarette smoking as a major risk factor for periodontitis, *J Periodontol* 64:16–23, 1993.

Hanes PJ, Schuster GS, Lubas S: Binding, uptake, and release of nicotine by human gingival fibroblasts, *J Periodontol* 62:147–152, 1991.

Hart TC, Kornman KS: Genetic factors in the pathogenesis of periodontitis, *Periodontol 2000* 14:202–215, 1997.

Heitz-Mayfield LJA: Disease progression: identification of high-risk groups and individuals for periodontitis, *J Clin Periodontol* 32:196–209, 2005.

Hersey P, Prendergost D, Edwards A: Effects of cigarette smoking on the immune system, *Med J Australia* 15:425–429, 1983.

Hilgert JB, Hugo FN, Bandeira DR, et al: Stress, cortisol, and periodontitis in a population aged 50 years and over, *J Dent Res* 85:324–328, 2006.

Hoge HW, Kirkham DB: Clinical management and soft tissue reconstruction of periodontal damage resulting from habitual use of snuff, *J Am Dent Assoc* 107:744 745, 1983.

Holla LJ, Fassmann A, Benes P, et al: polymorphisms in the transforming growth factor-beta 1 gene (TNF-beta 1) in adult periodontitis, *J Clin Periodontol* 29:336–341, 2002.

Holla LJ, Fassmann A, Stejskalova A, et al: Analysis of the interleukin-6 gene promoter polymorphisms in Czech patients with chronic periodontitis, *J Periodontol* 75:30–36, 2004.

Hollenbach KA, Barrett-Connor E, Edelstein SL, et al: Cigarette smoking and bone mineral density in older men and women, *Am J Public Health* 83:1265–1270, 1993.

Holm G: Smoking as an additional risk for tooth loss, *J Periodontol* 65:996–1001, 1994.

Holmes LG: Effect of smoking and/or vitamin C on crevicular fluid flow in clinically healthy gingiva, *Quintessence Int* 21:191–195, 1990.

Holt RG: Immune and inflammatory function in cigarette smokers, *Thorax* 42:241–249, 1987.

Horning GM, Hatch CL, Cohen ME: Risk indicators for periodontitis in a military treatment population, *J Periodontol* 63:297–302, 1992.

Houri-Haddad Y, Itzchaki O, Ben-Nathan D, et al: The effect of chronic emotional stress on the humoral response to Porphyromonas gingivalis in mice, *J Periodontal Res* 38:204–209, 2003.

Hugoson A, Ljungquist B, Breivik T: The relationship between some negative life events and psychological factors to periodontal disease in an adult Swedish population 50–80 years of age, *J Clin Periodontol* 29:247–253, 2002.

Hutchison DC: alpha1-Antitrypsin deficiency in Europe: geographical distribution of Pi types S and Z, *Respir Med* 92:367–377, 1998.

Imirzalio P, Uckan S, Alaaddino EE, et al: Cigarette smoking and apoptosis, *J Periodontol* 76:737–739, 2005.

International Agency for Research on Cancer, Chemistry and analysis of tobacco smoke, In *IARC Monographs on the Evaluation of the Carcinogenic Risk of Chemicals to Humans. Tobacco Smoking*, vol 8, Lyon, 1986, IARC, pp 86–89.

Ismail AI, Burt BA, Eklund SA: Epidemiologic patterns of smoking and periodontal disease in the United States, *J Am Dent Assoc* 106:617–621, 1983.

Izakovi L, Ová Hollá L, Jurajda M, et al: Genetic variations in the matrix metalloproteinase-1 promoter and risk of susceptibility and/or severity of chronic periodontitis in the Czech population, *J Clin Periodontol* 31:685–690, 2004.

Kim J-S, Park JY, Chung W-Y, et al: Polymorphisms in genes coding for enzymes metabolizing smoking-derived substances and the risk of periodontitis, *J Clin Periodontol* 31:959–964, 2004.

Jepsen S, Eberhard J, Fricke D, et al: Interleukin-1 polymorphisms and experimental gingivitis, *J Clin Periodontol* 30:102–106, 2003.

Jette AM, Feldman HA, Tennstedt SL: Tobacco use: a modified risk factor for dental disease among the elderly, *Am J Public Health* 83:1271–1276, 1993.

Johnson CK, Todd GL, Johnson WT, et al: Effects of topical and systemic nicotine on gingival blood flow in dogs, *J Dent Res* 70:906–909, 1991.

Johnson CK, Organ CC: Prostaglandin E2 and interleukin-1 concentrations in nicotine-exposed oral keratinocyte cultures, *J Periodontal Res* 32:447–454, 1997.

Johnson JD, Houchens DP, Kluwe WM, et al: Effects of mainstream and environmental tobacco smoke on the immune system in animals and humans. A review. *CRC Crit Rev Toxicol* 20:369–395, 1990.

Jones JK, Triplett RG: The relationship of cigarette smoking to intraoral wound healing: a review of evidence and implications for patient care, *J Maxillofac Surg* 50:237–239, 1992.

Kalra J, Chandhary AK, Prasad K: Increased production of oxygen free radicals in cigarette smokers, *Int J Exp Pathol* 72:1–7, 1991.

Kenny EB, Saxe SR, Bowles RD: The effect of cigarette smoking on anaerobiosis in the oral cavity, *J Periodontol* 46:82–85, 1975.

Kenny EB, Kraal JH, Saxe SR, et al: The effects of cigarette smoke on human polymorphonuclear leukocytes, *J Periodontal Res* 12:227–234, 1977.

Kinane DF, Radvar M: The effect of smoking on mechanical and antimicrobial periodontal therapy, *J Periodontol* 68:467–472, 1997.

Kobayashi T, Ito S, Yamamoto K, et al: Risk of periodontitis in systemic lupus erythematosus is associated with Fcgamma receptor polymorphisms, *J Periodontol* 74:378–384, 2003.

Kornman KS, Crane A, Wang HY, et al: The interleukin-1 genotype as a severity factor in adult periodontal disease, *J Clin Periodontol* 24:72–77, 1997a.

Kornman KS, Page RC, Tonetti MS: The host response to the microbial challenge in periodontitis: assembling the players, *Periodontology* 14:33–53, 1997b.

Koundouros E, Odell EW, Coward PY, et al: Soluble adhesion molecules in serum of smokers and non-smokers, with and without periodontitis, *J Periodontal Res* 31:596–599, 1996.

Kowolik MJ, Nisbet T: Smoking and acute ulcerative gingivitis, *Br Dent J* 154:241–242, 1983.

Krall EA, Dawson-Hughes B, Garvey AJ, et al: Smoking, smoking cessation, and tooth loss, *J Dent Res* 76:1653–1659, 1997.

Krall EA, Chancellor MB, Bridges RB, et al: Variations in the gingival polymorphonuclear leukocyte migration rate in dogs induced by autogenous serum and migration inhibitor from tobacco smoke, *J Periodontal Res* 12:242–249, 1977.

Kuschner WG, D'Alessandro A, Wong H, et al: Dose-dependent cigarette-smoking-related inflammatory responses in healthy adults, *Eur Respir J* 9:1989–1994, 1996.

Laine ML, Morré SA, Murillo LS, et al: CD14 and TLR4 gene polymorphisms in adult periodontitis, *J Dent Res* 84:1042–1046, 2005.

Lamster IB: The host response in gingival crevicular fluid: potential applications in periodontitis clinical trials, *J Periodontol* 63:1117–1123, 1992.

Lang NP, Cumming BR, Löe H: Toothbrushing frequency as it relates to plaque development and gingival health, *J Periodontol* 44:396–405, 1973.

Lannan S, McLean A, Drost E, et al: Changes in neutrophil morphology and morphometry following exposure to cigarette smoke, *Int J Exp Pathol* 73:183–191, 1992.

Lehner T, Wilton JMA, Challacombe S, et al: Sequential cell mediated immune responses in experimental gingivitis in man, *Clin Exp Immunol* 16:481–492, 1974.

Li QY, Zhao HS, Meng HX, et al: Association analysis between interleukin-1 family polymorphisms and generalized aggressive periodontitis in a Chinese population, *J Periodontol* 75:1627–1635, 2004.

Linden GJ, Mullally BH: Cigarette smoking and periodontal destruction in young adults, *J Periodontol* 65:718–723, 1994.

Linden G, Patterson C, Evans A, et al: Obesity and periodontitis in 60–70-year-old men, *J Clin Periodontol* 34:461–466, 2007.

Ling TY, Sims TJ, Chen HA, et al: Titre and subclass distribution of serum IgG reactive with Actinobacillus actinomycetemcomitans in localized juvenile periodontitis, *J Clin Immunol* 13:101–112, 1993.

Listgarten MA: Microbial testing in the diagnosis of periodontal disease, *J Periodontol* 63:332–337, 1992.

Listgarten MA, Levin S: Positive correlation between proportions of subgingival spirochaetes and motile bacteria and susceptibility of human subjects to periodontal deterioration, *J Clin Periodontol* 8:122–138, 1981.

Listgarten MA, Schifter CC, Sulivan P, et al: Failure of a microbial assay to reliably predict disease recurrence in a treated periodontitis population receiving regularly scheduled prophylaxes, *J Clin Periodontol* 13:768–773, 1986.

Listgarten MA, Slots J, Nowotny AH, et al: Incidence of periodontitis recurrence in treated patients with and without cultivable Actinobacillus actinomycetemcomitans, Porphyromonas gingivalis and Prevotella intermedia: a prospective study, *J Periodontol* 62:377–386, 1991.

Liu L, Wen X, He H, et al: Species-specific DNA probe for the detection of Porphyromonas gingivalis from adult Chinese periodontal patients and healthy subjects, *J Periodontol* 74:1000–1006, 2003.

Locker D: Stress in dental practice. In *An introduction to behavioural science*. Tavistock, 1989, Rutledge, pp 21–38.

Locker D, Leake JL: Risk indicators and risk markers for periodontal disease experience in a population of older adults living independently in Ontario, *J Dent Res* 72:9–17, 1993.

Löe H, Theilade E, Jensen SB: Experimental gingivitis in man, *J Periodontol* 36:177–187, 1965.

Löe H, Anerud A, Boysen H, et al: The natural history of periodontal disease in Man, *J Periodontol* 49:607–620, 1978.

Loesche WJ: The role of spirochaetes in periodontal disease, *Adv Dent Res* 2:275–283, 1988.

Loos BJ, Leppers-Van de Straat FGA, Van den de Winkel JGJ, et al: Fcgamma receptor polymorphisms in relation to periodontitis, *J Clin Periodontol* 30:595–602, 2003.

Loos BG, John RP, Laine ML: Identification of genetic risk factors for periodontitis and possible mechanisms of action, *J Clin Periodontol* 32:159–179, 2005.

López NJ, Jara L, Valenzuela CY: Association of interleukin-1 polymorphisms with periodontal disease, *J Periodontol* 76:234–243, 2005.

MacFarlane GD, Herzberg MC, Wolff LF, et al: Refractory periodontitis associated with abnormal polymorphonuclear leucocyte phagocytosis and cigarette smoking, *J Periodontol* 63:908–913, 1992.

Macgregor IDM: Toothbrushing efficiency in smokers and non-smokers, *J Clin Periodontol* 11:313–320, 1984.

Macgregor IDM: Survey of toothbrushing habits in smokers and non-smokers, *Clin Prev Dent* 7:27–30, 1985.

Macgregor IDM, Edgar WM, Greenwood AR: Effects of cigarette smoking on the rate of plaque formation, *J Clin Periodontol* 12:259–263, 1985.

Macgregor IDM: Smoking and periodontal disease, In Seymour RA, Heasman PA, editors: *Drugs, Diseases and the Periodontium*, Oxford, 1992, Oxford University Press, pp 118–119.

MacKenzie TD, Bartecchi CE, Schrier RW: The human costs of tobacco use, *N Engl J Med* 331:975–980, 1994.

Machtei EE, Dunford R, Hausmann E, et al: Longitudinal study of prognostic factors in established periodontal patients, *J Clin Periodontol* 24:102–109, 1997.

Mancini NM, Bene MC, Gerard H, et al: Effects of short-term cigarette smoking on the human lung: a study of bronchoalveolar fluids, *Lung* 171:277–291, 1993.

Marcenes WS, Sheiham A: The relationship between work stress and oral health status, *Soc Sci Med* 35:1511 1520, 1992.

Marcenes WS, Croucher R, Sheiham A, et al: The association between self reported oral symptoms and life-events, *Psychology and Health* 8:123–134, 1993.

Martinez-Canut P, Lorca A, Magan R: Smoking and periodontal disease severity, *J Clin Periodontol* 22:743–749, 1995.

Massler M, Ludwick W: Relation of dental caries experience and gingivitis to cigarette smoking in males 17 to 21 years old (at the Great Lakes Naval Training Center), *J Dent Res* 31:319–322, 1952.

McDevitt MJ, Wang H-Y, Knobelman C, et al: Interleukin-1 genetic association with periodontitis in clinical practice. *J Periodontol* 71:156–163, 2000.

McGuire MK, Nunn ME: Prognosis versus actual outcome. IV. The effectiveness of clinical parameters and IL-1 genotype in accurately predicting prognoses and tooth survival, *J Periodontol* 70:49–56, 1999.

McLaughlin WS, Lovat FM, Macgregor IDM, et al: The immediate effects of smoking on gingival fluid flow, *J Clin Periodontol* 20:448–451, 1993.

McSharry C, Banham SW, Boyd G: Effect of cigarette smoking on antibody response to inhaled antigens and the prevalence of extrinsic allergic alveolitis among pigeon breeders, *Clin Allergy* 15:487–494, 1985.

Meisel P, Schwahn C, Gesch D, et al: Dose-effect relation of smoking and the interleukin-1 gene polymorphism in periodontal disease, *J Periodontol* 75:236–242, 2004.

Meisel P, Schwahn C, Luedemann J, et al: Magnesium deficiency is associated with periodontal disease, *J Dent Res* 84:937–941, 2005.

Meuric VP, Gracieux Z, Tamanai-Shacoori J, et al: Expression patterns of genes induced by oxidative stress in Porphyromonas gingivalis, *Oral Medicine and Immunity* 23: 308–314, 2008.

Michalowicz BS, Aeppli D, Virag JG, et al: Periodontal findings in adult twins, *J Periodontol* 62:293–299, 1991.

Michalowicz BS: Genetic and heritable risk factors in periodontal disease, *J Periodontol* 65(Suppl 5):479–488, 1994.

Miller PD Jr: Root coverage with free gingival graft. Factors associated with incomplete coverage. *J Periodontol* 58:674–681, 1987.

Mohlin B, Ingervall B, Hedegård B, et al: Tooth loss, prosthetics and dental treatment habits in a group of Swedish men, *Community Dent Oral Epidemiol* 7:101–106, 1979.

Molloy J, Wolff LF, Lopez-Guzman A, et al: The association of periodontal disease parameters with systemic medical conditions and tobacco use, *J Clin Periodontol* 31:625–632, 2004.

Moore WEC, Moore LH, Ranney RR: The microflora of periodontal sites showing active destruction progression, *J Clin Periodontol* 18:729–739, 1991.

Moreira PR, de Sá AR, Xavier GM, et al: A functional interleukin-1 [beta] gene polymorphism is associated with chronic periodontitis in a sample of Brazilian individuals, *J Periodontal Res* 40:306–311, 2005.

Moreira PR, Costa JE, Gomez RS, et al: The IL1A (+889) gene polymorphism is associated with chronic periodontal disease in a sample of Brazilian individuals, *J Periodontal Res* 42:23–30, 2007.

Newman MG, Kornman KS, Holzman S: Association of clinical risk factors with treatment outcomes, *J Periodontol* 65:489–497, 1994.

Nibali L, Griffiths GS, Donos N, et al: Association between interleukin-6 promoter haplotypes and aggressive periodontitis, *J Clin Periodontol* 35:193–198, 2008.

Nibali L, Parkar M, Brett P, et al: NADPH oxidase (CYBA) and Fcgamma R polymorphisms as risk factors for aggressive periodontitis: A case-control association study, *J Clin Periodontol* 33:529–539, 2006.

Nibali L, Ready DR, Parkar M, et al: Gene polymorphisms and the prevalence of key periodontal pathogens, *J Dent Res* 86:416–420, 2007.

Nicolau B, Netuveli G, Kim J-WM, et al: A life-course approach to assess psychosocial factors and periodontal disease, *J Clin Periodontol* 34:844–850, 2007.

Nishida N, Tanaka M, Hayashi N, et al: Association of ALDH2 genotype and alcohol consumption with periodontitis, *J Dent Res* 83:161–165, 2004.

Norderyd O, Hugoson A: Risk of severe periodontal disease in a Swedish adult population. A cross-sectional study. *J Clin Periodontol* 25:1022–1028, 1998.

Nossal GVA: Life, death and the immune system, *Sci Am* (Sept):21–30, 1993.

Nowak D, Ruta U, Piasecka G: Nicotine increases human polymorphonuclear leukocytes' chemotactic response – possible additional mechanism of lung injury in cigarette smokers, *Exp Pathol* 39:37–43, 1990.

Offenbacher S, Weathers DR: Effects of smokeless tobacco on the periodontal and caries status of adolescent males, *J Oral Pathol* 14:169–181, 1985.

Österberg T, Mellstrom D: Tobacco smoking: a major risk factor for loss of teeth in three 70-year-old cohorts, *Community Dent Oral Epidemiol* 14:367–370, 1986.

Page RC, Schroeder HE: *Periodontitis in man and other animals*. Basel, 1986, Karger.

Palmer RM, *Tobacco smoking and oral health*, 1987, Health Education Authority, Occasional Paper No. 6.

Palmer RM, Wilson RF, Hasan AS, et al: Mechanisms of action of environmental factors tobacco smoking, *J Clin Periodontol* 32:180–195, 2005.

Pankow W, Neumann K, Ruschoff J, et al: Reduction in HLA-DR density on alveolar macrophages in smokers, *Lung* 169:255–262, 1991.

Papapanou PN, Wennström JJ, Gröndahl K, et al: A 10 year retrospective study of periodontal disease progression, *J Clin Periodontol* 16:403–411, 1989.

Papapanou PN, Baelam V, Luan WM, et al: Subgingival microbiota in adult Chinese: prevalence and relation to periodontal disease progression, *J Periodontol* 68:651–666, 1997.

Papapanou PN, Neiderud A-M, Sandros J, et al: Interleukin-1 gene polymorphism and periodontal status. A case control study. *J Clin Periodontol* 28:389–396, 2001.

Park O-J, Shin S-Y, Choi Y, et al: The association of osteoprotegerin gene polymorphisms with periodontitis, *Oral Dis* 14:440–444, 2008.

Payne JB, Johnson GK, Reinhardt RA, et al: Smokeless tobacco effects on monocyte secretion of PGE2 and IL-1β, *J Periodontol* 65:937–941, 1994.

Peacock ME, Sutherland DE, Schuster GS, et al: The effect of nicotine on reproduction and attachment of human gingival fibroblasts in vitro, *J Periodontol* 64:658–665, 1993.

Peruzzo DC, Bruno BB, Glaucia MB, et al: A systematic review of stress and psychological factors as possible risk factors for periodontal disease, *J Periodontol* 78:1491–1504, 2007.

Peterson RJ, Marsh CL: The relationship of a1-antitrypsin to inflammatory periodontal disease, *J Periodontol* 50:31–35, 1979.

Pindborg JJ: Tobacco and gingivitis. I. Statistical examination of the significance of tobacco in the development of acute ulceromembranous gingivitis and in the formation of calculus, *J Dent Res* 26:261–264, 1947.

Pindborg JJ: Tobacco and gingivitis. II. Correlation between consumption of tobacco, acute ulceromembranous gingivitis and calculus, *J Dent Res* 28:460–463, 1949.

Pontes CC, Gonzales JR, Novaes AB, et al: Interleukin-4 gene polymorphism and its relation to periodontal disease in a Brazilian population of African heritage, *J Dent* 32:241–246, 2004.

Preber H, Bergström J: Occurrence of gingival bleeding in smoker and non-smoker patients, *Acta Odontol Scand* 43:315–320, 1985.

Preber H, Bergström J: Cigarette smoking in patients referred for periodontal treatment, *Scand J Dent Res* 94:102–108, 1986a.

Preber H, Bergström J: The effect of non-surgical treatment on periodontal pockets in smokers and non-smokers, *J Clin Periodontol* 13:319–323, 1986b.

Preber H, Bergström J: Effect of cigarette smoking on periodontal healing following surgical therapy, *J Clin Periodontol* 17:324–328, 1990.

Preber H, Bergström J, Linder LE: Occurrence of periopathogens in smoker and non-smoker patients, *J Clin Periodontol* 19:667–671, 1992.

Preber H, Kant T: Effect of tobacco smoking on the periodontal tissue of 15-year old children, *J Periodontal Res* 8:278–283, 1973.

Preber H, Kant T, Bergström J, et al: Cigarette smoking, oral hygiene and periodontal health in Swedish army conscripts, *J Clin Periodontol* 7:106–113, 1980.

Price P, Calder DM, Witt CS, et al: Periodontal attachment loss in HIV-infected patients associated with the major histocompatibility complex 8.1 haplotype (HLA-A1, B8, DR3), *Tissue Antigens* 54:391–399, 1999.

Quappe L, Jara L, López NJ: Association of interleukin-1 polymorphisms with aggressive periodontitis, *J Periodontol* 75:1509–1515, 2004.

Quinn SM, Zhang JB, Gunsolley JC, et al: Influence of smoking and race on immunoglobulin G subclass concentrations in early-onset periodontitis patients, *Infect Immun* 64:2500–2505, 1996.

Ragnarsson E, Elíasson ST, Ólafsson SH: Tobacco smoking a factor in tooth loss in Reykjavic, Iceland, *Scand J Dent Res* 100:322–326, 1992.

Raulin LA, McPherson JC, McQuade MJ, et al: The effect of nicotine on the attachment of human fibroblasts to glass and human root surfaces in vitro, *J Periodontol* 59: 318–325, 1988.

Robertson MD, Boyd JE, Collins HPR, et al: Serum immunoglobulin levels and humeral immune competence in coal workers, *Am J Ind Med* 6:387–393, 1984.

Robertson PB, Walsh M, Greene J, et al: Periodontal effects associated with the use of smokeless tobacco, *J Periodontol* 61:438–443, 1990.

Roome AJ, Walsh SJ, Cartter ML, et al: Hepatitis B vaccine responsiveness in Connecticut public safety personnel, *JAMA* 270:2931–2934, 1993.

Ryder MI: Nicotine effects on neutrophil F-actin formation and calcium release: implications for tobacco use and respiratory disease, *Exp Lung Res* 20:283–296, 1994.

Ryder MI: Position paper Tobacco use and the periodontal patient, *J Periodontol* 67:51–56, 1996.

Sahingur S, Scharma A, Genco RG, et al: Association of increased levels of fibrinogen and the -455G/A fibrinogen gene polymorphism with chronic periodontitis, *J Periodontol* 74:329–337, 2003.

Sakai Y, Shimauchi H, Ito HO, et al: Porphyromonas gingivalis specific IgG subclass antibody levels as immunological risk indicators of periodontal bone loss, *J Clin Periodontol* 28:853–859, 2001.

Sakellari D, Koukoudetsos S, Arsenakis M, et al: Prevalence of IL-1α and IL-1β polymorphisms in a Greek population, *J Clin Periodontol* 30:35–41, 2003.

Saletu A, Pirker-Frühauf H, Saletu F, et al: Controlled clinical and psychometric studies on the relation between periodontitis and depressive mood, *J Clin Periodontol* 32:1219–1225, 2005.

Sasaki H, Okamatsu Y, Kawai T, et al: The interleukin-10 knockout mouse is highly susceptible to Porphyromonas gingivalis-induced alveolar bone loss, *J Periodontal Res* 39:432–441, 2004.

Scarel-Caminaga RM, Trevilatto PC, Souza AP, et al: Investigation of an IL-2 polymorphism in different levels of chronic periodontitis, *J Clin Periodontol* 29:587–591, 2002.

Scarel-Caminaga RM, Trevilatto PC, Souza AP, et al: Investigation of the IL-4 gene polymorphisms in individuals with different levels of chronic periodontitis in a Brazilian population, *J Clin Periodontol* 30:341–345, 2003.

Scarel-Caminaga RM, Trevilatto PC, Souza AP, et al: Interleukin 10 gene promoter polymorphisms are associated with chronic periodontitis, *J Clin Periodontol* 31:443–448, 2004.

Schei O, Waerhaug J, Lovdal A, et al: Alveolar bone loss as a function of tobacco consumption, *Acta Odontol Scand* 17:3–10, 1959.

Schmidt EF, Bretz WA, Hutchinson RA, et al: Correlation of the hydrolysis of benzoyl-arginine-naphthylamide (BANA) by plaque with clinical parameters and subgingival levels spirochaetes in periodontal patients, *J Dent Res* 67:1505–1509, 1988.

Scott DA, von Ahsen N, Palmer RM, et al: Analysis of two common a1-antitrypsin deficiency alleles (PI*Z and PI*S) in subjects with periodontitis, *J Clin Periodontol* 29:1118–1121, 2002.

Sculley C, Porter R, Mutlu S: Changing subject-based risk factors for destructive disease. In Johnson N, editor: *Risk Markers for Periodontal Diseases, Vol. 3. Periodontal Diseases*, Cambridge, 1991, Cambridge University Press, pp 139–179.

Selby C, Drost E, Brown D, et al: Inhibition of neutrophil adherence and movement by acute cigarette smoke exposure, *Exp Lung Res* 18:813–827, 1992.

Seymour GL: Importance of host response in the periodontium, *J Clin Periodontol* 18:421–426, 1991.

Sheiham A: Periodontal disease and oral cleanliness in tobacco smokers, *J Periodontol* 42:259–263, 1971.

Shimada Y, Tai H, Endo M, et al: Association of tumor necrosis factor receptor type 2 +587 gene polymorphism with severe chronic periodontitis, *J Clin Periodontol* 31:463–469, 2004.

Slots J: Bacterial specificity in adult periodontitis. A summary of recent work. *J Clin Periodontol* 13:912–917, 1986.

Slots J, Emrich LJ, Genco R: Relationship between some subgingival bacteria and periodontal pocket depth and gain or loss of attachment after treatment of adult periodontitis, *J Clin Periodontol* 12:540–552, 1985.

Slots J, Bragd L, Wikström M, et al: The occurrence of Actinobacillus actinomycetemcomitans, Bacteroides gingivalis and Bacteroides intermedius in destructive periodontal disease in adults, *J Clin Periodontol* 13:570–577, 1986.

Slots J, Listgarten MA: Bacteroides gingivalis, Bacteroides intermedius and Actinobacillus actinomycetemcomitans in human periodontal disease, *J Clin Periodontol* 15:85–93, 1988.

Socransky SS: Relationship of bacteria to the aetiology of periodontal disease, *J Dent Res* 49:203–222, 1970.

Socransky SS: Criteria for infectious agents in dental caries and periodontal disease, *J Clin Periodontol* 6:16–21, 1979.

Socransky SS, Haffajee AD: Microbial risk factors for destructive periodontal diseases. In Bader JD, editor: *Risk Assessment in Dentistry*, Chapel Hill, 1990, University of North Carolina Dental Ecology, pp 79–90.

Socransky SS, Tanner ACR, Haffajee AD, et al: Present status of studies on the microbial etiology of periodontal diseases, In Genco RJ, Mergenhagen SE, editors: *Host-Parasite Interactions in Periodontal Diseases*, Washington DC, 1982, American Society for Microbiology, pp 1–12.

Soga Y, Nishimura F, Ohyama H, et al: Tumor necrosis factor-alpha gene (TNF-alpha) -1031/-863, -857 single-nucleotide polymorphisms (SNPs) are associated with severe adult periodontitis [in Japanese], *J Clin Periodontol* 30:524–531, 2003.

Solis ACO, Lotufo RFM, Pannuti CM, et al: Association of periodontal disease to anxiety and depression symptoms, and psychosocial stress factors, *J Clin Periodontol* 31:633–638, 2004.

Solomon HA, Priore RL, Bross ID: Cigarette smoking and periodontal disease, *J Am Dent Assoc* 77:1081–1084, 1968.

Stammers A: Vincent's infection: observations and conclusions regarding the aetiology and treatment of 1,017 civilian cases, *Br Dent J* 76:147–155, 1944.

Stoltenberg JL, Osborn JB, Philstrom BL, et al: Association between cigarette smoking, bacterial pathogens and periodontal status, *J Periodontol* 64:1225–1230, 1993.

Struve J, Aronsson B, Frenning B, et al: Intramuscular versus intradermal administration of recombinant hepatitis B vaccine: a comparison of response rates and analyses of factors influencing the antibody response, *Scand J Infect Dis* 24:423–429, 1992.

Summers CJ, Oberman A: Association of oral disease with 12 selected variables: II, Edentulism. *J Dent Res* 47:594–598, 1968.

Swango PA, Kleinman DV, Konzelman JL: HIV and periodontal health. A study of military personnel with HIV. *J Am Dent Assoc* 122:49–54, 1991.

Tai H, Endo M, Shimada Y, et al: Association of interleukin-1 receptor antagonist gene polymorphisms with early onset periodontitis in Japanese, *J Clin Periodontol* 29:882–888, 2002.

Takeuchi-Hatanaka K, Ohyama H, Nishimura F, et al: Polymorphisms in the 5′ flanking region of IL12RB2 are associated with susceptibility to periodontal diseases in the Japanese population, *J Clin Periodontol* 35:317–323, 2008.

Tangada SD, Califano JV, Nakishima K, et al: The effect of smoking on the serum IgG2 reactive with Actinobacillus actinomycetemcomitans in early-onset periodontitis patients, *J Periodontol* 68:842–850, 1997.

Tanner ARC, Socransky SS, Goodson JM: Microbiota of periodontal pockets losing alveolar crestal bone, *J Periodontal Res* 19:279–291, 1984.

Tappia PS, Troughton KL, Langley-Evans SG, et al: Cigarette smoking influences cytokine production and antioxidant defences, *Clin Sci* 88:485–489, 1995.

Telivuo M, Murtomaa H, Lahtinen A: Observations and concepts of the oral health consequences of tobacco use of Finnish periodontists and dentists, *J Clin Periodontol* 19:15–18, 1992.

Tervonen T, Raunio T, Knuuttila M, et al: Polymorphisms in the CD14 and IL-6 genes associated with periodontal disease, *J Clin Periodontol* 34:377–383, 2007.

Tezal M, Grossi SG, Ho AW, et al: Alcohol consumption and periodontal disease the third National Health and Nutrition Examination Survey, *J Clin Periodontol* 31:484–488, 2004.

Theilade E: The non-specific theory in microbial etiology of inflammatory periodontal diseases, *J Clin Periodontol* 13:905–911, 1986.

Thomson WM, Broadbent JM, Welch D, et al: Cigarette smoking and periodontal disease among 32-year-olds: a prospective study of a representative birth cohort, *J Clin Periodontol* 34:828–834, 2007.

Totti N, McCuster KT, Campbell EJ, et al: Nicotine is chemotactic for neutrophils and enhances neutrophil responsiveness to chemotactic peptides, *Science* 227:169–171, 1994.

Trevilatto PC, Scarel-Caminaga RM, de Brito RB, et al: Polymorphism at position -174 of the IL-6 gene is associated with susceptibility to chronic periodontitis in a Brazilian population, *J Clin Periodontol* 30:438–442, 2003.

Umeda M, Chen C, Bakker I, et al: Risk indicators for harboring periodontal pathogens, *J Periodontol* 69:1111–1118, 1998.

van Palenstein Helderman WH: Microbial etiology of periodontal disease, *J Clin Periodontol* 8:261–280, 1981.

Van Winkelhoff AJ, Loos BJ, van der Reijden WA, et al: Porphyromonas gingivalis, Bacteroides forsythus and other putative periodontal pathogens in subjects with and without periodontal destruction, *J Clin Periodontol* 29:1023–1028, 2002.

Vettore M, Quintanilha RS, Monteiro da Silva AM, et al: The influence of stress and anxiety on the response of non-surgical periodontal treatment, *J Clin Periodontol* 32:1226–1235, 2005.

Wagner J, Kaminski WE, Aslanidis C, et al: Prevalence of OPG and IL-1 gene polymorphisms in chronic periodontitis, *J Clin Periodontol* 34:823–827, 2007.

Wennström JL, Dahlén G, Swensson J, et al: Actinobacillus actinomycetemcomitans, Bacteroides gingivalis and Bacteroides intermedius: Predictors of attachment loss? *Oral Microbiol Immunol* 2:158–163, 1987.

WHO: alpha1-Antitrypsin deficiency: memorandum from a WHO meeting, *Bull World Health Organ* 75:397–415, 1998.

Wilton J, Griffiths G, Curtis M, et al: Detection of high risk groups and individuals for periodontal disease. Systemic predisposition and markers of general health, *J Clin Periodontol* 15:339–346, 1988.

Wolff L, Dahlén G, Aeppli D: Bacteria as risk markers for periodontitis, *J Periodontol* 65:498–510, 1994.

Wouters FR, Salonen LF, Frithiof L, et al: Significance of some variables on interproximal alveolar bone height based on cross-sectional epidemiologic data, *J Clin Periodontol* 20:199–206, 1993.

Wray A, McGuirt E: Smokeless tobacco usage associated with oral carcinoma. Incidence, treatment and outcome, *Arch Otolaryngol Head Neck Surg* 119:929–933, 1993.

Yamamoto K, Kobayashi T, Grossi S, et al: Association of Fcgamma receptor IIa genotype with chronic periodontitis in Caucasians, *J Periodontol* 75:517–522, 2004.

Yamazaki K, Tabeta K, Nakajima T, et al: Interleukin-10 gene promoter polymorphism in Japanese patients with adult and early onset periodontitis, *J Clin Periodontol* 28:828–832, 2001.

Ylöstalo P, Suominen-Taipale L, Reunanen A, et al: Association between body weight and periodontal infection, *J Clin Periodontol* 35:297–304, 2008.

Zambon JJ: Microbial risk factors in human periodontal disease, In Bader JD, editor: *Risk Assessment in Dentistry*, Chapel-Hill, 1990, University of North Carolina, pp 91–93.

Zambon JJ, Grossi SG, Machtei EE, et al: Cigarette smoking increases the risk for subgingival infection with periodontal pathogens, *J Periodontol* 67:1050–1054, 1996.

Zhang L, Meng H, Zhao H, et al: Estrogen receptor-alpha gene polymorphisms in patients with periodontitis, *J Periodontal Res* 39:362–366, 2004.

Bacteria are the primary cause of periodontal disease but are rarely found in the tissues in chronic periodontitis except during abscess formation. Only in acute necrotizing ulcerative gingivitis are spirochaetes seen to invade the tissues on a regular basis and then only penetrate superficially. Intact crevicular epithelium is not permeable to bacteria but is permeable to bacterial antigens, metabolites and enzymes. It is assumed that inflammation and tissue destruction are brought about by these products. Plaque bacteria produce a number of factors which may operate on the tissues directly or indirectly by stimulating the immune and inflammatory reactions.

In periodontal disease, there appears to be a fine balance between health and disease dependent upon the nature of the bacterial flora and its virulence and the nature of the host response to it and whether this is predominantly protective or damaging.

The virulence of a microbe represents a combination of complex factors including the agent's transmissibility and the severity of the disease associated with infection and is also significantly influenced by the susceptibility of the colonized host (Curtis et al 2005). Virulence factors may be defined as those products of the organism which are required to complete the various stages of the life cycle leading to pathology in the host. The absence of an accurate experimental model for periodontal disease means that our understanding of the microbial virulence determinants and pathways in this disease remains hypothetical and based largely on observations *in vitro*. However, factors which enable the organism to persist in spite of the elevated immune and inflammatory pressure at sites of disease are liable to be critical. Periodontal bacterial genomics is liable to make a significant impact on the field through an increased appreciation of the role of gene acquisition and gene loss in the evolution of periodontal bacteria and of the consequences of strain variation in gene content on virulence potential.

Current evidence seems to indicate that individuals predisposed to periodontal disease have aberrant immune/inflammatory responses to plaque which is genetically determined (Fredriksson et al 1998). Mechanisms responsible could include inappropriate levels of polymorphonuclear leucocyte (PMN) recruitment, function or turnover. The resultant release of PMN enzymes and reactive oxygen species (ROS) are likely to be responsible for the tissue destruction but this would also be influenced by the genetically predetermined levels of enzyme inhibitors or scavenging antioxidants (Gustafsson et al 1997; Chapple 1996; Chapple et al 2002). Thus in the periodontal tissues there is a fine balance between factors determining health or disease (**Figs 5.1, 5.2**).

The first barrier encountered by the colonizing subgingival bacteria is the epithelium lining of the gingival crevice which protects the underlying connective tissue. These crevicular and junctional epithelia are capable of reacting to the oral bacteria by releasing signalling molecules initiating the host response such as interleukin (IL)-1, IL-8, prostaglandin PGE_2 and granulocyte-macrophage colony stimulating factor (GM-CSF) (see Table 3.1). These are pivotal in establishing the early inflammatory response through vascular changes and leucocyte recruitment and activation. The factors outlined above are considered in more detail below.

DIRECT EFFECTS OF BACTERIA

In order to cause damage bacteria must:

- Colonize the gingival crevice by evading host defences
- Damage the crevicular epithelial barrier
- Produce substances which can either directly or indirectly cause tissue damage.

These will be discussed separately below.

EVASION OF HOST DEFENCES

A number of the putative periodontal pathogens possess potent mechanisms of evading or damaging host defences, including the following:

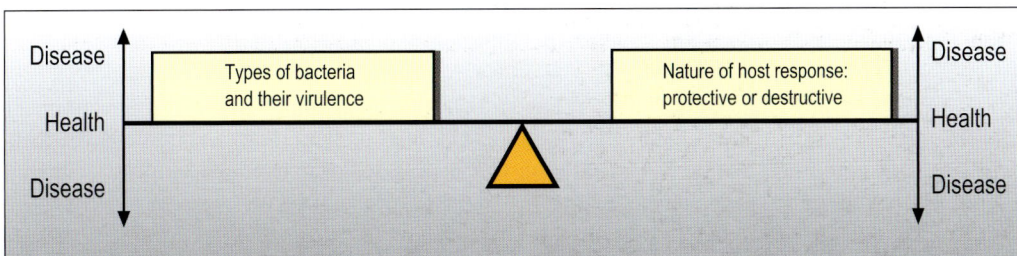

Fig. 5.1 The balance between periodontal health and disease.

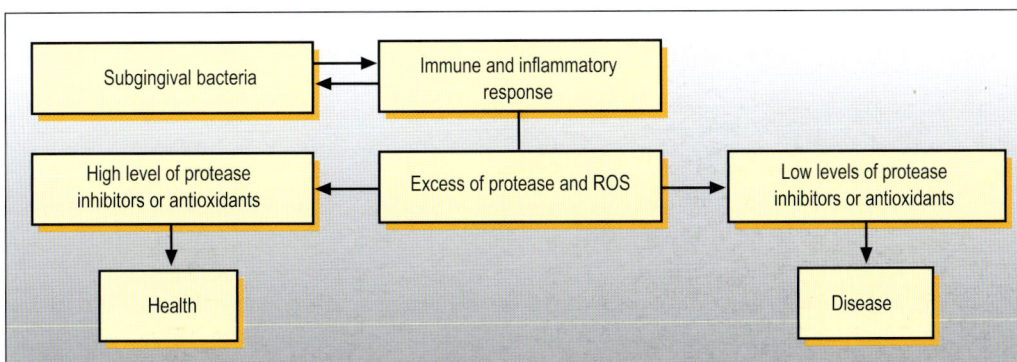

Fig. 5.2 The relationship between genetically determined protease inhibitor and antioxidant levels in the balance between health and disease.

ADHERENCE TO HOST CELLS

Direct damage to polymorphonuclear leucocytes (PMNs) and macrophages

The leucotoxin (see Ch. 23) produced by some strains of *Actinobacillus actinomycetemcomitans* (now *Aggregatibacter actinomycetemcomitans*) can damage PMNs and macrophages (Tsai et al 1979).

Porphyromonas gingivalis adheres to crevicular epithelial cells and this process signals changes in both these cells and the adhering bacteria. The bacteria are then able to initiate infection and colonization and also the epithelial cells will rally their defenses (Hosogi & Duncan 2005). These workers hypothesized that the expression of a defined set of *P. gingivalis* genes would be consistently upregulated during infection of human epithelial cells. *P. gingivalis* genome microarrays were used to compare the gene expression profiles of bacteria that adhered to human epithelial HEp-2 cells and bacteria that were incubated alone. Genes whose expression was temporally upregulated included those involved in the oxidative stress response and those encoding heat shock proteins that are essential to maintaining cell viability under adverse conditions. The results suggest that contact with epithelial cells induces in *P. gingivalis* stress-responsive pathways that promote the survival of the bacterium.

Actinobacillus actinomycetemcomitans (now *Aggregatibacter actinomycetemcomitans*) express a surface-exposed, outer membrane autotransporter protein, designated Aae, which has been implicated in epithelial cell binding (Fine et al 2005). These workers constructed a mutant strain of *A. actinomycetemcomitans* that contained a transposon insertion in the Aae structural gene (aae) and tested the mutant to determine its ability to bind to buccal epithelial cells isolated from healthy volunteers. Significantly fewer mutant cells than wild-type cells bound to these cells. A broad-host-range plasmid that contained an intact aae gene driven by a heterologous tac promoter restored the ability of the mutant strain to bind to buccal epithelial cells at wild-type levels. They also found that this plasmid also conferred upon *Escherichia coli* the ability to express the Aae protein on its surface and to bind to human buccal epithelial cells. Aae-expressing *E. coli* also bound to buccal epithelial cells isolated from six Old World primates but not to the cells isolated from four New World primates or nine other non-primate mammals. It also bound to human gingival epithelial cells but not to human pharyngeal, palatal, tongue, bronchial, or cervical epithelial cells. Their interesting findings indicate that Aae mediates the binding of *A. actinomycetemcomitans* to buccal epithelial cells from humans and Old World primates and that this process may contribute to the host range specificity and tissue tropism exhibited by this bacterium.

Reduced PMN chemotaxis

A number of bacterial species, including *P. gingivalis, A. actinomycetemcomitans* and *Capnocytophaga* species, can reduce PMN chemotaxis and decrease phagocytosis and intracellular killing (Slots & Genco 1984).

Degradation of immunoglobulins

A number of Gram-negative, black pigmented anaerobes and *Capnocytophaga* species produce proteases which can degrade IgG and IgA (Slots & Genco 1984; Kilian 1981; Jansen et al 1995).

Modulation of cytokine function

Cytokines are the major controlling factors of the inflammatory and immune systems (see Ch. 3). There is now growing evidence that infectious agents are able to modify cytokine networks to their advantage

(Henderson et al 1996b; Takahashi & Earnshaw 1996). There is also now evidence that some of the putative periodontal pathogens may have this ability. In this regard, the arginine specific trypsin-like proteinase (RgpA) (see below) of *P. gingivalis* can both cleave and activate certain pro and anti-inflammatory cytokines and activate others (Aduse-Opoku et al 1995, 1996; Rangarajan et al 1997a). The balance between these two opposing functions may influence the inflammatory status of the local cytokine network in the periodontal tissues.

Gingival epithelial cells are the first cells of the periodontium to encounter putative periodontal pathogens and these cells are able to secrete cytokines in response to these encounters which can influence the local host defence mechanisms such as inflammation and neutrophil migration (see above). It has been shown that most periodontal pathogens, including *Fusobacterium nucleatum* and *A. actinomycetemcomitans*, stimulate these cells to secrete IL-8 which is a potent chemoattractant and activator of PMNs and intercellular adhesion molecule 1 (ICAM-1) which is an adhesion molecule involved in leucocyte recruitment from the blood vessels into the tissues (Huang et al 1998; Huang et al 2001; Uchida et al 2001; Sfakianakis et al 2001). These effects involve the upregulation of the mRNA for IL-8 and ICAM-1 in gingival epithelial cells (Huang et al 1998; Huang et al 2001; Uchida et al 2001) and the activation of the p38 MARK MAP signal transducing pathway (Sfakianakis et al 2001). These effects have been shown to be independent of lipopolysaccharides (LPSs) from these bacteria (Sfakianakis et al 2001).

In complete contrast it has been shown that *P. gingivalis* stimulation of human gingival epithelium cells strongly inhibited secretion of both IL-8 and ICAM-1 (Darveau et al 1998; Huang et al 1998; Huang et al 2001). It has also been shown that co-culture of human gingival epithelium cells with *P. gingivalis* over the duration of their culture downregulated the expression of mRNA for IL-8 and ICAM-1 (Darveau et al 1998; Huang et al 2001). In addition, it has been shown that co-culture of *P. gingivalis* with human gingival epithelial cells can significantly reduce the upregulation of mRNA for IL-8 and ICAM-1 produced by other bacteria such as *F. nucleatum* (Huang et al 2001). While the effects of *P. gingivalis* at the protein level could be due to effects from this bacterium's proteases, its effects on the mRNA expression and the kinase signal pathways could not be caused by these proteases (Huang et al 2001).

These effects of *P. gingivalis* are only produced by the adherent stains of the bacterium and specifically effect human gingival epithelium cells. Thus this bacterium does not affect KB epithelial cells line because it does not support the adhesion and invasion of *P. gingivalis* (Darveau et al 1998).

Thus, while most periodontal pathogens stimulate leucocyte recruitment and inflammation *P. gingivalis* inhibits these mechanisms. These effects favour its colonization of the periodontal pocket and gingival epithelial cells by evading the local defence mechanisms.

Degradation of fibrin

Some Gram-negative, black pigmented anaerobes possess fibrinolytic activity (Slots & Genco 1984), which will reduce the trapping of bacteria by fibrin for surface phagocytosis.

Altered lymphocyte function

A number of Gram-negative bacteria and spirochaetes in the subgingival flora can alter lymphocyte function and produce immunosuppression (Schenker 1987). It has been suggested that these mechanisms could produce a temporary delay in the local immune response which might lead to enhanced colonization, possible invasion and tissue injury and account for the episodic nature of periodontal disease progression.

DAMAGE TO CREVICULAR EPITHELIUM

Many bacteria in the subgingival flora seem capable of directly or indirectly damaging crevicular epithelium. Factors directly toxic to epithelium are produced by *P. gingivalis*, *Prevotella intermedia*, *A. actinomycetemcomitans*, *Treponema denticola* and *Capnocytophaga* species (Slots & Genco 1984). This would increase the permeability of the crevicular epithelium to bacterial products and possibly to the bacteria themselves.

In this regard it has been shown (Jarnbring et al 2002) that although there are no differences in the number of proliferating and dying keratinocytes in most parts of the oral mucosa between gingivitis and periodontitis patients there are more apoptotic keratinocytes in periodontitis patients in the most apical part of the sulcular epithelium, close to the junctional epithelium. In these patients, only in this area does the number of apoptotic keratinocytes exceed the number of proliferating ones.

Production of volatile sulphur compounds

Volatile sulphur compounds comprise hydrogen sulphide, H_2S, methyl mercaptan, CH_3SH, dimethyl sulphide $(CH_3)_2S$ and dimethyl disulphide $(CH_3)_2S_2$. They are all thiols containing a characteristic -SH group which is formed when the oxygen atom in the hydroxyl group (-OH) is replaced by sulphur. Oral thiols are all toxic by-products of Gram-negative anaerobic bacterial metabolism of sulphur containing amino acids (cystine, cysteine and methionine) that reside in saliva, gingival crevicular fluid, the gingival and periodontal pocket and tongue surface. This bacterial metabolism is of a putrefactive nature and leads to oxygen depletion (Tonzetich & Carpenter 1971; Tonzetich & Catherall 1976; Tonzetich 1977; Nara 1977; Persson et al 1989; Kleinberg & Westbay 1992).

Porphyromonas gingivalis, *Prevotella intermedia*, *P. melaninogenica*, *Bacteroides forsythus*, *T. denticola* and *F. nucleatum* have all been shown to be capable of producing volatile sulphur compounds through their metabolic pathways (Sawyer et al 1962; Tonzetich & McBride 1981; Pianotti et al 1986; Claesson et al 1990; Persson et al 1989, 1990; Kleinberg & Westbay 1992). They are all strictly anaerobic Gram-negative bacteria.

It has been shown that volatile sulphur compounds and especially CH_3SH increase the permeability of the oral mucosa and crevicular epithelium (Ng & Tonzetich 1984). Furthermore, proteoglycans and glycoproteins in the extracellular matrix are held in an aggregated state via disulphide bonds and volatile sulphur compounds can induce their disaggregation by breaking these bonds (Ng & Tonzetich 1984).

Volatile sulphur compounds also impair oxygen utilization by host cells, react with cellular proteins, interfere with collagen maturation, increase collagen solubility, decrease DNA synthesis and proline transport and reduce the total protein content and collagen synthesis of fibroblasts (Horowitz & Folke 1972; Tonzetich & Lo 1978; Johnson & Tonzetich 1979, 1982; Johnson et al 1992a).

In addition, volatile sulphur compounds, especially CH_3SH incite the secretion of collagenase and prostaglandins from human fibroblasts, stimulate mononuclear cells to produce interleukin-1, augment the activity of cathepsin B and convert mature collagen to a product more susceptible to enzymic degradation (Johnson et al 1992b; Ratkay et al 1995). Volatile sulphur compounds, especially CH_3SH also reduce intracellular pH, inhibit cell growth periodontal ligament cell migration (L'Allemain et al 1984; Simchowitz & Cragoe 1986; Lancero et al 1996). Volatile sulphur compounds, thus have the capacity to contribute to periodontal pathology.

Finally, volatile sulphur compounds are also related to the production of oral malodour or halitosis. Although it had been previously assumed that indole and amines were the main malodorous components in mouth air (Fosdick et al 1953), it is now established that volatile sulphur compounds are the malodorous substances primarily responsible for unpleasant oral breath (Tonzetich & Kesterbaum 1969; Tonzetich 1971, 1978; Miyaki et al 1995; Scully et al 1997). However, it has also been postulated that another possible component of oral malodour may be cadaverine, a malodorous diamine produced from fish and meat by BANA-hydrolysing Gram-negative anaerobic bacteria (Goldberg et al 1994). Finally, the possible contribution of volatile fatty acids (butyrate, propionate, valerate) and putrescine (another diamine) to oral malodour remains unclear (Scully et al 1997).

DEGRADATION OF PERIODONTAL TISSUES BY BACTERIAL EFFECTS ON INFLAMMATORY CELLS

Periodontitis is a chronic inflammatory disease that results in extensive soft and hard tissue destruction of the periodontium. *Porphyromonas gingivalis* possesses an array of virulence factors and has been shown to induce expression of inducible nitric oxide synthase (iNOS) in inflammatory cells. Alayan et al (2006) investigated the effect of eliminating iNOS in a murine model of *P. gingivalis* infection. This was achieved by utilizing a *P. gingivalis*-induced skin abscess model, and an alveolar bone loss model employing an oral infection of *P. gingivalis* in iNOS knockout mice. The results indicated that iNOS knockout mice exhibited more extensive soft tissue damage and alveolar bone loss in response to *P. gingivalis* infection compared to wild-type mice. The local immune response to *P. gingivalis* in iNOS knockout mice was characterized by increased numbers of polymorphonuclear monocytes, while the systemic immune response was characterized by high levels of interleukin-12. They concluded that iNOS was required for an appropriate response to *P. gingivalis* infection.

Periodontal pathogenic bacteria are associated with elevated levels of interleukin-1α (IL-1α) but it is unclear if all species can induce cytokine production equally. *P. gingivalis* may also be able to antagonize IL-1α induced by other species through the activity of its proteases or lipopolysaccharide (LPS) (Bostanci et al 2007a). This group showed that co-stimulation of monocytes with *P. gingivalis* antagonized the ability of other bacterial species to induce IL-1α production and they also demonstrated that its LPS appeared to be the crucial component in this process. This study highlights the importance of mixed infections in the pathogenesis of periodontal disease because reduction of pro-inflammatory cytokine levels may impair the ability of the host to tackle infection.

DEGRADATION OF PERIODONTAL TISSUES BY BACTERIAL ENZYMES

The subgingival Gram-negative bacteria use proteins for their nutrition and therefore possess proteolytic enzymes to breakdown proteins to peptides and amino acids which they can absorb. A number of these proteases can degrade proteins essential to the host. In this respect, a number of the putative pathogens in the subgingival flora produce enzymes which can degrade components of the periodontal tissues and proteins essential to the defence system and these are described in detail below.

Proteolytic enzymes from putative periodontal pathogens

A number of the putative periodontal pathogens have been shown to produce proteases which are capable of degrading structural periodontal tissues and proteins involved in the inflammatory and immune reactions characteristic of chronic periodontitis. The main structural proteins of gingival connective tissue and periodontal ligament are collagen and proteoglycans. An early and persistent feature of periodontal disease is breakdown of connective tissue composed of these proteins which can be attacked by proteases of bacterial or host origin (Page & Schroeder 1976).

The bacteria associated with periodontal disease produce a variety of proteolytic enzymes which may participate in these processes. These include collagen degrading enzymes from *P. gingivalis*, *Actinobacillus actinomycetemcomitans* (now *A. actinomycetemcomitans*) and spirochaetes (Robertson et al 1982); an elastase-like enzyme from spirochaetes (Uitto et al 1986) and *Capnocytophaga* species (Gazi et al 1996; 1997); trypsin-like enzymes from *P. gingivalis*, *Bacteroides forsythus*, *T. denticola* and other spirochaetes (Suido et al 1986; Gazi et al 1997), chymotrypsin-like enzymes from *T. denticola* and *Capnocytophaga* species (Gazi et al 1997; Uitto et al 1989a), aminopeptidases from *Capnocytophaga* species (Suido et al 1986; Gazi et al 1997) and *T. denticola* (Mäkinen et al 1986; Gazi et al 1997) and dipeptidyl peptidases from *P. gingivalis*, *Prevotella intermedia* and *Capnocytophaga* species (Cox et al 1993; Gazi et al 1995, 1997) (Table 5.1).

The amount of enzyme produced by each bacterial species varies considerably. The bacterial proteases from cell sonicates of putative periodontal pathogens have been investigated using selective peptide substrates with appropriate inhibitors and activators (Cox et al 1993; Gazi et al 1994, 1996, 1997). Strong trypsin-like activity was found in *Porphyromonas gingivalis*, moderate activity from *T. denticola* and *C. gingivalis* and weak activity from *C. ochracea* and *C. sputigena* and *Prevotella intermedia*. The activity from *Porphyromonas gingivalis* and *Prevotella intermedia* had the characteristics of a cysteine proteinase and in the case of *Prevotella gingivalis* there appeared to be two separate cysteine proteinases, one cleaving arginine substrates and one lysine substrates (Gazi et al 1994, 1996, 1997) (see below). Weak chymotrypsin-like activity was found in *C. gingivalis*, *C. ochracea* and *T. denticola* (Gazi et al 1996, 1997). Weak elastase-like activity was only found in *C. sputigena* and very weak activity in *C. gingivalis* and *C. ochracea* (Gazi et al 1996). Moderate DPP-like activity was found in *P. gingivalis*, *Prevotella intermedia* and *C. gingivalis* and weak activity in *C. ochracea*, *C. sputigena* and *T. denticola* (Cox et al 1993; Gazi et al 1995, 1997) (Table 5.1).

These proteases can degrade all the components of periodontal connective tissue and the host defence systems. They may also inactivate key components of the plasma proteinase cascade systems involved in the inflammatory response and blood clotting and degrade the serum proteinase inhibitors, α1-proteinase inhibitor and α2-macroglobulin. Furthermore, some bacteria have fibrinolytic activity and some can also degrade haemoglobin (Kuramitsu 1998).

Tiranathanagul et al (2004) have also found that the supernatant from *A. actinomycetemcomitans* and *Porphyromonas gingivalis* could induce the activation of tissue-derived MMP-2 possibly through the imbalance of MT1-MMP and TIMP-2 in human periodontal ligament cells but each by different mechanisms. The imbalance of MT1-MMP and TIMP-2 may be another factor that is involved in the severity of periodontal disease (see below).

Table 5.1 *Bacterial proteases*

Bacteria	AminoP	DDP	Elastase	Trypsin	ChymoT	Collagenase
P. gingivalis	–	++	–	++++	–	++++
P. intermedia	–	++	–	±	–	±
A. actino	–	–	–	–	–	+
C. gingivalis	++	++	±	++	+	±
C. ochracea	++	+	+	+	±	–
C. sputigena	++	+	+	+	±	–
T. denticola	+	±	–	++	++	+
F. nucleatum	–	–	–	–	–	–
C. recta	+	–	–	–	–	–
E. corrodens	–	–	–	–	–	–

A. actino, *Aggregatibacter actinomycetemcomitans*; AminoP, aminopeptidase; DPP, dipeptidyl peptidase; ChymoT, chymotrypsin-like protease; Trypsin, trypsin-like protease; Elastase, elastase-like protease; ++++, Strong activity; ++, Moderate activity; +, Weak activity; ±, Very weak activity; –, No activity.

Hydrolytic enzymes from putative periodontal pathogens

These bacteria also produce enzymes capable of degrading the non-proteinaceous elements of the periodontal connective tissue. Hyaluronidase and chondroitinase activities are produced by *C. ochracea*, *F. nucleatum*, *P. gingivalis* and *T. denticola* (Steffan & Hengtes 1981; Tipler & Embery 1985; Fiehn 1986; Seddon & Shah 1989). These could hydrolyse the glycosaminoglycan components of proteoglycans in the extracellular matrix. Neuraminidase (sialidase) activity, which is found in *B. forsythus*, *Prevotella melaninogenicus* and *Porphyromonas gingivalis* (Moncla et al 1990), might attack sialoproteins in the epithelium, thereby increasing its permeability to bacterial products. Damage to the surface of epithelial and other cells could result from the action of phospholipases from *Porphyromonas*, *Prevotella* and *Bacteroides* species (Bulkacz et al 1979, 1981, 1985). Finally, strong acid and alkaline phosphatase activities are present in *Porphyromonas*, *Prevotella*, *Bacteroides* and *Capnocytophaga* species (Slots 1981; Laughton et al 1982a).

The proteolytic and hydrolytic enzymes from individual putative periodontal pathogens are described in more detail below.

P. gingivalis

Proteolytic enzymes

P. gingivalis produces by far the greatest proteolytic activity of any periodontal bacterium (Courant & Bader 1966; Eley & Cox 2003). It produces a variety of proteases which differ in size, pH optima, sensitivity to inhibitors, ability to hydrolyse specific substrates and location within or on the surface of the bacterial cell (Lawson & Meyer 1992). When separated by gel electrophoresis, a total of eight distinct bands of proteolytic activity have been seen, each with different properties (Grenier et al 1989b). All these proteases are produced in large quantities by this bacteria and are recognized as important virulence factors because of their potential to favour bacterial growth and cause damage to host tissues (Loesche et al 1985). The extracellular proteases of *P. gingivalis* are critical survival determinants and loss or reduction of these protease activities by the use of protease inhibitors or gene inactivation renders the bacteria susceptible to phagocytosis and killing by human neutrophils *in vitro* (Schenkein et al 1995; Kesavulu et al 1996). It also renders it avirulent in animal models of periodontitis (Schenkein et al 1995; Kesavulu et al 1996).

One group (Nakamura et al 1991) has separated the proteases in supernatants from *P. gingivalis* cultures into four separate activities which they called proteases A, B and C and a Gly-Pro dipeptidyl peptidase. Proteases B and C were found to be thiol-dependent cysteine proteinases and had trypsin-like activity. Protease A was neither a cysteine proteinase nor had trypsin-like activity. Protease C was the most abundant and had a large molecular size. They felt that it could have represented a mixture of two or three enzymes. All the collagenolytic activity from this bacteria was present in this fraction. However, they stated that this could result from either a separate enzyme or several enzymes acting together. These proteinases have been found to be produced in both cell associated and secretory forms (Grenier & McBride 1987).

Trypsin-like proteinases

In surveys of the proteolytic activity of oral bacteria *P. gingivalis* was found to have a particular ability to cleave peptide substrates with arginine terminal groups such as benzoyl-arginine-2-naphthylamide (BANA) or benzoyl-arginine-p-nitroanilide (BAPNA) and this activity was termed trypsin-like (Laughton et al 1982b; Slots 1981; Eley & Cox 2003). In cultures of *P. gingivalis* the relative amount of trypsin-like activity in bacterial cells and medium depends both on the stage of growth and growth rate. During high growth rates the enzymes are mainly associated with the cells, but as the culture ages or at low growth rates the proportion of activity released into the medium increases (Fujimura & Nakamura 1989; Minas & Greenman 1989; Suido et al 1986; Tokuda et al 1986). A significant proportion of the activity is associated with bacterial membranes (Fujimura & Nakamura 1989; Tsutsui et al 1987; Yoshimura et al 1984) and the enzymes are located at the inner cell membrane and cell surface (Lantz et al 1993). High activity has also been found in extracellular outer membrane vesicles (Grenier & Mayrand 1987; Smalley & Birss 1987) with the relative amount varying in similar way to that in the supernatant (Minhas & Greenman 1989).

The purified enzyme is inhibited by thiol blocking agents and enhanced by sulphydryl compounds (Fujimura & Nakamura 1987; Lantz et al 1993; Otsuka et al 1987; Shah et al 1991; Smalley & Birss 1987; Sorsa et al 1987; Suido et al 1987; Sundqvist et al 1987; Tsutsui et al 1987; Yoshimura et al 1984). It is similar in its actions to other common cysteine proteinases like papain and by analogy it has been proposed that it is either known as 'gingipain' or 'gingivain' (see below).

There have also been some conflicting reports on other properties of the trypsin-like activities. Some workers have found them sensitive to the serine protease inhibitors (Sorsa et al 1987; Suido et al 1987; Sundqvist et al 1987; Tsutsui et al 1987), while others have not (Fujimura & Nakamura 1987; Nilsson et al 1985; Lantz et al 1991a). Also some groups have found a requirement for metal ions (Yoshimura et al 1984; Fujimura & Nakamura 1987; Sorsa et al 1987; Sundqvist et al 1987; Tsutsui et al 1987) but others have found the opposite (Suido et al 1987; Okamoto et al 1998). Also, the quoted figures for pH optimum range from 6.0–8.5 (Yoshimura et al 1984; Fujimura & Nakamura 1987; Otsuka et al 1987; Suido et al 1987; Sundqvist et al 1987; Tsutsui et al 1987), while estimates for molecular weight range from 18–300 kDa (Fujimura & Nakamura 1987; Otsuka et al 1987; Lantz et al 1993; Smalley & Birss 1987; Sorsa et al 1987; Tsutsui et al 1987).

The most likely explanation for these variations is that there is more than one trypsin-like enzyme. In this regard, one study obtained four distinct factions of trypsin-like activity all of which appeared to be classifiable as cysteine proteinases (Fujimura & Nakamura 1989). Another group separated them into three cysteine proteinases, two of which cleaved arginine bonds, and one which cleaved lysine bonds and a fourth protease which behaved as a serine proteinase (Hinode et al 1991). Similar findings have been reported by other workers (Nakamura et al 1991). In addition, many reports on trypsin-like proteinases include descriptions of collagenase activity which may well be due to separate collagenolytic proteinases (see below).

One group (Shah et al 1991) has separated the trypsin-like activity from *P. gingivalis* from both outer membrane vesicles and culture supernatant. They showed that it was a thiol-dependent cysteine proteinase which cleaved synthetic arginine substrates. They proposed the name gingivain for this enzyme. A similar and probably identical proteinase was isolated from the culture supernatant by another group (Chen et al 1992) and they gave it the name of gingipain. They showed that it had a narrow spectrum of activity against peptide bonds containing arginine, was resistant to inhibition by serine proteinase inhibitors and was activated by glycine-containing dipeptidases. They found that it had a molecular weight of 50 kilo Daltons (kDa) and a pH optimum of 6.0. They suggested that this enzyme may be either referred to as arg-gingipain or gingipain-R.

This second group (Pike et al 1994) also separated the trypsin-like activity in *P. gingivalis* culture supernatants and found that there were two separate cysteine proteinase activities, one with arginine and one with lysine specificity, respectively. The arginine specific proteinase was a high molecular weight form of gingipain and proved to be 50 kDa gingipain complexed with 44 kDa of binding proteins which were shown to be haemagglutinins (Aduse-Opoku et al 1995; Curtis et al 1993b). The lysine specific activity had a molecular weight of 60 kDa and a pH optimum of

8.0–8.5 and was also complexed with haemagglutinin binding proteins (Curtis et al 1993b). This protease was named lys-gingipain but it is also referred to as gingipain-K. It was thought that these proteinase/ haemagglutinin complexes might be involved in the uptake of haemin, which is a vital metabolite for *P. gingivalis*, by haemagglutination and subsequent haemolysis of erythrocytes.

Another group of workers (Scott et al 1993) also isolated and identified this lysine specific activity and called the enzyme lys-gingivain. They showed that it was capable of cleaving high molecular weight kininogens to generate bradykinin and could also degrade fibrinogen. This protease has also been shown to be capable of activating fibroblast and neutrophil interstitial collagenases (matrix metalloproteinases (MMP) -1, -8) (De Carlo et al 1997; Sorsa et al 1992). Thus *P. gingivalis* appears to produce two cysteine proteinases with trypsin-like activity. One of these is arginine specific and is called either arg-gingipain or arg-gingivain and the other is lysine specific and is called either lys-gingipain or lys-gingivain.

The methods for cloning the major arginine and lysine protease genes have involved screening the *P. gingivalis* genomic DNA library in *E. coli* with oligonucleotides directed to the N-terminus or specific antisera (Curtis et al 1999). The first gene cloned and sequenced was arg-gingipain-1(*rgp-1*) from strain HG66 (99) and this was followed in rapid progression by protease polyprotein arg-1(*prp-1*) from W50 arg-gingipain-A (*rgp-A*) from strain 381, *prpR* from strain W50 and *prpH* from strain W83 (Aduse-Opoku et al 1995, 1996; Curtis et al 1993b; Fletcher et al 1994; Kerzbaum et al 1995; Lewis & Macrina 1998; Okamoto et al 1995; Pavloff et al 1995). There is now general agreement that all of these genes are very closely related and probably represent homologous loci from different bacterial strains (Curtis et al 1999) and it would therefore be legitimate to use a single descriptor for all of them, *rgpA*.

The deduced translation of this gene (**Fig. 5.3**) reveals (Curtis et al 1999) a N-terminal propeptide, a 50 kDa catalytic domain and a long C-terminal extension which codes for the haemagglutinin/adhesin (Aduse-Opoko et al 1995; Pike et al 1994). This gene structure can result in the translation of multiforms of arg-specific protease which have been described as dimers and multimers by different groups (Curtis et al 1999). Southern blotting also revealed regions of homology at multiple loci on the chromosome suggesting the presence of a family of sequence-related genes. DNA probes to the catalytic region hybridized to two separate loci suggesting the presence of a second closely related gene. Moreover, probes directed to the C-terminus extension also hybridized to multiple loci suggesting several sequence-related genes with haemagglutinin activity (Aduse-Opoko et al 1995; Barkocy-Gallagher et al 1999; Curtis et al 1996; Nakayama et al 1995).

The existence of a second arginine specific gene has now been proved by insertional gene inactivation studies. These showed that two insertions were necessary to abolish all this activity (Aduse-Opoko et al 1999; Curtis et al

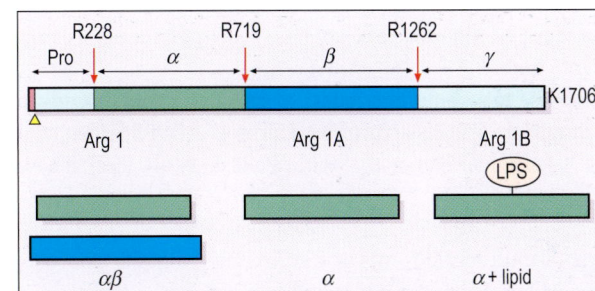

Fig. 5.3 A schematic representation of the prpR1 protein produced by the prpR1 gene of *P. gingivalis*. The protein consists of 1706 amino acids and is organized into four major domains: pro, α, β, and γ. The propeptide is preceded by a typical *E. coli* signal sequence. The presence of arginine residues at the junction of these domains suggests autolytic processing of the polyprotein I indicated by the vertical arrows to give either dimeric Arg 1(αβ) or monomeric Arg1A(α). The LPS annotation to Arg1B denotes extensive lipid modification to this form.

1999; Mortensen & Kilian 1984). The second gene was very closely similar to *rgpA* but lacked its C-terminus extension (Mikolajczyk-Pawlinska et al 1998; Nakayama 1997; Rangarajan et al 1997b; Slakeski et al 1998). It is possible that this second gene arose by a process of gene duplication. This second arginine specific gene has been named *rgpB* (Curtis et al 1999).

The first complete sequence for the lysine specific protease gene was produced from strain W12 and was termed *prpP* (Barkocy-Gallagher et al 1999). This was followed by five further sequences with lysine specific products which were placed in the database (Curtis et al 1999). These comprised *kgp* from strains HG66 and 381, *kgp(381)-hagD* from strain 381, *prpP* from W80 and *prtK* from W50 (Lewis & Macrina 1998; Okamoto et al 1996; Pavloff et al 1997; Slakeski et al 1999). In each case the genomic organization of these loci was found to be markedly similar to the arginine specific protease/haemagglutinin gene, *rgpA*.

Comparison of the lysine specific genes showed that they were all highly homogeneous, particularly in the pro-protein and the catalytic domains. However, the C-terminal extension had some rearrangements between strains (Curtis et al 1999). Southern hybridization experiments have confirmed that the catalytic domain is only present as one copy on the *P. gingivalis* chromosome (Barkocy-Gallagher et al 1999; Lewis and Macrina 1998). Therefore it has been concluded that the *kgp, prtK* and *prtP* genes all represent homologous loci in different strains which could be redefined under a single descriptor, *kgp*.

Purified *kgp* from strains HG66 and 33277 (Otsuka et al 1987) and *prtK* from strain W50 appear to be specific for lysine bonds, although cell-associated *prtK* has been found in non-covalent association with *prpR*, an arginine specific protease (Slakeski et al 1998). Conversely, the translated protease from the *prtP* gene from strain W12 has been suggested to have dual-specific activity for both arginine and lysine bonds (Ciborwski et al 1994). However, this controversy has now been resolved by gene inactivation experiments (Nakayama 1997; Nakayama et al 1995). First, inactivation of both arginine specific genes abolishes all the arginine protease activity of strains 33277 (Nakayama et al 1995) and W50 (Nakayama 1997) suggesting that these genes account for all this activity. Second, *prtP* protease from *Bacteroides* species has been found to have only lysyl activity (Barkocy-Gallagher et al 1999). Third, inactivation of the *prtP* gene in strain W12 (Barkocy-Gallagher et al 1999), the *kgp* gene in strain ATCC 33277 (Okamoto et al 1998) and the *prtK* gene in strain W50 (25) had no effect on arginine protease activity while the lysine protease activity was reduced to background levels. Thus, it appears that the lysine protease activity is derived from a single gene product which is entirely specific for lysyl peptide bonds (Curtis et al 1999).

The suggested nomenclature (Curtis et al 1999) is *rgpA* (arg gingipain A) and *rgpB* (arg gingipain B) for the two arginine specific gene and *kgp* (lys gingipain) for the lysine specific gene.

The gene organization is shown in **Figure 5.3** (Curtis et al 1999). It can be seen that while both *rgpA* and kgp genes contain propeptide, catalytic domain and a haemagglutinin/adhesin domains, *rgpB* only contains propeptide and catalytic domains.

These genes give rise to a complex process of translation which leads to the production of multiple protease isoforms (Curtis et al 1999; Chen et al 1992; Pike et al 1994; Rangarajan et al 1997b; Slakeski et al 1998). These are (**Fig. 5.3**):

- Heterodimeric or multimeric forms of RgpA comprising the catalytic chain in non-covalent association with adhesin and occasionally complexed with Kgp. This has been termed HRgpA
- Soluble, monomeric forms of the catalytic chains of Rgp or Kgp (~50 kDa). These have been termed RgpA(cat) and RgpB(cat)
- Membrane associated forms of these monomers containing large post-translational additions (~70–80 kDa) are known as mtRgpA(cat) and mtRgpB(cat).

The *Kgp* gene may also give rise to similar products but these have not yet been fully determined (Curtis et al 1999).

The polyproteins, RgpA and Kgp, are proteolytically processed into proteinases and adhesins. Veith et al (2004) have demonstrated that the RgpA and Kgp proteinases and adhesins are C terminally processed by carboxy-peptidase CPG70 by sequencing C-terminal peptides from both the wild type and an isogenic CPG70 mutant, using ion trap mass spectrometry.

An experimental study by Rangarajan et al (2005) has also suggested that RgpB is required for the normal posttranslational glycosylation of Arg-gingipains derived from rgpA and that this process is required for enzyme stabilization.

The regulation and activation of the *P. gingivalis* gingipains is poorly understood. However in this regard, Vanterpool et al (2004) have presented good evidence that the vimE gene downstream of vimA is independently expressed and is involved in modulating proteolytic activity in *P. gingivalis* W83.

The presence in the genome of *P. gingivalis* of two other members of the protease and haemagglutinin gene family has been suggested by the Southern hybridization of chromosomal DNA using *rgpA*-derived probes (Aduse-Opoko et al 1995; Barkocy-Gallagher et al 1996; Naskayama et al 1995). The first of these is gene for the surface protein haemagglutinin A (*hag A*) and this contains four direct repeats which share significant sequence homology with the haemagglutinin coding area of both *rgpA* and *kgp* (Han et al 1996). The second one is TonB-linked adhesin (tla) which codes for the surface protein involved in haemin capture and utilization. This has an internal region of 460 amino acids with 98% homology to the haemagglutinin domain of RgpA.

Gingipains from *P. gingivalis* strongly affect the host defense system by degrading some cytokines, components of the complement system, and several immune cell receptors. In this connection, Mezyk-Kope et al (2005) found that gingipains were able not only to cleave soluble TNF-α but also to destroy the membrane form of this cytokine. They felt that in this way it might additionally dysregulate the cytokine network. Arginine-specific gingipains have also been shown to stimulate production of hepatocyte growth factor (scatter factor) through protease-activated receptors in human gingival fibroblasts in culture (Uehara et al 2005). The mechanism(s) involved may actively participate in both inflammatory and reparative processes in periodontal diseases.

Yun et al (2006) provided evidence that *P. gingivalis* gingipains can reduce the functional expression of CD99 on endothelial cells, leading indirectly to the disruption of adhesion molecule expression and of leucocyte recruitment to inflammatory foci.

Sheets et al (2006) had shown previously that gingipains from *P. gingivalis* W83 can induce cell detachment, cell adhesion molecule cleavage, and apoptosis in endothelial cells but the specific roles of the individual gingipains were unclear. They used purified gingipains, and determined that each of the gingipains can cleave cell adhesion molecule to varying degrees with differing kinetics. Kgp and HRgpA worked together to quickly detach endothelial cells. In addition, in the absence of active caspases, both gingipain-active W83 extracts and purified HRgpA and RgpB induced apoptotic morphology, suggesting that the gingipains were able to induce both caspase-dependent and caspase-independent apoptosis.

Beikler et al (2005) studied the sequence variations in the active centre of the Arg-X-specific protease encoding genes rgpA and rgpB of *P. gingivalis* isolates and to analyse their prevalence in periodontitis patients before and 3 months after mechanical periodontal therapy. However, they found no specific variation within the rgpA sequence in these situations.

In spite of a comprehensive role of gingipains in the survival of *P. gingivalis* other workers have found additional related mechanisms. In this regard, Slaney et al (2006) investigated the role of the complement system in the host defence against infection and concluded that the production of surface anionic polysaccharide (a phosphorylated branched mannan) at the surface of *P. gingivalis* rather than Arg- and Lys-gingipain synthesis was the principal mechanism of serum resistance in *P. gingivalis*.

Collagenolytic proteinases

The reports of the collagenolytic activity of *P. gingivalis* trypsin-like proteinases (Smalley et al 1988a; Sorsa et al 1987; Tsutsui et al 1987; Eley & Cox 2003) may reflect contamination of the enzyme preparation with true collagenases (Fujimura & Nakamura 1987). However, there is some evidence that the breakdown of Type I collagen by *P. gingivalis* may involve the concerted action of both a collagenase and trypsin-like enzyme (McDermid et al 1988).

Collagenolytic activity has frequently been reported in *P. gingivalis* (Birkedal-Hansen et al 1988; Robertson et al 1982; Toda et al 1984). The activity is usually described as cell bound and has also been found in extracellular outer membrane vesicles (Grenier & Mayrand 1987). Unlike mammalian collagenase it degrades collagen into multiple fragments (Birkedal-Hansen et al 1988; Robertson et al 1982; Sundqvist et al 1987; Toda et al 1984) but the initial attack is in the triple helical region, indicating that it is a true collagenase (Birkedal-Hansen et al 1988). Further breakdown probably involves other proteases. The activity is activated by sulphydryl compounds and inhibited by thiol-blocking agents and metal chelating agents (Birkedal-Hansen et al 1988; Robertson et al 1982; Sundqvist et al 1987; Toda et al 1984). Thus, it appears to be a cysteine proteinase with a requirement for metal ions and it probably has a binding specificity for arginine residues (Birkedal-Hansen et al 1988; Toda et al 1984). Type IV collagen is also degraded by *P. gingivalis* but its activity is not affected by thiol blocking agents indicating that another enzyme is involved (Uitto et al 1988b).

The separate collagenolytic enzymes from *P. gingivalis* have been investigated by several workers and these separate proteinase activities have only recently been isolated. One group of workers (Lawson & Meyer 1992) purified the collagenolytic activities from *P. gingivalis* using electrophoretic techniques. They showed that the enzymes were present in the bacterial cell wall and were released into the culture medium. The purified enzyme was capable of cleaving basement membrane collagen Type IV and synthetic substrates for bacterial collagenases. The activity had the characteristics of a cysteine proteinase and appeared to exist as an active precursor protein of 94 kDa molecular weight which underwent proteolytic cleavage to 75, 56 and 19 kDa forms. It appeared to function also as an adhesin permitting the bacteria to attach to collagenous tissue.

Another group (Sojar et al 1993) purified the proteases from *P. gingivalis* which were capable of cleaving the bacterial collagenase substrate called the pZ-peptide. They showed that the purified enzyme activity was present in the bacterial cell wall and was also released into the culture medium. The purified enzyme was capable of hydrolysing salt-solubilized Type I collagen, kininogen and transferrin in the presence of both calcium and dithiothreitol (a reducing agent required by cysteine proteinases). It could also function as a gelatinase. However, it failed to degrade acid-soluble Type I or Type IV collagens and fibrinogen and also did not cleave either terminal arginine or lysine or glycyl-prolyl synthetic peptide substrates. It thus appeared to be a collagenolytic cysteine proteinase with no trypsin-like or dipeptidyl peptidase activities which had a calcium and salt requirement for its activity. The native enzyme had a molecular weight of 120 kDa and its range of activity suggested that it had specificity for the Pro-X-Gly sequence found on several proteins including collagen.

A gene (prt C) has been isolated from *P. gingivalis*. It was found to code for a protein with collagenolytic activity (Kato et al 1992). The gene was cloned into *E. coli* and the resultant protein was harvested. This was then purified by gel filtration and ion exchange chromatography. The purified enzyme had a molecular weight of 35 kDa and the active enzyme behaved as a dimer. It degraded soluble and reconstituted fibrillar Type I collagen, heat denatured Type I collagen but did not degrade gelatin or synthetic substrates for bacterial collagenases. Its activity was not dependent on reducing agents, was enhanced by calcium ions and inhibited by chelating agents. It was therefore not a cysteine proteinase and had some properties of a metalloproteinase.

The three collagenolytic proteinases described above (Kato et al 1992; Lawson & Meyer 1992; Sojar et al 1993) all differ from each other in important respects so it appears that at least 3 distinct collagenolytic proteinases are produced by *P. gingivalis*. These enzymes are also distinct from the three cysteine proteinases, arg-gingipain A and B and lys-gingipain and the dipeptidyl peptidase and probably also other proteinases degrading other proteins.

Studies have shown that *P. gingivalis* and host matrix metalloproteinases (MMPs) play important roles in the tissue destruction associated with periodontal disease. However, it is still unclear which MMPs or their inhibitors are regulated by *P. gingivalis* at the transcriptional and/or at the protein levels (Zhou & Windsor 2006). Therefore, this group investigated the effects *P. gingivalis* supernatant had on the collagen degrading ability of human gingival fibroblasts (HGFs) and how it regulated the activation, mRNA expression, and inhibition of MMPs.

They were able to show that *P. gingivalis* increased the collagen degrading ability of HGFs, in part, by increasing MMP activation and by lowering the TIMP-1 protein level, as well as by affecting the mRNA expression of multiple MMPs and TIMPs.

Other proteases

Two other protease coding genes, tpr and prtT, have been isolated from *P. gingivalis* and cloned into *E. coli* and it has been found that they translate to low level protease activities (Kuramitsu 1998; Eley & Cox 2003). The resultant enzyme from tpr had a molecular weight of 64 kDa and was active against general protein substrates but not collagen (Bourgeau et al 1992). In addition, two proteinases of 120 and 150 kDa which degraded fibrinogen (Kato et al 1992) and fibronectin (Lantz et al 1991a, 1991b) and a 70 kDa collagenase-like neutral protease (Sorsa et al 1987) have also been isolated from *P. gingivalis*. The 150 kDa fraction has been shown to be a cysteine proteinase with trypsin-like activity and to bind to both fibrinogen and fibronectin prior to degrading them (Lantz et al 1991b). It has also been shown to be located on the outer cell membrane and to mediate attachment of the bacteria to these proteins (Lantz et al 1991b). Since it cleaves fibrinogen in an identical way to plasmin it may also activate pro-collagenase and degrade fibrin and glycoproteins in the extracellular matrix and basement membrane.

Finally *P. gingivalis* produces dipeptidyl peptidase activity against glycyl-prolyl and alanyl-prolyl dipeptides (Cox et al 1993; Gazi et al 1995; Nakamura et al 1991; Suido et al 1986). Glycyl-prolyl arylamidase activities have also been studied by several groups (Abiko et al 1985; Barua et al 1989; Grenier & McBride 1987; Kay et al 1989; Suido et al 1987). These are serine proteases with a pH optima of 7.5–8.5. These activities are found in bacterial cells in association with the outer membrane and are also present in extracellular outer membrane vesicles (Grenier & McBride 1987; Kay et al 1989).

Hydrolytic enzymes

P. gingivalis also produces hyaluronidase and chondroitinase activities (Fiehn 1986; Seddon & Shah 1989; Steffan & Hengtes 1981; Tipler & Embery 1985) and these activities appear to be present in the outer membrane vesicles (Smalley et al 1988b). This bacteria also produces neuraminidase activity (Moncla et al 1990) and strong acid and alkaline phosphatase activities (Laughton et al 1982a; Slots et al 1986).

Effects of *P. gingivalis* enzymes on the host

Proteases

The proteases of *P. gingivalis* are all produced for the benefit of the bacteria and have been shown to have both internal and external effects (Kuramitsu 1998).

INTERNAL EFFECTS

This bacteria, like all the other Gram-negative bacteria inhabiting the periodontal pocket, derives its energy and nutrition from the breakdown of proteins. Therefore defective production of one or more of its major proteinases is likely to affect its growth and reproduction (Kuramitsu 1998; Imamura 2003). In this regard, it has been shown that mutations of the rgpA, prtT and tpr genes result in growth reductions (Pavloff et al 1995; Scott et al 1993; Tokuda et al 1998) and reductions in the production of fimbriae which are concerned with attachment (Tokuda et al 1996, 1998). These mutants also showed reduced levels of attachment to epithelial cells and other bacteria (Tokuda et al 1996, 1998). RgpA mutants also showed reduced production of haemagglutinins (Nakayama et al 1995; Yoneda & Kuramitsu 1996).

There are two different types of fimbriae concerned with *P. gingivalis* attachment (Umemoto & Hamada 2003) and these researchers produced constructed mutants to look at their role in attachment and invasion using a rat model. The invasion and attachment levels of *P. gingivalis* on human KB cells from both types of mutants were lower than those from the wild type. Also the alveolar bone loss in the rats infected by the mutant to filA was greater than to those infected with the mutant to mfa1. Moreover, the bone loss in rats infected with the double knock-out mutant was greater than the rats infected with the wild strain. Thus both types of fimbriae seem to play important roles in the pathogenesis of periodontal disease.

These fimbriae can bind to human salivary components, commensal bacteria, and a variety of host cells including epithelial cells, macrophages and fibroblasts (Amano 2003). They are also thought to be critically important in invasion of host cells. Recent clinical investigations (Amano 2003) have demonstrated a close relationship between the bacteria with type II Fim A and periodontitis development. Missailidis et al (2004) further reported that *P. gingivalis* fim types can be divided into six genotypes. They found that fim type II strains followed by type Ib were more prevalent in periodontitis patients from a multiracial Brazilian population suggesting an increased pathogenic potential of these types.

Nakagawa et al (2006) compared the efficiencies of *P. gingivalis* strains with distinct types of fimbriae for invasion of epithelial cells and for degradation of cellular focal adhesion components, paxillin, and focal adhesion kinase (FAK). Six representative strains with the different types of fimbriae were tested, and *P. gingivalis* with type II fimbriae (type II *P. gingivalis*) adhered to and invaded epithelial cells at significantly greater levels than the other strains. There were negligible differences in gingipain activities among the six strains; however, type II *P. gingivalis* apparently degraded intracellular paxillin in association with a loss of phosphorylation 30 min after infection. Degradation was blocked with cytochalasin D or in mutants with FimA disrupted. Paxillin was degraded by the mutant with Lys-gingipain disrupted, and this degradation was prevented by inhibition of Arg-gingipain activity by N-p-tosyl-L-lysine chloromethyl ketone. FAK was also degraded by type II *P. gingivalis*. Cellular focal adhesions with green fluorescent protein-paxillin macroaggregates were clearly destroyed, and this was associated with cellular morphological changes and microtubule disassembly. Furthermore, in an *in vitro* wound closure assay, type II *P. gingivalis* significantly inhibited cellular migration and proliferation compared to the cellular migration and proliferation observed with the other types. These results suggest that type II *P. gingivalis* efficiently invades epithelial cells and degrades focal adhesion components with

Arg-gingipain, which results in cellular impairment during wound healing and periodontal tissue regeneration.

Tamura et al (2005) showed that a limited number of Japanese children harbor *P. gingivalis*, and that the distribution of type II and IV FimA genotypes was extremely low. Furthermore, some adolescents were found to possess the type IV FimA genotype which has been shown to be possibly related to adult periodontitis, in contrast to types I, III, and V.

Noiri et al (2004) detected positive reactions with an anti-*P. gingivalis*-fimbriae serum, located in the cementum-attached plaque area in the deep pocket zones. In the so-called 'plaque-free zones' *P. gingivalis*-carrying fimbriae were immunocytochemically observed to reside in contact with the dental cuticle in six of the nine samples examined. These findings suggest that *P. gingivalis*-carrying fimbriae are strongly related to adherence to the root surface at the bottom of human periodontal pockets.

The FimA gene, which encodes fimbrillin (FimA), is found in *P. gingivalis* and has been classified into six genotypes based on nucleotide sequence. *P. gingivalis* that possesses the type II FimA gene is prevalent in adult periodontitis (Miura et al 2005). These workers investigated the prevalence of *P. gingivalis* FimA genotypes in Japanese aggressive periodontitis patients. They examined their virulence in subgingival samples from 18 Japanese aggressive periodontitis patients and 22 periodontally healthy young adults. *A. actinomycetemcomitans P. gingivalis* and *Tannerella forsythensis* detection, determination of the FimA genotype in *P. gingivalis*, and the quantification of *P. gingivalis* were analysed by polymerase chain reaction (PCR) methods. The proteolytic activities of the *P. gingivalis* FimA type I and FimA type II were also examined. They showed that *P. gingivalis* FimA type I strains were significantly higher than those of the FimA type II strains in the aggressive periodontitis subjects. Their results suggested that differences in virulence exist among different FimA genotypes. Co-adherence with other pathogens in *P. gingivalis* FimA type II-associated aggressive periodontitis and quantitative increases in *P. gingivalis* in FimA type I-associated aggressive periodontitis seemed to be related to this virulence.

Inaba et al (2008) studied the proteolytic activities of *P. gingivalis* clones with type II fimbria and found that their results suggested that pathogenic heterogeneity had relationships with the invasive and proteolytic activities of these clones. This same relationship was also found by Tachibana-Ono et al 2008.

P. gingivalis can adhere to and invade pocket epithelium and the ability of six capsular and non-capsular *P. gingivalis* serotypes to adhere to cultured monolayers from human periodontal pockets of chronic periodontitis patients has been investigated (Dierickx et al 2003). It was found that the non-capsular strains adhered significantly more than their capsulated variants. Capsulated type 4 (K-4) serotype adhered slightly better than the other capsulated K types. This indicates that the presence and type of capsule may influence adherence to epithelium.

P. gingivalis is known to invade oral epithelial cells in periodontal lesions, although the mechanism is unclear (Tamai et al 2005). These workers showed that goat polyclonal anti-intercellular adhesion molecule 1 (anti-ICAM-1) antibody inhibited the invasion of *P. gingivalis* into KB cells (human oral epithelial cells) and also that *P. gingivalis* fimbria bound to recombinant human ICAM-1, as shown by enzyme-linked immunosorbent assay. *P. gingivalis* was also found to co-localize with ICAM-1 on KB cells, as seen with an immunofluorescence microscope, and the knockdown of ICAM-1 in KB cells resulted in the inhibition of *P. gingivalis* invasion by RNA interference. In addition, methyl-β-cyclodextrin, a cholesterol-binding agent, inhibited the co-localization of *P. gingivalis* with ICAM-1 and invasion by the microorganism. The co-localization of caveolin-1, a caveolar marker protein, on KB cells with *P. gingivalis* was also shown, and the knockdown of caveolin-1 in KB cells caused a reduced level of *P. gingivalis* invasion. These results suggest that ICAM-1 and caveolin-1 were required for the invasion of *P. gingivalis* into human oral epithelial cells, and these molecules appeared to be associated with the primary stages of the development and progression of chronic periodontitis.

EXTERNAL EFFECTS

TRANSMISSION OF *P. GINGIVALIS*

P. gingivalis is usually recovered from diseased adult subjects, and transmission of this pathogen seems largely restricted to adult individuals (Van Winkelhoff & Boutaga 2005). Horizontal transmission of *P. gingivalis* may therefore be controlled by periodontal treatment involving elimination or significant suppression of the pathogen in diseased individuals and by a high standard of oral hygiene. Van Winkelhoff et al (2007) studied transmission of *P. gingivalis* in a population living in a remote area in Southern Java, Indonesia. They found that vertical transmission of *P. gingivalis* occurred within family units, most likely from parents to children. However, transmission of *P. gingivalis* between spouses could not be established.

INFLAMMATORY AND IMMUNE SYSTEMS

P. gingivalis proteinases are known to be able to degrade immunoglobulins A1, A2 and G (Grenier et al 1989a; Kilian 1981; Mortensen & Kilian 1984; Sato et al 1987). Refined RgpA (arg-gingipain) is able to degrade IgG but not IgA (Bedi & Williams 1994; Kadowaki et al 1994) and thus it appears that IgA is degraded by one of the other proteinases (Potempa et al 1995b). These functions may reduce the hosts response against these bacteria by reducing immune opsonization (Grenier 1992). *P. gingivalis* attenuates serum bactericidal activity (Grenier 1992) and RgpA could be responsible for this as a result of its degradation of immunoglobulins and complement (Kuramitsu 1998).

P. gingivalis proteinases have been shown to degrade complement components (Jagle et al 1996; Schenkein 1995; Scott et al 1993; Sundqvist et al 1985). RgpA (arg-gingipain) degrades C3 and this may also reduce its opsonization function (Schenkein 1995). This process eliminates the creation of C3-derived opsonins and renders *P. gingivalis* resistant to phagocytosis by neutrophils. RgpA and Kgp (lys-gingipain) have been shown to degrade C5 and to release C5a as a result. C5a is a neutrophil polymorphonuclear leucocyte (PMN) attractant and may thus stimulate inflammation (Schenkein 1995; Travis et al 1997). These combined effects result in a massive accumulation of neutrophils in the tissues which then produce an array of proteinases that can degrade connective tissue. The resulting production of peptides in turn allows these bacteria to thrive.

P. gingivalis proteinases are capable of modulating cytokine function (Fletcher et al 1997, 1998; Sharp et al 1998). In this regard, it has been shown that the arg-gingipain is capable of cleaving and inactivating certain pro- and anti-inflammatory cytokines (Fletcher et al 1997, 1998). In addition, a 16 kDa protein from the outer surface membrane of this bacterium has been found to have cytokine inducing function with regard to IL-6 (Sharp et al 1998). This protein shares the sequence of part of the catalytic chain of the RgpA protein and may be a cleaved fragment from this chain. Thus, the RgpA proteinase appears to have a dual action in both activating and inactivating certain cytokines. Gingipains also degrade macrophage CD14, thus inhibiting activation of leucocytes through the LPS receptor, and thereby facilitating sustained colonization of *P. gingivalis* (Imamura 2003).

The modulation of cytokine function could also be responsible for the observation that *P. gingivalis* can alter leucocyte recruitment (Potempa et al 1995b). This could result from the degradation of cytokines by *P. gingivalis* proteinases and they have been shown to degrade tumour necrosis factor alpha (TNF-α) (Catkins et al 1998), interleukin-1 (IL-1) (Darveau et al 1998), IL-6 (Fletcher et al 1997) and IL-8 (Huang et al 1998).

P. gingivalis has been shown to alter the C5α receptor on PMNs (Jagle et al 1996). This however is not a function of its cysteine proteinases and must be carried out by one of its other proteases (Jagle et al 1996). It also

attenuates the bactericidal activity of PMNs (Kadowaki et al 1994) possibly by effects on cell surface receptors.

In addition *P. gingivalis* inhibits PMN migration across epithelium (Madianos et al 1997) and this could involve proteinase degradation of IL-8 and intracellular adhesion molecule-1 (ICAM-1) on epithelial cells (Huang et al 1998). Thus *P. gingivalis* proteinases may both inhibit (Madianos et al 1997) and stimulate (Schenkein 1995) PMN migration into the gingival crevice. Furthermore, purified RgpA can attenuate the respiratory burst characteristic of PMN bacterial killing (Kadowaki et al 1994). Finally *P. gingivalis* cysteine proteinases can degrade lysozyme (Endo et al 1989) found in gingival crevicular fluid (GCF) and saliva.

P. gingivalis culture supernatant has been found to activate the production of MMP-2 by human periodontal ligament cells and this effect could be inhibited by MMP inhibitors (Puttamapun et al 2003). The supernatant was also found to upregulate the expression of MT1 MMP by these cells both in terms of transcription and translation and the bacterium's activation of MMP-2 might involve this mechanism.

P. gingivalis potently induces the production of pro-inflammatory cytokines by neutrophils, monocytes, and macrophages (Cohen et al 2004). It can also desensitize immune cells *in vitro* and *in vivo*. This group analysed the ability of *P. gingivalis* lipopolysaccharide (LPS) to induce endotoxin tolerance. Treatment of dendritic cells (DCs), the human macrophage cell line THP-1, and monocytes (antigen-presenting cells, APC) with *P. gingivalis* LPS inhibited APC maturation assessed by CD80 and CD86 expression, and inhibited the production of chemokines CCL3 and CCL5. Pre-treatment with glucocorticoids and interleukin-10 abolished the effect of *P. gingivalis* LPS on CD80, CD83, and CD86, and on CCL3 and CCL5 production. They also showed that *P. gingivalis* LPS enhanced the tolerogenic properties of APCs and upregulated ILT-3 and B7-H1 expression. Thus *P. gingivalis* appears to induce tolerance of APCs and this mechanism could possibly be an important factor implicated in periodontal disease parthenogenesis.

Mahanonda et al (2004) studied the possible hyper-responsiveness of monocytes to bacterial lipopolysaccharide (LPS) in aggressive periodontitis patients. They used whole-blood cultures to compare monocyte activation by *P. gingivalis* LPS between Thai subjects with generalized aggressive periodontitis and those without periodontitis. Upon stimulation with *P. gingivalis* LPS, expression of co-stimulatory molecules on monocytes and expression of CD69 on NK and γ and ΔT cells were analysed by flow cytometry. The production of interleukin-1β and prostaglandin E_2 was monitored by ELISA. LPS stimulation resulted in a dose-dependent upregulation of CD40, CD80, and CD86 on monocytes, and upregulation of CD69 on NK cells and γ and ΔT cells in both the periodontitis and non-periodontitis groups. The levels of activation markers and the mediator production after LPS stimulation were quite similar for both groups. Thus they did not observe hyper-responsiveness of monocytes to *P. gingivalis* LPS challenge in Thai patients with aggressive periodontitis.

Modulation of pro-inflammatory cytokine activity is a plausible therapeutic target in periodontal disease. Vasoactive intestinal peptide (VIP) has a role in immunoregulation, and has been identified as a molecule with therapeutically beneficial immunosuppressive effects in inflammatory and autoimmune conditions. In this regard, Foster et al (2005) investigated the effect of VIP on immune responses induced by *P. gingivalis* LPS *in vitro*. They found that VIP (10–8 M) significantly ($p<0.05$) inhibited TNF- production by human monocytic THP1 cells stimulated with *P. gingivalis* LPS and also that VIP inhibited nuclear translocation of NFβ and c-Jun in a time-dependent manner, but did not decrease the expression of CD14 receptors. Thus, VIP may have the potential as an immunomodulator of *P. gingivalis*-stimulated inflammatory pathways in human monocytes.

Walter et al (2004) showed that *in vitro* two strains of *P. gingivalis*, ATCC 53799 and DSMZ 20709, were able to infect endothelial cells and trigger signalling cascades leading to endothelial activation, which in turn may result in or promote severe local and systemic inflammation.

VASCULAR SYSTEM

P. gingivalis proteinases may degrade some key factors in the serum protein cascades, which in turn increase vascular permeability (Kaminishi et al 1993; Nilsson et al 1985; Travis et al 1997). RgpA and RgpB have been shown to activate the pre-kallikrein system leading to the formation of bradykinin which causes vasodilation (Imamura et al 1997). Both RgpA and RgpB activate prekallikrein while both in addition to Kgp may degrade high-molecular weight kininogen directly to bradykinin (Imamura et al 1997; Travis et al 1997). Thus both arg-gingipain and lys-gingipain appear to work in concert to produce vasodilation and an increase in vascular permeability. These processes increase gingival crevicular fluid production and thus provide continuous supply of nutrients for this bacterium, enhancing its growth and virulence.

P. gingivalis possesses several protease related properties that prevent blood clotting and hence promote bleeding (Imamura et al 1995). Its proteases can alter the clotting precipitator factor X (Imamura et al 1997; Nilsson et al 1985).

Fibrinogen is particularly susceptible to degradation by *P. gingivalis* proteinases (Grenier 1992; Schenkein et al 1995; Travis et al 1997; Imamura 2003) and this appears to be mainly caused by Kgp activity (Imamura et al 1995). Gingipains act as adhesins and have a strong binding affinity for fibrinogen. This interaction inhibits haemagglutination (Travis et al 1997). All the bound proteins are then easily degraded by the functional proteinase domain. Fibrinogen degradation increases the local clotting time leading to gingival bleeding. The bleeding of periodontal sites is of primary importance for the growth of *P. gingivalis* since it ensures a rich source of haem and iron that *P. gingivalis* requires for survival.

Finally purified protease preparation, mainly RgpA, can induce the aggregation of human platelets (Curtis et al 1999).

HOST TISSUE DESTRUCTION

As well as being essential for the nutrition of *P. gingivalis* its proteinases could be involved in periodontal tissue degradation (Eley & Cox 2003) and they have been shown to degrade protein substrates such as albumin (Fujimura & Nakamura 1987; Hinode et al 1992; Otsuka et al 1987; Tsutsui et al 1987) and iron-binding proteins (Carlsson et al 1984b).

Most tissue destruction in periodontitis seems to be mediated by host-derived enzymes (Sorsa et al 1992). However, it has been shown that *P. gingivalis* proteinases can influence these host systems (Potempa et al 1995b; Sorsa et al 1992). However, *P. gingivalis* has been shown to be capable of degrading type 1 collagen (Birkedal-Hansen et al 1988; Gibbons and MacDonald 1961; Tokuda et al 1998; Toda et al 1984). In some studies this has been attributed to arg-gingipain (Bedi & Williams 1994; Tokuda et al 1998) but this has more recently been questioned (Potempa et al 1995a). In this regard, collagenolytic proteinases have been isolated from *P. gingivalis* (Kato et al 1992; Lawson & Meyer 1992; Sojar et al 1993) including the products of the prt C gene (Kato et al 1992) and these proteases could be responsible for degrading collagen I.

However, purified protease preparation, mainly RgpA, has been shown to activate fibroblasts and PMNs to produce MMP-1 and MMP-8 respectively (Sorsa et al 1992) which would then lead to the degradation of collagen by host MMPs. In this respect it has also been shown that it can degrade the main MMP inhibitor, TIMP I into lower molecular weight fragments (Grenier & Mayrand 2001). Furthermore, this protease can also induce the secretion of plasminogen activator from fibroblasts (Uitto et al 1989a), which will lead to the formation of plasmin which can

also activate pro-collagenases. Finally, this protease has been shown to degrade the plasma proteinase inhibitors, α1-proteinase inhibitor and α2-macroglobulin (Carlsson et al 1984a; Potempa et al 1995b; Genier 1996), antichymotrypsin, antithrombin III, antiplasmin and cystatin C (Grenier 1996), which would lead to further connective tissue degradation.

RgpA has also been shown to degrade basement membrane type IV collagen (Potempa et al 1995b) and other components of the extracellular matrix including fibronectin, laminin and other cell surface glycoproteins (Lantz et al 1991a, 1991b; Potempa et al 1995b; Smalley et al 1988b; Uitto et al 1988b, 1989). Gingipains have a strong binding affinity for fibronectin and laminin which inhibits haemagglutination (Travis et al 1997). All the bound proteins are then easily degraded by the functional proteinase domain. By these processes these proteases may progressively attach to, degrade and detach from their target proteins. Since these proteinase-adhesin complexes are present on the surfaces of the vesicles and membranes of *P. gingivalis*, they may play an important role in the attachment of this bacterium to host cells (Kuramitsu 1998).

Thus *P. gingivalis* proteinases could play an important role in periodontal pathology as they have the potential to degrade connective tissues and basement membrane, to interfere with host defences by degrading immunoglobulins and complement and degrading or activating inflammatory proteins (Sojar et al 1993) and to activate host MMP 1 and 8 (Sorsa et al 1992).

All of the cysteine proteinases, collagenolytic proteinases, dipeptidyl peptidases and other proteases described above would appear to be located in the cell wall, to be concentrated in outer membrane vesicles and to be released into the surrounding environment in extracellular vesicles. Thus, they could enter the periodontal tissues and play a role in periodontal pathology. In summary, these proteases could:

- Degrade basement membrane and extracellular matrix proteins including collagens, proteoglycans and glycoproteins such as fibronectin. This would both destroy periodontal connective tissue and facilitate bacterial invasion of the host tissues
- Interfere with tissue repair by inhibiting clot formation or lysing the fibrin matrix in periodontal lesions
- Activate latent host tissue collagenases (MMP 1 and 8) which would enhance host tissue enzyme-mediated tissue destruction
- Inactivate proteins important in host defence.

Shelburne et al (2005) used restriction fragment differential display (RFDD) to identify and measure the genes of *P. gingivalis* expressed by surrogates of environmental stresses, heat and oxidative stress and were confirmed using quantitative reverse-transcription polymerase chain reaction. They selected 16 genes differentially induced from over 800 total expression fragments on the RFDD gels for further characterization. With primers designed from those fragments they found that a +5°C heat shock caused a statistically significant increase in expression compared with 12 of 18 untreated genes tested. The exposure of *P. gingivalis* to atmospheric oxygen resulted in statistically significant increases in five of the target genes. These genes are likely to be involved in transport and synthesis of components of the lipopolysaccharide biosynthetic pathway important in anchoring the Arg-gingipains required for virulence-related activities. They felt that these results emphasized the need for studies to measure the coordinated responses of bacteria like *P. gingivalis* which use a multitude of interrelated metabolic activities to survive the environmental hazards of the infection process.

Hydrolytic enzymes

The hydrolytic enzymes may also play a subsidiary role in host tissue degradation and in this regard hyaluronidase and chondroitinase activities could hydrolyse the glycosaminoglycan components of proteoglycan

(Fiehn 1986; Seddon & Shah 1989; Steffen & Hengtes 1981; Tipler & Embery 1985). The neuraminidase activity (Moncla et al 1990) might attack sialoproteins between the cells of epithelium increasing the permeability of the crevicular or pocket epithelium and lead to its ulceration.

Prevotella intermedia and *P. nigrescens*

Proteolytic enzymes

Prevotella intermedia and *nigrescens* proteases are capable of degrading a number of tissue, tissue fluid and immune proteins (Eley & Cox 2003). The proteases have been shown to have trypsin-like activity which has the properties cysteine proteases (Gazi et al 1997). This trypsin-like activity is however weak when compared with that produced by *Porphyromonas gingivalis* (Gazi et al 1994, 1996, 1997). Furthermore, these bacteria have been shown to have no aminopeptidase, chymotrypsin- or elastase-like activity (Laughton et al 1982a; Seddon & Shah 1989; Slots 1981; Suido et al 1988a,b). They do, however, produce moderate levels dipeptidyl peptidase activity (Cox et al 1993; Gazi et al 1995, 1997; Suido et al 1986).

Kim et al (2004) have shown that *Prevotella intermedia* lipopolysaccharide fully induced inducible nitric oxide synthase (iNOS) expression and NO production in a macrophage cell line in the absence of other stimuli. The ability of *P. intermedia* lipopolysaccharide to promote the production of NO may be important in the pathogenesis of inflammatory periodontal disease.

Hydrolytic enzymes

This bacteria also produces strong acid and alkaline phosphatase activity (Laughton et al 1982b; Slots 1981).

EFFECTS OF *P. INTERMEDIA* AND NIGRESCENS ENZYMES ON THE HOST

INFLAMMATORY AND IMMUNE SYSTEMS

Prevotella sp. trypsin-like proteases are able to degrade immunoglobulins particularly IgG (Jansen et al 1995; Kilian 1981) and fibrinogen (Smalley et al 1988a) and thus reduce the effectiveness of host immune and inflammatory defences.

Host tissue proteins

Prevotella sp. proteases are able to contribute to the degradation of a number of tissue proteins including collagen (Uitto et al 1989b) and fibronectin (Larjarva et al 1987; Wikström & Lindhe 1986). In this regard, proteolytic activity has been demonstrated against gelatin (Seddon & Shah 1989; Wikström & Lindhe 1986) and fibronectin (Larjarva et al 1987; Wikström & Lindhe 1986) and also it has been shown to activate host pro-collagenases (Sorsa et al 1992). However, these bacteria only produce relatively low levels of trypsin-like activity (Table 5.1), responsible for these actions (Gazi et al 1994, 1996, 1997).

Treponema species

The spirochaetes from the periodontal pocket that have been cultivated are *Treponema denticola, T. pectinovorum, T. socranskii* and *T. vincentii* and of these *T. denticola* seems to be the most virulent (Chen & McLaughlin 2000; Eley & Cox 2003).

The primary niche for oral spirochaetes is the gingival crevice/periodontal pocket and to prevent being washed away by GCF they must attach to a substrate. *T. denticola* has been shown to adhere to fibroblasts by lectin mediated binding and also to the basement membrane proteins fibronectin, laminin and type IV collagen and type I collagen, gelatin, fibrinogen (Chen & McLaughlin 2000). The major surface protein of *T. denticola* that is involved in this adherence is a 53 kDa protein.

Proteolytic enzymes

T. denticola has an outer cell envelope which contains a number of proteases important to its nutrition and these have been termed ectoenzymes (Makinen & Makinen 1996). These include the membrane-associated chymotrypsin-like protease which in addition to its proteolytic role can also mediate the adherence of this bacterium to hyaluronan (Chen & McLaughlin 2000).

T. denticola also can agglutinate and lyse red blood cells (RBCs) (Grenier 1991). This first involves the bacterium adhering to the RBC and then damaging its cell membrane. A 46 kDa haemolysin of *T. denticola* is responsible for these processes and is a product of its hly gene (Chen & McLaughlin 2000). Its main proteolytic enzyme, the chymotrypsin-like protease, can also produce haemolysis. It is a 30.4 kDa protein and is a product of its prtB gene.

T. denticola shows significant proteolytic activity against a range of host components such as collagens type IV, fibronectin, keratin and fibrin (Lantz et al 1991b; Larjarva et al 1987; Mikx & De Jong 1987; Smalley et al 1988b; Uitto et al 1988a,b; Wikström & Lindhe 1986). The gene coding for the *T. denticola* chymotrypsin-like activity has been isolated from this bacterium and has been inserted into *E. coli*. The protein product (the cloned enzyme) showed similar properties to the bacteria itself in its effects on some host proteins (Que & Kuramitsu 1990). However, there is evidence that the cloned chymotrypsin-like protease does not directly hydrolyse fibronectin, type IV collagen or laminin (Arakawa & Kuramitsu 1994).

T. denticola proteases have also been shown to be capable of activating fibroblast and neutrophil pro-collagenases (Sorsa et al 1992). The *T. denticola* chymotrypsin-like protease has also been shown to degrade $\alpha1$ proteinase inhibitor, anti-chymotrypsin, $\alpha2$ macroglobulin, antithrombin III, antiplasmin and cystatin (Grenier 1996) and IgA, IgG, serum albumin and transferrin and to convert angiotensin into angiotensin II and breakdown angiotensin II into tetrapeptides (Makinen et al 1995). *T. denticola* also hydrolyses a number of synthetic peptide substrates including those degraded by aminopeptidase, trypsin-, chymotrypsin- and bacterial collagenase-like activities (Laughton et al 1982b; Mäkinen et al 1986; Uitto et al 1988a,b) (Table 5.1).

The *T. denticola* chymotrypsin-like protease has also been shown to have potent cytotoxic effects on epithelial cells in culture (Chen & McLaughlin 2000). The purified protein was shown to be able to degrade endogenous pericellular fibronectin on epithelial cells and fibroblasts and this may be the source of its cytotoxic effects on these cells. The 53 kDa surface protein as well as functioning as an adhesin also acts as a porin.

Trypsin-like activity can be detected in strains of *T. denticola* and *T. pectinovorum* but not in strains of *T. socranskii* or *T. vincentii*. This protease differs from the enzyme from *Porphyromonas gingivalis* and appears to play a much lesser role in virulence (Chen & McLaughlin 2000).

In contrast *T. vincentii* has negligible trypsin- and chymotrypsin-like activities (Laughton et al 1982a; Mäkinen et al 1986; Uitto et al 1988a,b), although it does appear to possess collagenase-like and aminopeptidase-like activities (Mäkinen et al 1986). These proteases are also found in the outer sheath and extracellular vesicles from these bacteria (Rosen et al 1995).

The capacity of *T. denticola* to degrade proteins appears to be mostly associated with its chymotrypsin-like activity. The partially purified activity has a molecular weight of 95 kDa, a pH optimum of 7.5 and the characteristics of a cysteine proteinase (Uitto et al 1988a,b). However, the fully purified enzyme has a molecular weight of 30.4 kDa (Chen & McLaughlin 2000).

This enzyme has a broad range of proteolytic activity and extensively breaks down transferrin, fibrinogen and gelatin and produces a limited cleavage of α1 proteinase inhibitor and immunoglobulins. It has also been found to attack the basement membrane components including collagen type IV, fibronectin and laminin. This ability, together with its location on the outside of the cell envelope, indicates a possible role for this proteinase in destruction and invasion of the epithelium by *T. denticola* (Grenier et al 1990).

The trypsin-like proteinases of *T. denticola* are active against BANA and BAPNA substrates and there is evidence that two different enzymes cleave each of these substrates. Furthermore, these activities may vary in different strains of this bacterium. The protease active against BAPNA has a molecular weight in the range of 40–69 kDa and a pH optimum of about 8.5 (Ohta et al 1986). It had the characteristics of a serine proteinase but was not able to degrade haemoglobin or gelatin.

Both *T. denticola* and *T. vincentii* are able to cleave synthetic substrates for bacterial collagenase activity (Mäkinen et al 1988). Cell extracts from *T. vincentii* yielded two fractions active against this substrate with molecular weight of 23 and 75 kDa and pH optima of 7.0–8.0 and 6.5–7.5, respectively (Mäkinen et al 1988). Both activities have the characteristics of metalloproteinases and the 75 kDa fraction hydrolysed gelatin at a low rate.

The gene coding for the *T. denticola* collagenase-like activity has been isolated and inserted into *E. coli*. Furthermore, the cloned enzyme has been purified and characterized (Que & Kuramitsu 1990). This has a molecular weight of 36 kDa and a pH optimum of 7.5. Like the *T. vincentii* collagenase enzyme it has the characteristics of a metalloproteinase. However, it is unable to directly hydrolyse collagens types I and IV or gelatin.

T. denticola produces both an iminopeptidase and an aminopeptidase. The iminopeptidase has a molecular weight of 100 kDa, a pH optimum of 7.5 and the characteristics of a cysteine protease (Mäkinen et al 1986, 1987). As collagen is rich in proline, it is possible that the enzyme acts on collagen degradation products to provide nutrition for the organism. Some *T. denticola* strains also produce an aminopeptidase cleaving terminal aspartic acid residues (Mäkinen et al 1986). *T. vincentii* gave the highest aminopeptidase activity cleaving terminal arginine residues and this has a molecular weight of about 200 kDa and a pH optimum of 7.0–8.0 (Mäkinen et al 1988). Finally *T. denticola* has also been shown to produce dipeptidylpeptidase activity (Gazi et al 1997).

Hydrolytic enzymes

Hyaluronidase and chondroitinase activities are produced by *T. denticola* (Fiehn 1986; Seddon & Shah 1989; Steffan & Hengtes 1981; Tipler & Embery 1985).

EFFECTS OF *TREPONEMA* SPECIES ENZYMES ON THE HOST

INFLAMMATORY AND IMMUNE SYSTEMS

The chymotrypsin-like cysteine proteinase of *T. denticola* can degrade immunoglobulins and fibrinogen (Uitto et al 1988a,b; Eley & Cox 2003) and thus reduce the effectiveness of host immune and inflammatory defences.

McDowell et al (2005) investigated the ability of *T. denticola* to bind the complement regulatory proteins factor H and factor H-like protein 1 (FHL-1). The binding of these proteins had previously been demonstrated to facilitate evasion of the alternative complement cascade and/or to play a role in adherence and invasion. These workers showed that *T. denticola* specifically bound to FHL-1 via a 14-kDa, surface-exposed protein that they designated FhbB. Consistent with its FHL-1 binding specificity, FhbB bound only to factor H recombinant fragments spanning short consensus repeats (SCRs) 1–7 (H7 construct) and not to SCR constructs spanning SCRs 8–15

and 16–20. Binding of H7 to FhbB was inhibited by heparin. The specific involvement of SCR 7 in the interaction was demonstrated using an H7 mutant (H7AB) in which specific charged residues in SCR 7 were replaced by alanine. This construct lost FhbB binding ability. Analyses of the ability of FHL-1 bound to the surface of *T. denticola* to serve as a cofactor for factor I-mediated cleavage of C3b revealed that C3b was cleaved in an FHL-1/factor I-independent manner, perhaps by an unidentified protease. Based on this data they hypothesize that the primary function of FHL-1 binding by *T. denticola* might have been to facilitate adherence to FHL-1 present on anchorage-dependent cells and in the extracellular matrix.

Thomas et al (2006) showed that pre-treatment of human polymorphonuclear leucocytes (PMNs) with *Treponema denticola* major outer sheath protein (Msp) inhibited formyl-methionyl-leucyl-phenylalanine (fMLP)-induced chemotaxis, phagocytosis of immunoglobulin G-coated microspheres, fMLP-stimulated calcium transients, and actin assembly. Msp neither altered oxidative responses to phorbol myristate or fMLP nor induced apoptosis. Thus, Msp may selectively impair chemotaxis and phagocytosis by impacting the PMN cytoskeleton.

Host tissue proteins

The chymotrypsin-like cysteine proteinase of *T. denticola* can degrade a wide range of tissue proteins including transferrin, gelatin, α1-antiproteinase inhibitor and the basement membrane components type IV collagen, fibronectin and laminin (Uitto et al 1988a,b). This latter ability may aid its invasion of the epithelium (Grenier et al 1990). This proteinase has also been shown to activate latent neutrophil and fibroblast type collagenases and thus secondarily stimulate collagen degradation (Sorsa et al 1992). Its effects on α1-proteinase inhibitor will also alter the balance towards collagen degradation (Uitto et al 1988a,b).

The trypsin-like serine proteinases of *T. denticola* have only limited activity against degradation products and are unable to degrade intact gelatin (Ohta et al 1986). The iminopeptidase, aminopeptidase (Mäkinen et al 1986, 1987) and dipeptidylpeptidase activity (Gazi et al 1997) also act upon tissue degradation products. Likewise the bacterial collagenase activity from these bacteria are unable to degrade intact type I or IV collagen and therefore can only play a secondary role in collagen degradation (Mäkinen et al 1988; Que & Kuramitsu 1990).

Hydrolytic enzymes

The hyaluronidase and chondroitinase activities produced by *T. denticola* (Fiehn 1986; Seddon & Shah 1989; Steffan & Hengtes 1981; Tipler & Embery 1985) can hydrolyse the glycosaminoglycan components of proteoglycans.

CAPNOCYTOPHAGA SPECIES

Proteolytic enzymes

Capnocytophaga species show low to moderate activity against host proteins (Eley & Cox 2003) (Table 5.1) and may degrade types I and IV collagens and immunoglobulins (Kilian 1981; Seddon & Shah 1989). In a recent study both smooth and rough surfaced strains were found to possess weak to moderate activity against Type I collagen, gelatin, collagen polypeptides and synthetic bacterial collagenase substrates (Söderling et al 1991). The main fraction of the separated sample which contained these activities had a molecular weight of 54 kDa. The cleavage of IgA1 by *C. gingivalis*, *C. ochracea* and *C. sputigena* protease was inhibited by metal chelators, suggesting that metalloproteinases were involved.

Weak trypsin-like activity has been shown in *C. gingivalis*, *C. ochracea* and *C. sputigena* by a number of studies (Gazi et al 1994, 1996, 1997; Laughton et al 1982b; Nakamura & Slots 1982; Seddon & Shah 1989; Slots

1981; Söderling et al 1991; Suido et al 1986). However, more recently, this activity has been shown to consist of two separate proteases, one specific for arginine and the other for lysine substrates (Gazi et al 1997). Weak chymotrypsin-like activity has also been detected in various *Capnocytophaga* sp. (Gazi et al 1996, 1997). In addition, weak elastase activity has been found in *C. sputigena* and very weak activity in *C. gingivalis* and *C. ochracea* (Gazi et al 1996, 1997).

A number of studies have found that all *Capnocytophaga* strains and species possess high aminopeptidase (Slots 1981; Söderling et al 1991; Suido et al 1986) and dipeptidylpeptidase activity (Gazi et al 1997).

Hydrolytic enzymes

Hyaluronidase and chondroitinase activities are produced by *C. ochracea* (Fiehn 1986; Seddon & Shah 1989; Steffan & Hengtes 1981; Tipler & Embery 1985). Strong acid and alkaline phosphatase activities are also produced by *Capnocytophaga* species (Laughton et al 1982b; Slots 1981).

EFFECTS OF *CAPNOCYTOPHAGA* SPECIES ENZYMES ON THE HOST

Proteases

Immune system

Capnocytophaga species show low to moderate activity against immunoglobulins (Kilian 1981; Seddon & Shah 1989). This may involve both actions of both metallo- and cysteine proteinases from these species.

Host tissue proteins

Capnocytophaga species show low to moderate activity against host proteins including Types I and IV collagens and gelatins (Kilian 1981; Robertson et al 1982; Seddon & Shah 1989). The particular proteases responsible for these activities are not certain and this activity could be both direct and indirect.

Hydrolytic enzymes

Hyaluronidase and chondroitinase activities are produced by *C. ochracea* (Fiehn 1986; Seddon & Shah 1989; Steffan & Hengtes 1981; Tipler & Embery 1985) which may hydrolyse the glycosaminoglycan components of proteoglycans.

ACTINOBACILLUS ACTINOMYCETEMCOMITANS (NOW AGGREGATIBACTER ACTINOMYCETEMCOMITANS)

Proteolytic enzymes

Some studies have shown that *A. actinomycetemcomitans* is able to degrade native type I collagen (Robertson et al 1982; Rozanis & Slots 1982; Rozanis et al 1983) and a synthetic substrate for bacterial collagenases (Rozanis et al 1983) (Table 5.1). The activity is found both in bacterial cellular material and the culture medium (Robertson et al 1982; Rozanis & Slots 1982). This protease(s) (Eley & Cox 2003) produces multiple scissions in the collagen molecule (Robertson et al 1982). The activity has the characteristics of a metalloproteinase (Robertson et al 1982; Rozanis & Slots 1982; Rozanis et al 1983). Weak gelatinase activity has also been reported. However, surveys with a variety of other substrates have shown that this bacteria produces no trypsin-, chymotrypsin-, elastase-, dipeptidyl peptidase- or aminopeptidase-like activity (Laughton et al 1982a; Seddon & Shah 1989; Slots 1981; Suido et al 1986) (Table 5.1). However, unidentified alanine/lysine activity has been detected (Gazi et al 1997).

Cellular invasion

A. actinomycetemcomitans has been shown to be capable of invading the superficial gingival tissues in localized juvenile periodontitis (see Ch. 23). Two cell invasion-related loci, apiA and the two gene operon apiBC, have been isolated from this bacterium (Li et al 2004). The apiA gene encoded for a 32.5 kDa protein which facilitated the binding of this cell surface locus to collagen types II, III, and V and fibronectin. The apiB and apiC genes encoded for proteins of 130.1 and 70.6 kDa, respectively which increased the binding to collagen III. ApiB-deficient mutants exhibited a 4-fold diminished capacity to invade KB epithelial cells whereas apiA-deficient mutants showed increased cell invasion. Thus these genes and their proteins in loci on the surface of this bacterium are related to the ability of this bacterium to invade epithelial cells and to bind to cell-associated connective tissue proteins.

A. actinomycetemcomitans also adheres to the root surface probably by means of its fimbriae. The DNA sequence of the major fimbrial subunit gene (fip-1) has been investigated (Kaplan et al 2002) and has found to have seven variations in 43 samples of this bacterium isolated in Europe, Japan and the USA. This could be utilized to detect different genetic strains of this bacterium.

Effects of *A. actinomycetemcomitans* enzymes on the host

Collagenase

A. actinomycetemcomitans produces a collagenolytic proteinase which can attack type I collagen (Robertson et al 1982; Rozanis & Slots 1982; Rozanis et al 1983). This could contribute to degradation of collagen and connective tissue breakdown in the periodontal tissues.

In addition, an arginine- and lysin-specific protease of approximately 50 kDa in molecular weight has been purified from the culture supernatant of *A. actinomycetemcomitans* and this enzyme showed collagen degrading activity (Wang et al 1999).

This purified protease (Wang et al 1999) has also been shown to reduce the cell growth rate, DNA synthesis rate and fibronectin level of human gingival epithelial cells in a dose-dependent way *in vitro* (Wang et al 2001). Thus this protease may inhibit the proliferation of these cells.

Inflammatory and immune systems

Capsular polysaccharide from *A. actinomycetemcomitans* Y4 has been shown to inhibit the release of IL-6 and IL-8 from human gingival fibroblasts and this mechanism could modulate the inflammatory response (Ohguchi et al 2003). This effect was reversed by specific anti-*A. actinomycetemcomitans* Y4 antibodies which suggests an important relationship between this bacterium and the host humoral response.

FUSOBACTERIUM NUCLEATUM

Once established, early-colonizing bacterial species tend to persist in the mouth. To obtain detailed information on the population dynamics of early-colonizing oral anaerobes, one study (Haraldsson et al 2004) examined the clonal diversity and persistence of clones among oral *F. nucleatum* populations in infants during the first 2 years of life. Consecutive salivary samples from 12 infants were collected at 2, 6, 12, 18, and 24 months of age and they yielded a total of 546 *F. nucleatum* isolates for clonal typing with arbitrarily primed PCR (AP-PCR). Up to seven AP-PCR types were simultaneously detected in each sample. Furthermore, in 11 out of the 12 infants examined, AP-PCR types persisted for up to 1 year. Strain turnover rate was found to be high during the first year of life after which the occurrence of persistent clones increased. The results indicated a wide genetic diversity within this species and provided evidence for the increasing persistence of *F. nucleatum* clones in the oral cavity with age.

Proteolytic enzymes

F. nucleatum appears to have little ability to degrade proteins or synthetic substrates for trypsin-, chymotrypsin-, elastase-, dipeptidyl peptidase-, or aminopeptidase-like activity (Suido et al 1986) (Table 5.1).

Hydrolytic enzymes

Hyaluronidase and chondroitinase activities are produced by *F. nucleatum* (Fiehn 1986; Seddon & Shah 1989; Steffan & Hengtes 1981; Tipler & Embery 1985).

EFFECTS OF *F. NUCLEATUM* ENZYMES ON THE HOST

The ability of this bacteria to degrade structural or vascular proteins seems limited and its role in connective tissue degradation appears to be very limited since it appears to produce no proteases. This is probably why it is always found in association with many other bacteria and within the periodontal pocket it seems to rely on the proteolytic functions of other bacteria to provide it with a source of amino acids.

However, Gendron et al (2004) have investigated the ability of *F. nucleatum* subsp. *nucleatum* to increase its tissue-invasive potential by acquiring cell-associated human matrix metalloproteinase 9 (MMP-9) activity. They demonstrated the binding of pro-MMP-9 to fusobacteria by enzyme-linked immunosorbent assay and they also showed by zymography and a colorimetric assay that the bound pro-MMP-9 can be converted into a proteolytically active form. This therefore suggests that this bacterium may use this mechanism in tissue invasion and this was demonstrated using a reconstituted basement membrane.

LIPOPOLYSACCHARIDE

Grenier and Grignon (2006) assessed the response of human monocyte cells, differentiated into adherent macrophages to stimulation by *F. nucleatum* ssp. *nucleatum* lipopolysaccharide. Attachment of 3H-lipopolysaccharide to macrophage-like cells was partially inhibited by anti-CD14 and anti-TLR4 polyclonal antibodies. Fusobacterial lipopolysaccharide did not cause cell apoptosis or block apoptosis induced by camptothecin. Lipopolysaccharide upregulated the secretion of the pro-inflammatory cytokines and the chemokine interleukin-8 by macrophage-like cells. In addition, it increased phospholipase C and D activities, which may have contributed to the high levels of prostaglandin E_2 detected in the cell culture supernatant. Lastly, the amount of matrix metalloproteinase-9 produced by macrophage-like cells was significantly increased by the lipopolysaccharide treatment. Thus, the lipopolysaccharide of *F. nucleatum* ssp. *nucleatum* appeared to possess a large array of biological effects on macrophage-like cells. This monocytic responsiveness to lipopolysaccharide may be one of the regulators of periodontitis.

CAMPYLOBACTER RECTA

Proteolytic enzymes

C. recta produces aminopeptidases but so far no proteinases have been detected (Table 5.1) (Umemoto et al 1991).

Effects of C. recta enzymes on the host

The proteases of *C. recta* would seem to be active only against protein degradation products produced by other bacteria for nutritional purposes. These proteases have not been further characterized (Umemoto et al 1991).

EIKENELLA CORRODENS

Proteolytic enzymes

E. corrodens produces proteases connected with its nutritional use of protein (Table 5.1) but these have not yet been characterized (Umemoto et al 1991).

Effects of E. corrodens enzymes on the host

The lack of characterization of *E. corrodens* proteases makes this impossible to assess at this point in time (Umemoto et al 1991).

ANAEROBIC GRAM-POSITIVE BACTERIA

The uncertain taxonomy of oral anaerobic Gram-positive bacilli and their slow growing nature has limited the understanding of their role in periodontal disease. In view of this Booth et al (2004) used species-specific oligonucleotide probes to investigate the relationship of selected Gram-positive anaerobic bacilli to periodontal disease. Subgingival samples and clinical measurements were collected from 40 patients with periodontitis and from 40 matched controls *Mogibacterium timidum* and *Bulleidia extracta* were detected in only three and four samples, respectively. However, the level of both *Eubacterium nodatum* and *Slackia exigua* was significantly higher in deep compared to shallow pockets (Wilcoxon, $p<0.001$). The level of *E. nodatum*, but not *S. exigua*, was higher in patients than matched controls (Mann-Whitney U, $p<0.03$). Using an ordered logistic regression model, the probing depth of the sampled sites had the greatest influence on the level of both species and significant variations occurred between individuals. Bleeding also influenced the levels of both species, with supragingival plaque also influencing *S. exigua*. Thus, both *E. nodatum* and *S. exigua* were found to be associated with the clinical indicators of periodontal disease.

THE COMBINED EFFECTS OF BACTERIAL SPECIES

Kesavalu et al (2007) documented that *P. gingivalis*, *T. denticola*, and *Tannerella forsythia* not only existed as a consortium but were associated with chronic periodontitis. They also showed that their synergistic virulence resulted in the immunoinflammatory bone resorption which is characteristic of periodontitis.

VIRUSES AND PERIODONTAL DISEASE

There have been some reports of the presence of viruses in subgingival plaque and recent findings have begun to provide a basis for a causal link between herpesviruses and aggressive periodontitis. One theory is that herpes viruses cooperate with specific bacteria in the aetiopathogenesis of the disease. Yapar et al (2003) investigated the presence of the human cytomegalovirus (HCMV) and the Epstein–Barr virus (EBV) in subgingival plaque samples from 17 aggressive periodontitis patients and 16 healthy controls using the polymerase chain reaction (PCR). They also took samples before and after treatment of the periodontitis patients which was related to clinical parameters. They found that HCMV was present in 64.7% of aggressive periodontitis patients and none of the healthy controls ($p<0.001$) and that EBV was found in 70.6% of aggressive periodontitis patients and 6.3% of healthy controls ($p<0.0001$). Furthermore, co-infection with both viruses was found in 41.7% of the aggressive periodontitis patients and none of the healthy controls ($p<0.001$). There were also statistically significant decreases in clinical parameters and HCMV and EBV following treatment ($p<0.001$) and after treatment none of the patients harboured

HCMV and only one EBV. These findings indicate that the subgingival presence of HCMV and EBV appear to be strongly associated with aggressive periodontitis. Similar findings were also found by Kubar et al (2005) and Slots et al (2006).

Saygun et al (2004) investigated whether the presence of herpes viruses including human cytomegalovirus (HCMV), Epstein–Barr virus (EBV) type 1, herpes simplex virus (HSV) type 1 and 2 were associated with the presence of putative pathogenic bacteria (*P. gingivalis, Prevotella intermedia, T. forsythia, Campylobacter rectus, A. actinomycetemcomitans*) in aggressive periodontitis lesions. They compared 18 young adults with advanced periodontitis and 16 periodontally healthy subjects from Ankara, Turkey. Subgingival specimens pooled from two sites in each subject were collected with a periodontal curette. Qualitative polymerase chain reaction methodology was used to identify herpes viruses and bacteria. Chi-square tests were employed to determine statistical associations among herpes viruses, bacteria and periodontal disease. HCMV, EBV-1 and HSV-1 were each detected in 72–78% of the aggressive periodontitis patients. HSV-2 occurred in 17% of the periodontitis patients. EBV-1 was detected in one periodontally healthy subject. *Porphyromonas gingivalis, T. forsythia* and *C. rectus* occurred in 78–83% and *Prevotella intermedia* and *A. actinomycetemcomitans* in 44% of the aggressive periodontitis patients. All the test bacteria were only detected in a very small minority of the healthy patients. HCMV, EBV-1 and HSV-1 were positively associated with *Porphyromonas gingivalis, Prevotella intermedia, T. forsythia* and *C. rectus*, but not with *A. actinomycetemcomitans*. HSV-2 was not associated with any test bacteria. Another study (Ling et al 2004) reported similar results for herpes viruses and showed that HSV appeared to be related to the severity of periodontal diseases in terms of clinical attachment loss and also that coinfection of any two herpes viruses may also play roles. These results support the notion that the clinical outcome of some types of severe periodontal infection may be influenced by the co-presence of specific herpes viruses and bacterial pathogens. These findings would need to be supported by the testing of a variety of hypotheses regarding the deleterious aspects of combined herpes viral-bacterial infections in periodontal sites since at present studies only show associations.

A recent review of viruses and periodontal pathogenesis (Cappuyns et al 2005) concluded that the sampling methods and general methodology of many studies and the interpretation of their data cast doubts on the role of viruses in the aetiology of periodontal disease. Also another recent study (Konstantinidis et al 2005) utilizing RT-PCR detection of EBV showed negative findings.

BACTERIAL METABOLITES AND TOXIC FACTORS

There are many bacterial metabolites and toxic products which can damage the tissues or stimulate inflammation. They include ammonia, toxic amines, indole, organic acids, hydrogen sulphide, methylmercaptan and dimethyl disulphide (Slots & Genco 1984).

Gram-negative bacterial cell walls contain lipopolysaccharides (LPS, endotoxins) which are released when they die. Distinct LPSs are produced by individual species but they share common properties, including activating complement by the alternative pathway and stimulating bone resorption in tissue culture. Lipoteichoic acid and peptidoglycans present in Gram-positive bacterial cell walls also stimulate bone resorption (Meikle et al 1986). Extracts from Gram-negative bacteria isolated from periodontal pockets can cause polyclonal B-cell activation, which could contribute to periodontal pathology by inducing B lymphocytes to produce antibodies with determinants unrelated to the activating agent. They can also induce the release of lymphokines that mediate inflammation and bone resorption.

GRAM-NEGATIVE BACTERIAL LIPOPOLYSACCHARIDES

Lipopolysaccharides (LPS, endotoxins) are components of the Gram-negative bacterial cell wall which are released when these bacteria die or are lysed. They are also present in smaller amounts in capsular or surface-associated material (SAM) on the cell wall of many of these species and from there may find their way into the tissues. The genetic codes for LPSs are highly conserved and they have a number of common actions which are common to all Gram- negative species. They are key inflammatory mediators and their actions include activating complement by the alternative pathway and thus producing inflammation and stimulating bone resorption (see below). By these actions and by their antigenicity they are also able to alert the host of potential bacterial infection.

There are, however, some minor differences in LPS coding and thus some of their functions between species. In this regard *Porphyromonas gingivalis* LPS causes a highly significant host response (Bainbridge & Darveau 2001). It is an agonist for human monocytes but an antagonist for human vascular endothelial cells. Unlike other bacterial LPSs *P. gingivalis* LPS does not activate the p38 nor the ERK MAP kinase signal transducer pathway molecules in these cells which govern the recruitment of inflammatory cells from blood vessels into the tissues. Thus *P. gingivalis* LPS reduces the passage of these cells, in particularly PMNs, into the tissues by interfering with MAP kinase activation and this favours its survival in the periodontal pocket and on gingival epithelial cells. Nociti et al (2004) investigated whether *P. gingivalis* lipopolysaccharide (P-LPS) could regulate gene expression in murine cementoblasts by real-time (RT)-PCR and Northern blot analysis. They found that exposure of cementoblasts to P-LPS can alter cell function by regulating markers of osteoclastic activity (e.g. receptor activator of nuclear factor KB ligand (RANKL) and its natural inhibitor, osteoprotegerin (OPG) (see below), thereby potentially affecting the inflammation-associated resorption of mineralized tissues.

Cho et al (2005) investigated the role of *P. gingivalis, Treponema denticola*, and *T. socranskii* in inducing prostaglandin E_2 induction of osteoclastogenesis via its effect on the receptor activator (RANK) of nuclear factor-B. Their findings suggest that the osteoclastogenesis by *P. gingivalis, T. denticola*, and *T. socranskii* was mediated by a RANKL-dependent pathway and that PGE_2 was a main factor in the pathway by the enhancing of RANKL expression and the depression of osteoprotegerin, a RANKL inhibitor.

BACTERIAL ANTIGENS

Each bacterial species contains many antigens which can stimulate the immune system and lead to a variety of immune and hypersensitivity reactions which may contribute to both host protection and tissue damage. It has been established that patients with chronic inflammatory diseases have raised levels of serum antibodies to a variety of periodontopathic bacteria (Taubman et al 1992). One such bacteria, *A. actinomycetemcomitans*, has been found to have 13 major antigen bands which are recognized by sera from patients with juvenile periodontitis and rapidly progressing periodontitis (Watanabe et al 1989). Patients with juvenile periodontitis also produce serum antibodies against its leucotoxin (see Ch. 23).

It is known that many important antigen sites are located on or close to the bacterial outer cell membrane and it has been shown that components of the surface associated material (SAM) (see below) can provoke an immune response. It has been established that one of the main components of SAM from many bacteria is the chaperonins (Coates 1996) and these chaperonins, in particular chaperonin 60, are important immunodominant antigens in bacterial infections. In this regard it has been found that a proportion of localized juvenile periodontitis patients have serum anti-bodies to *A. actinomycetemcomitans* SAM which can inhibit the osteolytic activity of this material (Meghji et al 1993). It is probable that the immuno-determinant antigen in these cases is chaperonin 60. It is also known that about half of the patients with localized juvenile periodontitis also produce serum antibodies that neutralize the cell cycle inhibitory activity of gap statin (White et al 1995).

SITES OF PERIODONTAL INFECTIONS

The sites of periodontal infection are shown in **Figure 5.4** and listed below:

1. Supragingival plaque
2. Subgingival flora which are:
   a. Attached to the root surface
   b. Free within the pocket
   c. Within radicular cementum or dentine
   d. Attached to the lining of the pocket
   e. Within the soft tissue wall of the pocket.

In all stages of periodontitis, bacteria are present on the root surface, on the surface of the soft tissue wall of the pocket and free within the pocket. From these sites bacterial products may enter the tissues through the pocket epithelium which is often ulcerated.

BACTERIAL PENETRATION OF THE RADICULAR CEMENTUM AND DENTINE

Actinomyces species may penetrate small distances into cementum and bacterial products such as LPS may contaminate the cementum. However, the degree of penetration of these products into cementum appears superficial (Moore et al 1986).

Many Gram-negative bacteria have the ability to attach to Gram-positive bacteria and epithelial cells (Slots & Genco 1984). This ability is an impor-tant factor in their colonization of the subgingival environment and also allows them to colonize the surface cells of the pocket epithelium.

Bacterial invasion of the cementum and radicular dentine was thought by early investigators to be an important factor in the pathogenesis of perio-dontal disease and Miller (1890) described bacteria invading the radicu-lar dentine of periodontally diseased teeth. More recently, observations using light microscopy, scanning electron microcopy and bacterial culture have suggested that some bacteria invade cementum and radicular dentine and that the dentinal tubules may act as reservoirs of putative periodontal pathogens (Adriaens et al 1984; 1987; 1988a,b).

Another recent study (Giuliana et al 1997) attempted to determine the bacterial species which invaded the root dentine. Samples of the middle

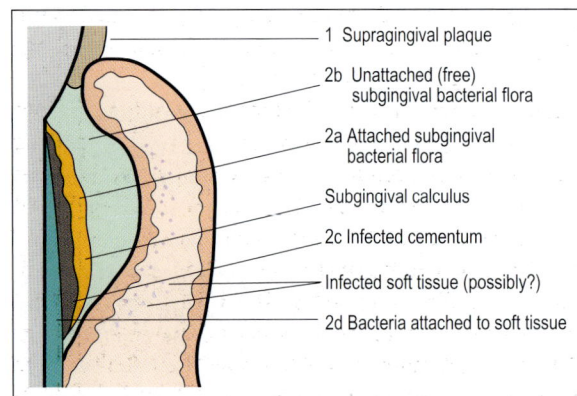

Fig. 5.4 Sites of periodontal infection.

layer of the radicular dentine of 26 periodontally diseased teeth and 14 healthy teeth were taken and these were further divided into outer, middle and inner parts. All of these samples were cultured anaerobically and the bacterial concentrations at these sites were expressed as colony forming units (CFU) per mg of tissue. Bacteria were detected in 14 (54%) of the periodontally diseased teeth and in none of the healthy teeth. The con-centrations of bacteria ranged from 831–11971 CFU/mg and the bacte-ria detected included many of the putative periodontal pathogens such as *Porphyromonas gingivalis, Prevotella intermedia, Bacteroides forsythus, Fusobacterium nucleatum, Peptostreptococcus micros* and *Streptococcus intermedius*.

Gonçalves et al (2008) stated that previous data demonstrated that root cementum may affect periodontal regeneration and carried out a study aimed to explore further possible mechanisms involved in this process. They found that it altered osteopontin in the adjacent tissue.

All these findings suggest that radicular dentine could act as a bacte-rial reservoir from which periodontal pathogens can recolonize treated periodontal pockets and could thus contribute to the recurrence of disease.

BACTERIAL INVASION

It can be shown from evidence of transient bacteraemias which can follow gingival trauma that, from time to time, bacteria penetrate into the soft tis-sues of the pocket. However, infection of the soft tissue appears to be rare because of the ability of the immune and inflammatory systems to destroy bacteria in the tissues.

Bacterial invasion of the tissues in periodontitis has mainly been described in cases of advanced chronic periodontitis (Takeuchi et al 1974; Frank 1980; Saglie et al 1982b, 1985; Manor et al 1984) and juvenile peri-odontitis (Gillett & Johnson 1982; Carranza et al 1983; Christersson et al 1987). Some studies have indicated that putative periodontal pathogens may penetrate epithelium, epithelial cells and connective tissue (Saglie et al 1986; 1988b; Wolinsky et al 1987; Papapanou et al 1994; Sandros et al 1994). On the other hand, another study of advanced chronic and juve-nile periodontitis (Liakoni et al 1987) has concluded that the few bacteria found in the tissues were more likely to result from passive entry in tissue processing than from active invasion.

It has been suggested that bacterial invasion could be a factor in the production of an acute episode of progression in chronic periodontitis (Pertuiset et al 1987; Saglie et al 1987, 1988c). In this regard, it has been suggested that the mechanism involved might be the production of local necrosis or microabscesses (Allenspach-Petrzilka & Guggenheim 1983).

Saglie et al (1987) attempted to test this hypothesis by monitoring 20 patients with advanced chronic periodontitis for episodic progression. When active sites were detected by significant attachment loss periodon-tal surgery was performed. Biopsies of the active sites and control inactive sites in the same patient with similar pocket depths were obtained. These tissues were examined by a number of electron microscope and immu-nocytochemical techniques. They found statistically significant higher numbers of bacteria in the gingival connective tissue in active as opposed to control sites. *Porphyromonas gingivalis* and *A. actinomycetemcomitans* were found most frequently at active sites.

Several recent studies have specifically identified bacterial species in the periodontal tissues of patients with advanced chronic periodontitis or juvenile periodontitis using immunofluorescent techniques or DNA probes (Ch. 14). These are listed in Table 5.2.

In these studies care was taken to avoid translocation of bacteria during the surgery and tissue processing. Saglie et al (1987) claimed that translo-cation was ruled out in their work because control biopsies did not contain bacteria, a pattern of invasion of the gingival connective tissue was seen in the intercellular spaces, bacteria were seen in the same plane as the tissue elements and bacteria were also seen within phagocytic cells.

The labels in Fig. 5.4 read:
1 Supragingival plaque
2b Unattached (free) subgingival bacterial flora
2a Attached subgingival bacterial flora
Subgingival calculus
2c Infected cementum
Infected soft tissue (possibly?)
2d Bacteria attached to soft tissue

Table 5.2 *Specific identification of bacteria in the gingival tissue*

Author/Year	Method	Bacteria	Disease
Courant & Bader (1966)	Immunofluorescence	*Bacteroides melaninogenicus*	Chronic periodontitis
Takeuchi et al (1974)	Immunofluorescence	*Bacteroides melaninogenicus Corynebacterium*	Chronic periodontitis
Saglie et al (1982a)	Immunoperoxidase	*Aggregatibacter actinomycetemcomitans Capnocytophaga sputigena*	Juvenile periodontitis Chronic periodontitis
Pekovic & Fillery (1984)	Immunofluorescence	*Actinomyces viscosus A. naeslundii Porphyromonas gingivalis Prevotella intermedia*	Chronic periodontitis
Saglie et al (1988b)	Immunoperoxidase	*Porphyromonas gingivalis Aggregatibacter actinomycetemcomitans Capnocytophaga Fusobacterium nucleatum Bacterionema matruchotii*	Chronic and juvenile periodontitis
Saglie et al (1988a)	DNA probes	*Mycoplasma pneumoniae*	Chronic and juvenile periodontitis
Christersson et al (1987)	Immunofluorescence	*Aggregatibacter actinomycetemcomitans*	Juvenile periodontitis
Wolinsky et al (1987)	Immunoperoxidase	*Treponema vincentii*	Chronic periodontitis

Animal studies using normal and immunosuppressed rats (Savani et al 1985) showed that bacterial invasion of the gingiva only occurred when virulent bacteria overcame normal host defences or when the host defences were compromised by immunosuppression.

Saglie et al (1988b) have also studied the cellular infiltration associated with bacterial invasion of the gingival connective tissue. On the basis of their findings they postulated that inactive periods were associated with T-helper lymphocytes, NK cells and macrophages and active periods with B lymphocytes, T-cytotoxic/suppressor lymphocytes, Langerhans cells, pan-lymphocytes and polymorphs. In addition, it has also been shown that bacteria in gingival connective tissue were always associated with specific antibodies and often also complement (Pekovic & Fillery 1984). This indicates that a strong immune reaction is mounted against bacteria invading the gingiva. In most situations the local defence mechanisms will rapidly kill invading bacteria and prevent any multiplication. It would seem that bacteria only multiply in the gingival tissues rarely and usually in advanced periodontitis. Multiplication of bacteria within the tissues may lead to the formation of a lateral periodontal abscess.

P. gingivalis has been shown *in vitro* to be able to invade gingival epithelial cells and grow intracellularly (Rautemaa et al 2004). This group attempted to detect *P. gingivalis* in gingival tissues from 13 chronic periodontitis patients by utilizing immunohistochemistry with monoclonal antibodies specific to a cell membrane-bound thiol proteinase of *P. gingivalis*. They also looked for the presence of *P. gingivalis* in gingival tissue by the polymerase chain reaction (PCR). Immunohistochemical analysis of the periodontal tissues revealed positive staining for *P. gingivalis* thiol proteinase in 11 of the 13 patients. This was mainly located intracellularly in the perinuclear region of the cytoplasm in the periodontal epithelial cells and it could be detected throughout the whole depth of both the pocket and oral epithelium. The sensitivity of immunohistochemistry was found to be comparable with that of PCR. These results have provided *in vivo* evidence of the ability of *P. gingivalis* to enter human gingival epithelial cells. Intracellular localization of *P. gingivalis* may contribute to its evasion of

the host immune surveillance and may also increase its resistance to conventional periodontal treatment.

In a study of the intracellular survival of *P. gingivalis* (Eick et al 2006) this bacterium was co-cultured with KB cells and the number of intracellular bacteria was determined up to 3 days after infection. They found that *P. gingivalis* survived well and that the invasion into these cells modulated its virulence properties as well as the inflammatory response of the cells.

Vitkov et al (2005) investigated the mechanism of the invasion of epithelial cells. Pocket epithelium biopsies from periodontitis patients were analysed using scanning and transmission electron microscopy with ultra-histochemical staining with ruthenium red for glycocalyx visualization. They demonstrated that oral bacteria adhered by fimbriae-mediated adhesion only. The bacterial internalization in periodontitis was produced by a fimbriae-induced zipper mechanism of the phagocytic cup. However, they found no sign of the trigger mechanism of internalization. In addition, they also frequently observed apoptosis in the phagocytizing epithelial cells. Fimbriae-mediated adhesion may be a prerequisite for bacterial invasion in periodontitis. As the internalization mechanism appears to induce apoptosis, the subsequent exfoliation might play a significant role in the clearance of periodontal pathogens.

The *P. gingivalis*-epithelial cell interactions in periodontitis have also been reviewed by Andrian et al (2006).

INDIRECT TISSUE DAMAGE

Patients at risk of progressive periodontitis are likely to have either an aberrant inflammatory or immune response to microbial plaque and this is considered in detail below.

IMMUNITY

The role of the immune system in protection and tissue damage

Bacteria and bacterial antigens may penetrate the crevicular epithelium to enter the tissue and stimulate immunity. Both arms of the immune system have the potential for host protection and tissue damage.

Activation of humoral immunity leads to an accumulation of plasma cells and the production of immunoglobulins. These antibodies activate the complement cascade which then stimulates inflammation and generation of prostaglandins. These processes support the immune system by delivering the protective antibodies at the infection site in the inflammatory exudate and by attracting a continuing supply of phagocytic cells, at first PMNs and later macrophages. These cells will then phagocytose the bacteria with the help of opsonizing antibodies, and kill them within their phagosomes. The protective antibodies thus kill bacteria either by facilitating their phagocytosis or by complement mediated lysis. They can also neutralize toxic products (see Ch. 3 and below). The accumulated inflammatory cells can also release tissue destructive enzymes, designed to kill bacteria within their phagosomes, into the tissues as a result of spillage from phagosomes or following PMN lysis (see below).

Stimulation of cellular immunity leads to the production of lymphokines from activated T lymphocytes which modulate macrophage activity leading to improved phagocytosis and intracellular killing. Activated macrophages (Ch. 3) release a number of cytokines and these can affect a number of other cell types. In some cases these interactions can lead to tissue damage. The cytokines released include interleukin-1 (IL-1), tumour necrosis factor (TNF), and gamma interferon (IFN-γ) (Table 5.3). IL-1 can induce the release of collagenase from a variety of connective tissue cells including fibroblasts and osteoblasts. Osteoclast activation factor has now been shown to be identical to IL-1 (Dewhirst et al 1985). Activated T-8 lymphocytes (Ch. 3) also release cytotoxic lymphokines known as perforans which disrupt cell

Table 5.3 *Host and bacterial factors involved in bone resorption*

Bacterial
Capsular and surface-associated material
Lipopolysaccharides
Lipoteichoic acids
Peptidoglycan
Muramyl dipeptide
Lipoprotein

Host

Inflammatory mediators
Prostaglandins, e.g. PGE$_2$
Leukotrienes
12-HETEs
Heparin
Thrombin
Bradykinin

Cytokines
Interleukin-1
Interleukin-6
Tumour necrosis factors
Transforming growth factor β
Platelet derived growth factor

It would seem that the more superficial areas of the lesion have features more consistent with the mucosal immune response while the deeper tissues resemble the systemic immune response. Thus, the areas adjacent to epithelium have more IgA secreting plasma cells while the deeper tissues have more IgG and IgM secreting cells.

Lappin et al (2003) used *in situ* hybridization and immunochemistry to detect the expression of chemokines, adhesion molecules and immunoglobulins in tissue sections from gingival and granulation tissue excised from periodontitis-affected sites and of healthy and gingivitis-affected tissue. Greater numbers of plasma cells were seen in gingival and granulation tissue from periodontitis lesions compared with gingivitis lesions. IgA1 expressing cells were predominant in all lesions while IgA2 and J-chain expressing cells were present in increasing proportions in gingival tissue compared with granulation tissue. Intracellular adhesion molecule-1 (ICAM-1) expression was higher in periodontitis than gingivitis and IL-8 mRNA was higher in lesions with a pronounced neutrophil infiltration. Vascular cell adhesion molecule-1 (VCAM-1) was localized to the deep connective tissue and indicated the presence of a systemic-type immune response in this region. Periodontal tissues did not appear to express the mucosal addressin adhesion molecule (MAdCAM-1). This appears to show that the systemic-type immune response is predominant in periodontal disease. Although the mucosal immune response is minor and limited to the superficial tissues it could still have an important role in the host defence to periodontal pathogens.

In periodontitis lesions, plasma cells are the most common cell type and represent about 50% of all cells, while B cells comprise about 18% (Berglundh & Donati 2005). The proportion of B cells is larger than that of T cells and Th cells occur in larger numbers than T cytotoxic cells. Polymorphonuclear cells and macrophages are found in fractions of less than 5% of all cells. Lesions in aggressive and chronic forms of periodontitis exhibit similar cellular composition. Differences in disease severity, however, may reflect increases in plasma cell and B cell densities. B cells serve as important antigen-presenting cells in periodontitis. The periodontitis lesion expresses a unique TCR gene repertoire that is different from that in blood. The role of superantigens in periodontitis is unclear. There are few studies using comparative designs and unbiased quantitative methods regarding Th-1 and Th-2 cells in periodontitis. The relative dominance of B cells and plasma cells in periodontitis lesions cannot entirely be explained by enhanced Th-2 functions but maybe because of an imbalance between Th-1 and Th-2. Autoimmune reactions are evident in periodontitis lesions. The role of autoantibodies in the regulation of host response in periodontitis, however, needs to be clarified. Autoreactive B cells occur in larger proportions in subjects with periodontitis than in healthy controls.

Papapanou et al (2004) examined serum immunoglobulin (IgG) responses to periodontal bacteria in patients with periodontitis and periodontitis-free individuals over a 30-month period. A total of 89 patients with chronic periodontitis and 42 control subjects with no deep periodontal pockets and no or minimal attachment loss (30–72 years old, 43% men) were included. Patients were examined at baseline, after completion of periodontal therapy, 4 months post-baseline, and at 30 months, and controls, at baseline and 30 months. IgG antibodies to 19 periodontal species were determined by checkerboard immunoblotting. On average, patients displayed at baseline up to 800-fold higher titres than controls to all but three bacterial species. Over the 30-month period, titres remained stable at low levels in controls. Over time, antibody titres showed a modest decline in patients, but remained significantly elevated at 30 months in comparison with controls. Antibody-level changes over time were not significantly different between subjects that did and did not receive adjunctive systemic antibiotics. Thus, conspicuous differences in IgG titres to periodontal bacteria exist between periodontitis patients and periodontally healthy controls. Despite successful periodontal therapy, titres remained elevated over a 30-month period, suggesting that serology may mark the history of past periodontal infection.

membranes and connective tissue cells close to activated T-8 cells could be damaged. Some clinical findings support the idea that immune responses take part in the pathogenesis of periodontal disease:

- Patients receiving immunosuppressive drugs or who have immunodeficiency diseases have less gingival inflammation than might be expected from their oral hygiene status
- When drugs which enhance the immune response are given the severity of gingivitis increases
- Patients with a deficiency of white cells (agranulocytosis) are prone to infection and have much more severe periodontal disease
- Patients with immunosuppression are prone to develop infections including acute necrotizing ulcerative gingivitis. This can occur as a complication of HIV infection and these patients are also prone to develop an aggressive form of periodontitis (Winkler et al 1988).

The type of humoral response is likely to be particularly important to the periodontal outcome since plasma cells dominate the gingivitis and periodontitis active lesions. The antibodies they produce are probably important in facilitating the removal of oral bacteria that may occasionally get into the tissues from the gingival crevice or periodontal pocket. They do this by the processes of opsonization and complement activation leading to phagocytosis and killing. In this regard they appear to be very successful since bacterial infection of the tissues is a rare event in all stages of periodontal disease.

The immunoglobulins (Igs) found in the periodontal tissues and in GCF are derived from both local and systemic sources (Kinane et al 1999a). This research group has shown that IgM, IgG and IgA antibody classes including IgA -J- linked antibody can be produced by local site plasma cells. Ig and IgA subclass specific plasma cells and specific Ig mRNA- expressing plasma cells have been localized in the periodontal lesion (Takahashi et al 1997). The predominant immunoglobulin produced is IgG and it has been shown that 65% of this is produced locally (Kinane et al 1999b; Takahashi et al 1997). These studies also show that most of the IgA is also produced locally and IgA1 and IgA2 plasma cells are found in the periodontal tissues. The IgA antibody levels in gingival tissue have been found to be 30.7% for IgA1 and 7.5% for IgA2. However, the proportion of IgA plasma cells is less in the deeper parts of the lesion than superficially (Kinane et al 1999b; Takahashi et al 1997).

It is also possible that autoimmune mechanisms may contribute to periodontal disease pathogenesis. This has been investigated by Rajapakse and Dolby (2004) who measured by ELISA the tissue antibodies against a self antigen of collagen type I, and antigens from the periodontal pathogens *P. gingivalis* (Pg), and *A. actinomycetemcomitans* (Aa) and *Bacteroides fragilis* (Bfr), a non-oral bacterium, in granulomatous tissue obtained from 13 chronic periodontitis patients undergoing periodontal surgery. They found that the level of tissue antibodies to collagen I was significantly higher than those in serum ($p<0.0001$). The tissue antibody level to Pg was also significantly higher than that in serum ($p<0.0271$) but those from Aa and Bfr were not. These findings appear to confirm the local production of antibodies to the autoantigen of collagen I and to bacterial antigens in chronic periodontitis and suggest that autoimmune processes could contribute to tissue breakdown.

ANTIBODY RESPONSE TO PERIODONTAL PUTATIVE PATHOGENS

P. gingivalis

The immune system responds to specific surface proteins to produce specific antibodies. Subjects suffering from adult periodontitis have elevated antibody levels to several *P. gingivalis* antigens and these are produced in much greater quantities than those produced against other associated bacteria (Lamster et al 1998; Kinane et al 1993). These antibodies have been shown to have both opsonizing and complement activating functions (Saito et al 1999). Proteolytic enzymes produced by *P. gingivalis* (see above) can degrade immunoglobulins and complement and can thus affect this response (Schenkein 1988). An important surface component of *P. gingivalis* is the RgpA-Kgp proteinase adhesin complex (see above). It has been shown that there is a specific IgG antibody response directed against this antigen and this antibody is significantly higher in adult periodontitis patients compared with healthy subjects (O'Brien-Simpson et al 2000). Antibodies have been also detected to Prp C, a collagenolytic protease (see above), in 34 maintenance periodontal patients (Beikler et al 2003). IgG antibodies were found in all 34 patients and IgA antibodies were found in 33.

Rams et al (2006) showed that serum levels of IgG antibodies against *A. actinomycetemcomitans* or *P. gingivalis* in periodontitis-stable patients were higher than those in patients with active periodontitis. These results suggested that elevated levels of IgG antibody against *A. actinomycetemcomitans* and *P. gingivalis* may have had a detectable protective effect against periodontal infections with these microorganisms.

The predominant IgG subgroup antibody response to this bacteria is IgG4 > IgG2 > IgG3 and IgG1 (O'Brian-Simpson et al 2000). This study also showed that while IgG2 levels positively correlated with indices of disease severity, IgG4 levels negatively correlated. Also IgG4 was found to be lower and IgG2 higher in diseased subjects compared with healthy ones. This shows that there may be some variations in the immune response to this bacterium in healthy and diseased subjects and although the cause of this is unknown it could be partly due to genetic differences.

There also appear to be differences in the immune response to *P. gingivalis* between patients with chronic periodontitis and juvenile periodontitis. Juvenile periodontitis subjects have an antibody response to this bacteria which resembles that found in healthy subjects (Hagewald et al 2000). Furthermore, the affinity of IgG antibodies towards *P. gingivalis* has been found to be much lower in subjects with a rapidly progressive periodontitis than those with either healthy gingivae or a more slowly progressing chronic periodontitis (Lamster et al 1998). Also in more severe cases of chronic periodontitis the antibody affinities towards *P. gingivalis* have been found to be lower (Kinane et al 1993). Thus a lower level of effective antibody to this bacterium may be a major factor in producing severe and rapidly progressive disease.

Other studies have also suggested that bacterial specific serum antibody levels and IgG subclass responses may relate to periodontal status. In this regard, antibodies to periodontal bacteria are known to vary according to IgG subclass (McArthur & Clark 1993). Furthermore, it has also been reported that a positive correlation may exist between IgG levels to *P. gingivalis* and the severity of chronic periodontitis (Gmür et al 1986; Lopatin & Blackburn 1992; Lamster et al 1998). In addition, elevations in *P. gingivalis* specific IgG2, IgG1 and IgG4 have been found in rapidly progressive and chronic periodontitis (Kinane et al 1999b).

An investigation (Sakai et al 2001) of *P. gingivalis* specific IgG subclasses in chronic periodontitis patients and controls has recently been completed. They examined three groups of subjects, 20 treated and maintained chronic periodontitis patients, 30 untreated chronic periodontitis patients and 19 periodontally healthy patients. The maintained group were seen over 5 years with measurements at both baseline and 5 years. Significantly higher IgG1 levels were found in both patient groups compared to controls. The untreated group also had significantly higher IgG2 responses compared to other groups. In addition, the IgG4 levels were significantly higher in the maintained patients compared to the untreated group. Furthermore, a statistically significant correlation was found in the maintained group between IgG2 levels and changes in bone levels. Subjects from this group with high IgG2 levels and low IgG4 levels showed greater bone loss than those with low IgG2 and high IgG4, in spite of the fact that the mean prevalence of *P. gingivalis* did not differ between the two groups. This work suggests that a persistently high *P. gingivalis* specific IgG2 level after periodontal treatment may be indicative of recurrent or persistent periodontal destruction.

Takeuchi et al (2006) analysed IgG subclass antibody levels of *P. gingivalis* in patients with both aggressive periodontitis and chronic periodontitis. They found that *P. gingivalis* infection elicited an IgG subclass antibody response in both periodontitis patients and healthy subjects, while higher anti-*P. gingivalis* IgG1 levels were found in the periodontitis groups compared with the healthy control group.

Booth et al (2006) showed that both IgG1 and IgG2 antibodies recognized a dominant antigen of 47 kDa, probably Arg-gingipain, of *P. gingivalis*. Much of the response to the carbohydrate antigen was found to be of the IgG2 subclass. they also showed that neither the level of IgG1 or the IgG2 antibody specific to *P. gingivalis* was related to the total IgG.

Haemagglutinin A (hagA) and outer membrane protein (OMP) are major virulence factors associated with colonization of *P. gingivalis* in the gingival crevice. Kobayashi et al (2006) carried out a clinical and laboratory study into the immune responses to these antigens. They found that serum IgG subclass distribution for patients and controls was IgG1 > IgG4 > IgG2 > IgG3 and that the serum IgG responses were to *P. gingivalis* OMP rather than to hag A. They also showed evidence that this response may be more active in chronic periodontitis than in health.

Two *P. gingivalis* outer membrane proteins, PG32 and PG33, have been shown in gene knockout studies to play an important role in bacterial growth (Ross et al 2004). Two truncated peptides of these proteins were produced in an insoluble form suitable for vaccine production. These were then shown to give high levels of protection in a *P. gingivalis* murine model of periodontal disease. They may be considered as potential candidates for vaccines for testing in human periodontal disease.

P. gingivalis binds to fibrinogen, fibronectin, haemoglobin, and collagen type V with a similar profile to that of its major virulence factor, the cell surface RgpA-Kgp proteinase-adhesin complex. O'Brien-Simpson et al (2005) used peptide-specific, purified antibodies in competitive inhibition ELISAs and epitope mapping assays to identify potential adhesin binding motifs (ABMs) of the RgpA-Kgp complex responsible for binding to host proteins. They then developed a vaccine by conjugating RgpA-Kgp complex, synthetic ABM and proteinase active site peptides to diphtheria toxoid. They then showed that this vaccine protected against *P. gingivalis*-induced periodontal bone loss in a murine perio dontitis model. The most efficacious peptide and protein vaccines were found to induce a high-titre IgG1 antibody response. Furthermore, mice protected in the periodontitis model had a predominant *P. gingivalis*-specific IL-4 response, whereas mice with disease had a predominant IFN- response. The peptide-specific antibodies directed to the ABM2 sequence protected against periodontal bone loss and inhibited binding of the RgpA-Kgp complex to fibrinogen, fibronectin, and collagen type V. Furthermore, the peptide-specific antibodies directed to the ABM3 sequence protected against periodontal bone loss and inhibited binding to haemoglobin. However, the most protective antibodies were those directed to the active sites of the RgpA and Kgp proteinases. The results suggest that when the RgpA-Kgp complex, or functional binding motif or active site peptides are used as a vaccine, they induce a Th2 response that blocks function of the RgpA-Kgp complex and protects against periodontal bone loss.

Outer membrane protein with a 53-kDa molecular weight (Ag53) isolated from *P. gingivalis* evokes strong humoral immune responses in many periodontitis patients. Regarding this, Kato et al (2005) showed that only Th cell lines with a high Th2/Th1 ratio induced Ag53-specific IgG production when cocultured with T-cell-depleted leucocytes They felt that the difference in Th2/Th1 balance might regulate the Ag53-specific IgG production.

Successive immunization of mice with *F. nucleatum* and *P. gingivalis* has been shown to modulate the specific serum IgG responses to these organisms. This was further investigated by examining the IgG subclasses (Gemmell et al 2004a). They demonstrated a systemic Th1/Th2 response in mice immunized with *P. gingivalis* and/or *F. nucleatum* with a trend towards a Th2 response in *P. gingivalis*-immunized mice and a significantly increased anti-*P. gingivalis* IgG2a (Th1) response in mice immunized with *F. nucleatum* prior to *P. gingivalis*. Further, the inhibition of neutrophil phagocytosis of immune serum-opsonized *P. gingivalis* was modulated by the presence of anti-*F. nucleatum* antibodies, while anti-*P. gingivalis* antibodies induced an inhibitory effect on the phagocytic response to *F. nucleatum*. Thus the type of immune response is modulated by sequence of exposure to these bacteria.

Califano et al (2004) has previously shown that patients with aggressive forms of periodontitis that were seropositive for *P. gingivalis* had less attachment loss than those that were seronegative which suggests that antibody reactive with antigens of *P. gingivalis* may be protective and may decrease disease severity and extent. Also recent studies in the murine abscess model and in the host antibody response in chronic periodontitis patients suggest that antibody reactive with *P. gingivalis* haemagglutinin may be an important protective antibody response. They therefore investigated the relationship between antibody reactive with *P. gingivalis* haemagglutinin and measures of periodontal attachment loss. They found IgG reactive with *P. gingivalis* haemagglutinin in both chronic periodontitis and generalized aggressive periodontitis patients and found that most of it was of the IgG1 and IgG3 subclasses. However, antibody reactive with *P. gingivalis* haemagglutinin was not found to have a significant relationship with measures of periodontal attachment loss.

Yonezawa et al (2005) previously demonstrated that a *P. gingivalis* rgpA DNA vaccine induced protective immune responses against *P. gingivalis* infection in mice. They have now shown that a reduction in lethality against infection by lethal doses of *P. gingivalis* was observed in the rgpA DNA vaccine-immunized mice. Cytokine levels in the mouse model with nonlethal doses of infection by *P. gingivalis* were also evaluated to analyse the mechanism of protection by immunization with the rgpA DNA vaccine. After nonlethal challenge with invasive *P. gingivalis* W50, production of interleukin (IL)-2, IL-4, IL-5 and IL-12 was elevated. However, interferon (IFN)⁻ was found to be lower in the serum of the DNA vaccine-immunized mice than in the serum of nonimmunized mice. The regulation of IFN⁻ production elicited by immunization with the rgpA DNA vaccine

may play a significant role in protection against *P. gingivalis* infection in mice and holds promise for a similar response in humans.

Koizumi et al (2008) recently investigated global gene expression in ST2 mouse stromal cells infected by the periodontal pathogen *P. gingivalis* using microarray technology, and found that the bacterium induces a wide range of pro-inflammatory gene expression. ST2 cells and primary calvarial osteoblasts from C3H/HeN, C57BL/6, and MyD88-deficient (MyD88−/−) mice were infected with *P. gingivalis* ATCC33277 and its gingipain-deficient mutant KDP136.

They found that various pro-inflammatory responses in *P. gingivalis*-infected stromal/osteoblast cells are NF-αβ-dependent, but not always dependent on the Toll-like receptor/MyD88 pathway, while some responses are related to the activation of protease-activated receptors. Thus *P. gingivalis* does not fully utilize well-established pathogen recognition molecules such as Toll-like receptors.

Lee et al (2006) showed that in rats *P. gingivalis* heat shock protein 60 (HSP60) could be used as a vaccine and showed that it inhibited multiple bacteria-induced alveolar bone loss (see Ch. 11 for further details).

The infectious aetiology of periodontitis is complex and no curative treatment modality exists (Persson 2005). Studies in non-human primate models using ligature-induced experimental periodontitis suggest that antibody responses by active immunization against *P. gingivalis* can safely be induced, enhanced, and obtained over time. Immune responses to whole bacterial cell and purified protein preparations considered as vaccine candidates have been evaluated in different animal models demonstrating that there are several valid vaccine candidates. Data suggest that immunization reduces the rate and severity of bone loss. It is also, temporarily, possible to alter the composition of the subgingival microflora. Natural active immunization by therapeutic interventions results in antibody titre enhancement and potentially improves treatment outcomes. Passive immunization of humans using *P. gingivalis* monoclonal antibodies temporarily prevents colonization of *P. gingivalis*. Pro biotic therapy may be an alternative approach. Regulatory and safety issues for human periodontal vaccine trials must be considered. Shared infectious aetiology between periodontitis and systemic diseases may enhance vaccine effort developments. The impact of natural immunization and passive immunization in humans should be explored and may, presently, be more feasible than active immunization studies.

Koizumi et al (2008) have previously reported that specific immunoglobulin G (IgG) antibodies induced by transcutaneous immunization (TCI) with a 40-kDa outer membrane protein (40k-OMP) of *P. gingivalis*, with cholera toxin (CT) as adjuvant, inhibited coaggregation by *P. gingivalis*. In this study, they further pursued the potential of the 40k-OMP as a transcutaneous vaccine.

TCI of rats administered 40k-OMP elicited significant 40k-OMP-specific serum IgG and IgA, as well as salivary IgG antibody plus. Importantly, these antibody responses were induced without adjuvant. Thus, both serum and saliva antibody titres induced by TCI with the 40k-OMP alone were identical to those of 40k-OMP plus cholera toxin as adjuvant. The serum antibody responses induced by 40k-OMP persisted for more than 140 days. On the other hand, salivary IgG anti-40k-OMP antibodies were gradually decreased. Analysis of antibody-forming cells (AFCs) confirmed the antibody titres by detecting high numbers of 40k-OMP-specific IgG AFCs in spleen and cervical lymph node. They concluded that since 40k-OMP-specific IgG inhibited the coaggregation of *P. gingivalis* with *Streptococcus gordonii*, and the hemagglutinin activity of *P. gingivalis*, TCI with the 40k-OMP may be important as an adjuvant-free immunogen for the prevention of chronic periodontitis.

Kato et al (2008) have previously reported that specific immunoglobulin G (IgG) antibodies induced by transcutaneous immunization (TCI) with a 40-kDa outer membrane protein (40k-OMP) of *P. gingivalis*, with cholera toxin (CT) as adjuvant, inhibited coaggregation by *P. gingivalis*. In their present study, they further pursue the potential of the 40k-OMP as a transcutaneous vaccine. TCI of rats administered 40k-OMP elicited significant 40k-OMP-specific serum IgG and IgA, as well as salivary IgG antibody titres. Importantly, these antibody responses were induced without adjuvant. Thus, both serum and saliva antibody titres induced by TCI with the 40k-OMP alone were identical to those of 40k-OMP plus cholera toxin as adjuvant. The serum antibody responses induced by 40k-OMP persisted for more than 140 days. On the other hand, salivary IgG anti-40k-OMP antibodies were gradually decreased. Analysis of antibody-forming cells (AFCs) confirmed the antibody titres by detecting high numbers of 40k-OMP-specific IgG AFCs in spleen and cervical lymph node. They concluded that since 40k-OMP-specific IgG inhibited the coaggregation of *P. gingivalis* with *S. gordonii*, and the hemagglutinin activity of *P. gingivalis*, TCI with the 40k-OMP may be important as an adjuvant-free immunogen for the prevention of chronic periodontitis.

One pathway by which *P. gingivalis* may affect the immune system is by its possible stimulation of some parts of the cytokine system (see below and Ch. 3). It is known that *P. gingivalis* can stimulate the production of interferon-γ (Kobayashi et al 2000). Also a surface molecule (CD69) found on the surface of *P. gingivalis* has been shown to stimulate monocytes and also to activate B and NK cells (Champaiboon et al 2000). This group also showed that *P. gingivalis* induced a dose-dependent stimulation of IL-10 production which in turn led to an increase in B-cell proliferation. De-Waal-Malefyt et al (1991) showed that monocytes were stimulated by IL-10 to suppress their production of IL-1, IL-6 and TNF-α. The body appears to produce more IL-10 in the presence of *P. gingivalis* and this may represent the body's attempt to reduce or prevent overactivation of the immune system by this bacteria. It has also been shown that IL-10 stimulates PMNs to decrease their production of IL-1α, IL-1β, IL-8 and TNF-α.

IL-10 is an anti-inflammatory cytokine secreted by stimulated Th2 lymphocytes that can downregulate inflammatory responses to bacterial challenge. Houri-Haddad et al (2007) hypothesized that local delivery of IL-10 using gene-transfer would downregulate inflammatory responses. They examined the effect of IL-10 plasmid injection on the local cytokine response. Two weeks after the implantation of chambers, either IL-10 plasmid or vector was injected into the mice. Four days later, they were challenged with an intra-chamber injection of *P. gingivalis*. The intra-chamber levels of IL-10, IFN, TNF, and IL-1β were evaluated after 2 and 24 h. Their results showed that local IL-10 gene delivery elevated the levels of IL-10 at both time periods. It also attenuated the levels of IFN and TNF at 2 h, and of IL-1β at 24 h. The results suggested the possibility of modulating the local inflammatory response to *P. gingivalis* by direct IL-10 gene transfer.

P. gingivalis has also been shown to increase the cytokine production by oral epithelial cells (Sandros et al 2000). It showed that the expression of IL-1, IL-6, IL-8 and TNF-α mRNA increased. The extent of the cytokine response was also shown to be positively correlated with the adhesive and invasive properties of various strains of *P. gingivalis*. It thus appears that these reactions may be stimulated by the adherence of these bacteria to oral epithelium (Sandros et al 2000).

Dye et al (2005) examined the relationship between serum antibodies against *P. gingivalis* and *A. actinomycetemcomitans*, and plasma fibrinogen and serum C-reactive protein (CRP) in a nationally representative sample. They found that both the high serum titre to *P. gingivalis* and the presence of periodontal disease were independently related to high CRP levels.

Zhou et al (2005) investigated the cytokine profile induced by live *P. gingivalis*, its lipopolysaccharides (LPS), and its major fimbrial protein, fimbrillin (FimA). They found that *P. gingivalis* LPS and FimA induced a similar profile of cytokine expression when exposed to mouse peritoneal macrophages but that this profile differed significantly in response to live

P. gingivalis. *In vitro*, mouse peritoneal macrophages were stimulated to produce IL-6, granulocyte colony-stimulating factor, and lymphotactin by live *P. gingivalis*, but not by *P. gingivalis* LPS or FimA, while RANTES, γ-interferon, IL-17, vascular cell adhesion molecule 1 (VCAM-1), and vascular endothelial growth factor were induced by *P. gingivalis* LPS or FimA, but not by live *P. gingivalis*. *In vivo*, IL-6 mRNA was strongly induced only by live *P. gingivalis* while monocyte chemoattractant protein 1 mRNA was strongly induced only by *P. gingivalis* LPS and FimA in mouse calvarial scalp, further confirming the differences of cytokine profile induced *in vitro*. They also found that the cytokines induced by *P. gingivalis* LPS or FimA signalled through TLR2, while most of cytokines induced by live *P. gingivalis* signalled through both TLR2 and TLR4. Interestingly, the activation of TLR2 by live *P. gingivalis* inhibited the release of RANTES, VCAM-1, and IL-1α from mouse peritoneal macrophages. These results indicate that host immune cells sense live *P. gingivalis* and its components differently, which translates into the expression of different inflammatory cytokine profiles.

To characterize the roles of *P. gingivalis* and its components in disease processes, Zhou and Amar (2006) investigated the cytokine profiles induced by live *P. gingivalis*, its lipopolysaccharide (LPS), and its major fimbrial protein, fimbrillin (FimA). A cytokine antibody array revealed that human monocyte-derived macrophages were induced to produce chemokines such as monocyte chemoattractant protein 1, macrophage inflammatory protein 1β (MIP-1β), and MIP-3 as early as 1 h after exposure to *P. gingivalis*, with production declining after 24 h of exposure. There was also an extensive repertoire of inflammatory mediators increased subsequent to infection, most predominantly tumour necrosis factor alpha (TNF-α), interleukin 1b (IL-1β), IL-6, IL-10, and granulocyte-macrophage colony-stimulating factor. The induction of cytokines by *P. gingivalis* was not triggered simply by bacterial cell surface components, since purified *P. gingivalis* LPS and FimA both induced similar patterns of cytokines, while the pattern of cytokines induced by live *P. gingivalis* was significantly different. This indicated that the host defense system senses live bacteria differently than it does the cell surface components LPS and FimA. To further understand the mechanisms by which live *P. gingivalis* and its components exert their effects, these workers used a high-throughput immunoblot screening approach (Becton–Dickinson PowerBlot) to analyse intracellular proteins involved in *P. gingivalis* infection in human macrophages. Exposure of human macrophages to either live *P. gingivalis*, its LPS, or its FimA protein led to the upregulation of 12, 8, and 10 proteins and the downregulation of 15, 8, and 17 proteins, respectively. The expression of proteins involved in gene transcription (e.g. monocyte enhancer factor 2D (MEF2D), signal transducer and activator of transcription 1 (STAT1), STAT3, STAT6, and IL enhancer binding factors, ILF3), of protein kinases (e.g. mitogen-activated protein kinase 3 (MAPK3), MAP3K8, double-stranded RNA-activated protein kinase (PRKR), and MAP2K4. It also involved proteins involved in immune responses (e.g. TNF super family member 6 (TNFSF6) and interferon-induced protein with tetratricopeptide repeat 4 (IFIT4), apoptosis (e.g. genes associated with retinoid interferon-induced mortality 19 [GRIM19]), and other fundamental cellular processes (e.g. clathrin heavy-chain polypeptide, calreticulin). The Ras-associated protein RAB27A) was found to be modulated differentially by *P. gingivalis*, LPS, and FimA. These differential changes were interpreted as preferential signal pathway activation in host immune/inflammatory responses to *P. gingivalis* infection.

Ohno et al (2008) recently investigated global gene expression in ST2 mouse stromal cells infected by the periodontal pathogen *P. gingivalis* using micro array technology, and found that the bacterium induced a wide range of pro-inflammatory gene expression. Their results suggest that various pro inflammatory responses in *P. gingivalis*-infected stromal/osteoblast cells are nuclear factor-γB I. This suggests that various pro-inflammatory responses in *P. gingivalis*-infected stromal/osteoblast cells are NF-γB-dependent, but not always dependent on the Toll-like receptor/MyD88 pathway, while some responses are related to the activation of protease-activated receptors. Thus *P. gingivalis* does not fully utilize well-established pathogen recognition molecules such as Toll-like receptors.

A. Actinomycetemcomitans

The serum antibody response to *A. actinomycetemcomitans* has been shown to correlate with its presence in the gingival crevice or periodontal pocket (Kinane et al 1993). There are three serotypes of this bacterium and patients may vary in their antibody response to each of them (Nakashima et al 1998). Patients also show a humoral antibody response to this bacterium's lipopolysaccharide (LPS) and leucotoxin (Califano et al 1997a). Patients suffering from localized juvenile periodontitis (see Ch. 23) have raised IgG antibody responses to both of these factors (Califano et al 1997; Farida et al 1986). In the case of LPS the dominant antigenic site is the o-chain of this molecule (Page et al 1991). Both localized juvenile and rapidly progressive periodontitis patients have been shown to have increased IgG antibodies directed against this site of LPS (Gu et al 1998). 80% of these LPS antibodies are directed against the carbohydrate component and only 20% against the protein component of this molecule. Patients harbouring the serotype b strain have increased antibodies to this strain and these have been shown to be present in the IgG2 fraction.

The antibodies directed against the leucotoxin are capable of neutralizing this toxin and are thus protective (Califano et al 1997a). In this regard it has been shown that individuals with lower titres of this specific antibody exhibit significantly greater amounts of attachment loss than individuals with higher titres (Califano et al 1997a). Another study (Sakellari et al 1997) found that the serum antibody levels to serotype b in adult periodontitis patients averaged 124 μg/mL and this was in broad agreement with concentrations quoted in other studies. It has also been shown (Kinane et al 1993) that antibody levels to this bacterium are significantly higher in healthy patients than those with periodontitis which is suggestive of a protective role.

Tannerella forsythensis (B. forsythus)

There is evidence that the presence of *T. forsythensis* (*B. forsythus*) in the gingival crevice of patients makes them five times more likely to lose periodontal attachment at least one site within their mouths (Tran et al 2001). However, in this study the site losing attachment did not always harbour *T. forsythensis* but more commonly *P. gingivalis* and/or *A. actinomycetemcomitans* suggesting some form of interaction between these different species. Although *T. forsythensis* was found to be present in 53% of periodontal pockets in excess of 6 mm there were significantly fewer seropositive results for this bacterium compared with *P. gingivalis* (Califano et al 1997b).

Another study examined the presence of *T. forsythensis* in the subgingival flora of a group of adolescents over 3 years by PCR (Hamlet et al 2004) and related it to loss of attachment. The prevalence of *T. forsythensis* in sites that lost attachment increased to 86% compared with baseline levels of 64%. In contrast sites which did not lose attachment always had a significantly lower prevalence of 25–36%. They also found that the odds of loss of attachment were 8.16 times greater in subjects infected with *T. forsythensis* at each of the three examinations over the time period.

P. gingivalis and *T. forsythia* are often isolated simultaneously from active periodontitis sites and these bacteria may interact in the periodontal environment. In this connection, Yoneda et al (2005) examined whether *T. forsythia* stimulated the growth of *P. gingivalis*. They added cell extracts of *T. forsythia* to nutrition-decreased medium of *P. gingivalis* and examined the effect on growth. They concluded that a product or component of *T. forsythia* seemed to stimulate growth of *P. gingivalis* under nutrition-limited

conditions. Gingipains were also considered to play an important role in the digestion or uptake of this growth-promoting factor. The interaction between *T. forsythia* and *P. gingivalis* in growth may be in part related with a synergistic virulence between them.

In this regard, Inagaki et al (2006) showed that epithelial cell attachment and invasion by *T. forsythia* was dependent on the BspA surface protein. They also showed that *P. gingivalis* or its outer membrane vesicles enhanced the attachment and invasion of *T. forsythia* to epithelial cells. They concluded that interactions between these two bacteria may play important roles in virulence by promoting host cell attachment and invasion.

Persson et al (2000) showed considerable variation in the antibody response to this bacterium between individuals and showed that they were independent of health status. Thus, the exact role of this bacterium in the disease process is uncertain.

The fact that *T. forsythia* is difficult to cultivate from mixed infections has impeded precise estimates of its distribution within a given population. Narayanan et al (2005) determined the distribution of *T. forsythia* in an adult and in an adolescent population. In order to discern *T. forsythia* alone from the mixed infection of plaque, the use of sensitive 16S ribosomal RNA-based polymerase chain reaction (PCR) detection was necessary. In the adolescent population, 25% were found to carry *T. forsythia*, albeit in relatively low numbers. In the adult population, a total of 37.8% and 11% were found to carry the organism with primer 2 and primer 1, respectively, suggesting that around 27% had between 103 and 107 organisms. There was no significant increase in their number with increasing age. However, *T. forsythia* positive male smokers showed increased disease severity compared with *T. forsythia* negative subjects. This study has shown that at least 25% of the adolescent population carry low numbers of *T. forsythia*, whereas at least 37% of adults carry the organism, with some 11% having relatively high numbers. The relationship between *T. forsythia* and disease progression in these populations, however, remains to be determined.

IMMUNOREGULATION IN PERIODONTAL DISEASE

Although chronic periodontitis is primarily caused by bacteria, patient susceptibility is also of the utmost importance to its rate of progression (see Ch. 4). Furthermore the host immune response to periodontal bacteria is also of fundamental importance to its outcome (Seymour 1987). A review of the evidence that genetic factors help to control the immune response in periodontal diseases has been carried out by Baker (2005) and the evidence suggested that susceptibility and resistance are heritable traits and also that strain differences in basal mRNA expression correlate with differences in susceptibility. It also showed that genes that change expression in response to infection also correlated with differences in susceptibility.

Histological studies show that the periodontal lesion consists predominately of lymphocytes and inflammatory cells (see Ch. 8) and that whereas T lymphocytes predominate in the stable lesion, the number of B lymphocytes and plasma cells dramatically increase in the progressive lesion (Seymour 1987, 1991). Immunological studies also suggest that cell mediated responses may be suppressed in active periodontal disease. Therefore the active lesion of chronic periodontitis seems to be a predominantly B-lymphocyte mediated response (Cole et al 1986, 1987; Taubman et al 1984; Seymour et al 1985; Seymour & Gemmell 2001).

In many chronic inflammatory diseases, IgG glycans are galactose-deficient and thus capable of complement activation through the lectin pathway. Novak et al (2005) investigated whether IgG in serum and gingival crevicular fluid, and IgG locally produced by plasma cells in gingiva of periodontal disease patients, displayed altered glycosylation. They developed a lectin-ELISA to measure levels of galactose-deficient IgG in the fluids and immunofluorescence staining to detect galactose-deficient IgG-producing cells in gingiva. Their results indicated higher levels of galactose-deficient IgG in sera and gingival crevicular fluid from periodontal disease patients, compared with levels in healthy controls. Furthermore, gingivae from periodontal disease patients was found to exhibit infiltration of IgG-producing plasma cells. Many of them were found to contain galactose-deficient IgG in the cytoplasm. These results suggested that IgG secreted by B cells was aberrantly glycosylated and resulted in the production of pro-inflammatory galactose-deficient IgG.

THE ROLE OF CYTOKINES IN THE IMMUNOREGULATION OF PERIODONTAL DISEASE

Cytokines are recognized as being vital in the immunoregulation of many diseases and the production of appropriate cytokine(s) appears to be essential for the development of protective immunity. Conversely, if inappropriate cytokines are produced then progressive disease may result (Kelso 1990). The release of the appropriate cytokine itself depends on the activation of the appropriate gene which in turn depends on the nature of the subject's genome (see Ch. 3).

The majority of this immune process is directed by the cellular release of cytokines. Some cytokines are produced by a restricted cell type, such as IL-2 produced only by T lymphocytes, whereas others, such as IL-1 and IL-6 are produced by many cells (Seymour & Gemmell 2001) (see Table 3.1).

Many cytokines are pleiotropic and have multiple activities on different target cells. The response of a cell to a given cytokine also depends on its local concentration, the cell type stimulated, and the other regulating cytokines to which the cell has been previously exposed (Seymour & Gemmell 2001). In addition, cytokines only persist in the tissues for short time periods before they are degraded.

Cytokines interact in a network first by inducing each other, second by transmodulating cell surface receptors and third by synergistic, additive, or antagonistic interactions on cell function (Balkwill & Burke 1989; Seymour & Gemmell 2001). There appears to be a particularly complex network of interactions in the control of the immune system and this complexity may be essential to overcome the various defence strategies of microorganisms which evolve more rapidly than their mammalian hosts (Mosmann 1991).

Cytokines are key factors in the immune response to periodontal pathogens. In this regard, Tanaka et al (2006) found that the cytokines IL-1β, IL-1α, IFN-α, IL-12, and PGE$_2$ were all necessary for optimal production of human anti-*A. actinomycetemcomitans* and the need for pro-inflammatory cytokines including the T-helper 1 (Th1) cytokines was consistent with a response with a significant IgG2 component.

IL-1 AS A MEDIATOR OF TISSUE DESTRUCTION

Uncontrolled production IL-1 appears to be a major mediator of tissue destruction in periodontal disease and other inflammatory diseases (Page et al 2000). While its normal major source is from macrophages, this seems unlikely in chronic periodontitis since only a few of these cells are present in the progressive periodontal lesion (Seymour & Gemmell 2001). The most likely source of IL-1 in periodontal disease seems to be B lymphocytes which are present in large numbers in the progressive lesion (Seymour & Gemmell 2001). Furthermore, it has been shown that *P. gingivalis* can induce the release of IL-1 from B lymphocytes (Gemmell & Seymour 1998).

As with all inflammatory reactions it is the balance of cytokines that determines the ultimate outcome. In this regard, a number of cytokines such as IL-10 and IL-11 are known to downregulate IL-1 production and it has been shown that the subcutaneous injection of recombinant IL-11 significantly

reduced periodontal attachment loss in a beagle dog, ligature induced periodontitis model (Martuscelli et al 2000). Thus, it is possible that periodontal tissue destruction may be the result of unregulated production of IL-1 by B cells in the periodontal lesion (Seymour & Gemmell 2001).

Ejeil et al (2003a) grew healthy and mildly, moderately and severely inflamed gingival tissue specimens in organ culture for 72 h. They measured the levels of cytokines released into the media and histologically measured the area occupied by collagen in the specimens. The area occupied by collagen decreased progressively from the healthy to the severely inflamed tissue. Compared with controls, there were significant increases in IL-1β levels and a significant decreases in the levels of IL-4 and no change in the level of EGF. The area occupied by collagen was significantly correlated with the amounts of IL-4 and inversely significantly correlated with the amounts of IL-1β. Thus the relative levels of these two cytokines could be related to periodontal progression.

Another group (Hou et al 2003) carried out an immunocytochemical study of the diseased tissue adjacent to deep pockets in chronic periodontitis patients and corresponding tissue from healthy control sites. They used antibodies to detect IL-1β and PMNs (neutrophil elastase) and monocyte/macrophage cells (CD68). The clinical sites were classified using the GI and PPD and the biopsied sites were histometrically analysed to determine the percentage of inflammatory cell infiltration (PICI). The amount of IL-1β was measured by ELISA in tissue extracts. Total tissue IL-1β and IL-1β concentration and PICI were significantly higher in diseased sites than in healthy ones. PMNs and macrophages dominated the infiltrates and total tissue IL-1β correlated with GI and the PICI. Thus the amount of IL-1β in the tissues seems to relate to the severity of inflammation indicating that it may play a significant role in the mechanisms producing it.

Dayan et al (2004) showed that transgenic mice that overexpress the 17-kDa form of IL-1α in the basal layer of oral mucosal epithelium develop a syndrome that possesses all of the cardinal features of periodontal disease, including epithelial proliferation and apical migration, loss of attachment, and destruction of cementum and alveolar bone. In this model, bacterial colonization and infection were not required, since levels of periodontal bacteria were equivalent in transgenic and wild-type mice, and continuous treatment with antibiotics from birth did not ameliorate the disease. Their findings therefore indicated that elevated levels of IL-1α in the oral micro-environment can mediate all of the clinical features of periodontal disease.

IL-1 and tumour necrosis factor (TNF) are pro-inflammatory cytokines that stimulate a number of events in periodontal disease (Graves & Cochrane 2003; Takashiba et al 2003). These include stimulation of matrix metalloproteinases and bone resorption (see below). The use of antagonists to IL-1 and TNF in experimental periodontitis have demonstrated a cause and effect relationship between their activity and the spread of the inflammatory front into the deeper areas of the connective tissue, the loss of connective tissue attachment, osteoclast formation and alveolar bone resorption. Furthermore, the loss of fibroblasts during inflammation may be partly mediated by TNF. Thus, much of the tissue damage that occurs in periodontal disease activity may represent an over-reaction of the host response to periodontal pathogens caused by expressive production of IL-1 and TNF.

It has also be shown that IL-4 can inhibit the IL-1β induction of matrix metalloproteinase-3 expression in human gingival fibroblasts (HGF) from chronic periodontitis patients (Jenkins et al 2004). Similar effects of this cytokine on human skin and synovial fibroblasts and articular chondrocytes have been previously reported. The effect of IL-4 on HGF was shown to be independent of PGE$_2$ and inhibition of DNA binding of known transcription factors to the MMP-3 promoter.

Ide et al (2004) measured the acute phase protein response to short-term periodontal treatment and found that the circulating levels of TNF-α and IL-6 significantly increased following an episode of subgingival scaling.

The degree of change in TNF-α correlated with the severity of periodontal breakdown. This may account for anecdotal reports of pyrexia after subgingival scaling and may be significant in the relationship between periodontal disease and bacteraemia and cardiovascular disease (see Chs 6 and 18).

Interleukin-11 and IL-17 are cytokines that modulate the inflammatory process. Interleukin-17 (IL-17) is exclusively produced by activated T cells, and this cytokine can induce inflammatory responses, support immune responses (Th1), and stimulate osteoclastic bone resorption in combination with receptor activator of NF-κB (RANK) and RANK ligand (RANKL). These biological functions may be relevant to the aetiopathogenesis of periodontitis.

Their concentrations in normal and inflamed human gingival tissue have been compared (Johnson et al 2004). Biopsies of healthy and inflamed gingival tissue were obtained and homogenized. IL-11,17, IL-6 and RANTES concentrations were measured by ELISA assays and compared in the different types of tissue. IL-11 concentration was highest in gingivitis tissue and IL-17 concentration was highest in early periodontitis tissue. The concentrations of both of these cytokines were significantly higher than at other sites ($p<0.001$). However, the concentrations of both these cytokines were significantly lower in advanced periodontitis tissue. RANTES concentrations were significantly higher in advanced periodontitis tissue compared to other tissue types ($p<0.001$). IL-11, IL-6 and RANTES concentrations were significantly correlated with probing depth. This suggests that the concentrations of these cytokines may change as a consequence of the progression of gingivitis to periodontitis and may play a role in this process.

Keiso et al (2005) investigated whether IL-17 is produced in periodontal lesions and also assessed the relationship of gene expression between IL-17 and other cytokines in order to determine the effect of IL-17 on IL-6 production in human gingival fibroblasts (HGF). IL-17 was detected and measured in periodontal tissue biopsies obtained during periodontal surgery and in the cell-free culture supernatants cultured *ex vivo*, by using Western immunoblotting and enzyme-linked immunosorbent assay, respectively. IL-17 and other cytokine gene expressions were also investigated by RT-PCR. The contribution of IL-17 to IL-6 production by HGF was finally studied. IL-17 protein was moderately detected in periodontal tissues. In contrast, IL-17 mRNA was expressed only in nine of 23 periodontitis tissue samples by RT-PCR. The IL-17 mRNA-positive samples simultaneously expressed mRNAs encoding IFN-γ, IL-2, RANK, and RANKL, but not IL-4. IL-10 (Th2 cytokine). This was also detected more frequently in the samples than IFN-γ and IL-2 (Th1 cytokine). Recombinant human IL-17 induced IL-6 production from HGF in a dose- and time-dependent fashion. These results appear to indicate that IL-17 is produced in periodontal lesions, and may be involved in Th1 modulation. It may also enhance inflammatory reactions via gingival fibroblast-derived mediators in periodontal disease. Thus, IL-17, together with other cytokines, has a potential role in the aetiopathogenesis of periodontal disease.

IL-17 has been shown to upregulate IL-1β and tumour necrosis factor-alpha (TNF-α). Beklen et al (2007) hypothesized that it is increased in periodontitis and upregulates these cytokines and tissue-destructive matrix metalloproteinases (MMP) in local migrant and resident cells. Using immunocytochemistry they disclosed elevated IL-1β, TNF-, and IL-17 levels in periodontitis. These cytokines induced proMMP-1 and especially MMP-3 in gingival fibroblasts, whereas MMP-8 and MMP-9 were not induced. IL-17 was less potent as a direct MMP inducer than IL-1β and TNF-, but it induced IL-1β and TNF- production from macrophages, and IL-6 and IL-8 from gingival fibroblasts. Immunocytochemistry also disclosed that MMP-1 and MMP-3 were increased in periodontitis. Thus, gingival fibroblasts may play an important role in tissue destruction in periodontitis via cytokine-inducible MMP-1 and MMP-3 production, in which IL-17 plays a role as a key regulatory cytokine.

Since the presence of interleukin (IL)-23 has not been reported within inflamed gingivae before Lester et al (2007) evaluated its concentration within tissue from normal sites and sites of chronic periodontal disease. They obtained gingival tissue prior to extraction of teeth and grouped it according to clinical attachment loss (CAL) as follows: 0–2 mm (normal), 3–4 mm (moderate), and >5 mm (severe). Tissues were solubilized, and IL-12, -23, -6, -17, and -1b; interferon-gamma (IFN-γ) and tumour necrosis factor-alpha (TNF-α) concentrations were assessed by enzyme-linked immunosorbent assay and the data was statically analysed. Gingival concentrations of IL-23, -17, -1β, and -6 and IFN-α were significantly greater at moderate CAL sites than at normal CAL sites. Gingival concentrations of IL-23, -1β, -17, and -6 and TNF-α were significantly greater at severe CAL sites than at normal CAL sites. In addition, the gingival concentrations of IL-23, -17, and -6 and TNF-α were significantly greater and the gingival concentrations of IL-12 and IFN-α were significantly lower at severe CAL sites than at moderate CAL sites. Gingival concentrations of IL-23, -17, -6, and -1β and TNF-α correlated positively with CAL. The IL-23 gingival concentration correlated significantly with IL-17, -1β, and -6 and TNF-α concentrations and correlated negatively with IL-12 and IFN-α concentrations. These results suggested the possibility that the IL-23/IL-17 immune response was active within chronically inflamed gingival tissue and this is host response may be an important factor in the chronic nature of the disease.

Suzuki et al (2006) carried out a study to assess the effects of a tumour-necrosis factor-alpha (TNF-α) antagonist on inflammatory bone resorption and osteoclast formation in the periodontal pathogen-infection model. They found that the TNF-α antagonist peptide significantly prevented the *P. gingivalis*-induced reduction in the bone mineral density at the calvariae. Their histomorphometric assessments revealed the inhibitory effects of the TNF-α antagonist peptide on the *P. gingivalis*-induced increase in the number of the inflammatory cells and in the area of sagittal suture at the calvariae. Furthermore, there was also an inhibitory effect on the *P. gingivalis*-induced increase in the number of osteoclasts per unit bone surface at the calvariae. These results also suggested that the low molecular size of the TNF-α antagonists might be beneficial for the treatment of local inflammatory bone loss induced by periodontal-pathogen infection.

Vernal et al (2005) investigated the presence of IL-17 in gingival crevicular fluid (GCF) samples and in the culture supernatants of gingival cells from patients with chronic periodontitis. GCF samples were collected during 30 s from two sites in 16 patients from periodontally affected sites. A comparison with healthy controls was carried out by collecting GCF samples from eight healthy volunteers. ELISA was performed to determine the total amount of IL-17. Supernatant cellular cultures of gingival cells were obtained from periodontal biopsies taken from 12 periodontitis patients and from eight healthy control subjects during the surgical removal of wisdom teeth. Spontaneous and phytohaemagglutinin (PHA)-stimulated levels of IL-17 were determined by ELISA. The total amount of cytokine IL-17 was significantly higher in the periodontitis group than the control group ($p=0.005$). Significantly higher GCF volume and amount of total proteins were obtained from periodontitis patients as compared with control subjects ($p=0.0005$). A higher concentration of IL-17 was detected in culture supernatants from periodontitis patients compared with healthy subjects, either with or without stimulation ($p=0.01$). Treatment with PHA induced a significant increase in the production of IL-17 in healthy subjects and periodontitis patients ($p=0.001$). Thus the total amount of cytokine IL-17 in GCF samples and in the culture supernatants of gingival cells appear to be significantly increased in periodontal disease.

Another study (Oda et al 2003) found that *P. gingivalis* antigen (outer membrane protein) stimulated T cells to express IL-17 but not the receptor activator of nuclear factor KB ligand (RANKL) in both gingivitis and periodontitis patients.

Johnson and Serio (2005) showed that periodontal inflammation may not successfully resolve because of accumulation of IL-6 and IL-18, and decreased concentrations of IL-12, within diseased gingiva.

Lester et al (2007) evaluated the concentration of interleukin (IL)-23 within gingiva from normal sites and sites of chronic periodontal disease. Their results suggested the possibility that the IL-23/IL-17 immune response was present within chronically inflamed gingiva. This is a host response that had not been reported previously in periodontal disease and may be another important factor in the chronic nature of the disease.

THE BALANCE BETWEEN Th1 AND Th2 IMMUNE RESPONSES IN PERIODONTAL DISEASE

It has been suggested (Seymour & Gemmell 2001) that the development of the progressive lesion of periodontal disease is related to a shift from a T helper lymphocyte 1 (Th1) to a Th2 response (see Ch. 3). The stable lesion is small in area and consists of a T-lymphocyte/macrophage response. The T lymphocytes in this lesion have been shown not to express CD25 which seems to indicate that they are not proliferating locally within the tissues (Seymour et al 1988).

It is suggested that a strong innate immune response would lead to the production of IL-12, which in turn would turn on the Th1 response (Seymour & Gemmell 2001). The consequential production of IFN-γ would then enhance the activity of both macrophages and PMNs to contain the infection. In the periodontal tissues the stable lesion persists because of the continual presence of bacterial plaque.

The dominance of B-lymphocytes and plasma cells in the progressive lesion suggests that the change from Th1 to a Th2 response may lead to the possibility of tissue destruction as a result of unregulated release of IL-1 from plasma cells. In this regard if the innate response to a pathogen is poor it will fail to control the infection which may then result in polyclonal activation of B cells and the subsequent production of IL-4. This would then stimulate the development of a Th2 response (Seymour & Gemmell 2001). If the antibodies generated by this response are protective and successfully clear the infection then disease will not progress. If, however, they are non-protective the lesion will persist and continued B-lymphocyte activation may then lead to unregulated production of IL-1 with possible subsequent tissue destruction (Gemmell & Seymour 1988, 1994; Seymour et al 1993).

The Th1 to Th2 shift in periodontal disease is supported by evidence from a majority of the studies attempting to delineate the Th1/Th2 profile in periodontal tissue from chronic periodontitis patients (Seymour & Gemmell 2001). In this regard, a number of studies have reported decreased Th1 responses (Fujihashi et al 1991; Sigushi et al 1998) and/or increased Th2 responses (Aoyagi et al 1995; Yamazaki et al 1994, Reinhardt et al 1989; Tokoro et al 1997; Manhardt et al 1994; Gemmell & Seymour 1988) in periodontal disease. However, in contrast to these studies, there are some investigations that have indicated either an increase in Th1 response (Ebersole & Taubman 1994; Salvi et al 1998) or the joint involvement of Th1, Th2 and Th0 cells in a continuum of responses (Fujihashi et al 1994, 1996; Takeichi et al 1994; Prabhu et al 1996) in periodontal disease.

Studies on T-cell lines and clones have also produced some conflicting results. Flow cytometry and RT-PCR have been used to show the CD4 and CD8 lymphocytes derived from a *P. gingivalis*-positive gingivitis patient and a *P. gingivalis*-positive periodontitis patient produced IL-4, IL-10 and IFN-γ (Gemmell et al 1995). In contrast, a further study by the same group using a number of cell lines, produced from a number of *P. gingivalis*-positive gingivitis and periodontitis patients, demonstrated highly variable cytokine profiles (Gemmell et al 1999). However, another group (Wassenar et al 1995) established T-cell lines from gingival tissue from four adult chronic periodontitis patients and found that 80% of the CD4 clones had Th2 profiles and produced high levels of IL-4 and low levels of IFN-γ.

CD4+/CD25+ regulatory T (Tr) cells appear to be critical in regulating the immune response and thereby may play an important role in the defense against infection and control of autoimmune diseases. Nakajima et al (2005) identified the CD4+CD25+ Tr cells in periodontitis tissues and compared them with those in gingivitis tissues. Immunohistological analysis of CD4, CD25, and CTLA-4 and the gene expression analysis of FOXP3, TGF-β1, and IL-10 on gingival biopsies revealed the presence of CD4+CD25+ Tr cells in all tissues. In periodontitis, the percentage of CD4+CD25+ Tr cells increased with increasing proportions of B cells relative to T cells. FOXP3, a characteristic marker for CD4+CD25+ Tr cells, TGF-β1 and IL-10 were expressed more highly in periodontitis compared with gingivitis. These findings suggest that CD4+CD25+ Tr cells and possibly other regulatory T-cell populations do exist and may play regulatory roles in periodontal diseases.

Caution must be applied in interpreting all these studies since it is very difficult in many cases to be sure that the tissue used for the samples was either at a truly active or truly stable phase in the disease process at the time of sampling.

In addition, emanating from a number of studies on the cytokine profile in periodontal disease, is the concept that the production of IL-10 may be of fundamental importance in the control of periodontal disease progression (Gemmell et al 1997). One group (Yamamoto et al 1997) were able to show two distinct cytokine patterns in cells from periodontal tissues. One showed the presence of IFN-γ, IL-6, IL-10 and IL-13 mRNA, while the other was similar but lacked IL-10. This suggests that those lesions producing high levels of IL-10 remain stable, while those with low levels may progress. These findings are supported by evidence that mice lacking in both IL-10 genes had accelerated levels of alveolar bone loss compared with normal (IL-10+/+) control mice (Al-Rasheed et al 2003). In a further study using the same model this group (Al-Rasheed et al 2004) found that the accelerated alveolar bone loss in the IL-10 (−/−) mice occurred after 9 months and thus appeared to be a late-onset condition. The results also suggested that lack of IL-10 may have an effect on bone homeostasis (see also Ch. 4).

Sasaki et al (2004) tested the hypothesis that endogenous IL-10 is a potent suppressor of *Porphyromonas gingivalis*-induced alveolar bone loss *in vivo*. IL-10 knockout ([−]/[−]) and wild-type mice were inoculated intraorally with *P. gingivalis*. Non-infected animals served as negative controls. Alveolar bone loss, gingival cytokine levels, and gingival gene expression were assessed using morphometric analysis, enzyme-linked immunosorbent assay, and semiquantitative reverse transcription polymerase chain reaction, respectively. *P. gingivalis*-infected IL-10 [−]/[−] mice exhibited severe alveolar bone loss compared to non-infected IL-10 [−]/[−] and wild-type mice by day 42. Surprisingly, bone resorptive cytokines IL-1α and TNF-α were not upregulated in gingival tissues by *P. gingivalis*-infection. They concluded that the IL-10 [−]/[−] mouse is highly susceptible to bone loss induced by the periodontal pathogen *P. gingivalis*, which is mediated via an IL-1-independent pathway.

However, caution must again be exercised in interpreting cytokine data since the in-built redundancy within cytokine networks ensures that if one cytokine is absent another with similar activity may take its place (Seymour & Gemmell 2001). In this regard, IL-6 and IFN-γ have many of the functions of IL-1 and IL-13 can replace IL-4 and in many respects IL-11 may replace IL-10.

THE ROLE OF THE ANTIGEN PRESENTING CELL (APC)

The nature of the APC may also be of fundamental importance in determining whether a Th1 or a Th2 cytokine profile is produced following contact with the antigen (Seymour & Gemmell 2001). The development of a Th1 response depends primarily on the production of IL-12 which may be secreted by APCs, monocytes, macrophages and PMNs. In contrast, a Th2 cytokine profile is dependent on IL-4 secretion which is produced by Th2-lymphocytes, mast cells and transformed B lymphocytes (Seymour & Gemmell 2001). Thus, the response may depend on a number of different factors including the genetic status which determines the APC response, the local cytokine response and the nature of the infective agent(s).

It is generally held that Th0 cells following activation by antigen differentiate into either Th1 or Th2 cells. However, it has been also proposed (Kelso 1995) that Th1 and Th2 cells form a continuum and a particular clone can secrete either ThI or Th2 cytokine or both depending on the nature of the stimulus. In this regard it has also been shown (Gemmell et al 1999) that when peripheral blood mononuclear cells were used to present *P. gingivalis* antigens to *P. gingivalis* specific T cells it resulted in the production of highly varied cytokine profiles. This could be due to a number of cells including dendritic APCs, monocytes and B cells all acting as antigen-presentation cells within the peripheral blood. Using the same cell lines this group have shown that when *P. gingivalis* antigens were presented to autogenous EBV-transformed B cells, the cytokine profiles were predominantly IL-4 positive, with low numbers of IFN-γ positive T cells and very few IL-10 positive T cells and these profiles were consistent for all the T-cell lines examined (Seymour & Gemmell 2001). While these results are suggestive of a Th0, Th1, Th2 continuum they do not definitely prove it. It does, however, indicate that APCs are of fundamental importance in directing the appropriate response for the antigen they bind and present (Hart 1997). In this regard, it has be shown (Choi et al 2000) that T-cell clones derived from mice immunized with Fusobacterium nucleatum followed by *P. gingivalis* demonstrated a Th2 profile, while those from mice immunized with *P. gingivalis* alone all demonstrated a Th1 profile. Although these results have not yet been confirmed independently they do suggest that complexes of organisms, such as are regularly seen in periodontal diseases, are necessary to promote a Th2 response and a polyclonal B-cell activator such as *F. nucleatum* could be critical in stimulating this type of response.

Different APC sub-populations may activate different T-cell subsets. One group (Gemmell et al 2002) has utilized an immunoperoxidase technique to investigate the presence of CD1a+, CMRF-44+, CMRF-58+ and CD83+ dendritic cells, CD14+ macrophages or dendritic precursors and CD19+ B cells in gingival biopsies from 21 healthy or gingivitis and 25 periodontitis subjects. The samples were also divided into three groups according to the size of infiltrate. The presence of large numbers of CD1a+ Langerhans cells was found in the epithelium of all the groups with no differences between them. The percentage of CD83+ dendritic cells was higher than the proportion of CD1a+, CMRF-44+ or CMRF-58+ dendritic cells in the infiltrates. Endothelial cells positive for CD83 were found predominantly in areas adjacent to infiltrating cells. Many CD83+ dendritic cells were found adjacent to CD 83+ endothelial cells. The percentage of CD14+ macrophages was similar to that of the CD83+ dendritic cells in the infiltrates. CD19+ B cells were the predominant APC in the larger infiltrate groups and the percentage of B cells was increased in the periodontitis group compared to the healthy/gingivitis group. The precise role of the APC subgroups in periodontal pathology still remains unclear.

Bodineau et al (2006) found that Langerhans cells expressed matrix metalloproteinases 2 and 9, and tissue inhibitors of matrix metalloproteinases 1 and 2 in both healthy and diseased gingival tissues. The MMP-positive Langerhans cells were mainly observed in the upper epithelial layers. MMP 9-positive Langerhans cells were observed especially during periodontitis and in the basal epithelial layer or crossing the basement membrane. They felt that during periodontal disease, changes in the expression of matrix metalloproteinases and their tissue inhibitors by gingival Langerhans cells could have been implicated in the migration of the cells towards the connective tissue. (Further information on the immunoregulation in periodontal disease can be seen in a series of reviews of this subject in Periodontology 2000, details in the Further Reading section below.)

INFLAMMATION

Inflammation leads to the accumulation of PMNs, macrophages and mast cells which are very important in protecting against infection. They do, however, contain destructive enzymes within lysosomes, normally used to degrade phagocytosed material and these are capable of damaging tissue if released. Such enzymes may be released by inflammatory cells during function or when they degenerate and die. PMNs and macrophages also produce reactive oxygen species (ROS) to destroy phagocytosed bacteria but these may also be released into the tissues. Both these sources of potential tissue damage will be considered separately below.

Bacterial components/virulence factors may be involved in modulating inflammatory responses and include: lipopolysaccharides (LPS), peptidoglycans, lipoteichoic acids, fimbriae, proteases, heat-shock proteins, formyl-methionyl peptides, and toxins (Madianos et al 2005). Potential host cell receptors involved in recognizing bacterial components and initiating signalling pathways that lead to inflammatory responses include: Toll-like receptors (TLRs), CD14, nucleotide-binding oligomerization domain proteins (Nod) and G-protein-coupled receptors, including formyl-methionyl peptide receptors and protease-activated receptors. Of the above bacterial and host molecules, evidence from experimental animal studies implicate LPS, fimbriae, proteases, TLRs, and CD14 in periodontal tissue or alveolar bone destruction. However, evidence verifying the involvement of any of the above molecules in periodontal tissue destruction in humans does not exist.

The association between genetic variability and the inflammatory response induced by periodontal infection is currently unclear (Shapira et al 2005). To date, there is no clear correlation between any of the gene polymorphisms and clinical indicators of inflammation. The powering of studies to reveal associations between single or multiple nucleotide polymorphisms and inflammatory parameters will need to involve a much larger number of subjects than were used in the past. The available data (including the interleukin-1 composite genotype) do not currently support the utility of such tests in the diagnosis and prognostic assessments of periodontal diseases.

REACTIVE OXYGEN SPECIES (ROS)

Inflammatory cells and in particular PMNs once stimulated produce reactive oxygen species (ROS) via the metabolic pathway of the respiratory burst, which occurs in the process of phagocytosis. These include the super oxide anion (O_2-) and hydrogen peroxide (H_2O_2) which further react together in the presence of transitional metal ions to produce the hydroxyl radical (OH). PMNs also produce hyperchlorous acid via myeloperoxidation. The production of these highly reactive oxygen species enable inflammatory cells to kill phagocytosed pathogens. However, evidence suggests that ROS can cause connective tissue destruction (Freeman & Crapo 1982), resulting in the loss of structural integrity and function of the periodontal tissues, when these substances leak into the tissues. Epithelial and connective tissue cells are highly susceptible to damage from ROS which produces DNA damage, lipid peroxidation, protein damage and oxidation of important enzymes such as protease inhibitors. The generation of ROS during periodontal disease could be associated with degradation of gingival connective tissue. In this regard, ROS released by PMNs have been shown to damage proteoglycans (Moseley et al 1995). Cells and tissues in the vicinity of inflammatory cells will be damaged by these processes (Fredriksson et al 1998; Chapple 1997; Battino et al 1999, Bartold et al 1984; Waddington et al 2000) and this type of damage around these cells is known as bystander damage. ROS damage to cells also results in pro-inflammatory cytokine release.

ROS can also be produced by osteoclasts and osteoblasts they may play a role in bone resorption during normal turnover and disease. Bone cells are probably involved in the pathological destruction of the mineralized matrix as a consequence of their altered metabolic activity during active disease, following stimulation by factors from bacteria and mediators such as prostaglandins and IL-1 from gingival fibroblasts and circulating monocytes (Hausmann 1974; Reynolds et al 1994). Osteoclasts, stimulated with parathyroid hormone and IL-1 have been shown to produce superoxide anions (Garrett et al 1990). Moreover, bone resorption by osteoclasts was inhibited by superoxide dismutase, an enzyme which scavenges superoxide (see below).

ANTIOXIDANT DEFENCE SYSTEMS

The tissues are protected against the effects of ROS by antioxidants. These are substances which when present in low concentrations can delay or inhibit oxidation of large amounts of substrates. Important antioxidants are the 'chain breaking' antioxidant vitamins E, C and A and urate, bilirubin and substances containing sulphydryl (SH, thiol) groups (Halliwell & Gutterridge 1990). All these antioxidants work in concert with each other through redox cycling and they regenerate each other through chain breaking antioxidant reactions (Chapple 1997). Using a chemiluminescence assay capable of measuring the total antioxidant capacity (TAOC) one group (Chapple et al 1997; Brock et al 2004) has shown that patients with periodontitis have significantly reduced TAOC both peripherally in plasma and locally in GCF compared with healthy age and sex matched controls. They also showed that the oxidant capacity of GCF differed from that of serum and saliva in that the predominant active component was glutathione (GSH) which was present at levels 1000-fold higher than those in serum (Chapple et al 2002). The only other areas of the body where GSH is present in such quantities are the lining fluids of the lung alveoli (Cantin et al 1987) and the uterine cervix (Cope et al 1999). In the lung, it is known that GSH plays a major role in redox balance within epithelial cells (Cantin et al 1987; Pacht et al 1991). If this balance is upset then important transcription factors such as NF-κB are activated which lead to the production of pro-inflammatory cytokines (IL-1, IL-6, IL-8, PGE_2, TNF-α) which in turn initiate an inflammatory response. In this regard it is known that patients suffering from pulmonary fibrosis and acute respiratory distress syndrome are deficient in GSH level in their alveolar epithelial cells (Cantin et al 1987; Pacht et al 1991). Since GSH seem to be the principal antioxidant in GCF a similar mechanism might underlie some cases of high susceptibility to periodontitis.

Brock et al (2004) carried out a cross-sectional study to determine both local (saliva and gingival crevicular fluid, GCF) and peripheral (plasma and serum) antioxidant capacity in periodontal health and disease. A total of 20 non-smoking volunteers with chronic periodontitis were sampled together with 20 age- and sex-matched, non-smoking controls. After overnight fasting, saliva (whole unstimulated and stimulated) and blood were collected and the total antioxidant capacity (TAOC) was determined using an enhanced chemiluminescence method. GCF antioxidant concentration was significantly lower in periodontitis subjects compared to healthy controls ($p<0.001$). Although mean levels of peripheral and salivary TAOC were also lower in periodontitis the difference was only significant for plasma ($p<0.05$). Healthy subjects' GCF antioxidant concentration was also significantly greater than from paired serum or plasma ($p<0.001$). Data stratified for gender did not alter the findings and a male bias was revealed in all clinical samples except GCF. These findings suggest that the antioxidant capacity of GCF is both qualitatively and quantitatively distinct from that of saliva, plasma and serum. Whether changes in the GCF compartment in periodontitis reflect predisposition to or the results of ROS-mediated damage remains unclear. Reduced plasma total antioxidant defence could result from low-grade systemic inflammation induced by the host response to periodontal bacteria, or may be an innate feature of periodontitis patients.

Soory (2008) in a review of non-antimicrobial actions of tetracyclines in combating oxidative stress in periodontal and metabolic disease showed that tetracyclines had diverse mechanisms of overcoming oxidative stress and enhancing matrix synthesis (see also Ch. 17).

In order to understand the possible roles of enzymes and ROS in periodontal pathology it is necessary also to consider collagen and proteoglycan degradation processes (see below).

Inflammatory markers

Severe periodontitis is associated with elevated inflammatory markers in otherwise healthy populations. A recent study (D'Aiuto et al 2004) assessed whether the degree of response to periodontal therapy was associated with changes in the serological markers of systemic inflammation. A total of 94 systemically healthy subjects with severe generalized periodontitis were recruited into a prospective 6-month, blind, intervention trial. Periodontal parameters and inflammatory markers (C-reactive protein (CRP) and IL-6) were evaluated prior to and 2 and 6 months after periodontal therapy; 6-month after treatment, significant reductions in serum IL-6 ($p=0.001$) and CPR ($p=0.001$) were observed. Decreases in inflammatory markers were also significant in subjects with an above average clinical response to therapy after correction for possible confounders. Thus periodontitis may add to the systemic inflammatory burden of affected individuals.

Another group (Joshipura et al 2004) evaluated the cross-sectional association between periodontal disease and the serum levels of CRP, fibrinogen, factor VII, tissue plasminogen activator (t-PA), low density lipoprotein-C (LDL-C), von Willebrand factor and soluble tumour necrosis factor receptor 1 and 2. The study group was 468 men, aged 47–80 years free of cardiovascular disease (CVS), diabetes and cancer. They used a multivariate regression model controlling for age, cigarette smoking, alcohol intake, physical activity and aspirin intake. Periodontal disease was associated with significantly higher levels of CPR, t-PA and LDL-C. This data suggests that periodontal disease may be associated with the biomarkers of endothelial dysfunction and dyslipidemia, which may potentially mediate the suggested association between periodontitis and CVD (see Ch. 4).

Collagen degradation

Collagen degradation is a multistage process (**Fig. 5.5**). Each collagen molecule consists of two distinct regions. The larger (96% by weight) is the triple helical region which is resistant to attack by most proteinases except collagenase. The smaller terminal regions consist of peptides known as the terminal peptides, which contain the sites of intra- and intermolecular cross-links. These areas can be attacked by a number of proteinases. Collagen fibrils, with intermolecular cross links are resistant to the action of collagenases and under physiological conditions a number of enzymes may act in concert (Harris & Cartwright 1977). Mammalian collagenases are metalloproteinases which act at neutral pH, in the presence of metal ions to cleave the triple helix into two fragments. They cannot cleave the molecule further but expose it to the action of other proteinases in the tissues or within cells. Collagenases now known as matrix metalloproteinases (MMPs) 1 and 8 are present in many cells and tissues as latent enzymes either as pro-enzymes or enzyme inhibitor complexes (Meikle et al 1986; Birkedal-Hansen 1993; Reynolds et al 1994; Reynolds 1996) and need to be activated by other proteinases. Under physiological conditions the tissues are at neutral pH and neutral proteinases are most likely to be involved.

The evidence for the possible role of MMPs, and particularly inflammatory cell derived MMPs, MMP-8,9, is quite strong (Ryan et al 1996; Birkedal-Hansen et al 1993a,b; Vernillo et al 1994). This includes the production of elevated levels by diseased gingival tissue in culture, the detection of active rather than latent collagenase in GCF and extracts of adjacent

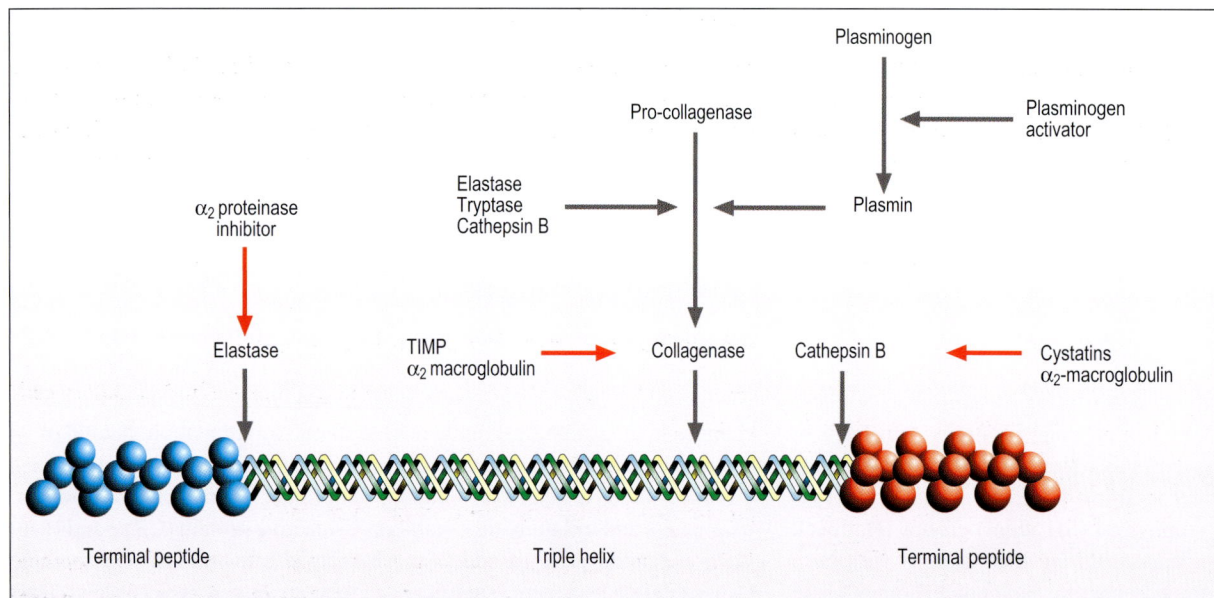

Fig. 5.5 A diagram of collagen degradation showing the proteolytic enzymes and inhibitors involved.

gingival tissue in patients with chronic periodontitis (Fullmer & Gibson 1966; Golub et al 1985; Lee et al 1995) and the presence of MMP messenger RNA in the cells of the periodontal lesion as well as periodontal ligament and gingival fibroblasts, keratinocytes, endothelial cells, osteoblasts and osteoclasts. Inflammatory cells, particularly PMNs, are thought to play a major role in the MMP-mediated destructive lesion (Lee et al 1995; Golub et al 1989, 1995, 1998). Additional evidence for this pathogenic pathway is the presence of elevated MMP protein in periodontal lesions shown by immunocytochemical studies (Birkedal-Hansen et al 1993b; Ryan et al 1996). Moreover, the ability of MMP inhibitors such as doxycycline to retard periodontal breakdown (see Ch. 17) further supports the possible pathogenic role of these proteinases.

Other proteinases such as the serine proteinase elastase could also play a role in these processes (Eley & Cox 1996a; Booth et al 2007). Furthermore, in inflammatory states the tissues surrounding inflammatory cells may be acidified and could also provide suitable conditions for the action of acid proteinases such as cathepsin B (Burleigh 1977; Eley & Cox 1996b).

In this regard, Cox et al (2006a) showed in a tissue culture model of gingival fibroblasts that fibroblast MMP 1 was most likely responsible for collagen dissolution in the model, while cathepsin B might have been part of the activation process. A number of metallo-, cysteine and serine proteases probably contribute to extracellular matrix destruction in inflamed gingival tissue, where they may activate each other in proteolytic cascades.

Proteoglycan degradation

When connective tissue is degraded in disease, the catabolism of collagen is often preceded by that of proteoglycans. Proteoglycans are composed of a central protein core to which is attached a variable number of highly anionic glycosaminoglycan (GAG) chains (Bartold 1987). The structure of proteoglycans (**Fig. 5.6**) depends on the type of GAG chains attached to its protein core (see Ch. 1). Several interactions occur between individual proteoglycans and cell surfaces, basal lamina and collagen. The most common GAG in the gingiva and periodontal ligament is hyaluronic acid (hyaluronan) and large amounts of this GAG are found in gingiva. The main proteoglycans in these tissues are small dermatan sulphate proteoglycans and a larger molecular weight chondroitin sulphate proteoglycan, versican, which is capable of interacting with hyaluronan (Embery et al 1979, 1987; Larjava et al 1992; Pearson & Pringle 1986; Purvis et al 1984). In bone and cementum the principal proteoglycans are two small molecular

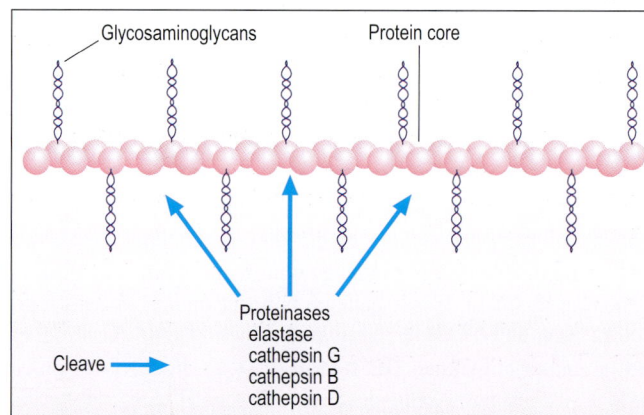

Fig. 5.6 A diagram of proteoglycan degradation showing the proteolytic enzymes involved.

weight chondroitin sulphate (CS) proteoglycans named decorin and biglycan which contain one and two CS chains, respectively (Waddington & Embery 1991).

In proteoglycan degradation (**Fig. 5.6**) protein cleavage occurs first to release GAGs from the protein core. A number of metallo-, serine and cysteine proteinases can do this. The metalloproteinases with this function (Birkedal-Hansen 1993; Reynolds et al 1994; Reynolds 1996) are known as stromelysins (MMP-3,10,11). The released GAG usually remains intact but may be further degraded. The role of the hydrolytic enzymes such as hyaluronidase, chondroitinases, aryl sulphatase and glucuronidases, in degrading proteoglycans is confusing since none of them are proteolytic. They could be involved in the subsequent degradation of the released GAGs but observations of GAGs isolated from inflamed gingiva indicate that they remain intact despite the abundance of hydrolytic enzymes in the tissues.

Reactive oxygen species (ROS) have also been shown to damage proteoglycans (Moseley et al 1995). Both ROS generated by chemical means and from stimulation of isolated polymorphonuclear leucocytes in vitro have been shown to produce chain depolymerization, modification of hexuronic acid and hexuronic residues and limited desulphation. OH radicles and non-sulphated GAGs were more susceptible than sulphated GAGs to this damage.

Proteolytic enzymes

Proteolytic enzymes can be classified as to the biochemistry of their active site (serine, metallo-, cysteine or aspartic), their predominant substrate or their pH optima (Owen & Campbell 1999; Uitto et al 2003). The proteases active at neutral pH can take part in both intracellular and extracellular activity in both physiological and pathological conditions. Those active at acid pH are best suited to intracellular, lysosomal activity but may still carry out limited extracellular activity in close proximity to the cell surface.

Serine proteinases

These are active at neutral pH and their activity depends on the catalytic triad of aspartic acid, histidine and serine which are widely separated in the primary sequence but come together in the active site when the molecule folds into its tertiary structure (Owen & Campbell 1999; Uitto et al 2003). The principle enzymes in this group are human leucocyte elastase (HLE), cathepsin G, proteinase 3, plasminogen activator, tryptase, chymase and granzymes A and B. Collectively, they can degrade elastin, fibronectin, laminin, vitronectin, proteoglycans, collagens III, IV, VII, fibrin, fibrinogen, complement components, clotting factors, heat shock protein and immunoglobulins. They can also activate pro-collagenases, cleave CD 2, 4 and 8 receptors and pro-IL1β and TNF-α, -β and convert angiotensin I to angiotensin II which mediates the vascular changes of inflammatory hyperaemia. Furthermore, they can activate lymphocytes and platelets and induce the secretion of cytokines and chemoattractants from mononuclear phagocytes, fibroblasts, endothelial and epithelial cells. Finally, the granzymes A and B prime cytotoxic lymphocytes to function and process the secreted perforin molecule.

Seine proteinase inhibitors include α1- proteinase inhibitor, α1-antichymotrypsin, α2-plasmin inhibitor, antithrombin III, plasminogen activator inhibitors, C1 inhibitor, secretory leucocyte proteinase inhibitor (SLPI) and skin-derived anti-leucoproteinase (SKALP) (see below).

Matrix metalloproteinases (MMP)

MMPs are dependent upon intrinsic Zn2+ and extrinsic Ca2+ for their activity at neutral pH. They can be divided into true collagenases (MMP 1, 8, 13), gelatinases (MMP 2, 9), stromelysins (MMP 3, 10, 11, 19), matrilysins (MMP 7, 26), metalloelastase (MMP 12) and membrane anchored MMPs or MT-MMPs (MMP 14, 15, 16, 17, 24 and 25). MMP 1, 8, 13 are the only proteinases that can cleave the triple helix of collagens at neutral pH (Werb 1997; Owen & Campbell 1999; Uitto et al 2003). The MMP family can collectively degrade all the components of the extracellular matrix including collagens I, II, III, IV V, VII, IX X, XI, gelatin, elastin, fibronectin, laminin, entactin and proteoglycans. The stromelysins (MMP 3, 10, 11) can also activate pro-MMP-1, -8, -9. MMPs are inhibited by tissue inhibitors of MMPs (TIMPs) and α2-macroglobulin (α2M) (see below).

Imbalance of their secretion, activity, inhibition and functions may play a key role in oral and periodontal disease (Sorsa et al 2004).

Cysteine proteinases

These depend on the presence of cysteine and histidine at the active site in the tertiary structure. They include cathepsins B, L and K. They are all active at acid pH and are adapted to play a major role in intracellular, lysosomal degradation of phagocytosed proteins. Cathepsin B also plays an important role in priming the MHC class II antigen receptor. They can also activate a number of pro-enzymes. They also play an essential role in breaking down bone collagen in bone resorption, particularly cathepsin K (see below). They are inhibited by α2M and the cystatins (see below).

Aspartic proteinases

These proteinases are all active at acid pH and within inflammatory cells and the most prominent one is cathepsin D. They are also most suited to intracellular, lysosomal degradation of proteins. Like cathepsin B, cathepsin D can also prime the MHC class II antigen receptor. Since there is a lack of known serum inhibitors for these enzymes they could also function in the pericellular area where the pH may be sufficiently low to allow cathepsin D to function.

Proteolytic enzymes in inflammatory cells

Most of these proteinases are stored in the lysosomes of inflammatory cells (**Fig. 5.7**).

Neutrophil polymorphonuclear leucocytes

PMNs synthesize proteinases at the pro-myelocyte stage of development and then store them in their lysosomes (**Fig. 5.7A**). After cellular activation these enzymes may translocate on to their cell surface where they may become active.

PMNs appear to be hyperactive in periodontal disease. In this regard, Fredriksson et al (2003) studied PMNs extracted from the venous blood from patients with severe periodontitis and matched healthy controls. The PMNs were activated and the total release of oxygen radicals was measured by luminal-enhanced chemiluminescence. The PMNs from the periodontitis patients had significantly higher chemiluminescence than controls when activated via the FcγR pathway and this suggests that their enhanced activity in periodontitis may be due to the greater responsiveness of this receptor.

In a study of the venous blood of 23 adult patients with moderate to advanced chronic periodontitis, Restaíno et al (2007) also showed that peripheral neutrophils of periodontitis-affected patients were more reactive. This was suggested by their significantly higher response toward periodontal pathogen extracts and other stimulating agents.

PMNs contain and release acid and neutral proteinases (Baggiolini et al 1980). Four distinct types of cytoplasmic body – azurophilic, specific, C-particles and secretory vacuoles – are formed during polymorph maturation.

The azurophil granules contain neutral serine proteinases, the most important of which are elastase, cathepsin G and small amounts of acid proteinases. The specific granules contain collagenases principally collagenase-2 (MMP-8) (Kiili et al 2002) and other metalloproteinases, known as gelatinases and stromelysins, which can degrade collagen further once it has been cleaved by collagenase. They also contain basement membrane collagenases and proteoglycans. Of these PMNs contain (Birkedal-Hansen 1993; Reynolds et al 1994; Reynolds 1996) gelatinase B (MMP-9) and some stromelysins (MMP-3 and possibly also MMP-10 and 11). The C granules contain the acid hydrolases cathepsins B and D (Rawlings & Barrett 2000; Dickinson 2002). Plasminogen activator is stored in secretory vacuoles. While the granule-bound proteinases are only released during phagocytosis, plasminogen activator is secreted. Proteinases can leak from the cells into the tissues during the process of phagocytosis and are also released when cells degenerate. They may also have surface bound, membrane associated MMPs mainly MMP 14 which becomes activated and then can degrade pericellular collagenous matrix during cell migration (Werb 1997; Uitto et al 2003).

Elastase can only occasionally be detected in PMNs in inflamed human gingiva using histochemical peptide substrates which only detect active enzyme (Kennett et al 1995). In contrast elastase can be immunocytochemically detected in all gingival PMNs using a monoclonal antibody which can

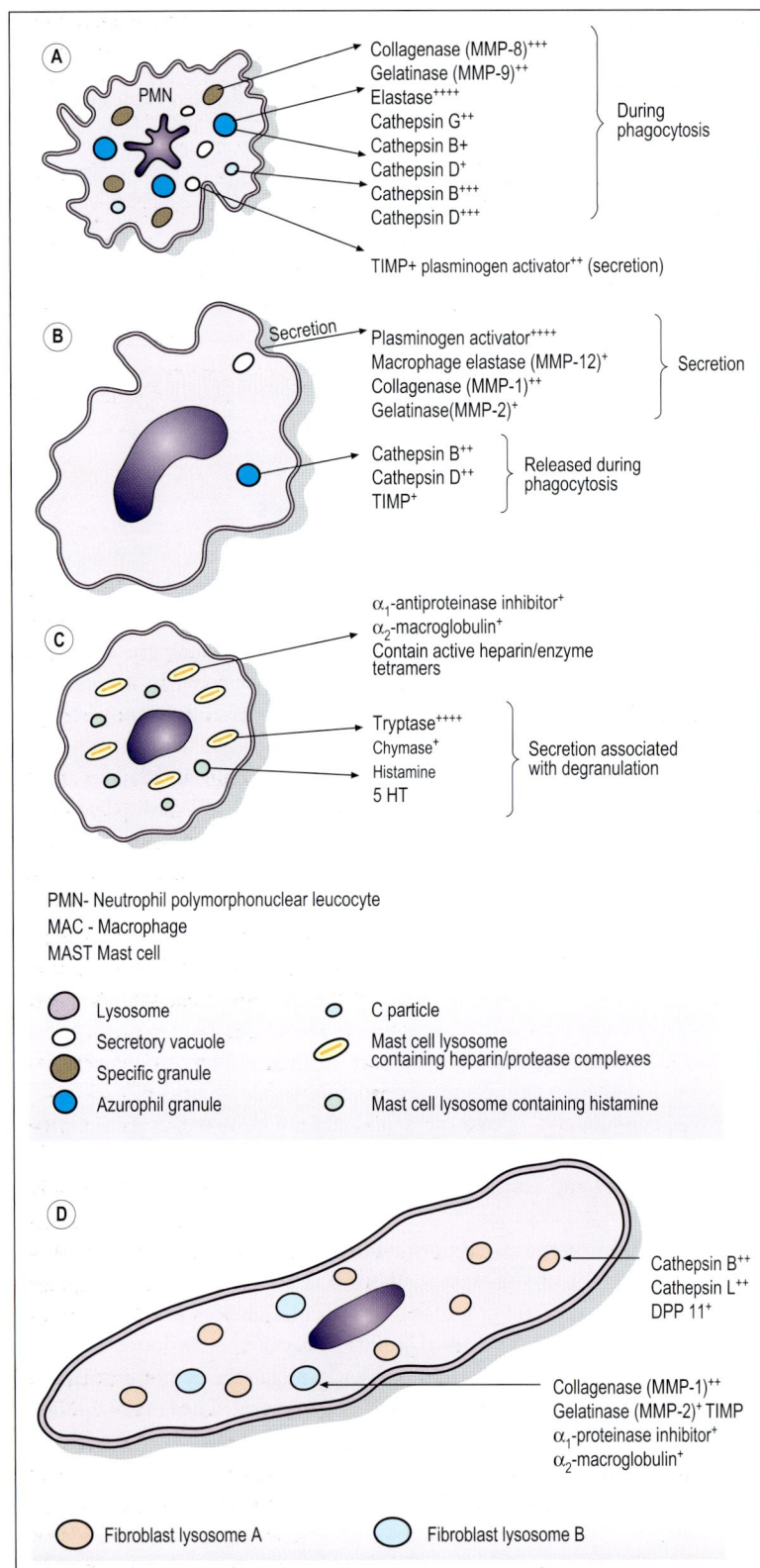

Fig. 5.7 Release of proteolytic enzymes and vasoactive substances from inflammatory cells: (A) neutrophil polymorphonuclear leucocyte, (B) macrophage, (C) mast cell, (D) fibroblast.

the junctional epithelium and at the active front of the lesion and could have been associated with disease activity.

The uncontrolled proteolytic activity in secretions during inflammatory diseases might be due to the resistance of membrane-bound proteases to inhibition (Korkmaz et al 2005). These workers have used a fluorogenic neutrophil elastase substrate to measure the activity of free and membrane-bound human neutrophil elastase in the presence of alpha 1-proteinase inhibitor (α1-PI). Fixed and unfixed neutrophils bore the same amounts of active elastase at their surface. However, the elastase bound to the surface of unfixed neutrophils was fully inhibited by stoichiometric amounts of α1-PI, unlike that of fixed neutrophils. In the presence of α1-PI, membrane-bound elastase is almost entirely removed from the unfixed neutrophil membrane to form soluble irreversible complexes. They concluded that elastase activity at the surface of human neutrophils is fully controlled by α1-PI when the cells are in suspension. Pericellular proteolysis could be limited to zones of contact between neutrophils and subjacent protease substrates where natural inhibitors cannot penetrate.

PMNs also produce reactive oxygen species (ROS) via the metabolic pathway of the respiratory burst, which occurs in the process of phagocytosis (Freeman & Crapo 1982). These can leak out of these cells during phagocytosis or when these cells die and degenerate and can be one cause of bystander damage (see above).

Figueredo et al (2005) compared the activity of neutrophilic granulocytes in patients with severe periodontitis and patients with gingivitis alone. The free elastase activity and the neutrophil activity, estimated as the ratio between elastase and lactoferrin, were significantly higher in the samples from the periodontitis patients. These differences were also observed in shallow pockets in periodontitis patients compared to similar pockets in patients with gingivitis. This may explain some of the tissue destruction seen in periodontitis.

Johnstone et al (2007) examined neutrophil function in a unique population of patients diagnosed with refractory aggressive periodontitis (RAP). They found that a larger receptor-independent respiratory burst and higher phagocytotic activity in PMNs derived from patients with RAP compared to PMNs derived from CP patients and periodontally healthy controls. They speculated that the higher intrinsic intracellular activity of the nicotinamide adenine dinucleotide phosphate oxidase system may account for the continued periodontal breakdown, despite ongoing periodontal therapy in these challenging patients (see also Ch. 23).

Receptors for the Fc part of IγG (FcγRIIa) on polymorphonuclear leucocytes (PMN) mediate phagocytosis and cell activation. Previous studies have showed that one of the genetic variants of the FcγRIIa, the 131 H/H, is associated with more periodontal breakdown than the R/R. This may be due to hyper-reactivity of the H/H-PMNs upon interaction with bacteria. Nicu et al (2007) genotyped a cohort of 98 periodontitis patients in order to study whether the FcγRIIa genotype modifies the PMN reactivity in periodontitis patients. From these, 10 H/H and 10 R/R consented to participate. PMNs were incubated with immune serum-opsonized *A. actinomycetemcomitans* (Aa). Phagocytosis, degranulation (CD63 and CD66b expression), respiratory burst and elastase release were assessed. Patients of the H/H genotype were found to show more bone loss than those with the H/R or R/R genotype ($p=0.038$). H/H-PMNs phagocytosed more opsonized Aa than did R/R-PMNs ($p=0.019$). The H/H-PMNs also expressed more CD63 and CD66b than did the R/R-PMNs ($p=0.004$ and 0.002, respectively) and released more elastase ($p=0.001$).

The genotyping results seemed to confirm previous reports that more periodontal destruction occurs in the H/H genotype than in the H/R or R/R genotype. The functional studies indicate a hyper-reactivity of the H/H-PMN in response to bacteria, which may be one of several pathways leading to more periodontal breakdown (see also Ch. 4).

detect both active and inactive enzyme. This suggests that the vast majority of gingival PMNs contain inactive elastase. Using immunocytochemistry, PMNs containing elastase are found throughout the periodontal lesion and in the junctional epithelium migrating into the crevice. Numerous PMNs containing elastase can also be found in the crevice (Kennett, et al 1997a). Occasional PMNs containing active elastase were only seen in a few individuals with severe periodontitis (Kennett et al 1995) and were found in

Macrophages

Macrophages (**Fig. 5.7B**) synthesize a variety of proteinases (Baggiolini et al 1980). The levels are usually low compared with those in PMNs but the amounts produced become sizable with time.

Acid and neutral proteinases are confined to different intracellular compartments. Acid proteinases (cathepsins B and D) are found in lysozymes and neutral proteinases in secretory vacuoles (Rawlings & Barrett 2000; Dickinson 2002). The major neutral proteinase of activated inflammatory macrophages is plasminogen activator. The other neutral proteinases are present in small amounts and include the serine proteinase elastase and the metalloproteinases collagenase-1(MMP-1) and gelatinase (MMP-9). Collagenase-3 (MMP 13) has also been localized by immunocytochemistry within macrophages (Kiili et al 2002). In addition, they contain metalloelastase (MMP 12) which is also known as macrophage elastase (Uitto et al 2003; Owen & Campbell 1999). They may also have membrane associated MMPs on their surfaces which when activated can degrade pericellular collagenous matrix during cell migration (Werb 1997; Uitto et al 2003).

Monocytes contain many serine proteinases (**Fig. 5.7**) with marked variation between subgroups (Uitto et al 2003; Owen & Campbell 1999). They usually also express these enzymes on the cell surface. A subgroup, known as pro-inflammatory monocytes contain larger amounts of human leucocyte elastase (HLE) and cathepsin G both in their lysosomes and on their surfaces. All monocytes have a very limited ability to secrete MMPs. However, when monocytes mature into macrophages they progressively lose their serine proteinases and increasingly express and secrete MMPs. Macrophages may secondly acquire serine proteinases within their lysosomes by phagocytosing dead PMNs and extracellular proteins.

The acid lysosomal proteinases (Dickinson 2002) are released during phagocytosis and although small quantities may leak out during this process they are generally confined to the cell. The neutral proteinases are all secreted. Enzyme secretion, in particular of plasminogen activator, is a characteristic property of activated macrophages.

Cathepsin B can be detected in both macrophages and fibroblasts in human gingiva either histochemically using peptide substrates detecting only active enzyme and immunocytochemically using an antibody which detects both active and inactive enzyme (Kennett et al 1994). This suggests that lysosomal cathepsin B in gingival cells is in an active form. Ultrastructural studies have also shown this proteinase localized within lysosomes and associated with the surface membrane of macrophages (Kennett et al 1997b). In addition, cathepsin B was seen on the surface of collagen fibrils in the adjacent connective tissue to these cells and this suggests that it could play a role in connective tissue degradation around these infiltrating cells. In this connection, macrophages containing the enzyme were seen in areas of inflammatory cellular infiltration and also within the junctional epithelium migrating into the crevice. Furthermore, cells containing these enzymes are present in the crevice (Kennett et al 1997a).

Macrophages also produce reactive oxygen species (ROS) in the process of phagocytosis (Freeman & Crapo 1982) which may leach from the cells to cause bystander damage. Less ROS is released from these cells than PMNs. Macrophages live for much longer than PMNs and therefore the release of ROS from dying and degenerating macrophages is much less.

Macrophages also contain $\alpha1$ antiproteinase inhibitor, $\alpha2$-macroglobulin and tissue inhibitor of metalloproteinases (TIMP) (**Fig. 5.7D**). All of these enzymes and inhibitors may be secreted by these cells when suitably stimulated.

Blood monocytes are a heterogeneous population, with phenotypes that can change on activation or differentiation (Nagasawa et al 2004). Most of these cells express the lipopolysaccharide (LPS) receptor (CD 14) intensely, and do not express the Fcγ receptor III, CD16 (CD14++ CD16−). However, monocytes expressing CD16 with reduced expression of CD14

increase in number in inflammatory diseases, sepsis and bacteraemia (CD14+ CD16+). In addition, CD45A is also expressed in activated monocytes and is regarded as an activation marker. Nagasawa et al (2004) investigated the phenotype and functional alteration of monocytes in periodontitis patients (33 aggressive periodontitis, 55 chronic periodontitis and 30 healthy subjects). They found that the percentage of CD14+ CD16+ monocytes was significantly increased in chronic periodontitis patients and the percentage of CD45A+ monocytes was significantly increased in aggressive periodontitis patients compared to healthy subjects. Both CD16+ and CD16− monocytes produced IL-6 in response to LPS from either *E. coli* or *A. actinomycetemcomitans*. However, the percentage of IL-6 producing cells was higher in CD16+ monocytes than CD16− monocytes. This suggests that the CD14+ CD16+ monocytes represent a hyper-reactive phenotype and these predominate in chronic periodontitis while activated CD45A+ monocytes predominate in aggressive periodontitis.

Mast cells

Mast cells (**Fig. 5.7C**) are important in inflammation since they release histamine and other vasoactive compounds. They also contain heparin and a number of proteinases, which are associated with heparin as active tetramers. In the absence of heparin the enzymes dissociate into inactive monomers. The principal proteolytic enzymes are tryptase and a chymotrypsin-like enzyme.

Mast cells are found abundantly below and within several types of mucosal epithelia (Steinsvoll et al 2004). On the basis of their proteinase content they are divided into connective tissue and mucosal phenotypes. The connective tissue phenotype produces both tryptase and chymase while the mucosal phenotype produces only tryptase. Mast cells are able to phagocytose, process and present antigens as effectively as macrophages.

Tryptase can be histochemically detected in mast cells in the healthy and inflamed human gingiva using synthetic peptide substrates (Kennett et al 1993). Mast cells are mainly present in the lamina propria but are also found in the junctional epithelium migrating into the crevice. Greater numbers of these cells are found in inflamed as compared to healthy gingiva. Mast cells containing tryptase are also found in the gingival crevice (Kennett et al 1997a).

Recently mast cells have been found in high numbers in chronically inflamed gingival tissue from chronic periodontitis subjects (Steinsvoll et al 2004). The number of mast cells was found to be even higher in HIV-positive patients with chronic periodontitis. Mast cells also strongly express matrix metalloproteinases. Mast cells may release preformed cytokines directing local innate and adaptive immune responses.

Also recently, mast cells have been shown to produce cytokines which can direct the development of T-cell subsets (Gemmell et al 2004b). They studied the relationship between mast cells and the Th1/Th2 response in human periodontal disease. They found that tryptase+ mast cell numbers were decreased in chronic periodontitis tissues compared with healthy/gingivitis lesions. Lower numbers of c-kit+ cells, which remained constant regardless of clinical status, indicate that there may be no increased migration of mast cells into periodontal disease lesions. While there were no differences in IgG2+ or IgG4+ cell numbers in healthy/gingivitis samples, there was an increase in IgG4+ cells compared with IgG2+ cells in periodontitis lesions, numbers increasing with disease severity. This suggests a predominance of Th2 cells in periodontitis, although mast cells may not be the source of Th2-inducing cytokines.

Fibroblasts

Fibroblasts (**Fig. 5.7D**) are found throughout the connective tissues and are the main cells secreting and degrading collagen under physiological conditions (Everts et al 1996). Small amounts of collagen are phagocytosed and degraded intracellularly primarily by cysteine proteinases (see Ch. 1). Larger amounts of collagen may be degraded by these cells extracellularly as a result of their secretion of metalloproteinases. They contain two forms of lysosomes one containing cathepsin B, cathepsin L, dipeptidylpeptidase (DPP) II and the other collagenase (MMP-1), other MMPs (MMP-2, MMP-3, 10, 11). They also have surface bound membrane associated MMPs mainly MMP 14 which becomes activated and then can degrade pericellular matrix during cell migration (Uitto et al 2003). Intracellular collagen degradation may be mediated by either cysteine proteinases in acid lysosomes or MMPs in neutral ones. Extracellular degradation of extracellular matrix involves many secreted and surface associated proteinases acting together.

IL-6 is abundantly present in inflammatory lesions and activates fibroblasts in the presence of soluble IL-6 receptor. It also stimulates gingival fibroblasts to produce collagenolytic enzymes resulting in tissue destruction (Takashiba et al 2003).

Lipopolysaccharide-binding protein (LBP) participates in the interaction of lipopolysaccharide (LPS) with CD14 to modulate the expression of cytokines (Ren et al 2005). This group has shown that LBP may downregulate the expression of IL-6 by human gingival fibroblasts.

Matrix metalloproteinase-1 (MMP-1) plays an important role in inflammatory diseases including periodontitis, which is characterized by tissue destruction and dense infiltration of mononuclear cells. Domeij et al (2006) investigated the effect of cell interactions between human gingival fibroblasts and human monocytes on the production of MMP-1 in a coculture model. They demonstrated that monocytes stimulated the production of MMP-1 in gingival fibroblasts by cell interactions, which may contribute to the maintenance of MMP-mediated tissue destruction in periodontitis.

Sulcular and junctional epithelial cells

When gingival connective tissue is degraded below the apical margin of the junctional epithelium, junctional epithelial cells proliferate and migrate apically. The sulcular and junctional epithelial cells themselves are equipped with a wide range of proteolytic enzymes which could be released when they are stimulated (Werb 1997). Collagenase-2 (MMP-8) and collagenase-3 (MMP-13) have been localized to cells in gingival sulcular and junctional epithelia (Kiili et al 2002) and the expression of MMP-13 is stimulated by TNF-α and keratinocyte growth factor (KGF) (Uitto et al 2003). Ilgenli et al (2006) showed that in chronic periodontitis patients the GCF levels of 29–30 kDa fragment of MMP-13, total MMP-13, and activated form of MMP-13 were significantly higher than in the healthy, gingivitis and aggressive periodontitis patients. This would seem to indicate that elevated GCF MMP-13 levels may play an important role in the pathogenesis of chronic periodontitis. Sulcular cells also contain gelatinases A and B (MMP 2, 9) and matrilysin (MMP 7) and have membrane associated MMPs on their surfaces (Werb 1997). All these enzymes could aid their migration.

They also contain and secrete urokinase-type plasminogen activator (uPA) and have lysosomes containing elastase-like serine proteinases, cysteine and aspartate proteases and DPP I (cathepsin C) (Uitto et al (2003). Interestingly, cathepsin C must be an important enzyme in some essential process in the immune response since a defect of the gene for this enzyme leads to rapid perinodal breakdown (Uitto et al 2003).

Endothelin-1 (ET-1) is a peptide which expresses on cell surfaces during inflammation. It has been found (Yamamoto et al 2003) by RT-PCR, ELISA and immunocytochemistry that ET-1 was strongly induced in KB epithelial cells by infection with *P. gingivalis*. Furthermore, ET-1 was more strongly expressed in gingival epithelial and vascular endothelial cells in inflamed in comparison to healthy gingival tissue. The level of ET-1 mRNA was also greater in inflamed than in healthy gingival tissue. The expression of ET-1 therefore appears to reflect the level of inflammation in these tissues.

Human gingival epithelial cells produce chemoattractant factors, IL-8 and monocyte chemoattractant protein 1, when stimulated by *P. gingivalis* (Kusumoto et al 2004). These workers have shown that this mechanism is mediated by Toll-like receptors (TLRs) on the surface of the epithelial cells. These cells have been shown to express TLR 2, TLR 4, TLR 5 and TLR 9 and this mechanism appears to be mediated by TLR 2. This mechanism is more effective when stimulated by *P. gingivalis* sonicate than when stimulated by lipopolysaccharide or *P. gingivalis* fimbriae. TRL 2 appears to participate in the signalling pathway to induce chemokine production by gingival epithelial cells when stimulated by *P. gingivalis*.

Vankeerberghen et al (2005) investigated the possible role of beta-defensins from primary human diseased gingival epithelial cell cultures from periodontitis patients in gingival health and periodontal disease. They showed that a correlation could be found in diseased oral epithelium between the defensin profiles that are induced and the pathogenicity of the oral bacterial strains.

Ji et al (2007) have previously reported different susceptibilities of periodontopathic and non-periodontopathic bacteria to antimicrobial peptides and phagocytosis by neutrophils. Differences between the two groups of bacteria may exist also in their ability to induce immune responses from the host. They, therefore evaluated the effects of various oral bacteria on innate immune responses by gingival epithelial cells. HOK-16B cells were cocultured with live or lysed non-periodontopathic ($n = 3$) and periodontopathic ($n = 5$) bacterial species. The levels of human β-defensin-1, -2 and -3, and of the cathelicidin, LL-37, were examined by real-time reverse transcription-polymerase chain reaction, and the accumulated interleukin-8 and interleukin-1α were measured by enzyme-linked immunosorbent assay. Non-periodontopathic bacteria were found to upregulate some antimicrobial peptides without affecting the levels of cytokines. In the periodontopathic group, the orange-complex (non-periodontopathic) bacteria induced antimicrobial peptides and interleukin-8 efficiently, but the red-complex (periodontopathic) bacteria often demonstrated suppressive effects. In contrast to live bacteria, bacterial lysates had no suppressive effects. In addition, some bacterial lysates demonstrated a reduced ability to induce antimicrobial peptides compared with live bacteria. These findings indicated that non-periodontopathic, the orange-complex, and the red-complex bacteria had different effects on the innate immune responses from gingival epithelial cells, which may affect the outcome of their host–microbial interaction in gingival sulcus.

Other cells

MMP-8 has also been localized within gingival tissue plasma cells by double staining immunocytochemistry (Kiili et al 2002). In addition, eosinophils contain HLE and MMP-1 but in much smaller amounts than PMNs (Uitto et al 2003; Owen & Campbell 1999). Lymphocytes and natural killer cells (NKC) contain granzymes A and B and can release them. Granzymes A and B can process the perforin molecule secreted by cytotoxic T lymphocytes.

Proteinase inhibitors

The proteinase inhibitors can be divided into serine-, cysteine-, aspartate- and metallo-proteinase inhibitors (Barrett 1980). In addition to these there is another important general proteinase inhibitor, α2- macroglobulin, which can bind all proteinases but does not react with exopeptidases, non-proteolytic hydrolases or inactivate proteinases (Barrett & Starky 1973; James 1990).

The proteolytic enzymes released by inflammatory cells and putative periodontal pathogens fall into three main classes, metallo-, cysteine- and serine-proteinases. The effect that they have on the tissues does not just depend on their release but rather on the enzyme/inhibitor balance present within the tissues. For these reasons, it is pertinent to also consider the nature and distribution of the inhibitors to these classes of proteinase.

Metalloproteinase inhibitors

The inhibitors of MMPs play an important role in regulation of the connective tissues since an imbalance between the amount of activated enzyme and their inhibitors can lead to pathological breakdown of extracellular matrix. The natural inhibitors of MMPs are the tissue inhibitors of MMPs (TIMPs) and α2-macroglobulin (α2M) (Ryan et al 1996). TIMPs probably function mainly pericellularly, whereas α2M functions as a regulator in body fluids. However, during inflammation, it is possible for this large molecular weight protein to leave the blood vessels in the exudate and thus find its way into the tissues. α2M functions by entrapment of the susceptible proteinase followed by cleavage of a peptide bond in the bait region, a venus fly trap-like mechanism (Birkedal-Hansen 1993b).

The TIMPs are expressed by fibroblasts, keratinocytes, endothelial cells, monocytes and macrophages and are also widely distributed in tissue fluids (Ryan et al 1996). They are capable of inactivating all the MMPs by binding strongly to their catalytic domains and they may also prevent the activation of some latent MMPs.

TIMP-1 is a glycoprotein and TIMP-2 is its non-glycosylated counterpart. TIMP-3 has only just been isolated and is not yet fully characterized. TIMPs can be inactivated by reduction and alkylation and by cleavage by some serine proteinases.

TIMP-1 binds more commonly to MMP-1, -9 while TIMP-2 mainly binds to MMP-2. TIMP function is under the control of the hormone and cytokine systems and TIMP-1 is upregulated by retinoids, glucocorticoids, IL-1, EGF, TGF-β, and TNF-α whereas TIMP-2 is downregulated by TGF-β.

Cysteine proteinase inhibitors

The two groups of inhibitors which act on cysteine proteinases are the general proteinase inhibitor α2-macroglobulin, described above, and the cystatins (Henskens et al 1996a; Turk & Bode 1991; Turk et al 2000; Dickinson 2002).

The cystatins are tissue-derived specific inhibitors of cysteine proteinases and are small molecular weight proteins which have been divided into three families.

Family 1, previously known as the Stefin family, is comprised of proteins with 100 amino-acid residues and a molecular mass of 11 kDa. The human cystatins in this group comprise cystatins A and B (Henskens et al 1996a; Turk & Bode 1991; Turk et al 2000). Cystatin A is an acid protein which is found in whole saliva, liver, spleen, placenta, oral mucosa, other epithelial cells and PMNs. It is also the main cystatin present in GCF. It appears to have a mainly defensive role against cysteine proteinases produced by invading pathogens. Cystatin B has a pI of 5.7–6.3 and a molecular mass of 11.2 kDa. It is widely distributed in cells and tissues including liver, spleen, placenta, epithelial cells, lymphocytes and monocytes. It appears to have a general defensive role.

Family 2 consists of proteins with 115–120 amino-acid residues and molecular masses of 13–14 kDa (Henskens et al 1996a; Turk & Bode 1991). They also have two disulphide loops near their carboxyl termini. They comprise cystatins C, D, S, SA and SN. Cystatin C is found in most biological fluids such as plasma, saliva, seminal fluid, tears and GCF. It is thought to play both a regulatory and defensive role against host- and pathogen-derived cysteine proteinases. Cystatins S, SA and SN were first isolated from saliva (Henskens et al 1996a) and originate mainly from the submandibular and sublingual salivary glands. Cystatin D originates only from the parotid salivary gland and also passes into saliva. These cystatins are thought to protect the oral cavity and eyes from cysteine proteinases produced by bacteria, viruses and host inflammatory cells.

Family 3 comprises the plasma kininogens which are multifunctional proteins which contain 3 cystatin-like domains. They are synthesized in the liver and pass into plasma. Two of them, L and H kininogens probably function as cysteine proteinase inhibitors in the plasma (Henskens et al 1996a).

In terms of their protective role in the oral cavity cystatins A, C, D, S, SA and SN are present in saliva and the oral cavity and cystatins A and C are also present in GCF (Henskens et al 1996a). Furthermore, salivary cystatin levels have been found to be higher in chronic periodontitis patients than healthy controls and to reduce following periodontal treatment (Henskens et al 1993a,b, 1996b,c). It has also been shown (Henskens et al 1994, 1996b) that saliva from healthy patients mainly contains cystatin S while that from chronic periodontitis patients contains additionally cystatin C (see also Ch. 13).

Serine proteinase inhibitors

The main serine proteinase inhibitors are known as serpins and are small glycoproteins with a single polypeptide chain and a variable number of oligosaccharide side chains. They are formed into a well conserved tertiary structure and the reactive centre of each serpin is specific to the amino-acid sequence of the protein it binds (Loebermann et al 1984). They are suicidal proteins which form 1:1 complexes with their target proteinase. The complexes are then removed from the circulation and subsequently catalysed. Serpins are thought to function by exposing their reactive centre as a result of changing their shape. This is then presented to the proteinase and attaches by a lock and key mechanism (Carrell & Boswell 1986).

The most important serpin is α1-proteinase inhibitor (α1PI) which is also known as α1-antitrypsin. This inhibits various serine proteinases including neutrophil elastase (Ohlsson et al 1974), trypsin (Schulze et al 1962), chymotrypsin (Schwick et al 1966), cathepsin G (Travis et al 1978), plasmin and thrombin (Rimon et al 1966) and tissue kallikrein (Hirano et al 1984). However, the kinetics of the association of α1PI with elastase is more favourable by several orders of magnitude than those for the other proteinases (Travis & Salvensen 1983).

The α1PI-elastase complex is chemotactic for PMNs (Banda et al 1988a,b). Also elastase increases α1PI synthesis in monocytes and macrophages but the response is dependent on the presence of α1PI-elastase complex (Perlmutter et al 1988; Perlmutter & Pierce 1989).

The normal concentration of α1PI in human plasma is between 1.5 and 5.0 mg/mL (Fragerhol & Laurell 1970). The daily production rate is 34 mg/kg body weight and one-third of this is degraded each day (Permutter & Pierce 1989). The production of α1PI increases 3-fold during the host response to injury and inflammation (Aronsen et al 1972), probably reflecting the increased production and release of elastase by inflammatory cells, in particular PMNs.

Other low molecular weight inhibitors of elastase have been described in other tissues and more recently these have been shown to be also present in gingival tissue (Cox et al 2001). One such low molecular weight inhibitor, secretory leucocyte protease inhibitor (SLPI) has been found in saliva (Wahl et al 1997) and human mast cells (Westin et al 1999), large numbers of which are a feature of healthy and inflamed gingival tissue.

The molar concentrations of elastase, cathepsin B, α1PI and SLPI have been found to be significantly higher in the GCF than the saliva and that of the α1PI was higher than SLPI (Cox et al 2006b). For GCF α1PI was found to be the major elastase inhibitor, but in the saliva SLPI was also found to reduce its activity. The inflamed gingiva was found to be an additional source of SLPI in the oral cavity, but here it was also found to be cleaved by GCF cysteine proteinases, such as cathepsin B.

Connective tissue mast cells also show immunoreactivity for bikunin, the anti-proteinase portion of inter-α-trypsin inhibitor (IαI) family (Odum & Nielsen 1994). Both bikunin and α1-microglobulin are located on the same gene but separate on translation as separate protein products (Salier et al 1996). A least four genes are involved in the synthesis of the inter-α-trypsin inhibitor family members. These genes code for the heavy chains of the final protein and are known as H1–H4. Each of these heavy chain products can then associate with bikunin to form a functional inhibitor.

There are also further possibilities for other low molecular weight gingival elastase inhibitors and these currently are 12 kDa skin-derived anti-leucoproteinase (SKALP) (Molhuizen & Schalkwijk 1995) and 27–31 kDa serpins which are associated with extracellular matrix and fibroblasts (Rao et al 1995). SKALP has been found in oral epithelial cells and gingival tissue (Cox et al 2003). Recent studies confirmed the presence of SLPI in parotid saliva and showed that it was also released by gingival epithelial cells (Cox et al 2001). Furthermore, Booth et al (2006) found that proteases and inhibitors in GCF and saliva were better related to elastase activity in these fluids than the clinical variables. and concluded that SLPI may be an important inhibitor of elastase activity in the periodontium.

The presence of a multiplicity of elastase inhibitors and their production in large amounts probably reflect the potential tissue destructive capability of elastase on host tissues. This can be clearly seen by the high susceptibility to pulmonary emphysema seen in patients genetically deficient in α-1-antiproteinase (Perlmutter & Pierce 1989).

The α1PI gene has been fully characterized and the human forms of α1PI genetic deficiency have also been characterized. It is attributable to two mutant alleles, PI*Z and PI*S (Crystal 1994). Compared with the wild-type (PI*M), the PI*Z allele is characterized by a G to A mutation in exon 5, which encodes a glutamine to lysine change at position 342 (Nukiwa et al 1986). The PI*S is characterized by an A–T substitution in exon 3, of 7 exons, encoding a glutamine to valine change at position 264 (Long et al 1984).

Genetic deficiencies of α1PI are known to predispose to cirrhosis of the liver and inflammatory diseases such as chronic obstructive pulmonary disease, panniculitis and possibly inflammatory bowel disease (Mahadeva & Lomas 1998; Smith et al 1989; WHO 1998; Yang et al 2000). Even mild or intermediate deficiencies (PI*M, PI*S and PI*Z allele-containing heterozygotes) have been associated with reduced lung function compared to PI*M homozygotes (Dahl et al 2001). In PI*ZZ subjects an imbalance between proteolytic enzymes and their inhibitors at sites of inflammation is thought to be responsible for the pulmonary tissue destruction and the onset of emphysema (Steenbergen 1993).

It has recently been hypothesized that a protease:inhibitor imbalance could also be of relevance to rate of progression of chronic periodontitis (Cox 1995; Fokkema et al 1998). In this connection Fokkema et al (1998) compared the periodontal status of subjects with severe α1PI deficiency to that of normal controls and found a significant increase in the proportion of deep pocket depths in the α1PI deficient subjects. Previously, Peterson and Marsh (1979) had reported a 34% prevalence of the α1PI deficient phenotype in 50 subjects with severe periodontitis. This appears to represent a dramatic increase in mild and intermediate α1PI deficiencies in this condition compared to either a periodontally healthy control group or the regional USA background level. This proportion is also higher than the reported levels of the α1PI deficient phenotypes in the healthy worldwide population (Hutchison 1998; WHO 1998). However, another recent investigation (Scott et al 2002) could not find an association between mutant PI* alleles and periodontitis in a small, controlled study. It is therefore likely that larger controlled studies will be necessary to resolve fully this issue.

Petropoulou et al (2003) compared the levels of native and inactivated forms of α1PI in human extracellular inflammatory fluids. They found that in GCF from chronic periodontitis subjects had $73.5 \pm 16.6\%$ of inactivated α1PI compared to normal human plasma ($8.4 \pm 4.9\%$), knee-joint synovial fluid from rheumatoid arthritis patients ($8.0 \pm 1.2\%$) and osteoarthritis patients (8.6 ± 8.2) and plasma from osteoarthritis patients $95.7 \pm 4.8\%$. The high levels of inactivated α1PI in periodontitis subjects could be the result of bacterial proteases in the periodontal pocket. If this situation occurs in the gingival tissue then it would allow serine proteinases in to take part in tissue breakdown in chronic periodontitis. However, the situation in the gingival tissues is probably different.

Control of proteolytic enzymes

Macrophages and fibroblasts and the extracellular environment contain the proteinase inhibitors alpha-1-proteinase inhibitor (α1PI) and α2-macroglobulin (α2M) (Kennett et al (1995). Also cystatins A and B are present in PMNs and monocytes respectively (Henskens et al 1996a; Turk & Bode 1991; Turk et al 2000), TIMPs in epithelial cells and macrophages (Ryan et al 1996) and SLPI and SKALP in epithelial cells and mast cells (Cox et al 2001; Westin et al 1999; Odum & Nielsen 1994). Thus, there is a ready supply of all the necessary proteinase inhibitors in gingival tissue. Therefore, active enzyme in the tissues can only cause damage if there is an enzyme/inhibitor imbalance. This could take place in the close environment of these cells where bystander damage could occur. It might also be a local feature of episodic periodontal disease activity.

The control of the synthesis and secretion of proteinases and inhibitors in both health and disease is controlled by the activation of the appropriate gene(s) by the cellular messenger system which itself is under the control of the activation of cell surface receptors by the appropriate growth factor or cytokine. Transcription of these enzymes in inflammatory cells is upregulated by pro-inflammatory cytokines (Uitto et al 2003; Owen & Campbell 1999) (see **Fig. 3.1**). In this regard, it has recently been shown that interleukin (IL)-1β can upregulate MMP-3, at both the mRNA and protein level, in periodontal ligament cells (Nakaya et al 1997) and may control the release of this proteinase in both health and disease. MMPs (Uitto et al 2003; Owen & Campbell 1999) are also upregulated by a number of growth factors (see **Fig. 3.1**). They are secreted as pro-enzymes that have to be activated by cleavage of the pro-sequence before becoming functional. In addition, IL-1β and tumour necrosis factor TNF-α have also been shown to stimulate the release of cathepsin B (Hussain et al 1997) and TNF-α dipeptidyl peptidase IV (Kennett et al 1997c) from cultured gingival fibroblasts.

The migration of proteinases to the cell's surface membrane is also mediated by cytokines, phagocytosis and exposure to immune complexes and opsonized substrates. Serine proteinases in particular become bound to the cell's surface membrane and in this situation become active.

In order to function in proteolysis these proteinases must circumvent the activities of their inhibitors which are present in abundant amounts in the serum and tissue fluid. They may achieve this by several mechanisms (Uitto et al 2003; Owen & Campbell 1999). First, inhibitors may be inhibited themselves by cleavage by some proteinases or by ROS released by inflammatory cells. Second, the binding of proteinases to the surface membrane of the cell may prevent the inhibitor from gaining access to the enzyme. Third, when cells come into close contact with its substrate the area of activity between them may become compartmentalized between the surface membrane and its attached, active proteinase and the substrate. This would severely limit the ingress of inhibitor molecules. Finally, the tight binding that occurs between serine proteinases and MMPs and their substrates may also prevent ingress of inhibitor molecules.

Connective tissue degradation by inflammatory cell proteinases

Proteoglycans can be degraded at neutral pH by elastase and cathepsin G (serine proteinases, SP) and at acid pH by cathepsin B (cysteine proteinase, CP) and cathepsin D (carboxylproteinase).

Collagenases (matrix metalloproteinases, MMPs) can be activated at neutral pH by tryptase and plasmin (SP) and at acid pH by cathepsin B

(CP). The terminal peptide regions of collagen can be cleaved at neutral pH by elastase and at acid pH by cathepsin B.

The triple helix of collagen is specifically cleaved by specific collagenases (MMP-1, 8) and further degraded at neutral pH by gelatinases (MMP-3, 9) and elastase (SP) and at acid pH by cathepsin B (CP).

Proteoglycans, basement membrane collagens (type IV, X and XI), laminin and fibronectin can be degraded at neutral pH by stromelysins (MMP-3, 10, 11) and elastase (SP) and at acid pH by cathepsins B and L (CP).

Tryptase (SP) can also cleave complement to generate C3α and thus increase vascular permeability; mast cell chymase (SP) can attack basal lamina, increasing epithelial permeability.

The degradation products of proteoglycans (GAGs) have been found in crevicular fluid (Embery et al 1982); MMPs, elastase, cathepsins B, D and G, tryptase, chymotrypsin and aminopeptidases have been found in gingival tissue and/or crevicular fluid (Cox & Eley 1987, 1989a,b,c; Meikle et al 1986; Uitto et al 2003). The activity of a number of crevicular fluid proteases have been positively correlated with the severity of chronic periodontitis and also significantly decrease following basic periodontal treatment and periodontal surgery (Cox & Eley 1992; Eley & Cox 1992a,b,c). To date elastase, cathepsin B and dipeptidylpeptidases-II and IV have been shown to be predictors of disease activity in longitudinal studies (Eley & Cox 1995, 1996a,b) (see also Ch. 14).

Ejeil et al (2003b) have grown gingival tissue specimens from healthy controls, patients with mild gingival inflammation and patients with severe inflammation in organ culture for 3 days. They then measured the release of MMPs and TIMPs into the medium. The gingival specimens were then subjected to histological processing and examination to determine the area occupied by collagen fibres. The area occupied by collagen decreased progressively and this correlated with a similar pattern of increase in the levels of MMP-1, 2, 9 and 13 and the active forms of MMP-2 and 9. This indicates their probable involvement in connective tissue breakdown in periodontitis.

Ma et al (2003) designed a small study to show that the collagenases produced by host cells in chronic periodontitis do act to cleave collagen fibres in that condition. They used a polyclonal antibody linked to avidin-biotin-peroxidase to detect a specific collagen-cleaved product on gingival tissue sections from 10 chronic periodontitis patients and 10 healthy control subjects. They found considerably greater positive staining in the chronic periodontitis patients compared with the controls and when this was subjected to statistical testing it was found to be significant ($p<0.01$). This would seem to indicate that host cell collagenases contribute to tissue destruction and attachment loss in chronic periodontitis.

Protease-activated receptors

Proteolytic enzymes from inflammatory cells and subgingival bacteria may also act by processing and thus activating protease-activated receptors (PARs) on cell surfaces and thus influence cell function (Schmidlin & Bunnett 2001). They accomplish this by signalling directly to cells by cleaving the PAR which are members of the G-protein-coupled receptor family. The proteases capable of this function are proteins generated during blood coagulation such as thrombin and activated clotting factors, VIIa and Xa, trypsin secreted by gastrointestinal epithelium and mast cell tryptase and cathepsin G from PMNs (Schmidlin & Bunnett 2001).

The first PAR (PAR1) was discovered in 1991(Schmidlin & Bunnett 2001) and since then four have been cloned (PAR1, 2, 3 and 4). Thrombin activates PAR1, PAR3 and PAR4 with a potency PAR1>PAR3>PAR4. Factor Xa also activates PAR1 and trypsin activates PAR2 and PAR4 (PAR2>PAR4). Mast cell tryptase and factors VIIa, Xa and membrane-type serine protease 1 can also activate PAR2 (Camerer et al 2000; Compton et al 2001; Schmidlin & Bunnett 2001). PMN cathepsin G can also activate PAR4 (Sambrano et al 2000).

PARs 1, 2 and 3 are present as receptors on the surface of platelets, endothelial cells, leucocytes, fibroblasts, myocytes and neurones (Schmidlin & Bunnett 2001). PAR 2 is expressed by epithelial cells of the gastrointestinal (GI) tract, pancreatic cells, liver cells, cells of the airway, prostate cells, ovarian cells, ocular cells and is also found on epithelial cell lines, smooth muscle cells, fibroblasts, endothelial cells, T-cell lines, neutrophils, tumour cells and neurones.

Once activated PARs can couple to several heterotrimeric G proteins and thereby trigger a cascade of signalling events that result in marked phenotypic changes in the stimulated cells (Schmidlin & Bunnett 2001). This coupling activates signalling pathways that alter cell motility, adhesion and migration, secretion, growth and survival (Coughlin 2000; Macfarlane, et al 2001).

PARs are disposable, 'one-shot' receptors and once the receptor is activated it cannot be reactivated again (Schmidlin & Bunnett 2001). Once having served its function the PAR is internalized and targeted to the cell's lysosomes for degradation. A new PAR is then fabricated by the cell to take its place.

Thrombin is generated following tissue injury and via its activation of PARs1, 3 and 4 it stimulates platelet aggregation, the generation of neurogenic inflammatory stimuli, PMN adhesion to vascular endothelium prior to migration, myocyte contraction, which is involved in some of the inflammatory vascular changes, and fibroblast proliferation. PAR1 and 4 can also be activated by gingivain produced by *P. gingivalis* and PAR4 by cathepsin G from PMNs (Sambrano et al 2000; Loubakos, et al 2001).

Mast cell tryptase is one of the major activators of PAR2 (Compton et al 2001; Schmidlin & Bunnett 2001) and by this mechanism it can produce neurogenic inflammatory stimuli, fibroblast proliferation and myocyte proliferation and contraction. Tryptase can also stimulate vascular endothelial cells to induce leucocyte adhesion and migration (Compton et al 1999), almost certainly as a result of cleaving PAR 2 receptors on these cells (Compton et al 2001; Schmidlin & Bunnett 2001).

All of these mechanisms could play a significant role in the generation and maintenance of the inflammatory lesion of chronic inflammatory periodontal diseases.

BONE RESORPTION

The host and bacterial factors involved in bone resorption are summarized in Table 5.3. An understanding of how these work requires a knowledge of the physiology of bone resorption which is briefly described in this section.

Bone resorption is probably the most critical factor in periodontal attachment loss leading to eventual tooth loss. Substances produced by the subgingival bacterial flora and the tissues during inflammation and immune reactions may affect bone turnover by either causing the differentiation and stimulation of osteoclasts or by inhibiting bone formation by osteoblasts.

HOST AND BACTERIAL FACTORS INVOLVED IN BONE RESORPTION

The factors thought to be involved in bone resorption have been studied with tissue culture systems using embryonic bone labelled with radioactive calcium and bone loss can be detected and measured by the release of this marker. The substances which can induce resorption in periodontal disease come from two sources:

- Subgingival bacteria
- Periodontal tissues.

Bacterial factors

Substances from bacteria include lipopolysaccharides (LPS) from Gram-negative bacteria (Hausmann et al 1970; Hausmann 1974), lipoteichoic acid from *Actinomyces viscosus* (Hausmann 1974; Hausmann et al 1975), peptidoglycan (Lensgraf et al 1979), muramyl dipeptide (MDP) (Dewhirst 1982), bacterial lipoprotein (Millar et al 1986) and capsular or surface associated material (SAM) from Gram-negative bacteria (Wilson et al 1985) can stimulate bone resorption *in vitro* using the murine calvaria model. The potency to cause resorption *in vitro* varies with each source and LPS is 10 times more potent than lipoteichoic acid and capsular material is 1000 times more potent than the corresponding LPS (Hopps & Sisney-Durrant 1991). Peptidoglycan, MDP and bacterial lipoprotein are all less potent than the three materials above.

There are also differences in effect from different bacterial sources of these materials. In this regard, LPS from *P. gingivalis* is more active than those from *Aggregatibacter actinomycetemcomitans, C. ochracea* or *F. nucleatum*. Some bacterial LPS, such as that from *E. corrodens*, also release cytokines such as IL-1 and/or IL-6 from osteoblasts and fibroblasts but most do not (Reddi et al 1995a; Wilson 1995). However, LPS is known to activate the complement cascade by the alternative pathway which in turn generates prostaglandins.

It has been shown during the last decade that proteins associated with the outer surfaces of some but not all periodontopathogens, are potent inducers of cell and tissue pathology *in vitro* (Wilson et al 1985, 1993; Meghji et al 1992a; Wilson & Henderson 1995). Capsular material or surface-associated material (SAM) can stimulate the production of prostaglandin E_2 (PGE$_2$) and collagenase from bone cells (Harvey et al 1987).

The SAMs from *P. gingivalis* and *E. corrodens* appear to achieve this by first releasing IL-1 which then stimulates the release of PGE$_2$ and collagenase (Henderson & Blake 1992). Inhibition of bone DNA and collagen production by osteoblasts in murine calvaria is produced by low titres of SAM from *P. gingivalis* and *E. corrodens* and this may be due to this mechanism because it is blocked by indomethacin, an inhibitor of prostaglandins (Meghji et al 1992a).

The SAM from *A. actinomycetemcomitans*, is most potent in stimulating bone resorption *in vitro*. However, it appears to produce this effect by mimicking the action of IL-1. The main cytokine released from connective tissue and bone cells by SAMs is IL-6 and it seems that this release may either be stimulated by IL-1 or stimulated directly. This is of particular relevance because IL-6 has been shown to stimulate the formation of osteoclasts (Löwick et al 1989).

The constituents of the SAM from *A. actinomycetemcomitans* have been recently characterized (Wilson & Henderson 1995). This SAM is made up of a number of proteins and peptides with potent biological actions which are relevant to the pathology of both chronic periodontitis and juvenile periodontitis (Wilson & Henderson 1995). These include first, a protein with potent osteolytic activity which has close homology to the molecular chaperone from *Escherichia coli* known either as chaperonin 60 or GroEL (Meghji et al 1994; Kirby et al 1995); second, a protein with anti-mitotic activity which has been termed, gapstatin (White et al 1995); and third, a potent cytokine inducing peptide which acts by stimulating IL-6 gene transcription (Nair et al 1996). This cytokine is pro-inflammatory and plays a role in the differentiation and maturation of T and B lymphocytes (see Ch. 3 and Table 3.1). These proteins are active in the picogram to nanogram per mL concentration range and it is presumed that their actions are important in the pathogenesis of chronic periodontitis and juvenile periodontitis by stimulating alveolar bone resorption (Wilson et al 1985, 1993; Reddi et al 1995b; Kirby et al 1995), inhibiting bone and periodontal ligament regeneration and repair (Kamin et al 1986; Wilson et al 1988; Meghji et al 1992b) and by promoting B-lymphocyte and plasma cell proliferation (Reddi et al 1995c, 1996a,b; Wilson et al 1996; Henderson et al 1996a).

Host factors

The main host-derived bone-resorbing factors appear to be the eicosanoids and cytokines which are generated in the gingiva and periodontium during the inflammatory and immune reactions.

Eicosanoids

Prostaglandins, hydroxyeicosatetraenoic acids (HETEs) and leukotrienes are inflammatory mediators derived from cell membrane phospholipids by the action of cyclo-oxygenase or lipo-oxygenase on arachidonic acid. These compounds are secreted by cells involved in inflammatory and immune reactions such as macrophages, PMNs and endothelial cells. These are also released by some cells during normal function such as fibroblasts and osteoblasts. Many of these compounds have been implicated in the pathogenesis or periodontal diseases (Seymour & Heasman 1988).

The prostaglandins (PG) were the first mediators of local bone resorption to be discovered and may be one of the most important factors in periodontal bone loss. PGE$_1$, PGE$_2$ and prostacyclin (PGI$_2$) all stimulate bone resorption in tissue culture systems but PGE$_2$ is the most potent and stimulates increasing resorption in concentrations ranging from 1 nM–10 μM (Dietrich et al 1975). The levels of PGE$_2$ found in inflamed gingival tissue (Ohm et al 1984) and GCF from inflamed sites (Offenbacher et al 1984) fall well within the levels stimulating bone resorption *in vitro*. The GCF levels of PGE$_2$ also correlate with the periodontal disease status and have been claimed to predict periodontal attachment loss (Offenbacher et al 1986).

The role of prostaglandins in alveolar bone loss is supported by numerous experiments in which the effects of non-steroidal anti-inflammatory drugs (NSAIDs) on periodontal bone loss have been studied. Drugs such as indomethacin and flurbiprofen, which inhibit the synthesis of prostaglandins, markedly reduce bone loss in experimental periodontitis in animals induced by ligaments (Nyman et al 1979; Weakes-Dybvig et al 1982; Williams et al 1988) or diet (Lasfargues & Saffir 1983).

In addition, lipo-oxygenase products of arachidonic acid also stimulate bone resorption in tissue culture experiments (Meghji et al 1988). Leukotrienes and 12-HETE are potent stimulators of bone resorption at picomolar or nanomolar concentrations. Relatively high levels of leukotrienes and HETEs are present in inflamed gingival tissue (Sighagen et al 1982; El Attar & Lin 1982) and diseased periodontal pocket tissue (El Attar et al 1986). These experiments also showed that gingival tissue in culture metabolized arachidonic acid mainly through the lipo-oxygenase pathway and if this also occurs *in vivo* then these would be important bone resorbing factors.

Prostaglandin E$_2$ (PGE$_2$) exerts its biological actions via EP receptors (EP1, EP2, EP3, EP4,). A recent study (Ruwanpura et al 2004) investigated whether PGE$_2$ regulated IL-1β induced matrix metalloproteinase (MMP)-3 production in human gingival fibroblasts (HGF) derived either from periodontally healthy subjects or periodontally diseased patients. PGE$_2$ was downregulated by IL-1β -induced MMP-3 production in HGF from healthy gingiva, whereas it was upregulated by it in HGF from periodontally diseased patients. Both EP2 and EP4 agonists suppressed IL-1β induced MMP-3 production, while an EP1 agonist mimicked the PGE$_2$ effects in HGF from healthy and periodontally diseased tissue, respectively. This data suggests that in HGF from healthy gingiva IL-1β induced MMP-3 production is downregulated by PGE$_2$, via EP2 and EP4 receptors, whereas in cells from periodontally diseased tissue, IL-1β induced MMP-3 production is upregulated by PGE$_2$ via EP1 receptors. Thus, different regulation of IL-1β induced MMP-3 production by PGE$_2$ between healthy and periodontally diseased tissue may be involved in the pathogenesis of periodontal disease.

Other products of inflammation

Heparin from mast cell can enhance bone resorption in tissue culture systems induced by LPS and lipoteichoic acid, but cannot induce bone resorption on its own. Thrombin, an inflammatory mediator and end product of the blood coagulation cascade is a potent bone resorbing agent (Dziak 1993). Another inflammatory agent, bradykinin, evokes similar effects and in both cases these effects are independent of prostaglandin production.

Cytokines and other mediators

Several cytokines produced during inflammation stimulate bone resorption *in vitro* and these represent a potentially important major group of host derived bone resorbing factors which may play a role in alveolar bone loss in periodontal disease. The cytokines which have been shown to stimulate bone resorption *in vitro* include interleukin (IL)-1α and β (Gowen & Mundy 1986), Tumour necrosis factor (TNF)-α and -β (Bertolini et al 1986), transforming growth factor (TGF) (Tashjian et al 1985) and platelet derived growth factor (PDGF) (Tashjian et al 1982). In addition, IL-6 produced by fibroblasts, endothelial cells and osteoblasts may stimulate the formation of osteoclasts from precursor cells (Löwick et al 1989). Out of all these cytokines, IL-1 and TNF are the most potent stimulators of bone resorption and are the only ones so far to be implicated in periodontal pathology (Hopps & Sisney-Durrant 1991). IL-1 has widespread effects on non-immune cells and these are shown in Table 5.4.

IL-1 is 100 times more potent than TNF and can produce resorption in picomolar concentrations. Osteoclast activation factor (OAF) has now been shown to be identical with IL-1β (Dewhirst et al 1985). IL-1β has been found in significant amounts in inflamed gingiva but has not been detected in healthy gingiva (Hönig et al 1989). Both IL-1α and β have been found in GCF from diseased sites in nanomolar concentrations which are sufficient to cause bone loss *in vitro* (Masada et al 1990). TNF-α has also been detected in GCF but in low levels which are below those necessary for bone resorption *in vitro* (Rossomando et al 1990).

Two key mediators of osteoclastic activity which regulated their differentiation are receptor activator of nuclear factor κB ligand (RANKL) and its natural inhibitor, osteoprotegerin (OPG). The levels of these mediators in inflamed connective tissue adjacent to the bone from periodontitis patients have been compared with tissue from healthy subjects (Crotti et al

2003) using immunocytochemistry with specific monoclonal antibodies. The sections were also double labelled with cell identification antibodies. *In situ* hybridization was also used to detect cells expressing RANK mRNA. Significantly higher levels of RANKL protein was found in the periodontal in comparison to the healthy tissue ($p<0.05$). Conversely, OPG protein was found to be significantly lower in periodontal compared to healthy tissue ($p<0.05$). RANKL protein was associated with lymphocytes and macrophages and OPG protein with vascular endothelium in both tissues. Many lymphocytes were also found to express RANK mRNA in periodontitis tissue. The change in levels of these key regulators of osteoclast differentiation may play a major role in the bone loss seen in periodontitis.

Another study (Ogasawara et al 2004) examined by *in situ* hybridization the expression of RANKL, RANK, osteoprotegerin and cytokines in rat periodontal tissue osteoclasts, osteoblasts and periodontal ligament cells during tooth movement. They found that both RANKL and RANK were concomitantly expressed in some osteoclasts. RANKL was also positive in osteoblasts and periodontal ligament cells. Osteoprotegerin was expressed in nearly all osteoblasts and periodontal ligament cells but there were no osteoprotegerin-positive osteoclasts. During tooth movement the number of osteoclasts expressing RANKL and RANK increased and some osteoclasts also expressed IL-1β and TNF-α. This suggests that an autocrine mechanism of RANKL-RANK exists in osteoclasts and that this is heightened during pathological bone resorption. These autocrine mechanisms therefore seem to regulate osteoclast function in both physiological and pathological conditions.

Another study (Mogi et al 2004) has investigated the concentrations of RANKL and the RANKL decoy receptor, osteoprotegerin (OPG), in gingival crevicular fluid (GCF) of periodontal subjects with severe, moderate and mild periodontitis and healthy controls. They found an increased concentration of RANKL and a decreased concentration of OPG in periodontitis patients compared with healthy controls ($p<0.05$). The ratio of the concentration of RANKL to OPG in the GCF was also found to be significantly higher for periodontitis patients than for healthy subjects ($p<0.01$). Taken together, these results suggest that RANKL and OPG contribute to osteoclastic destruction in periodontal disease.

Receptor activator of nuclear factor-κB ligand (RANKL) is responsible for the induction of osteoclastogenesis and bone resorption, whereas its decoy receptor, osteoprotegerin, can directly block this action (Bostanci et al 2007a). These two cytokines seem to be crucial for regulating the bone remodelling process and imbalances in their expression may cause a switch from the physiological state to enhanced bone resorption or formation. Bostanci et al (2007b) investigated the mRNA expression of RANKL and osteoprotegerin, as well as their relative ratio, in the gingival tissues of patients with various forms of periodontal pathology. Gingival tissue was obtained from nine healthy subjects and patients who had either chronic gingivitis, chronic periodontitis or generalized aggressive periodontitis, or were chronic periodontitis patients receiving immunosuppressant therapy. Quantitative real-time polymerase chain reaction was used to evaluate the mRNA expression of RANKL and osteoprotegerin in these tissues. Compared with healthy individuals, patients in all periodontitis groups, but not those with gingivitis, exhibited stronger RANKL expression and a higher relative RANKL:osteoprotegerin ratio. In addition, osteoprotegerin expression was weaker in patients with chronic periodontitis. When patients with generalized aggressive periodontitis and chronic periodontitis were compared, the former exhibited stronger RANKL expression, whereas the latter exhibited weaker osteoprotegerin expression, but there was no difference in their relative ratio. When chronic periodontitis patients were compared with chronic periodontitis patients receiving immunosuppressant therapy, osteoprotegerin, but not RANKL, expression was stronger in the latter. This study appears to demonstrate that RANKL and osteoprotegerin expression are differentially regulated in various forms of periodontitis, and

Table 5.4 *Action of IL-1 on non-immune cells*

Tissue/cell type	Prostaglandin synthesis	Proliferation	Protein synthesis	Other effects
Brain	+	−	−	Fever
Synovial cells	+	−	Collagenase	Proteolytic enzyme release
Bone/osteoblasts	−	−	Collagenase	−
Cartilage/chondrocytes	+	−	Plasminogen activator	−
Muscle cells	+	−	−	Proteolytic enzyme release
Fibroblasts	+	+	Collagenase	−
Endothelium	+	+	Pro-coagulant activity	Boosts macrophage and PMN adhesion
Epithelium	−	−	Type IV collagen	−
Liver/hepatocytes	−	−	Acute phase proteins	−

the relative RANKL:osteoprotegerin ratio appears to be indicative of the severity of disease. This information could be of diagnostic and therapeutic value in periodontal treatment.

Nuclear (adenosine diphosphate (ADP)-ribose) polymerase (PARP) enzyme is a downstream mediator of nitric oxide toxicity. The role of this enzyme in ligature-induced periodontitis in mice has been reported (Lohinai et al 2003). They used a pharmacological inhibitor of PARP and a group of genetically PART-1 deficiency mice and a group of genetically normal mice. Ligature-induced periodontitis was produced on one side of the mandible of each group of mice and the other side served as control. The gingival tissues on the ligature-induced periodontitis side became inflamed and alveolar bone loss was produced. Using immunocytochemistry it was shown that the periodontitis-induced side had a marked increase in nuclear staining for PARP compared with the control side. PARP inhibition in genetically normal mice considerably reduced the tissue inflammation and bone loss. Furthermore, the genetically PART-1 deficiency mouse group also had considerably reduced the tissue inflammation and bone loss compared to controls. Thus, PARP activation may contribute to periodontal tissue damage during periodontal disease activity.

THE MECHANISM OF BONE RESORPTION

The account below is based upon a wealth of experimental evidence reviewed in articles by Vaes (1988), Dziak (1993), Meghji (1992), Delaissé et al (2000).

Bone is continually remodelled by the combined activities of osteoblasts and osteoclasts and in pathological situations like chronic periodontitis there may be a preponderance of bone resorption over formation due to a variety of factors discussed in the previous section. The bone loss in periodontal disease occurs at local sites but it is regulated by both systemic and local factors.

Osteoclasts are the main effector cells in the resorptive process but it has been shown in tissue culture experiments that bone resorption cannot occur without the presence of both osteoblasts and osteoclasts. All systemic and local bone resorbing factors exert their influence by stimulating the osteoblast (**Fig. 5.8**). Osteoblasts are involved in the regulation of osteoclast function at several levels. Osteoblasts have receptors for systemic factors such as parathormone (PTH) and 1, 25(OH)$_2$ (vitamin D$_3$) which affect general remodelling, and locally produced factors such as prostaglandins, leukotrienes and cytokines which affect local changes and all exert their influence by stimulating the osteoblast in a specific way (Meikle et al 1986). In distinction, the systemic hormone, calcitonin, which favours bone deposition directly inhibits osteoclasts and causes their disaggregation into mononuclear cells. Osteoclasts have numerous receptors for calcitonin (**Fig. 5.8**).

As explained in the previous section several of the locally produced factors are increased by the inflammatory and immune reactions of chronic periodontitis and some are produced by subgingival bacteria (Table 5.4). Osteoblasts stimulated by these factors (**Fig. 5.8**) mediate their response through a series of intracellular secondary messenger systems. One

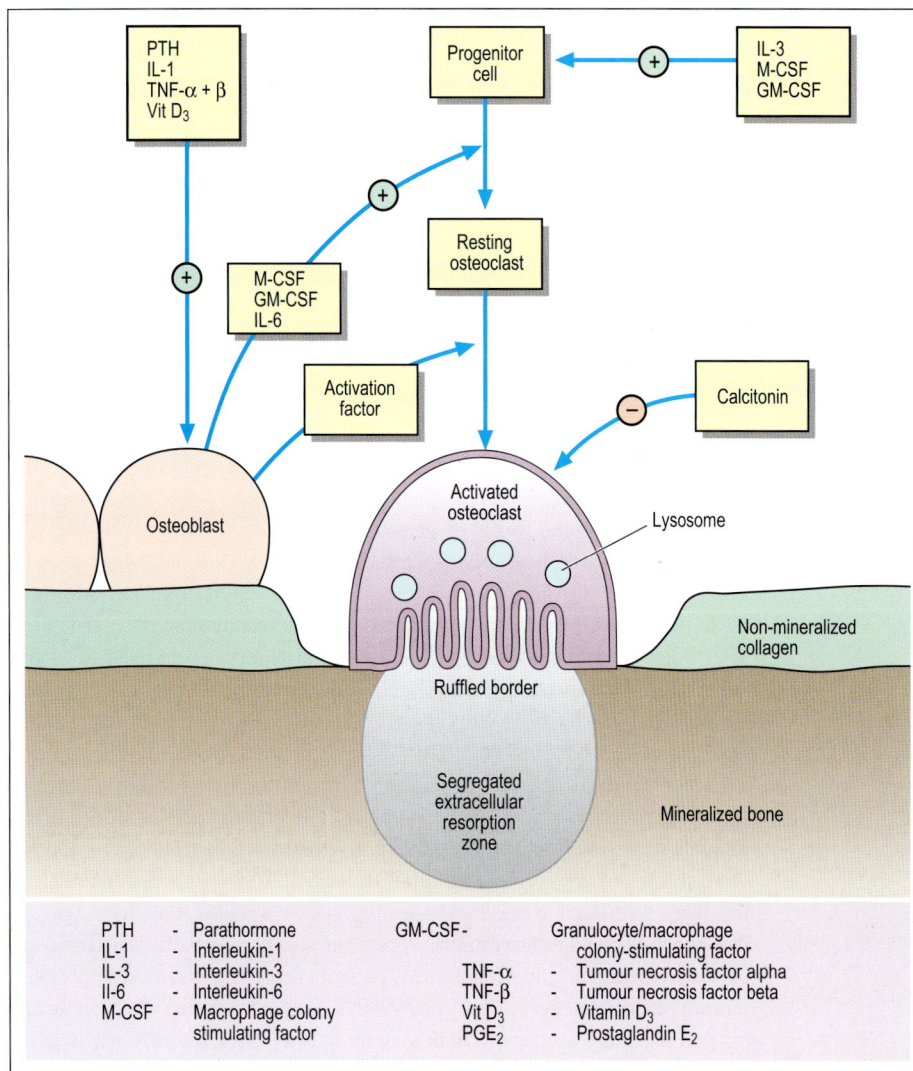

Fig. 5.8 Regulation of bone resorption.

PTH	- Parathormone	GM-CSF-	Granulocyte/macrophage colony-stimulating factor
IL-1	- Interleukin-1		
IL-3	- Interleukin-3	TNF-α	- Tumour necrosis factor alpha
II-6	- Interleukin-6	TNF-β	- Tumour necrosis factor beta
M-CSF	- Macrophage colony stimulating factor	Vit D$_3$	- Vitamin D$_3$
		PGE$_2$	- Prostaglandin E$_2$

pathway involves cyclic AMP and a second involves membrane phospholipids, diacylglycerol, protein kinase C and systolic calcium. Both of these mechanisms are stimulated by PGE_2 and prostacyclin (PGI_2) and thrombin and bradykinin. The leukotrienes and cytokines (IL-1, TNFs) do not appear to affect these intracellular mechanisms and must involve others at present unknown. In response to this stimulus osteoblasts secrete factors which both prepare the bone surface for osteoclastic resorption and stimulate the development of functional osteoclasts.

The role of the immune system in bone resorption in periodontal diseases and the evidence for this has been reviewed by Taubman et al (2005).

Osteoclast production involves the formation of precursor cells from stem cells in the bone marrow and the migration of these to the bone surface where they remain as pre-osteoclasts until they receive the appropriate stimulus (**Fig. 5.8**). Osteoblasts stimulate osteoclast formation by the secretion of cytokines and cell to cell contact. Osteoblasts and other cells such as lymphocytes and macrophages secrete growth factors, in particular granulocyte/macrophage colony stimulating factor (GM-CSF) and macrophage colony stimulating factor (M-CSF) and IL-6. IL-6 secretion is stimulated by IL-1 attachment to its osteoblast receptor. Secreted IL-6, GM-CSF and M-CSF in the presence of IL-3 can then stimulate the development of precursor cell in the marrow. Receptor activator of nuclear factor κB ligand (RANKL) from lymphocytes and macrophages stimulates the differentiation and maturation of these cells into functioning osteoclasts (Crotti et al 2003). Its natural inhibitor, osteoprotegerin, is secreted by vascular endothelium. IL-6 can also stimulate the differentiation and maturation of these cells into osteoclasts but cannot, however, stimulate the mature osteoclast.

Stimulated osteoblasts secrete a protein made of two components (activation factor) which is responsible for activating the mature osteoclast (**Fig. 5.8**). Prostaglandins also modulate osteoclast function. The pre-osteoclasts divide and fuse into multinucleated osteoclasts and spread over the bone surface prior to resorption. Stimulated osteoblasts also secrete pro-collagenase and plasminogen activator. Plasminogen activator generates plasmin from plasminogen and this activates pro-collagenase. This is then responsible for removing the non-mineralized collagenous surface layer which covers most bone surfaces in preparation for osteoclastic resorption.

Osteoclastic resorption involves firstly a solubilization of the mineral phase and secondly a dissolution of the organic matrix and these processes take place extracellularly (**Fig. 5.9**). The resorption area is defined beneath the ruffled border of the osteoclast. This is a highly specialized region of cytoplasmic infolding of the plasma membrane below which is outlined a sealing or clear zone. This contains podosomes, which are specialized protrusions of the ventral membrane of the osteoclast, which adhere directly to the bone surface being broken down.

The mineral is dissolved by acid secretion which is brought about by an electrogenic hydrogen ion transporting system. This is an ATPase-driven proton pump (**Fig. 5.9**). Intracellular pH regulation is achieved by carbonic anhydrase, which is abundant in the osteoclast cytoplasm. Bicarbonate, generated by carbonic anhydrase appears to be secreted from the basal outer membrane via HCO_3^-/Cl^- exchange. The hydrogen ions are released into the functionally extracellular lysosomal compartment and here they solubilize the mineral.

Osteoclasts also produce reactive oxygen species (ROS) which may play a role in the pathological demineralization of bone during disease

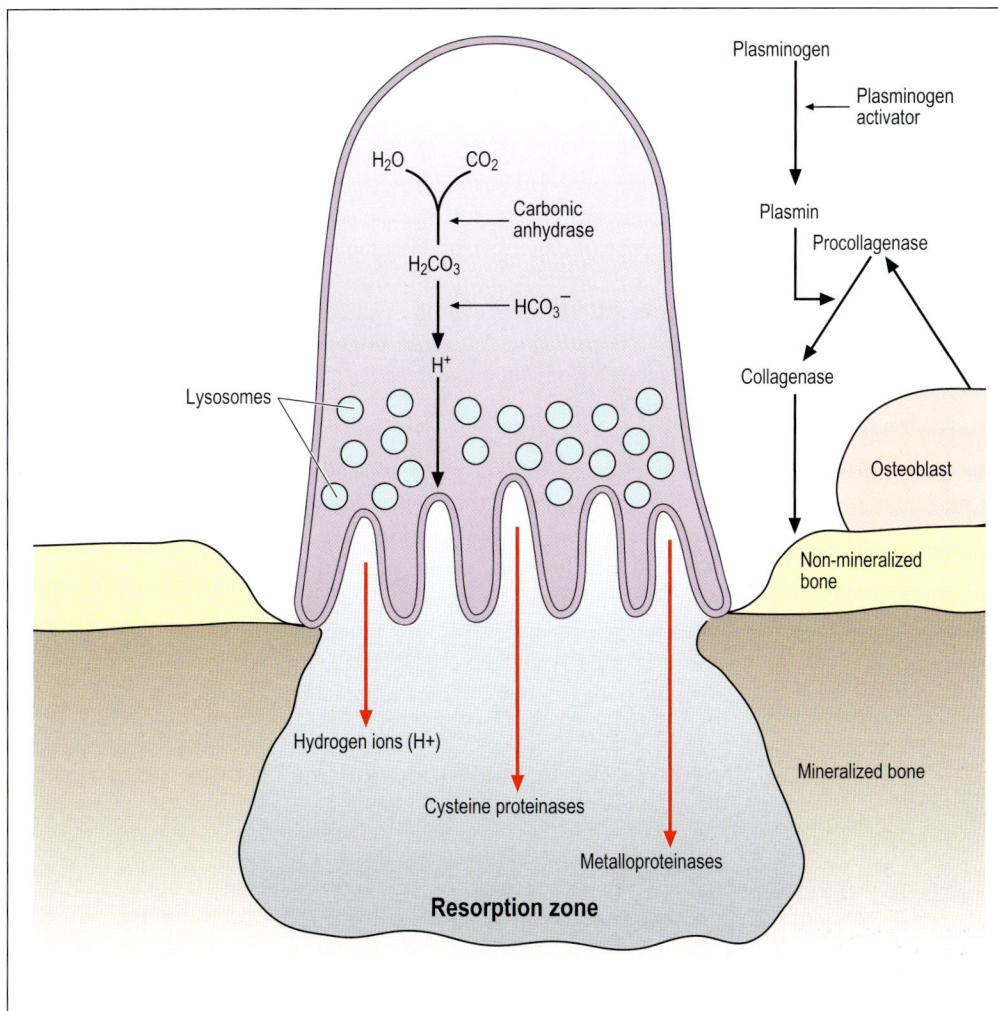

Fig. 5.9 Osteoclastic function in bone resorption.

(Garrett et al 1990). Osteoclasts involved in the pathological destruction of the mineralized matrix may have altered metabolic activity during active disease, following stimulation by factors from bacteria and inflammatory mediators such as prostaglandins and IL-1 released by gingival fibroblasts and circulating monocytes (Hausmann 1974; Reynolds et al 1994). In this regard, osteoclasts stimulated with parathyroid hormone and IL-1 have been shown to produce superoxide anions (Garrett et al 1990). In addition, bone resorption by osteoclasts has been shown to be inhibited by superoxide dismutase, an enzyme which scavenges superoxide.

Hydrogen ions and/or ROS create a suitable pH for the lysosomal cysteine proteinase enzyme activity which is involved in the first stage of the degradation of the demineralized bone matrix. This involves the secretion of acid cysteine proteinases including cathepsins B L, N and K which have been shown to be capable of degrading collagen and proteoglycans under these conditions (**Fig. 5.9**). However, recently it has been shown that the degradation of the demineralized organic matrix of bone by osteoclasts may involve the production, secretion and function of both cysteine- and metalloproteinases (Everts et al 1992, 1994). Using a bone tissue culture system, they showed that when selective inhibitors of either cysteine proteinases or metalloproteinases were separately added to the system, bone demineralization occurred but there was no degradation of the remaining organic bone matrix. Therefore, degradation of the organic matrix may involve both cysteine- and metalloproteinases (**Fig. 5.9**). It seems likely that the cysteine proteinases are responsible for the first and most important stage of degradation when the environment within the bone resorbing compartment below the ruffled border of the osteoclast is acid. They appear to degrade the proteoglycans of the bone matrix and attack the helical and non-helical terminal portions of the collagen molecules. Furthermore, at this acid pH, the key role in bone protein degradation is probably carried out by the cysteine proteinase, cathepsin K (Dickinson 2002), which is very highly expressed in osteoclasts and can cleave the triple helix area of native collagens (see below). In addition, later in the process cysteine proteinases may also function to activate the metalloproteinase pro-enzymes and as the pH in this environment increases the metalloproteinases may become functional and then also attack the helical portion of the remaining collagen molecules.

The central role of cathepsin K in bone resorption

The rabbit and human cDNA of an apparently novel cysteine proteinase has been recently cloned from an osteoclast cDNA library by differential screening (Inaoka et al 1995; Drake et al 1996). A section known as OC-2 was found to encode for this proteinase which was termed cathepsin K. The rabbit protein had 329 amino acid residues and showed 94% homology with the human protein. It has also been shown that cathepsin K has significant homology to members of the papain cysteine proteinase superfamily which also includes cathepsins B L, and S (Bossard et al 1996; Dickinson 2002). The mRNA for cathepsin K has been shown to be mainly expressed in osteoclasts (Drake et al 1996; Littlewood-Evans et al 1997) and osteoclast precursor cells (James et al 1996). It has also been observed in some hypertrophic chondrocytes of growth cartilages (Rantakakko et al 1996). It is thus primarily found in bony tissues and is absent from most other tissues. During embryogenesis in the mouse the mRNA for this proteinase was strongly expressed in osteoclasts, preosteoclasts and osteoclast precursor cells in sites of cartilage and bone remodelling (Dodds et al 1998).

Cathepsin K is first secreted as a proenzyme and this is activated by autocatalysis by mature, active cathepsin K which cleaves off the pre-sequence (McQueney et al 1997; Delaissé et al 2000; Dickinson 2002). The main substrates for cathepsin K appear to be collagen and osteonectin (Bossard et al 1996). In this regard, cathepsin K has been shown to cleave the triple helix area of the molecule of native collagens I and II at pH 5–5.5 (Kafienah et al 1998). This is a unique property for cysteine proteinases

and the only other enzymes with this property are the MMPs. Cathepsin K cleaves native collagens close to the N-terminal end of the triple helix region (Kafienah et al 1998).

This enzyme is now thought to play a central role in bone resorption by osteoclasts (Inaoka et al 1995; Sanishige et al 1995; Bossard et al 1996; Mano et al 1996; Inui et al 1997; Volta et al 1997; Dodds et al 1998; Lazner et al 1999; Delaissé et al 2000; Dickinson 2002). It appears to be responsible for the degradation of bone proteins, particularly collagen, in the acid environment below the ruffled border of the osteoclast (**Fig. 5.9**).

Its key role in bone resorption is clearly shown by several different areas of evidence (Lazner et al 1999; Delaissé et al 2000; Dickinson 2002). First, vitamin A derivatives such as retinoic acid (RA) are mediators of key steps in vertebrate metabolism. RA receptors are expressed on osteoclasts and RA stimulates a dose dependent increase in bone resorption in bone cultures (Saneshige et al 1995). In this regard, RA has been shown to regulate the gene expression of cathepsin K/OC-2 at the transcriptional level in mature osteoclasts. Second, osteoclasts also have a receptor for oestrogen and oestrogen decreases bone resorption in a dose dependent manner. It appears to do this by downregulating the expression of cathepsin K mRNA in osteoclasts (Mano et al 1996). This may be one of the mechanisms underlying the protective effects of oestrogen on osteoporosis. Third, it has been shown that the insertion of an antisense oligonucleotide for cathepsin K into osteoclasts inhibited the bone resorption process (Inui et al 1997). Fourth, the application of peptide-aldehyde inhibitors of cathepsin K to bone cultures strongly inhibited bone resorption by osteoclasts (Votta et al 1997). Finally, a nonsense mutation of the cathepsin K gene occurs as an autosomal recessive trait in humans and the resulting condition is known as pycnodysostosis (Johnson et al 1996; Gelb et al 1996a,b). This condition is characterized by short stature, wide open cranial sutures and increased bone density and fragility which are caused by disordered bone remodelling. It appears that this condition is totally caused by the defective cathepsin K gene.

Interleukin-1α is also a powerful activator of osteoclast cells but the underlying mechanism for this is unknown. In this regard, Kamolmatyakul et al (2004) showed that IL-1α upregulated the expression of cathepsin K protein by 5-fold. Northern blot analysis and promoter analysis showed that this induction occurred at the transcriptional level, in a dose-responsive and time-dependent manner. However, no increase in expression occurred in the presence of either pyrrolidine dithiocarbamate, a selective inhibitor of NF-κB, or genistein, a protein tyrosine kinase inhibitor and this suggests that the IL-1α upregulation of cathepsin K may be via the tyrosine kinase-NF-κB pathway. Antisense oligonucleotides to p65, but not the p50 subunit of NF-κB suppressed the IL-1α -induced expression of cathepsin K. They therefore concluded that IL-1α upregulates the cathepsin K gene expression at the transcription level, and this regulation may be via the tyrosine-kinase-NF-κB pathway. Thus, there is overwhelming evidence for the central role of cathepsin K in bone resorption.

Mogi and Otogoto (2007) reported that the *in vivo* concentrations of cathepsin-K and RANKL in the gingival crevicular fluid (GCF) were significantly increased in patients with periodontitis compared with healthy control subjects. Also, they found a positive correlation between cathepsin-K and RANKL levels suggesting that both of them contribute to osteoclastic bone destruction in periodontal disease.

The role of the immune mechanisms on bone resorption

Host immune responses to periodontal pathogens may contribute to the alveolar bone destruction in periodontitis. However, the role of B lymphocytes in the pathogenesis of periodontal bone loss is not clear. Harada et al (2006) examined the effect of adoptive transfer of antigen-specific B cells from rat spleens on experimental periodontal bone resorption. Donor rats were immunized intraperitoneally with formalin-killed *A. actinomycetemcomitans*. Antigen-specific B cells were prepared from splenocytes by first binding CD43+ cells to Petri dishes coated with anti-CD43 antibody to remove T cells, and non-binding cells were passed through a nylon wool column to deplete accessory cells. The retained cells were then collected and bound to *A. actinomycetemcomitans*-coated Petri dishes for enrichment of *A. actinomycetemcomitans*-binding B cells (AAB). *A. actinomycetemcomitans* non-binding B cells (ANB) and B cells from non-immunized donor rats (NIB) were also collected from these procedures. Each type of B cell was injected into a group of recipient rats that were then orally infected with live *A. actinomycetemcomitans*.

At termination, the antibody levels to *A. actinomycetemcomitans* in serum and gingival wash fluids were significantly higher in the recipients transferred with AAB when compared with the recipients transferred with ANB or NIB. A markedly elevated number of antibody-forming cells were observed in the spleens of the recipients transferred with AAB, and these recipient rats also exhibited significantly increased bone resorption when compared to the other groups. These results suggested that B cells can contribute to periodontal bone resorption and that antigen-triggering of B cells is required for the bone resorption.

Kawai et al (2007) examined whether induction of an adaptive immune response to orally colonizing non-pathogenic *Pasteurella pneumotropica* by immunization with the phylogenetically closely related bacterium, *A. actinomycetemcomitans*, could result in periodontal bone loss in mice. They showed that the induction of this adaptive immune response resulted in RANKL-dependent periodontal bone loss in mice.

REFERENCES

Abiko Y, Hayakawa M, Murai S, et al: Glycylprolyl dipeptidyl aminopeptidase from Bacteroides gingivalis, *J Dent Res* 64:106–111, 1985.

Adriaens PA, Claeys GW, De Boever JA: Colonization of human dentin by a mixed flora of oral bacteria in vitro, *Caries Res* 18:160, Abstr. 21, 1984.

Adriaens PA, Loesche WJ, De Boever JA: Bacteriology of the flora present in the roots of periodontally diseased teeth, *J Dent Res* 66:338, Abstract 1855, 1987.

Adriaens PA, De Boever JA, Loesche WJ: Bacterial invasion in root cementum and radicular dentin of periodontally diseased teeth in humans, *J Periodontol* 59:222–230, 1988a.

Adriaens PA, Edwards CA, De Boever JA, et al: Ultrastructural observations on bacterial invasion in cementum and radicular dentin of periodontally diseased human teeth, *J Periodontol* 59:493–503, 1988b.

Aduse-Opoku J, Muir J, Slaney JM, et al: Characterization, genetic analysis and expression studies of a protease antigen (PrpR1) of Porphyromonas gingivalis W50, *Infect Immun* 63:4744–4754, 1995.

Aduse-Opoku J, Slaney JM, Rangarajan M, et al: Characterization of an adherence and antigen determinant of the Arg 1 protease Porphyromonas gingivalis which is present on multiple gene products, *Infect Immun* 64:2532–2539, 1996.

Allenspach-Petrzilka GE, Guggenheim B: Bacterial invasion of the periodontium; an important factor in the pathogenesis of periodontitis? *J Clin Periodontol* 10:609–617, 1983.

Al-Rasheed A, Scheerens H, Rennick DM, et al: Accelerated alveolar bone loss in mice lacking interleukin-10, *J Dent Res* 82:632–635, 2003.

Al-Rasheed A, Scheerens H, Srivastava AK, et al: Accelerated alveolar bone loss in mice lacking interleukin-10: late onset, *J Periodontal Res* 39:194–198, 2004.

Alayan J, Ivanovski S, Gemmell E, et al: Deficiency of inos contributes to Porphyromonas gingivalis-induced tissue damage, *Oral Microbiol Immunol* 21:360–365, 2006.

Amano A: Molecular interaction of Porphyromonas gingivalis with host cells: implications for the microbial pathogenesis of periodontal disease, *J Periodontol* 74:90–96, 2003.

Andrian E, Grenier D, Rouabhia M: Porphyromonas gingivalis-epithelial cell interactions in periodontitis, *J Dent Res* 85:392–403, 2006.

Aoyagi T, Sugawara- Aoyagi M, Yamazaki K, et al: Interleukin-4 (IL-4) and IL-6-producing memory T- cells in peripheral blood and gingival tissues in periodontitis patients with high serum antibody titres to Porphyromonas gingivalis, *Oral Microbiol Immunol* 10:304–310, 1995.

Arakawa S, Kuramitsu H: Cloning and sequence analysis of the chymotrypsin-like protease from Treponema denticola, *Infect Immun* 62:3424–3433, 1994.

Aronsen KF, Ekelund G, Kindmark CO, et al: Sequential changes in plasma proteins after myocardial infarction, *Scand J Clin Lab Invest* 29:127–134, 1972.

Baggiolini M, Schnyder J, Bretz U, et al: Cellular mechanisms of proteinase release from inflammatory cells and degradation of extracellular proteins, In Evered D, Whelan J, editors: Protein degradation in health and disease. Ciba Foundation Symposium 75, 1980, pp 105–121.

Baker PJ: Genetic control of the immune response in pathogenesis, *J Periodontol* 76:2042–2046, 2005.

Balkwill FR, Burke F: The cytokine network, *Immunol Today* 9:299–304, 1989.

Banda MJ, Rice AJ, Griffin GL, et al: a-1-proteinase inhibitor is a neutrophil chemoattractant after proteolytic inactivation by macrophage elastase, *J Biol Chem* 363:4481–4484, 1988a.

Banda MJ, Rice AJ, Griffin GL, et al: The inhibitory complex of human a-1-proteinase inhibitor and human leukocyte elastase is a neutrophil chemoattractant, *J Exp Med* 167:1608–1615, 1988b.

Barkocy-Gallagher GA, Han N, Patti JM, et al: Analysis of the prtP gene encoding porphypain, a cysteine proteinase of Porphyromonas gingivalis, *J Bacteriol* 176:2734–2741, 1996.

Barkocy-Gallagher GA, Foley WF, Lantz MS: Activities of the Porphyromonas gingivalis prtP proteinase determined by construction of prtP deficient mutants and expression of the gene in Bacteroides species, *J Bacteriol* 181:246–255, 1999.

Barrett AJ: Introduction: the classification of proteinases, *Ciba Found Symp* 75:1–13, 1980.

Barrett AJ, Starky PM: The interaction of alpha2-macroglobulin with proteases, characteristics and specificity of reaction, and a hypothesis concerning its molecular mechanism, *Biochem J* 133:709–724, 1973.

Bartold PM: Proteoglycans in the periodontium. Structure, role and function, *J Periodontal Res* 22:431–444, 1987.

Bartold PM, Wiebkin OW, Thonard JC: The effect of oxygen-derived free radicals on gingival proteoglycans and hyaluronic acid, *J Periodontal Res* 19:390–400, 1984.

Barua PK, Neiders ME, Topolnyeky A, et al: Purification of an 80:000 Mr glycylprolyl peptidase from Bacteroides gingivalis, *Infect Immun* 57:2522–2528, 1989.

Battino M, Bullon P, Wilson M, et al: Oxidative injury and inflammatory periodontal diseases: the challenge of anti-oxidants to free radicals and reactive oxygen species, *Crit Rev Oral Biol Med* 10:458–476, 1999.

Bedi GS, Williams T: Purification and characterization of a collagen-degrading protease from Porphyromonas gingivalis, *J Biol Chem* 269:599–606, 1994.

Beikler T, Ehmke B, Wittstock M, et al: Serum antibody reactivity against recombinant PrtC of Porphyromonas gingivalis following periodontal therapy, *J Periodontal Res* 38:276–281, 2003.

Beikler T, Peters U, Prior K, et al: Sequence variations in rgpA and rgpB of Porphyromonas gingivalis in periodontitis, *J Periodontal Res* 40:193–198, 2005.

Beklen A, Ainola M, et al: mmps, IL-1, and TNF are regulated by IL-17 in periodontitis, *J Dent Res* 86:347–351, 2007.

Berglundh T, Donati M: Aspects of adaptive host response in periodontitis, *J Clin Periodontol* 32:87–107, 2005.

Birkedal-Hansen H, Moore W, Bodden M, et al: Matrix metalloproteinases: a review, *Crit Rev Oral Biol Med* 4:197–250, 1993a.

Birkedal-Hansen H: Role of matrix metalloproteinases in human periodontal diseases, *J Periodontol* 64:474–484, 1993b.

Birkedal-Hansen H, Taylor RE, Zambon JJ, et al: Characterization of collagenolytic activity from strains of Bacteroides gingivalis, *J Periodontal Res* 23:258–264, 1988.

Bodineau A, Godeau G, Brousse N, et al: Langerhans cells express matrix metalloproteinases 9 and 2 and tissue inhibitors of metalloproteinases 1 and 2 in healthy human gingival tissue and in periodontitis, *Oral Microbiol Immunol* 21:197–200, 2006.

Booth V, Downes J, Van den Berg J, et al: Gram-positive anaerobic bacilli in human periodontal disease, *J Periodontal Res* 39:213–220, 2004.

Booth V, Solakoglu Ö, Bavisha N, et al: Serum IgG1 and IgG2 antibody responses to Porphyromonas gingivalis in patients with periodontitis, *Oral Microbiol Immunol* 21:93–99, 2006.

Booth V, Cox SW, Rodriguez Gonzalez EM, et al: Elastase activity in GCF and saliva relates to both clinical parameters and protease inhibitor levels in patients with severe periodontitis, *Periodontal Practice Today* 4:129–138, 2007.

Bossard MJ, Tomaszek TA, Thompson SK, et al: Proteolytic activity of human osteoclast cathepsin K: Expression, purification, activation and substrate identification, *J Biol Chem* 271:12517–12524, 1996.

Bostanci N, Allaker R: Johansson U, et al: Interleukin-1a stimulation in monocytes by periodontal bacteria: antagonistic effects of Porphyromonas gingivalis, *Oral Microbiol Immunol* 22:52–60, 2007a.

Bostanci N, Ilgenli T, Emingil G, et al: Differential expression of receptor activator of nuclear factor-kappab ligand and osteoprotegerin mRNA in periodontal diseases, *J Periodontal Res* 42:287–293, 2007b.

Bourgeau G, Laponte H, Péloquin P, et al: Cloning, expression and sequencing of a protease gene (tpr) from Porphyromonas gingivalis W83 in Escherichia coli, *Infect Immun* 60:3186–3192, 1992.

Brock GR, Butterworth CJ, Matthews JB, et al: Local and systemic total antioxidant capacity in periodontitis and health, *J Clin Periodontol* 31:515–521, 2004.

Bulkacz J, Newman MG, Socransky SS, et al: Phospholipase A activity of microorganisms from dental plaque, *Microbiology Letters* 10:79–88, 1979.

Bulkacz J, Erbland JF, MacGregor J: Phospholipase A in supernatants from cultures of Bacteroides melaninogenicus, *Biochim Biophys Acta* 664:148–155, 1981.

Bulkacz J, Schuster GS, Singh B, et al: Phospholipase A activity of extracellular products from Bacteroides melaninogenicus on epithelial tissue cultures, *J Periodontal Res* 20:146–153, 1985.

Burleigh MC: Degradation of collagen by non-specific proteinases, In Barrett AJ, editor: *Proteinases in Mammalian Cells and Tissues*, Amsterdam, 1977, Elsevier/North-Holland Biomedical Press, pp 185–209.

Califano JV, Pace Gunsolly JC, et al: Antibody reactive with Actinobacillus actinomycetemcomitans leukotoxin in early onset periodontitis, *Oral Microbiol Immunol* 12:20–26, 1997a.

Califano JV, Gunsolly JC, Schenkein HA, et al: A comparison of igg antibody reactive with Bacteroides forsythus and Porphyromonas gingivalis in adult and early onset periodontitis, *J Periodontol* 68:734–738, 1997b.

Califano JV, Chou D, Lewis JP, et al: Antibody reactive with Porphyromonas gingivalis hemagglutinin in chronic and generalized aggressive periodontitis, *J Periodontal Res* 39:263–268, 2004.

Camerer E, Huang W, Coughlin SR: Tissue factor and factor X dependent activation of protease-activated receptor-2 by factor VII, *Proc N Y Acad Sci* 97:5255–5260, 2000.

Cantin A, North SA, Hubbard RC: Normal alveolar epithelial lining fluid contains high levels of glutathione, *J Appl Physiol* 63:152–157, 1987.

Cappuyns I, Gugerli P, Mombelli A: Viruses in periodontal disease – a review, *Oral Dis* 11:219–229, 2005.

Carlsson J, Hofling JF, Sundqvist GK: Degradation of albumin, haemopexin, heptoglobin and transferrin by black-pigmented Bacteroides species, *J Med Microbiol* 18:39–46, 1984b.

Carlsson J, Hermann BF, Hofling JF, et al: Degradation of the human proteinase inhibitors alpha-1-antitrypsin and alpha-2-macroglobulin by Bacteroides gingivalis, *Infect Immun* 43:644–648, 1984a.

Carranza FA, Saglie FR, Newman MG, et al: Scanning and transmission electron microscopic study of tissue-invading microorganisms in localised juvenile periodontitis, *J Periodontol* 54:598–617, 1983.

Carrell RW, Boswell DR: The serpins: the superfamily of plasma serine proteinase inhibitors. In Barrett AJ, Salvensen G, editors: *Proteinase Inhibitors. Research Monographs in Cell and Tissue Physiology*, vol 12, 1986, pp 403–420.

Catkins CC, Platt K, Potempta J, et al: Inactivation of tumor necrosis factor alpha by proteinases (gingipains) from the periodontal pathogen, Porphyromonas gingivalis. Implications of immune evasion, *J Biol Chem* 273:6611–6614, 1998.

Champaiboon C, Yongvanitchit K, Pichyangkul S, et al: The immune modulation of B-cell responses by Porphyromonas gingivalis and interleukin-10, *J Periodontol* 71:468–475, 2000.

Chapple LC: The role of free radicals and antioxidants in the pathogenesis of the inflammatory periodontal diseases, *J Cell Mol Pathol* 49:M247-M255, 1996.

Chapple ILC: Reactive oxygen species and antioxidants in inflammatory diseases, *J Clin Periodontol* 24:287–296, 1997.

Chapple ILC, Brock G, Eftimiadi C, et al: Glutathione in gingival crevicular fluid and its relationship to local antioxidant capacity in periodontal health and disease, *J Mol Pathol* 55:367–373, 2002.

Chapple ILC, Mason GM, Matthews JB, et al: Enhanced chemiluminescence assay for measuring the total antioxidant capacity of serum, saliva and crevicular fluid, *Ann Clin Biochem* 34:412–421, 1997.

Chen ECS, McLaughlin R: Taxonomy and virulence of oral spirochetes, *Oral Microbiol Immunol* 15:1–9, 2000.

Chen Z, Potempta J, Polanowski A, et al: Purification and characterization of a 50-kDa cysteine proteinase (gingipain) from Porphyromonas gingivalis, *J Bio Chem* 267:18896–18901, 1992.

Choi JI, Borrello MA, Smith ES, et al: Polorization of Porphyromonas gingivalis-specific helper T-cell subsets by prior immunization with Fusobacterium nucleatum, *Oral Microbiol Immunol* 15:181–187, 2000.

Choi BK, Moon SY, Cha JA, et al: Prostaglandin E(2) is a main mediator in receptor activator of nuclear factor-kappaB ligand-dependent osteoclastogenesis induced by Porphyromonas gingivalis, Treponema denticola, and Treponema socranskii, *J Periodontol* 76:813–820, 2005.

Christersson LA, Wikesjö UMA, Albini B, et al: Tissue localization of Actinobacillus actinomycetemcomitans in human periodontitis. 1. Light, immunofluorescent and electron microscopic studies, *J Periodontol* 58:529–539, 1987.

Ciborwski P, Nishikata M, Allen RD, et al: Purification and characterization of two forms of high molecular weight cysteine proteinase (porphypain) from Porphyromonas gingivalis, *J Bacteriol* 176:4549–4557, 1994.

Claesson R, Edlund MB, Persson S, et al: Production of volatile sulphur compounds by various Fusobacterium species, *Oral Microbiol Immunol* 5:137–142, 1990.

Coates ARM: *The Chaperonins*, London, 1996, Academic Press, pp 267–296.

Cohen N, Morisset J, Emilie D: Induction of tolerance by Porphyromonas gingivalis on apcs: A mechanism implicated in periodontal infection, *J Dent Res* 83:384–387, 2004.

Cole KC, Seymour GJ, Powell RN: The autologous mixed lymphocyte relations (AMLR) using periodontal lymphocytes, *J Dent Res* 65:473, 1986.

Cole KC, Seymour GJ, Powell RN: Phenotype and functional analysis of T-cells extracted from chronically inflamed human periodontal tissues, *J Periodontol* 58:569–573, 1987.

Compton SJ, Cairnes JA, Holgate ST, et al: Interaction of mast cell tryptase with endothelial cells to stimulate inflammatory recruitment, *Int Arch Allergy Immunol* 118:204–205, 1999.

Compton SJ, Renaux B, Wijesuriya SJ, et al: Glycosylation and activation of protease-activated receptor-2(PAR$_2$) by human mast cell tryptase, *Br J Pharmacol* 134:705–718, 2001.

Cope G, Thorpe G, Holder R, et al: Serum and tissue antioxidant capacity in cervical intraepithelial neoplasia investigated by an enhanced chemiluminescence reaction, *Ann Clin Biochem* 36:86–93, 1999.

Coughlin SR: Thrombin signalling and protease-activated receptors, *Nature* 407:258–264, 2000.

Courant P, Bader H: Bacteroides melaninogenicus and its products in the gingiva of man, *Periodontics* 4:131–136, 1966.

Cox SW: Extending their scope of gingival crevicular fluid elastase research, *Oral Dis* 1:103–105, 1995.

Cox SW, Eley BM: Preliminary studies on cysteine and serine proteinase activities in inflamed human gingiva using different 7-amino-4-trifluoromethyl coumarin substrates and protease inhibitors, *Arch Oral Biol* 32:599–605, 1987.

Cox SW, Eley BM: Identification of a tryptase-like enzyme in extracts of inflamed human gingiva by effector and gel filtration studies, *Arch Oral Biol* 34:219–221, 1989a.

Cox SW, Eley BM: Tryptase-like activity in crevicular fluid from gingivitis and periodontitis patients, *J Periodontal Res* 24:41–44, 1989b.

Cox SW, Eley BM: The detection of cathepsin B and L-, elastase-, tryptase-, trypsin-, and dipeptidyl peptidase IV-like activities in crevicular fluid from gingivitis and periodontitis patients with peptidyl derivatives of 7-amino-4-trifluoromethyl coumarin, *J Periodontal Res* 24:353–361, 1989c.

Cox SW, Eley BM: Cathepsin B/L-, elastase-, tryptase-, trypsin- and dipeptidylpeptidase IV-like activities in gingival crevicular fluid: a comparison of levels before and after basic periodontal treatment, *J Clin Periodontol* 19:333–339, 1992.

Cox SW, Gazi MI, Clark DT, et al: Host tissue and Porphyromonas gingivalis dipeptidyl peptidase activities in gingival crevicular fluid, *J Dent Res* 72:705, 1993.

Cox SW, Eley BM, Proctor GB, et al: Elastase inhibitors from gingival homogenates, gingival epithelial cells and saliva, *J Dent Res* 80:1153, Abstract 94, 2001.

Cox SW, Eley BM, Carpenter GH, et al: Skin antileukoproteinase in gingival tissue homogenates and epithelial cell media, *J Dent Res* 82:C-51, Abstract 281, 2003.

Cox SW, Eley BM, Kiili M, et al: Collagen degradation by interleukin-Ib-stimulated gingival fibroblasts is accompanied by release and activation of multiple matrix metalloproteinases and cysteine proteinases, *Oral Dis* 12:34–40, 2006a.

Cox SW, Rodriguez-Gonzalez EM, Booth V, et al: Secretory leukocyte protease inhibitor and its potential interactions with elastase and cathepsin B in gingival crevicular fluid and saliva from patients with chronic periodontitis, *J Periodontal Res* 41:477–485, 2006b.

Crystal RG: Impact of cell and molecular biology on pulmonary disease. In Isslebacher KJ, Braunwald E, Wilson JD, et al, editors: *Harrison's Principles of Internal Medicine*, ed 13, New York, 1994, McGraw Hill, pp 1147–1151.

Curtis MA, Ramakrishnan M, Slaney JM: Characterization of the trypsin-like enzymes of P. Gingivalis W83 using a radio-labelled active-site-directed inhibitor, *J Gen Microbiol* 139:949–955, 1993.

Curtis MA, Aduse-Opoku J, Slaney JM, et al: Characterization of an adherence and antigenic determinant of the R1 protease of Porphyromonas gingivalis which is present on multiple gene products, *Infect Immun* 64:2532–2539, 1996.

Curtis MA, Kuramitsu HK, Lantz M, et al: Molecular genetics and nomenclature of proteases of Porphyromonas gingivalis, *J Periodontal Res* 34:464–472, 1999.

Curtis MA, Slaney JM, Aduse-Opoku J: Critical pathways in microbial virulence, *J Clin Periodontol* 32:28–38, 2005.

D'Aiuto F, Parkar M, Andreou G, et al: Periodontitis and systemic inflammation: control of the local infection is associated with a reduction in serum inflammatory markers, *J Dent Res* 83:156–160, 2004.

Dahl M, Nordestgaard BG, Lange P, et al: Molecular diagnosis of intermediate and severe a1-Antitrypsin deficiency: MZ individuals with chronic obstructive pulmonary disease may have lower lung function than MM individuals, *Clin Chem* 47:56–62, 2001.

Darveau RP, Belton CM, Reife RA, et al: Local chemokine paralysis, a novel pathogenic mechanism for Porphyromonas gingivalis, *Infect Immun* 66:1660–1665, 1998.

Dayan S, Stashenko P, Niederman R, et al: Oral epithelial over expression of IL-1α causes periodontal disease, *J Dent Res* 83:786–790, 2004.

De Carlo AA Jr, Windsor LJ, Bodden NK, et al: Activation and novel processing of matrix metalloproteinases by a thiol-proteinase from the oral anaerobe Porphyromonas gingivalis, *J Dent Res* 76:1260–1270, 1997.

Delaissé JM, Engsig MT, Everts V, et al: Proteinases in bone resorption: obvious and less obvious roles, *Clinica Chimica Acta* 291:223–234, 2000.

De-Waal-Malefyt R, Haanen J, Splits H, et al: Interleukin-10 and viral IL-10 strongly reduced antigen-specific human T cell proliferation by diminishing the antigen-presenting capacity of monocytes via complex expression, *J Exp Med* 174:915–924, 1991.

Dewhirst FE: N-acetyl muramyl dipeptide stimulation of bone resorption in tissue culture, *Infect Immun* 35:133–137, 1982.

Dewhirst FE, Stashenko PP, Mole JE, et al: Purification and partial sequence of osteoclast-activation factor: identity with interleukin-1-beta, *J Immunol* 135:2562–2568, 1985.

Dickinson DP: Cysteine peptidases of mammals: their biological roles and potential effects in the oral cavity and other tissues in health and disease, *Crit Rev Oral Biol Med* 13:238–275, 2002.

Dierickx K, Pauwels M, Laine ML, et al: Adhesion of Porphyromonas gingivalis serotypes to pocket epithelium, *J Periodontol* 74:844–848, 2003.

Dietrich FE, Goodson JM, Raisz LG: Stimulation of bone resorption by various prostaglandins in organ culture, *Prostaglandins* 10:231–240, 1975.

Dodds RA, Connor JR, Drake F, et al: Cathepsin K mrna detection is restricted to osteoclasts during fetal mouse development, *J Bone Miner Res* 13:673–682, 1998.

Domeij H, Yucel-Lindberg T, Modéer T: Cell interactions between human gingival fibroblasts and monocytes stimulate the production of matrix metalloproteinase-1 in gingival fibroblasts, *J Periodontal Res* 41:108–117, 2006.

Drake FH, Dodds RA, James IE, et al: Cathepsin K, but not cathepsins B L, or S is abundantly expressed in human osteoclasts, *J Biol Chem* 271:12511–12516, 1996.

Dye BA, Choudhary K, Shea S, et al: Serum antibodies to periodontal pathogens and markers of systemic inflammation, *J Clin Periodontol* 32:1189–1199, 2005.

Dziak R: Biochemical and molecular mediators of bone metabolism, *J Periodontol* 64:407–415, 1993.

Ebersole JL, Taubman MA: The protective nature of the host responses in periodontal diseases, *Periodontol 2000* 5:112–141, 1994.

Eick S, Reismann A, Rödel J, et al: Porphyromonas gingivalis survives within KB cells and modulates inflammatory response, *Oral Microbiol Immunol* 21:231–237, 2006.

Ejeil AL, Gaultier F, Igondjo-Tchen S, et al: Are cytokines linked to collagen breakdown during periodontal disease progression, *J Periodontol* 74:196–201, 2003a.

Ejeil A-L, Igondjo-Tchen S, Ghomrasseni S, et al: Expression of matrix metalloproteinases (MMPs) and tissue inhibitors of metalloproteinases (TIMPs) in healthy and diseased human gingiva, *J Periodontol* 74:188–195, 2003b.

El Attar TMA, Lin HS: Relative conversion of arachidonic acid through lipo-oxygenase and cyclo-oxygenase pathways by homogenates of diseased periodontal tissues, *J Oral Pathol* 12:7–10, 1982.

El Attar TMA, Lin HS, Killoy WJ, et al: Hydroxy fatty acids and prostaglandins formation in diseased periodontal pocket tissue, *J Periodontal Res* 21:169–176, 1986.

Eley BM, Cox SW: Cathepsin B/L-, elastase-, tryptase-, trypsin- and dipeptidylpeptidase IV-like activities in gingival crevicular fluid: correlation with clinical parameters in untreated chronic periodontitis patients, *J Periodontal Res* 27:62–69, 1992a.

Eley BM, Cox SW: Correlation of gingival crevicular fluid proteases with clinical and radiological measurements of periodontal attachment loss, *J Dent* 20:90–99, 1992b.

Eley BM, Cox SW: Cathepsin B/L-, elastase-, tryptase-, trypsin- and dipeptidylpeptidase IV-like activities in gingival crevicular fluid: a comparison before and after periodontal surgery, *J Periodontol* 63:412–417, 1992c.

Eley BM, Cox SW: Correlation between gingival crevicular fluid dipeptidyl peptidase II and IV and periodontal attachment loss, *Oral Dis* 1:201–213, 1995.

Eley BM, Cox SW: A 2-year longitudinal study of elastase in gingival crevicular fluid and periodontal attachment loss, *J Clin Periodontol* 23:681–692, 1996a.

Eley BM, Cox SW: The relationship between gingival crevicular fluid cathepsin B and periodontal attachment loss in chronic periodontitis patients. A 2-year longitudinal study, *J Periodontal Res* 31:381–392, 1996b.

Eley BM, Cox SW: Proteolytic and hydrolytic enzymes from putative periodontal pathogens: characterization, molecule genetics, effects on host defenses and tissues and detection in gingival crevice fluid, *Periodontol 2000* 31:105–124, 2003.

Embery G, Oliver WM, Stanbury JB: The metabolism of proteoglycans and glycosaminoglycans in inflamed human gingiva, *J Periodontal Res* 14:512–519, 1979.

Embery G, Picton D, Stanbury JB: Biochemical changes in the periodontal ligament ground substance associated with short-term intrusive loading in adult monkeys, *Arch Oral Biol* 32:545–549, 1987.

Embery G, Olivier WM, Stanbury JB, et al: The electrophoretic detection of acid glycosaminoglycans in human gingival sulcular fluid, *Arch Oral Biol* 27:177–179, 1982.

Endo J, Otsuka M, Ohara E, et al: Cleavage action of a trypsin-like protease from Bacteroides gingivalis 381 on reduced egg-white lysozyme, *Arch Oral Biol* 34:911–916, 1989.

Everts V, Creemers L, Beertsen W: The use of selective inhibitors in the study of collagen breakdown, *Proceedings of Royal Microscopical Society* 29:216, Abstract 7c, 1994.

Everts V, Delaissé JM, Korper W, et al: Degradation of collagen in the bone-resorbing compartment of the osteoclast involves both cysteine-proteinase and matrix metalloproteinases, *Journal of Cell Physiology* 150:221–231, 1992.

Everts V, Van der Zee E, Creemers L, et al: Phagocytosis and intracellular digestion of collagen, its role in turnover and remodelling, *Histochem J* 28:229–245, 1996.

Farida R, Wilson M, Ivanyi L: Serum IgG antibodies to lipopolysaccharide on various forms of periodontal disease in Man, *Arch Oral Biol* 31:711–715, 1986.

Fiehn N-E: Enzyme activities from eight small-sized oral spirochaetes, *Scand J Dent Res* 94:132–140, 1986.

Figueredo CMS, Fischer RGA, Gustafsson A: Aberrant neutrophil reactions in periodontitis, *J Periodontol* 76:951–955, 2005.

Fine DH, Velliyagounder K, Furgang D, et al: The Actinobacillus actinomycetemcomitans autotransporter adhesin Aae exhibits specificity for buccal epithelial cells from humans and old world primates, *Infect Immun* 73:1947–1953, 2005.

Fletcher HM, Schenkein HA, Macrina FL: Cloning and characterization of a new protease gene (prtH) from Porphyromonas gingivalis, *Infect Immun* 62:4279–4286, 1994.

Fletcher J, Reddi K, Poole S, et al: Interactions between periodontopathic bacteria and cytokines, *J Periodontal Res* 32:200–205, 1997.

Fletcher J, Nair S, Poole S, et al: Cytokine degradation by biofilms of Porphyromonas gingivalis, *Curr Microbiol* 36:216–219, 1998.

Fokkema SJ, Timmerman MF, Van der Weijden FA, et al: A possible association of a1- antitrypsin deficiency with the periodontal condition in adults, *J Clin Periodontol* 25:617–623, 1998.

Fosdick LS, Blackwell RQ, Carter WJ: Chemical studies on periodontal disease, *J Dent Res* 32:646–651, 1953.

Foster N, Cheetham J, Taylor JJ, et al: VIP inhibits Porphyromonas gingivalis LPS-induced immune responses in human monocytes, *J Dent Res* 84:999–1004, 2005.

Fragerhol MK, Laurell CB: The Pi system variants of serum alpha-1-antitrypsin, *Prog Med Genet* 7:96–111, 1970.

Frank RM: Bacterial penetration in the apical pocket wall of advanced human periodontitis, *J Periodontal Res* 15:563–573, 1980.

Fredriksson M, Gustafsson A, Asman B, et al: Hyper-reactive peripheral neutrophils in adult periodontitis: generation of chemiluminescence and intracellular hydrogen peroxide after in vitro priming and FCgammaR-stimulation, *J Clin Periodontol* 25:394–398, 1998.

Fredriksson MI, Gustafsson AK, Bergström KG, et al: Constitutionally hyperreactive neutrophils in periodontitis, *J Periodontol* 74:219–224, 2003.

Freeman BA, Crapo JC: Biology of disease. Free radicals and tissue injury. *Lab Invest* 47:421–426, 1982.

Fujihashi K, Komo Y, Yamamoto M, et al: Interleukin production by gingival mononuclear cells isolated from adult periodontitis patients, *J Dent Res* 70:550, 1991.

Fujihashi K, Yamamoto M, McGhee JR, et al: Type 1/Type 2 cytokine production by CD4+ T-cells in adult periodontitis, *J Dent Res* 73:204, 1994.

Fujihashi K, Yamamoto M, Hiroi T, et al: Selected Th1 and Th2 cytokine mrna expression by CD4(+) T-cells isolated from inflamed human gingival tissues, *Clin Exp Immunol* 103:422–428, 1996.

Fujimura S, Nakamura T: Isolation and characterization of a protease from Bacteroides gingivalis, *Infect Immun* 55:716–720, 1987.

Fujimura S, Nakamura T: Multiple forms of proteases of Bacteroides gingivalis and their cellular location, *Oral Microbiol Immunol* 4:227–229, 1989.

Fullmer H, Gibson W: Collagenolytic activity of gingivae of man, *Nature* 209:728–729, 1966.

Garrett IR, Boyce BF, Oreffo ROC, et al: Oxygen-derived free radicals stimulate osteoclastic bone resorption in rodent bone in vitro and in vivo, *J Clin Invest* 85:632–639, 1990.

Gazi MI, Cox SW, Clark DT, et al: Cathepsin B, tryptase and Porphyromonas gingivalis trypsin-like activities in gingival crevicular fluid, *J Dent Res* 73:799, 1994.

Gazi MI, Cox SW, Clark DT, et al: Comparison of host tissue and bacterial dipeptidylpeptidases in human gingival crevicular fluid by analytical isoelectric focusing, *Arch Oral Biol* 40:731–736, 1995.

Gazi MI, Cox SW, Clark DT, et al: A comparison of cysteine and serine proteinases in human gingival crevicular fluid with host tissue, saliva and bacterial enzymes by analytical isoelectric focusing, *Arch Oral Biol* 41:393–400, 1996.

Gazi MI, Cox SW, Clark DT, et al: Characterization of protease activities in Capnocytophaga spp., Porphyromonas gingivalis, Prevotella spp., Treponema denticola and Actinobacillus actinomycetemcomitans, *Oral Microbiol Immunol* 12:240–248, 1997.

Gelb BD, Shi G-P, Chapman HA, et al: Pycnodysostosis, a lysosomal disease caused by cathepsin K deficiency, *Science* 273:1236–1239, 1996a.

Gelb BD, Moissoglu K, Zhang J, et al: Isolation and characterization of the murine cDNA and genomic sequence of the homologue of the human pycnodysostosis gene, *Biochem Mol Med* 59:200–206, 1996b.

Gemmell E, Seymour GJ: Modulation of immune responses to periodontal bacteria, *Curr Opin Periodontol* 94:28–38, 1994.

Gemmell E, Carter CL, Hart DNJ, et al: Antigen-presenting cells in human periodontal disease tissue, *Oral Microbiol Immunol* 17:388–393, 2002.

Gemmell E, Kjeldsen M, Yamazaki K, et al: Cytokine profiles of Porphyromonas gingivalis-reactive T-lymphocyte line and clones derived from P. Gingivalis-infected subjects, *Oral Dis* 1:139–146, 1995.

Gemmell E, Seymour GJ: Cytokine profiles of cells extracted from humans with periodontal diseases, *J Dent Res* 77:16–26, 1998.

Gemmell E, Marshall RI, Seymour GJ: Cytokines and prostaglandins in immune homeostasis and tissue destruction in periodontal disease, *Periodontol 2000* 14:112–143, 1997.

Gemmell E, Grieco DA, Cullinan MP, et al: The proportion of interleukin-4, interferon -10-positive cells in Porphyromonas gingivalis-specific T-cell lines established from P. Gingivalis-positive subjects, *Oral Microbiol Immunol* 14:267–274, 1999.

Gemmell E, Carter CL, Seymour GJ: Mast cells in human periodontal disease, *J Dent Res* 83:384–387, 2004b.

Gemmell E, Bird PS, Ford PJ, et al: Modulation of the antibody response by Porphyromonas gingivalis and Fusobacterium nucleatum in a mouse model, *Oral Microbiol Immunol* 19:247–251, 2004a.

Gendron R, Plamondon P, Grenier D: Binding of pro-matrix metalloproteinase 9 by Fusobacterium nucleatum subsp. nucleatum as a mechanism to promote the invasion of a reconstituted basement membrane, *Infect Immun* 72:6160–6163, 2004.

Gibbons RJ, MacDonald JB: Degradation of collagenous substrates by Bacteroides melaninogenicus, *J Bacteriol* 81:614–621, 1961.

Gillett R, Johnson NW: Bacterial invasion of the periodontium in a case of juvenile periodontitis, *J Clin Periodontol* 9:93–100, 1982.

Giuliana G, Ammatuna P, Pizzo G, et al: Occurrence of invading bacteria in radicular dentin of periodontally diseased teeth: microbiological findings, *J Clin Periodontol* 24:478–485, 1997.

Gmür R, Hrodek K, Saxen UP, et al: Double-blind analysis of relation between adult periodontitis and systemic host responses to suspected periodontal pathogens, *Infect Immun* 52:768–776, 1986.

Goldberg S, Kozlovsky A, Gordon D: Caderverine as a putative component of oral malodour, *J Dent Res* 73:1168–1172, 1994.

Golub L, Wolff M, Lee H, et al: Further evidence that tetracyclines inhibit collagenase activity in human crevicular fluid and other mammalian sources, *J Periodontal Res* 20:12–23, 1985.

Golub L, Sorsa T, Lee HM, et al: Doxycycline inhibits neutrophil (PMN)-type matrix metalloproteinases in human adult periodontitis gingiva, *J Clin Periodontol* 21:1–9, 1989.

Golub L, Sorsa T, Lee HM, et al: Doxycycline inhibits neutrophil (PMN)-type matrix metalloproteinases in human adult periodontitis gingiva, *J Clin Periodontol* 22: 100–109, 1995.

Golub L, Lee HM, Ryan ME, et al: Tetracyclines inhibit connective tissue breakdown by multiple non-antimicrobial mechanisms, *Adv Dent Res* 12:12–26, 1998.

Gonçalves PF, Lima LL, Sallum EA, et al: Root cementum may modulate gene expression during periodontal regeneration: a preliminary study in humans, *J Periodontol* 79:323–331, 2008.

Gowen M, Mundy GR: Actions of recombinant interleukin 1, interleukin 2 and interferon g on bone resorption in vitro, *J Immunol* 136:2478–2482, 1986.

Graves DT, Cochrane D: The contribution of interleukin-1 and tumor necrosis factor to periodontal disease destruction, *J Periodontol* 74:391–401, 2003.

Grenier D: Characteristic of hemolytic and hemagglutinating activities of Treponema denticola, *Oral Microbiol Immunol* 6:246–249, 1991.

Grenier D: Inactivation of human serum bactericidal activity by a trypsin-like protease isolated from Porphyromonas gingivalis, *Infect Immun* 60:1854–1857, 1992.

Grenier D: Degradation of host protease inhibitors and activation of plasminogen by enzymes from Porphyromonas gingivalis and Treponema denticola, *Microbiology* 142:955–961, 1996.

Grenier D, McBride B: Isolation of membrane-associated Bacteroides gingivalis glycylprolyl protease, *Infect Immun* 55:3131–3136, 1987.

Grenier D, Mayrand D: Functional characterization of extracellular vesicles produced by Bacteroides gingivalis, *Infect Immun* 55:111–117, 1987.

Grenier D, Mayrand D: Degradation of tissue inhibitor of metalloproteinases-1 (TIMP-1) by Porphyromonas gingivalis, *FEMS Microbiol Lett* 203:161–164, 2001.

Grenier D, Chao D, McBride BC: Characterization of sodium dodecyl sulfate-stable Bacteroides gingivalis proteases by polyacrylamide gel electrophoresis, *Infect Immun* 57:95–99, 1989a.

Grenier D, Mayrand D, McBride BC: Further studies on the degradation of immunoglobulins and black-pigmented Bacteroides, *Oral Microbiol Immunol* 4:12–18, 1989b.

Grenier D, Uitto VJ, McBride BC: Cellular location of a Treponema denticola chymotrypsin-like protease and the importance of the protease in migration through basement membrane, *Infect Immun* 58:347–351, 1990.

Grenier D, Grignon L: Response of human macrophage-like cells to stimulation by Fusobacterium nucleatum ssp. Nucleatum lipopolysaccharide, *Oral Microbiol Immunol* 21:190–196, 2006.

Gu K, Bainbridge B, Daveau R, et al: Antigenic components of Actinobacillus actinomycetemcomitans lipopolysaccharide recognized by sera from patients with localised juvenile periodontitis, *Oral Microbiol Immunol* 13:150–157, 1998.

Gustafsson A, Asman B, Bergström K: Priming response to inflammatory mediators in hyperreactive peripheral neutrophils from adult periodontitis, *Oral Dis* 3:167–171, 1997.

Hagewald S, Bernimoulin JP, Kottgen E, et al: Total IgA and Porphyromonas gingivalis-reactive IgA in the saliva of patients with generalized early onset periodontitis, *Eur J Oral Sci* 108:147–173, 2000.

Halliwell G, Gutterridge JM: The antioxidants of human extracellular fluids, *Arch Biochem Biophys* 280:1–8, 1990.

Hamlet S, Ellwood R, Cullinan M, et al: Persistent colonization with Tannerella forsythensis and loss of attachment in adolescents, *J Dent Res* 83:232–235, 2004.

Han N, Whitlock J, Progulske-Fox J: The hemagglutinin gene A (hagA) of Porphyromonas gingivalis 381 contains four large, contiguous, direct repeats, *Infect Immun* 64:4000–4007, 1996.

Harada Y, Han X, Yamashita K, et al: Effect of adoptive transfer of antigen-specific B cells on periodontal bone resorption, *J Periodontal Res* 41:101–107, 2006.

Haraldsson G, Holbrook WP, Könönen E: Clonal persistence of oral Fusobacterium nucleatum in infancy, *J Dent Res* 83:500–504, 2004.

Harris ED, Cartwright EC: Mammalial collagenases. In Barrett AJ, editor: *Proteinases in Mammalian Cells and Tissues*, Amsterdam, 1977, Elsevier/North-Holland Biomedical Press, pp 247–283.

Hart DN: Dendritic cells: unique leukocyte population that control the primary immune response, *Blood* 90:3245–3287, 1997.

Harvey W, Kamin S, Meghji S, et al: Interleukin 1-like activity in capsular material from Haemophilus actinomycetemcomitans, *Immunology* 60:415–418, 1987.

Hausmann E: Potential pathways for bone resorption in human periodontal disease, *J Periodontol* 45:338–343, 1974.

Hausmann E, Raisz LG, Miller WA: Endotoxin: stimulation of bone resorption in tissue culture, *Science* 168:862–864, 1970.

Hausmann E, Ludereitz EO, Knox K, et al: Structural requirements for bone resorption by endotoxin and lipoteichoic acid, *J Dent Res* 54:94–99, 1975.

Henderson B, Blake S: Therapeutic potential of cytokine manipulation, *Trends Pharmacol Sci* 13:145–152, 1992.

Henderson D, Poole S, Wilson M: Bacterial modulins: a novel class of virulence factors which cause host tissue pathology by inducing cytokine synthesis, *Microbiol Rev* 60:316–341, 1996a.

Henderson D, Poole S, Wilson M: Microbial/host interactions in health and disease: who controls the cytokine network? *Immunopharmacology* 35:1–21, 1996b.

Henskens YM, van der Velden U, Veerman EC, et al: Protein, albumin and cystatin concentrations in saliva of healthy subjects and of patients with gingivitis or periodontitis, *J Periodontal Res* 28:43–48, 1993a.

Henskens YM, van der Velden U, Veerman EC, et al: Cystatin C levels of whole saliva are increased in periodontal patients, *Ann N Y Acad Sci* 694:280–282, 1993b.

Henskens YM, Veerman EC, Mantel MS, et al: Cystatins S and C in human whole saliva in glandular salivas in periodontal health and disease, *J Dent Res* 73:1606–1614, 1994.

Henskens YM, Veerman EC, Nieuw-Amerongen AV: Cystatins in health and disease, *Biol Chem* 377:71–86, 1996a.

Henskens YM, van den Keijbus PA, Veerman EC, et al: Protein composition of whole and parotid saliva in healthy and periodontitis subjects, *J Periodontal Res* 31:57–65, 1996b.

Henskens YM, Van der Weijden GA, Van den Keijbus PA, et al: Effects of periodontal treatment on the protein composition of whole and parotid saliva, *J Periodontol* 67:205–212, 1996c.

Hinode D, Hayashi H, Nakamura R: Purification and characterization of three types of proteases from culture supernatants of Porphyromonas gingivalis, *Infect Immun* 59:3060–3068, 1991.

Hinode D, Nagata A, Ichimiya S, et al: Generation of plasma kinin by three types of protease isolated from Porphyromonas gingivalis 381, *Arch Oral Biol* 37:859–861, 1992.

Hirano K, Okamura Y, Hayakawa S, et al: Inhibition of human tissue kallikrein by a-1-proteinase inhibitor, *Hoppe Seyer Zeitschrift Physiologica Chemie* 365:27–32, 1984.

Hönig J, Rordorf-Adam C, Siegmund C, et al: Increased interleukin-1-beta (IL-1β) concentration in gingival tissue from periodontitis patients and healthy controls, *J Periodontal Res* 24:362–367, 1989.

Hopps RM, Sisney-Durrant HJ: Mechanisms of alveolar bone loss in periodontal disease. In Hamada S, Holt SC, McGhee JR, editors: *Periodontal Disease Pathogens and Host Immune Response*, Tokyo, 1991, Quintessence, pp 307–320.

Horowitz A, Folke EA: Hydrogen sulphide and periodontal disease, *Periodontal Abstr* 2:59–62, 1972.

Hosogi Y, Duncan MJ: Gene expression in Porphyromonas gingivalis after contact with human epithelial cells, *Infect Immun* 73:2327–2335, 2005.

Hou LT, Liu CM, Liu BY, et al: Interleukin-1beta, clinical parameters and matched histopathologic changes in biopsied gingival tissue from periodontitis patients, *J Periodontal Res* 38:247–254, 2003.

Houri-Haddad Y, Soskolne WA, Halabi A, et al: IL-10 Gene transfer attenuates P. Gingivalis-induced inflammation, *J Dent Res* 86:560–564, 2007.

Huang GT, Kinder Haake S, Kim J, et al: Differential expression of interleukin-8 and intracellular adhesion molecule-1 by human gingival epithelial cells in response to Actinobacillus actinomycetemcomitans or Porphyromonas gingivalis infection, *Oral Microbiol Immunol* 13:301–309, 1998.

Huang GT, Kim D, Lee JK, et al: Interleukin-8 and intercellular adhesion molecule 1 regulation in oral epithelial cells by selected periodontal bacteria: multiple effects from Porphyromonas gingivalis via antagonistic mechanisms, *Infect Immun* 69:1364–1372, 2001.

Hussain A, Kennett CN, Allaker R, et al: Stimulation of cathepsin B activity in cultured gingival fibroblasts by host and bacterial factors, *J Dent Res* 76:1048, Abstract 235, 1997.

Hutchison DC: alpha1-Antitrypsin deficiency in Europe: geographical distribution of Pi types S and Z, *Respir Med* 92:367–377, 1998.

Ide M, Jagdev D, Coward PY, et al: The short-term effects of treatment of chronic periodontitis on circulating levels of endotoxin, c-reactive protein, tumor necrosis factor-alpha, and interleukin-6, *J Periodontol* 75:420–428, 2004.

Ilgenli T, Vardar-Sengul S, Gürkan A, et al: Gingival crevicular fluid matrix metalloproteinase-13 levels and molecular forms in various types of periodontal diseases, *Oral Dis* 12:573–579, 2006.

Inaba H, Nakano K, Kato T, et al: Heterogenic virulence and related factors among clinical isolates of Porphyromonas gingivalis with type II fimbriae, *Oral Microbiol Immunol* 23:29–35, 2008.

Inagaki S, Onishi S, Kuramitsu HK, et al: Porphyromonas gingivalis vesicles enhance attachment, and the leucine-rich repeat BspA protein is required for invasion of epithelial cells by Tannerella forsythia, *Infect Immun* 74:5023–5028, 2006.

Imamura T: The role of gingipains in the pathogenesis of periodontal disease, *J Periodontol* 74:111–118, 2003.

Imamura T, Potempa J, Pike RN, et al: Effect of free and vesicle-bound cysteine proteinases of Porphyromonas gingivalis on plasma clot formation: implications for bleeding tendency at periodontitis sites, *Infect Immun* 63:4877–4882, 1995.

Imamura T, Potempa J, Tenase S, et al: Activation of blood coagulation factor X by arginine-specific cysteine proteinase (gingipain R) from Porphyromonas gingivalis, *J Biol Chem* 272:16062–16067, 1997.

Inaoka T, Bilbe G: Ishibashi O, et al: Molecular cloning of human cDNA for cathepsin K: novel cysteine proteinase predominantly expressed in bone, *Biochem Biophys Res Commun* 206:89–96, 1995.

Inui T, Ishibashi O, Inaoka T, et al: Cathepsin K antisense oligonucleotide inhibits osteoclastic bone resorption, *J Biol Chem* 272:8109–8112, 1997.

Jagle MA, Ember JA, Travis J, et al: Cleavage of the C5a receptor by proteinase derived from Porphyromonas gingivalis. In Suzuki K, Bond J, editors: *Intracellular protein catabolism*, New York, 1996, Plenum Press, pp 155–164.

James IE, Dodds RA, Lee-Rykaczewski E, et al: Purification and characterization of fully functional human osteoclast precursors, *J Bone Miner Res* 11:1608–1618, 1996.

James K: Interactions between cytokines and alpha 2-macroglobulin, *Immunol Today* 11:163–166, 1990.

Jansen HJ, Grenier D, Van der Hoeven JS: Characterization of immunoglobulin G-degrading proteases of Prevotella intermedia and Prevotella nigrescens, *Oral Microbiol Immunol* 10:138–145, 1995.

Jarnbring F, Somogyi E, Dalton J, et al: Quantitative assessment of apoptotic and proliferative gingival keratinocytes in oral and sulcular epithelium in patients with gingivitis or periodontitis, *J Clin Periodontol* 29:1065–1071, 2002.

Jenkins K, Javadi M, Carter Borghaei R: Interleukin-4 suppresses IL-1-induced expression of matrix metalloproteinase-3 in human gingival fibroblasts, *J Periodontol* 75:283–291, 2004.

Ji S, Kim Y, Min B et al, Innate immune responses of gingival epithelial cells to nonperiodontopathic and periodontopathic bacteria, *J Periodontal Res* 42:503–510, 2007.

Johnson MR, Polymeropoulos MH, Vos HL, et al: A nonsense mutation in the cathepsin K gene observed in a family with pycnodysostosis, *Genome Res* 6:1050–1055, 1996.

Johnson PW, Tonzetich J: Solubilization of acid-soluble collagen by H_2S, *J Dent Res* 58:283, Abstract 763, 1979.

Johnson PW, Tonzetich J: Effect of H_2S on protein synthesis by gingival fibroblasts, *J Dent Res* 61:260. Abstract 736, 1982.

Johnson PW, Ng W, Tonzetich J: Modulation of human gingival fibroblast cell metabolism by methyl mercaptan, *J Periodontal Res* 27:476–483, 1992a.

Johnson PW, Yaegaki K, Tonzetich J: Effects of volatile sulphur compounds on protein metabolism by human gingival fibroblasts, *J Periodontal Res* 27:553–561, 1992b.

Johnstone AM, Koh A, Goldberg MB, et al: A hyperactive neutrophil phenotype in patients with refractory periodontitis, *J Periodontol* 78:1788–1794, 2007.

Johnson RB, Wood N, Serio FG: Interleukin-11 and IL-17 and the pathogenesis of periodontal disease, *J Periodontol* 75:37–43, 2004.

Johnson RB, Serio FG: Interleukin-18 concentrations and the pathogenesis of periodontal disease, *J Periodontol* 76:785–790, 2005.

Joshipura KJ, Wand HC, Merchant AT, et al: Periodontal disease and biomarkers related to cardiovascular disease, *J Dent Res* 83:151–155, 2004.

Kadowaki T, Yoneda M, Okamoto K, et al: Purification and characterization of a novel arginine-specific cysteine proteinase (arg-gingipain) involved in the pathogenesis of periodontal disease from the culture supernatants of Porphyromonas gingivalis, *J Biol Chem* 269:21371–21378, 1994.

Kafienah W, Bromme D, Buttle DJ, et al: Human cathepsin K cleaves native type I and II collagens at the N-terminal end of the triple helix, *Biochem J* 331:727–732, 1998.

Kamin S, Harvey W, Wilson M, et al: Inhibition of fibroblast proliferation and collagen synthesis by capsular material from Actinobacillus actinomycetemcomitans, *J Med Biol* 22:245–249, 1986.

Kaminishi H, Cho T, Itoh T, et al: Vascular permeability enhancing activity of Porphyromonas gingivalis protease in guinea pigs, *FEMS Microbiol Lett* 114:109–114, 1993.

Kamolmatyakul S, Chen W, Yang S, et al: IL-1alpha stimulates cathepsin K expression in osteoclasts via the tyrosine kinase-NF-kappaB pathway, *J Dent Res* 83:791–796, 2004.

Kaplan JB, Kokeguchi S, Murayama Y, et al: Sequence diversity in the major fimbrial subunit gene (fip-1) of Actinobacillus actinomycetemcomitans, *Oral Microbiology and Immunity* 17:354–359, 2002.

Kato T, Takahashi N, Kuramitsu H: Sequence analysis and characterization of the Porphyromonas gingivalis ptrC gene, which expresses a novel collagenase activity, *J Bacteriol* 174:3889–3895, 1992.

Kato N, Ohyama H, Nishimura F, et al: Role of helper T cells in the humoral immune responses against 53-kDa outer membrane protein from Porphyromonas gingivalis, *Oral Microbiol Immunol* 20:112–117, 2005.

Kato T, Tsuda T, Inaba H, et al: Porphyromonas gingivalis gingipains cause G1 arrest in osteoblastic/stromal cells, *Oral Microbiol Immunol* 23:158–164, 2008.

Kawai T, Paster BJ, Komatsuzawa H, et al: Cross-reactive adaptive immune response to oral commensal bacteria results in an induction of receptor activator of nuclear factor-kappaB ligand (RANKL)-dependent periodontal bone resorption in a mouse model, *Oral Microbiol Immunol* 22:208–215, 2007.

Kay HM, Birss AJ, Smalley JW: Glycylprolyl dipeptidase activity of Bacteroides gingivalis W50 and the avirulent variant W50/DE1, *FEMS Microbiol Lett* 57:93–96, 1989.

Keiso T, Takashi A, Hitoshi M, et al: The potential role of interleukin-17 in the immunopathology of periodontal disease, *J Clin Periodontol* 32:369–374, 2005.

Kelso A: Cytokines in infectious disease, *Australian Microbiology* 11:372–376, 1990.

Kelso A: Th1 and Th2 subsets: paradigms lost? *Immunol Today* 16:374–379, 1995.

Kennett CN, Cox SW, Eley BM, et al: Comparative histochemical and biochemical studies of mast cell tryptase in human gingiva, *J Periodontol* 64:870–877, 1993.

Kennett CN, Cox SW, Eley BM: Comparative histochemical, biochemical and immunocytochemical studies of cathepsin B in human gingiva, *J Periodontal Res* 29:870–877, 1994.

Kennett CN, Cox SW, Eley BM: Localization of active and inactive elastase, alpha-1-proteinase inhibitor and alpha-2-macroglobulin in human gingiva, *J Dent Res* 74: 667–674, 1995.

Kennett CN, Cox SW, Eley BM: Investigations into the cellular contribution to host tissue protease activity in gingival crevicular fluid, *J Clin Periodontol* 24:424–431, 1997a.

Kennett CN, Cox SW, Eley BM: Ultrastructural localization of cathepsin B in gingival tissue from chronic periodontitis patients, *Histochem J* 29:727–734, 1997b.

Kennett CN, Hussain A, Allaker R, et al: Stimulation of DPP IV activity in cultured gingival fibroblasts by host and bacterial factors, *J Dent Res* 76:1048, Abstract 235, 1997c.

Kerzbaum L, Sotiropoulos C, Jackson C, et al: Complete nucleotide sequence of a gene prtR of Porphyromonas gingivalis W50 encoding a 132 kDa protein that contains an arginine specific thiol endopeptidase domain and a haemagglutinin domain, *Biochem Biophys Res Commun* 207:424–431, 1995.

Kesavulu L, Holt SC, Ebersole JL: Trypsin-like protease activity of Porphyromonas gingivalis as a potential virulence factor in murine lesion model, *Microbial Pathogen* 20:1–10, 1996.

Kesavalu L, Sathishkumar S, Bakthavatchalu V, et al: Rat model of polymicrobial infection, immunity, and alveolar bone resorption in periodontal disease, *Infect Immun* 75:1704–1717, 2007.

Kiili M, Cox SW, Chen HY, et al: Collagenase-2 (MMP-8) and collagenase-3 (MMP-13) in adult periodontitis: molecular forms and levels in gingival crevicular fluid and immunolocalization in gingival tissue, *J Clin Periodontol* 29:224–232, 2002.

Kilian M: Degradation of immunoglobulins A1, A2 and G by suspected principal periodontal pathogens, *Infect Immun* 34:757–765, 1981.

Kim SJ, Ha MS, Choi EY, et al: Prevotella intermedia lipopolysaccharide stimulates release of nitric oxide by inducing expression of inducible nitric oxide synthase, *J Periodontal Res* 39:424–431, 2004.

Kinane DF, Mooney J, MacFarlane T, et al: Local and systemic antibody response to putative periodontal pathogens in patients with chronic periodontitis. Correlation with clinical indices, *Oral Microbiol Immunol* 8:65–68, 1993.

Kinane DF, Lappin DF, Koulouri O, et al: Humoral immune responses in periodontal disease may have mucosal and systemic immune features, *Clinical and Experimental Immunity* 115:534–541, 1999.

Kinane DF, Mooney J, Ebersole JL: Humoral immune response to Actinobacillus actinomycetemcomitans and Porphyromonas gingivalis in periodontal disease, *Periodontology 2000* 20:289–340, 1999.

Kirby AC, Meghji S, Nair SP, et al: The potent bone-resorbing mediator of Actinobacillus actinomycetemcomitans is homologous to the molecular chaperone GroEL, *J Clin Invest* 96:1185–1194, 1995.

Kleinberg I, Westbay G: Salivary and metabolic factors involved in oral malodour formation, *J Periodontol* 63:768–775, 1992.

Kobayashi H, Nagasawa T, Aramaki M, et al: Individual diversities in interferon gamma production by human peripheral blood mononuclear cells stimulated by periodontopathic bacteria, *J Periodontal Res* 35:319–328, 2000.

Kobayashi T, Kaneko S, Tahara T, et al: Antibody responses to Porphyromonas gingivalis hemagglutinin A and outer membrane protein in chronic periodontitis, *J Periodontol* 77:364–369, 2006.

Koizumi Y, Kurita-Ochiai T, Yamamoto M: Transcutaneous immunization with an outer membrane protein of Porphyromonas gingivalis without adjuvant elicits marked antibody responses, *Oral Microbiol Immunol* 23:131–138, 2008.

Konstantinidis A, Sakellari D, Papa A, et al: Real-time polymerase chain reaction quantification of Epstein–Barr virus in chronic periodontitis patients, *J Periodontal Res* 40:294–298, 2005.

Korkmaz B, Attucci S, Jourdan ML, et al: Inhibition of neutrophil elastase by alpha1-protease inhibitor at the surface of human polymorphonuclear neutrophils, *J Immunol* 175:3329–3338, 2005.

Kubar A, Saygun I, Özdemir A, et al: Real-time polymerase chain reaction quantification of human cytomegalovirus and Epstein–Barr virus in periodontal pockets and the adjacent gingiva of periodontitis lesions, *J Periodontal Res* 40:187–191, 2005.

Kuramitsu HK: Proteases of Porphyromonas gingivalis: what don't they do? *Oral Microbiol Immunol* 13:263–270, 1998.

Kusumoto Y, Hirano H, Saitoh K, et al: Human gingival epithelial cells produce chemoattractant factors interleukin-8 and monocyte chemoattractant protein-1 after stimulation with Porphyromonas gingivalis via toll-like receptor 2, *J Periodontol* 75:370–379, 2004.

L'Allemain G, Franchi A, Gragoe E, et al: Blockage of the Na+/H+ antiport abolishes growth factor-induced DNA synthesis in fibroblasts, *J Biol Chem* 259:4313–4319, 1984.

Lamster IB, Kaluszhner-Shapira CE, Herrera-Abreu M, et al: Serum igg antibody response to Actinobacillus actinomycetemcomitans and Porphyromonas gingivalis: implications for periodontal diagnosis, *J Clin Periodontol* 25:510–516, 1998.

Lancero H, Niu J, Johnson PW: Exposure of periodontal ligament cells to methyl mercaptan, *J Dent Res* 75:1994–2002, 1996.

Lantz MS, Allen RD, Duck RD, et al: Porphyromonas gingivalis surface components bind and degrade connective tissue proteins, *J Periodontal Res* 26:283–285, 1991a.

Lantz MS, Allen RD, Vail TA, et al: Specific cell components of Bacteroides gingivalis mediate binding and degradation of human fibrinogen, *J Bacteriol* 173:495–504, 1991b.

Lantz MS, Allen RD, Chiorowski P, et al: Purification and immunolocalization of a cysteine protease from Porphyromonas gingivalis, *J Periodontal Res* 28:467–469, 1993.

Lappin DF, McGregor AMP, Kinane DF: The systemic immune response is more prominent than the mucosal immune response in the pathogenesis of periodontal disease, *J Clin Periodontol* 30:778–786, 2003.

Larjava H, Häkkinen L, Rahemtulla F: A biochemical analysis of human periodontal tissue proteoglycans, *Biochem J* 284:267–274, 1992.

Lasfargues JJ, Saffir JL: Effect of indomethacin on bone destruction during experimental periodontal disease on the hamster, *J Periodontal Res* 18:110–117, 1983.

Laughton BE, Syed SA, Loesche WJ: API ZYM system for the identification of Bacteroides spp., Capnocytophaga spp, and spirochaetes of oral origin, *J Clin Microbiol* 15:97–102, 1982a.

Laughton BE, Syed SA, Loesche WJ: The rapid identification of Bacteroides gingivalis, *J Clin Microbiol* 15:345–346, 1982b.

Lawson DA, Meyer TF: Biochemical characterization of Porphyromonas (Bacteroides) gingivalis collagenase, *Infect Immun* 60:1524–1529, 1992.

Lazner F, Gowen M, Pavasovic D, et al: Osteopetrosis and osteoporosis: two sides of the same coin, *Hum Mol Genet* 8:1839–1846, 1999.

Lee W, Aitken S, Sodek J, et al: Evidence for a direct relationship between neutrophil collagenase activity and periodontal disease destruction in vivo; the role of active enzyme in human periodontitis, *J Periodontal Res* 30:23–33, 1995.

Lee JY, Yi NN, Kim US, et al: Porphyromonas gingivalis heat shock protein vaccine reduces the alveolar bone loss induced by multiple periodontopathogenic bacteria, *J Periodontal Res* 41:10–14, 2006.

Lensgraf EJ, Greenblatt JJ, Bowden JW: Effect of group A streptococcal peptidoglycan and group A streptococcal cell wall on bone in tissue culture, *Arch Oral Biol* 24: 495–498, 1979.

Lester SR, Bain JL, Johnson RB, et al: Gingival concentrations of interleukin-23 and -17 at healthy sites and at sites of clinical attachment loss, *J Periodontol* 78:1545–1550, 2007.

Lewis JP, Macrina FL: IS195, an insertional sequence-like element associated with protease genes in Porphyromonas gingivalis, *Infect Immun* 66:3035–3042, 1998.

Li L, Matevski D, Aspiras M, et al: Two epithelial cell invasion-related loci of the oral pathogen Actinobacillus actinomycetemcomitans, *Oral Microbiology and Immunity* 19:16–25, 2004.

Liakoni H, Barber P, Newman HN: Bacterial penetration of pocket soft tissues in chronic adult and juvenile periodontitis cases. An ultrastructural study, *J Clin Periodontol* 14:22–28, 1987.

Ling LJ, Ho C-C, Wu CY, et al: Association between human Herpesviruses and the severity of periodontitis, *J Periodontol* 75:1479–1485, 2004.

Littlewood-Evans A, Kokubo T, Ishibashi, et al: Localization of cathepsin K in human osteoclasts by in situ hybridization and immunocytochemistry, *Bone* 20:81–86, 1997.

Loebermann H, Tokuoka R, Diesenhofer J, et al: Human alpha-1-proteinase inhibitor: crystal structure analysis of two crystal modifications, molecular model and preliminary analysis of the implications for function, *J Mol Biol* 177:531–556, 1984.

Loesche WJ, Syed SA, Schmidt E, et al: Bacterial profiles of subgingival plaques in periodontitis, *J Periodontol* 56:447–456, 1985.

Lohinai Z, Mabley JG, Fehér E, et al: Role of the activation of the nuclear enzyme poly (ADP-ribose) polymerase in the pathogenesis of periodontitis, *J Dent Res* 82:987–992, 2003.

Long GL, Chandra T, Woo SL, et al: Complete sequence of the cDNA for human alpha1-antitrypsin and the gene for the S variant, *Biochemistry* 23:4828–4837, 1984.

Lopatin DE, Blackburn E: Avidity and titre of immunoglobulin G subclasses to Porphyromonas gingivalis in adult periodontitis patients, *Oral Microbiol Immunol* 7:332–337, 1992.

Loubakos A, Yuan YP, Jenkins AL, et al: Activation of protease-activated receptors by gingipains from Porphyromonas gingivalis leads to platelet aggregation: a new trait in microbial pathogenicity, *Blood* 97:3790–3797, 2001.

Löwick CWGM, van der Pluijm G, Bloys H, et al: Parathyroid hormone (PTH) and PTH-like protein (PLP) stimulate interleukin-6 production by osteogenic cells: a possible role of interleukin-6 in osteoclastogenesis, *Biochem Biophys Res Commun* 162: 1546–1552, 1989.

Ma J, Sorsa T, Billinghurst CR, et al: Direct evidence of collagenolysis in chronic periodontitis, *J Periodontal Res* 38:564–567, 2003.

Macfarlane SR, Seatler MJ, Kanke T, et al: Protease-activated receptors, *Pharmacology Reviews* 53:245–282, 2001.

McArthur WP, Clark WB: Specific antibodies and their potential role in periodontal diseases, *J Periodontol* 64:807–818, 1993.

McDermid AS, McKee AS, Marsh PD: Effect of pH on enzyme activity and growth of Bacteroides gingivalis W50, *Infect Immun* 56:1096–1100, 1988.

McDowell JV, Lankford J, Stamm L, et al: Demonstration of factor H-like protein 1 binding to Treponema denticola, a pathogen associated with periodontal disease in humans, *Infect Immun* 73:7126–7132, 2005.

McQueney MS, Amegadzie BY, D'Alessio K, et al: Auto catalytic activation of human cathepsin K, *J Biol Chem* 272:13955–13960, 1997.

Madianos PN, Papanou PN, Sandros J: Porphyromonas gingivalis infection of oral epithelium inhibits neutrophil trans-epithelial migration, *Infect Immun* 65:3983–3990, 1997.

Madianos PN, Bobetsis YA, Kinane DF: Generation of inflammatory stimuli: how bacteria set up inflammatory responses in the gingiva, *J Clin Periodontol* 32:57–71, 2005.

Mahadeva R, Lomas DA: a1 Antitrypsin deficiency, cirrhosis and emphysema, *Thorax* 53:501–505, 1998.

Mahanonda R, Sa-Ard-Iam N, Charatkulangkun O, et al: Monocyte activation by Porphyromonas gingivalis LPS in aggressive periodontitis with the use of whole-blood cultures, *J Dent Res* 83:540–545, 2004.

Mäkinen KK, Syed SA, Mäkinen PL: Benzylarginine peptidase and immunopeptidase profiles of Treponema denticola strains isolated from the human periodontal pocket, *Curr Microbiol* 14:85–89, 1986.

Mäkinen KK, Syed SA, Mäkinen PL, et al: Dominance of immunopeptidase activity in the human oral bacterium Treponema denticola ATCC 35405, *Curr Microbiol* 14:341–346, 1987.

Mäkinen KK, Syed SA, Loesche WJ, et al: Proteolytic profile of Treponema denticola ATCC 35580 with special reference to collagenolytic and arginine aminopeptidase activity, *Oral Microbiol Immunol* 3:121–128, 1988.

Makinen KK, Makinen PL: The peptidolytic capacity of the spirochete system, *Med Microbiol Immunol (Berlin)* 185:1–10, 1996.

Makinen KK, Makinen PL, Syed S: Role of the chymotrypsin-like protease from Treponema denticola ATCC 35405 in inactivation of human bioactive peptides, *Infect Immun* 63:3567–3575, 1995.

Manhardt SS, Reinhardt RA, Payne JB, et al: Gingival cell IL-2 and IL-4 in early-onset periodontitis, *J Periodontol* 65:807–813, 1994.

Mano H, Yuasa T, Kameda T, et al: Mammalian mature osteoclasts and estrogen target cells, *Biochem Biophys Res Commun* 223:637–642, 1996.

Manor A, Lebendiger M, Shiffer A, et al: Bacterial invasion of the periodontal tissues in advanced periodontitis in humans, *J Periodontol* 55:567–573, 1984.

Martuscelli G, Fiorellini JP, Crohin CC, et al: The effect of IL-11 on the progress of ligature-induced periodontal disease in the beagle dog, *J Periodontol* 71:573–578, 2000.

Masada MP, Persson R, Kenney JS, et al: Measurement of interleukin-1alpha and -1beta in gingival crevicular fluid: implications for the pathogenesis of periodontal disease, *J Periodontal Res* 25:156–163, 1990.

Meghji S: Bone remodelling, *Br Dent J* 172:235–242, 1992.

Meghji S, Sandy JR, Scutt AM, et al: Stimulation of bone resorption by lipo-oxygenase metabolites of arachidonic acid, *Prostaglandins* 36:139–149, 1988.

Meghji S, Henderson B, Nair S, et al: Inhibition of bone DNA and collagen production by surface-associated material from bacteria implicated in the pathology of periodontal disease, *J Periodontol* 63:736–742, 1992a.

Meghji S, Wilson M, Henderson B, et al: Anti proliferative and cytotoxic activity of surface associated material from periodontopathic bacteria, *Arch Oral Biol* 37: 637–644, 1992b.

Meghji S, Henderson B, Wilson M: High titre antisera from patients with periodontal disease inhibit bacterial-capsule-induced bone breakdown, *J Periodontal Res* 28: 115–121, 1993.

Meghji S, Barber P, Wilson M, et al: Bone resorbing activity of surface-associated material from Actinobacillus actinomycetemcomitans and Eikenella corrodens, *J Med Microbiol* 41:197–203, 1994.

Meikle MC, Heath JK, Reynolds JJ: Advances in understanding cell interactions in tissue resorption, Relevance to the pathogenesis of periodontal diseases and a new hypothesis. *J Oral Pathol* 15:239–250, 1986.

Mezyk-Kope R, Bzowska M, Potempa J, et al: Inactivation of membrane tumor necrosis factor alpha by gingipains from Porphyromonas gingivalis, *Infect Immun* 73: 1506–1514, 2005.

Mikolajczyk-Pawlinska J, Kordula T, Pavoff N, et al: Genetic variation of Porphyromonas gingivalis genes encoding gingipains, cysteine proteinases with arginine or lysine specificity, *J Biol Chem* 379:205–211, 1998.

Mikx FH, De Jong MH: Keratinolytic activity of cutaneous and oral bacteria, *Infect Immun* 55:621–625, 1987.

Millar SJ, Goldstein EJ, Levine MJ, et al: Lipoprotein: a Gram negative cell wall component that stimulates bone resorption, *J Periodontal Res* 21:256–259, 1986.

Miller WD: *The Microorganisms of the Human Mouth. The Local and General Diseases Which are Caused by Them*, Philadelphia, 1890, SS White Dental Manufacturing.

Minhas T, Greenman J: Production of cell-bound and vesicle-associated trypsin-like protease, alkaline phosphatase and N-acetyl-beta-glucosaminidase by Bacteroides gingivalis W50, *J Gen Microbiol* 135:564–577, 1989.

Missailidis CG, Umeda JE, Ota-Tsuzuki C, et al: Distribution of FimA genotypes of Porphyromonas gingivalis in subjects with various periodontal conditions, *Oral Microbiol Immunol* 19:224–229, 2004.

Miura M, Hamachi T, Fujise O, et al: The prevalence and pathogenic differences of Porphyromonas gingivalis FimA genotypes in patients with aggressive periodontitis, *J Periodontal Res* 40:147–152, 2005.

Miyaki H, Sakao S, Katoh Y, et al: Correlation between volatile sulphur compounds and certain oral health measurements in the general population, *J Periodontol* 66:679–684, 1995.

Mogi M, Otogoto J, Ota N, et al: Differential expression of RANKL and osteoprotegerin in gingival crevicular fluid of patients with periodontitis, *J Dent Res* 83:166–169, 2004.

Mogi M, Otogoto J: Expression of cathepsin-K in gingival crevicular fluid, *Arch Oral Biol* 52:894–898, 2007.

Molhuizen HO, Schalkwijk J: Structural, biochemical, and cell biological aspects of the serine proteinase inhibitor SKALP/Elafin/ESI, *Biol Chem* 376:1–7, 1995.

Moncla BL, Braham P, Hillier SL: Sialidase (neuraminidase) activity among Gram-negative anaerobic and capnophilic bacteria, *J Clin Microbiol* 28:422–425, 1990.

Moore J, Wilson M, Kieser JB: The distribution of bacterial lipopolysaccharide (endotoxin) in relation to periodontally involved root surfaces, *J Clin Periodontol* 13:748–751, 1986.

Mortensen SB, Kilian M: Purification and characterization of immunoglobulin A1 protease from Bacteroides melaninogenicus, *Infect Immun* 45:550–557, 1984.

Moseley R, Waddington RJ, Evans P, et al: The chemical moderation of glycosaminoglycan structure by oxygen-derived species in vitro, *Biochim Biophys Acta* 1244:245–252, 1995.

Mosmann TR: Cytokines: is there biological meaning, *Curr Opin Immunol* 3:311–314, 1991.

Nagasawa T, Kobayashi H, Aramaki M, et al: Expression of CD14, CD16 and CD45A on monocytes from periodontitis patients, *J Periodontal Res* 39:72–78, 2004.

Nair SP, Meghji S, Wilson M, et al: Bacterially induced bone destruction: mechanisms and misconceptions, *Infect Immun* 64:2371–2380, 1996.

Nakagawa I, Inaba H, Yamamura T, et al: Invasion of epithelial cells and proteolysis of cellular focal adhesion components by distinct types of Porphyromonas gingivalis fimbriae, *Infection and Immunity* 74:3773–3782, 2006.

Nakajima T, Ueki-Maruyama K, Oda T, et al: Regulatory T-cells infiltrate periodontal disease tissues, *J Dent Res* 84:639–643, 2005.

Nakamura R, Hinode D, Terai H, et al: Extracellular enzymes of Porphyromonas (Bacteroides) gingivalis in relation to periodontal destruction. In Hamada S, Holt SC, McGhee JR, editors: *Periodontal Disease: Pathogens and Host Immune Responses*, Tokyo, 1991, Quintessence, pp 129–141.

Nakamura M, Slots J: Aminopeptidases of *Capnocytophaga*, *J Periodontal Res* 17: 597–603, 1982.

Sheets SM, Potempa J, Travis J, et al: Gingipains from Porphyromonas gingivalis W83 synergistically disrupt endothelial cell adhesion and can induce caspase-independent apoptosis, *Infect Immun* 74:5667–5678, 2006.

Shelburne CE, Gleason RM, Coulter WA, et al: Differential display analysis of Porphyromonas gingivalis gene activation response to heat and oxidative stress, *Oral Microbiol Immunol* 20:233–238, 2005.

Sighagen B, Hamberg M, Fredholm BB: Formation of 12L-hydroxyeicosatetraenoic acid (12 HETE) by gingival tissue, *J Dent Res* 61:761–763, 1982.

Sigushi B, Klinger G, Glockmann E, et al: Early-onset and adult periodontitis associated with abnormal cytokine production by activated T-lymphocytes, *J Periodontol* 69:1098–1104, 1998.

Shapira L, Wilensky A, Kinane DF: Effect of genetic variability on the inflammatory response to periodontal infection, *J Clin Periodontol* 32:72–86, 2005.

Simchowitz I, Cragoe E: Regulation of human neutrophil chemotaxis by intracellular pH, *J Biol Chem* 261:6492–6500, 1986.

Slakeski N, Bhogal PS, O'Brien-Simpson N, et al: Characterization of a second cell-associated Arg-specific cysteine proteinase of Porphyromonas gingivalis and identification of an adhesin-binding motif involved in association of the ptrR and prtK proteinase and adhesins into large complexes, *Microbiology* 144:1583–1593, 1998.

Slakeski N, Cleal SM, Bhogal PS, et al: Characterization of a Porphyromonas gingivalis gene, prtK that encodes a lysine specific cysteine proteinase and three sequence-related adhesins, *Oral Microbiol Immunol* 14:92–97, 1999.

Slaney JM, Gallagher A, Aduse-Opoku J, et al: Mechanisms of resistance of Porphyromonas gingivalis to killing by serum complement, *Infect Immun* 74: 5352–5361, 2006.

Slots J: Enzymatic characterization of some oral and non-oral Gram-negative bacteria with the API ZYM system, *J Clin Microbiol* 14:288–294, 1981.

Slots J, Genco RJ: Black pigmented Bacteroides species, Capnocytophaga species and Actinobacillus actinomycetemcomitans in human periodontal disease: virulence factors in colonization, survival and tissue destruction, *J Dent Res* 63:412–421, 1984.

Slots J, Saygun I, Sabeti M, et al: Epstein–Barr virus in oral diseases, *J Periodontal Res* 41:235–244, 2006.

Smalley JW, Birss AJ: Trypsin-like enzyme activity of the extracellular membrane vesicles of Bacteroides gingivalis W50, *J Gen Microbiol* 133:2883–2894, 1987.

Smalley JW, Birss AJ, Suttleworth CA: Degradation of type I collagen and human plasma fibrinogen by trypsin-like enzyme and extracellular membrane vesicles of Bacteroides gingivalis W50, *Arch Oral Biol* 33:323–329, 1988a.

Smalley JW, Birss AJ, Suttleworth CA: Effect of the outer membrane fraction of Bacteroides gingivalis W50 on the glycosaminoglycan metabolism by human fibroblasts, *Arch Oral Biol* 33:547–553, 1988b.

Smith KC, Su WP, Pittelkow MR, et al: Clinical and pathologic correlations in 96 patients with panniculitis, including 15 patients with deficient levels of alpha1-antitrypsin, *J Am Acad Dermatol* 21:1192–1196, 1989.

Söderling E, Mäkinen PL, Syed SA, et al: Biochemical comparison of proteolytic enzymes present in rough- and smooth-surfaced Capnocytophaga isolated from the subgingival plaque of periodontitis patients, *J Periodontal Res* 26:17–23, 1991.

Sojar HT, Lee JY, Bedi GS, et al: Purification and characterization of a protease from Porphyromonas gingivalis capable of degrading salt-solubilized collagen, *Infect Immun* 61:2369–2376, 1993.

Soory M: A role for non-antimicrobial actions of tetracyclines in combating oxidative stress in periodontal and metabolic diseases, *Open Dentistry Journal* 2:5–12, 2008.

Sorsa T, Uitto VJ, Suomalainen K, et al: A trypsin-like protease from Bacteroides gingivalis. Partial purification and characterization. *J Periodontal Res* 22:375–380, 1987.

Sorsa T, Ingman T, Suomalainen K, et al: Identification of proteases from periodontopathic bacteria as activators of latent human neutrophil and fibroblast type interstitial collagenases, *Infect Immun* 60:4491–4495, 1992.

Sorsa T, Tjäderhane L, Salo T: Matrix metalloproteinases (MMPs) in oral diseases, *Oral Dis* 10:311–318, 2004.

Steenbergen W: α_1-Antitrypsin deficiency: an overview, *Acta Clin Belg* 48:171–189, 1993.

Steffan EK, Hengtes DJ: Hydrolytic enzymes of anaerobic bacteria isolated from human infections, *J Clin Microbiol* 14:153–156, 1981.

Steinsvoll S, Helgeland K, Schenck K: Mast cells – a role in periodontal diseases? *J Clin Periodontol* 31:413–419, 2004.

Suido H, Nakamura M, Mashimo PA, et al: Arylaminopeptidase activities of oral bacteria, *J Dent Res* 65:1335–1340, 1986.

Suido H, Neiders ME, Barua PK, et al: Characterization of the N-CBz-glycyl-glycyl-arginyl peptidase and glycyl-prolyl peptidase of Bacteroides gingivalis, *J Periodontal Res* 22:412–418, 1987.

Suido H, Eguchi T, Nakamura M: Investigation of periodontopathic bacteria based upon their peptidase activities, *Adv Dent Res* 2:304–309, 1988a.

Suido H, Zambon JJ, Mashimo PA, et al: Correlations between gingival crevicular fluid enzymes and the subgingival microflora, *J Dent Res* 67:1070–1074, 1988b.

Sundqvist G, Carlsson J, Hänström L: Collagenolytic activity of black-pigmented Bacteroides species, *J Periodontal Res* 22:300–306, 1987.

Sundqvist G, Carlsson J, Herrmann B, et al: Degradation of human immunoglobulins G and M and complement factors C3 and C5 by black pigmenting Bacteroides, *J Med Microbiol* 19:85–94, 1985.

Suzuki Y, Aoki S, Saito H, et al: A tumor necrosis factor-alpha antagonist inhibits inflammatory bone resorption induced by Porphyromonas gingivalis infection in mice, *J Periodontal Res* 41:81–91, 2006.

Tachibana-Ono M, Yoshida A, Kataoka T, et al: Identification of the genes associated with a virulent strain of Porphyromonas gingivalis using the subtractive hybridization technique, *Oral Microbiol Immunol* 23:84–87, 2008.

Takashiba S, Naruishi K, Murayama Y: Perspective of cytokine regulation for periodontal treatment: fibroblasts biology, *J Periodontol* 74:103–110, 2003.

Takahashi A, Earnshaw W: ICE-related proteases in apoptosis, *Current Opinions in Genetic Development* 6:50–55, 1996.

Takahashi K, Mooney J, Franson EV, et al: IgG and IgA subclass mRNA-bearing plasma cells in periodontitis gingival tissue and immunoglobulin levels in gingival crevicular fluid, *Clin Exp Immun* 107:158–165, 1997.

Takeuchi H, Sumitani M, Tsubakimoto K, et al: Oral organisms in the gingiva of individuals with periodontal disease, *J Dent Res* 53:132–136, 1974.

Takeuchi Y, Aramaki M, Nagasawa T, et al: Immunoglobulin G subclass antibody profiles in Porphyromonas gingivalis-associated aggressive and chronic periodontitis patients, *Oral Microbiol Immunol* 21:314–318, 2006.

Takeichi H, Taubman MA, Haber J, et al: Cytokine profiles of CD4 and CD8 T-cells isolated from adult periodontitis gingivae, *J Dent Res* 73:205, 1994.

Tamai R, Asai Y, Ogawa T: Requirement for intercellular adhesion molecule 1 and caveolae in invasion of human oral epithelial cells by Porphyromonas gingivalis, *Infect Immun* 73:6290–6298, 2005.

Tamura K, Nakano K, Nomur R, et al: Distribution of Porphyromonas gingivalis fimA Genotypes in Japanese Children and Adolescents, *J Periodontol* 76:674–679, 2005.

Tanaka S, Fakher M, Barbour SE, et al: Influence of proinflammatory cytokines on Actinobacillus actinomycetemcomitans specific IgG responses, *J Periodontal Res* 41:1–9, 2006.

Tashjian AH, Hohmann EL, Antoniades HN, et al: Platelet derived growth factor stimulates bone resorption via a prostaglandin-mediated mechanism, *Endocrinology* 111:118–124, 1982.

Tashjian AH, Voelkel EF, Lazzaro M, et al: alpha and beta human transforming growth factors stimulate prostaglandin production and bone resorption in cultured mouse calvaria, *Proc Natl Acad Sci USA* 82:4535–4538, 1985.

Taubman MA, Stoufi ED, Ebersole JL, et al: Phenotypic studies of cells from periodontal disease tissue, *J Periodontal Res* 19:587–590, 1984.

Taubman MA, Haffajee AD, Socransky SS, et al: Longitudinal monitoring of humoral antibodies in subjects with destructive periodontal disease, *J Periodontal Res* 27: 511–521, 1992.

Taubman MA, Valverde P, Han X, et al: Immune response: the key to bone resorption in periodontal disease, *J Periodontol* 76:2033–2041, 2005.

Thomas BP, Sun CX, Bajenova E, et al: Modulation of human neutrophil functions in vitro by Treponema denticola major outer sheath protein, *Infect Immun* 74:1954–1957, 2006.

Tipler LS, Embery G: Glycosaminoglycan depolymerising enzymes produced by anaerobic bacteria isolated from the human mouth, *Arch Oral Biol* 30:391–396, 1985.

Tiranathanagul S, Pattamapun K, Yongchaitrakul T, et al: MMP-2 activation by Actinobacillus actinomycetemcomitans supernatant in human PDL cells was corresponded with reduction of TIMP-2, *Oral Dis* 10:383–388, 2004.

Toda K, Otsuka M, Ishikawa Y, et al: Thiol-dependent collagenolytic activity in culture media of Bacteroides gingivalis, *J Periodontal Res* 19:372–381, 1984.

Tokoro Y, Matsuki Y, Yamamoto T, et al: Relevance of local Th2-type cytokine mRNA expression in immunocompetent infiltrates in inflamed gingival tissue to periodontal diseases, *Clin Exp Immunol* 107:166–174, 1997.

Tokuda M, Duncan M, Cho MI, et al: Role of Porphyromonas gingivalis protease activity in the colonization of oral surfaces, *Infect Immun* 64:4067–4073, 1996.

Tokuda M, Karunakaran T, Duncan M, et al: Role of Arg-gingipain A in virulence of Porphyromonas gingivalis, *Infect Immun* 66:1159–1166, 1998.

Tonzetich J: Direct gas chromatographic analysis of sulphur compounds in mouth air in man, *Arch Oral Biol* 16:587–597, 1971.

Tonzetich J: Production and origin of oral malodour. A review of mechanisms and methods of analysis, *J Periodontol* 48:13–20, 1977.

Tonzetich J: Oral malodour: an indicator of health status and oral cleanliness, *Int Dent J* 28:309–319, 1978.

Tonzetich J, Kesterbaum RG: Odour production by human salivary fractions and plaque, *Arch Oral Biol* 14:815–821, 1969.

Tonzetich J, Carpenter PAW: Production of volatile sulphur compounds from cystine, cysteine and methionine by human dental plaque, *Arch Oral Biol* 16:599–607, 1971.

Tonzetich J, Catherall DM: Metabolism of thiosulphate and thiocyanate by human saliva and dental plaque, *Arch Oral Biol* 22:125–131, 1976.

Tonzetich J, Lo KKC: Reaction of H_2S with proteins associated with the human mouth, *Arch Oral Biol* 23:875–880, 1978.

Tonzetich J, McBride BC: Characterization of volatile sulphur production by pathogenic and non-pathogenic strains of oral Bacteroides, *Arch Oral Biol* 26:963–969, 1981.

Tran SD, Rudney JD, Sparks BS, et al: Persistent presence of Bacteroides forsythus as a risk factor in a population of low prevalence and severity of adult periodontitis, *J Periodontol* 72:1–10, 2001.

Travis J, Baugh R, Giles PJ, et al: Human leukocyte elastase and cathepsin G. Isolation, characterization and interaction with plasma proteinase inhibitors. In Haverman H, Janoff A, editors: *Neutral Proteases of Human Polymorphonuclear Leukocytes*, Baltimore, 1978, Schwartzenberg, pp 118–135.

Travis J, Salvensen GS: Human plasma proteinase inhibitors, *Annu Rev Biochem* 52: 655–709, 1983.

Travis J, Pike R, Imamura T, et al: Porphyromonas gingivalis proteinases as virulence factors in the development of chronic periodontitis, *J Periodontal Res* 32:120–125, 1997.

Tsai CC, McArthur WP, Baehni PC, et al: Extraction and partial characterization of a leukotoxin from plaque-derived Gram-negative microorganisms, *Infect Immun* 25:427–439, 1979.

Tsutsui H, Kinouchi T, Wakano Y, et al: Purification and characterization of a protease from Bacteroides gingivalis, *Infect Immun* 55:420–427, 1987.

Turk V, Bode W: The cystatins: protein inhibitors of cysteine proteinases, *Fed Eur Biochem Soc* 285:213–219, 1991.

Turk B, Turk D, Turk V: Lysosomal cysteine proteinases: more than scavengers, *Biochim Biophys Acta* 1477:98–111, 2000.

Uchida Y, Shiba H, Komatsuzawa H, et al: Expression of IL-1β and IL-8 by human gingival epithelial cells in response to Actinobacillus actinomycetemcomitans, *Cytokine* 14:152–161, 2001.

Uehara A, Muramoto K, Imamura T, et al: Arginine-specific gingipains from Porphyromonas gingivalis stimulate production of hepatocyte growth factor (scatter factor) through protease-activated receptors in human gingival fibroblasts in culture, *J Immunol* 175:6076–6084, 2005.

Uitto VJ, Chan EC, Quee TC: Initial characterization of neutral proteinases from oral spirochaetes, *J Periodontal Res* 21:95–100, 1986.

Uitto VJ, Grenier D, Chan ECS, et al: Isolation of a chymotrypsin-like enzyme from Treponema denticola, *Infect Immun* 56:2717–2722, 1988a.

Uitto VJ, Haapasalo M, Laakso T, et al: Degradation of basement membrane collagen by proteases from some anaerobic oral microorganisms, *Oral Microbiol Immunol* 3:97–102, 1988b.

Uitto VJ, Grenier D, McBride BC: Effect of Treponema denticola on periodontal epithelial cells, *J Dent Res* 68:894, Abstract 223, 1989a.

Uitto VJ, Larjava H, Heino J, et al: A protease of Bacteroides gingivalis degrades cell surface and matrix glycoproteins of cultured gingival fibroblasts and induces secretion of collagenase and plasminogen activator, *Infect Immun* 57:213–218, 1989b.

Uitto VJ, Overall CM, McCulloch C: Proteolytic host cell enzymes in gingival crevicular fluid, *Periodontology* 2000 31:77–104, 2003.

Umemoto T, Watanabe K, Kumada H, et al: The role of motile rods in periodontal disease. In Hamada S, Holt SC, McGhee JR, editors: *Periodontal Disease: Pathogens and Host Immune Responses*, Tokyo, 1991, Quintessence, pp 65–76.

Umemoto T, Hamada N: Characterization of biologically active cell surface components of a periodontal pathogen. The roles of the major and minor fimbriae of Porphyromas gingivalis, *J Periodontol* 74:119–122, 2003.

Vaes G: Cellular biology and biochemical mechanism of bone resorption, *Clin Orthop Relat Res* 23:239–271, 1988.

Van Winkelhoff AJ, Boutaga K: Transmission of periodontal bacteria and models of infection, *J Clin Periodontol* 32:16–27, 2005.

Van Winkelhoff AJ, Rijnsburger MC, Abbas F, et al: Java project on periodontal diseases: a study on transmission of Porphyromonas gingivalis in a remote Indonesian population, *J Clin Periodontol* 34:480–484, 2007.

Vankeerberghen A, Nuytten H, Dierickx K, et al: Differential induction of human beta-defensin expression by periodontal commensals and pathogens in periodontal pocket epithelial cells, *J Periodontol* 76:1293–1303, 2005.

Vanterpool E, Roy F, Fletcher HM: The vimE gene downstream of vimA is independently expressed and is involved in modulating proteolytic activity in Porphyromonas gingivalis W83, *Infect Immun* 72:5555–5564, 2004.

Veith PD, Chen Y-Y, Reynolds EC: Porphyromonas gingivalis rgpA and Kgp proteinases and adhesins are C terminally processed by the carboxypeptidase CPG70, *Infect Immun* 72:3655–3657, 2004.

Vernal R, Dutzan N, Chaparro A, et al: Levels of interleukin-17 in gingival crevicular fluid and in supernatants of cellular cultures of gingival tissue from patients with chronic periodontitis, *J Clin Periodontol* 32:383–389, 2005.

Vernillo A, Ramamurthy N, Golub L, et al: The non-antimicrobial properties of tetracyclines for the treatment of periodontal disease, *Curr Opin Periodontol* 2:111–118, 1994.

Vitkov L, Krautgartner WD, Hannig M: Bacterial internalization in periodontitis, *Oral Microbiol Immunol* 20:317–321, 2005.

Votta BJ, Levy MA, Badger A, et al: Peptide aldehyde inhibitors of cathepsin K inhibit bone resorption both in vitro and in vivo, *J Bone Miner Res* 12:1396–1406, 1997.

Waddington RJ, Embery G: Structural characterization of human alveolar bone proteoglycans, *Arch Oral Biol* 36:859–866, 1991.

Waddington RJ, Moseley R, Embery G: Reactive oxygen species: potential role in the pathogenesis of periodontal diseases, *Oral Dis* 6:138–151, 2000.

Wahl SM, McNeely TB, Janoff EN, et al: Secretory leukocyte protease inhibitor (SLPI) in mucosal fluids inhibits HIV-1, *Oral Dis* 3(Suppl i):564–569, 1997.

Walter C, Zahlten J, Schmeck B, et al: Porphyromonas gingivalis strain-dependent activation of human endothelial cells, *Infect Immun* 72:5910–5918, 2004.

Wang P-L, Shirasu S, Daito M, et al: Purification and characterization of a trypsin-like protease from the culture supernatant of Actinobacillus actinomycetemcomitans Y4, *Eur J Oral Sci* 106:1–7, 1999.

Wang P-L, Azuma Y, Shinohara M, et al: Effect of Actinobacillus actinomycetemcomitans protease on the proliferation of gingival epithelial cells, *Oral Dis* 7:233–237, 2001.

Wassenar A, Reinhardus C, Thepen T, et al: Cloning, characterization, and antigen specificity of T-lymphocyte subsets extracted from gingival tissue of chronic adult periodontitis patients, *Infect Immun* 63:2147–2153, 1995.

Watanabe H, Marsh PD, Ivanyi L: Antigens of Actinobacillus actinomycetemcomitans identified by immunoblotting with sera from patients with localised human juvenile periodontitis and generalised severe periodontitis, *Arch Oral Biol* 34:649–656, 1989.

Weakes-Dybvig M, Sanavi F, Zander H, et al: The effect of indomethacin on alveolar bone loss in experimental periodontitis, *J Periodontal Res* 17:90–100, 1982.

Werb Z: ECM and cell surface proteolysis: regulating cellular ecology, *Cell* 91:439–442, 1997.

Westin U, Polling A, Ljungkrantz I, et al: Identification of SLPI (secretory leukocyte protease inhibitor) in human mast cells using immunohistochemistry and in situ hybridization, *Biol Chem* 380:489–493, 1999.

White PA, Wilson M, Nair SP, et al: Characterization of an anti-proliferative surface-associated protein from Actinobacillus actinomycetemcomitans which can be neutralised by sera from a portion of patients with localised juvenile periodontitis, *Infect Immun* 63:2612–2618, 1995.

WHO: alpha1-Antitrypsin deficiency: memorandum from a WHO meeting, *Bull World Health Organ* 75:397–415, 1998.

Wikström M, Lindhe A: Ability of oral bacteria to degrade fibronectin, *Infect Immun* 51:707–711, 1986.

Williams RC, Jeffcoat MK, Howell TC, et al: Ibuprofen: an inhibitor of alveolar bone resorption in beagles, *J Periodontal Res* 23:225–229, 1988.

Wilson M: Bacterial activities of lipopolysaccharides from oral bacteria and their relevance to the pathogenesis of chronic periodontitis, *Scientific Progress* 78:19–34, 1995.

Wilson M, Kamin S, Harvey W: Bone resorbing activity from purified capsular material from Actinobacillus actinomycetemcomitans, *J Periodontal Res* 20:484–491, 1985.

Wilson M, Meghji S, Harvey W: Effect of capsular material from H. Actinomycetem-comitans on bone collagen synthesis in vitro, *Microbios* 54:181–185, 1988.

Wilson M, Meghji S, Barber P, et al: Biological activities of surface associated material from Porphyromonas gingivalis, *FEMS Immunol Med Microbiol* 6:147–155, 1993.

Wilson M, Henderson B: Virulence factors of Actinobacillus actinomycetemcomitans relevant to the pathogenesis of inflammatory periodontal diseases, *FEMS Microbiol Rev* 17:365–379, 1995.

Wilson M, Reddi K, Henderson D: Cytokine-inducing components of periodontopathic bacteria, *J Periodontal Res* 31:393–407, 1996.

Winkler JR, Grassi M, Murray PA: Clinical description and aetiology of HIV-associated periodontal diseases.In Robertson PB, Greenspan JS, editors: *Oral Manifestations of AIDS*, Littleton, MA, 1988, PSG Publishing, pp 49–70.

Wolinsky LE, Saglie FR, Carranza FA, et al: The identification of Treponema vincentii in the gingival tissue of humans with adult periodontitis, *J Periodontol* 58:337, 1987.

Yamamoto M, Fulihashi K, Hiroi T, et al: Molecular and cellular mechanisms for periodontal diseases: role for Th1 and Th2 type cytokines in induction of mucosal inflammation, *J Periodontal Res* 32:115–119, 1997.

Yamazaki K, Nakajima T, Aoyagi T, et al: Immunohistological analysis of memory T-lymphocytes and activated B-lymphocytes in tissues with periodontal disease, *J Periodontal Res* 28:324–334, 363, 1994.

Yamamoto E, Awano S, Koseki T, et al: Expression of endothelin-1 in gingival epithelial cells, *J Periodontal Res* 38:417–421, 2003.

Yang P, Tremaine WJ, Meyer RL, et al: alpha1-Antitrypsin deficiency and inflammatory bowel diseases, *Mayo Clin Proceed* 75:450–455, 2000.

Yapar M, Saygun I, Ozdemir A, et al: Prevalence of human herpesviruses in patients with aggressive periodontitis, *J Periodontol* 74:1634–1640, 2003.

Yoneda M, Kuramitsu HK: Genetic evidence for the relationship of Porphyromonas gingivalis cysteine proteinase and hemagglutinin activity, *Oral Microbiol Immunol* 11:129–134, 1996.

Yoneda M, Yoshikane T, Motooka N, et al: Stimulation of growth of Porphyromonas gingivalis by cell extracts from Tannerella forsythia, *J Periodontal Res* 40:105–109, 2005.

Yonezawa H, Kato T, Kuramitsu HK, et al: Immunization by Arg-gingipain A DNA vaccine protects mice against an invasive Porphyromonas gingivalis infection through regulation of interferon-production, *Oral Microbiol Immunol* 20:259–266, 2005.

Yoshimura F, Nishikata M, Suzuki T, et al: Characterization of a trypsin-like protease from the bacterium Bacteroides gingivalis isolated from human dental plaque, *Arch Oral Biol* 29:559–564, 1984.

Yun PLW, DeCarlo AA, Hunter N: Gingipains of Porphyromonas gingivalis modulate leukocyte adhesion molecule expression induced in human endothelial cells by ligation of CD99, *Infect Immun* 74:1661–1672, 2006.

Zhou J, Windsor LJ: Porphyromonas gingivalis affects host collagen degradation by affecting expression, activation, and inhibition of matrix metalloproteinases, *J Periodontal Res* 41:47–54, 2006.

Zhou Q, Desta T, Fenton M, et al: Cytokine profiling of macrophages exposed to Porphyromonas gingivalis, its lipopolysaccharide, or its FimA protein, *Infect Immun* 73:935–943, 2005.

Zhou Q, Amar S: Identification of proteins differentially expressed in human monocytes exposed to Porphyromonas gingivalis and its purified components by high-throughput immunoblotting, *Infect Immun* 74:1204–1214, 2006.

6

The effect of systemic factors on the periodontal tissues

The systemic conditions which can potentially affect the periodontal tissues are numerous and will be described under the following headings:

- Physiological changes
- Systemic diseases
- Infections
- Drug reactions
- Dietary and nutritional factors.

PHYSIOLOGICAL CHANGES

THE SEX HORMONES

Oestrogens and progesterone are the predominant female sex hormones and are controlled by the ovary. Oestrogens produce the physiological changes in women at puberty and progesterone prepares the female reproductive tract for fertilization. The androgen, testosterone, is the predominant male hormone which produces the male characteristics at puberty and also promotes protein synthesis. Synthetic hormones which mimic the effects of the endogenous female hormones are used as oral contraceptives.

These hormones can affect the periodontal tissues. Oestrogens can promote keratinization and increase the mucopolysaccharide content of the connective tissue. Progesterone can increase the permeability of gingival blood vessels. Changes in the periodontal tissues may become clinically apparent principally at puberty (Hart et al 2000), during pregnancy and during the use of oral contraceptives when there may be an exaggerated response to plaque products.

The changes seen in puberty, menstruation and pregnancy are summarized below and reviewed recently (Mascarenhas et al 2003; Guncu et al 2005).

PUBERTY

The increasing levels of the sex hormones in the circulation at puberty have been linked to the increased prevalence and severity of gingivitis at this time and this is supported by the observation that gingivitis peaks earlier in girls (11–13) than boys (13–14). However, a 6-year longitudinal study failed to show any increase in gingivitis at puberty in 18 hormonally stable girls, and a significant increase of gingivitis was seen in girls experiencing precocious puberty.

It would appear that a small amount of plaque which at a different age might cause minimal gingival inflammation, produces an obvious inflammation with gingival swelling and bleeding at puberty. When puberty is passed the inflammation tends to subside but does not disappear until adequate plaque control is achieved.

MENSTRUATION

With pre-existing gingivitis, gingival crevicular exudate increases at the time of ovulation in the menstrual cycle owing to the increased production of oestrogens and progesterone. However, no such increase was seen in healthy tissues. This may explain why in a few women a deterioration of a pre-existing gingivitis may occur at this time in their menstrual cycle.

PREGNANCY

Folklore has always associated pregnancy with gingivitis and tooth loss but where the mouth is clean, gingivitis does not occur in pregnancy. However, as in puberty an otherwise low-grade plaque-induced inflammation will become more severe in pregnancy (**Fig. 6.1**).

The incidence of gingivitis in pregnancy has been reported as between 30% and 100%. The changes usually start about the 3rd month of gestation and the severity of the inflammation gradually increases during pregnancy, with partial or complete resolution after parturition. Gingivitis has also been reported to peak at 6 months' gestation and remain the same in the third trimester. The gingivae may become bright red, swollen, sensitive and bleed spontaneously. There is also an increase in gingival exudate and tooth mobility which may be due to the level of inflammation. The relevance of the effects of gestational hormones on tissues of the periodontium has been reviewed extensively (Mascarenhas et al 2003; Guncu et al 2005). Increased gingivitis amongst pregnant women was shown in a more recent study of a rural population of Sri-Lankan women (Tilakaratne et al 2000a) compared with matched non-pregnant controls, more significant in the second and third trimester of pregnancy despite plaque levels remaining unchanged. The level of gingival inflammation at 3 months after parturition was comparable with that seen in the first trimester of pregnancy, indicating a direct correlation between raised levels of gestational hormones and gingivitis with regression after parturition. The values for loss of attachment remained unchanged throughout the period.

Increasing levels of progesterone produce an increase in vascularity with alterations in the walls of the gingival vessels which makes them more permeable. It has also been shown that the numbers of black-pigmented anaerobic bacteria in the subgingival flora increase as pregnancy progresses (Kornman & Loesche 1980). The raised levels of oestrogen and progesterone in the bacteria due to increased steroid uptake in pregnancy may be due to oestrogen being a substitute for methadione, which is a growth requirement for these bacteria.

Despite the elevated levels of gestational hormones and gingival inflammation, pregnancy gingivitis rarely progresses to periodontitis and resolves

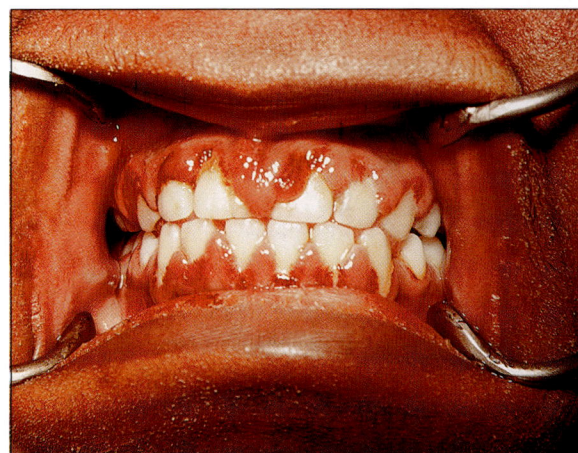

Fig. 6.1 Severe hyperplastic and oedematous gingivitis caused by poor oral hygiene, pre-existing gingivitis and the effects of the hormonal changes of pregnancy. The exaggerated tissue response results from the increase in sex hormones.

post partum. In this context, an *in vitro* cell culture study using fibroblasts has shown that interleukin-1β upregulated the release of matrix metalloproteinases in the absence of progesterone and downregulated their release in the presence of progesterone (Lopp et al 2003). Thus, the reduced levels of MMPs may reduce the breakdown of gingival connective tissue and may therefore prevent the progression of pregnancy gingivitis to periodontitis, although other vascular effects of progesterone maintain gingival inflammation.

To control gingivitis in the pregnant patient or in the adolescent, it is important to explain the nature of the condition and the special care which she needs to take during this period. Regular scaling and instruction in home care are essential; at the same time all plaque retentive factors should be eliminated.

Pregnancy epulis (pyogenic granuloma of pregnancy)

The pregnancy epulis is a soft pedunculated granuloma which often arises from an inflamed gingival papilla and can present as an average to large granulomatous lesion, associated with the second trimester of pregnancy. It is typically deep red in colour and bleeds easily and may cause the patient great concern (**Fig. 6.2A**), being most prevalent in the anterior region of the mouth. It is inclined to regress partially or completely after parturition. In addition to the presence of plaque, it is often associated with plaque retentive factors such as a carious cavity, poor tooth contact or an overhanging restoration.

Histologically it resembles a pyogenic granuloma (**Fig. 6.2B**). It is composed of numerous, wide-spaced and thin-walled blood vessels within a delicate connective tissue stroma, which can intensify with age. A moderate to dense inflammatory infiltrate is present with numerous PMNs. The covering epithelium is thin and in areas of ulceration a thin fibrin exudate covers the surface.

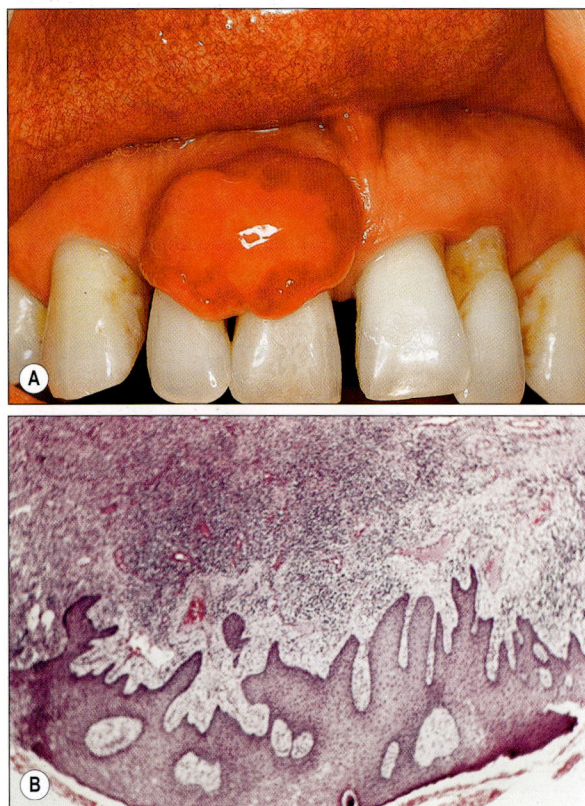

Fig. 6.2 (A) A pyogenic granuloma (pregnancy granuloma) in a pregnant patient. (B) The histopathology of a pregnancy epulis. The main features are large vascular channels, marked infiltration with PMNs and epithelial hyperplasia.

An epulis should only be surgically removed in pregnancy if it is being traumatized by opposing teeth or restorations causing bleeding. The lesion can bleed profusely when excised and electrocautery of the base of the lesion may be necessary to control this. The excised lesion should be placed in formol saline and sent for histological examination to confirm the diagnosis. Any secondary irritating factor associated with the lesion should also be corrected. There is a high recurrence rate of these lesions and for this reason removal should be delayed until after parturition whenever possible. At this stage the lesion usually regresses considerably and becomes more fibrous, making it easier to remove the residual lesion with less likelihood of recurrence due to the return of normal hormone levels.

It has been proposed that the absence of vascular endothelial growth factor (VEGF) and angiopoietin-2 (Ang-2) cause blood vessels to regress (Yuan & Lin 2004). This group have investigated their possible role in the regression of pregnancy pyogenic granulomata after parturition. They showed that TNF-α upregulated the expression of Ang-2 in all the endothelial cell lines investigated. They also demonstrated that levels of Ang-2 were highest in the pregnancy granulomata investigated, followed by those taken after parturition and were lowest in the normal gingival specimens. The protein levels of VEGF were very high in the granulomata from pregnant women and were almost undetectable after parturition. More apoptotic cells were also seen in specimens taken after parturition. These findings suggest that the lack of VEGF after parturition causes apoptosis of vascular endothelial cells leading to vascular regression and the regression of the pyogenic granulomata.

ORAL CONTRACEPTIVES

The hormonal oral contraceptive pill contains progesterone, often combined with an oestrogen. Hormonal contraceptives reduce the likelihood of ovulation/implantation by utilizing synthetic formulations of the gestational hormones oestrogen and progesterone. Hormonal contraceptive users sometimes present with similar effects to those seen in pregnancy gingivitis, but less pronounced and associated with increased inflammation and gingival exudate (Mariotti 1994). The degree of inflammation seems to be related to the length of time the woman is taking 'the pill'. As with pregnancy these changes do not affect healthy tissues in a clean mouth and the effect is to exaggerate a pre-existing gingivitis and is secondary to irritation from plaque. The exogenous hormones can also enhance the development of an anaerobic plaque in which black-pigmented anaerobic rods predominate (Kornman & Loesche 1980).

The long-term use of hormonal contraceptives has been linked to significant cardiovascular thromboembolic episodes (Westhoff 1996). Arterial and venous effects are attributed to oestrogen while progesterone affects mainly arterial responses. Raised levels of the clotting factors VIIc and XIIc are seen in women using oral contraceptives, in response to the dose of oestrogen increasing the risk of coagulation. In men these factors demonstrate a significant positive correlation with ischaemic heart disease. However, the contraceptive formulation used would determine the level of risk involved. There may not be a consistent biological basis for this in all users (Davis 2000).

The different formulations of hormonal contraceptives (Davis 2000) include the following:

1. Combined oral contraceptives containing artificial analogues of oestrogen and progesterone
2. Progesterone based mini-pill
3. Slow release progesterone implants placed subdermally that last up to 5 years (e.g. Norplant)
4. Depo Provera, a very effective progestin injection given by a doctor every 3 months.

The hormonal contraceptive formulations used in earlier periodontal studies contained higher concentrations of gestational hormones comprising 50–100 μg oestrogen and 4–5 mg progestin compared with later formulations with low doses of oestrogens and progestins of 50 μg/day and 1.5 mg/day respectively (Mariotti 1994). This could affect the results of earlier studies which showed greater periodontal destruction in 1.5 years compared with the control group comparable for age and oral hygiene. However a more recent study on a matched population of rural Sri-Lankan women (Tilakaratne et al 2000b) showed significantly higher levels of gingivitis in contraceptive users (0.03 mg estradiol and 0.15 mg of a progestin) than in non-users. In those who used the progesterone depot preparation of 150 mg 3 monthly for 2–4 years, there was also significant periodontal breakdown, when compared with those who used it for less than 2 years. These findings have some bearing on the duration of use and tissue catabolism caused by progesterone resulting in increased periodontal attachment loss. However, if low plaque levels are established and maintained for the duration of use, these effects could be minimized. The lack of correlation between dosing and gingival inflammation or periodontitis is reinforced in a recent cross-sectional study (Taichman & Eklund 2005).

Duration of use may be a more important factor.

EFFECT ON TISSUES

It has been suggested that oestrogen can interact with progesterone resulting in the mediation of effects characteristic of progesterone. Receptors for progesterone and oestrogen in human gingivae indicate that gingivae are a target tissue for both gestational hormones. *In vitro* studies of gingival fibroblasts in culture showed that oestrogen enhanced the formation of anabolic androgen metabolites, while progesterone decreased yields. The combined effect of both gestational hormones on the yield of androgens was less pronounced than with oestrogen alone, implying a more catabolic role for progesterone (Tilakaratne & Soory 1999).

Progesterone contributes to increased vascular permeability. However, the main effects of oestrogen are in controlling blood flow. Hence, the combination of oestrogen and progesterone in the contraceptive pill can affect vascular changes in the gingivae. The resultant gingivitis can be minimized by establishing low plaque levels prior to commencing oral contraceptive therapy.

SYSTEMIC DISEASES

ENDOCRINES

Diabetes mellitus

Diabetes mellitus is a metabolic disorder characterized by glucose intolerance. It can be classified into two major categories, Type I or insulin-dependent diabetes mellitus (IDDM) and type II or non-insulin-dependent diabetes (Soory 2002).

IDDM has a sudden onset and occurs usually before the age of 25. Symptoms include thirst, polyuria, hunger and weight loss and it is controlled by daily injections of insulin. It is a primary disease of the cells of the islets of Langerhans. Type II has a gradual onset and mainly affects obese middle-aged people. It is associated with insulin resistance and is controlled by diet and hypoglycaemic drugs (Soory 2002, 2004).

The precise aetiology of IDDM is unclear but it appears to involve genetic factors relating to the HLA system and has some features of an autoimmune condition. Peptide sequence mimicry of islet cells by Coxsackie 6B virus and the presence of antibodies to it in IDDM patients would damage or kill the islet cells. This would probably only occur in a group of susceptible individuals with representative antigens of the peptide sequence from the virus (Ch. 3). Approximately 2% of the population has IDDM and the numbers appear to be increasing.

It is possible to screen for the presence of suspected diabetes with a glucose stick self-monitoring device using fingertip capillary blood. It has also been shown that this can also be accomplished with gingival blood produced by periodontal probing and the levels produced from both these sources correlate well (Beikler et al 2002).

IDDM may produce atherosclerotic changes in the arterioles, capillaries and venules of a wide range of organs and the complications of long-term diabetes are retinopathy, macrovascular disease, nephropathy, neuropathy and impaired healing. These complications can be prevented by establishing glycaemic control by administering insulin for type I or hypoglycaemic agents for type II with personal blood glucose monitoring. The risk of hypoglycaemia also needs to be protected against.

Some of the direct effects of chronic hyperglycaemia are elevated levels of sorbitol and fructose due to aldose reductase activity. Furthermore, increased production of diacylglycerol results in activation of the protein kinase C system. These events have been linked to some of the diabetic complications (Soory 2002).

Formation of glycation end products

Reducing sugars resulting from chronic hyperglycaemia form reversible products with blood and tissue proteins by non-enzymic glycation and oxidation (Mealey & Ocampo 2007). These include glycated haemoglobin A1, which can be used as a sensitive index of glycaemic control. These reversible compounds undergo irreversible structural changes to become advanced glycation end products (AGEs). Accumulation of AGEs is associated with the onset of diabetic complications. AGEs produce significant alterations in cellular composition, synthesis and secretion of growth factors and basement membrane structure and function (Nishimura et al 2007). They also affect barrier functions, cell attachment and mitosis. It is also interesting that activation of the PMN myeloperoxidase system in an inflammatory environment can result in the formation of AGEs in the absence of hyperglycaemia.

Increased secretion of growth factors has been found following activation of their secretion pathways by AGEs (Soory 2000, 2004; Chiarelli et al 2000; Rahman & Soory 2006). AGE activation of cellular receptors can also lead to microvascular changes and secretion of pro-inflammatory cytokines and reactive oxygen species by inflammatory cells. The main cytokines affected are insulin like growth factor (IGF)-1, transforming growth factor (TGF)-β, vascular cell adhesion molecule (VCAM)-1, IL-1β, IL-6 and TNF-α. Most of these effects are caused by AGEs attaching to specific cellular receptors (RAGE). These receptors are present at low levels during physiological conditions but increase in critical target tissue during inflammatory conditions and in diabetes (Nassar et al 2007).

The binding of AGEs to vascular endothelial cells has been shown to increase vascular permeability and to increase the production of ICAM-1. Similar interactions of AGEs with fibroblast and smooth muscle cell receptors result in impaired remodelling of connective tissue and vascular wall damage. Their interactions with monocytes and macrophages stimulate the release of pro-inflammatory cytokines such as IL-1β, IL-6 and TNF-α. They also stimulate the secretion of reactive oxygen radicals from inflammatory cells which can produce tissue damage (Jakus 2000) including vessel wall damage leading to cardiovascular disease (Jakus 2000). The increase in the secretion of reactive oxygen radicals can in turn trigger aldose reductase production and the formation of diacylglycerol leading to the activation of protein kinase C which can further stimulate the formation of AGEs (Nishikawa et al 2000).

It has also been found that periodontal ligament cells are susceptible to hyper- and hypoglycaemia and these effects appear to be mediated via the integrin system (Nishimura et al 2007). Hyperglycaemia produces an increased expression of fibronectin receptor and results in reduced cellular adhesion and motility and hence probable tissue impairment. Hypoglycaemia lowers the expression of fibronectin receptor which lowers cell viability and ultimately results in cell death and hence tissue impairment.

Oral effects

Poorly controlled diabetic patients may complain of diminished salivary flow and burning mouth or tongue. Diabetics taking oral hypoglycaemic agents may suffer from xerostomia and this may be complicated by oral *Candida albicans* infections.

Periodontal effects

Diabetes mellitus is a complex metabolic disease with or without systemic complications and its course depends on effective control of hyperglycaemia. As a result epidemiological studies on the relationship between periodontal disease and diabetes show conflicting results. However, there is good evidence to support an association between poorly controlled diabetes and periodontitis especially in the longstanding and severe cases (**Fig. 6.3**). Diabetic children have more severe gingivitis than healthy children. However, opinion is somewhat divided with regard to susceptibility of adult diabetics to periodontitis. In both Type 1 and Type 2 DM, a range of positive and negative correlations have been shown which are likely to be confounded by the degree of control of the diabetic condition, environmental, genetic and host factors. The mechanisms described can potentially contribute to a correlation which may not manifest in all cases for the above reasons. The influence of periodontal diseases on diabetes and that of diabetes on oral health has been reviewed recently (Mealey & Ocampo 2007).

Takeda et al (2006) showed that the serum level of AGEs was significantly associated with the deterioration of chronic periodontitis in Type 2 diabetes patients. A recent *in vitro* study in a hyperglycaemic cell culture model of fibroblasts demonstrated the importance of AGE and nicotine as oxidative agents using radiolabelled markers of oxidative stress. These effects were overcome by the antioxidants glutathione and the growth factor IGF, which also has antioxidant properties (Rahman & Soory 2006). This demonstrates the importance of oxidative damage in the progression of inflammatory diseases, compounded by smoking.

Promsudthi et al (2005) examined the effect of periodontal therapy on glycemic control in 52 Thai, older type 2 diabetic patients. The treatment group received mechanical periodontal treatment combined with systemic doxycycline, 100 mg/day for 14 days. The control group received neither periodontal treatment nor systemic doxycycline. They showed that the test group significantly improved in 3 months whereas the control group rapidly deteriorated.

The consensus from these studies would seem to be that the well controlled diabetic is at no greater risk from periodontal destruction than the normal population. However, several studies have shown that longstanding diabetics and particularly those who show systemic complications do appear to have greater rates of periodontal progression than age-matched

healthy people (Safkan-Seppälä et al 2006). In addition, there is good evidence of poorly controlled diabetic patients with associated prolonged periods of hyperglycaemia being far more susceptible to progressive periodontitis (Mealey & Ocampo 2007), with a greater likelihood of damage occurring during these spells, partly dependent on age and duration of diabetes.

The importance of hyperglycaemia in this scenario is also supported by the Hisayama study (Saito et al 2004). This community-based study examined the relationship between periodontitis severity and the glucose tolerance status. Increased severity of periodontitis was found to be significantly associated both with the development of impaired glucose tolerance in previously non-diabetic patients and its presence in diabetic patients.

Diabetic patients with advanced periodontal disease also seem to suffer more frequently with complications such as lateral abscesses. Their occurrence can increase insulin resistance. The factors most likely to account for this association include impaired host response, excessive release of pro-inflammatory cytokines and tissue degrading enzymes. It is relevant that periodontal treatment in Type 2 diabetics has been shown to improve their glycaemic control (Stewart et al 2001). These aspects have been reviewed recently (Mealey & Ocampo 2007).

Obesity is associated with hypertension, hyperlipidaemia, type II diabetes and periodontal disease (Nishimura et al 2003). Adipose tissue of obese subjects produces large quantities of biologically active molecules such as leptin, an important molecule regulating energy expenditure and body weight. Furthermore, adipocyte-derived active molecules called adipocytokines may account for the close association between obesity and related conditions such as type II diabetes and periodontal disease. The pro-inflammatory cytokine tumour necrosis factor-α (TNF-α) is produced by adipocytes, monocytes/macrophages in inflammatory diseases and its blood concentration is elevated in obese patients declining with weight loss. TNF-α suppresses insulin action via its specific receptor and thus exacerbates insulin resistance. Therefore, TNF-α from adipose tissue may act as a risk factor for both periodontal disease and type II diabetes and this is a possible mechanism for the 2-way relationship between these two conditions. Metabolic syndrome, a clustering of related risk factors for CVD and Type 2 diabetes is linked to obesity which has reached global epidemic proportions. Abdominal or visceral fat associated with waist circumference has a stronger correlation as a risk factor than peripheral fat (Ritchie 2007; Saito & Shimazaki 2007).

Effects on host response

Patients with DM are prone to infection partly due to phagocyte dysfunction and impaired PMN superoxide generation. Low zinc levels may also be associated with respiratory burst dysfunction in diabetics (Larijani et al 2007). In addition, impaired chemotactic response of PMNs in the gingival crevice due to an altered chemokine gradient (Engebretson et al 2006) has been demonstrated in diabetic patients with severe periodontitis and in families with a history of diabetes. It has been suggested that the defect is at the cellular level and may involve inhibition of the glycolytic pathway, abnormal cyclic nucleotide metabolism, which disrupts the organization of microtubules and microfilaments, or a reduction in leucocyte membrane receptors. One explanation of these effects may be that they are mediated by hyperglycaemia via glycosylation of proteins and the binding of AGEs to RAGE on these cells. Increased PMN secretion of collagenase (Soory 2000) and elastase (Piwowar et al 2000) have also been found in diabetic patients.

Poorly controlled diabetics also have higher levels of GCF IL-1β and PGE$_2$ in comparison to controlled diabetics with similar levels of periodontal disease. Increased release of these cytokines and TNF-α by inflammatory cells has been shown in diabetics compared with healthy controls. The binding of AGEs to RAGE (receptor for AGE) on these cells could be responsible for these effects.

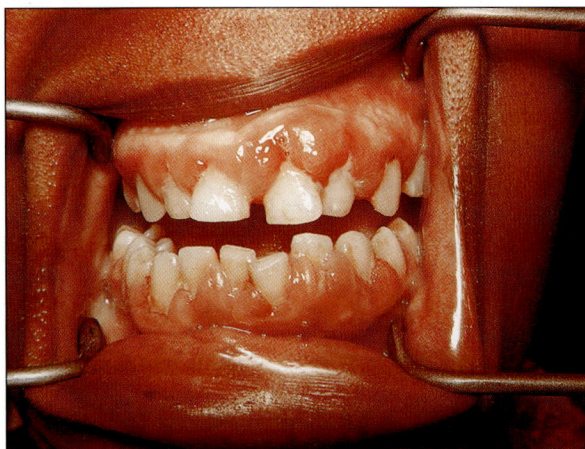

Fig. 6.3 Severe chronic periodontitis, marked gingival inflammation and multiple lateral periodontal abscesses in a patient with poorly controlled insulin-dependant diabetes mellitus.

Effects on connective tissue

Diabetes enhanced inflammation causes dysregulation of the cellular environment, formation of AGEs and excessive release of cytokines such as TNF-α. The resultant apoptosis results in enhanced loss of fibroblasts and osteoblasts which could contribute to limited repair of damaged tissue (Graves et al 2006). The hyperglycaemic environment can reduce tissue growth and matrix synthesis by fibroblasts and osteoclasts. AGE/RAGE interactions also lead to oxidative damage with adverse effects on cell/matrix interactions and vascular integrity. This contributes to delayed wound healing compounding the direct effects of hyperglycaemia mentioned above and explains impaired periodontal treatment responses in uncontrolled diabetics.

Periodontal treatment

Strict control of periodontal disease with treatment, patient motivation on plaque control measures and a stringent maintenance programme are essential for good metabolic control of diabetes mellitus.

The use of adjunctive antibiotics may be considered in poorly controlled diabetics with severe periodontitis (Rees 2000) which fail to respond to subgingival scaling alone. In these cases, the combination of subgingival scaling with systemic tetracycline has been found to have better results than scaling alone and also resulted in improved glycaemic control. Periodontal wound healing has been shown to be accelerated in response to doxycycline hyclate in diabetic mice (Kol & Palattella 2006) and humans with Type 1 diabetes (Llambes et al 2006).

GENETIC CONDITIONS

A number of conditions of genetic origin can affect the periodontal tissues and these are listed below:

- Down's syndrome
- Hypophosphatasia
- Papillon–Lefèvre syndrome
- Ehlers–Danlos syndrome
- Hereditary gingival fibromatosis
- Mucopolysaccharidoses
- Hyperoxaluria
- Cyclic neutropenia
- Familial neutropenias
- Chediak–Higashi syndrome.

Down's syndrome

Down's syndrome results from trisomy of chromosome 21 caused by non-dysjunction during oogenesis. A few cases of the syndrome have a normal number of 46 chromosomes but have a reciprocal translocation of chromosomes groups 13–15 and groups 21–22. The overall incidence of Down's syndrome is about 1 in 700 births but increases to 1:100 if the mother is 45 or over. People with the syndrome have a variable degree of mental handicap and typical mongoloid facial features.

Orally, they typically have a Class III occlusion, an anterior open bite, a large tongue and a lack of lip seal. They are prone to infections and their incidence of leukaemia is 20 times greater than the normal population. This is probably related to the presence on chromosome 21 of the genes for leucocyte development.

If living at home with their family or in a well-ordered community, they usually have a very happy and trusting personality and if they receive an appropriate education they can develop reasonable levels of skill.

It is now well established by a large number of epidemiological studies that cases of Down's syndrome are far more prone to destructive periodontitis than either the normal population or cases of other forms of mental handicap (Morgan 2007). The overall incidence of periodontitis is in excess of 90% but tends to be less in those living at home rather than in institutions. The distribution of disease is uneven with the lower permanent incisors most commonly involved and these teeth often have short conical roots, followed by upper incisors and first molars, the deciduous molars, premolars and canines. The commonest clinical presentation is mobility of the lower incisors with radiographic evidence of advanced alveolar bone loss (**Fig. 6.4**). They also have an increased susceptibility to ANUG. In this regard numerous black-pigmented anaerobic rods and spirochaetes can be frequently isolated from the subgingival flora of Down's cases.

The susceptibility to periodontitis is most likely to be related to many abnormalities that have been reported in PMNs from Down's cases. Impaired chemotaxis, reduced phagocytosis and intracellular killing have been reported. This last feature may be related to disturbances in the intracellular oxidative metabolism in PMNs. In the first 5 years of life, a progressive trend has been observed with decreased CD4 lymphocytes, plasma Zinc levels and increased CD8 cells but within a normal range. Decreased plasma levels of Zinc have been observed (Cocchi et al 2007). Monocyte function is also impaired but less so than PMNs. There may be a premature ageing of B lymphocytes in Down's syndrome. T-lymphocyte function is profoundly affected and their numbers are reduced with impaired maturation, possibly due to a defect in thymic processing associated with structural abnormalities in the thymus. There are also some vascular changes in people with Down's syndrome. They suffer from circulatory problems due to abnormally thin and narrow peripheral arterioles and capillaries resulting in local tissue hypoxia. Capillary fragility is high in comparison to normal children or children with other forms of mental handicap. This could be due either to a connective tissue disorder or diminished platelet activity. These vascular changes could lead to local tissue anoxia.

Patients with Down's syndrome need special care if dental problems are to be avoided or kept under control. They need frequent monitoring with prompt treatment of any problem. Good plaque control must be established to combat periodontal problems and scaling needs to be carried out frequently. Patient cooperation and acceptance of treatment and the support of the family and carers are of paramount importance. If the patient lacks the dexterity necessary for immaculate oral hygiene then these functions will need to be carried out by relatives or carers and they will need to be trained in this function and informed about dental disease and its control and the increased susceptibility in Down's syndrome. These functions are considerably more difficult to carry out in an institution than in the home environment.

Hypophosphatasia

Hypophosphatasia is a rare condition with an autosomal recessive mode of inheritance. There is a deficiency of the enzyme alkaline phosphatase and urinary excretion of phosphoethanolamine. It is characterized by abnormal mineralization of bones and dental tissues. In the infantile form which appears at birth there is softening of bones, fever, anaemia,

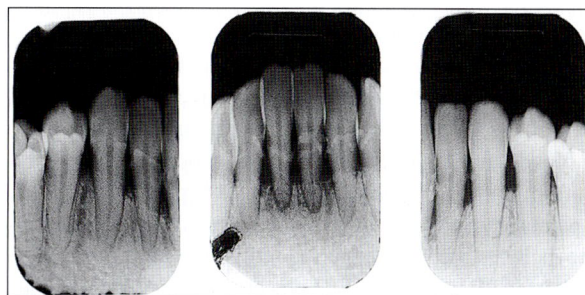

Fig. 6.4 Radiographs of the lower incisors, canines and premolars of a 14-year-old boy with Down's syndrome. They show advanced alveolar bone loss.

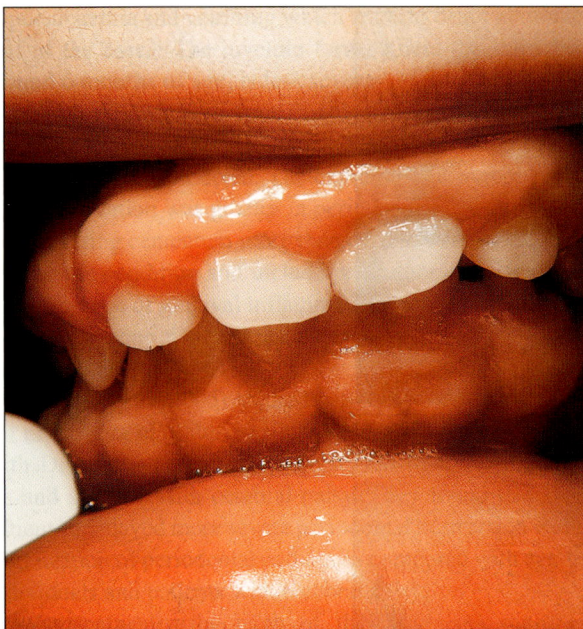

Fig. 6.6 Hereditary gingival fibrous overgrowth in a 13-year-old boy. Regrowth of this tissue followed gingivectomies on two occasions.

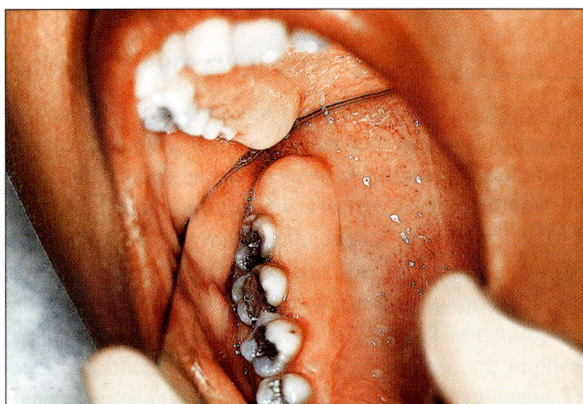

Fig. 6.7 Hereditary gingival fibrous overgrowth of the lingual gingivae and retromolar area of a 25-year-old man. This tissue also recurred after several gingivectomies.

All cells expressed *c-myc* mRNA at quiescence and up to 1 h after serum stimulation. Expression of *c-myc* in quiescent HGF from hereditary gingival fibromatosis tissue was elevated, peaked and remained higher after serum stimulation than in NGF. There was significant inhibition of HGF proliferation by *c-myc* antisense ODN and not by *c-myc* sense ODN with reversal in response to hybridized *c-myc* antisense and sense ODNs. This suggests that the elevated proliferation of the HGF cell line from hereditary gingival fibromatosis tissue was related to elevated *c-myc* expression. A simultaneous decrease in apoptosis could contribute to gingival overgrowth (Kantarci et al 2007).

Mucopolysaccharidoses

The mucopolysaccharidoses (MPS) are a group of inherited disorders characterized by disturbances of lysosomal enzymes that break down glycosaminoglycans resulting in increased storage of these substances in various tissues (Ponder & Haskins 2007). They include Hurler's syndrome (MPS I), Hunter's syndrome (MPS II), I-cell disease and MPS III, IV, V and VI. Hurler's syndrome is inherited as an autosomal recessive trait, while Hunter's syndrome is an X-linked recessive trait and I-cell disease probably represents the homozygous state of a recessive mutation. Hurler's syndrome manifests in early childhood and children usually die before 10 years of age from respiratory infection or cardiac disease secondary to

deposition of mucopolysaccharides in the heart valves and intima of the coronary arteries. The main clinical features of this syndrome are mental retardation, dwarfism, hernia, deformed head, typical facies, short neck and spinal deformities. Hunter's syndrome is less severe and the survival rate is greater. In both syndromes there are increased levels of chondroitin sulphate B and heparin sulphate in the urine.

Dental manifestations can be severe with unerupted teeth, dentigerous cyst like follicles, malocclusion, condylar defects and gingival overgrowth (Alpoz et al 2006).

Hyperoxaluria and oxalosis

Primary hyperoxaluria is a rare autosomal recessive inherited disease of glycoxalate metabolism and is due to an enzyme deficiency. It results in the deposition of calcium oxalate in various tissues throughout the body. Its clinical features are nephrolithiasis, nephrocalcinosis, acute arthritis, heart block and peripheral neuropathy. The life expectancy is poor and death is usually due to renal failure. New therapeutic approaches include recombinant gene therapy for enzyme replacement (Babrowski & Langman 2006). Secondary hyperoxaluria can also occur in chronic renal failure where oxalate deposits in the kidney possibly due to recurrent dialysis failing to remove all the calcium oxalate.

The main oral changes of oxalosis (Wysocki et al 1982) are root resorption, both external and internal, associated with deposits of calcium oxalate crystals; and pain resulting from the inflammatory granulomatous foreign body reaction in the periodontal ligament or pulp which could account for root resorption.

The only effective treatment of the root resorption appears to be extraction of the grossly involved teeth.

GRANULOMATOUS CONDITIONS

Crohn's disease

Crohn's disease or regional enteritis is a chronic inflammatory condition primarily of the terminal ileum and was first described by Crohn et al (1932). It affects the submucosa of the gastrointestinal tract and produces stenosis, necrotic breakdown and scarring of the mucosa. All areas of the tract including the mouth can be affected but the initial lesion is in the terminal ileum. Symptoms include abdominal pain, pyrexia, intermittent diarrhoea, joint pains and generalized malaise. The overall incidence is about 15 per 100 000 but is higher in Jews and siblings of affected patients. Some cases present with mucocutaneous findings and are subsequently diagnosed as Crohn's disease (Galbraith et al 2005).

The aetiology is unknown but intolerance to certain foods particularly those containing gluten may be an important factor and there is a familial tendency. A gluten-free diet is recommended for these subjects.

The oral manifestations of Crohn's disease are aphthous-like ulceration and a cobblestone appearance of the oral mucosa (**Fig. 6.8**), labial and buccal gingival swellings, mucosal tags, fissuring of the midline of the lip and angular cheilitis (Galbraith et al 2005).

The characteristic gingival lesion is diffuse, erythematous, granular enlargement of the attached gingiva. The cobblestone appearance of the oral mucosa is mainly confined to the buccal mucosa and the lesions are lobulated, oedematous and fissured and ulceration may be present. The tag-like lesions in the mucobuccal fold resemble denture granulomata. Gingival overgrowth is one of the early manifestations of Crohn's disease (Ruocco et al 2007); severe periodontitis has been seen in patients with this condition. Dense lymphocyte infiltrates and non caseating giant cell granulomas are typically seen in the submucosa (Galbraith et al 2005; Bogenrieder et al 2003). Patients with active bowel disease have been reported to have high levels of circulating immune complexes and metabolically active PMNs

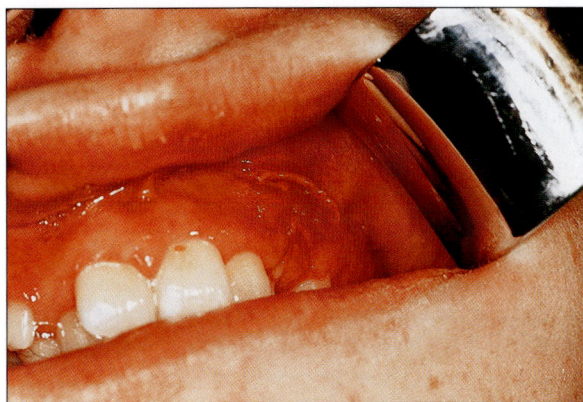

Fig. 6.8 Appearance of the gingivae in Crohn's disease (Courtesy of Professor C. Scully).

compared with healthy controls. It has also been found that the PMNs from these patients had elevated levels of alkaline phosphatase which is an indication of early release of these cells from the marrow. In addition, it has been found that these patients had low circulating B-lymphocyte numbers and high numbers of T-lymphocytes. All of these factors could exacerbate an existing periodontal condition or accelerate its progress. These patients usually respond well to conventional periodontal treatment.

Sarcoidosis

Sarcoidosis is a granulomatous condition of uncertain aetiology, which may affect the lymph nodes, lungs, liver, spleen, skin, eyes, phalangeal bones and parotid glands. The worldwide prevalence is 20 per 100 000 with higher levels in blacks than whites. Its prognosis is good with most cases showing spontaneous healing which can be accelerated by the administration of corticosteroids (Suresh & Radfar 2005).

Oral lesions occur rarely with swelling of the parotid glands and cervical lymph nodes as the most common and gingival involvement as least common. It may also affect the minor salivary glands (Suresh & Radfar 2005). The histopathology is a collection of monocyte-derived epithelioid cells with T-lymphocytes and occasional plasma cells. Several cases of sarcoid gingivitis have been reported. The gingivae have a hyperplastic, granulomatous appearance and may have superficial ulceration. Histologically there is an infiltration of macrophages and their polykaryons.

Scleroderma

Scleroderma or systemic sclerosis is a connective tissue disorder of uncertain aetiology. It produces inflammatory, vascular and fibrotic changes in the skin and other organs and structures. The changes may be limited to the skin or generalized and in the latter form the prognosis is poor particularly if there is involvement of the lungs, heart and kidneys.

The main change in the periodontium brought about by this condition is widening of the periodontal ligament space at the expense of alveolar bone (Alpoz et al 2007). The changes affect the posterior teeth more than the anterior teeth. The teeth remain firm and the apical level of the junctional epithelium is unaffected. There is a proportional increase in collagen and oxytalan fibres and the fibrous tissue contains areas of degeneration with sclerosis and hyalinization.

HAEMATOLOGICAL CONDITIONS (BLOOD DISEASES)

Blood diseases do not appear to cause gingivitis but they do bring about tissue changes which alter the tissue response to plaque. The dentist has a special responsibility in relation to these diseases as severe gingival bleeding is a common feature of acute leukaemia and the dentist may be the first person to examine the patient. Delay in the control of such a disease could be fatal.

Red blood cell (RBC) disorders

Anaemia

Anaemia is defined as a reduction in the concentration of haemoglobin in the blood below the normal level. This is usually accepted for males as 12.5–18.0 g/dL and for females as 12.0–16.5 g/dL. There are a large number of causes of anaemia, including haemorrhage, chemical damage and disease, but the most common form is iron-deficiency anaemia which is found in about 10% of the female population. Anaemia lowers the oxygen-carrying capacity of the blood so that the patient may feel tired and faint and may have difficulty in breathing and tingling of the fingers and toes. There could be pallor of the mucosa, the tongue may lose its normally rough papillated surface and become smooth. There may be recurrent aphthous ulcers and angular cheilitis in some cases. If anaemia is suspected blood examination is necessary.

Aplastic anaemia

Aplastic anaemia can be caused by drugs, chemicals, radiation, infections or neoplasia. The resultant anaemia, leucopenia and thrombocytopenia produce weakness, fatigue, recurrent infections, pyrexia, epistaxis and retinal haemorrhage. The main oral effects are gingival bleeding and infections.

A rare autosomal recessive inherited form of aplastic anaemia with a poor prognosis is called Fanconi's anaemia. Orally, it produces a rapidly progressive destructive periodontitis with early tooth loss (Opinya et al 1988).

Acatalasia

This is a rare inherited disease caused by the absence of the enzyme catalase in RBCs and WBCs. Catalase converts hydrogen peroxide to oxygen and water. High concentrations of hydrogen peroxide can be toxic, affecting cell signalling, proliferation and apoptosis, resulting in gangrene (Goth et al 2004) and necrosis of gingival tissue. A case report of two siblings with this condition described gingival necrosis and severe destructive periodontitis.

White blood cell (WBC) disorders

Neutrophils (PMNs) and monocytes are essential cells in the defence system of the periodontium. Reductions in their numbers or their function can have a profound effect on the periodontal tissues. The term leucopenia means an absolute reduction in numbers of WBCs and neutropenia means reduction in the number of PMNs. The leukaemias are a group of neoplastic conditions in which there is uncontrolled proliferation of the affected group of WBCs.

Neutropenia

Neutropenia may be genetic, familial, idiopathic or secondary to viral, bacterial or protozoan infections or systemic disease. All forms of neutropenia profoundly affect periodontal health. The main primary neutropenias are:

- Cyclic neutropenia
- Chronic benign neutropenia
- Familial neutropenias
- Chronic idiopathic neutropenia.

The periodontal manifestations of neutrophil dysfunction (Deas et al 2003) and other immunodeficient states including a protocol for management (Pattni et al 2000) have been extensively reviewed recently, some of which are summarized below.

Cyclic neutropenia

This is a rare autosomal dominant inherited condition. It produces a cyclical depression of PMNs in the peripheral blood at intervals varying from 15–55 days with occasional longer periods of neutropenia lasting 1–2 months. The main clinical manifestations are pyrexia, oral ulceration and skin infections. The condition appears to be due to periodic stem cell failure in the bone marrow related to a disorder of haemopoietic feedback control.

The main oral and periodontal features of this condition are oral ulceration, severe gingivitis, rapid periodontal breakdown and alveolar bone loss. In the permanent dentition the bone loss is most obvious around the teeth that erupt first, the first molars and lower incisors. Patients with this condition require regular periodontal maintenance for careful supra- and subgingival scaling and meticulous oral hygiene should be encouraged. Antibiotic therapy will be necessary to control acute episodes and antiseptic mouthwashes will help when oral ulceration is present.

Chronic benign neutropenia of childhood

The onset of this condition is usually between 6 and 20 months. There is a moderate neutropenia with an absolute lymphocytosis and monocytosis. The bone marrow appears normal and the neutropenia may be due to increased peripheral destruction.

Pyogenic infections of the skin and mucous membranes are a feature of this condition. However, the increased numbers of monocytes in this condition can compensate for the neutropenia and may provide a reasonable resistance to infections.

Several case reports of the oral and periodontal features of this condition have appeared and most of these relate to boys aged 4–12 years. There is a bright red, hyperplastic, oedematous gingivitis, which affects the free and attached gingivae and the gingivae bleed easily. There appears to be premature loss of primary teeth due to bone loss. Some older children show a rapidly progressive periodontitis in the permanent dentition with generalized bone loss. In most reports attempts to control the condition with periodontal treatment have been unsuccessful and early loss of primary and permanent teeth seems difficult to prevent.

Benign familial neutropenia

Benign familial neutropenia is an autosomal dominant inherited condition. There is a moderate neutropenia and an accompanying monocytosis. The bone marrow appears normal and the condition may be due to an anomaly in the marrow release mechanism.

The first case report of this condition described the oral and periodontal changes in a 14-year-old boy with this condition; described as a bright red, hyperplastic, oedematous gingivitis and the tissues that bled profusely. There was also marked bone loss around the first molars suggesting a rapidly progressive periodontitis. The treatment was plaque control, scaling and antiseptic mouthwashes but no long-term follow-up of the patient's condition was reported. Other reports of 34 cases and 11 controls gave a similar description of the clinical picture and also showed that although regular treatment and excellent oral hygiene helped to control the periodontal condition, these measures did not prevent its progression.

Severe familial neutropenia

This is more severe than the benign form and is inherited as an autosomal dominant trait. There is a more marked neutropenia and some monocytosis. Children are susceptible to repeated infections. The oral and periodontal changes are similar to those described above but more severe and the prognosis is poor.

Chronic idiopathic neutropenia

Chronic idiopathic neutropenia appears to occur mainly in females. There is a persistent neutropenia from birth which is not cyclical and there is no family history of the condition. There are persistent recurrent infections throughout the life of the sufferers. The cause of the condition is uncertain but there does appear to be a maturation abnormality of granulocytes in the bone marrow which could be related to an autoimmune disorder.

The periodontal features have been reported in two case reports. There is a severe, oedematous, inflammatory gingival enlargement with early bone loss and the condition does not respond well to treatment.

Leukaemia

Leukaemias are malignant neoplastic diseases of the white blood cell forming tissues. They usually result in an increased number of leucocytes in the circulation including developing blast cells and an infiltration of leukaemic cells into other tissues, particularly lymph nodes. The condition may affect granulocytes (myeloid), monocytes (monocytic) or lymphocytes (lymphocytic) and can be either chronic or acute. In acute forms large numbers of neoplastic primitive stem and blast cells proliferate in the marrow and enter the circulation. The acute forms of leukaemia are more common in children and young adults and the chronic forms in adults over 40 years.

The clinical signs and symptoms are due to reduced numbers of other marrow cells such as red cells and megakaryocytes which are crowded out by the proliferation of neoplastic cells and from the lack of normal function from the leukaemic cells themselves. Early symptoms include tiredness, lethargy and fatigue due to anaemia, malaise, sore throat, oral ulceration and skin infections due to infection from reduced white cell function and lymph nodes, splenic and hepatic enlargement due to leukaemic infiltration. Chronic leukaemias have a slow, insidious onset with tiredness, weight loss, fatigue, pyrexia and splenic enlargement being the main features.

The oral and periodontal features may reflect both the condition and its treatment with radiotherapy and chemotherapy. They include oral ulceration, petechiae and ecchymoses, gingival enlargement, gingival bleeding and bacterial, viral and fungal infections. Oropharyngeal lesions may be the initial complaint in over 10% of acute leukaemias. The gingival enlargement (**Fig. 6.9**) is due to infiltration of leukaemic cells

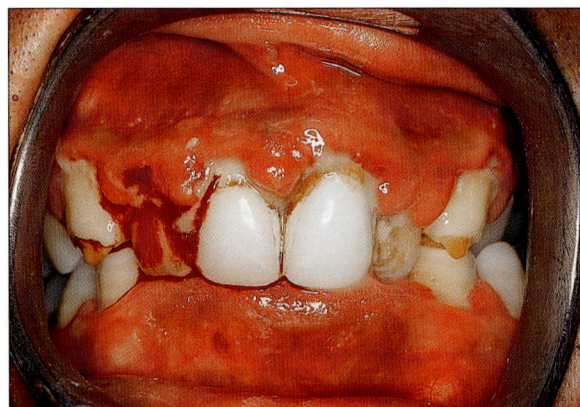

Fig. 6.9 Gingival inflammation, spontaneous gingival bleeding and oedematous gingival enlargement in a patient with myeloid leukaemia during an acute exacerbation of the condition.

(Ozcan et al 2007) and is most common in monocytic leukaemia. Gingival bleeding is secondary to the accompanying thrombocytopenia and may present as oozing or frank bleeding. It is most marked when the platelet count drops below 10 000 per mL.

Infections may be due either to an exacerbation of an existing condition or to susceptibility to a range of bacterial, viral and fungal infections. Existing periodontitis can be exacerbated by the leukaemia or by chemotherapy. A variety of infections can occur for similar reasons and include acute necrotizing ulcerative gingivitis (ANUG), acute herpetic gingivostomatitis and fungal infections such as candidiasis.

Leukaemic patients need careful hygiene care during acute episodes of the disease or during treatment with radiotherapy and chemotherapy. Regular gentle professional cleaning and swabbing with chlorhexidine can be very beneficial.

Every effort should be made to treat any periodontal condition during phases of remission of the disease and to encourage immaculate plaque control during this time. Oral and periodontal infections may need to be treated with the appropriate antibiotic. The patient's physician should always be consulted before any treatment is carried out so that an appropriate regime can be discussed and agreed.

DISORDERS OF WHITE CELL FUNCTION

These conditions affect the ability of PMNs to phagocytose and destroy bacteria intracellularly. Primary functional disturbances that affect the periodontal tissues are the Chediak–Higashi syndrome and the lazy leucocyte syndrome.

Chediak–Higashi syndrome

Chediak–Higashi syndrome is a rare autosomal recessive inherited disease. Clinical features include albinism with photophobia and nystagmus and frequent pyogenic infections and febrile illnesses. Later a lymphoma-like condition develops with accompanying neutropenia, anaemia and thrombocytopenia. Death usually results from infection or haemorrhage. Circulating leucocytes have large abnormal lysosomes in their cytoplasm and show defective migration and phagocytic degranulation and grossly diminished intracellular killing. The disease gives rise to a very severe gingivitis and periodontitis, and premature loss of the primary and permanent teeth. The condition does not appear to respond well to periodontal treatment.

Lazy leucocyte syndrome

Lazy leucocyte syndrome is associated with a defect in PMN chemotaxis and random mobility. A severe gingivitis has been described in two children with this condition.

Chronic granulomatous disease

Chronic granulomatous disease is an inherited condition transmitted as an autosomal recessive trait in females and as an X-linked recessive trait in males. It is characterized by the inability of phagocytes to destroy certain infective bacteria. The PMNs of subjects with this condition are unable to generate hydrogen peroxide possibly because of the absence of the enzyme NADPH oxidase. A granulomatous response occurs to inflammation and involves the lymph nodes, spleen, liver, skin and lungs. People with this condition are very prone to osteomyelitis, liver abscesses and pneumonia and their prognosis is poor.

Case reports (Buduneli et al 2001) have described severe pre-pubertal periodontitis. This responds to periodontal treatment with adjunctive antibiotics.

IMMUNOLOGICAL CONDITIONS

Hypogammaglobulinaemia

This can, rarely, occur as an X-linked recessive inherited disease. More commonly, it is secondary to chronic lymphatic leukaemia and myeloma. Patients are highly susceptible to infection, particularly of the respiratory tract. There have been some reports of severe destructive periodontitis but other reports have been inconclusive regarding periodontal disease and caries.

Multiple myeloma

This is a multifocal malignant neoplasm of plasma cells. Deposits can occur in the mandible and maxilla. Lesions have also been reported involving the periodontium and gingiva (Petit & Ripamonti 1990). The oral lesions described are gingival ulceration and bleeding and the condition may produce a rapidly growing, retromolar myelomatous mass with multiple foci of alveolar bone destruction.

AUTOIMMUNE CONDITIONS

Systemic lupus erythematosus

Systemic lupus erythematosus (SLE) is a systemic autoimmune condition which affects multiple body organs including the skin and oral mucosa. There is a high prevalence of chronic periodontitis (CP) in SLE and in one study (Kobayashi et al 2003) there was CP in 70% of their studied cases. The leucocyte Fc receptor for immunoglobulin G (IgG) (FcγR) plays a major role in handling pathogens and immune complexes in both SLE and CP. Thus polymorphisms of the gene for this receptor could be associated with both conditions and this has been investigated by Kobayashi et al (2003). A total of 42 SLE patients with CP (SLE/P), 18 SLE patients without CP (SLE/H) and 42 healthy subjects without CP (H/H) were compared among non-related Japanese non-smokers. They found a significant difference in FcγRIIa genotypes between the SLE/P and H/H groups ($p = 0.004$). There was also a significant over-expression of the FcγRIIa-R131 allele in SLE/P compared with H/H subjects ($p = 0.001$). This allele was also significantly over-expressed in the SLE/P compared with the SLE/H subjects ($p = 0.01$). Thus, the FcγRIIa-R131 allele seems to be associated with a high risk of CP in SLE patients.

Immunosuppressive drugs

Immunosuppressive drugs are often given to combat autoimmune disease or to prevent rejection of transplants. They include corticosteroids, azathioprine and ciclosporin. Corticosteroids and azathioprine reduce the inflammatory response and may reduce gingivitis. Ciclosporin may produce gingival fibrous hyperplasia (see below).

DERMATOSES

A number of skin diseases have oral manifestations which can occur on the gingivae. Some of these diseases are moderately common such as lichen planus and some are extremely rare such as pemphigus vulgaris.

Lichen planus

This disease is estimated to occur in 1% of the population. It is an inflammatory disease of doubtful aetiology which occurs in the skin and mucous membranes. It is more frequently observed in conjunction with diseases of immunity, e.g. ulcerative colitis, myasthenia gravis and hypogammaglobulinaemia, and there is increasing evidence that lichen planus is immunologically mediated. Lichen planus can occur in families and there is an increasing frequency of HLA-B7 in the MHC (see Ch. 3). The oral lesion can occur either in the absence of skin lesions or with minimal or widespread skin lesions and there is no difference in the oral lesion with or without skin involvement. The disease may be manifest in various forms.

The classification of lichen planus has evolved over the years. Andreasen (1968) proposed a scheme based on recognition of reticular, papular, plaque-like, atrophic, ulcerative and bullous forms of the lesion. The most recent classification by Eisen (2002) describes three main categories comprising: (1) a reticular lesion with white lines, plaques and papules, (2) an atrophic or erythematous presentation and (3) an erosive form with ulcerations and bullae.

The reticular form is the most common and consists of an interlacing network of white lines, plaques and papules found frequently on the cheeks, vestibule and gingiva (**Fig. 6.10**). Either erosive or reticular lesions can occur on the gingivae (**Fig. 6.11**) and it is the most common cause of erosive (desquamative) gingivitis. The lesion may be symptomless or painful and sore, the latter being more common with the erosive form. The lesions are sensitive to spicy and acid foods.

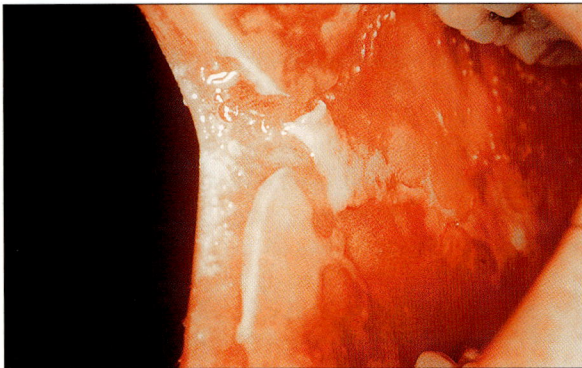

Fig. 6.10 Reticular and erosive lichen planus of the buccal mucosa.

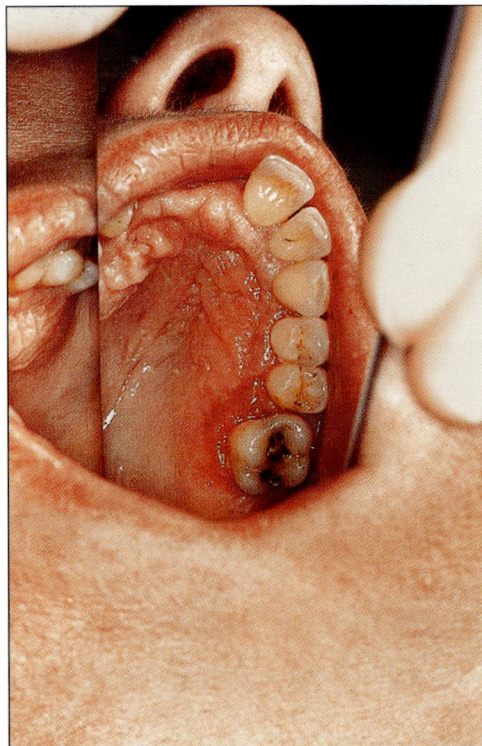

Fig. 6.11 Erosive lichen planus of the palatal gingivae in a 45-year-old female patient.

A semi-quantitative scoring system has been proposed for monitoring the severity of reticular/hyperkeratotic, erosive/erythematous and ulcerative lesions of oral lichen planus and chronic graft versus host disease following allogenic bone marrow transplantation (Piboonniyom et al 2005). It has the advantage of combining the clinical presentation and degree of involvement at different sites and enables monitoring of disease progression and response to therapy, for comparison between patients.

Some reports have suggested that some cases of oral lichenoid lesions in contact with amalgam restorations (contact lesions) may be caused or aggravated by an allergy to mercury from the amalgam (Eley 1993). Mercury deposits have been found in lysosomes of fibroblasts and macrophages from contact lesions. Some of these cases show remission following the replacement of amalgam restorations with alternative restorative materials and this may support the theory that mercury allergy may be a causative or aggravating factor in certain cases of oral lichen planus.

Treatment of lichen planus is symptomatic and topical applications of triamcinolone paste (Adcortyl A in Orabase) 2–4 times per day may alleviate symptoms.

Benign mucous membrane pemphigoid

This is a disease of mucous membranes caused by an immunological disorder. Usually it occurs in older adults. The lesion is a bulla (**Fig. 6.12**) which breaks down quickly to form an ulcer with an inflamed surrounding area; this heals to form scarring (Shklar & McCarthy 1959). It is most often seen in women at the menopause or after, but is not confined to women.

The disease may affect the gingivae and it is an uncommon cause of erosive gingivitis. There is diffuse erythema of the gingivae with grey patches of desquamated epithelium. The involved areas are very sensitive and patients complain of soreness aggravated by spicy foods. The condition is chronic with periods of remission.

Treatment is symptomatic. Irritant foods or drinks or mouthwashes should be avoided. Topical applications of triamcinolone paste (Adcortyl A in Orabase) may help but Orabase alone is often just as effective. The patient needs to be reassured that the condition is benign, unless there is ocular involvement, when scarring may impair vision.

Pemphigus vulgaris

This is an autoimmune disease in which antibody and T cells react with cells of mucous membranes thus destroying the cells. If widespread involvement occurs the disease may be fatal. The oral lesions often occur before skin lesions appear and the dentist has a special diagnostic responsibility. Most cases develop in middle age, often in patients of Jewish or Italian extraction.

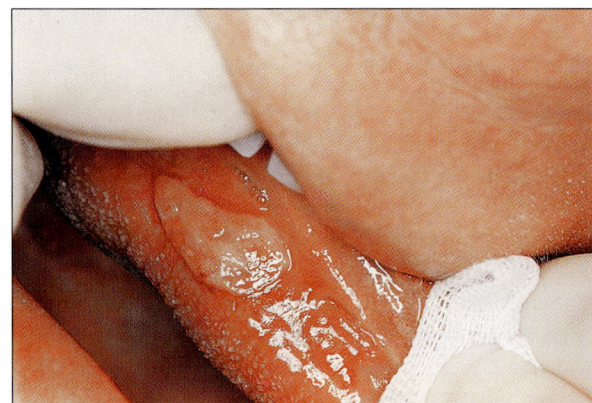

Fig. 6.12 Sub-epithelial bulla on the lower buccal mucosa of a patient with benign mucous membrane pemphigoid.

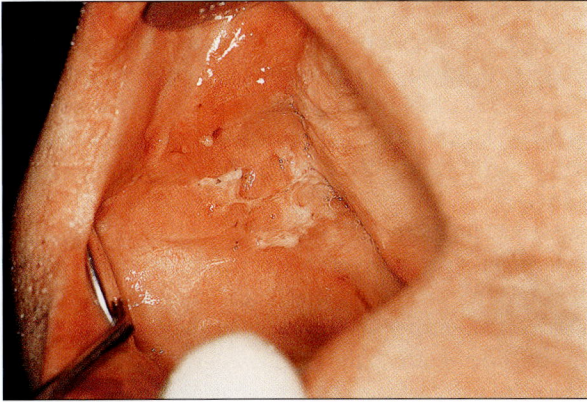

Fig. 6.13 Intraepithelial bullae on the buccal mucosa of a patient with pemphigus vulgaris (Courtesy of Professor S. Warnkulsuriya).

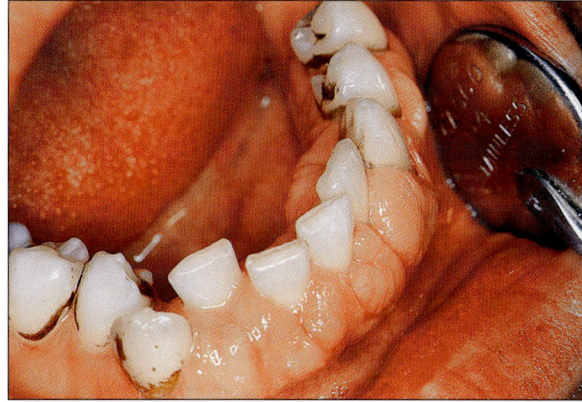

Fig. 6.14 Fibrous gingival overgrowth in an epileptic patient controlled with phenytoin (epanutin).

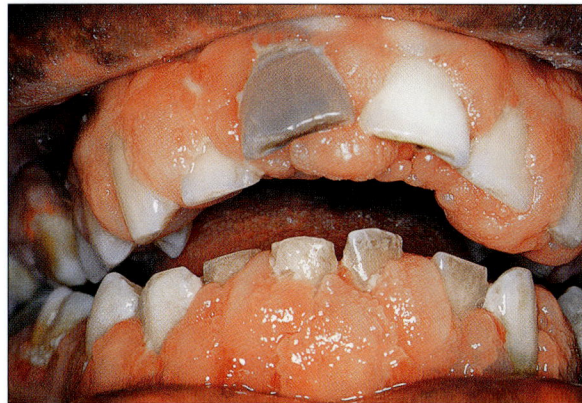

Fig, 6.15 Marked generalized fibrous gingival overgrowth in a kidney transplant patient controlled with the immunosuppressant ciclosporin.

The disease is characterized by the formation of bullae (large vesicles or blisters) in any part of the oral mucosa (**Fig. 6.13**), including the gingivae. The bullae break down rapidly to form ragged ulcers which may heal slowly. There is pain and swelling and if the lesions involve the palate and throat, swallowing is difficult.

Sometimes it is possible to make a diagnosis by using the 'Nikolsky sign', in which sliding pressure with the finger over apparently intact mucosa dislodges the mucosa. Definitive diagnosis is made by histological examination of biopsy specimens. If pemphigus is suspected immediate referral to a physician is essential. The condition may be controlled by systemic corticosteroids. Scully and Felix (2005) have reviewed the more serious causes of oral mucosal ulceration.

INFECTIONS

Localized or generalized infections may involve the oral mucosa or periodontal tissues. Localized infections include acute necrotizing ulcerative gingivitis (Ch. 25) and acute lateral periodontal abscess (Ch. 22). Generalized infections include herpes simplex infections, herpes varicella/zoster infections, measles, tuberculosis, syphilis and *Candida albicans* infections (Ch. 24) and acquired immune deficiency syndrome (AIDS) (Ch. 7).

DRUG REACTIONS

In recent years, it has been established that drugs which alter the haemopoietic system or the immune system, either to decrease or to enhance its activity, alter the response of the gingivae to plaque. As stated in Chapter 3, these findings support the idea of the involvement of the immune system in the pathogenesis of periodontal disease. However, the most common response of the gingiva to drugs is gingival overgrowth described below.

DRUG-RELATED GINGIVAL OVERGROWTH

The anticonvulsant drug phenytoin (Epanutin, Dilantin, DPH) given to epileptics, the immunosuppressive drug ciclosporin and the calcium channel blocking drug nifedipine, given to treat cardiac angina, arrhythmias and hypertension, can produce fibrous overgrowth of the gingivae (Seymour 2006), not directly related to drug dose. Phenytoin stabilizes neuronal membranes by reducing their permeability to calcium and can contribute to folic acid depletion.

Some degree of gingival enlargement occurs in a large percentage of epileptics taking phenytoin (**Fig. 6.14**), especially those under 40 years. The condition is less common in patients on ciclosporine (Savage et al 1987)

but when it occurs it may be very severe (**Fig. 6.15**). Nifedipine induced gingival overgrowth is less firm than the other two and contains a higher proportion of ground substance.

The gingivae on the labial surface of the anterior teeth are usually more severely affected than the posterior teeth, and appear firm, pink and lobulated, aggravated by poor plaque control. With superimposed inflammation, the gingival swelling can become soft and red and bleed when provoked. The gingival enlargement can almost cover the teeth and the condition may add to the social handicap that the epileptic patient may suffer.

Both inflammation and the effects of the drugs on androgen metabolism seem to be important in causing the fibrous overgrowth in both sexes. Testosterone is converted by 5α-reductase into 5α-dihydrotestosterone (DHT) which is its main biologically active metabolite. Specific receptors for androgens are present in the gingivae (Huang et al 2003) and these increase in number by 2–3-fold in inflamed and enlarged gingival tissue. These DHT receptors are located on gingival epithelial cells and fibroblasts and phenytoin has been found to stimulate 5α-reductase activity in fibroblasts from inflamed gingival tissue (Soory 2000). DHT stimulates gingival fibroblasts to produce and secrete collagen and proteoglycan. During inflammation gingival tissue metabolizes testosterone to the same extent in males and females (Ojanatko et al 1980). Phenytoin stimulates the biosynthesis of DHT from testosterone in gingival fibroblasts. Ciclosporin and nifedipine also carry out this function (Soory 2000).

These drugs, probably as a result of the production of DHT, may also select a subpopulation of fibroblasts which produce large amounts of collagen with the production of an inactive form of collagenase. This subgroup of cells may be more responsive to DHT stimulation. Hyland et al (2003) have grown gingival fibroblasts in culture in the presence or absence of pharmacologically related concentrations of ciclosporin. They determined the levels of the mRNA for MMP-1 and MMP-1 released into the medium.

They showed that ciclosporin inhibited MMP-1mRNA production and MMP-1 release into the medium. These results supported the hypothesis that the accumulation of collagen seen in ciclosporin overgrowth is, at least in part, due to reduced collagenolytic activity.

It has also been found by experiments on rats (Paik et al 2004) that ciclosporin A decreases collagen degradation by lowering the phagocytic activity of rat gingival fibroblasts. Clinically ciclosporin A (CsA)- induced gingival overgrowth in rats can be reduced by additional administration of azithromycin and this appears to be due to compensation for decreased phagocytic activity by this agent.

Cotrim et al (2003) have incubated normal gingival fibroblasts with increasing concentrations of either ciclosporin A or transforming growth factor beta-1 (TGF-β1). They found that both these agents increased the rate of proliferation of these cells. They also found that if the cells were simultaneously treated with ciclosporin and an antisense oligonucleotide against the translation-start site of the TGF-β1 mRNA the proliferative effects were abolished. This suggests that ciclosporin has an autocrine stimulatory effect on TGF-β1.

Apoptosis plays a critical role in the regulation of inflammation and the host immune response. In a recent investigation, Alaaddinolu et al (2005) showed that the extent of keratinocyte apoptosis in the gingiva of kidney recipients with CsA-induced gingival overgrowth was similar to that observed in inflamed gingiva of healthy individuals, implying other mechanisms for gingival overgrowth. Only a percentage of patients undergoing treatment with ciclosporin A (CsA) show gingival overgrowth (GO). Ruggeri et al (2005) previously showed that CsA induced over-expression of phospholipase C (PLC)β1 in fibroblasts of patients with clinical GO, in cells from both enlarged and clinically healthy gingival sites. Their more recent study investigated whether the exaggerated fibroblast response to CsA and associated increase in PLCβ1 expression could also be detected in CsA-treated patients without clinical signs of GO. They found a reduced response. These findings supported the concept of a multi-factorial origin of gingival overgrowth, including specific changes within the gingival tissues orchestrating fibroblastic hyper-responsiveness as a consequence of a long-term *in vivo* exposure to ciclosporin A.

A study on rats and human epithelial cells (Chin et al 2006) suggested that CsA could upregulate the gene and protein expression of epidermal growth factor (EGF) and EGF-receptor, and the upregulation might then play a role in gingival overgrowth.

Another study on 121 Italian renal transplant recipients (Vescovi et al 2005) showed that gingival enlargement as a result of all immunosuppressive drugs was predominantly related to genetic predisposition, duration of immunosuppressive treatment and oral hygiene status. The inflammatory response associated with the latter results in a pool of growth mediating agents which could exacerbate medication induced gingival overgrowth. This may have some support from the study of Dannewitz et al (2006) who showed elevated gene expression for collagen and decorin in human gingival overgrowth subjects.

Bostanci et al (2006) investigated the relationship between IL-1A polymorphisms and gingival overgrowth in renal transplant recipients on Ciclosporin A (CsA). They found an association of this gene polymorphism as a risk factor for CsA-induced gingival overgrowth in renal transplant patients and demonstrated that IL-1A polymorphism might alter individual susceptibility to CsA. However, there was no association between GCF cytokine levels and the presence of gingival overgrowth or patient IL-1A genotype.

Huang et al (2003) compared the expression of the androgen receptor (AR) and the Th1/Th2 cytokine profile in gingival cells from tissue obtained from healthy (H), periodontitis (P) subjects and subjects with nifedipine gingival overgrowth (N) by immunocytochemistry. AR and IL-1, IFN-γ, IL-4, IL-10 and IL-13 were intensely expressed in the nuclei of inflammatory cells and fibroblasts in gingival connective tissue. There was much stronger expression of AR and IL-1 and IFN-γ (Th1) in the nifedipine group (N) than the other groups (H,P). The numbers of AR+ gingival fibroblasts were significantly higher in the N group than the others (H,P) ($p < 0.05$). The trend of the N group towards a Th1 profile was highly significant ($p < 0.0001$). Thus, nifedipine appears to elevate AR expression in cells in susceptible tissue such as the gingiva and strongly promotes a Th1 immune profile.

Treatment aimed at patient motivation to improve plaque control measures and thorough supra- and subgingival debridement improves the clinical presentation of gingival overgrowth. Local removal of gingival overgrowth may be carried out by gingivectomy or inverse bevel gingivectomy in some cases. Recurrence of the overgrowth is common but may be reduced if immaculate oral hygiene can be maintained. Laser excision of gingival overgrowth has been shown to reduce the rate of recurrence at 6 months when compared with conventional gingivectomy procedures (Mavrogiannis et al 2006).

A macrolide molecule known as tacrolimus has recently been introduced as an alternative immunosuppressant drug to ciclosporin A and it has performed well in clinical trials. Despite major differences in chemical structure, tacrolimus and ciclosporin A have several intracellular effects in common. A recent study (James et al 2001) compared 25 renal transplant recipients on tacrolimus immunosuppression for at least 18 months with 26 controls. Neither group showed clinically significant gingival overgrowth and this seems to indicate that tacrolimus has no adverse effects on gingival tissue.

A regression of nifedipine-induced gingival overgrowth has been shown to occur when patients have been switched on to other drugs in the same class of calcium channel blockers (Westbrook et al 1997). They found that 60% of patients placed on the alternative calcium channel blocker, Isradipine, had regression of their nifedipine-induced gingival hyperplasia. Furthermore, no patients placed primarily on Isradipine developed gingival overgrowth.

DIETARY AND NUTRITIONAL FACTORS

Epidemiological studies have demonstrated that at any given age, there is more severe periodontal disease in African and Asian populations than in Europeans. This could be due either to nutritional deficiency or poor oral hygiene, both of which reflect socioeconomic status. There is no evidence to support the supplementation of an already balanced diet with extra vitamins for improved outcome. It is relevant that health professionals should identify deficient nutrition as an aggravating risk factor in conditions with an inflammatory pathogenesis such as periodontal diseases (Riley 2007) and its implications on management.

Recent literature has demonstrated the efficacy of antioxidants found in plant extracts in treating diseases with an inflammatory pathogenesis. Plant derived substances such as lycopene in tomatoes (Wood & Johnson 2004), flavonoid extracts of Ginkgo biloba (Mozaffarieh & Flammer 2007), green tea (Hirasawa et al 2002; Sakanaka & Okada 2004), soy isoflavones (Nielsen & Williamson 2007), Coenzyme Q10 in mitochondria of cells (Battino et al 2005) and Pycnogenol (Baumann 2005) derived from French maritime pine bark and rich in proanthocyanidins have been shown to have potent antioxidant effects in reducing free radical damage relevant to periodontal and metabolic diseases.

A correlation has been shown between chronic periodontal disease and risk of congestive heart failure in adult participants (Wood & Johnson 2004). A high monthly consumption of tomatoes associated with elevated levels of serum lycopene seemed to reduce this risk in periodontitis subjects with decreased levels of CRP and a reduced WBC (Wood & Johnson 2004). Lycopene seems to be the most effective carotenoid in reducing adhesion of monocytes to human aortic endothelial cells as well as cell surface expression of adhesion molecules (Martin et al 2000).

Oxidative stress can be reduced at a mitochondrial level by Ginkgo biloba; polyphenolic flavonoids found in tea, dark chocolate and red wine also have antioxidant properties (Mozaffarieh & Flammer 2007). The bactericidal effect of green tea catechin against *Porphyromonas gingivalis* and *Prevotella* spp. was shown at an MIC of 1.0 mg/mL; the *in vivo* study on periodontal patients using hydroxypropyl cellulose strips impregnated with green tea catechin as a slow release device as an adjunct to mechanical debridement showed improvement in periodontal status (Hirasawa et al 2002). At a concentration of 1–2 mg/mL polyphenolic compounds isolated from green tea have also been shown to inhibit the production of n-butyric acid and propionic acid by *Porphyromonas gingivalis* suggestive of an application in the adjunctive management of periodontal disease (Sakanaka & Okada 2004). Soy isoflavones also demonstrate antioxidant, antiatherosclerotic and anti-cancer properties. They bind to oestrogen receptor and act as moderate phytoestrogens (Nielsen & Williamson 2007) without the side effects of oestrogenic hormones.

An *in vitro* investigation was done to study the oxidant/antioxidant effects of nicotine, coenzyme Q10, Pycnogenol and phytoestrogens in oral periosteal fibroblasts and osteoblasts, using a steroid marker to detect oxidative stress (Figuero et al 2006). The oxidative effects of nicotine were significantly overcome by CoQ10, Pycnogenol and phytoestrogens suggestive of an application for these antioxidants in overcoming the catabolic effects of nicotine. They may be used as adjunctive agents in the management of periodontal patients particularly those with a smoking habit or coexisting diabetes mellitus.

PERIODONTAL DISEASE AS A POSSIBLE RISK FACTOR FOR OTHER SYSTEMIC CONDITIONS

In the early part of the twentieth century, the medical profession held a general belief that severe systemic infection could result from local site infection and from this the theory of focal injection was developed. With increasing understanding of disease processes and local and systemic defence mechanisms this concept was progressively rejected with the exception of bacterial endocarditis (see Ch. 18).

More recently, this concept has re-emerged with the notion that periodontal infection could play a role in cardiovascular disease (Beck et al 1998; Nakib et al 2004) and pre-term low birth weight pregnancies depending on the size of the inflammatory burden incurred by the severity and distribution of periodontal disease and the type of population studied. The evidence needs to be considered in the context of an association with the risk factor rather than a cause and effect relationship. This is more difficult to prove in view of several studies being cross-sectional and retrospective.

CARDIOVASCULAR DISEASE

For over a decade periodontal disease has been found to be significantly correlated to cardiovascular disease as well as to cerebral infarction (Syrjanon et al 1989) in case control and follow-up studies. Recently, Renvert et al (2004) demonstrated that a combination of five periodontal parameters comprising BOP, probing depths >6 mm, tooth loss, bone loss and smoking status in a pentagon risk diagram added predictive value to the association and suggested that this should be used in future studies. Radiographic bone loss was found to be the best individual parameter. A systematic review and meta-analysis of cohort studies of this relationship with 100 or more subjects, carried out between 1980 and 2001, showed that subjects with chronic periodontitis average a 19% increased risk of future CVD in comparison to subjects who were periodontally healthy (Janket et al 2003). This increase was more marked in the 44% of subjects who were under 65 years of age. However, this average increase was modest in comparison to other major risk factors for CVD.

Significant reduction in levels of inflammatory markers such as C-reactive protein and oxidized LDL also implicated in cardiovascular atherosclerotic diseases has been reported 3 months after treating periodontal disease in patients with cardiovascular disease (Montebugnoli et al 2004). Chronic infections can increase plasma levels of very-low-density lipoprotein which can lead to a potent atherogenic small, dense low-density lipoprotein. Prevalence of the atherogenic lipoprotein profiles in healthy controls, localized aggressive periodontitis subjects and generalized aggressive periodontitis subjects was 8.3%, 33.3% and 66.6%, respectively (Rufail et al 2007). These findings were significant and may account for increased risk of cardiovascular disease in periodontitis patients. Similarly D'Aiuto et al (2004) studied the systemic effects of treating severe generalized periodontitis in a population of otherwise healthy individuals by examining treatment associated changes in the serum inflammatory markers that are also implicated in cardiovascular atherosclerotic diseases. These patients were enrolled on a prospective single blind longitudinal intervention trial with a 6 month follow-up. The potential impact of specific polymorphisms in cytokine genes known to influence both periodontitis and cardiovascular diseases was also examined. Serum C-reactive protein (CRP) and interleukin-6 (IL-6) levels were assessed by high-sensitivity assays. Serological and clinical periodontal parameters were evaluated at baseline, 2 and 6 months after completion of non-surgical periodontal therapy. There were improvements in all clinical periodontal parameters in the 94 subjects that completed this trial. There were also significant reductions in serum IL-6 and CRP concentrations. Serum CRP levels were significantly associated with the outcome of periodontal treatment after correcting for potential covariates (age, body mass index, gender, smoking and polymorphisms in the IL-6 (-174 C/G) and IL-1A (-889) genes). Subjects with above average response to periodontal therapy accounted for most of the observed improvement in serum CRP. This shows that both severe generalized periodontitis and atherosclerosis cause systemic inflammation and implies a possible association between periodontitis and cardiovascular atherosclerotic diseases.

These findings were reinforced in a subsequent randomized trial (D'Aiuto et al 2005) on 65 systemically healthy subjects suffering from severe generalized periodontitis. Two months after periodontal therapy, there were highly significant reductions in serum C-reactive protein and IL-6 compared with the untreated control group independent of age, gender, body mass index, and ethnicity. In another study looking at slightly different parameters, the possible association of chronic periodontitis and biomarkers of cardiovascular disease has been evaluated in 468 men aged 47–80 free of self-reported CVD, diabetes and cancer (Joshipura et al 2004). Periodontitis was compared with levels of c-reactive protein (CRP), fibrinogen, factor VII, tissue plasminogen activator (t-PA), LDL-C, von Willebrand's factor and soluble tumour necrosis factor receptors 1 and 2. They used multivariate analysis models controlling for age, cigarette smoking, alcohol intake, physical activity and aspirin intake. Self-reported chronic periodontitis was associated with significantly higher levels of CRP (30%), t-PA (11%), LDL-C (11%). This data showed that periodontal disease showed significant associations with biomarkers of endothelial dysfunction and dyslipidaemia. This could potentially mediate the association between chronic periodontitis, cardiovascular disease and diabetes. These results may indicate that periodontitis causes moderate systemic inflammation in systemically healthy subjects. Other studies may not have demonstrated a correlation due to variables such as genetic predisposition of the population studied, host response, severity of the inflammatory burden and smoking habit.

The presence of *P. gingivalis* in the periodontal pocket and the high levels of gingipain activity detected in gingival crevicular fluid could implicate a role for gingipains in the destruction of the highly vascular periodontal tissue. In order to explore the effects of these proteases on endothelial cells, Sheets et al (2005) exposed bovine coronary artery endothelial cells and human microvascular endothelial cells to gingipain-active extracellular protein preparations and/or purified gingipains from *P. gingivalis*. They found that treated cells exhibited a rapid loss of cell adhesion properties that was followed by apoptotic cell death. These results might indicate that gingipains from *P. gingivalis* may alter cell adhesion molecules and induce endothelial cell death, which could have implications for the pathogenicity of this organism and propensity for atherosclerotic plaque formation. These findings have been reinforced by Lee et al (2006) demonstrating another mechanism for cardiac cell apoptosis. The results of a cell culture study on cultured cardiac cells was suggestive of apoptosis directly induced by *P. gingivalis* medium. Their findings suggested that the development of *P. gingivalis*-related H9c2 cell apoptosis was mainly found to be co-activated by p38 and ERK pathways and may have been involved in death receptor-dependent (caspase 8) and mitochondria (caspase 9)-dependent apoptotic pathways. *P. gingivalis*-related cardiac cell apoptosis was also found to be partially mediated by PI3K or calcineurin signalling pathways, whereas the JNK pathway might have played a protective role in *P. gingivalis*-related cardiac cell apoptosis.

Oral bacteria including putative periodontal pathogens have been found in atheromatous plaques (Haraszthy et al 2000) and they are likely to play a role in the pathogenesis of atherosclerosis and coronary vascular disease. Fiehn et al (2005) confirmed that DNA of periodontal pathogens was detected in atherosclerotic plaques including consistency of *Prevotella intermedia* although viable oral bacteria could not be isolated from the atheromas. However, in this regard, more recently Padilla et al (2006) has isolated several periodontal pathogens from the atherosclerotic plaques of 9 out of 12 patients studied and these included *Aggregatibacter actinomycetemcomitans*. Interestingly, each of these subjects had different bacterial species.

In connection with the possible association of periodontitis and atherosclerosis it has been reported (Miyakawa et al 2004) that macrophages stimulated by *Porphyromonas gingivalis* form foam cells in the presence of low density lipoproteins (LDL). This appears to be at least in part due to the aggregation of the protein component of LDL by *P. gingivalis* proteases.

Rodrigues and Progulske-Fox (2005) identified the genes of *P. gingivalis* W83, which were differentially expressed during their invasion of primary human coronary artery endothelial cells, the majority being downregulated. Haemagglutinins may function as adhesins and are required for virulence of several bacterial pathogens. Song et al (2005) studied the role of haemagglutinin B (hagB) in the adherence of *P. gingivalis* to human coronary artery endothelial (HCAE) cells. When the attachment of *P. gingivalis* and the hagB mutant were compared, no statistical significance was observed between the two groups ($p = 0.331$), which was thought to be due to the expression of the *hagB* homologue *hagC*. However *Escherichia coli*-hagB was found to adhere significantly better to HCAE cells than did *E. coli*-pUC9, the control strain, confirmed with competitive assays using antibodies to hagB. These results indicate that hagB may be involved in the adherence of *P. gingivalis* to human primary endothelial cells.

A recent systematic review of the relationship between periodontal disease and coronary heart disease (Madianos et al 2002) was unable to carry out a meta-analysis because of the extensive heterogeneity of the included studies. It, however, reported that 50% of the cohort studies, 75% of the case control studies and 50% of the cross-sectional studies showed a significant association between them. However, it concluded that there was very limited evidence linking periodontal disease and coronary heart disease and that there was a clear need for better designed and larger observational and intervention studies to try to resolve this contentious issue. However, periodontal disease can potentially constitute systemic exposure and play a central role in atheroma formation due to a sequence of events associated with endothelial cell expression of adhesion molecules, oxidative stress induced development of a fatty streak leading to maturation and rupture of the atheroma. Controlling the release of surrogate markers of inflammation in this context has not been fully established in reducing the risk of myocardial infarction (Paquette et al 2007). Further studies along the lines mentioned above are required in order to establish a definitive cause and effect relationship.

RHEUMATOID ARTHRITIS

Periodontal disease and rheumatoid arthritis share many common pathophysiologic features, but a clinical relationship between the two conditions remains controversial, in part because of the confounding effects of anti-inflammatory drug therapy universally used in the latter disease (Ramamurthy et al 2005). These workers further explored this issue. Inflammatory arthritis was induced in rats to determine the effect on gingival biomarkers of inflammation and tissue destruction and to investigate the effect of a therapeutic intervention devoid of conventional anti-inflammatory properties. Adjuvant arthritis was induced in Lewis male rats by injecting mycobacterium cell wall in complete Freund's adjuvant using standard techniques. One group of animals was treated by induction of systemic tissue inhibitor of matrix metalloproteinases (TIMP-4). At 3 weeks, arthritis severity was recorded and both paw and gingival tissues were collected for matrix metalloproteinase activity (MMP) and cytokine analysis. In addition, the maxillary jaws were removed for assessment of periodontal bone loss. The development of arthritis was associated with elevated joint tissue MMPs, tumour necrosis factor alpha (TNF-α), and interleukin-1 (IL-1) levels compared to control rats. In the gingival tissue of the untreated arthritic rats, gelatinase, collagenase, TNF-α, and IL-1 were also elevated compared to control rats. Periodontal bone loss and tooth mobility were also increased significantly ($p < 0.05$) in untreated arthritic rats. All parameters improved after TIMP-4 gene therapy. This appears at the time of writing to be the first study to report an association between experimental systemic arthritis in rats and elevated gingival tissue MMPs, cytokine levels, and periodontal disease. Reversal of these changes with TIMP-4 gene therapy strengthens the pathophysiologic correlation between systemic and local disease. A recent review provides a comprehensive account of the parallels in disease progression and therapeutic scope for rheumatoid arthritis and periodontal diseases, detailing pathogenic mechanisms for potential coexistence of the two diseases in the same individual, driven by an inflammatory stimulus (Soory 2007).

PRE-TERM LOW BIRTH WEIGHT BABIES

Pre-term low birth weight deliveries share a number of common risk factors with periodontal disease including smoking, alcohol consumption, drug use, socioeconomic class, age and nutrition; other risk factors include the level of prenatal care and the prevalence of genito–urinary infections. It is therefore difficult to determine the true level of risk for each of these factors. It also has to be said that all the studies on this subject so far have been cross-sectional cohort or case control studies which can only show associations. They have no power to resolve whether such an association is inconsequential or causal.

There have been a number of such studies recently. Premature low birth weight (PLBW) is defined as those babies weighing less that 2500 g before the 37th week of gestation. A total of 200 periodontal patients were randomly assigned to treatment (during gestation) and treatment after parturition (controls). A multiple regression model showed a significantly better outcome in the group treated during pregnancy, with regard to pre-term and low birth weight (PTLBW) babies (Tarannum et al 2007). They concluded that periodontal treatment could reduce the risk of PTLBW babies in mothers presenting with periodontal disease. Another study on 3576 Turkish women showed that maternal periodontal disease was a risk factor linked to PTLBW and abnormal births (Toygar et al 2007).

A case control study was done on 48 pregnant women in which GCF PGE_2 and IL-Iβ levels were compared (Offenbacher et al 1998). Subgingival plaque samples were also taken for detection of *P. gingivalis*, *A. actinomycetemcomitans*, *Bacteroides forsythus* and *Treponema denticola* by the use of DNA probes and these were also compared in PLBW cases and controls. GCF levels of PGE_2 and IL-Iβ were found to be significantly higher in PLBW cases ($p = 0.02$) and higher levels of the bacteria were also found. These mechanisms, i.e. LPS stimulation of PGE_2 and IL-Iβ may also be postulated for cardiovascular disease and atherogenic plaque formation.

Another group (Dasanayake 1998) carried out a case control study of 55 matched pairs of PLBW and NBW babies. Similar logistic regression analysis was undertaken and showed odds ratios and correlation indices below the level of significance and hence showed no association between periodontal disease and PLBW. The population under investigation, severity and distribution of periodontal disease and the size of the inflammatory burden are likely to impact on the results from diverse population studies.

A prospective follow-up study of 227 rural Sri Lankan prima-gravida (first pregnancy) women who were free of tobacco, alcohol, and drug use was carried out by Rajapakse et al (2005). Their results were only suggestive of a low level of association between periodontal disease and pre-term low birth weight, possibly indicating that previously reported associations may have been subjected to residual confounding due to tobacco, alcohol and drug use.

Moreu et al (2005) investigated the influence of periodontal status on low birth weight pre-term delivery in 96 pregnant women in their first, second and third trimester. Their results suggested an association between periodontal disease and low birth weight but not pre-term delivery. Budunel et al (2005) also investigated the possible link between periodontal infections and PLBW collecting clinical and microbiological data in postpartum women with a low socioeconomic level. They used checkerboard DNA-DNA hybridization for 12 common putative periodontal pathogens. They studied 181 women (53 cases and 128 controls) within 3 days postpartum. Their findings showed that when subgingival bacteria were evaluated together, *Peptostreptococcus micros* and *Campylobacter rectus* may have had a role in increasing the risk for PLBW, although no single bacteria exhibited any relation with the risk of PLBW.

A prospective study (Moore et al 2004) recruited 3738 pregnant subjects in the 10–15th week of their pregnancy. They had a mean age of 29.8 ± 5.5, a good ethnic mix and low levels of attachment loss (Moore et al 2001) similar to that seen in the Adult Dental Health Survey 1998 (Kelly et al 2000). The patients completed a questionnaire and received a periodontal examination including PPD, PAL, Pl.I and GBI (Moore et al 2004). Subsequently pregnancy outcome data was collected. Regression analysis showed the expected relationships between pregnancy outcome and obstetric risk factors but there were no statistically significant relationships between pregnancy outcome and the severity of periodontal disease. There were relationships between miscarriage and the mean probing depth ($p = 0.023$) and increasing attachment loss ($p = 0.053$). However, the regression coefficients in these analyses were low suggesting their limited ability to explain variations in pregnancy outcome. There was thus no evidence of a relationship between pregnancy outcome and markers of periodontal disease severity.

A small intervention study (Jeffcoat et al 2003) on 366 pregnant women with chronic periodontitis divided into three study groups found that standard periodontal treatment significantly reduced the rate of pre-term delivery. It also found that the adjunctive use of oral metronidazole in one of the study groups significantly increased its rate in comparison to the group receiving periodontal treatment alone. This shows the inadvisability of unnecessary administration of antibiotics during pregnancy.

Another study (Wood et al 2006) found no evidence that clinical periodontal disease is associated with spontaneous pre-term birth. However, elevated gingival crevicular fluid levels of elastase were associated with pre-term birth but further research is needed before this can be assumed to be a causal relationship.

Since then, there have been further similar studies which have been evenly balanced between those with evidence of a slight association (Martins Moliterno et al 2005) and those which had negative findings (Noack et al 2005; Bassani et al 2007).

A recent systematic review (Madianos et al 2002) of the relationship between periodontal disease and PLBW only included one cohort and two case control studies. The cohort study and one of the case control studies showed a significant association between them. However, it concluded that the evidence linking periodontal disease and PLBW was very limited and that there was a clear need for better designed and larger observational and intervention studies to further resolve this issue. A variety of studies suggest some evidence linking periodontal disease and pre-term birth weight. But there is no compelling evidence to indicate a causal relationship and it is likely to be a coincident finding (Michalowicz & Durand 2007). As mentioned above further work is required.

POST-IMPLANTATION SEPTICAEMIA

Septicaemia is a cause of death in haematopoietic stem cell transplant (HSCT) recipients. Extraction of teeth with advanced periodontitis has been advocated before HSCT to prevent septicaemia in myeloablated hosts. A study (Akintoye et al 2002) was designed to determine the impact of chronic periodontitis, as measured by radiographic alveolar bone loss, on septicaemia and transplant mortality. A retrospective design was used to study 77 subjects who received pre-transplantation dental evaluation, panoramic radiography, and full myeloablative allogeneic HSCT to treat haematologic malignancies. Radiographic crestal alveolar bone loss was measured with a Schei ruler on all teeth. Microorganisms isolated from positive blood cultures within the first 100 days after transplant were categorized as of likely origin from periodontal, oral, or any body sites. The associations between positive blood cultures, mean subject whole-mouth percentage radiographic crestal alveolar bone loss, and 100-day survival were statistically assessed. Radiographic crestal alveolar bone loss per subject averaged $13\% \pm 7\%$, with 18.2% exhibiting bone loss of 20% or greater. During the initial 100 days after transplant, 63.6% subjects yielded septicaemia-associated positive blood cultures and *Staphylococcus epidermidis*, *Streptococcus mitis*, *Enterococcus faecalis*, *Streptococcus sanguis*, *Staphylococcus aureus* and *Escherichia coli* were the most common isolates recovered. No statistically significant associations were found between mean subject radiographic alveolar bone loss and septicaemia of likely periodontal or oral origin. Thus this preliminary study found no relationship between radiographic periodontal status and septicaemia or mortality for 100 days after transplantation.

REFERENCES

Akintoye SO, Brennan MT, Graber CJ, et al: A retrospective investigation of advanced periodontal disease as a risk factor for septicemia in hematopoietic stem cell and bone marrow transplant recipients, *Oral Surg Oral Med Oral Pathol Oral Radiol Endod* 94:581–608, 2002.

Alaaddinolu EE, Karabay G, Bulut S, et al: Apoptosis in cyclosporin A-induced gingival overgrowth: a histological study, *J Periodontol* 76:166–170, 2005.

Alpoz E, Cankaya H, Guneri P: Facial subcutaneous calcinosis and mandibular resorption in systemic sclerosis: a case report, *Dentomaxillofacial Radiology* 36:172–174, 2007.

Alpoz AR, Coker M, Celen E, et al: The oral manifestations of Maroteaux Lamy syndrome (mucopolysaccharidosis VI): A case report, *Oral Surg Oral Med Oral Pathol Oral Radiol Endod* 101:632–637, 2006.

Andreasen JO: Oral lichen planus. 1. A clinical evaluation of 115 cases, *Oral Surg Oral Med Oral Pathol* 25:31–42, 1968.

Babrowski AE, Langman CB: Hyperoxaluria and systemic oxalosis: current therapy and future directions, *Expert Opin Pharmacother* 7:1887–1896, 2006.

Baumann L: How to prevent photoaging? *J Invest Dermatol* 125:12–13, 2005.

Baer PN, Brown NC, Hammer JE: Hypophosphatasia: report of two cases with dental findings, *Periodontics* 2:209–215, 1964.

Bassani DG, Olinto MTA, Kreiger N: Periodontal disease and perinatal outcomes: a case-control study, *J Clin Periodontol* 34:31–39, 2007.

Battino M, Bompadre S, Politi A, et al: Antioxidant status (CoQ10 and Vit. E levels) and immunohistochemical analysis of soft tissues in periodontal diseases, *Biofactors* 25:213–217, 2005.

Beck JD, Offenbacher S, Williams R, et al: Periodontitis: a risk factor for coronary heart disease? *Ann Periodontol* 1:127–141, 1998.

Beikler T, Kuczek A, Petersilka G, et al: In-dental-office screening for diabetes mellitus using gingival crevicular blood, *J Clin Periodontol* 29:216–218, 2002.

Bogenrieder T, Rogler G, Vogt T, et al: Orofacial granulomatosis as the initial presentation of Crohn's disease in an adolescent, *Dermatology* 206:273–278, 2003.

Bostanci N, Ilgenli T, Pirhan DC, et al: Relationship between IL-1A polymorphisms and gingival overgrowth in renal transplant recipients receiving Cyclosporin A, *J Clin Periodontol* 33:771–778, 2006.

Buduneli N, Baylas H, Aksu G, et al: Prepubertal periodontitis associated with chronic granulomatous disease, *J Clin Periodontol* 28:589–593, 2001.

Buduneli N, Baylas H, Buduneli E, et al: Periodontal infections and pre-term low birth weight: a case-control study, *J Clin Periodontol* 32:174–181, 2005.

Chiarelli F, Santilli F, Mohn A: Advanced glycation end products in adolescent and young adults with diabetic angiopathy, *Horm Res* 53:53–63, 2000.

Chin Y-T, Chen Y-T, Hsiao-Pei T, et al: Upregulation of the expression of epidermal growth factor and its receptor in gingiva upon cyclosporin-A treatment, *J Periodontol* 77:647–656, 2006.

Cocchi G, Mastrocola M, Capelli M, et al: Immunological pattern in young children with Down's syndrome: is there a temporal trend? *Acta Paediatrica* 96:147–182, 2007.

Cotrim P, Martelli-Junior H, Graner E, et al: Cyclosporin A induces proliferation in human gingival fibroblasts via induction of transforming growth factor-beta1, *J Periodontol* 74:1625–1633, 2003.

Crohn BB, Ginzburg L, Oppenheimer GD: Regional ileitis, a pathological and clinical entity, *JAMA* 99:1323–1329, 1932.

D'Aiuto F, Parkar M, Andreaou G, et al: Periodontitis and atherogenesis: causal association or simple coincidence? *J Clin Periodontol* 31:402–411, 2004.

D'Aiuto F, Nibali L, Parkar M, et al: Short-term effects of intensive periodontal therapy on serum inflammatory markers and cholesterol, *J Dent Res* 84:269–273, 2005.

Dannewitz B, Edrich C, Tomakidi P, et al: Elevated levels of gene expression for collagen and decorin in human gingival overgrowth, *J Clin Periodontol* 33:510–516, 2006.

Dasanayake AP: Poor periodontal health of the pregnant woman as a risk factor for low birth weight, *Ann Periodontol* 3:206–212, 1998.

Davis AJ: Advances in contraception (review), *Obstet Gynecol Clin North Am* 27:597–610, 2000.

Deas DE, Mackey SA, Mc Donnell HT: Systemic disease and periodontitis: manifestation of neutrophil dysfunction, *Periodontol 2000* 32:82–104, 2003.

De Coster PJ, Martens LC, De Paepe A: Oral health in prevalent types of Ehlers–Danlos syndromes, *J Oral Pathol Med* 34:298–307, 2005.

Dickinson DP: Cysteine peptidases of mammals: their biological roles and potential effects in the oral cavity and other tissues in health and disease, *Crit Rev Oral Biol Med* 13:238–275, 2002.

Doufexi A, Mina M, Ioannidou E: Gingival overgrowth in children: epidemiology, pathogenesis and complications. A literature review, *J Periodontol* 76:3–10, 2005.

Eisen D: The clinical features, malignant potential and systemic associations of oral lichen planus: a study of 723 patients, *J Am Acad Dermatol* 46:207–214, 2002.

Eley BM: *Dental Amalgam: A Review of Safety*, London, 1993, British Dental Association, pp 49–51.

Engebretson SP, Vossughi F, Hey-Hadavi J, et al: The influence of diabetes on gingival crevicular fluid beta-glucuronidase and interleukin-8, *J Clin Periodontol* 33:784–790, 2006.

Fiehn NE, Larsen T, Christiansen N, et al: Identification of periodontal pathogens in atherosclerotic vessels, *J Periodontol* 76:731–736, 2005.

Figuero E, Soory M, Cerero R, et al: Oxidant/antioxidant interactions of nicotine, Coenzyme Q10, Pycnogenol and phytoestrogens in oral periosteal fibroblasts and MG63 osteoblasts, *Steroids* 71:1062–1072, 2006.

Galbraith SS, Drolet BA, Kugathasan S, et al: Asymptomatic inflammatory bowel disease presenting with mucocutaneous findings, *Paediatrics* 116:439–444, 2005.

Goth L, Rass P, Pay A: Catalase enzyme mutation and their association with diseases, *Mol Diagn* 8:141–149, 2004.

Graves DT, Liu R, Alikhani M, et al: Diabetes-enhanced inflammation and apoptosis-impact on periodontal pathology, *J Dent Res* 85:15–21, 2006.

Guncu GN, Tozum TF, Caglayan F: Effects of endogenous sex hormones on the periodontium - review of the literature, *Aust Dent J* 50:138–145, 2005.

Haraszthy VI, Zambon JJ, Trevisan M, et al: Identification of periodontal pathogens in atheromatous plaques, *J Periodontol* 71:1554–1560, 2000.

Hart TC, Hart PS, Bowden DW, et al: Mutations of the cathepsin C gene are responsible for Papillon Lefèvre syndrome, *J Med Genet* 36:881–887, 1999.

Hart TC, Hart PS, Michalec MD, et al: Localization of a gene for prepubertal periodontitis to chromosome 11q14 and identification of a cathepsin C mutation, *J Med Genet* 37:95–101, 2000.

Hirasawa M, Takada K, Makimura M, et al: Involvement of periodontal status by green tea catechin using a local delivery system: a clinical pilot study, *J Periodontal Res* 37:433–438, 2002.

Huang W-T, Lu H-K, Chou H-H, et al: Immunocytochemical analysis of the Th1/Th2 cytokine profiles and androgen receptor expression in the pathogenesis of nifedipine-induced gingival overgrowth, *J Periodontal Res* 38:422–427, 2003.

Hyland PL, Traynor PS, Myrillas TT, et al: The effects of cyclosporin on the collagenolytic activity of gingival fibroblasts, *J Periodontol* 74:437–445, 2003.

Jakus V: Role of free radicals, oxidant stress and anti-oxidant systems in diabetic vascular disease, *Bratislavski Lekarsky Listy* 101:541–551, 2000.

James JA, Jamal S, Hull PS, et al: Tacrolimus is not associated with gingival overgrowth in renal transplant patients, *J Clin Periodontol* 28:848–852, 2001.

Janket SJ, Baird A, Chang E, et al: Meta-analysis of periodontal disease and risk of coronary heart disease and stroke, *Oral Surg Oral Med Oral Pathol Oral Radiol Endod* 95:559–669, 2003.

Jeffcoat MK, Hauth JC, Geurs NC, et al: Periodontal disease and pre-term birth: results of a pilot intervention study, *J Periodontol* 74:1214–1218, 2003.

Joshipura KJ, Wand HC, Merchant AT, et al: periodontal disease and biomarkers related to cardiovascular disease, *J Dent Res* 83:151–155, 2004.

Kantarci A, Augustin P, Firatli E, et al: Apoptosis in gingival overgrowth tissues, *J Dent Res* 86:888–892, 2007.

Kelly M, Steele J, Nutall N, et al: *Adult Dental Health Survey. Oral health in the United Kingdom 1998*, London, 2000, Office for National Statistics.

Kobayashi T, Ito S, Yamamoto K, et al: Risk of periodontitis in systemic lupus erythematosus is associated with Fcγ receptor polymorphisms, *J Periodontol* 74:378–384, 2003.

Kol R, Palattella A: The use of doxycycline in periodontology. Histologic in vivo study on mice affected by diabetes mellitus, *Minerva Stomatol* 55:77–86, 2006.

Kornman KS, Loesche WJ: The subgingival microflora during pregnancy, *J Periodontal Res* 15:111–122, 1980.

Larijani B, Shooshtarizadeh P, Mosaffa N, et al: Polymorphonuclear leucocyte respiratory burst activity correlates with serum zinc level in type 2 diabetic patients with foot ulcers, *Br J Biomed Sci* 64:13–17, 2007.

Lee SD, Wu CC, Kuo WW, et al: Porphyromonas gingivalis-related cardiac cell apoptosis was majorly co-activated by p38 and extracellular signal-regulated kinase pathways, *J Periodontal Res* 41:39–46, 2006.

Llambes F, Silvestre FJ, Hernandez-Mijares A, et al: Effect of non-surgical periodontal treatment with or without doxycycline on the periodontium of type 1 diabetic patients, *J Clin Periodontol* 32:915–920, 2006.

Lobao DS, Silva LC, Soares RV, et al: Idiopathic gingival fibromatosis: a case report, *Quintessence Int* 38:699–704, 2007.

Loos BG, John RP, Laine ML: Identification of genetic risk factors for periodontitis and possible mechanisms of action, *J Clin Periodontol* 32:159–179, 2005.

Lopp CA, Lohse JE, Dickinson DP, et al: The effects of progesterone on matrix metalloproteinases in cultured human gingival fibroblasts, *J Periodontol* 74:277–288, 2003.

Lundgren T, Renvert S: Periodontal treatment of patients with Papillon-Lefèvre syndrome: a 3-year follow-up, *J Clin Periodontol* 31:933–938, 2004.

Madianos PN, Bobetis GA, Kinane DF: Is periodontitis associated with an increased risk of coronary heart disease and pre-term and/or low birth weight births, *J Clin Periodontol* 29(Suppl 3):22–36, 2002.

Mariotti A: Sex steroid hormones and cell dynamics in the periodontium, *Crit Rev Oral Biol Med* 5:27–53, 1994.

Martin K, Wu D, Meydani M: The effect of carotenoids on the expression of cell surface adhesion molecules and binding of monocytes to human aortic endothelial cells, *Atherosclerosis* 150:265–274, 2000.

Martins Moliterno LF, Monteiro B, Silva Figueredo CM, et al: Association between periodontitis and low birth weight: a case-control study, *J Clin Periodontol* 32:886–890, 2005.

Mascarenhas P, Gapski R, Al-Shammari K, et al: Influence of sex hormones on the periodontium, *J Clin Periodontol* 30:671–681, 2003.

Mavrogiannis M, Ellis JS, Seymour RA, et al: The efficacy of three different surgical techniques in the management of drug-induced gingival overgrowth, *J Clin Periodontol* 33:677–682, 2006.

Mealey BL, Ocampo GL: Diabetes mellitus and periodontal disease, *Periodontol 2000* 44:127–153, 2007.

Michalowicz BS, Durand R: Maternal periodontal disease and spontaneous pre-term birth, *Periodontol 2000* 44:103–112, 2007.

Miyakawa H, Honma K, Qi M, et al: Interaction of Porphyromonas gingivalis with low-density lipoproteins: implications for the role of periodontitis in atherosclerosis, *J Periodontal Res* 39:1–9, 2004.

Montebugnoli L, Servidio D, Miaton RA, et al: Poor oral health is associated with coronary heart disease and elevated inflammatory and haemostatic factors, *J Clin Periodontol* 31:25–29, 2004.

Moore S, Ide M, Wilson RF, et al: Periodontal health of London women during early pregnancy, *Br Dent J* 191:570–573, 2001.

Moore S, Ide M, Coward PY, et al: A prospective study to investigate the relationship between periodontal disease and adverse pregnancy outcome, *Br Dent J* 197:251–258, 2004.

Moreu G, Téllez L, González-Jaranay M: Relationship between maternal periodontal disease and low birth weight pre-term infants, *J Clin Periodontol* 32:622–627, 2005.

Morgan I: Why is periodontal disease more prevalent and more severe in people with Down's syndrome, *Spec Care Dentist* 27:196–201, 2007.

Mozaffarieh M, Flammer J: A novel perspective on natural therapeutic approaches in glaucoma therapy, *Expert Opin Emerg Drugs* 12:195–198, 2007.

Nakib SA, Pankow JS, Beck JD, et al: Periodontitis and coronary artery calcification: the atherosclerosis risk in communities (ARIC) Study, *J Periodontol* 75:505–510, 2004.

Nassar H, Kantarci A, Van Dyke TE: Diabetic periodontitis: A model for activated innate immunity and impaired resolution of inflammation, *Periodontol 2000* 43:233–244, 2007.

Nielsen IL, Williamson G: Review of the factors affecting bioavailability of soy isoflavones in humans, *Nutr Cancer* 57:1–10, 2007.

Nishikawa T, Edelstein D, Brownlee M: The missing link: a simple unifying mechanism for diabetic complications, *Kidney Int* 77:526–530, 2000.

Nishimura F, Iwamoto Y, Soga Y, et al: The periodontal host response with diabetes, *Periodontol 2000* 43:245–253, 2007.

Nishimura F, Iwamoto Y, Mineshiba J, et al: Periodontal disease and diabetes mellitus: the role of tumor necrosis factor-α in a 2-way relationship, *J Periodontol* 74:97–102, 2003.

Noack B, Klingenberg J, Weigelt J, et al: Periodontal status and pre-term low birth weight: a case control study, *J Periodontal Res* 40:339–345, 2005.

Offenbacher S, Jared HL, O'Reilly PG, et al: Potential pathogenic mechanisms of periodontitis associated pregnancy complications, *Ann Periodontol* 3:233–250, 1998.

Ojanatko A, Neinstedt W, Harri MP: Metabolism of testosterone by human healthy and inflamed gingiva (in vitro), *Arch Oral Biol* 25:481–484, 1980.

Opinya GN, Kaimenyi JT, Meme JS: Oral findings in Fanconi's anaemia, *J Periodontol* 33:266–269, 1988.

Ozcan A, Ali R, Ozkalemkas F, et al: Acute myeloblastic leukaemia (AML-M1) presenting with prominent gingival hypertrophy, *Eur J Haematol* 78:547, 2007.

Padilla C, Lobos O, Hubert E, et al: Periodontal pathogens in atheromatous plaques isolated from patients with chronic periodontitis, *J Periodontal Res* 41:350–353, 2006.

Paik J-W, Kim C-S, Cho K-S, et al: Inhibition of cyclosporin A-induced gingival overgrowth by azithromycin through phagocytosis: an in vivo and in vitro study, *J Periodontol* 75:380–387, 2004.

Papillon MM, Lefèvre P: Deux cas de keratodermie palmaire et plantaire symétrique familiale (maladie de Meteda) chez le frère et la soeur. Coexistence dans les deux cas d'altérations dentaire grave, *Bull Soc Fr Dermatol Syphilgr* 31:82–87, 1924.

Paquette DW, Brodala N, Nichols TC: Cardiovascular disease, inflammation, and periodontal infection, *Periodontol 2000* 44:113–126, 2007.

Pattni R, Walsh LJ, Marshall RI, et al: Periodontal implications of immunodeficient states: manifestations and management, *J Int Acad Periodontol* 2:79–93, 2000.

Petit JC, Ripamonti U: Multiple myeloma of the periodontium. A case report, *J Periodontol* 61:132–137, 1990.

Pham CTN, Ivanovich JL, Raptis SZ, et al: Papillon-Lefèvre Syndrome: correlating the molecular, cellular, and clinical consequences of cathepsin C/dipeptidyl peptidase I deficiency in humans, *J Immunol* 173:7277–7281, 2004.

Piboonniyom S, Treister N, Pitiphat W: Scoring system for monitoring oral lichenoid lesions: A preliminary study, *Oral Surg Oral Med Oral Pathol Oral Radiol Endod* 99:696–703, 2005.

Piwowar A, Knapik-Kordecka M, Warwas S: Concentration of leukocyte elastase in plasma and polymorphonuclear extracts in type 2 diabetes, *Clin Chem Lab Med* 38:1257–1261, 2000.

Ponder KP, Haskins ME: Gene therapy for mucopolysaccharidosis, *Expert Opin Biol Ther* 7:1333–1345, 2007.

Promsudthi A, Pimapansri S, Deerochanawong C, et al: The effect of periodontal therapy on uncontrolled type 2 diabetes mellitus in older subjects, *Oral Dis* 11:293–298, 2005.

Rahman ZA, Soory M: Antioxidant effects of glutathione and IGF in a hyperglycaemic cell culture model of fibroblasts: Some actions of advanced glycaemic end products (AGE) and nicotine, *Endocr Metab Immune Disord Drug Targets* 6:279–286, 2006.

Rajapakse PS, Nagarathne M, Chandrasekra KBA, et al: Periodontal disease and prematurity among non-smoking Sri Lankan women, *J Dent Res* 84:274–277, 2005.

Ramamurthy NS, Greenwald RA, Celiker MY, et al: Experimental arthritis in rats induces biomarkers of periodontitis which are ameliorated by gene therapy with tissue inhibitor of matrix metalloproteinases, *J Periodontol* 76:229–233, 2005.

Rees TD: Periodontal management of the patient with diabetes mellitus, *Periodontol 2000* 23:63–73, 2000.

Renvert S, Ohlsson O, Persson S, et al: Analysis of periodontal risk profiles in adults with or without a history of myocardial infarction, *J Clin Periodontol* 31:19–24, 2004.

Riley M: Incorrect nutrition as a risk factor for periodontal disease, *Alpha Omegan* 100:85–88, 2007.

Ritchie CS: Obesity and periodontal disease, *Periodontol 2000* 44:154–163, 2007.

Rodrigues PH, Progulske-Fox A: Gene expression profile analysis of Porphyromonas gingivalis during invasion of human coronary artery endothelial cells, *Infect Immun* 73:6169–6617, 2005.

Rufail ML, Schenkein HA, Koertge TE, et al: Atherogenic lipoprotein parameters in patients with aggressive periodontitis, *J Periodontal Res* 42:495–502, 2007.

Ruggeri Jr A, Montebugnoli L, Matteucci A, et al: Cyclosporin A specifically affects nuclear PLCβ1 in immunodepressed heart transplant patients with gingival overgrowth, *J Dent Res* 84:747–751, 2005.

Ruocco E, Cuomo A, Salerno R, et al: Crohn's disease and its mucocutaneous involvement, *Skinmed* 6:179–185, 2007.

Safkan-Seppälä B, Sorsa T, Tervahartiala T, et al: Collagenases in gingival crevicular fluid in type 1diabetes mellitus, *J Periodontol* 77:189–194, 2006.

Saito T, Shimazaki Y: Metabolic disorders related to obesity and periodontal disease, *Periodontol 2000* 43:254–266, 2007.

Saito T, Shimazaki Y, Kiyohara Y, et al: The severity of periodontal disease is associated with the development of glucose intolerance in non-diabetics: The Hisayama Study, *J Dent Res* 83:485–490, 2004.

Sakanaka S, Okada Y: Inhibitory effects of green tea polyphenols on the production of a virulence factor of the periodontal-disease-causing anaerobic bacterium Porphyromonas gingivalis, *J Agric Food Chem* 52:1688–1692, 2004.

Sakellari D, Arapostathis KN, Konstantinidis A: Periodontal conditions and subgingival microflora in Down's syndrome patients. A case-control study, *J Clin Periodontol* 32:684–690, 2005.

Savage NW, Seymour GJ, Robinson MF: Cyclosporin-A-induced gingival enlargement – a case report, *J Periodontol* 58:475–480, 1987.

Scully C, Felix DH: Oral medicine – update for the dental practitioner. Mouth ulcers of more serious connotation, *Br Dent J* 199:339–343, 2005.

Seymour RA: The management of drug-induced gingival overgrowth, *J Clin Periodontol* 33:434–439, 2006.

Sheets SM, Potempa J, Travis J, et al: Gingipains from Porphyromonas gingivalis W83 induce cell adhesion molecule cleavage and apoptosis in endothelial cells, *Infect Immun* 73:1543–1552, 2005.

Shklar G, McCarthy PL: Oral manifestations of benign mucous membrane pemphigus (mucous membrane pemphigoid), *Oral Surg Oral Med Oral Pathol* 12:950–966, 1959.

Song H, Bélanger M, Whitlock J, et al: Hemagglutinin B is involved in the adherence of Porphyromonas gingivalis to human coronary artery endothelial cells, *Infect Immun* 73:7267–7273, 2005.

Soory M: Targets for steroid hormone mediated actions of periodontal pathogens, cytokines and therapeutic agents: Some implications on tissue turnover in the periodontium, *Curr Drug Targets* 1:309–325, 2000.

Soory M: Hormone mediation of immune responses in the progression of diabetes, rheumatoid arthritis and periodontal diseases, *Curr Drug Targets Immune Endocr Metabol Disord* 2:13–25, 2002.

Soory M: Biomarkers of diabetes mellitus and rheumatoid arthritis associated with oxidative stress, applicable to periodontal diseases, *Current Topics in Steroid Research* 4:1–17, 2004.

Soory M: Periodontal diseases and rheumatoid arthritis: a coincident model for therapeutic intervention? *Curr Drug Metab* 8:750–757, 2007.

Stewart JD, Wagner KA, Friedlander AH, et al: The effect of periodontal treatment on glycemic control in patients with type 2 diabetes mellitus, *J Clin Periodontol* 28:23–30, 2001.

Suresh L, Radfar L: Oral sarcoidosis: a review of literature, *Oral Dis* 11:138–145, 2005.

Syrjanon J, Peltola JM, Valtonen VV: Dental infections in association with cerebral infarction in young and middle aged men, *J Intern Med* 255:179–184, 1989.

Taichman LS, Eklund SA: Oral contraceptives and periodontal diseases: rethinking the association based upon analysis of national health and nutrition examination survey data, *J Periodontol* 76:1374–1385, 2005.

Takeda M, Ojima M, Yoshioka H, et al: Relationship of serum advanced glycation end products with deterioration of periodontitis in type 2 diabetes patients, *J Periodontol* 77:15–20, 2006.

Tarannum F, Faizuddin M: Effect of periodontal therapy on pregnancy outcome in women affected by periodontitis, *J Periodontol* 78:2095–2103, 2007.

Tilakaratne A, Soory M: Modulation of androgen metabolism by oestradiol-17β and progesterone, alone and in combination, in human gingival fibroblasts in culture, *J Periodontol* 70:1017–1025, 1999.

Tilakaratne A, Soory M, Ranasinghe AW, et al: Periodontal disease status during pregnancy and 3 months post-partum, in a rural population of Sri-Lankan women, *J Clin Periodontol* 27:787–792, 2000a.

Tilakaratne A, Soory M, Ranasinghe AW, et al: Effects of hormonal contraceptives on the periodontium, in a population of rural Sri-Lankan women, *J Clin Periodontol* 27:753–757, 2000b.

Tipton DA, Howell KJ, Dabbous MK: Increased proliferation, collagen and fibronectin production by hereditary gingival fibromatosis fibroblasts, *J Periodontol* 68:524–530, 1997.

Tipton DA, Woodard ES, Baber MA, et al: Role of the c-myc proto-oncogene in the proliferation of hereditary gingival fibromatosis fibroblasts, *J Periodontol* 75:360–369, 2004.

Toygar HU, Seydaoglu G, Kurklu S, et al: Periodontal health and adverse pregnancy outcome in 3576 Turkish women, *J Periodontol* 78:2081–2094, 2007.

van den Bos T, Handoko G, Niehof A, et al: Cementum and dentine in hypophosphatasia, *J Dent Res* 84:1021–1025, 2005.

Vescovi P, Meleti M, Manfredi M, et al: Cyclosporin-induced gingival overgrowth: a clinical and epidemiological evaluation of 121 Italian renal transplant recipients, *J Periodontol* 76:1259–1264, 2005.

Wani AA, Devkar N, Patole MS, et al: Description of Two New Cathepsin C Gene Mutations in Patients With Papillon-Lefèvre Syndrome, *J Periodontol* 77:233–237, 2006.

Westbrook P, Bednarczyk EM, Carlson M, et al: Regression of nifedipine-induced gingival hyperplasia following switch to same class calcium channel blocker, Isradipine, *J Periodontol* 68:645–650, 1997.

Westhoff CL: Oral contraceptives and venous thromboembolism: should epidemiological associations drive clinical decision making? *Contraception* 54:1–3, 1996.

Wood N, Johnson RB: The relationship between tomato intake and congestive heart failure risk in periodontitis subjects, *J Clin Periodontol* 31:574–580, 2004.

Wood SL, Frydman A, Cox SW, et al: Periodontal disease and spontaneous premature birth: A case control study, *BMC Pregnancy and Childbirth* 6:24, 2006.

Wysocki GP, Fay WP, Ulrichsen RF, et al: Oral findings in primary hyperoxaluria and oxalosis, *Oral Surg Oral Med Oral Pathol* 53:267–272, 1982.

Yuan K, Lin MT: The roles of vascular endothelial growth factor and angiopoietin-2 in the regression of pregnancy pyogenic granuloma, *Oral Dis* 10:179–185, 2004.

7

Acquired immunodeficiency syndrome (AIDS)

The acquired immunodeficiency syndrome (AIDS) is one of the principal threats to health worldwide; the number of people infected with the human immunodeficiency virus (HIV) is about 19.5 million and the great majority of these will probably die of this condition.

THE HUMAN IMMUNODEFICIENCY VIRUS

The HIV is a retrovirus which is roughly spherical and is one ten-thousandths of a millimetre across. Its outer coat or envelope consists of a double layer of lipid molecules and this is studded with proteins (**Fig. 7.1**). One of these appears like a spike in electron microscope (EM) photographs and is a glycoprotein (gp). The outer part is known as gp120 (the number stands for the mass of the protein in Daltons) and the inner part embedded in the membrane as gp41. Below this is a matrix protein (p17) which surrounds the core or capsid, made of another protein (p24), in the shape of a hollow cone. This holds the genetic material in the form of RNA of about 9200 nucleotide bases. Molecules of the enzyme reverse transcriptase, which transcribes the RNA to DNA once the virus enters the cell, lie on the surface of the strands. Also present within the capsid are integrase, protease and ribonuclease enzyme proteins.

The gp120 protein can bind tightly to CD4 molecules present on several types of immune cells (**Fig. 7.2**). When the virus binds to the cell, the membranes fuse, a process governed by the gp41 envelope protein, and the virus core and its contents are brought into the cell. The viral core then partially disintegrates releasing the RNA. The reverse transcriptase then transcribes a DNA copy with the aid of the other viral enzymes. When activated, the viral integrated DNA can code for viral RNA which leaves the nucleus, codes for structural and other proteins and buds new virus from the cell surface to infect other cells.

PATHOGENESIS OF HIV INFECTION AND AIDS

Some CD4 bearing cells, known as dendritic cells, are present throughout the body's mucosal surfaces and it is possible that these are the first cells infected in sexual transmission. Macrophages and monocytes also carry the CD4 molecule and are similarly vulnerable. They may carry HIV to other parts of the body including the lymphoid organs and brain. The principal targets of the HIV virus are CD4 bearing T-helper lymphocytes which help to activate other parts of the immune system including the T4-effector cells, the T8-killer cells and the B cells. In patients who are about to commence antiretroviral therapy, measurement of HIV-1 viral load in conjunction with a CD4 count provides an accurate risk assessment of the likelihood of developing AIDS (Phillips 2004).

An infected person first mounts a vigorous defence when first infected. As a result of this, B cells produce antibodies to neutralize virus and killer T cells multiply and destroy the virus infected cells. Although it is possible that the immune system may successfully fight off HIV at a very early stage by the time antibodies to the virus have appeared in the blood the infection is generally permanent. The clinical picture is first a mild flu-like illness with fever and muscle aches lasting no more than a few weeks and throughout this stage, large amounts of virus are present in the blood-stream and transmission is easy. The immune system mounts its response and begins to eliminate infected cells and circulating virus. However, a proportion of infected cells remain by eluding these defences and the virus continues to replicate in low numbers for as long as a decade and for most of this period of chronic infection the patient is quite well. It is only after several years when the virus has significantly damaged the immune system that opportunist infections and malignancies begin to appear.

At first it was thought that the damage to the immune system was due to the progressive decline in the numbers of T4 cells in the blood as a result of the killing of these cells by the virus. In support of this is evidence that the numbers of these cells decline from 1000/mm³ to ≤100/mm³ during the long subclinical phase of the illness. However, even in the late stages of the

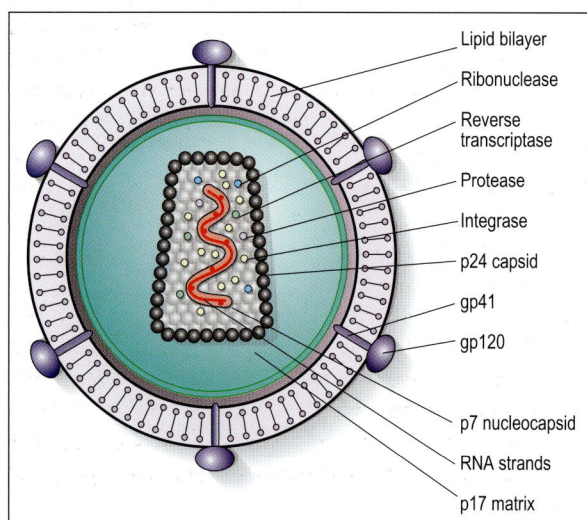

Fig. 7.1 A diagram of the human immunodeficiency virus.

Lipid bilayer
Ribonuclease
Reverse transcriptase
Protease
Integrase
p24 capsid
gp41
gp120
p7 nucleocapsid
RNA strands
p17 matrix

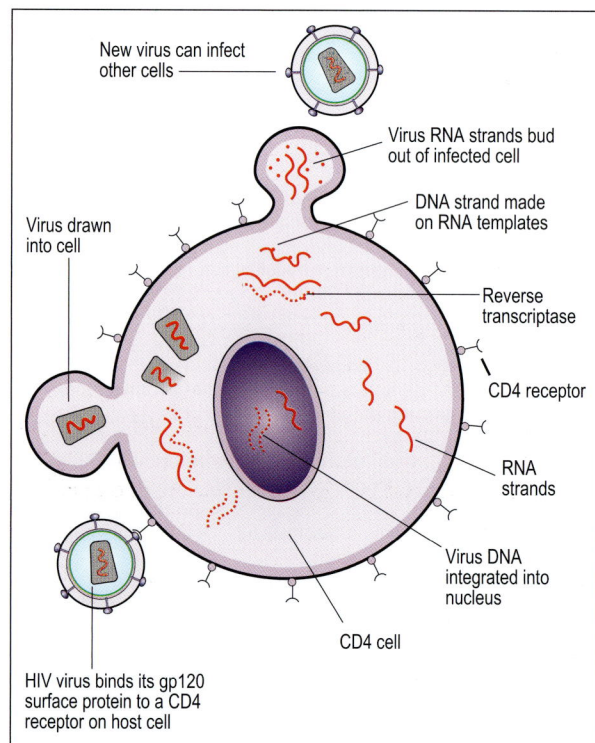

Fig. 7.2 The life cycle of the human immunodeficiency virus.

New virus can infect other cells
Virus RNA strands bud out of infected cell
DNA strand made on RNA templates
Virus drawn into cell
Reverse transcriptase
CD4 receptor
RNA strands
Virus DNA integrated into nucleus
CD4 cell
HIV virus binds its gp120 surface protein to a CD4 receptor on host cell

disease when there are very low numbers of T4 cells in the blood, the proportion of these cells producing virus is only 1 in 40 cells. In fact, in the early stages of the disease only about 1 in 1000 T4 cells in the blood produce virus. One reason for the decline in T4 cells could be that the unaffected T8 killer cells could progressively destroy infected cells. Another possibility is that antibodies recognizing the viral gp120 and gp41 proteins on the viral envelope might also interfere with the MHC on healthy cells. A further theory supported by experimental evidence is that HIV might precipitate a widespread apoptosis (programmed death) of healthy immune cells.

Recent experimental evidence suggests that the most likely reason is that HIV infection gradually and progressively destroys the lymphoid organs, particularly the lymph nodes. There is evidence that in the long chronic asymptomatic phase HIV replicates mainly in the lymph nodes and this gradually increases the body burden of infected cells in these organs. Thus, it seems that in the lymph nodes the viral burden is substantial and increases steadily throughout the chronic phase. The abrupt rise in the blood levels of the virus in the late stages of the disease is most likely due to the burning out of the lymph nodes. Loss of follicular dendritic, T4 helper and memory cells probably leads to a rapid loss of immune function and the virus spills out into the blood. The patient, now with a paralysed immune system dies, from recurrent opportunistic infections and neoplasms.

CLINICAL FEATURES OF AIDS

GENERAL

The main clinical features of AIDS are lymphadenopathy, weight loss, unexplained diarrhoea, opportunistic infections and neoplasms. The infections include:

- Oral and pharyngeal candidiasis
- Mucocutaneous herpes simplex
- *Pneumocystis carinii* pneumonia
- *Mycobacterium tuberculosis*
- Atypical mycobacterial infections
- Salmonellosis
- Cryptococcal meningitis
- Cryptosporidiosis
- Toxoplasma encephalitis
- Cytomegalovirus disease.

The neoplasms include:

- Kaposi's sarcoma
- B-cell lymphoma
- Hodgkin's lymphoma.

ORAL

AIDS has a variety of oral manifestations and these have been classified by Pindborg (1989). The commonest of these are candidiasis, hairy leukoplakia, Kaposi's sarcomata and periodontal infections and subjects with these lesions are likely to be HIV seropositive. However a variety of oral lesions can occur and these include:

Fungal infections

- Candidiasis
- Histoplasmosis
- Cryptococcus
- Geotrichosis.

Bacterial infections

- Acute necrotizing ulcerative gingivitis (ANUG)
- Rapid periodontal destruction
- *Mycobacterium avium intracellulare*
- Actinomycosis
- Cat-scratch disease
- *Klebsiella pneumoniae*
- *Enterobacteriaceae*
- *Escherichia coli*
- Exacerbation of chronic abscesses
- Sinusitis
- Submandibular cellulitis.

Viral infections

- Herpes simplex stomatitis
- Cytomegalovirus
- Ebstein–Barr (EB) virus
- Varicella-zoster virus
- Papillomavirus.

Neoplasms

- Kaposi's sarcoma
- Non-Hodgkin's lymphoma
- Squamous cell carcinoma.

Neurological disturbances

- Trigeminal neuropathy
- Facial palsy.

Unknown causes

- Recurrent aphthous ulceration
- Progressive necrotizing ulceration
- Toxic epidermolysis (Lyell's syndrome)
- Delayed wound healing
- Idiopathic thrombocytopenia
- Salivary gland enlargement
- Xerostomia
- Oral mucosa hypopigmentation.

Lesions such as oral candidiasis (OC), oral hairy leukoplakia (OHL) and acute necrotic ulcerative gingivitis (ANUG) may be the first signs of an HIV infection or its progression. Almost all HIV infected patients will have oral manifestations. Dentists play an important role in its early detection. In addition to the above Kaposi's sarcoma (KS), non-Hodgkin's lymphoma (NHL) and necrotizing ulcerative periodontitis may be present in up to 50% of patients with HIV infection and up to 80% of those with AIDS. The prevalence of OC, OHL and HIV-associated periodontal disease has decreased in adults with the advent of highly active antiretroviral therapy (HAART) (Reichart 2006).

Kendpon et al (2004) assessed the prevalence of the oral manifestations of HIV disease and related them to the CD4 status of subjects in Northern and Southern Thailand. They found that oral candidiasis, hairy leukoplakia and HIV-related periodontal disease were the most common oral lesion in both areas. They also found that the most significant association was between oral candidiasis, particularly the pseudomembranous type, and CD4 immunological status.

PERIODONTAL

The main periodontal infections associated with AIDS are ANUG and rapidly progressive atypical periodontitis. Two types of periodontal disease, HIV gingivitis (HIV-G) and HIV periodontitis (HIV-P) have been described in HIV patients (Yin et al 2007).

HIV-related ANUG and ANUP

More aggressive forms of gingivitis and periodontitis occur amongst HIV patients (Yin et al 2007). It can also result in soft tissue ulceration (Salama et al 2004). Concurrent manifestation of ANUG, ANUP, oro-facial herpes infection, pseudomembranous candidiasis and atypical oral ulceration in an HIV-seropositive patient has been reported. Despite very low CD4+ T-cell counts the patient responded well to standard periodontal treatment in the absence of HAART, with no recurrence of oral lesions at the 3 month follow-up (Feller et al 2006).

HIV gingivitis (HIV-G)

HIV-G (linear erythema) manifests as a distinct erythema of the free and attached gingiva and sometimes the alveolar mucosa. It bleeds easily on toothbrushing and gently probing. The gingival margins often shows a well circumscribed band of erythema patients (Yin et al 2007).

It may fail to respond to conventional treatment such as plaque control and scaling if the CD4 cell levels are low (see below).

HIV periodontitis (HIV-P)

HIV-P (necrotizing ulcerative periodontitis) involves extensive soft tissue necrosis and marked loss of periodontal attachment. Soft tissue destruction can be rapid and is often accompanied by interdental necrosis and ulceration which can expose bone. Unlike chronic periodontitis, there is no deep pocket formation but rather marked recession, ulceration and exposure and sometimes sequestration of bone. Localized pain is a feature of this condition and it is deeper seated than that associated with ANUG. These conditions usually occur when the CD4 cell levels are low and hence HIV infection is converting to full blown AIDS. The incidence has decreased with the advent of HAART (Ryder 2002).

Is there a link between HIV infection and the severity of chronic periodontitis?

A 6-month longitudinal study of attachment loss in HIV-infected patients demonstrated significantly higher levels of interferon-γ, neutrophil elastase and β-glucuronidase in sites with 2 mm loss of attachment (Alpagot et al 2003). Elevated levels of pro-inflammatory cytokines have been detected in the gingival crevicular fluid of HIV-positive patients (Baqui et al 2000) and when compared with non-infected controls with periodontal disease (Yin et al 2007), which could contribute to its pathogenesis in HIV-infected patients.

Sites with progressive periodontal disease in HIV positive subjects were found to be colonized with *Fusobacterium nucleatum*, *Prevotella intermedia* and *Aggregatibacter actinomycetemcomitans* (Alpagot et al 2004). Detection of *Candida* may indicate an opportunistic presence associated with a weakened host response. However, it could contribute to the pathogenesis of periodontal disease by damaging the sulcular and junctional epithelium, resulting in the ingress of pathogens into underlying tissues. *Candida* has been shown to trigger a significant pro-inflammatory cytokine response (Dongari-Bagtzoglou and Fidel 2005). This could contribute to progression of attachment loss in HIV-infected patients. In a study on British subjects (Robinson et al 1997), the differences in periodontal attachment loss were compared in HIV subjects and controls and were also related to CD4 counts. There were significantly greater amounts of periodontal attachment loss in the HIV subjects and the amounts increased as the CD4 count decreased. Other studies have been reported regarding increased probability of developing necrotizing ulcerative gingivitis and periodontitis with decreasing CD4 counts (Yin et al 2007).

However, it has also been shown that long term periodontal maintenance treatment can maintain attachment levels in HIV subjects providing that good oral hygiene is maintained by the subjects themselves (Feller et al 2006).

The microbiology of HIV-G (linear erythema) and HIV-P (necrotizing ulcerative periodontitis NUP)

The microbiology of necrotizing ulcerative periodontitis in HIV-infected subjects was compared with that of ANUG in HIV-negative subjects by electron microscopy (Cobb et al 2003). In addition to the typical presentation of spirochaetes, zones of PMN aggregates and necrotic cells, *Candida* invasion was a typical feature of the necrotizing ulcerative periodontitis lesions in HIV-positive subjects; this indicates the relevance of *Candida* in its aetiology. The presence of *Candida* in both linear gingival erythema and necrotizing ulcerative periodontitis may imply that linear erythema is a precursor to the development of necrotizing ulcerative periodontitis. Although the microbial profile of NUP was similar to the putative periodontal pathogens in HIV-negative subjects, typical species detected in NUP using a PCR-based, reverse capture, checker board DNA-DNA hybridization assay were: *Bulleidia extructa*, *Dialister*, *Fusobacteria*, *Selenomonas*, *Peptostreptococcus* and *Veillonella*. It is relevant that *Porphyromonas gingivalis* was not detected in NUP, using this assay (Paster et al 2002).

CHANGES IN DEFENCE MECHANISMS OF AIDS PATIENTS

Often HIV patients with normal levels of CD4 lymphocytes and good oral hygiene have healthy gingiva and do not differ from normal patients in their response to plaque. Thus it would seem that it is the disruption of immune function by HIV infection that increases the pathogenicity of subgingival bacteria. The mechanisms involved have been reviewed by Ryder (2002). It has also been shown that HIV-positive subjects with chronic periodontitis have significantly lower serum IgG antibody levels to putative periodontal pathogens than HIV-negative chronic periodontitis patients.

PMNs harvested from HIV-positive patients have been shown to have increased phagocytosis, oxidative bursts and F-actin formation when compared with those from normal controls. This would seem to suggest that PMNs from HIV patients show increased activity and this is in contrast to the decrease in activity of these cells seen in rapidly progressing periodontitis. In chronic periodontitis the PMNs form the first line of defence and as the disease progresses they are increasingly replaced by macrophages and lymphocytes. In HIV subjects with low levels of CD4 lymphocytes this change is unlikely to occur and thus the PMNs have a more important role in protecting the tissues in these subjects.

PMNs from AIDS patients are possibly primed because of their prolonged exposure to opportunistic fungal and bacterial infections and the failure of CD4-lymphocyte and macrophage response. They could also be primed as the result of the transient bacteraemia which can occur from chewing in the presence of periodontal disease. These hyperactive PMNs could produce local tissue damage.

Thus, the main factors which contribute to severe periodontal destruction seen in HIV patients would seem to be:

- Primed or hyperactive PMNs
- Failure of the CD4 lymphocyte and macrophage response
- Increase pathogenicity of bacteria species in the subgingival flora due to immunodeficiency.

TREATMENT OF HIV-G (LINEAR ERYTHEMA) AND HIV-P (NECROTIZING ULCERATIVE PERIODONTITIS)

The management of periodontal lesions in HIV-infected patients has not changed very much since they were first diagnosed (Ryder 2002). Very careful cross-infection control must be used with all these patients as all periodontal procedures produce blood in the mouth.

Patients are normally treated by conventional periodontal therapy, i.e. plaque control, scaling and root planing. This may be supplemented by the use of chlorhexidine mouthwashes or local irrigation. The treatment is usually very successful in HIV infection but not in AIDS.

Three treatment approaches have been evaluated in HIV-associated periodontitis. These were: (1) conventional therapy i.e. plaque control, scaling and subgingival scaling and root planing, (2) conventional therapy supplemented with a local irrigation of a 10% povidone iodine (Betadine) and (3) conventional therapy plus rinsing twice a day with a 0.12% chlorhexidine solution. All patients were assessed at 1 and 3 months after scaling and root planing. Patients treated with conventional therapy and 0.12% chlorhexidine solution showed a significant improvements in the clinical measurements, i.e. plaque index, gingival index and pocket depth and complete resolution of spontaneous gingival bleeding. Patients using the 10% povidone iodine solution appeared to benefit from its topical anaesthetic effects.

Responses to treatment in motivated HIV patients with good oral hygiene is usually good when the CD4 cell levels are good. However, the response to treatment is likely to fall as the CD4 cell levels decrease. Thus, a failure to respond to treatment and the presence of opportunistic infections such as candidiasis and hairy leukoplakia, may be indicative of a progression to AIDS.

HIV-RELATED ANUG

The incidence of ANUG is higher in HIV patients than the rest of the population (Reichart 2006). The microbiology of this condition in HIV subjects is the same as that seen in non-infected subjects and thus its severity appears to be due to the decreased immunocompetence. The condition becomes more prevalent and more resistant to treatment as the CD4 cell levels decrease.

The condition is treated in a similar way to ANUG in normal subjects. Thus, oxygenating mouthwashes such as Bocasan can be used to supplement local swabbing and scaling. The infection is treated by the appropriate antimicrobials such as metronidazole or amoxicillin.

OTHER HIV-ASSOCIATED LESIONS ON THE GINGIVA

Other HIV-associated lesions may occur on the gingiva and these include herpetic gingivostomatitis, candidiasis, human papillomavirus (HPV) causing multiple condylomas of the gingival margin and gingival ulceration due to infection with *Mycobacterium avium* intracellulare. Kaposi's sarcoma is the commonest oral tumour and it can involve the gingival margin. Non-Hodgkin's lymphoma has been found in AIDS patients and may appear as a diffuse gingival swelling, epulis or nodule (Reichart 2006; Feller et al 2006).

TREATMENT OF HIV INFECTION

There are four main classes of antiretroviral agents:

1. Nucleoside and nucleotide analogue reverse transcriptase inhibitors
2. Non-nucleoside analogue reverse transcriptase inhibitors

3. Protease inhibitors
4. Entry (fusion) inhibitors.

Due to early establishment of a pool of latently infected CD4 cells it is not easy to eradicate HIV with currently available therapeutic regimens (DHHS 2006). The goals of therapy are based on optimal suppression of viral load, maintenance of immune responses and improvement of the quality of life, mortality and morbidity.

1. The nucleotide analogue reverse transcriptase inhibitors are effective against both HIV-1 and HIV-2 and were the first class of antiretroviral agents to be developed. Lactic acidosis/hepatic steatosis is a complication of therapy with this class of drugs and potentially life-threatening. The onset may be insidious with gastrointestinal symptoms which could lead to hepatic failure, pancreatitis and respiratory failure (Cote et al 2002).
2. Non-nucleoside analogue reverse transcriptase inhibitors block the action of HIV-1 reverse transcriptase by binding and locking the active site into an inactive configuration; although very potent, resistance can occur rapidly due to a single step mutation with cross resistance to other drugs in this class. Drug interactions with other HIV agents could also occur. They are not effective against HIV-2. The occurrence of serious skin manifestations with one drug in this class could preclude the use of others in this category (DHHS 2006).
3. Protease inhibitors are a class of antiretrovirals that are effective against both HIV-1 and HIV-2. They bind to the active site of the enzyme and inhibit the HIV protease at a late stage of viral replication, preventing the cleavage of precursor polyproteins. This results in the formation of noninfectious virions. Many potential drug interactions occur between this class and other HIV agents. Recognized adverse effects of protease inhibitors are the development of visceral adiposity, insulin resistance, hyperlipidaemia including total cholesterol, low density lipoprotein and triglyceride.
4. The only approved fusion inhibitor Enfuvirtide, binds to a transmembrane glycoprotein of HIV and prevents virus-cell fusion. It is administered by subcutaneous injection and a major adverse effect is the development of pruritic indurations and it is usually used as a last resort.

Combined antiretroviral therapy has had a tremendous impact on the management and course of HIV infection by reducing transmission and improving the quality of life. Therapy is recommended for all symptomatic HIV patients and those with CD4 cell counts ≤ 200 cells/mm^3 (Yeni et al 2004). Therapeutic intervention at this stage could overcome potentially life-threatening complications seen in patients with moderately advanced immunodeficiency. Antiretroviral therapy initiated in the early stages has been shown to improve viral and immune status in the short-term compared with no therapy. But there is no evidence to suggest that early intervention can prevent or alter its course in the future compared with treatment efficacy at a later stage of intervention (Smith et al 2004).

REFERENCES

Alpagot T, Duxgunes N, Wolff LF, et al: Risk factors for periodontitis in HIV patients, *J Periodontal Res* 39:149–157, 2004.
Alpagot T, Font K, Lee A: Longitudinal evaluation of GCF IFN-gamma levels and periodontal status in HIV+ patients, *J Clin Periodontol* 30:944–948, 2003.
Baqui AA, Meiller TF, Jabra-Rizk MA, et al: Enhanced interleukin 1 beta, interleukin 6 and tumor necrosis factor alpha in gingival crevicular fluid from periodontal pockets of patients infected with human immunodeficiency virus 1, *Oral Microbiol Immunol* 15:67–73, 2000.
Cobb CM, Ferguson BL, Keselyak NT, et al: A TEM/SEM study of the microbial plaque overlying the necrotic gingival papillae of HIV-seropositive, necrotising ulcerative periodontitis, *J Periodontal Res* 38:147–155, 2003.
Cote HC, Brumme ZL, Craib KJ, et al: Changes in mitochondrial DNA as a marker of nucleoside toxicity in HIV-infected patients, *N Engl J Med* 346:811–820, 2002.

DHHS: *Guidelines for the use of antiretroviral agents in HIV-1 infected adults and adolescents*. Washington DC, 2006, Department of Health and Human Services (DHHS), pp 1–121.

Dongari-Bagtzoglou A, Fidel PL Jr: The host cytokine responses and protective immunity in oropharyngeal candidiasis, *J Dent Res* 84:966–977, 2005.

Feller L, Wood NH, Raubenheimer E: Complex oral manifestations of an HIV-seropositive patient, *J Int Acad Periodontol* 8:10–16, 2006.

Kendpon D, Pongsiriwet S, Pongsomboon K, et al: Oral manifestations of HIV infection in relation to clinical and CD4 immunological status in northern and southern Thai patients, *Oral Dis* 10:138–144, 2004.

Paster BJ, Russell MK, Alpagot T, et al: Bacterial diversity in necrotising ulcerative periodontitis in HIV-positive subjects, *Ann Periodontol* 7:8–16, 2002.

Phillips A: Short-term risk of AIDS according to current CD4 cell count and viral load in antiretroviral drug-naïve individuals and those treated in the monotherapy era, *AIDS* 18:51–58, 2004.

Pindborg JJ: Classification of oral lesions associated with HIV infection, *Oral Surg Oral Med Oral Pathol* 67:292–295, 1989.

Reichart P: US1 HIV – changing patterns in HAART era, patients' quality of life and occupational risks, *Oral Dis* 12:S3, 2006.

Robinson PJ, Sheiham A, Challacombe SE, et al: Periodontal health and infection, *Oral Dis* 3(Suppl 1):149–152, 1997.

Ryder MI: An update on HIV and periodontal disease, *J Periodontol* 73:1071–1078, 2002.

Salama C, Finch D, Bottone EJ: Fusospirochetosis causing necrotic oral ulcers in patients with HIV infection, *Oral Surg Oral Med Oral Pathol* 98:321–323, 2004.

Smith DE, Walker BD, Cooper DA, et al: Is antiretroviral treatment of primary HIV infection clinically justified on the basis of current evidence? *AIDS* 18:709–718, 2004.

Yeni PG, Hammer SM, Hirsch MS, et al: Treatment for adult HIV infection: 2004 recommendation of the International AIDS Society-USA Panel, *JAMA* 292:251–265, 2004.

Yin MT, Dobkin JF, Grbic JT: Epidemiology, pathogenesis and management of human immunodeficiency virus infection in patients with periodontal disease, *Periodontol 2000* 44:55–81, 2007.

In health, the gingivae are firm, pink, knife-edged and do not bleed on probing. There is a shallow gingival crevice or sulcus and the junctional epithelium is attached to the enamel (**Fig. 8.1**). The gingival fibre system is well organized. A few PMNs are present in the junctional epithelium as they pass through from the gingival vessels into the gingival crevice and into the mouth (**Fig. 8.2A**). In the subjacent connective tissue isolated inflammatory cells, mainly lymphocytes with the occasional plasma cell and macrophage, may also be seen. The picture manifests the quiet but dynamic balance of health.

GINGIVITIS

Because plaque accumulation is greatest in the sheltered interdental region, gingival inflammation tends to start in the interdental papilla and spreads from there around the neck of the tooth.

The histopathology of chronic gingivitis has been described chronologically by Page and Schroeder (1976) in a number of stages: the initial lesion at 2–4 days followed by an early gingivitis which at 2–3 weeks becomes an established gingivitis. These changes were described by examining biopsies of experimental gingivitis lesions at different time intervals.

THE INITIAL LESION

The first observed change occurs around the small gingival blood vessels apical to the junctional epithelium. These vessels begin to leak and perivascular collagen disappears to be replaced by a few inflammatory cells, plasma cells and lymphocytes – mainly T lymphocytes – tissue fluid and serum protein. There is increased migration of leucocytes through the junctional epithelium and exudation of tissue fluid from the gingival crevice. Other than the increased flow of fluid exudate and PMNs there may be no clinical signs of tissue change at this stage.

EARLY GINGIVITIS

If plaque deposition persists, the initial inflammatory changes continue with an increased flow of gingival fluid and migration of PMNs (**Fig. 8.3**). Changes occur in both the junctional and crevicular epithelia where there are signs of cell separation and some proliferation of basal

cells. Fibroblasts begin to degenerate and the collagen bundles of the dentogingival fibre groups break up so that the seal of the marginal cuff of gingiva is weakened. There is a small increase in the number of inflammatory cells, 75% of which are lymphocytes. There are also a few plasma cells and

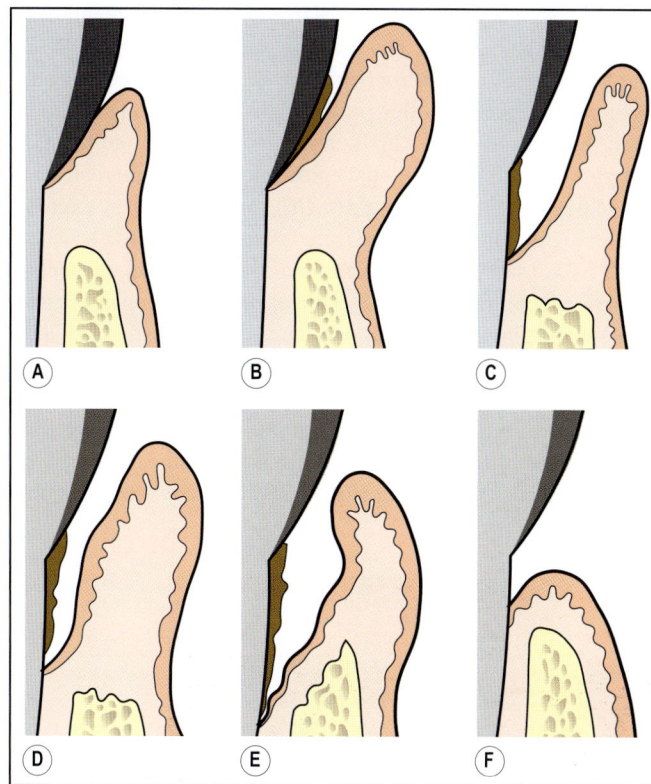

Fig. 8.2 Diagram to show the various forms of periodontal pathology. (A) Gingival health and shallow gingival crevice. (B) Gingival swelling with production of a 'false' or gingival pocket. (C) 'True' or periodontal pocket with apical migration of junctional epithelium, detachment of crevicular epithelium and associated resorption of the alveolar crest to form a 'suprabony' pocket. (D) A suprabony pocket plus gingival hyperplasia producing a deep pocket but with little bone loss. (E) An 'intrabony' pocket where the epithelial attachment is apical to the alveolar crest. (F) Gingival recession, i.e. equal apical movement of gingival margin and alveolar crest.

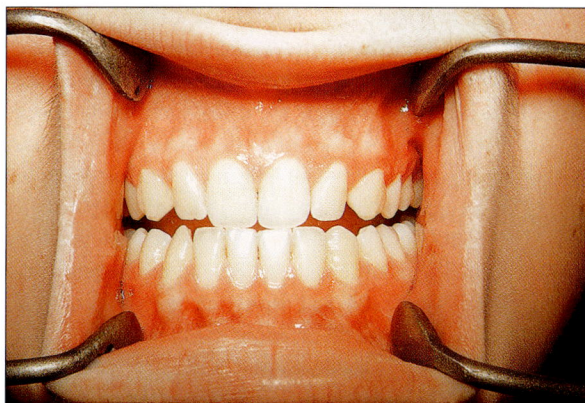

Fig. 8.1 A healthy mouth.

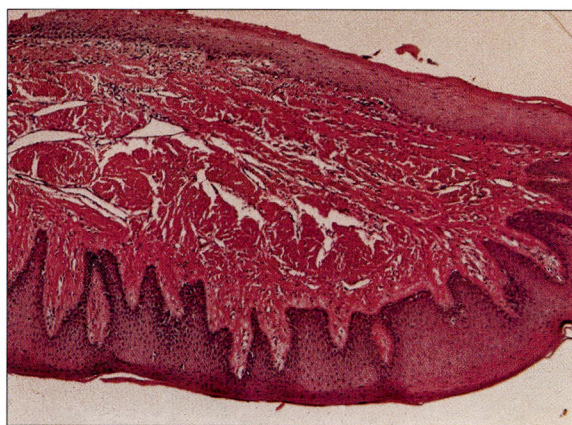

Fig. 8.3 A photomicrograph showing early gingivitis. The junctional epithelium is intact and adherent to the cervical part of the crown. Most of the gingival collagen bundles are intact and there is a mild infiltration of the gingival corium with inflammatory cells.

macrophages. The clinical signs at this stage are few and the gingivae often appear clinically healthy. This is because the lesion, which has become more 'chronic' in nature, occupies a very small area of the gingiva. Also the signs of acute inflammation reduce as the lesion becomes chronic. This stage is probably classed as gingival health in clinical dentistry.

ESTABLISHED GINGIVITIS

If satisfactory oral hygiene is not re-established, clinically obvious gingivitis becomes established within 7–14 days. Clinical signs of inflammation appear and the interdental papillae may become swollen and bleed on probing (**Figs 8.4, 8.5**). The number of lymphocytes increases and B lymphocytes become more dominant. Many of these cells mature and develop into plasma cells which manufacture specific antibodies to the many plaque antigens. Some macrophages appear but there is a secondary stimulation of acute inflammation produced by complement activation. This results in the emigration of PMNs from blood vessels, and many of these also migrate through the junctional epithelium into the gingival crevice. The flow of gingival crevicular fluid (GCF), an inflammatory exudate, increases. Immunoglobulins, mainly IgG, are found in the gingival connective tissue and GCF. Mast cells are also found in the gingival connective tissue and junctional epithelium. These changes result in clinical gingival inflammation and the gingivae are red, swollen and bleed easily (**Fig. 8.5**). The lesion increases in size and occupies a larger volume within the gingival connective tissue.

With the increased destruction of collagen and inflammatory swelling the gingival margin can be separated easily from the tooth surface giving rise to 'gingival' or 'false' pocketing (**Fig. 8.2B**). If there is considerable

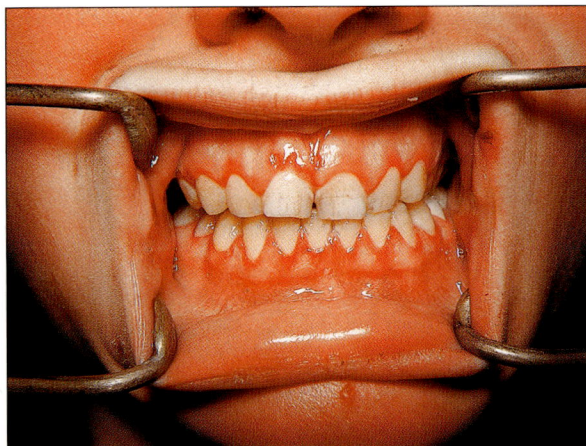

Fig. 8.4 Early signs of chronic marginal gingivitis showing distinct redness around gingival margins due to vascular hyperaemia.

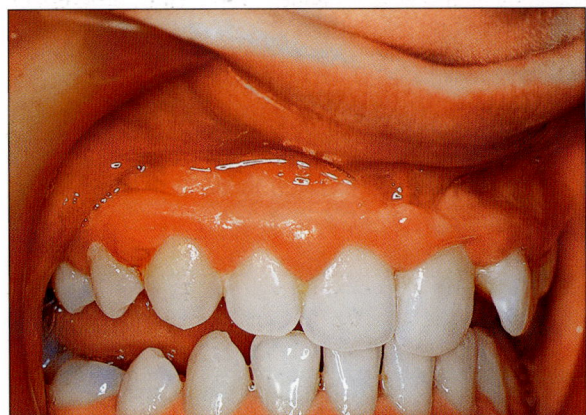

Fig. 8.5 Established gingivitis with oedematous papillary swelling.

inflammatory oedema and gingival swelling the gingival pocket can be quite deep. There is now degeneration of the cells of the junctional epithelium and some proliferation of its basal layers into the underlying connective tissue but at this stage there is no significant migration of epithelial cells on to the root surface.

As the inflammation spreads along the trans-septal fibres there may be some resorption of the alveolar crest. This is reversible on resolution of the inflammation.

One interesting feature of the disease is that no bacteria are found either in the epithelium or in the connective tissue.

As fibrous tissue is destroyed within the site of active inflammation, at more distant sites there is some proliferation of fibrous tissue and formation of new blood vessels. This productive or repair activity is a very important characteristic of the chronic lesion and where the irritation and inflammation are longstanding the fibrous tissue element can become the predominant component of the tissue change.

Thus, destruction and repair continue side by side and the proportion of each affects the colour and shape of the gingivae. If the inflammation dominates, the tissues are red, soft and bleed easily; if fibrous tissue production dominates, the gingivae can be firm and pink, although swollen, and there may be little or no bleeding. The systemic factors which determine the tissue response to plaque irritation are discussed in Chapter 6.

Effective treatment of gingivitis will remove the cause of irritation and the condition will resolve and turn back into a small lesion resembling the 'early' lesion with a small number of lymphocytes occupying a small area of gingival connective tissue subjacent to the junctional epithelium. The gingiva then appears clinically healthy.

The lesions described so far have been described as 'contained' because they are limited to the gingiva and are largely reversible on removal of the plaque. They may remain contained for many years; on the other hand, an established gingivitis lesion may spread into the deeper tissues to become a destructive chronic periodontitis. This progression is not inevitable, and some longitudinal studies indicate that the incidence of conversion to periodontitis is very low (Albander et al 1986; Listgarten 1988). There is considerable debate as to whether this progression is determined by the nature of the bacterial plaque or by host factors or by both. Plasma cells appear to be related to more aggressive lesions and it is possible that the proliferation of plasma cells may be provoked by particular plaque constituents.

CHRONIC PERIODONTITIS

With continuing plaque irritation and inflammation the integrity of the junctional epithelium is increasingly damaged. The epithelial cells degenerate and separate and the attachment to the tooth completely breaks down. At the same time, the junctional epithelium proliferates into the connective tissue and down the root surface as the dentogingival fibres and alveolar crest fibres are destroyed. Apical migration of the junctional epithelium continues and as this epithelium separates from the root surface, a 'periodontal' or 'true' pocket is formed (**Figs 8.2C, 8.6**). This seems to be an irreversible change.

Once a true pocket is formed, plaque is in contact with the cementum. The connective tissue is oedematous; vessels are dilated and thrombosed; vessel walls break down with haemorrhage into the surrounding tissues. There is a massive inflammatory infiltrate of plasma cells, lymphocytes and macrophages. IgG is the predominant immunoglobulin but some IgM and IgA are present. The epithelium of the pocket wall may be intact or ulcerated. This appears to make no difference as plaque products diffuse through the epithelium. The flow of GCF and migration of PMNs continue and it is likely that the fluid flow helps to promote the deposition of subgingival calculus.

Extension of the inflammation into the alveolar crest is marked by the infiltration of some inflammatory cells into trabecular spaces, and these may

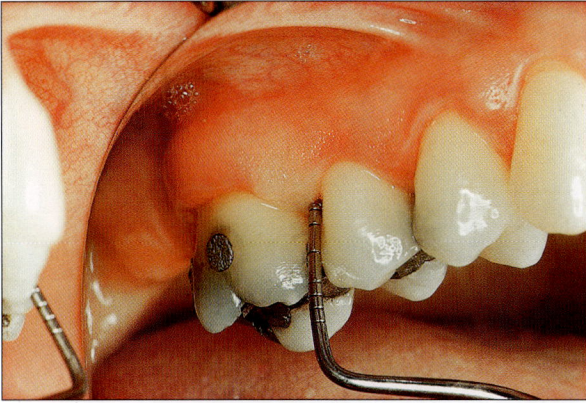

Fig. 8.6 Clinical features of a periodontal pocket distal to upper left second premolar demonstrated with a periodontal probe.

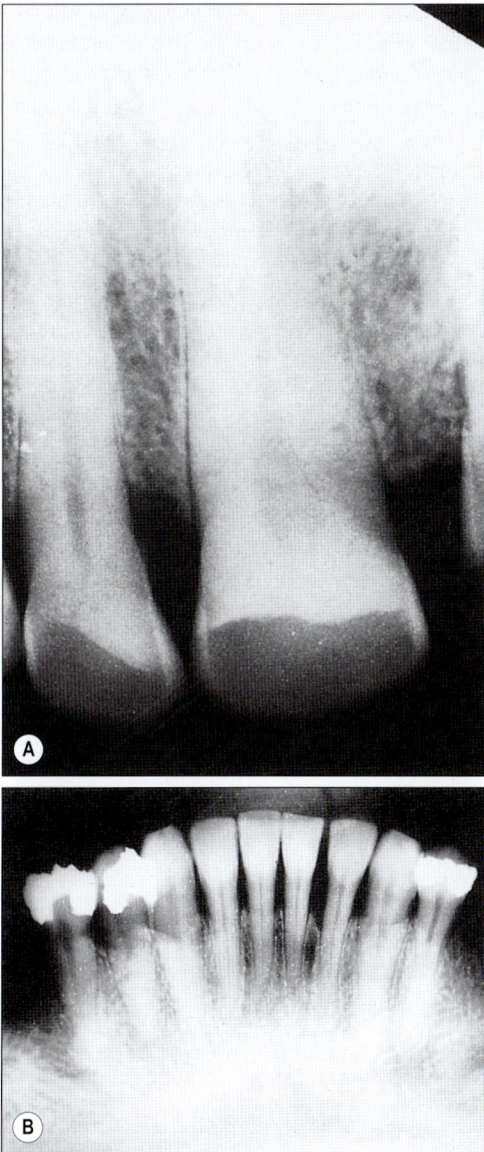

Fig. 8.7 (A) Early resorption of interproximal alveolar crest. (B) More advanced and more generalized bone loss.

increase in size. Bone resorption tends to be compensated for by deposition further away from the inflammatory zone so that the bone is remodelled but shows a net loss. Bone resorption usually starts interproximally so that where the table of interproximal bone is broad, as it is between molars, an interdental crater is formed and then as the resorption process spreads laterally the entire alveolar crest is resorbed (**Fig. 8.7**).

The periodontal lesion also appears to be 'contained' because as it advances and connective tissue is destroyed the trans-septal fibres are continually reformed and seem to separate the main inflammatory infiltrate from the underlying bone.

The progression of the lesion is not continuous, periods of advance and remission take place, and fibrosis is a constant feature, especially in the latter phase.

With destruction of periodontal ligament and alveolar crest resorption the pocket deepens. At a later stage in the disease there may be varying degrees of suppuration and abscess formation. Finally, the teeth become loose, migrate and are lost.

DISEASE PROGRESSION

At one time it was believed that periodontitis, once established, progresses continuously and inevitably, with a simple straight-line age correlation. This led to the notion that tooth-loss was part of the ageing process. So strong was this belief that many dentists recommended full extractions in middle age when the patient was still 'adaptable' to dentures, rather than waiting to a time when the elderly person, having lost most or all teeth, would find such adaptation difficult or impossible.

This belief about the pattern of disease progression was supported by clinical studies which reduced measurements of pocket depth or alveolar bone loss to average values for a given mouth, thus eliminating intra-oral variation and obscuring both sites of little or no disease, and sites of worst disease. Epidemiological studies on various populations also used average values for age groups, and these findings also supported the belief in a straightforward age-correlated linear progression. In this way ideas about longitudinal change were derived from the compilation of misleading findings from cross-sectional studies.

However, detailed measurement of loss of attachment at specific sites over time, i.e. valid longitudinal study, contradicts the idea of continuous and inevitable disease progression, and indicates that:

1. As stated above, gingivitis, even when persistent and untreated, does not inevitably progress to periodontitis
2. Even when established, periodontal destruction is not continuous but progresses in an episodic manner with 'bursts' of destructive activity alternating with periods of quiescence, and possibly repair
3. There is great individual variation in the pattern of destruction, which also varies over time in the same individual.

Some research workers believe that the bursts of activity occur at random (Goodson et al 1982; Socransky 1984), and that a past history of persistent and severe gingivitis or of periodontal destruction does not indicate future destructive activity. Thus, progress is unpredictable. Other workers find that progress is not random, and that there is a correlation between the initial degree of bone loss and the subsequent rate of bone loss (Papapanou et al. 1989; Albander 1990). Thus, progression is to some extent predictable. Others have suggested that prognosis is affected by the site of disease, i.e. whether related to incisors, molars or distributed generally.

Many studies show that, once initiated the average rate of bone loss is very slow, 0.05–0.1 mm per year (Suomi et al 1971; Sheiham et al 1986; Albander 1990). However, this is not always the case; in some people rapid bone loss occurs early in life, and in others rapid bone loss may follow years of little or very slow tissue destruction.

It must be recognized that the amount of probing attachment loss (PAL) that can be reliably measured depends upon the threshold for the probing method used (see Ch. 13). Most of the clinical longitudinal studies which led to the development of the 'burst' theory of periodontal progression (Goodson et al 1982; Lindhe et al 1983; Haffajee & Socransky 1986) used manual probing, which cannot reliably measure changes in

PAL of less than 2.5–3 mm. They would therefore only detect rapidly progressive attachment loss (RAL) losing this amount or more and would not detect gradual attachment loss (GAL) losing much smaller amounts possibly over a longer time period. They therefore lead to the notion that all periodontal progression occurs in bursts of activity over short time periods.

More recently, electronic probes have been developed which will measure PAL more reliably and accurately and have thresholds of 0.3–0.8 mm (see Ch. 13). Using an electronic probe which detects and measures from the cement-enamel junction (CEJ) with a threshold of 0.25 mm, Jeffcoat et al (1991) monitored 30 patients with moderate–advanced chronic periodontitis for 6 months. Using a threshold of 0.4 mm they found 29% of sites with attachment loss (AL) and using one of 2.4 mm, they found AL at only 2% of sites. This latter figure is similar to the percentage in the studies above which used manual probing. This indicated that using large thresholds only RAL will be detected while using smaller thresholds will detect both RAL and GAL with a higher proportion of GAL sites. Thus, it appears that both RAL, progressing by 'bursts', and GAL occur during the progression of chronic periodontitis. GAL could either result from small 'mini-bursts' of activity producing AL of less than 0.5 mm or from slow progressive AL or both. It is likely that patients susceptible to periodontal disease will tend to progress more by bursts of RAL whilst those with lesser susceptibilities would progress more slowly and gradually.

It has also been shown that in patients with moderate chronic periodontitis that further attachment loss mostly occurred at sites with previous probing depths >5 mm (Gribic & Lamster 1991, 1992).

At present, we are handicapped in making precise diagnoses and prognoses by two important limitations:

1. We have no reliable markers for present disease activity (see Ch. 14)
2. We have no reliable criteria for identifying the 'at-risk' individual.

BONE DEFECTS

The pattern of alveolar resorption can vary from one tooth to the next and on different aspects of the same tooth.

It is believed that inflammation spreads from the gingiva into the deeper tissues along three pathways: through the alveolar bone, the attached gingiva and the periodontal ligament. The primary pathway appears to be through the alveolar bone in which inflammation tracks via perivascular and perineural channels into trabecular spaces. It may then travel laterally from bone into periodontal ligament and attached gingiva. If resorption of the alveolar crest is even, the base of the pocket remains coronal to the crest of the bone and a simple 'suprabony' pocket is formed, i.e. a pocket entirely surrounded by soft tissue (**Fig. 8.2C**). If resorption of the alveolar crest proceeds more rapidly in one part than another, the base of the pocket becomes apical to the crest of the bone. This is known as an 'intrabony' pocket (**Figs 8.2E, 8.8**).

As cancellous bone is more vascular and less dense than cortical bone, it is likely that, as stated above, the central cancellous part of a broad alveolar septum will resorb more rapidly than the lateral parts made up of cortical bone so that an intrabony pocket is formed in relation to an interdental 'crater'.

The variety of bone defects is infinite, but for purposes of description they have been classified according to their morphology as marginal defects, intra-alveolar defects, perforation and furcation defects. These are very rough groupings with considerable overlap. In chronic inflammation the formative bone response may more than compensate for the bone resorption so that a thickened or bulbous alveolar margin is formed. Intra-alveolar defects, i.e. defects within the alveolar process, are commonly classified according to the number of bone walls, that is, one-, two- or three-walled (**Fig. 8.9**). This group also includes interdental craters and hemisepta.

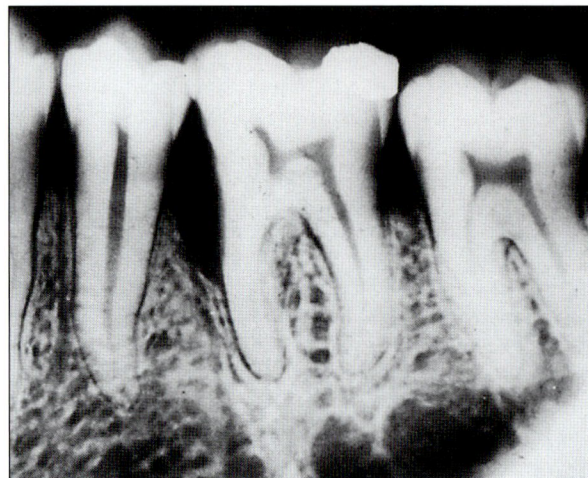

Fig. 8.8 Radiographical appearance of bone defect associated with an intrabony pocket mesial to the lower left first molar. The bone defect is frequently described as an 'intrabony' defect. *Note* early alveolar resorption in other areas that are related to suprabony pockets.

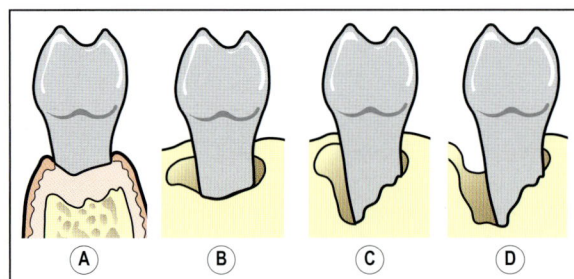

Fig. 8.9 Diagram to show some forms of bone defects: (A) interdental crater, (B) three-walled defect, (C) two-walled defect, (D) one-walled defect or hemisepta.

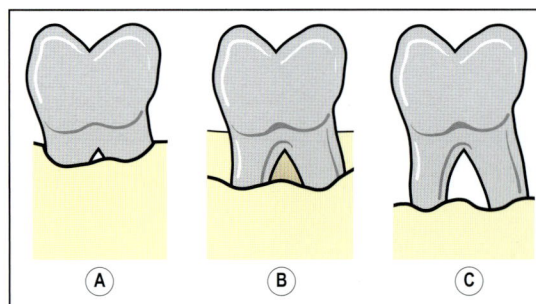

Fig. 8.10 Diagram to show furcation defects. (A) Class 1, (B) Class 2, (C) Class 3.

Furcation defects have been classified according to the degree of bone loss in the furcation measured in a horizontal plane (**Fig. 8.10**). An early or Class 1 defect is one which penetrates <2 mm into the furcation; a Class 2 defect is one where the bone loss is >2 mm into the inter-radicular area but does not go completely through the furcation so that one aspect of the bone is intact; in a Class 3 defect so much inter-radicular bone has been lost that a probe can be passed between the roots from one side to the other (**Fig. 8.11**).

There has been much speculation about the factors which might determine the pattern of bone resorption. Two factors appear to play an important role: the original morphology of the bone, and excessive occlusal stress. Variations in original bone morphology must influence the type of bone defects in disease. A thin alveolar plate of bone is more likely to be completely resorbed than a thick plate of bone; a thin interdental septum between incisors may be completely destroyed while an interdental crater will form in the septum between molars. A split or dehiscence may be formed where bone coronal to a developmental defect, a perforation or fenestration is resorbed by progressive inflammation.

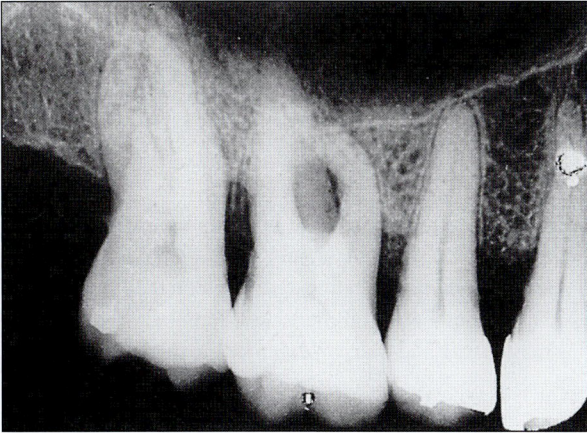

Fig. 8.11 Radiographical appearance of a trifurcation Class 3 defect.

OCCLUSAL TRAUMA

Considerable debate has centred on the role of occlusal forces in the development and progress of periodontal disease, as well as on the influence of these forces on the rate and form of alveolar bone destruction. Functional stresses on all parts of the skeleton tend to strengthen, while lack of function tends to weaken the tissues. Experimental rats fed on a coarse diet have thicker and heavier jaws than those fed on a soft diet, and the periodontal ligament is composed of more and thicker collagen bundles in the former group than in the latter.

Many experiments have been carried out on animals to determine the results of overloading teeth. A basic problem in such studies is to distinguish the effects of plaque-induced inflammation from those produced by occlusal stresses, and great care must be taken to maintain a high standard of oral hygiene in the experimental animals. A number of experiments demonstrate the kind of tissue changes produced in the tooth-supporting tissues when overloaded, e.g. when pressures are applied to teeth by different types of appliance or when a high restoration is placed so that it interferes with the occlusion.

The pattern of changes in the periodontium depends on whether the forces applied to the teeth are uni- or multidirectional. The reactions of the tissues to both of these are described below.

Orthodontic-type trauma

This is brought about by single directional forces applied to a normal periodontium such as occurs in orthodontic tooth movement. This type of trauma has been investigated in animal studies by histological examination of blocks of teeth and periodontium after varying time periods (Reitan 1951; Mühlemann & Herzog 1961; Ewan & Stahl 1962; Warhaug & Hansen 1966; Karing et al 1982). The crown of the tooth is tilted in the direction of the force and the tooth moves about its fulcrum at the apical third of the root producing pressure and tension zones within the marginal and apical parts of the periodontium. On the pressure side, the tissues become crushed and this produces disruption and disorganization of the periodontal fibres leading to hyaline degeneration and necrosis of connective tissues. The blood vessels are damaged and haemorrhage and thrombosis are present. If the magnitude of the forces is within certain limits, the periodontal ligament cells remain vital and osteoclasts appear on the adjacent bone surface leading to bone resorption. This is known as direct bone resorption. However, if the force is greater, then damage to the ligament cells prevents this from occurring. In this situation, osteoclasts develop in the marrow spaces below the bone surface and this leads to undermining or indirect bone resorption. This bone is resorbed until it reaches the hyalinized periodontium when the tooth is able to move away from the pressure force. Macrophages and osteoclasts

remove the damaged tissues after which they become revascularized allowing new periodontal tissues to form. Bone deposition then occurs in the tension zones to compensate for the increased width of the periodontium in this area. Once the tooth has moved the pressure is nullified and the full healing of the periodontal tissues takes place in both the pressure and tension zones.

Bodily movement of the teeth with fixed orthodontic appliances produce the same changes except that the pressure and tension zones are more extended in the apical-coronal direction. If excessive forces are used root cementum and dentine may also be resorbed.

These changes affect only the intra-alveolar periodontal ligament and do not involve the supra-alveolar connective tissues and therefore cannot affect the marginal periodontal tissues.

Jiggling-type trauma

The kind of stress that is transmitted to the tooth in occlusal trauma is not unidirectional but rather multidirectional. Cuspal interference imposes intermittent loading on opposing teeth and this is usually resisted by soft tissue forces or secondary cuspal contacts. This produces alternating or 'jiggling' forces on the teeth. These have been investigated by a number of animal studies which have sought to reproduce these 'jiggling' forces (Wentz et al 1958; Glickman & Smulow 1968; Svanberg & Lindhe 1973; Meitner 1975; Ericsson & Lindhe 1982). These forces produce alternating pressure and tension zones within the intra-alveolar periodontium and these exhibit the same changes described above for the pressure zones in unidirectional forces. The direct or indirect bone resorption associated with this process leads to a generalized widening of the periodontal ligament space and as a result of this the tooth or teeth involved display progressive increasing mobility. When the effect of the forces is compensated by the increased width of the ligament space, the damaged tissues are removed and the widened periodontium heals. The tooth remains mobile within this widened periodontium.

As with unidirectional forces, these changes affect only the intra-alveolar periodontal ligament and do not involve the supra-alveolar connective tissues. Therefore, they cannot affect the marginal periodontal tissues.

Jiggling-type trauma applied to a reduced periodontium

The effects of these forces on a reduced but healthy periodontium has been studied in dogs by Ericsson and Lindhe (1977). The same changes as have been described above were produced around the whole intra-alveolar periodontium which increased in width. The affected teeth became progressively mobile over several weeks, after which the enlarged space compensated for the forces. The bone resorption then ceased and the periodontal tissues in the enlarged space healed. The teeth remained hypermobile but were surrounded by periodontal tissues, which had adapted to the increased functional forces. The supra-alveolar connective tissues and marginal periodontium were again unaffected by the changes.

Jiggling-type trauma superimposed on inflammatory chronic periodontitis

Older studies

The relation between occlusal trauma and inflammatory periodontal disease has often been discussed in connection with human case reports and autopsy material. On the basis of this, Glickman (1964, 1965, 1967, 1971) claimed that the path along which the plaque-associated inflammatory lesion spread was affected by the presence of occlusal trauma. In this connection, it was suggested that occlusal trauma changed the vascular pattern so that the inflammatory lesion passed into the periodontal ligament space rather than into the alveolar crest (Macapanpan & Weinmann 1954). Glickman and Smulow (1962, 1965, 1968) claimed from the results of human autopsy and animal experiments that occlusal trauma imposed on inflammatory periodontitis produced angular bone resorption and intrabony pocketing. However, Warhaug (1979) examined human autopsy material and reported that angular bony defects and intra-bony pockets usually occurred in areas unaffected by occlusal trauma. His findings supported the observations of Prichard (1965) and Manson (1976), which showed that the pattern of alveolar bone loss resulted from an interplay between the form of the alveolar bone and the apical extension of the subgingival plaque on the root surface. Furthermore, these findings did not support the concept of Glickman (1964, 1971) which described a zone of co-destruction within the periodontium which could be affected by the combined effects of marginal inflammation and occlusal trauma. These matters have now been largely resolved by the later studies described below.

Later studies

Experiments on humans and other animals described in the previous sections have shown that trauma from occlusion cannot induce changes in the supra-alveolar marginal tissues. The effects of jiggling trauma superimposed on progressive destructive periodontitis have been studied by a number of research groups (Lindhe & Svanberg 1974; Meitner 1975; Nyman et al 1978; Ericsson & Lindhe 1982). In these experiments, destructive periodontitis was first initiated in dogs or monkeys and then the teeth were subject to jiggling trauma. The periodontal tissues in the combined pressure/tension zones were damaged as described before. The intra-alveolar periodontium showed signs of inflammation with hyperaemia, exudation, thrombosis and migration of inflammatory cells. Numerous osteoclasts differentiated on the adjacent bone surface and bone was resorbed. This process gradually increased the width of the periodontal ligament space and as a result the teeth became increasingly mobile. Angular bone resorption could be seen on radiographs of the affected area. The forces became nullified by the increased width of the periodontal ligament space and at this point the bone resorption ceased. The periodontium regenerated its normal tissues and within this increased space the tooth mobility stopped increasing. The angular bone resorption persisted but histological examination revealed that no further apical migration of the junctional epithelium had resulted from the imposition of occlusal trauma. This indicates that occlusal forces which allow adaptive alterations within the ligament will not aggravate inflammatory periodontal disease.

However, if this jiggling occlusal trauma generated greater forces and these were maintained for long time periods so that the periodontium could not become adapted, then the injury persisted and in some cases became permanent (Lindhe & Svanberg 1974). In these cases, the pressure/tension zones displayed continuing inflammation and damage over several months. The osteoclasts residing in the alveolar wall persisted producing continuing bone resorption and the angular bone defects remained. These changes produced gradual progressive widening of the periodontal ligament space and progressively increased tooth mobility. Under these circumstances, the marginal inflammatory lesion merged with the 'trauma' lesion in the periodontium. The junctional epithelium proliferated apically and the destructive periodontal disease was aggravated.

In another set of experiments in the dog (Ericsson & Lindhe 1982) prolonged jiggling forces for 10 months were applied to some teeth with established chronic periodontitis and these were compared with other control teeth also with established chronic periodontitis in the same dog which were not jiggled. The traumatized teeth showed an increased rate of progression compared with control teeth.

Conclusion

Unidirectional or jiggling forces applied to the healthy periodontium will not result in loss of attachment as trauma from occlusion cannot affect the marginal tissues. It does, however, produce tooth mobility within an adapted, widened periodontium. All of these changes are reversible on the removal of the trauma.

However, in teeth with established chronic periodontitis, superimposed prolonged and severe jiggling trauma may cause persistent damage within the periodontium such that adaptive changes are prevented from developing. Under these circumstances, the marginal periodontal and intra-alveolar 'trauma' lesions may merge and this can enhance the rate of periodontal disease progression.

The causes of excessive occlusal stress are discussed in Chapter 27. Loads can become excessive in two situations: (1) where there is an actual alteration in occlusal load, and (2) where there is a reduced capacity of the tooth-supporting tissues to absorb stress. Tissue damage caused by applying excessive occlusal loads to a previously healthy periodontium has been called primary occlusal trauma. Damage caused by normal functional stress applied to an impaired periodontium has been called secondary occlusal trauma. The division into primary and secondary trauma is rather artificial as, more often than not, excessive loads are applied to an already impaired periodontium. However, it remains a useful conceptual distinction as primary trauma is completely reversible (as in orthodontic treatment) while the tissue changes associated with secondary trauma may be only partly reversible.

GINGIVAL RECESSION

Gingival atrophy (**Figs 8.2F, 8.12, 8.13**) results in apical movement of the gingival margin to produce gingival recession and exposure of the root of the tooth. Recession involves some destruction of the periodontal tissues and it may accompany chronic periodontitis, but it is not necessarily a feature of this disease. Gingival recession is one of those tissue changes which are usually caused by the wear and tear of use and which lie between health and active pathology. Like tooth attrition gingival recession represents a departure from normal anatomy, which is not necessarily a sign of disease. It is extremely common and frequently the cause of patient concern.

A number of factors acting singly or in combination produce or affect gingival recession and these are described below.

Physical abuse

Both healthy gingiva and the gingival wall of a periodontal pocket can atrophy under the stress of toothbrush friction, especially when an overzealous horizontal brushing technique is used. The sheltered interdental gingiva

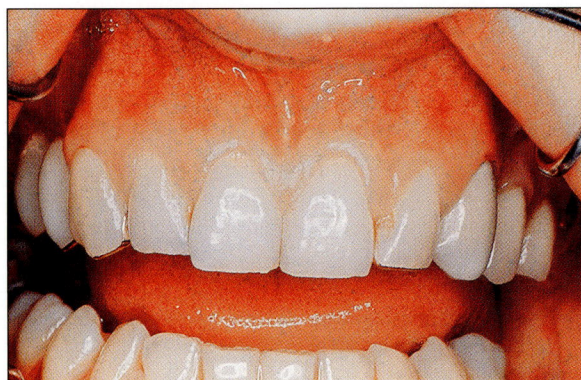

Fig. 8.12 Early gingival recession in a clean mouth and heathy gingiva due to toothbrush abrasion.

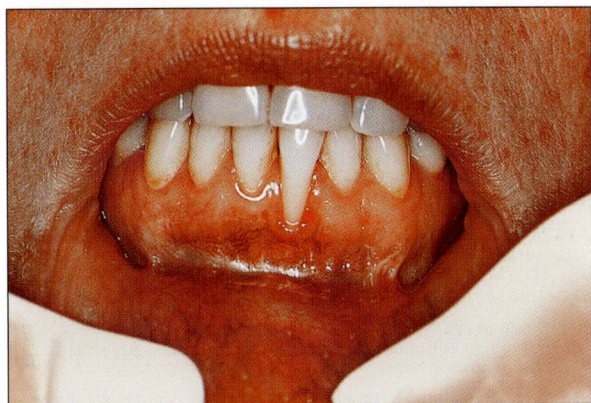

Fig. 8.13 Local gingival recession extending close to the mucogingival junction on the lower left central incisor.

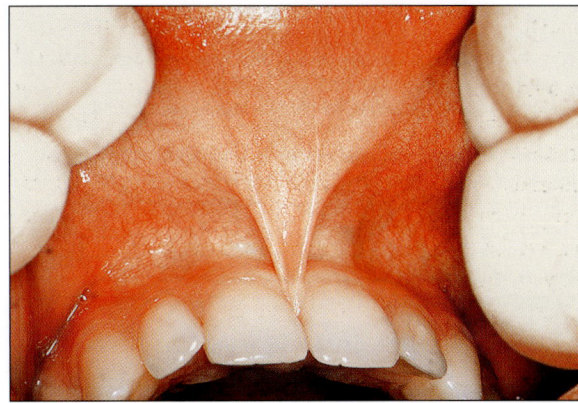

Fig. 8.14 Large frenum and healthy gingiva in 40-year-old man.

may escape this treatment so that the recession is restricted to labial tooth surfaces which may also suffer abrasion. The maxillary canines and first premolars which form the corner of the arch receive the brunt of this form of aggression and usually display the worst recession. The interdental gingiva may not escape the enthusiastic use of various interdental oral hygiene aids; some patients use woodsticks and floss like a hacksaw, and although gingiva and the underlying bone are remarkably resilient, they will atrophy in the face of determined attack.

Physical damage can also result from a variety of dental procedures – the carelessly applied matrix band or temporary crown, uncontrolled condensation of an interproximal or cervical restoration, pressure from a badly designed denture clasp or denture ('gum stripping') – or from strange habits, such as pressing a pencil into the gum!

Another physical factor is that associated with deep overbite where the incisal edge of an upper incisor impinges on the lower labial gingiva or where a lower incisor strikes the palatal tissue.

Alveolar defects

The presence of an underlying alveolar margin defect, e.g. dehiscence, means that the overlying gingiva is unsupported and less able to withstand irritation. The Northern European skull is often dolichocephalic, i.e. long-headed, the jaws narrow and overcrowded and alveolar plates thin; developmental defects, dehiscence and fenestration are common, especially on the labial surface of canines, lower incisors and first molars. Defects of alveolar plates are frequently related to tooth position and root morphology.

Tooth position

The position of the tooth in the arch is a determinant of the thickness of bone overlying the root. A displaced tooth may be accompanied by some compensating thickness of overlying bone but there is a limit to such accommodation and where teeth are placed in, say, a labial position the labial alveolar margin is displaced apically or is deficient (dehiscence).

Furthermore, teeth can be moved through alveolar bone by uncontrolled orthodontic forces and excessive occlusal stress, with resultant bone perforation and gingival recession.

Root morphology

Where roots diverge, as they do especially on first upper molars or where the root is markedly convex as it may be on both upper and lower canines, the overlying bone may be very thin or deficient. This may not manifest in health but where some tissue destruction has taken place a divergent palatal root of an upper first molar can be related to gross recession.

Soft-tissue attachment

The presence of a frenum or muscle attachment does not influence healthy gingiva (**Fig. 8.14**) but, in the presence of inflammation and pocketing, tension from these anatomical structures may result in retraction of the gingiva and recession. This is often the case where the zone of attached gingiva is narrow or absent. However, the mere presence of a frenum never justifies surgical intervention; only when an anatomical feature is obviously related to progressive pathology is surgical modification indicated.

Disease

Acute necrotising ulcerative gingivitis (see Ch. 25) can destroy gingival tissue which may not be reformed when the disease has resolved. If sufficient tissue is destroyed, recession results. In addition, the gingival wall of a periodontal pocket may move apically as the disease progresses or as inflammation subsides, to produce root exposure. Recession also follows pocket reduction surgery for the treatment of chronic periodontitis. The treatment of all forms of gingival recession and its complications is considered in Chapter 21.

REFERENCES

Albander JM, Rise J, Gjermo P, et al: Radiographic quantification of alveolar bone level changes, *J Clin Periodontol* 13:195–200, 1986.

Albander JM: A 6-year study on the pattern of periodontal disease progression, *J Periodontol* 17:467–471, 1990.

Ericsson I, Lindhe J: Lack of effect of trauma from occlusion on the recurrence of experimental periodontitis, *J Clin Periodontol* 4:115–127, 1977.

Ericsson I, Lindhe J: The effect of longstanding jiggling on experimental marginal periodontitis in the beagle dog, *J Clin Periodontol* 9:497–503, 1982.

Ewan SJ, Stahl SS: The response of the periodontium to chronic gingival irritation and long-term tilting forces in adult dogs, *Oral Surg Oral Med Oral Pathol* 15: 1426–1433, 1962.

Glickman I: Trauma from occlusion in the etiology of periodontal disease. In *Clinical Periodontology*, ed 3, Philadelphia, 1964, W B Saunders, Ch. 24, pp 286–299.

Glickman I: Clinical significance of trauma from occlusion, *J Am Dent Assoc* 70:607–618, 1965.

Glickman I: Occlusion and the periodontium, *J Dent Res* 49(Suppl. 1):5, 1967.

Glickman I, Smulow JB: Alterations in the pathway of gingival inflammation into the underlying tissues induced by excessive occlusal forces, *J Periodontol* 33:7–13, 1962.

Glickman I, Smulow JB: Effects of excessive occlusal forces upon the pathway of gingival inflammation in humans, *J Periodontol* 36:141–147, 1965.

Glickman I, Smulow JB: Adaptive alteration in the periodontium of the Rhesus monkey in chronic trauma from occlusion, *J Periodontol* 39:101–105, 1968.

Glickman I: Role of occlusion in the etiology and treatment in periodontal disease, *J Dent Res* 50:199–204, 1971.

Goodson JM, Tanner ACR, Haffajee AD, et al: Patterns of progression and regression of advanced destructive periodontal disease, *J Clin Periodontol* 9:472–481, 1982.

Gribic JT, Lamster IB: Risk indicators for future clinical attachment loss in adult periodontitis. Patient variables. *J Periodontol* 62:322–329, 1991.

Gribic JT, Lamster IB: Risk indicators for future clinical attachment loss in adult periodontitis. Tooth and site variables, *J Periodontol* 63:262–269, 1992.

Haffajee AD, Socransky SS: Attachment level changes in destructive periodontal disease, *J Clin Periodontol* 13:461–472, 1986.

Jeffcoat MK, Reddy MS: Progression of probing attachment loss in adult periodontitis, *J Periodontol* 62:185–189, 1991.

Karing T, Nyman S, Thilander B, et al: Bone regeneration in orthodontically produced alveolar bone dehiscences, *J Periodontal Res* 17:309–315, 1982.

Lindhe J, Svanberg G: Influence of trauma from occlusion on progression of experimental periodontitis in the beagle dog, *J Clin Periodontol* 1:3–14, 1974.

Lindhe J, Haffajee AD, Socransky SS: Progression of periodontal disease in adult subjects in the absence of periodontal therapy, *J Clin Periodontol* 10:433–442, 1983.

Listgarten MA: Why do epidemiological data have no diagnostic value? In Guggenheim B, editor: *Periodontology Today*, Basel, 1988, Karger, pp 59–67.

Macapanpan LC, Weinmann JP: The influence of injury to the periodontal membrane on the spread of gingival inflammation, *J Dent Res* 33:263–272, 1954.

Manson JD: Bone morphology and bone loss in periodontal disease, *J Clin Periodontol* 3:14–22, 1976.

Meitner SW: *Co-destructive factors of marginal periodontitis and repetitive mechanical injury*, Thesis. Rochester, 1975, Eastman Dental Center and The University of Rochester.

Mühlemann HR, Herzog H: Tooth mobility and microscopic tissue changes produced by experimental occlusal trauma, *Helvetica Odontologica Acta* 5:33–39, 1961.

Nyman S, Lindhe J, Ericsson I: The effect of progressive tooth mobility on destructive periodontitis in the dog, *J Clin Periodontol* 7:351–360, 1978.

Page RC, Schroeder HE: Pathogenesis of inflammatory periodontal disease. A summary of current work, *Lab Invest* 3:235–249, 1976.

Papapanou PN, Wennstrom JL, Grondahl K: A 10-year study of periodontal disease progression, *J Clin Periodontol* 16:403–411, 1989.

Prichard JF: *Advances in Periodontal Disease*, Philadelphia, 1965, W B Saunders.

Reitan K: The initial tissue reaction incident to orthodontic tooth movement as related to the influence of function, *Acta Odontol Scand* 6(Suppl):1–240, 1951.

Sheiham A, Smales FC, Cushing AM, et al: Changes in periodontal health in a cohort of British workers over a 14-year period, *Br Dent J* 160:125–127, 1986.

Socransky SS, Haffajee AD, Goodson JM, et al: New concepts of destructive periodontal disease, *J Clin Periodontol* 11:21–32, 1984.

Suomi JD, Greene JC, Vermillion JR, et al: The effect of controlled oral hygiene procedures on the progression of periodontal disease in adults: results after third and final year, *J Periodontol* 42:152–160, 1971.

Svanberg G, Lindhe J: Experimental tooth hypermobility in the dog. A methodological study, *Odontol Revy* 24:269–282, 1973.

Warhaug J: The infrabony pocket and its relationship to trauma from occlusion and subgingival plaque, *J Periodontol* 50:355–365, 1979.

Warhaug J, Hansen ER: Periodontal changes incident to prolonged occlusal overload in monkeys, *Acta Odontol Scand* 24:91–105, 1966.

Wentz FM, Jarabak J, Orban B: Experimental occlusal trauma imitating cuspal interferences, *J Periodontol* 29:117–127, 1958.

Classification of periodontal diseases   9

ON CLASSIFICATIONS

Many forms of classification have been devised in attempting to provide the clinician with some rationale for making a differential diagnosis, and arriving at a reasonable prediction of how the tissues will respond to treatment. Some classifications have used variation in clinical presentation as parameters; others in trying to provide some understanding of the causes of disease have included both aetiological factors and clinical features. Often the results have been confusing rather than clarifying.

A classification should be a systematic arrangement of groups (plants, animals, diseases etc.) that possess common attributes. This arrangement should provide insight into the relationship between groups, and between members of the same group. This requires some form of homogeneity within the group and clear delineation between groups. A very simple example of this process is to put dogs and cats in different animal groups because dogs of all kinds can interbreed but cannot mate with cats of any kind.

In the host–parasite interaction which results in periodontal pathology, many factors enter the equation to produce a variety of tissue changes and therefore clinical features. On one side lie the rich oral flora plus any 'secondary' factors described in subsequent chapters; on the other side of the equation are a multiplicity of host or systemic factors. Also there are wide quantitative variations rather than a simple present or absent situation in the different parameters connected with periodontal diseases. Thus, clear correlations between the severity of periodontal tissue destruction and, for example, specific bacterial species, or deficiencies in neutrophil activity, or even oral hygiene status, become difficult to define. Establishing a simple cause and effect relationship is impossible, and drawing the lines that a classification demands becomes a matter of approximation, and therefore of probable confusion. Given our present knowledge, this may not necessarily help to bring rationality to bear on our clinical problems.

ATTEMPTS AT CLASSIFICATION

Classification of disease is necessary to try to separate conditions into distinct categories so as to aid clinical and laboratory diagnosis and specific treatment. The criteria for separating diseases in this way should ideally be aetiology, histopathology and, where appropriate, genetics rather than age of onset and rates of disease progression. Over the last two decades there have been three major attempts to classify periodontal disease. Although they all had obvious merits they all did not produce totally universally acceptable results mainly because of the imprecise nature of our knowledge on the specific bacterial aetiology of periodontal diseases.

The first of these was by the 1st World Workshop in Clinical Periodontics in 1989 (American Academy of Periodontology 1989). This introduced the concept of periodontal diseases as distinct from periodontal disease and separated periodontitis into three categories: chronic periodontitis, rapidly progressive periodontitis and refractory periodontitis, on the basis of rate of progression and response to treatment. It also included separate entities of early-onset disease separating them into localized and generalized juvenile periodontitis and prepubertal periodontitis. Acute necrotizing gingivitis was also recognized as a separate entity.

The second attempt was made by the 1st European Workshop in Periodontics in 1993 (Attström & van der Velden 1994), which replaced chronic periodontitis with adult periodontitis, and introduced a broad category of early onset periodontitis, which contained localized and generalized juvenile periodontitis and prepubertal periodontitis.

The third attempt was started by the American Academy of Periodontology in 1997, who organized the International Workshop for a Classification of Periodontal Diseases and Conditions in 1999. At this workshop, a new classification was agreed upon (Armitage 1999). This attempted to develop a comprehensive classification of gingival diseases (Mariotti 1999; Holmstrup 1999), periodontal diseases (Femmig 1999; Tonetti & Mombelli 1999; Kinane 1999), necrotizing ulcerative gingivitis/periodontitis (Rowland 1999; Novak 1999), periodontal abscesses (Meng 1999a), periodontitis associated with an endodontic lesion (Meng 1999b), developmental or acquired deformities and conditions (Blieden 1999), mucogingival deformities and conditions (Pini Prato 1999) and occlusal trauma (Hallmon 1999). This classification includes both separate conditions and a number of other factors which may affect their severity or clinical presentation and is shown in Tables 9.1 and 9.2.

The main changes in this classification are:

1. The addition of a comprehensive section on gingival diseases.
2. The replacement of the term adult periodontitis with chronic periodontitis since epidemiological evidence (Papapanou et al 1989; Papapanou 1996) suggests that chronic periodontitis may also be seen in some adolescents.
3. The elimination of separate categories of rapidly progressive periodontitis and refractory periodontitis because of the lack of evidence that they represent separate conditions but rather describe the rate of progression of chronic periodontitis or its response to treatment that result from differences in patient susceptibility.
4. Replacement of the term 'early onset periodontitis' with 'aggressive periodontitis', largely because of the clinical difficulties in determining the age of onset in many of these cases. The authors of this new classification also question the use of the term juvenile periodontitis for the same reasons. They have replaced them with the terms localized aggressive periodontitis and generalized aggressive periodontitis. They have also largely discarded the term prepubertal periodontitis and have included those cases which are not directly caused by systemic disease in the appropriate aggressive periodontitis category.
5. A new classification group of 'periodontitis as a manifestation of systemic disease' has been created and this includes those cases of prepubertal periodontitis directly resulting from known systemic disease.
6. There are also new group categories on periodontal abscesses, periodontic–endodontic lesions and developmental or acquired deformities or conditions.

This new system of classifications has some merits but also some features that may not easily gain general acceptance. On the merit side, the removal of rapidly progressive periodontitis and refractory periodontitis is to be supported since these conditions simply reflect a chronic periodontitis case in a susceptible patient resulting in earlier onset, more rapid progression and more resistance to treatment. However, if one limits oneself to the

As described in Chapter 8, there has recently been a radical change in our ideas about the natural history of periodontal diseases. There has also been a parallel reappraisal of their prevalence and the methods by which they are studied. Until recently, periodontal disease was regarded as the main cause of tooth loss, and a WHO report of 1978 stated that 'almost all the adult population has experienced gingivitis, periodontitis or both'. These ideas are out-of-date and are now seen as the result of invalid methods of data collection and interpretation.

There has been a reduction in disease prevalence, and the reasons for the improvement in periodontal health which has taken place in the industrialized countries are probably related to better personal and oral hygiene, improved standards of living, reduction in cigarette smoking, decrease in the use and dosage of oral contraceptives, plus the effects of fluoride, fewer proximal restorations and overhanging margins (Sheiham 1990).

In order to measure the prevalence of the disease, its severity, and its relationship to other factors, such as age, oral hygiene status, nutrition and so on, special indices have been devised which attempt to provide an objective measure or score to specific identifiable features so that reliable comparisons can be made. Using these indices and applying the appropriate statistical tests should allow the interested observer to make a valid comparison of, for example, the periodontal condition of young adults in the USA, with the periodontal condition of individuals of any age anywhere in the world. Also, if successful public health measures are to be implemented, and personnel trained and recruited, the character and size of the problems to be tackled need to be defined.

INDICES

All indices should be appropriate to the nature of the investigation, and the circumstances under which this is being undertaken. Thus, the assessment of the gingival condition and oral hygiene status of 10–12-year-old children in an inner city area in Britain will require a very different approach from a study of the periodontal status of an East African nomadic cattle-breeding tribe, such as the Masai or Dinka. The application of any particular index needs to meet several criteria:

1. It must be practical and acceptable to the subject. The method of examination must not be painful or more uncomfortable than the individual can reasonably tolerate, e.g. taking six pocket measurements on every tooth in a child's mouth is impractical. Any examination in the absence of adequate illumination or sterilization facilities is not acceptable.
2. It must reflect the reality of the situation, thus pocket measurement on the buccal aspects of teeth may be irrelevant and misleading when the main site of periodontal destruction is interproximal. Also, pocket depth is an indicator of past pathology, and cannot validly be used as an indicator of current disease activity.
3. It should be sufficiently standardized and reliable to allow comparison between different examiners, and between examinations at different times, as in longitudinal studies.
4. It should allow numerical quantification and therefore statistical analysis. Assessment of gingival inflammation by degree of redness is subjective and quantifiable only in the grossest terms.

5. It should be sufficiently sensitive to detect small changes. Thus, bleeding on probing the pocket may or may not indicate the presence of active disease and does not tell us about the strength of that activity; biochemical assessment of crevicular fluid might be sufficiently sensitive for that purpose.

Indices of the gingival condition use colour, change of contour, readiness to bleed on gentle probing, bleeding time, measurement of gingival fluid exudate, counts of white cells in gingival fluid and gingival histology. Indices of periodontal destruction depend largely on probing depth and probing attachment level measurements. Some of the tests require special equipment and special skills and are used therefore only in sophisticated laboratory studies. Conditions in the field usually do not permit, other than the most simple, tests to be used, especially where large numbers of individuals are inspected. The most commonly used indices of gingival inflammation are the Gingival Index (Löe and Silness 1963) and the Bleeding on Probing Index (Löe 1967), which have a number of variations (Barnett et al 1980). The three periodontal indices to be described, the Periodontal Index (Russell 1956), the Periodontal Disease Index (Ramfjord 1959) and the Community Periodontal Index of Treatment Needs (CPITN; Ainamo et al 1983), score both gingival inflammation and periodontal destruction.

GINGIVITIS INDICES

Gingival Index (GI)

The severity of the condition is indicated on a scale of 0 to 3:

0 Normal gingivae
1 Mild inflammation, slight change in colour, slight oedema. No bleeding on probing
2 Moderate inflammation, redness, oedema and glazing. Bleeding on probing
3 Severe inflammation, marked redness and oedema, ulceration. Tendency to spontaneous bleeding.

The mesial, buccal, distal and lingual gingival units are scored separately. This index is particularly sensitive in the early stages of gingivitis.

The gingival index is reversible, as its values return to zero with the disappearance of the disease. By contrast, indices of chronic periodontitis measure the amount of periodontal destruction which is irreversible. Furthermore, as the progression of chronic periodontitis tends to be phasic, a periodontal index does not measure active disease.

Bleeding on Probing Index

0 Normal gingivae.
1 Signs of gingival inflammation but no bleeding on gentle probing.
2 Bleeding on probing.
3 Spontaneous gingival bleeding.

The mesial, buccal, distal and lingual gingival units are scored separately.

PERIODONTAL DESTRUCTION INDICES

Periodontal Index (PI)

All teeth are examined; the scores used in this index (Russell 1956) are as follows:

0 Negative: there is neither overt inflammation in the investing tissues nor loss of function due to destruction of supporting tissues

1 Mild gingivitis: there is an overt area of inflammation in the free gingivae, but this area does not circumscribe the tooth

2 Gingivitis: inflammation completely circumscribes the tooth, but there is no apparent break in the gingival attachment

6 Gingivitis with pocket formation: the epithelial attachment has been broken and there is a pocket (not merely a deepened crevice due to swelling in the free gingivae). There is no interference with normal masticatory function; the tooth is firm in its socket, and has not drifted

8 Advanced destruction with loss of masticatory function: the tooth may be loose, may have drifted, may sound dull on percussion with metallic instrument, may be depressible in its socket.

Rule: When in doubt, assign the lesser score.

This index has been applied with success to large population groups. Its limitation is that its score for periodontal destruction is so heavily weighted that it is not possible to distinguish the early stages of chronic periodontitis.

Periodontal Disease Index (PDI)

The periodontal disease index introduced by Ramfjord (1959) is a development of the Russell index. The Ramfjord index is particularly designed for assessing the extent of pocket deepening below the cemento-enamel junction. Scoring is as follows:

0 Healthy

1 Mild to moderate inflammatory change not extending all around tooth

2 Mild to moderate inflammatory change extending all around tooth

3 Severe gingivitis, characterized by marked redness, tendency to bleed, ulceration

4 3 mm apical extension of pocket base from enamel-cement junction.

5 3–6 mm extension

6 Over 6 mm extension.

Another feature of the PDI is that only six teeth, 6/14 / 41/6 are selected for examination and measurement. The data from these teeth have been found to be representative of the dentition as a whole, and their average score is the score of the patient.

Community Periodontal Index of Treatment Needs (CPITN)

If an attempt is made to provide an adequate dental service for a particular community, it is necessary to assess its treatment need. The CPITN (Ainamo et al 1983) has become the most widely employed system for this purpose and uses the following method:

1. A specially banded probe with a ball head (**Fig. 10.1**) has been designed for use with the index. It is to be used as an extension of the examiner's fingers in the gentle manipulation of the gingivae. The sensing force should correspond to about 20 g or less, and pain during probing indicates that too much pressure is being applied. A pressure guided probe has been designed to produce a standard force but it is difficult to see the relevance of such sensitive instrumentation in the context of CPITN.

2. The dentition is divided into six segments or sextants (four posterior and two anterior) in which there are two or more teeth present and not indicated for extraction. When only one tooth remains in a sextant, it is included in the adjacent sextant.

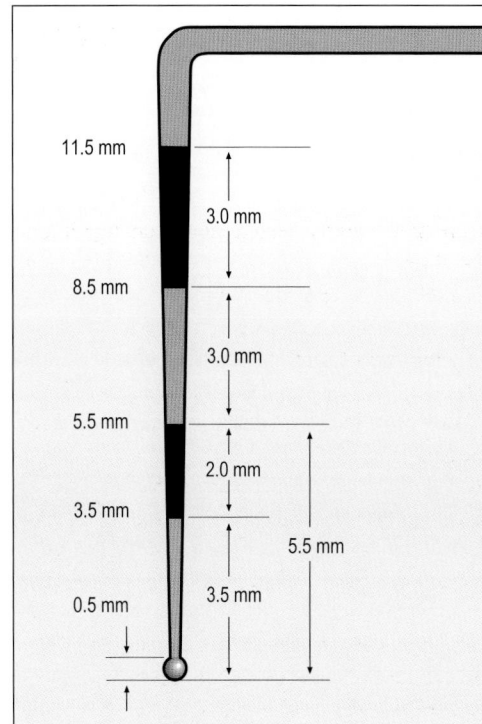

Fig. 10.1 The CPITN probe.

3. The scoring system is:

Code 0 Health: no pocketing or gingival bleeding on probing

Code 1 Gingival bleeding on probing

Code 2 The presence of calculus or other plaque-retentive factors such as overhanging margins of restorations that can be seen or felt on probing

Code 3 Pocketing of 4–5 mm, that is, when the gingival margin is on the black area of the probe

Code 4 Pocketing of 6 mm or more, i.e. when the black area of the special probe is no longer visible

Code X When only one tooth or no teeth are present in a sextant. Third molars are excluded unless they function in the place of second molars.

4. When used for epidemiological purposes (alternative 1), ten specific teeth are examined, these are 761/67 / 76/167 and the worst of the two molar scores is recorded, thus making six scores. When used for treatment purposes (alternative 2), for children and adolescents six index teeth 61/6 / 6/16 are examined, while for adults (20 years and older) all teeth are examined.

5. It is suggested that an appropriate treatment plan can be worked out on the following basis:

Code 0   Requires no treatment

Code 1   Requires improvement in home care

Codes 2 and 3   Require supra- and subgingival scaling and improvement in home care

Code 4   Requires more complicated treatment, i.e. supra- and subgingival scaling and root planing, improvement in home care and surgery.

The CPITN has proved to be a very useful broad screening tool, and as such, has been usefully employed in many WHO surveys throughout the world. A good example of its use is illustrated in **Figure 10.2**. This shows, on a three-dimensional bar diagram, the mean number of sextants according to CPITN scores of 2784 people in a 1986 Dutch National Dental

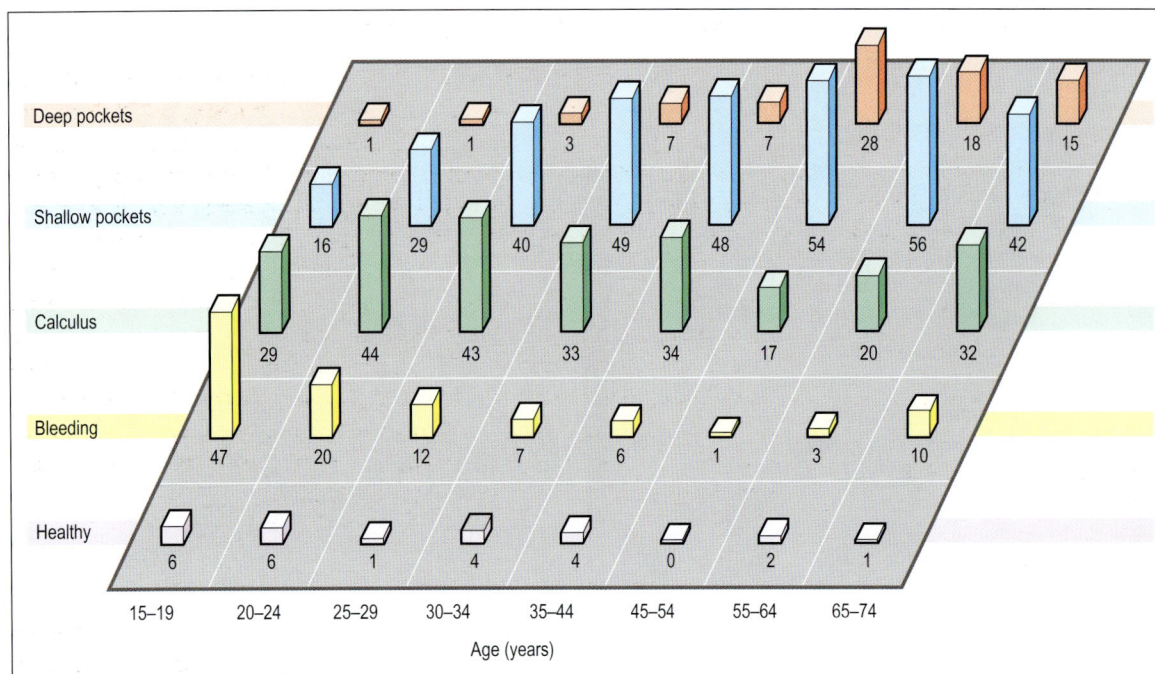

Fig. 10.2 CPITN scores in Dutch National Survey (Reproduced from Taco & Lewis 1992 Guidelines for Community Periodontal Care, by kind permission of FDI World Dental Press Ltd.).

Survey (reported in the FDI Guidelines for Community Periodontal Care; Taco & Lewis 1992). In a comparison of the Periodontal Index (PI) and CPITN, Cuttress et al (1986) demonstrated that although a partial recording index CPITN is more sensitive than PI.

However the CPITN is too insensitive to be used to produce a detailed diagnosis, prognosis and treatment plan for the individual patient in practice, or to monitor the individual patient on a regular basis.

INDICES ASSESSING EXTENT OF DISEASE

An index to measure the extent and severity of periodontitis has been proposed by Carlos et al (1986) and is denoted the Extent and Severity Index.

Extent and Severity Index (ESI)

This has two components:

1. Extent – proportion of tooth sites in the subject with destructive periodontitis
2. Severity – mean value of attachment loss at diseased sites.

An attachment loss threshold of >1 mm was set as the criteria to qualify as disease affected. By the use of this arbitrary figure, it distinguishes the fraction of the dentition affected by disease and prevents non-affected sites from contributing to the subject mean attachment loss value. It obviously depends on the use of an accurate and reliable measurement of attachment loss from the cemento-enamel junction and this is difficult to attain. It is biphasic in expression and gives a detailed description of attachment loss patterns. For example an ESI of 90,2.5 indicates a generalized early periodontitis whereas an ESI of 20,7.0 indicates a severe localized advanced periodontitis.

The same principles have been applied to the development of a partial index system based on radiographic assessment of alveolar bone loss (Papapanou et al 1991a,b) suitable for radiographic surveys of chronic periodontitis.

LIMITATION OF INDICES

All periodontal indices have the following limitations:

1. The criteria are subjective to some degree, and there is considerable variation in examiner assessment of degrees of inflammation and pocket depth or loss of attachment.

2. The scoring systems are arbitrary. Thus, a lesion scoring Russell PI 6 is not actually three times as severe as a lesion scoring PI 2; indeed gingivitis and periodontitis cannot be compared numerically in this way.

3. Although a gingivitis score measures present inflammation, pocket measurement is a reflection of past disease. If we accept the well-established idea that periodontal breakdown is episodic, pocket depth gives us no indication of disease activity at the time of measurement. The production of bleeding on careful probing of the pocket with a blunt probe has been regarded as an indicator of disease activity, but as Nevins et al (1989) point out, 'At best, bleeding on probing has a predictive value of 30%'. In this regard, the absence of bleeding on probing appears to be a good indicator of periodontal stability, whereas bleeding on probing is a very poor indicator of disease activity (Lang et al 1990). It also seems more likely that the provocation of bleeding on probing is a factor of the enthusiasm or clumsiness of the examiner than of current disease activity. However, as the mechanisms involved in tissue destruction are clarified, parameters of current disease activity are being defined. Also, some indicators of those individuals at risk from advanced periodontal disease, e.g. juvenile periodontitis, are being unravelled (see Ch. 23).

ORAL HYGIENE

The most commonly used indices of oral hygiene status are the oral hygiene index (Greene & Vermillion 1960) and the plaque index (Silness & Löe 1964).

Oral Hygiene Index

This is a composite index which scores debris and calculus deposition either on all or on selected tooth surfaces.

Oral debris is any soft foreign matter which is attached to the tooth. Oral debris and calculus are scored separately. The oral debris scoring is as follows:

0 No debris or stain present
1 Soft debris covering not more than one-third of the tooth surface

2 Soft debris covering more than one-third but not more than two-thirds of the tooth surface

3 Soft debris covering more than two-thirds of the tooth surface.

The calculus scores are assigned according to the same criteria with the addition that individual flecks of subgingival calculus are given score 2 and a continuous heavy band of subgingival calculus is scored 3.

The debris and calculus scores are added and divided by the number of surfaces examined to give the oral hygiene score.

Plaque Index (PI)

Criteria for scoring are:

0 No plaque

1 Film of plaque visible only by removal on probe or by disclosing

2 Moderate accumulation of plaque which can be seen by the naked eye

3 Heavy accumulation of soft material filling the niche between the gingival margin and the tooth surface. The interdental region is filled with debris.

This index has been used with the Gingival Index to provide precise evidence of the causal relationship between plaque and gingival inflammation. Variations of these indices measure the amount of calculus and plaque retention factors such as overhanging margins of fillings.

PROBLEMS WITH ACCURATELY ASSESSING THE PREVALENCE OF PERIODONTAL DISEASE

It is difficult to determine the prevalence, severity, extent and progression of periodontal disease because of poor correlation between the signs and symptoms of the disease and the disease process itself. Periodontal disease is a chronic inflammatory disease, induced by bacterial irritation, which is recognized by a number of signs and symptoms which in order of increasing severity include visual inflammation, bleeding on probing, gingival enlargement, pocket formation, loss of periodontal attachment and alveolar bone, tooth mobility and tooth loss. Therefore, it is probable that disease definitions based on single or in combinations of several symptoms and signs will result in different prevalence estimates. Periodontal disease is site specific and the number of sites involved varies from patient to patient and this adds another quantitative variable to disease definition. Also, many of the measurements made to assess the severity of disease such as probing depth, probing attachment loss and radiographic assessment of alveolar bone loss are far from reliably accurate and are subject to many technique variables (see Ch. 13). This makes precise disease level definitions difficult. This is particularly the case in epidemiological studies, where large numbers of patients are often examined in short periods of time and often under far from ideal conditions. Furthermore, it is necessary to define what level of attachment loss is required to consider periodontitis as an important oral health problem, and whether this should be uniform for the whole dentition or depend on tooth type or root length or the age of the patient. These are all very important questions to consider in determining disease definition.

Both cross-sectional and longitudinal studies have used different diagnostic criteria and examination methodologies and are therefore often difficult to compare. Finally, some studies have used partial mouth recording systems and these may seriously underestimate the extent of disease present. They are, therefore, difficult to compare with studies using whole mouth recording.

PREVALENCE OF GINGIVITIS

The prevalence of gingival inflammation varies significantly with age.

THE DECIDUOUS DENTITION

The gingivae around deciduous teeth appear to be remarkably resistant to plaque-induced inflammation. Even when toothbrushing is withdrawn for 3 weeks, there is a significant difference in tissue response to that in the adult. Early studies of American and English children under 5 years old recorded little or no gingival inflammation, but using more rigid criteria Poulsen and Moller (1972) found a 25% prevalence in Danish 3-year-olds. In a study of 128 5–6-year-old Australian children, Spencer et al (1983) found a high prevalence of mild inflammation around the deciduous teeth, little severe inflammation, and little correlation between the oral hygiene status and the severity of inflammation. It seems likely that this finding reflects a difference in the intensity of the immunological response in the young child, or in the microflora of the gingival crevice. The prevalence of spirochaetes and of *Bacteroides melaninogenicus* is lower at 3–7 years old than in the adult (de Araujo & MacDonald 1964).

THE TRANSITIONAL PERIOD

This period covers the mixed dentition from about the age of 5 or 6, through to puberty. It is marked by tooth irregularity and hormonal changes. Chronic gingivitis has been found in 80% of children under 12 years and approaches 100% by the age of 14 years (WHO 1978). This high prevalence was also found in a UK study of 1015 11–12-year-old children, in which Addy et al (1986) recorded that all the children had some inflammation as demonstrated by bleeding on probing, at one or more sites, with a good correlation between plaque and gingivitis scores.

In older studies, the prevalence of inflammation, i.e. the number of individuals in whose mouth some inflammation was present, was recorded, but not the fact that this was restricted to a few teeth. Therefore, the figures greatly exaggerated the size of the problem.

After about 14 years, there is a decrease in the severity of inflammation; a sexual difference also appears. Before 14 the severity of inflammation for girls is higher than for boys, the girls' scores peaking at about 12 years old; boys' scores peaked at 14 and were found to be higher than those for girls. This could be related to changing patterns in oral hygiene habits but in fact, in a study of the gingival status at puberty, Sutcliffe (1972) found that the increased severity of inflammation was not related to an increase in plaque deposition. One must conclude that in puberty, the tissues react more vigorously to any given amount of plaque; after puberty, the severity of inflammation does diminish.

THE ADULT

After the post-puberty decline in inflammation its prevalence appears to increase and has been recorded as high as 100% of young men of 17–22. But as indicated above, such figures need to be interpreted with caution. A study of 15–19-year-olds in New Zealand (Cuttress et al 1983) showed that although 79% of mouths had some gingival inflammation, only 34% of tooth sites were inflamed, and in this group, only 1% showed some periodontal breakdown. In a detailed analysis of data obtained in 1981 from the examination of 7078 people aged 19 years and older in 48 states of the USA (therefore regarded as representative of 147 million Americans), Brown et al (1989) found that 15% were free of any kind of periodontal disease, and that gingivitis without periodontitis occurred in 50% of the remaining people. The prevalence of gingivitis declined from 54% in the group aged 19–44 years to 44% at 45–64 years, and to 36% in people of 65 years. In most people, the gingivitis was restricted to a few teeth.

There is evidence that the transition from chronic gingivitis to chronic periodontitis takes place at an earlier age in Asiatic people than in Europeans or people of European origin. Although it is possible that genetic factors influence tissue vulnerability to plaque products (as appears to be the case in juvenile periodontitis), it is more likely that this difference may be explained by differences in oral hygiene habits which relate to educational and income levels. The role of nutrition in the gingival condition is uncertain, but it is likely that in the well-nourished people of developed countries nutritional factors play little or no part (Ch. 6).

Acute ulcerative gingivitis has a very low prevalence in rich countries and a higher one in poorer countries often affecting malnourished children (Ch. 25).

PREVALENCE OF PERIODONTITIS

CHILDREN AND ADOLESCENTS

Periodontal breakdown in children is often associated with some fault in the host response, as in Down's syndrome, hypophosphatasia, juvenile diabetes, etc. (see Ch. 6), but early destructive periodontal disease, i.e. juvenile periodontitis (see Ch. 23), has been reported by Cogen et al (1992) in healthy Alabama children. This radiographic study of 4757 children, 3172 Black and 1585 White, under the age of 15 revealed a prevalence of juvenile periodontitis of 1.5% in black children and 0.3% of white children. Among the black children, the male:female ratio with JP was almost equal, while among the white children it was 1:4. A further finding was that in 71.4% of the Black children with JP, previous radiographs also revealed bone loss around deciduous teeth.

The result of more than 100 WHO surveys in over 60 countries of adolescents, i.e. 15–19 years, using the CPITN have been reported by Miyazaki et al (1991a). The most frequently observed condition was score 2 (calculus with or without gingival bleeding), which was much more prevalent in non-industrialized countries than in industrialized countries. Some shallow pocketing of 4–5 mm was present in two-thirds of all populations observed, but it usually affected only a minority in the sample, and then only in one or two sextants. Some of this was probably due to false pockets due to gingivitis and gingival oedematous or fibrous enlargement.

In a more recent clinical study, 360 Brazilian public school children were examined for evidence of chronic periodontitis and 44 were found to have clinical attachment loss of ≥4 mm (Costa et al 2007). These were considered the reference sample and were recalled for a second examination after 1 year and received no dental care over this time. They showed a significant increase in the number of sites with attachment loss over this period. This indicates that early chronic periodontitis may be present in a small number of older children and adolescents and in these it has a tendency to progress to some sites in their mouths.

ADULTS

There is considerable palaeontological evidence of periodontal disease in early Man, and past epidemiological studies have emphasized the general prevalence of the disease. Hence the widespread belief that all adults would at some time during their lifetime experience deterioration of the periodontal tissues, and that a large proportion of edentulousness was due to periodontal disease. Indeed, many regarded periodontal breakdown as inevitable and part of the ageing process.

The earlier epidemiological surveys carried out between 1950 and 1970 mostly employed radiographical evidence of alveolar bone loss as a means of distinguishing between gingivitis and periodontitis. The influential study by Marshall-Day et al (1955) involving 1187 dentate subjects was representative in demonstrating that by the age of 40, 90% of adults had some periodontal disease. Findings from other epidemiological surveys of this period (Schour & Massler 1948; Belting et al 1953; Sandler & Stahl 1954; Bossert & Marks 1956; Russell 1957; Shei et al 1959; Gupta 1962; Littleton 1963; Johnson et al 1965; Ramfjord et al 1968; Sheiham & Hobdell 1969),

despite some differences in design, have also shown a very high prevalence of periodontitis in the adult population with a clear increase in prevalence with age. In 1964, Sherp reviewed the epidemiological literature at that time and concluded that periodontal disease appears to be a major global health problem affecting the majority of the adult population after the age of 35–40 years. This work indicated that the disease appears to start as gingivitis in youth which if left untreated progresses to periodontitis with more than 90% of the variance of severity in the population explainable by age and oral hygiene.

Such findings set the tone of attitudes to the conservation of the dentition. The question: Why go to all this trouble if I am going to lose my teeth?, reflected many people's attitudes to restorative dentistry. As stated earlier in the text, such notions were based on imperfect methods of data collection and interpretation. As Pilot (1992) points out, 'we have been brain-washed by averages; reports on mean attachment loss per year do not show those sites that are breaking down at a much faster rate than average, nor are persons indicated who have many of those sites and are in fact in the high risk category of losing their teeth at an early stage. Persons and sites with no attachment loss at all are also obscured in mean figures' and, 'in the early epidemiological surveys on periodontal conditions, any deviation from the ideal was recorded and implicitly considered as disease'.

Epidemiological surveys in the 1980s provided a more thorough description of the high variation in the periodontal conditions between different populations and individuals. Hugoson and Jordon (1982) examined 600 randomly selected subjects in Sweden, aged 20–70 years, by clinical and radiological means. Reporting on data relating to 1973, they found that in the age group of 30 and 40 years, 96% and 85%, respectively, of the subjects had no signs of alveolar bone loss. Severe periodontal destruction affected about 8% of subjects between 40 and 70 years. The same research group (Hugoson et al 1992) reported on the data from 597 subjects of a similar age, examined 10 years later and relating to 1983. Some 98% of the 20-year-olds and 77% of the 30-year-olds were classified as either periodontally healthy or gingivitis patients. In the entire sample, a higher percentage of subjects (11%) were placed in the severe periodontitis group than in their previous study. However, this apparent increase was accompanied by retention of more teeth and a decrease in the percentage of edentulous subjects (16% versus 12%, in ages 40–60).

Recently, the same group (Hugoson et al 1998) compared the distribution of periodontal disease in Swedish adults in 1973, 1983 and 1993 using their previous data and a new survey in 1993. The subjects were divided into five groups namely: healthy (group 1); gingivitis (group 2); moderate alveolar bone loss, i.e. up to one-third loss (group 3); severe alveolar bone loss, i.e. ranging from one-third to two-thirds loss (group 4); and angular bony defects and/or furcation defects (group 5). During these 20 years, the subjects in groups 1 and 2 increased from 49% in 1973 to 60% in 1993. In addition, there was a decrease in the number of subjects in group 3 with moderate periodontitis. The subjects with severe periodontitis in groups 4 and 5 comprised 13% of the population and showed no change from 1983 to 1993. However, the subjects in these groups had more teeth than their counterparts in 1983. In 1973, the numbers in these groups were smaller because greater numbers had become edentulous because of lack of suitable periodontal care at the time. In 1993, the subjects in groups 3–5 were divided according to the percentage of surfaces with gingivitis only or periodontal pockets ≥4 mm. At this time, 20%, 42% and 67% of individuals in groups 3, 4 and 5, respectively were classified as in need of periodontal treatment with more than 20% of sites bleeding on probing and more than 10% of sites with periodontal pockets ≥4 mm. Recently, they have reviewed their cross-sectional studies over 30 years from 1973 to 2003 (Hugoson et al 2005a,b) and they showed similar findings and trends with general improvements in periodontal and oral health.

There has also been a 20-year longitudinal study of marginal bone loss in the county of Stockholm (Jansson et al 2002). They found that the mean loss over the period was about 10% of the root length. They also found that this loss correlated with the subject's age and that the mean number of teeth in 1970 was 24.7 compared with 21.8 in 1990.

Thus, over this period there has been an increase in the number of individuals with no marginal bone loss and a decrease in the number with moderate alveolar bone loss. Although the numbers of subjects in the severe disease group remained the same the number of teeth retained by each individual increased.

Douglass et al (1983) compared data on periodontal disease from the US National Center for Health Statistics for the years 1960–1962 and 1971–1974, and found a definite downward trend in the prevalence of both gingivitis and periodontitis in younger adults.

Data taken from the UK 1988 Adult Dental Health Survey shows that 75% of the UK population at that time, aged between 35 and 45, had shallow pockets and 17% of the dentate population of 45 years and older had deep pockets. A similar pattern of prevalence was found in the large American survey reported by Brown et al (1989) and cited above. The prevalence of periodontitis increased with age from 29% at age 19–44 years, up to about 50% in people 45 years and older. Moderate periodontitis, i.e. at least one pocket of 4–6 mm deep, occurred in 28% of all people, while only 8% had advanced disease, that is at least one pocket >6 mm, and only 10% had six or more teeth with pocketing 4–6 mm. Pocketing over 6 mm deep was found in only one in 12 people, and then only around one or two teeth. The need for extraction was found in only 4%, while less than 20% of all missing teeth were listed as missing due to periodontal disease.

Baelum et al (1988a) carried out a cross-sectional study of plaque, calculus, gingivitis, periodontitis and tooth loss in a sample of adult Tanzanians aged 30–69 years and reported a tooth site frequency of plaque of >90%, calculus of 50–65%, gingival bleeding of 30–40%, pockets deeper than 3 mm of <10%, attachment loss of ≥4 mm of <35% and attachment loss >6 mm of <10%. None of the subjects were edentulous and very few had experienced any major loss of teeth. It was also shown that 75% of the tooth sites with attachment loss of ≥7 mm were found in 31% of subjects. Thus, in this population, attachment loss was found at a small number of tooth sites and was often associated with gingival recession rather than pocking. Furthermore, it was shown that a small subset of the population studied was responsible for most of the attachment loss found.

The same group (Baelum et al 1988b) also reported a similar study on 1131 Kenyan subjects aged 15–65 years, which confirmed their previous findings. Poor oral hygiene in the subject group was reflected by high plaque, calculus and gingivitis scores. However, significant attachment loss showed a skewed distribution and was found in only a small proportion of individuals. Furthermore, in these individuals, significant attachment loss was found at <20% of their tooth sites. This suggests that in these subjects, destructive periodontal disease was not an inevitable consequence of gingivitis but rather a feature of individual differences in susceptibility. Similar findings were also reported by Lembariti (1983).

Yoneyama et al (1988) described probing depth, probing attachment level and recession data from 319 randomly selected Japanese adults aged 20–79 years. The percentage of sites with deep pockets (≥6 mm) was small, ranging from 0.2% at the age of 30–39 years to 1.2% at the age of 70–79 years. However, the percentage of sites with advanced attachment loss (≥5 mm) ranged from 1% in the younger group to 12.4% in the older group and this discrepancy was attributed to gingival recession. They also found that relatively small groups of individuals accounted for substantial amounts of the observable attachment loss but the number of these individuals increased with age and was markedly increased after the age of 60. Therefore, destructive periodontitis was much more prevalent and widespread in older subjects. Furthermore, this study showed a similar pattern of destructive periodontitis to that found in Tanzania and Kenya by Baelum et al (1988a,b).

Lai et al (2007) estimated the prevalence and severity of periodontal disease (PD) in a Taiwanese population aged 35–44 years and also investigated the association between demographic factors and chronic periodontitis (CP).

Between 2003 and 2005, residents of Keelung of the appropriate age were invited to screening. Of 8462 enrollees, 94.8% had some signs of CP, of whom 29.7% had periodontal pockets >3 mm and 35% LA >3 mm. Calculus was the most common problem in terms of both prevalence (49.6%) and severity (affecting an average of 3.0 sextants per person). Risk factors for poor periodontal status were older age, male gender, low education level and being a manual worker. The prevalence of CP in 35–44-year-olds was found to be high in this large community-based study of screening. Poorer periodontal health was observed in males, the less educated and manual workers.

The results of the 1985–86 National Survey of Oral Health in the United States was published by Brown et al (1990). The sample included 15 132 employed males and females aged 18–64 years who were examined with respect to gingivitis, gingival recession and probing pocket depths at the mesial and buccal sites of all teeth in two randomly selected quadrants, one upper and one lower. The findings revealed that destructive periodontitis was very uncommon in the sample. Gingivitis was found in 44% of subjects and occurred at an average of 2.7 sites per subject and <6% of the sites examined. Its frequency decreased slightly with age. Periodontal pockets of 4–6 mm were found at 1.3% of the sites assessed, occurring in an average of 13.4% of the subjects ranging from 6% (18–24 years) to 18% (55–64 years). Pockets ≥7 mm were only found at 0.03% of all sites, were observed in only 0.6% of all subjects and were most frequent in subjects of 55–64 years (1.1%). Gingival recession of ≥3 mm occurred in 17% of subjects (range 3–46%) and when it occurred it was not extensive, affecting an average of between one and two sites per subject.

Much higher prevalence figures were reported by another study performed in the USA (Horning et al 1990) which employed full mouth circumferential probing in a sample of 1984 males and females, aged 13–84 years, at a military dental clinic. The prevalence of subjects with at least one 4 mm deep pocket was 63% and with at least one ≥7 mm deep pocket was 17%. Part of the discrepancy between the two US surveys may be because of population differences and the fact that a dental clinic population is more selective for subjects with disease than a random population sample. It could also have been affected by the use of partial recording methods by Brown et al (1990), which may have underestimated the true prevalence.

Röthlisberger et al (2007) compared the periodontal conditions of Swiss Army recruits in 2006 with those of previous surveys in 1996 and 1985.

A total of 626 Swiss Army recruits were examined for their periodontal conditions, caries prevalence, stomatological and functional aspects of the masticatory system and halitosis. A total of 2% of all teeth bled on probing. The mean PPD was 2.16 mm. Only 3.8% of the recruits showed at least one site of PPD of ≥5 mm, and 1.4% yielded more than one site with PPD of ≥5 mm. A significant improvement of the periodontal conditions of young Swiss males was demonstrated to have taken place between 1985 and 1996, but no further changes during the last decade were noticed in periodontal health among 35-year-olds in Oslo, 1973–2003.

Skudutyte-Rysstad et al (2007) investigated trends in periodontal health and oral hygiene using data available from four epidemiological studies on 35-year-olds in Oslo performed from 1973 to 2003. Periodontal status of randomly selected 35-year-olds was assessed clinically and radiographically. The proportion of persons with CPITN score 4 decreased from 21% in 1984 to 8.1% in 2003. In addition, the mean number of sextants with deep pockets per person was considerably lower in 2003 than previously. The proportion of persons without recorded bone loss increased from 46% in 1973 to 76% in 2003. An improvement in oral hygiene scores was also observed during this period. These results suggest that periodontal health and oral hygiene have been improving among 35-year-olds in Oslo during the last 30 years.

Figures from the WHO Global Oral Dental Bank based on CPITN data from over 50 countries have been published (Miyazaki et al 1991b). They have been carried in the age groups 35–44 and 45–74 years (**Fig. 10.3**). They found that calculus and shallow pocketing were the most frequently observed conditions and with a few exceptions, the percentages of persons (5–20%) and the mean number of sextants per person with deep pockets were small to very small with a tendency to increase with age. The assumed differences between industrialized and non-industrialized countries with regard to the prevalence and severity of periodontal diseases were not reflected in the survey data examined. Marked differences between two groups of countries were only seen for the estimated national levels of edentulousness, which was very low for the non-industrialized countries (perhaps a reflection of a smaller dentist:population ratio?).

From these data it appears that the progression of periodontal disease with age is not shown by an increase in CPITN scores but by an increasing number of missing teeth, which could be the result of factors other than periodontal disease. In the age group 65–74 years, this results, on average, in almost half of all sextants being excluded. Of the remaining sextants, approximately half had both shallow and deep pockets.

All studies show that poor oral hygiene is an important factor affecting both the prevalence and severity of gingivitis which may progress to periodontitis. Other factors already discussed in relation to gingivitis have, as one would expect, a similar relationship to chronic periodontitis.

Socioeconomic factors, in particular educational level and economic status, bear a significant relationship to prevalence and severity. This could well explain some observed ethnic differences but others are probably due to genetic variation. If one compares equal age groups in Asian and European populations (Löe et al 1978) the transition from gingivitis

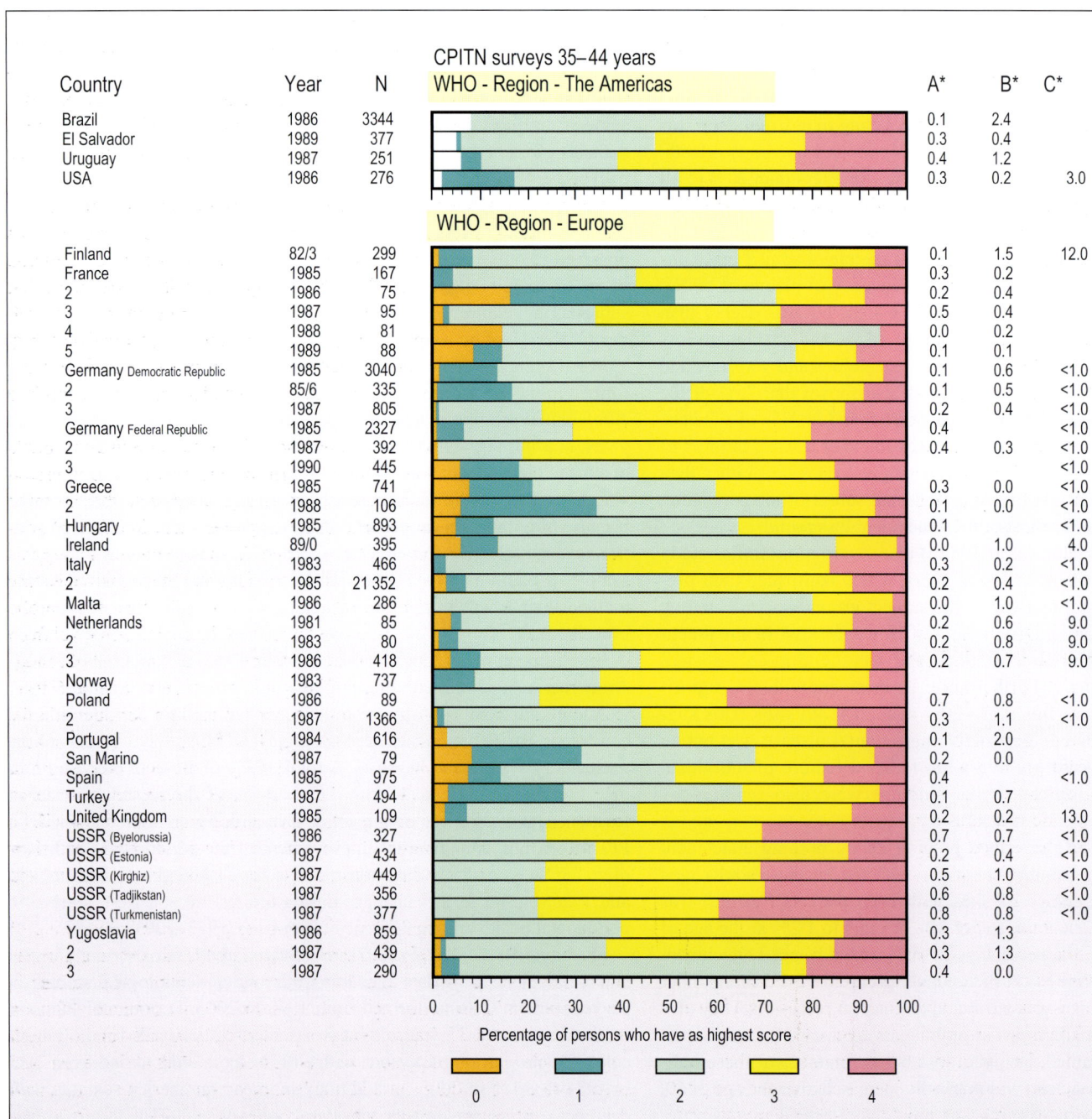

Fig. 10.3 The observed periodontal conditions measured by CPITN in America and Europe at age 35–44 years, from WHO Global Data Bank, 1 August 1990. Column A*: mean number of sextants with CPITN score 4 = pockets = 6 mm; Column B*: number of sextants with CPITN score X = sextants excluded, less than two teeth; Column C*: percentage edentulous (From Miyazaki et al 1991b. © Butterworth-Heinemann for Fédération Dentaire Internationale).

to periodontitis appears to be earlier and the severity of destruction greater in the Asian group than in the European group. Both oral hygiene habits and nutritional status were better in the latter group, and this probably reflected educational and income levels. If one compares different ethnic groups with equivalent income and educational levels the disease profile is very similar.

The onset of periodontal destruction, when it occurs, appears to take place most commonly in the young adult, and then both prevalence and severity may increase with age becoming clinically significant in the fourth decade of life. However, for the large majority of most of the observed populations the progress of periodontal diseases seems to be compatible with the retention of the natural dentition into older age.

Recent epidemiological studies seem to indicate that progression from gingivitis to periodontitis seems to take place in a much smaller proportion of individuals than was previously believed (Papapanou 1994). Unfortunately, we cannot yet predict which individual will progress from gingivitis to periodontitis and much current research is directed towards trying to define the person who is 'at risk'. A great deal of epidemiological and clinical research in the past decade has also highlighted considerable variation in clinical features and rates of disease progression of chronic periodontitis (Papapanou 1994).

Trends in periodontal diseases in the USA have been documented for years. However, the results have been mixed, mostly due to different periodontal assessment protocols. In this connection, Borrell et al (2005) examined the change in the prevalence of periodontitis between the NHANES III and the NHANES 1999–2000, and differences in the prevalence of periodontitis among racial/ethnic groups in the USA. Analysis was limited to non-Hispanic black, non-Hispanic white, and Mexican-American adults aged 18+ years in the NHANES III ($n = 12\,088$) or the NHANES 1999–2000 ($n = 3214$). The prevalences of periodontitis for the NHANES III and the NHANES 1999–2000 were 7.3% and 4.2%, respectively. In multivariable analyses, Blacks were 1.88 times (95% CI: 1.42, 2.50) more likely to have periodontitis than whites surveyed in the NHANES III. However, the odds of periodontitis for blacks and Mexican-Americans did not differ from those for Whites surveyed in the NHANES 1999–2000. Their findings indicated that the prevalence of periodontitis has decreased between the NHANES III and the NHANES 1999–2000 for all racial/ethnic groups in the USA.

NATURAL HISTORY OF PERIODONTAL DISEASE AS SHOWN BY LONGITUDINAL STUDIES OF DISEASE PROGRESSION

An accurate assessment of the natural history of any disease requires extensive knowledge of its aetiology and pathology, the population's attitudes towards the disease, the availability of a healthcare system and the effect of preventive and therapeutic measures and this is a complicated matter. Furthermore the study of the natural history and progression of chronic periodontitis requires a longitudinal study over many years. The studies suitable for this purpose are longitudinal studies of periodontal disease progression in which the periodontal conditions of subjects exposed to little or no therapeutic intervention are monitored for relatively long periods.

Lindhe et al (1983) studied the progression of periodontal disease in the absence of treatment in two subject groups consisting of 64 Swedish and 36 American subjects. The Swedish group included subjects with moderate periodontal attachment loss at entry and was monitored for attachment level changes at baseline, 3 months and 6 years. The American group consisted of subjects with advanced periodontitis at entry and was monitored at baseline and 1 year. Out of 4101 tooth sites examined at baseline and 3 years in the Swedish group, only 158 sites (3.9%) showed attachment loss of >2 mm. Out of 4097 sites examined at baseline and 6 years,

523 sites (11.6%) showed progressive attachment loss of the same magnitude. Approximately half the sites that showed no measurable change in the first 3-year period showed loss in the second 3-year period, while two-thirds of the sites with disease progression between baseline and the 3-year examination were stable during the second monitoring period.

In the US group, 102 out of 3210 sites (3.2%) showed attachment loss of 2 mm or more during 1 year of monitoring. When the association between initial and progressive attachment loss was examined by linear regression analysis, the hypothesis that sites with advanced attachment loss were more prone to exhibit disease progression than sites with less initial loss could not be supported.

Based on the results of this and other studies, the same research group challenged the concept of slow, continuous progressive attachment loss until treatment or tooth loss and suggested instead that periodontal disease progressed in recurrent acute episodes (Socransky et al 1984). They further suggested that these bursts of activity occurred in short periods of time at individual sites and were followed by relatively long periods of remission. Once a burst has occurred, certain sites may show no further activity while others may experience several additional bursts at later time periods. It was also suggested (Haffajee & Socransky 1986) that the random nature of the burst hypothesis should not be interpreted to suggest that episodes of disease activity may occur irrespective of microbiological, anatomical, clinical or other conditions of the particular site but rather as random bursts with respect of time.

The possible three models of periodontal progression (see also Chs 8 and 15), namely constant slow progression, instantaneous increments of progression (random burst) and variable non-instantaneous progression (asynchronous multiple burst) have been mathematically modelled so that longitudinal data can be loaded in to a computer program to see which model it best fits (Sterne et al 1992). Using available longitudinal data they found a better fit for the burst models over the continuous model but were unable to distinguish between the random burst and asynchronous multiple burst models.

However, it is apparent that the ability to reliably measure small amounts of attachment loss, such as would occur in the constant slow progression model, is not possible at present so that it is quite possible that all three types of progression may occur in different patients and in different situations in the same patient (see Ch. 8). There is some evidence to support this concept with the development of electronic probes which will measure probing attachment level more reliably and accurately. One such probe (Jeffcoat et al 1991), which detects and measures the attachment level from the cemento-enamel junction has been claimed to have a threshold ranging from 0.3–0.8 mm (see Ch. 14). Using this probe, Jeffcoat et al (1991) monitored 30 patients with moderate–advanced chronic periodontitis for 6 months. Using a threshold of 0.4 mm, they found 29% of sites with attachment loss and using one of 2.4 mm, they found attachment loss at only 2% of sites. This indicated that using large thresholds, only rapid attachment loss, either random burst or asynchronous multiple burst will be detected, while using smaller thresholds will detect both rapid and slow constant attachment loss with a higher proportion of slow constant attachment loss sites.

One of the few longitudinal studies to investigate the initiation, rate of progression of periodontal disease and consequent tooth loss in a population never exposed to any dental treatment or preventive programmes is that carried out in Sri-Lanka by Löe et al (1986). They examined 480 male tea labourers in Sri Lanka, aged between 14 and 30, initially in 1970 with respect to plaque, calculus, gingivitis and attachment loss at the mesial and buccal aspects of all their teeth. Five subsequent examinations were carried out up to 1985 when the study was terminated. At this stage, 161 individuals from the initial examination remained. The subjects did not practise any conventional oral hygiene measures and had uniformly large aggregates of plaque and calculus and inflammation was present at virtually every gingival site. Based on the measured rates of attachment loss and tooth loss, three subgroups of subjects were identified namely individuals with rapid progression (RP) of periodontitis (8% of the sample), those with moderate progression (MP) (81% of the sample) and those with no progression (NP) (11% of sample). At 35 years of age, subjects in the RP group showed a mean attachment loss of 9 mm, the subjects in the MP group an average of 4 mm and subjects in the NP group less than 1 mm. At 45 years of age, there was a mean loss of 13 mm in the RP group in comparison to 7 mm in the MP group. The annual progression rate ranged between 0.1 and 1 mm; in the MP group between 0.05 and 0.5 mm and in the NP group between 0.04 and 0.09 mm. Since these subjects were entirely caries-free, all missing teeth were lost due to periodontal disease. There was an average loss of 12 teeth at age 35 and 20 teeth at age 40 in the RP group, while in the MP group only an average of seven teeth were lost at age 45. The NP group showed no tooth loss.

In a later publication (Löe et al 1992) this data was re-analysed in respect of gingival recession and it was reported that more than 30% of the subjects exhibited gingival recession before the age of 20 years, while in ages over 40 years gingival recession was present in 100% of subjects, affecting 70% or more of the buccal surfaces, 50% or more of the lingual surfaces and 40% of the interproximal surfaces.

The overall rates of progression in this study are higher than those found in populations practising oral hygiene due to the much higher levels of plaque and calculus. However, the study also clearly shows different levels of susceptibility in this population which are very similar in percentage terms to those found in other population groups. It also shows that gingival recession is a major reflector of attachment loss in these subjects. It is important to realize that gingival recession as a reflector of attachment loss will not show up in some methods of data collection, such as the CPITN and this could severely limit its usefulness.

Papapanou et al (1989) reported on the progression of periodontitis assessed radiographically over 10 years in a group of 201 Swedish subjects aged 25–70 years. Tooth loss expressed as a percentage of the number of teeth present at the initial examination, varied between 3% and 28% and was highest in the subjects initially over 50 years old. The mean annual bone loss varied between 0.07 and 0.14 mm in ages between 25 and 65 years but was twice as high (0.28 mm) in individuals of 75 years at the completion of the study. A mean bone loss of ≥0.5 mm was found in 75% of the subjects, while 7% showed a loss of ≥3 mm. The same pattern was found on a tooth site level, with the majority of the sites showing small degrees of bone loss, but with relatively few sites showing greater magnitudes of bone loss. In this regard, about 15% of patients accounted for half of the observed sites with advanced bone loss (≥6 mm). While the subjects most affected by bone loss at entry were the ones most prone to develop further disease progression, the same trend could not be found at the tooth site level.

Ismail et al (1990) reported from a longitudinal study carried out between 1959 and 1987 in Michigan, USA. Out of an initial sample of 526 subjects who participated in the baseline examination, 167 dentate subjects remained at the completion of the study. Over the 28-year period 11% of the teeth initially present in these subjects were lost. A total of 22 subjects (13%) showed an average attachment loss of ≥2 mm, five subjects (3%) of ≥3 mm and two subjects (1.2%) of ≥4 mm.

A recent study (Griffiths et al 2001) of the progression of chronic periodontitis in young adults examined 100 male subjects, 16–20 years old, over 3 years. They measured amounts of attachment loss from the cemento-enamel junction at baseline and 1 and 3 years. Loss of 2 mm of attachment over this period was seen in about 10% of subjects and that of 3 mm in less than 1%. This data suggests that the onset and progression of chronic periodontitis can be measured in young adults. However, in this study, true progression above the threshold was only seen in less than 1% of these subjects. In this small subgroup gingival bleeding and subgingival calculus were also statistically associated with attachment loss.

Thus, all the longitudinal studies reported appear to show that there is a small subgroup of patients who have high susceptibility to periodontitis and a small subgroup of patients who are resistant to this condition and this holds true irrespective of plaque levels.

It has also been shown that professional plaque control programmes (see also Ch. 11) can significantly reduce the amount of tooth loss due to chronic periodontitis and have been also shown to be effective over 30 years (Axelsson et al 2004, 2006).

Furthermore, it has been shown in a 10-year and a 30-year prospective study in Sweden (Paulander et al 2004; Gabre et al 2006) that tooth loss was more common in the molar than in the anterior tooth regions, while periodontal bone loss had a random distribution in the dentition. It also showed that prevalence of dental caries had decreased in recent years (Gabre et al 2006). The predominant risk factors identified with regard to further radiographic bone loss were 'probing pocket depth of 6 mm' and 'smoking'.

SUMMARY

Worldwide epidemiological studies have shown that gingival inflammation is present in most populations, but that the more severe stages of periodontal disease, while not as prevalent as previously believed, are still of significant magnitude, affecting up to 15–20% of most populations over the age of 35. Although gingivitis is very common, it does not inevitably progress to periodontitis. Oral hygiene and therefore periodontal health in the majority of people is improving in industrialized countries.

REFERENCES

Addy M, Dummer PMH, Griffiths G, et al: Prevalence of plaque, gingivitis and caries in 11–12-year-old children in South Wales, *Community Dent Oral Epidemiol* 14:115–118, 1986.

Ainamo J: Assessment of periodontal treatment needs. Adaptation of the WHO Community Periodontal Index of Treatment Needs (CPITN) to European conditions. In Frandsen A, editor: *Public Health Aspects of Periodontal Disease in Europe*, Berlin, 1983, Quintessence Verlag.

Axelsson P: The effect of a needs-related caries preventive program in children and young adults – results after 20 years, *BMC Oral Health* 6:S7, 2006.

Axelsson P, Nystrom B, Lindhe J: The long-term effect of a plaque control program on tooth mortality, caries and periodontal disease in adults. Results after 30 years of maintenance, *J Clin Periodontol* 31:749–757, 2004.

Baelum V, Fejerskov O, Karring T: Oral hygiene, gingivitis and periodontal breakdown in adult Tanzanians, *J Periodontal Res* 21:221–232, 1988a.

Baelum V, Fejerskov O, Manji F: Periodontal diseases in adult Kenyans, *J Clin Periodontol* 15:445–452, 1988b.

Barnett M, Ciancio SG, Mather ML: The modified papillary bleeding index during the resolution of gingivitis, *J Prev Dent* 6:135–138, 1980.

Belting CM, Massler M, Schour I: Prevalence and incidence of alveolar bone disease in men, *J Am Dent Assoc* 17:190–197, 1953.

Borrell LN, Burt BA, Taylor GW: Prevalence and trends in periodontitis in the USA: from the NHANES III to the NHANES, 1988 to 2000, *J Dent Res* 84:924–930, 2005.

Bossert WA, Marks HH: Prevalence and characteristics of periodontal disease in 12,800 persons under periodic dental observation, *J Am Dent Assoc* 53:429–442, 1956.

Brown LJ, Oliver RC, Löe H: Periodontal diseases in the US in 1981: prevalence, severity, extent and role in tooth mortality, *J Periodontol* 60:363–380, 1989.

Brown LJ, Oliver RC, Löe H: Evaluating periodontal status of US employed adults, *J Am Dent Assoc* 121:226–232, 1990.

Carlos JP, Wolfe MD, Kingman A: The extent and severity index: a simple method for use in epidemiological studies of periodontal disease, *J Clin Periodontol* 13:500–505, 1986.

Cogen RB, Wright T, Tate AL: Destructive periodontal disease in healthy children, *J Periodontol* 63:761–765, 1992.

Costa FO, Cota LOM, Costa JE, et al: Periodontal disease progression among young subjects with no preventive dental care: a 52-month follow-up study, *J Periodontol* 78:198–203, 2007.

Cuttress TW, Hunter PBV, Hoskins DIH: *Adult oral health in New Zealand 1976–1982*. Wellington N Z, 1983, Dental Research Unit, Medical Research Council of New Zealand.

Cuttress TW, Hunter PBV, Hoskins DIH: Comparison of the Periodontal Index (PI) and Community Periodontal Index of Treatment Needs (CPITN), *Community Dent Oral Epidemiol* 14:39–42, 1986.

de Araujo WC, MacDonald JB: Gingival crevice microbiota of pre-school children, *Arch Oral Biol* 9:227–228, 1964.

Douglass C, Gillings D, Solecito W, et al: The potential for increase in the periodontal needs of the aged population, *J Periodontol* 54:721–730, 1983.

Gabre P, Berring E, Gahnberg L: A 20-year study of dentists' and dental hygienists' assessment of dental caries lesions in bite-wing radiographs, *Swed Dent J* 30:35–42, 2006.

Greene JC, Vermillion JR: The oral hygiene index. A method for classifying oral hygiene status, *J Am Dent Assoc* 61:172–179, 1960.

Griffiths GS, Duffy KA, Eaton KA, et al: Prevalence and extent of lifetime cumulative attachment loss (LCAL) at different thresholds and association with clinical variables: changes in a population of young male military recruits over 3 years, *J Clin Periodontol* 28:961–969, 2001.

Gupta OP: Epidemiological studies of dental disease in the state of Kerala. I, Prevalence and severity of periodontal disease, *J All India Dent Assoc* 34:45–50, 1962.

Haffajee AD, Socransky SS: Attachment level changes in destructive periodontal diseases, *J Clin Periodontol* 13:461–472, 1986.

Horning GM, Hatch CL, Lutskus J: The prevalence of periodontitis in a military treatment population, *J Am Dent Assoc* 121:616–622, 1990.

Hugoson A, Jordon T: Frequency distribution of individuals aged 20–70 years according to severity of periodontal disease, *Community Dent Oral Epidemiol* 10:187–192, 1982.

Hugoson A, Koch G, Gothberg C, et al: Oral health of individuals aged 3–80 years in Jonkoping, Sweden during 30 years (1973–2003). I, Review of findings on dental care habits and knowledge of oral health, *Swed Dent J* 29:125–138, 2005a.

Hugoson A, Koch G, Gothberg C, et al: Oral heath of individuals aged 3–80 years in Jonkoping, Sweden during 30 years (1973–2003) II. Review of clinical and radiographic findings, *Swed Dent J* 29:139–155, 2005b.

Hugoson A, Laurell L, Lundgren D: Frequency distribution of individuals aged 20–70 years according to severity of periodontal disease experience in 1973 and 1983, *J Clin Periodontol* 19:227–232, 1992.

Hugoson A, Norderyd O, Slotte C, et al: Distribution of periodontal disease in a Swedish adult population 1973:1983 and 1993, *J Clin Periodontol* 25:542–548, 1998.

Ismail AI, Morrison EC, Burt BA, et al: Natural history of periodontal disease in adults: findings from the Tecumseh periodontal disease study, 1959–1987, *J Dent Res* 69:430–435, 1990.

Jansson L, Lavstedt S, Zimmerman M: Marginal bone loss and tooth loss in a sample from the County of Stockholm – a longitudinal study over 20-years, *Swed Dent J* 26:21–29, 2002.

Jeffcoat MK, Reddy MS: Progression of probing attachment loss in adult periodontitis, *J Periodontol* 62:185–189, 1991.

Johnson ES, Kelly JE, Van Kirk LE: *Selected dental findings in adults by age, race and sex. United States 1960–1962*, U S, Department of Health Education and Welfare, National Center for Health Statistics. Series 11, No. 7:1, 1965.

Lai H, Lo M-T, Wang P-E, et al: A community-based epidemiological study of periodontal disease in Keelung, Taiwan: a model from Keelung community-based integrated screening programme (KCIS No. 18), *J Clin Periodontol* 34:851–859, 2007.

Lang NP, Alder R, Joss A, et al: Absence of bleeding on probing. An indicator of periodontal stability, *J Clin Periodontol* 17:714–721, 1990.

Lembariti BS: *Periodontal Diseases in Urban and Rural Populations in Tanzania*, Tanzania, 1983, Dar es Salaam University Press.

Lindhe J, Haffajee AD, Socransky SS: Progression of periodontal disease in adult subjects in the absence of periodontal therapy, *J Clin Periodontol* 10:433–442, 1983.

Littleton NW: Caries and periodontal disease among Ethiopian civilians, *Dent Abstr* 8:763–764, 1963.

Löe H: The gingival index, the plaque index and the retention index systems, *J Periodontol* 38:610–616, 1967.

Löe H, Anerud A, Boysen H: The natural history of periodontal disease in man: prevalence, severity and extent of gingival recession, *J Periodontol* 63:489–495, 1992.

Löe H, Anerud A, Boysen H, et al: The natural history of periodontal disease in man. Rapid, moderate and no loss of attachment in Sri Lankan labourers 14 to 46 years of age, *J Clin Periodontol* 13:431–440, 1986.

Löe H, Anerud A, Boysen H, et al: The natural history of periodontal disease in man. The rate of periodontal destruction before 40 years of age, *J Periodontol* 49:607–620, 1978.

Löe H, Silness J: Periodontal disease in pregnancy. I Prevalence and severity, *Acta Odontol Scand* 21:532–551, 1963.

Marshall-Day CD, Stephens RG, Quigley LF: Periodontal disease: prevalence and incidence, *J Periodontol* 26:185–191, 1955.

Miyazaki H, Pilot T, Leclercq MH, et al: Profiles of periodontal conditions in adolescents measured by CPITN, *Int Dent J* 41:67–73, 1991a.

Miyazaki H, Pilot T, Leclercq, et al: Profiles of periodontal conditions in adults measured by CPITN, *Int Dent J* 41:74–80, 1991b.

Nevins M, Becker W, Korman K: *Proceedings of the World Workshop in Clinical Periodontics*, Princeton, NJ, 1989, American Academy of Periodontology, pp 1–24.

Papapanou PN: Epidemiology and natural history of periodontal disease. In Lang NP, Karring T, editors: *Proceedings of the 1st European Workshop on Periodontology*, London, 1994, Quintessence Publishing, pp 23–41.

Papapanou PN, Wennström JL, Gröndahl K: A 10-year retrospective study of periodontal disease progression, *J Clin Periodontol* 16:403–411, 1989.

Papapanou PN, Wennström JL, Johnsson T: Extent and severity index based on assessments of radiographic bone loss, *Community Dent Oral Epidemiol* 19:313–317, 1991a.

Papapanou PN, Wennström JL, Johnsson T: Evaluation of a radiographic partial recording system assessing the extent and severity of periodontal destruction, *Community Dent Oral Epidemiol* 19:318–320, 1991b.

Paulander J, Axelsson P, Lindhe J, et al: Intra-oral pattern of tooth and periodontal bone loss between the age of 50 and 60 years. A longitudinal prospective study, *Acta Odontol Scand* 62:214–222, 2004.

Pilot T: Implications of the high risk strategy and of improved diagnostic methods for health screening and public health planning in periodontal diseases. In Johnson NW, editor: *Risk Makers for Oral Diseases, Vol. 3. Periodontal Diseases*, Cambridge, 1992, Cambridge University Press, pp 441–453.

Poulsen S, Moller IJ: The prevalence of dental caries, plaque and gingivitis in 3-year-old Danish children, *Scand J Dent Res* 80:94–103, 1972.

Ramfjord SP: Indices for prevalence and incidence of periodontal disease, *J Periodontol* 30:51–59, 1959.

Ramfjord SP, Emslie RD, Greene JC, et al: Epidemiological studies of periodontal diseases, *Am J Public Health* 58:1713–1722, 1968.

Röthlisberger B, Kuonen P, Salvi GE, et al: Periodontal conditions in Swiss army recruits: a comparative study between the years 1985, 1996 and 2006, *J Clin Periodontol* 34:860–866, 2007.

Russell AL: A system of classification and scoring for prevalence surveys of periodontal disease, *J Dent Res* 35:350–359, 1956.

Russell AL: Some epidemiological characteristics in a series of urban populations, *J Periodontol* 28:286–293, 1957.

Sandler HC, Stahl SS: The influence of generalized diseases on clinical manifestation of periodontal disease, *J Am Dent Assoc* 49:656–667, 1954.

Schour I, Massler M: Prevalence of gingivitis in young adults, *J Dent Res* 27:733–738, 1948.

Shei O, Waerhaug J, Lövidal A, et al: Alveolar bone loss as related to oral hygiene and age, *J Periodontol* 30:7–16, 1959.

Sheiham A: *Public Health Approaches to the Promotion of Periodontal Health*. In: Joint Department of Community Dental Health and Dental Practice, Monograph Series No. 3, London, 1990, University College, pp 2.

Sheiham A, Hobdell MH: Decayed, missing and filled teeth in a British adult population, *Br Dent J* 126:401–404, 1969.

Sherp HW: Current concepts in periodontal disease research: epidemiological contributions, *J Am Dent Assoc* 68:667–675, 1964.

Silness J, Löe H: Periodontal disease in pregnancy. II. Correlation between oral hygiene and periodontal condition, *Acta Odontol Scand* 22:121–135, 1964.

Skudutyte-Rysstad R, Eriksen HM, Hansen BF: Trends in periodontal health among 35-year-olds in Oslo, 1973–2003, *J Clin Periodontol* 34:867–872, 2007.

Socransky SS, Haffajee AD, Goodson JM, et al: New concepts of destructive periodontal disease, *J Clin Periodontol* 11:21–32, 1984.

Spencer AJ, Beighton D, Higgins TJ: Periodontal disease in five and six-year-old children, *J Periodontol* 54:19–22, 1983.

Sterne JAC, Kingman A, Löe H: Assessing the nature of periodontal disease progression – an application of covariance structure estimation, *Applied Statistics* 41:539–552, 1992.

Sutcliffe P: A longitudinal study of gingivitis and puberty, *J Periodontal Res* 7:52–58, 1972.

Taco P, Lewis DP: *Guidelines for Community Periodontal Care*, London, 1992, FDI World Dental Press.

WHO: *Epidemiology, Etiology and Prevention of Periodontal Diseases*, Technical Report Series No. 621. Geneva, 1978, World Health Organization.

Yoneyama T, Okamoto H, Lindhe J, et al: Probing depth, attachment loss and gingival recession. Findings from a clinical examination in Urhiku, Japan, *J Clin Periodontol* 15:581–591, 1988.

The essential requirement for the prevention of a disease is an understanding of its cause. Chapter 4 describes the cause of chronic periodontal disease but the prevalence of the disease bears sad witness to our inability to apply that knowledge to the full. Many factors, social and economic, are beyond the influence of the dental profession but the profession has certain undeniable obligations. These are: to educate the patient in good oral hygiene habits; to attempt to motivate the patient to apply advice given; to provide a regular service for professional cleaning; to apply fluoride to young teeth and if disease occurs, to practise sound dentistry which does not lead to further disease.

These ideas are also discussed in the treatment of chronic gingivitis (see Ch. 15), but patients without disease represent a different starting point from the patient with established disease. Both the patient and the practitioner are faced with a slightly different psychological situation and unfortunately, it is one which few dentists by training or experience are properly equipped to deal with. Conversion to the philosophy of prevention involves nothing less than a revolutionary reorientation of thoughts and attitudes of every dentist.

Patient education and motivation cannot be a once and for all process but must involve a continuing commitment to the patient. Such a commitment can be fulfilled only when dental personnel are organized to that end (Sims 1968). A preventive service can be provided in a general dental practice which is largely devoted to treatment, but it is possible that better results are obtained when both therapist and patient are freed from the constraints of the conventional dental surgery situation. In a therapeutic situation, the patient adopts a passive attitude in the face of professional authority. In providing a preventive service, the patient's active participation is essential; indeed, even the word 'patient' seems inappropriate in this situation – perhaps 'pupil' would be better.

In situations where the patient has to take responsibility for their own welfare, as in the control of diabetes or periodontal disease, the patient is accountable for both the success, and of great importance, the failure of what he or she does. In the latter case, people used to being passive and putting the burden on to the professional person, now have only themselves to blame.

At the same time, the professional person may find him or herself in an ambiguous situation. There is a conflict between the professional as expert and authority, which reflects the traditional patient–professional relationship, and the professional person as teacher and counsellor. In the preventive situation, the professional sets out to help the patient help himself, and he or she needs to recognize from the outset that the professional is separated from the patient in a number of respects – the most important of which are knowledge, values and language.

Many professional people, not just doctors and dentists but lawyers, accountants, etc. seem to overlook the fact that they possess specialist knowledge, particular attitudes to the problems of their patients or clients, and an exclusive vocabulary that they have learned and now take for granted. These factors create a gap which must be bridged by the professional person so that a creative dialogue can be pursued. The values and attitudes of the dentist do not necessarily coincide with those of the patient; the latter wants to eat in comfort and look nice, while the dentist wants a plaque score of zero and a balanced occlusion. These different levels of aspiration need to be approximated, and two factors become essential. The first is the provision of information in language the patient can understand, and second, the generation of motivation, i.e. an explanation of the real advantages that will result from taking the professional advice, as well as the disadvantages of ignoring it.

Unfortunately, many dentists do not feel they can give the time to this, or are ill-equipped to deal with these challenges, and become impatient and even patronising. The problem can be solved by having someone in an ancillary capacity, the practice nurse or hygienist, who has the time, the training and the personal motivation to take on the responsibility of undertaking the preventive programme.

The provision of information and instruction in home care can take place inside or outside the dental surgery: it may be applied to an individual or a group; it can be carried out by an informed patient or schoolteacher as well as by dental personnel. Information can be given through a variety of media, films, slides, lectures and printed material. The one-to-one relationship between therapist and patient is likely to be the most effective system but where this is not possible, group instruction is better than no instruction at all. Ancillary personnel, in particular the dental hygienist, have an extremely valuable role to play in prevention. Hygienist training includes a much greater emphasis on prevention than does the conventional dental undergraduate course, and in the patient's mind, she is often associated with this aspect of dentistry.

Certain groups are more receptive to information and instruction than others: adolescents with a developing awareness of self and interest in their general appearance and wellbeing; expectant and nursing mothers, and young couples whose sense of responsibility is sharpened by new parenthood. This is not to imply that the older person is beyond reach; the message that teeth can and should last for life is a powerful incentive for a mature person who has knowledge of the problems suffered by less fortunate members of his or her peer group.

Regular guidance and encouragement are essential and for the young patients, the application of topical fluorides can be included in their periodic check-ups. The long-term studies in Sweden by Axelsson and Lindhe (1974) provide overwhelming evidence of the benefits of an organized programme of regular professional care.

Prior to instituting a preventive programme, one must establish that disease is not already present. One cannot take it for granted in any individual that periodontal disease is not present; careful examination of every mouth is essential. Health is the starting point of a preventive programme, the aim of which is the maintenance of that state by the control of plaque deposition. By far the major part in plaque control must be played by the individual. The responsibilities of professional personnel are:

1. To provide information about dental health
2. To provide information and guidance about the techniques of plaque control
3. To attempt to change the individual's evaluation of dental health; in jargon terms, to motivate the patient.

PROVIDING INFORMATION

Providing a patient with the necessary information takes time and some insight into the limitations of the patient's understanding. It also requires the ability to express oneself in simple language. As stated, too often dentists do not have the time to provide patients with sufficient information, and sometimes patients do not appreciate the value of time spent in giving advice. Too frequently, adequate knowledge is taken for granted and when a description is provided, it is expressed in technical terms quite incomprehensible to the patient. It is useless to tell a patient that 'bacterial plaque in proximity to the dentogingival junction provokes gingival inflammation'.

The patient may not know what plaque or the dentogingival junction is, may not know that the mouth is full of bacteria or that gingiva means gum.

In addition, information provided in abstract may be only partly understood and quickly forgotten. Information needs to be given by demonstration in the patient's own mouth, and before any treatment is carried out. It is useful to give the patient a hand-mirror so that he or she can follow some of the examination; plaque and calculus are pointed out and the relationship to disease explained. At this time, it is demonstrated that the principal cause of disease, the bacterial plaque, is almost invisible but can be revealed by using a disclosing agent. This is a completely harmless dye, e.g. 4% Erythrosine, usually pink or blue, which is absorbed by the bacterial plaque (**Fig. 11.1**). To emphasize the harmful nature of the plaque a little of the stained deposit can be scraped off the tooth with a probe and shown to the patient with some remark about its bacterial content.

The patient is then given a toothbrush (if he has brought his own so much the better) and told to attempt to remove all the stained plaque. At this stage, no attempt should be made to instruct the patient in any particular brushing technique. The difficulties of the operation become apparent to the patient right away and he is thus more receptive to advice and instruction. Once the patient is aware of the problems in removing all the plaque he may be allowed to develop his own technique, but initially it is a good idea to demonstrate a formal technique as a basis for developing the necessary skill.

In starting treatment, it is very important to avoid confusing the patient with too much detail about toothbrushes and other oral hygiene aids, or to make the whole exercise seem too difficult or time consuming. Over-enthusiasm at this stage can be counterproductive but it must be made quite clear that the job of cleaning the mouth needs to be carried out methodically, section by section, and that frantic activity with the toothbrush is likely to do more harm to the gingiva than good.

MECHANICAL METHODS OF PLAQUE REMOVAL

TOOTHBRUSHING TECHNIQUES

A large number of toothbrushing techniques have been advised but the requirements of a satisfactory method of toothbrushing are few:

1. The technique should clean all tooth surfaces, in particular the area of the gingival crevice and the interdental region. A scrubbing technique will clean the tooth convexities well and yet leave plaque in more sheltered places.
2. The movement of the brush should not injure the soft or hard tissues. Vertical and horizontal scrubbing methods can produce gingival recession and tooth abrasion.
3. The technique should be simple and easy to learn. A technique which one person finds easy to use may be difficult for someone else; therefore each person needs individual guidance.
4. The method must be well organized so that each part of the dentition is brushed in turn and no area overlooked. The mouth can be divided into a number of sections depending on the size of the dental arch and the size of the toothbrush.

Toothbrushing techniques can be demonstrated both on a model and in the patient's mouth.

The Roll technique

The Roll technique (**Fig. 11.2A**) is a relatively gentle technique which was once popular. The side of the toothbrush is placed against the side of the tooth with the bristles pointing apically and parallel to the axis of the tooth; the back of the brush is at the level of the occlusal surface of the teeth. The brush is then rotated deliberately down in the upper jaw and up in the lower jaw so that bristles sweep across the gum and tooth. About 10 strokes are given to each section and the brush is moved in turn from one section to the

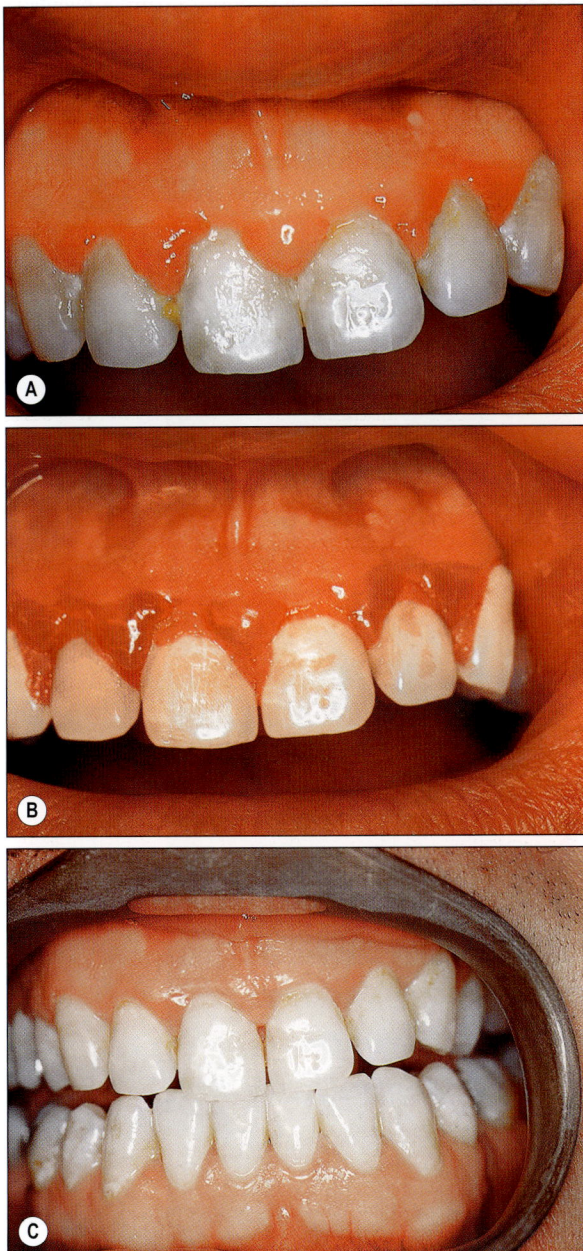

Fig. 11.1 Deposits of bacterial plaque (A) before and (B) after staining with a disclosing agent, which makes the plaque obvious to the patient. (C) Plaque free with resolution of gingivitis after oral hygiene instruction and scaling.

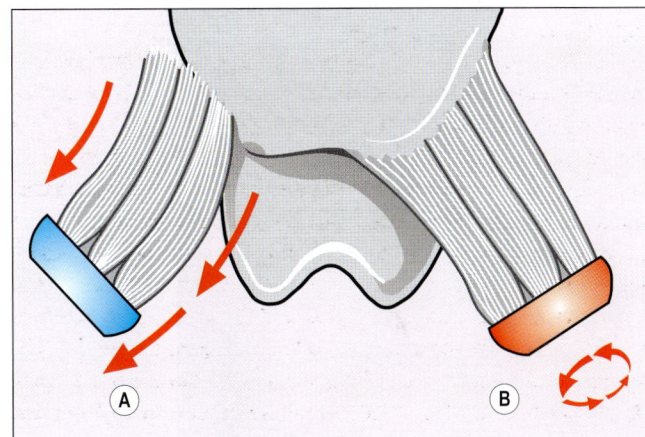

Fig. 11.2 Tooth brushing techniques: (A) The Roll technique. (B) The Bass technique.

next. If the arch in anterior segments is narrow, the brush can be used vertically. When all buccal and lingual surfaces have been brushed, the biting surfaces can be brushed with a rotary movement. This technique is no longer recommended for general use because it fails to clean the most important areas of the tooth, i.e. the junction of the tooth with the gingival margin and the gingival crevice and has been superseded by the Bass technique below.

The Bass technique

This brushing technique (**Fig. 11.2B**) aims to clean the gingival crevice and to this end the brush is held so that the bristles are about 45° to the axis of the teeth, the end of the bristle pointing into the gingival crevice (**Fig. 11.3**). The brush is pressed towards the gingiva and moved with a small circular motion so that the bristles go into the crevice and are also forced between the teeth. This may be uncomfortable if the tissues are inflamed and sensitive and thus will alert patients to this situation. It has been shown to be a most effective method for the removal of plaque, particularly from the gingival area of the tooth and gingival crevice. Therefore, it can be recommended as the method of choice for general use. It must be carried out with a suitable soft toothbrush, i.e. one with soft, flexible, rounded bristles in its brush head which can penetrate into the gingival crevice without causing trauma.

REQUIREMENTS OF A SATISFACTORY TOOTHBRUSH

There are now a large number of toothbrushes on the market of different sizes and shapes with bristles of various materials, textures, length and density. Overwhelmed by available choices, the man in the street is as likely to choose a brush that matches his bathroom tiles as one that he thinks will work well. Even a dentist may well be confused on this issue since a great many studies have been carried out on the specifications of a satisfactory toothbrush (Frandsen 1972) with contradictory results on almost every characteristic examined.

The bristles of toothbrushes are usually arranged in about 40 tufts in 3 or 4 rows (**Fig. 11.4**). Hard brushes should never be recommended as they can lacerate the gingiva, encourage gingival recession and cause tooth abrasion, particularly of exposed root surfaces. Furthermore, the bristle diameter of hard brushes is too large to penetrate into the gingival crevice. Soft toothbrushes should be recommended for all patients since they minimize gingival and tooth abrasion and maximize the efficiency of cleaning procedures particularly around the gingival margin and into the gingival crevice. Toothbrushes for children should be smaller and should relate to the mouth size at various ages. The bristles of children's toothbrushes should always be soft (0.1 mm–0.15 mm).

Certain basic requirements need to be met:

1. The brush head should be small enough to be manipulated effectively everywhere in the mouth, yet not be so small that it has to be used with extreme care in order to obtain complete coverage of the dentition. A length of about 2.5 cm is satisfactory for an adult; about 1.5 cm is suitable for a child.

2. The bristles should be of even length so that they function simultaneously. A convex or concave brush with bristles of different lengths will not clean a flat surface without undue pressure on some bristles. Short bristles will fail to reach interdental sites and may also be so rigid that they injure the tissues.

3. The texture should allow effective use without causing damage to either soft or hard tissues. Stiffness depends on the diameter and length of the filament and its elasticity. It also depends on whether the brush is used wet or dry, and on the temperature of the water. The bristles should be capable of penetrating into the gingival crevice without causing trauma.

4. The brush should be easy to keep clean. Densely packed tufts tend to retain debris and toothpaste at the base of the bristle. Modern synthetic fibre filaments are much more hygienic than natural bristle.

5. The toothbrush handle must rest comfortably and securely in the hand. It should be broad and thick enough to allow a firm grip and good control.

The main requirements of a satisfactory toothbrush are best summarized as:

- Good cleaning ability
- Minimal damage to soft and hard dental tissues
- Have a reasonable lifespan, i.e. have good wear characteristics
- Be hygienic
- Be non-toxic.

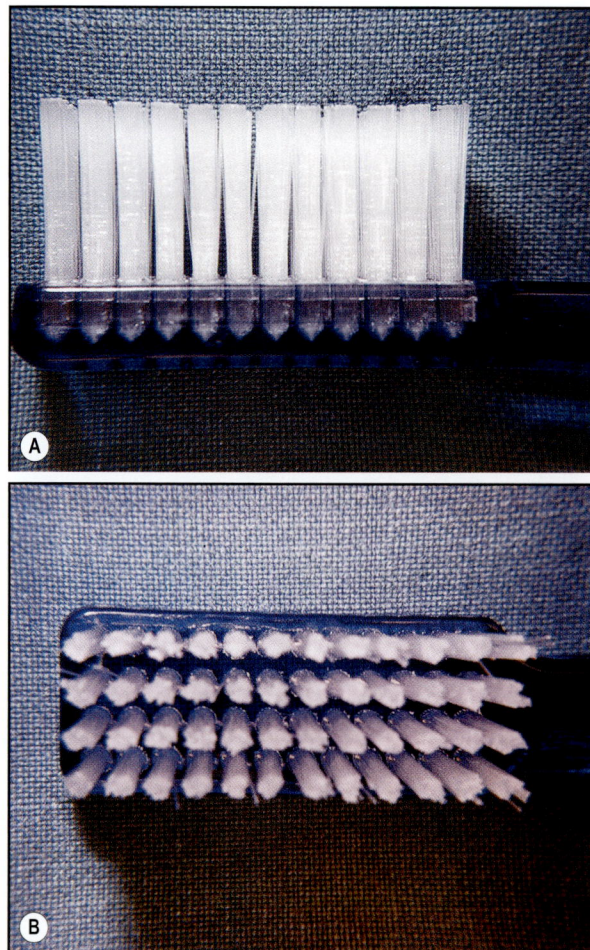

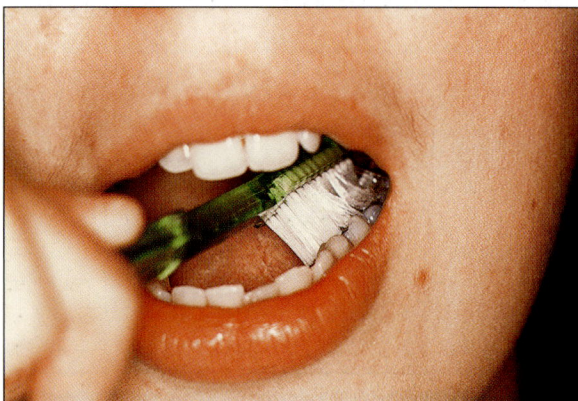

Fig. 11.3 A toothbrush positioned for lingual cleaning using the Bass technique.

Fig. 11.4 A toothbrush head viewed from (A) the side and (B) from above, showing its upper surface.

User performance is a huge variable and a balance must be achieved between this and the first three requirements. However, many of the factors involved in the brush head design can be defined reasonably precisely.

The handle

This is made of a variety of materials such as acrylic and polypropylene. Its flexibility, size and shape must be convenient for manual use in the mouth but details are more often a matter of styling rather than utility.

The toothbrush handle must rest comfortably and securely in the hand. It should be thick enough to allow a firm grip and good control. As the stiffness of the handle is one of the factors affecting the force applied to the teeth and gingiva during use, toothbrushes are now also made with flexible (stress breaking) handles (Ko et al 1995).

The brush head (Fig. 11.4)

The shape of the brush head may have a utility aspect but is often the result of styling. It should be small enough to be manipulated effectively everywhere in the mouth, yet not so small that it has to be used with extreme care to obtain complete coverage of the dentition. A length of about 2.5 cm is satisfactory for an adult; about 1.5 cm is suitable for a child.

The filaments (bristles)

Material

Today toothbrush bristles are either polyester or nylon. In 1938, DuPont created nylon and its first application was the toothbrush bristle, gradually replacing pig bristle. Initially, Nylon 66 (Exon) was used, but this was replaced first by Nylon 610 and then Nylon 612 (Tynex). Polyester and nylon are polymers with good chemical resistance and are inert so that they will pass through the body unchanged if swallowed. Nylon is said to wear less rapidly than polyester, and because of its antistatic properties, is more hygienic.

Diameter

The diameter of the filaments varies considerably from 0.064 mm to 1.524 mm but those used for toothbrushes fall into three categories:

1. Soft – 0.15–0.18 mm (0.006–0.007 in).
2. Medium – 0.18–0.23 mm (0.007–0.009 in).
3. Hard/extra hard – 0.23–0.28 mm (0.009–0.011 in).

Bristle stiffness also depends upon the length of the filament, its elasticity, whether the brush is used wet or dry, and the temperature of the water. In general, nylon loses 30% of stiffness when wet.

The bristles of children's brushes should always be soft (0.1–0.15 mm). Hard brushes should never be recommended as they can lacerate the gingiva, encourage gingival recession and cause tooth abrasion. Furthermore, the bristle diameter of hard bristles is too large to reach into the gingival crevice; soft brushes if used properly can clean effectively around the gingival margin and into the crevice, and minimize gingival and tooth abrasion.

Bristles should be of even length so that they function simultaneously. A convex or concave brush with bristles of different lengths will not clean a flat surface without undue pressure on some bristles. Short bristles will fail to reach into interdental sites and are also more rigid causing gingival and tooth abrasion. Bristles in a adult toothbrush are usually about 10–11 mm long (**Fig. 11.4A**).

End shape

To be as non-abrasive as possible, the end of the bristle should be round. It is essential that this applies to at least 90% of the bristles.

The tufts (Fig. 11.4)

The toothbrush bristle density is the number of bristles divided by the brush head area and there is some evidence that the greater this is, the better the plaque removing ability (Pretara-Spanedda et al 1989). However, forcing too many filaments into the tuft hole stresses the filaments against the tuft-hole wall so that the filaments curl over in the direction of the stress. On the other hand, too few bristles in the tuft-hole leaves them free to work loose. Many factors contribute to the balance between effectiveness, lack of tissue damage and wear and these are as follows:

Hole pattern in the brush head

Wisdom brushes lay the hole pattern from centre to centre at a minimum spacing of 2.3 mm lengthwise by 2.1 mm widthwise. Closer spacing than this tends to weaken the handle. The hole pattern is spread out in the brushes specifically designed for interdental penetration.

Tuft-hole diameter

This is usually about 1.6–1.7 mm but can be as high as 2.0 mm.

Number of tufts in the brush head

This varies greatly. Wisdom brushes use 42–45 and some larger American brushes use 60. These are arranged in 3–4 rows (**Fig. 11.4B**).

The density of the filaments in the tuft

This varies widely but 18–26 filaments per tuft appears to provide good wear performance. The brush should be easy to keep clean and densely packed tufts tend to retain debris and toothpaste at the base of the bristle.

Tuft length

This is usually about 10 mm (**Fig. 11.4A**). Wear performance deteriorates as tuft length increases.

Optimal packing factor

Optimal wear performance is controlled by putting the right number of filaments in the tuft hole to produce the correct packing factor. This is the ratio of the filament cross-section area minus the anchor wire area. The optimal packing factor is 0.63–0.74. The chosen dimensions of the diameters of the tuft-hole and the filament are not arrived at arbitrarily but need to produce this packing factor.

Anchor wire thickness

The anchor wire is the metal clip which holds the tuft of bristles in the tuft hole and this usually has a thickness of 0.20 0.35 mm.

Tuft knot retention

According to the BSI standard, this must exceed 17 Newtons. Many European manufacturers do not use a minimum standard.

Single strand filament retention: according to the BSI, this must exceed 1 Newton (N).

ELECTRIC TOOTHBRUSHES

The electric toothbrush is now a well-accepted part of the home care armamentarium. There are a number of designs available with different forms of movement: arcuating, vibrating and reciprocating.

There have been many studies comparing the effectiveness of the hand and automatic brush and the results indicate that the subject's control is more important than the appliance. These studies can be divided into two groups: those which have shown no added benefit of electric brushes over manual ones in respect of plaque levels and gingival health (Niemi 1987; Murray et al 1989; Walsh et al 1989; Ainamo et al 1991; Van der Weijden et al 1991) and those which have (Killoy et al 1989; Stoltze & Bay 1994; Van der Weijden et al 1993, 1994; Ainamo et al 1997), and in some cases the same research group has produced both results at different times. Some studies have also suggested that some electric toothbrushes produce less gingival abrasion than manual ones (Niemi 1987; Niemi et al 1986).

The most recent electric toothbrushes have reciprocating, rotating circular heads which are designed to clean each tooth surface separately. The head should be placed on each tooth surface in turn using an ordered process so that all facial and lingual surfaces are cleaned. The most apical bristles must be placed at the gingival margin so that the crevice is cleaned. Larger tooth surfaces such as molars need cleaning in two stages, i.e. distal and mesial. These brushes have pressure controls to limit gingival trauma and some also have a 2 min timer. In this regard, it takes about 4 min to clean all the surfaces effectively with these brushes, so the timer will operate as you start cleaning the second arch. There is also a Phillips Sonicare® model which has a more conventional shaped head and a reciprocating action. The Braun/Oral B® is rechargeable from the mains and is thus suitable for home use. The Colgate Actibrush® operates by replaceable batteries as does another Braun/Oral B® model and are thus also suitable for travel.

Properly used, the manual brush and automatic brush can both remove plaque effectively. As many people do not use the conventional brush properly the automatic brush may be beneficial in their hands. For the uninstructed patient, the automatic brush is as effective if not more effective than the manual brush. The small head allows access to difficult areas and many people find the sensation of the moving brush very pleasant.

The automatic brush is especially useful to the handicapped person; indeed it may be the only oral hygiene aid which can be used with a fair degree of success either by the individual, parent, care worker or a nurse.

The Braun/Oral B® electric brush has been compared with a conventional manual toothbrush with respect to plaque removal on 48 subjects in a single-blind, randomized, split mouth study (Sharma et al 2001). The brushes were used twice daily at home following instruction and a period of abstaining from brushing for 1 day. Plaque levels reduced with both brushes but the Braun/Oral B® model performed significantly better than the manual brush, particularly at accessible approximal sites.

The effect of the Braun/Oral B® model has been compared with the Colgate Actibrush® on changes in the plaque and gingival indices using a 3-month single blind, parallel group study (Putt et al 2001). The plaque index was reduced significantly more in the Braun/Oral B® group than the Colgate Actibrush® group but no differences were seen with respect to changes in the gingival index. The Braun/Oral B®, Phillips Sonicare® and Phillips Sensiflex brushes were also compared in an experimental gingivitis, split mouth study on 32 subjects (Van der Weijden et al 2002). This showed that all three electric brushes were similar in their ability to reduce plaque levels but that the Braun/Oral B® brush was slightly, albeit significantly better than the other two in reducing gingival bleeding.

The effect of the Braun/Oral B® and Phillips Sonicare® brushes using a normal toothpaste were compared with a conventional manual toothbrush using a tartar control toothpaste in respect of the rate of calculus and stain formation. The study used a cross-over design with 81 subjects (Sharma et al 2002). All three brushes reduced calculus and stain formation rates but in this respect, the Braun/Oral B® brush and the conventional manual brush performed significantly better than the Phillips Sonicare® brush. Recent publications (Siclia et al 2002; Heanue et al 2003) reported systematic reviews of studies comparing manual and electric toothbrushes and came to the same conclusions as those stated above. However, a recent systematic review (Deery et al 2004) found no significant differences of the efficiency of manual and powered toothbrushes.

Thus, the Braun/Oral B® electric brush seems to perform slightly better than the other electric and manual toothbrushes in terms of plaque, stain

and calculus control and in resolving gingivitis. However, it must be noted that the differences between them were small and that all brushes, electric and manual, when used correctly are both safe and effective.

INTERDENTAL CLEANING

As the interdental region is the most common site of plaque retention and the most inaccessible to the toothbrush, special methods of cleaning are needed. These include the use of floss, tape, dental woodsticks, the interspace brush and the miniature interproximal brush. Once again it needs to be stated that during the first stages of instruction in home care, the technique advised must be fairly easy for the patient to carry out. If it is not easy, discouragement will soon set in. The point of the exercise is the removal of plaque without injuring the soft tissues and the use of woodsticks or floss where inappropriate may be harmful.

A further word of caution needs to be given about supplying the patient with too many gadgets; two implements at the most, e.g. a toothbrush and floss or a woodstick, will suffice to get the patient off the mark.

Interdental plaque control with either floss or interproximal brushes has been found to be effective in removing interdental plaque and in resolving clinical signs of interdental gingival inflammation and bleeding (Gjermo & Flotra 1970; Bergenholtz & Olsson 1984; Caton et al 1993; Iacono et al 1998; Schmage et al 1999). Interdental plaque control has also been shown to be superior to the use of a chlorhexidine mouthwash in these respects (Caton et al 1993). Furthermore, it has also been shown to resolve the histological features of inflammation in a clinical and histological study (Bouwsma et al 1988).

DENTAL FLOSS

Dental floss either waxed or unwaxed can be very effective in removing interproximal plaque. To be effective, the floss should be pulled around the tooth curvature so that close contact with the tooth surface is made. It needs to be used with control so that the gingiva is not cut (**Fig. 11.5**); many people find it difficult to use in posterior segments. A floss-threader is necessary to clean bridge abutments. As with all oral hygiene aids, the use of floss must be demonstrated in the patient's mouth, after which the patient repeats the performance under supervision. Comprehensive flossing should be carried out once per day.

A number of different designs of floss holder are available on the market, some of which allow floss to be applied in the recommended way (**Fig. 11.6**). Suitably designed floss-holders may make the task easier and quicker for some people and thus make it more likely to be carried out every day. Oral B have also recently marketed a battery powered flossholder with replacement heads. The floss undergoes gently vibrating movements.

THE INTERSPACE BRUSH

This is a single-tuft brush designed for cleaning areas with difficult access for a normal toothbrush, such as around irregular teeth, in a space where a tooth is missing and around bridge abutments and pontics. The automatic rotating brush has proved to be very effective in these situations, as well as for general interproximal cleaning.

INTERPROXIMAL BRUSH

The interproximal brush is an important device for cleaning between molar teeth and furca, particularly after surgery. The proximal furrow in the root is not adequately cleaned by floss or woodsticks but will accommodate an interproximal brush well.

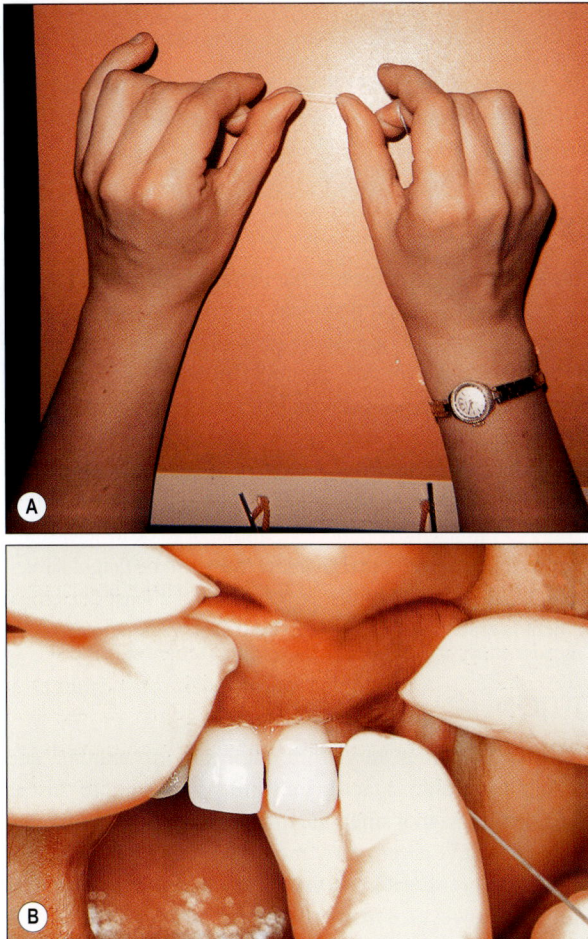

Fig. 11.5 Using dental floss. (A) Handling dental floss so that it can be used with control when being placed against an interproximal tooth surface. Note that the floss is wound round the fingers to stop slipping. (B) Floss in position on the mesial surface of the upper left second incisor (hidden by controlling finger).

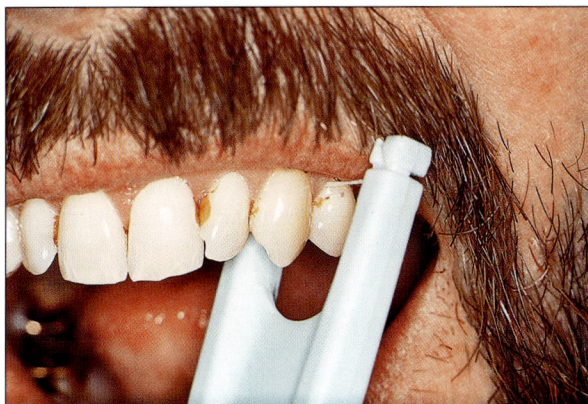

Fig. 11.6 A floss holder in use. The floss has been applied to the mesial surface of the left upper first premolar and can be used in the conventional way to clean the gingival crevice and the proximal surface.

THE DENTAL WOODSTICK

Once upon a time it was believed that bacterial invasion was better resisted by well-keratinized gingivae, and therefore that regular gingival massage was beneficial. The definition of the junctional epithelium as the portal of entry of bacterial products has undermined the rationale for this kind of exercise. The woodstick is used not to keratinize the gingivae but to clean the interdental dentogingival junction. There must be an adequate interdental space to use a woodstick effectively and without damaging the tissues. If a woodstick is rubbed on inflamed gingiva, it is more likely to stimulate the inflammation than aid its resolution.

IRRIGATING DEVICES (WATER-PIK)

An irrigating device can be a useful supplement to the toothbrush, particularly where there is fixed bridgework; however, it needs to be made clear to the patient that irrigation can remove food debris but it cannot remove plaque. In the immediate postoperative phase after periodontal surgery, irrigation with warm or even a fairly hot and weak saline solution can be very soothing. It is unlikely that the addition of antiseptics, e.g. chlorhexidine, to the irrigating fluid is of much benefit because the solution will be too dilute to affect the oral flora. On the other hand, if the taste is pleasant, it might encourage the patient to use the device frequently and therefore help to make the home care process more enjoyable and less of a chore. Using the device on full strength may be hazardous. It is possible for the impact of the fluid to drive pocket bacteria into the tissues and produce a periodontal abscess.

FREQUENCY OF BRUSHING

Theoretically one could clean the teeth once every other day and prevent plaque from accumulating to the point where it would provoke some gingival inflammation. However, few people clean their teeth so well at one time that all the plaque is removed; therefore more frequent brushing is essential. In addition, the presence of food debris or plaque build-up on the teeth is unpleasant, especially to people who are sensitive to the state of their mouth.

It has become the convention to clean teeth morning and night and certainly, the establishment of regular oral hygiene habits is essential; however, the rush to start the day or the fatigue of day's end do not provide the best climate for effective home care. In advising patients about the pattern of home care it seems wise to take into account the kind of life they lead. Many people do have both the time and energy as well as access to a washbasin to spend time on cleaning their teeth in the middle of the day. These days, so many people work where good toilet facilities exist that the habit of keeping a toothbrush at the place of work is one to encourage.

The essential requirement is the acquisition of an awareness of the state of the mouth. Once an individual knows what a clean mouth feels like, a dirty mouth becomes intolerable and the need to use a toothbrush is encouraged. Splaying of the bristles is the most obvious sign of toothbrush wear. This is influenced more by the quality, i.e. resilience of the bristle than by small differences in toothbrush design. Renewal of a toothbrush is usually recommended after 3 months' use. Market research indicates that women change their brush more frequently than men.

TOOTHPASTE

Essentially, toothpastes contain mild abrasives, which enhance the efficiency of the toothbrush in removing plaque deposits, as well as antibacterial agents which help retard the regrowth of plaque deposits (De La Rosa et al 1979). Many contain fluoride to retard enamel demineralization and promote remineralization, and thus help prevent and reduce caries. Some also contain chemicals to help desensitize exposed and sensitive dentine.

There is a large variety of toothpaste formulations, which can be very complicated. Typical constituents are as follows:

- Abrasives: Calcium carbonate, calcium pyrophosphate, aluminium silicate, diatomaceous earth, etc.
- Antibacterial agents: Sodium lauryl sulphate, zinc citrate trihydrate, triclosan, metal ions, etc.
- Anti-caries agents: Sodium monofluorophosphate, sodium fluoride, stannous fluoride
- Desensitizing agents: Strontium salts, sodium fluoride, formalin, etc.
- Fillers and thickeners, e.g. Sodium carboxymethyl cellulose
- Humectants to keep the paste moist, e.g. glycerine
- Detergents, e.g. sodium-lauryl sulphate. Flavouring agents, often mint
- Colouring agents
- Sweeteners, e.g. Sodium saccharin.

In the De La Rosa et al (1979) study, after prophylaxis, subjects brushed their teeth for 2 min with and without toothpaste over a 28-day period. Plaque levels were measured immediately after brushing and then after 24 h. After each brushing, about 40% of the plaque was removed leaving 60% to promote plaque regrowth. The regrowth rate for the group brushing with toothpaste was 27% lower than that for the group brushing without toothpaste. In subsequent studies, Rustogi et al (1984) compared the effects of brushing with tap water for 1 min with that of brushing with various abrasives, including silicon dioxide and sodium bicarbonate, and found that brushing with the abrasives removed 59–69% of 48-hour-old plaque compared with only 27–33% after brushing with tap water. Other chemotherapeutic agents are discussed in Chapter 16.

CHEMICAL CONTROL OF PLAQUE DEPOSITION

Mechanical methods of plaque removal require time and manual dexterity, and therefore a high level of patient motivation. These problems have stimulated the research for a chemical cleaner to supplement or replace mechanical cleaning. The central difficulty has been to find a substance that is both effective and harmless to the tissue.

Chemical control may be achieved in a number of ways:

1. Suppression of the oral flora
2. Inhibition of bacterial colonization of the tooth surface
3. Inhibition of plaque forming factors, e.g. binding carbohydrates such as dextran
4. Dissolution of established plaque
5. Prevention of mineralization of plaque.

These are discussed more fully in Chapter 16.

MOUTHWASHES

Mouthwashes have been used for a number of purposes, clearing the mouth of food debris, as carriers of antibacterial agents to prevent or reduce plaque accumulation, containing anti-caries fluorides, and to reduce the activity of odour-producing microorganisms.

The simplest and most frequently used mouthrinse has been a dilute saline solution, and when warm, is especially useful in postoperative care, but much more complicated formulations are now available to achieve the above objectives.

Mouthwashes are commonly mixtures of:

- An antibacterial agent; 0.2% chlorhexidine gluconate appears to be the most effective, but its powerful taste and tendency to stain teeth are disadvantages. Quaternary ammonium salts, e.g. cetylpyridinium chloride, are frequently used
- Alcohol; to enhance antibacterial activity and taste, and to help keep flavouring agents in solution
- A humectant; e.g. sorbitol, to prevent drying-out
- A surfactant; to help keep ingredients in solution
- Flavourings, colouring agents, preservatives, and water; as the vehicle.

There is evidence that the activity of the antibacterial agent is prolonged by absorption to the hydroxyapatite of tooth enamel (Jensen 1978).

It is usually recommended that the mouthwash is used for about 30 s twice a day, before or after toothbrushing, or independently of brushing. However, the evidence of many studies (Lobene et al 1979; Ashley et al 1984) supports the use of mouthwashes in conjunction with regular toothbrushing. Binney et al (1993) tested five commercial mouthwashes as pre-brushing rinses, and found that they were of no greater use than water, nor did they enhance the efficiency of subsequent toothbrushing; but the benefits of their use as adjuncts to normal hygiene procedures has been demonstrated.

PROBLEMS TO BE OVERCOME

Satisfactory plaque control is not easy. If the practitioner is to guide the patient towards this goal, he must be aware of all the problems that the patient might encounter.

MANUAL DEXTERITY

By training and experience, dentists achieve a high level of manual skill and it may be difficult for them to understand that many individuals are not so well endowed. Manual dexterity does not necessarily go with intellect and some of the brightest patients prove to be extremely clumsy. The extent of the patient's difficulty can be recognized by witnessing the patient's performance and directing his efforts with patience and tact. It is necessary to find out which technique the patient can best perform. It is useless to insist on a technique which the patient finds difficult. The scrubbing technique is probably the easiest to perform and if it is the only technique the patient can command, so be it, at least initially, but some effective form of interdental cleaning must also be taught. Given time and persistence, skills do come to most people, even the least dexterous. Positive encouragement is essential: criticism can be counterproductive.

ORAL PERCEPTION

Visual, oral and olfactory faculties vary from one person to another, and there is also considerable variation in tactile sensibility in the mouth. Just as some people are tone deaf or cannot smell the difference between curry and garlic, so some people can have a very dirty mouth without being aware of the condition, while others are sensitive to the presence of the smallest foreign body in the mouth. However, sensibility can be developed, although in some people it can be a slow process. The tongue is the most powerful instrument of oral tactile sensation and the patient can be instructed to run the tongue over the teeth before and after brushing and to recognize the glass-like feeling of clean teeth.

TOOTH POSITION

Malalignment is one of the most common causes of difficulty. Where teeth have been extracted and neighbouring teeth have tilted, a triangular space forms which can be difficult to clean. Areas of crowding can produce special problems as any form of interdental cleaning, even with floss, may be difficult and even harmful. Areas of special difficulty should be defined and techniques devised for those areas.

THE FORM OF TOOTH CONTACT

The contact point or area takes many forms depending on tooth shapes and relationships. The smaller the area of contact, the easier it is to clean. As attrition and interdental wear take place, the contact area increases in size. If the teeth are rectangular in shape, the contact area can be extremely wide. If the related embrasure space is filled by healthy gingiva, interdental cleaning may not be necessary but if inflammation is present, interdental cleaning is essential and floss or tape may be the only effective aid.

RESTORATIVE AND PROSTHETIC DENTISTRY

As emphasized in the text, badly executed restorative dentistry is an extremely common cause of plaque retention. The overhanging margin of the interproximal restoration creates a zone of plaque retention which is totally inaccessible to the patient's best efforts, and if possible, should be removed before subgingival scaling is undertaken. Badly designed contact areas, over-contoured crowns, subgingival crown margins, badly designed bridge pontics, especially the ridge-lap pontic, extracoronal precision attachments placed too close to the gingiva, etc. create problems of plaque control which can be extremely difficult to correct. It is in these latter cases that chemical cleaning can be beneficial in the short term.

It is obviously much more satisfactory to avoid creating these problems in the first place, and all restorative and prosthetic work must be undertaken with its effect on the periodontium in mind.

DIET

Few health topics exercise people's concern as much as their diet. More myths and more neuroses cloud the subject of nutrition than most other topics, and its relation to dental health is no exception. 'How does diet affect my gums?' is a constant question and a satisfactory answer should cover two aspects of this subject:

1. Nutritional deficiencies do not cause gum disease. However, if plaque-induced disease is already present, nutritional deficiency might affect its development; therefore a balanced diet is necessary.
2. Both the chemical composition and the physical character of food are important. Although some tooth surfaces can be cleaned by using hard and fibrous foods, it has been clearly demonstrated that foods, such as apples, carrots, celery, etc. have no effect on plaque deposits in the sheltered gingival crevice, especially in the interdental regions. On the other hand, hard fibrous foods do not encourage the deposition of plaque and are therefore beneficial as substitutes for soft, sticky foods which do encourage plaque deposition. The consumption of sugar in any form is to be discouraged particularly between meals.

For the concerned person, a simple 5-day diet analysis can be extremely revealing. All food and drinks, including between-meal snacks, are recorded, and in going through the list with the patient, all refined carbohydrate is underlined. Even a superficial analysis of this sort can shed light on the idiosyncrasies and limitations of the individual's diet, and seeing their total consumption in black and white can be a salutary experience. In dealing with young people the cooperation of the parents is essential and even the help of teachers is useful.

Unfortunately, there are pressures from all sides to promote the consumption of refined carbohydrate and sugar. The weight of convention and the pressure of advertising tend to limit the effectiveness of diet control advice and basic changes should not be anticipated or aimed for in the short term. Control over between-meal snacks can be achieved and can effect significant benefits.

Such an exercise must be an uphill task but in one regard dental personnel should be successful and that is in setting an example by their own performance and their own dental health.

SMOKING

The prevalence and severity of chronic periodontitis and acute ulcerative necrotizing gingivitis is greater in current smokers when compared with patients who have never smoked and patients who have quit smoking (Haber & Kent 1992; Bolin et al 1993; Haber et al 1993; Grossi et al 1994, 1995). This implies that quitting smoking may slow down or halt the progress of periodontal disease. Periodontists in the USA, UK and other countries are more likely to give advice regarding stopping smoking than other specialists or general dentists (Telivuo et al 1992). They also found that 'healthy' smokers are more likely to visit their dentist than their physician. Thus, anti-smoking advice from the dentist may be beneficial to the smoking patient from a number of different health aspects.

Another concern is that 90% of regular smokers start smoking before the age of 18 (MacKenzie 1994). Dentists can give advice to this young population on all aspects of its effects including those on periodontal disease.

One recent study (MacGregor 1996) has shown that dental hospital periodontal patients given advice regarding the dangers of smoking were much more likely to cease smoking or reduce the number of cigarettes smoked than patients who had expressed a wish to reduce tobacco consumption but were given periodontal treatment without this advice. After being told that smoking was a major risk factor in periodontal disease and a factor likely to prevent a good response to treatment, subjects were asked to set a target for their daily cigarette consumption and this was recorded. They also kept a record of their actual consumption. They were followed for periods ranging from 3 months to 1 year. In the group given the anti-smoking advice, 65% had reduced their smoking up to 50% and 13% had quit smoking. In the control group not given the advice, the proportions were 30% and 5%, respectively. Subjects in both groups had expressed a desire to stop smoking and of all the patients interviewed for participation in the study, only 8% did not want to stop or cut down their smoking. Thus it seems good practice to routinely provide dental patients with anti-smoking advice.

Anti-smoking advice should cover all the well-known medical risks from tobacco products as well as informing them of the strong link between smoking and periodontal disease. It should also inform them of the various available aids to quit smoking and outline a reasonable regime to undertake. Such a regime of quitting smoking should only be suggested to patients who have expressed a desire to quit smoking.

PATIENT MOTIVATION

In motivating a patient in good home care, one has to bring about change – change in knowledge and understanding, change in attitude and thus change in habit.

In the provision of any form of treatment, some explanation of the patient's problem is essential, and this is especially the case in the control of periodontal disease where the patient must take on the responsibility for his or her own wellbeing. In this respect, the periodontal patient is similar to the diabetic patient – both must look after themselves if the disease is to be controlled, and that control is likely to be effective if the patient has a clear understanding of the rationale behind the discipline.

In providing an explanation of the patient's problem, as already stated, certain rules must be followed:

1. Do not take any prior knowledge for granted; assume that the patient knows very little about dental matters and what information he or she may have garnered is likely to be a compound of gossip, old wives' tales and pseudo-science. For example, few patients realize that teeth are held in bone and that the gum is simply a cover for the bone; many people believe that plaque is degraded food.
2. Give information in simple everyday language and avoid jargon. To say 'You have a plaque-induced gingival infection exacerbated by iatrogenic retention factors' will be meaningless to most patients. Thus, use the word 'bacteria' not 'microorganism', 'gum' instead of 'gingiva', 'stick' instead of 'adhere', 'swollen' not 'hyperplastic', etc.
3. Do not give too much information at one time, and repeat everything that you have said. When the light dawns it may dawn very slowly.

CHANGE IN ATTITUDE TO DENTAL HEALTH

Periodontal health is important: teeth are worth keeping for life. The patients must believe this; otherwise any change in habit as an immediate response to the dentist's admonitions will be short-lived.

Telivuo M, Murtomaa H, Lahtinen A: Observations and concepts of the oral health consequences of tobacco use of Finnish periodontists and dentists, *J Clin Periodontol* 19:15–18, 1992.

Van der Weijden GA, Danser MM, Nijboer A, et al: The plaque removing efficiency of a resiproque rotating toothbrush, *J Dent Res* 70:557, 1991.

Van der Weijden GA, Danser MM, Nijboer A, et al: The plaque removing efficacy of an oscillating/rotating toothbrush. A short-term study, *J Clin Periodontol* 20:273–278, 1993.

Van der Weijden GA, Timmerman MF, Reijerse E, et al: The long-term effect of an oscillating/rotating toothbrush on gingivitis. An 8-month study, *J Clin Periodontol* 21:139–145, 1994.

Van der Weijden GA, Timmerman MF, Piscair MI, et al: A clinical comparison of three powered toothbrushes, *J Clin Periodontol* 29:1042–1047, 2002.

Walsh M, Heckman B, Leggott, et al: Comparison of a manual and powered toothbrushing with and without adjunctive oral irrigation for controlling plaque and gingivitis, *J Clin Periodontol* 16:419–427, 1989.

Wennström JL, Serino G, Lindhe J, et al: Periodontal conditions of adult regular care attendants. A 12-year longitudinal study, *J Clin Periodontol* 20:714–722, 1993.

Yonezawa H, Kato T, Kuramitsu HK, et al: Immunization by Arg-gingipain A DNA vaccine protects mice against an invasive Porphyromonas gingivalis infection through regulation of interferon-production, *Oral Microbiol Immunol* 20:259–266, 2005.

CHRONIC GINGIVITIS

The manifestations of gingival inflammation vary considerably between individuals and from one part of the mouth to another. This variation reflects the aetiological factors at work and the tissue response to these factors. This response is essentially a mixture of inflammation and fibrous tissue repair. When the former predominates, signs and symptoms are more obvious; when the fibrous tissue component predominates, clinical manifestations can be much more subtle and recognized only by careful examination.

In making a diagnosis it is important to keep in mind the appearance of health, departures from which may indicate disease. Clinical features are:

1. Altered gingival appearance
2. Gingival bleeding
3. Discomfort and pain
4. Unpleasant taste
5. Halitosis.

ALTERED GINGIVAL APPEARANCE

Changes in appearance are usually described according to colour, shape, size, consistency and surface characteristics.

Healthy gingivae are pale pink and the margin is knife-edged and scalloped; a streamlined papilla is often grooved by a sluice-way and the attached gingiva is stippled.

Because the interdental embrasure is the site of greatest plaque stagnation gingival inflammation usually starts in the interdental papilla and spreads around the margin. As the blood vessels dilate the tissue becomes red and swollen with inflammatory exudate. The knife-edged margin becomes rounded, the interdental sluice-way is lost and the surface of the gingiva becomes smooth and glossy (**Fig. 12.1**). As the gingival fibre bundles are broken up by the inflammatory process, the gingival cuff loses tone and comes away from the tooth surface, so that a shallow pocket is formed. If the inflammation becomes more diffuse and spreads into the attached gingiva the stippling disappears. If inflammation is severe, it can spread across the attached gingiva to the alveolar mucosa and so obliterate the normally well-defined mucogingival junction.

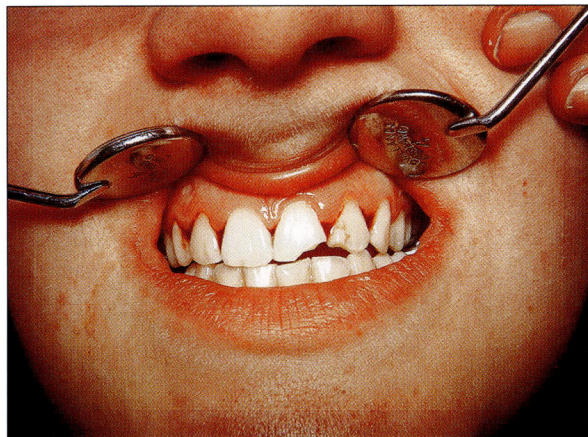

Fig. 12.1 Chronic marginal gingivitis showing slight papillary swelling and marked bleeding following brushing.

Usually, the most pronounced inflammatory swelling is seen in adolescents and young adults so that 'false pocketing' is formed. It is called false as opposed to real or periodontal pocketing, which is formed by apical migration of the crevicular epithelium as the periodontal ligament is destroyed by inflammation. Where several aetiological factors combine, e.g. plaque deposition plus lack of lip-seal plus the endocrinal changes of puberty, gingival swelling, especially papillary swelling, can be pronounced.

If plaque irritation is longstanding and low grade, the main tissue reaction will be fibrous tissue production so that the gingiva may remain firm and pink but become thickened and lose its streamlined shape.

GINGIVAL BLEEDING

Gingival bleeding (**Fig. 12.1**) is probably the most frequent patient complaint. Unfortunately, gingival bleeding is so common that people may not take it seriously and even believe it to be normal; however, unless bleeding obviously follows an episode of acute trauma, bleeding is always a sign of pathology. It occurs most frequently on toothbrushing. Bleeding may be provoked by eating hard food, apples, toast, etc. as well as by probing the gingival crevice or pocket on periodontal examination. 'Bleeding on probing' has been used as a sign of disease activity, but as stated earlier, this is an unreliable indicator of disease activity, and may be the result of injudicious examination. When gingivae are extremely soft and spongy, bleeding can occur spontaneously. Blood may be tasted by the patient and may be smelt on the patient's breath.

If the tissue response is fibrous overgrowth, there is no bleeding even with vigorous toothbrushing.

DISCOMFORT AND PAIN

These are uncommon features of chronic gingivitis and this is probably the main reason for the disease being overlooked. The gingivae may feel sore when the patient brushes his teeth and because of this he brushes more lightly and less frequently so that plaque accumulates and the condition is perpetuated.

This relative absence of pain is one of the symptoms which differentiates a chronic gingivitis from an acute ulcerative gingivitis.

UNPLEASANT TASTE

Patients may notice the taste of blood, particularly if they suck at an interdental space. Unfortunately, the senses are quickly blunted and a disagreeable taste is a relatively infrequent complaint.

HALITOSIS

'Bad breath' frequently accompanies gingival disease and is a common cause of a visit to the dentist. The smell derives from blood and poor oral hygiene and must be distinguished from smells from different sources.

Halitosis has a number of causes, both intra-oral and extra-oral. Oral disease and residual food deposits, especially those of a volatile nature, such as peppermint, garlic, curry, etc., represent the most common cause of halitosis. Pathology of the respiratory tract, nose, sinuses, tonsils and lungs can cause an embarrassing smell, as can diseases of the digestive tract. Some items of diet, e.g. garlic, are absorbed by the intestines, taken into the intestinal bloodstream and finally exhaled by the lungs so that they can be smelt a long time after they have been eaten. Mouth odour is common on waking and between meals, when it is associated with food stagnation and reduced salivary flow. Metabolic diseases, diabetes and uraemia give characteristic smells to the breath. Halitosis can increase with age.

CHRONIC PERIODONTITIS

The clinical features of chronic periodontitis are:

1. Gingival inflammation and bleeding
2. Pocketing
3. Gingival recession
4. Tooth mobility
5. Tooth migration
6. Discomfort
7. Alveolar bone loss
8. Halitosis and offensive taste.

Of these, only pocketing and alveolar bone loss are essential features of chronic periodontitis.

GINGIVAL INFLAMMATION AND BLEEDING

Although gingival inflammation is a necessary precursor to periodontitis, obvious manifestations of inflammation become less apparent with the progression of periodontitis. Frequently, the gingivae are pink and firm, the contours may be almost normal, there may be no bleeding on careful probing and the patient may not complain of bleeding on brushing. It is as though with the development of the pocket the disease has gone underground.

The presence and severity of gingival inflammation depend upon oral hygiene status; where this is poor, gingival inflammation is evident and bleeding or brushing, or even spontaneous bleeding, is noticed by the patient. When the patient's toothbrushing is good enough to control plaque but where subgingival deposits, because of inadequate scaling, persist, the presence of periodontal disease may not be apparent on superficial examination. If a careful history is taken, many such patients report a history of past bleeding which stopped when their toothbrushing technique improved. Periodontal destruction in the average adult is the product of past neglect, not the result of present oral hygiene habits. Royzman et al (2004) have shown that patients with gingivitis taking aspirin regularly have significantly more bleeding on probing (BOP) than those taking a placebo. While the effect is small, it could affect treatment outcomes and also the outcomes of clinical research studies when BOP is included as a variable.

POCKETING

Pocket measurement is an essential part of periodontal diagnosis but must be interpreted together with gingival inflammation and swelling, and radiographic evidence of alveolar bone loss. Theoretically, if there is no gingival swelling, a pocket over 2 mm deep indicates some apical migration of crevicular epithelium but inflammatory swelling is so common especially in the younger individual that pocketing of 3–4 mm may be entirely gingival or 'false'. Pocketing of 4 mm is likely to indicate an early chronic periodontitis (**Fig. 12.2**).

The precise measurement of pockets is difficult because:

1. Probing the pocket can be uncomfortable and even painful if there is frank inflammation.
2. Pocket depth is extremely variable around a tooth. Interproximal pocketing is usually deepest because that is the site of greatest plaque accumulation, while pocketing on the facial aspect of the tooth is usually most shallow, as this is where the toothbrush makes the

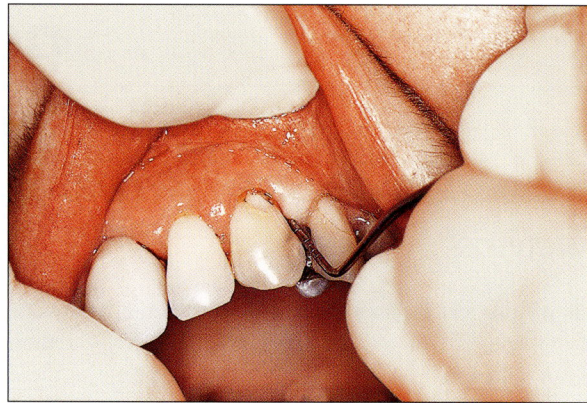

Fig. 12.2 Pocket measuring probe has been inserted into pocket and guided to the deepest point beneath the contact point.

greatest impact and may even produce gingival recession. This means that four or more measurements may be required on each tooth to give an accurate picture.

3. Where present oral hygiene is good, the gingival cuff may be so tight around the neck of the tooth as to resist the insertion of an ordinary periodontal probe without causing pain. The measurement of pockets in anaesthetized tissue often produces quite different results from previous measurement made in sentient tissue.
4. Tooth contour and angulation, subgingival calculus or restorations, as well as carious cavities, may impede the insertion of the probe. The deepest aspect of interproximal pockets usually lie below the contact area. Therefore the probe has to be inclined inwards to reach this point in molar or premolar teeth. Compensation should be made for the effect of this angulation on the probing depth measured, and it is usual to subtract 1 mm from the measurement value in these circumstances.

Other factors which affect the accuracy of the measurement of probing depth are discussed in Chapter 13.

There are many designs of pocket-measuring probe, some of which are too thick to provide accurate measurement, and some of which are sharp so that the tissue is penetrated unless great care is taken. The special CPITN probe has been described in Chapter 10. There are also probes which can control the pressure of probing and these are described in Chapter 13.

It has been shown that pockets of over 3 mm are measured with diminishing reliability, and it is unfortunate that much periodontal research is based upon such an unreliable criterion.

Sometimes a purulent discharge can be expressed from the pocket by pressure on the pocket wall.

GINGIVAL RECESSION

Gingival recession and root exposure may accompany chronic periodontitis but are not necessarily a feature of the disease. In this regard, localized gingival recession affecting only the facial aspect of the gingiva is usually not associated with chronic periodontitis (see Chs 8 and 24), whereas generalized recession involving all aspects of the tooth is invariably associated with periodontitis (**Fig. 12.3**). Where recession occurs pocket depth measurement is only a partial representation of the total amount of periodontal destruction and both should be recorded when carrying out periodontal charting. The other causes of gingival recession are discussed in Chapter 8.

TOOTH MOBILITY

Some tooth mobility in a labiolingual plane can be elicited in healthy single-rooted teeth, especially lower incisors, being more mobile than multirooted teeth. Increasing tooth mobility is produced by:

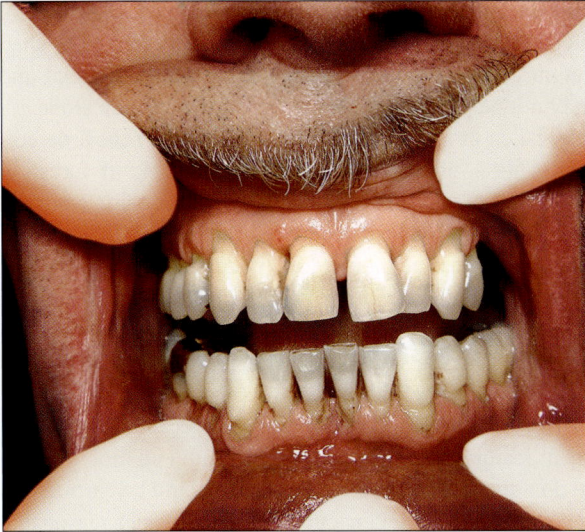

Fig. 12.3 Chronic periodontitis exhibiting generalized gingival recession which affects all aspects of the teeth.

1. Increased width of periodontal ligament with no loss of alveolar bone or other supporting tissue
2. Increased width of periodontal ligament plus loss of alveolar bone or other supporting tissue
3. Loss of alveolar bone or other supporting tissue without an increased width of periodontal ligament.

These tissue changes may be produced by:

1. Spread of inflammation from the gingiva into the deeper tissues
2. Loss of supporting tissue
3. Occlusal trauma.

Mobility also increases after periodontal surgery and in pregnancy. In periodontal pathology tissue destruction is always accompanied by inflammation and frequently by occlusal trauma. Mobility which is produced by inflammation and occlusal trauma is reversible, as demonstrated by the reduction in mobility following scaling and occlusal adjustment; mobility associated with destruction of supporting tissue is not reversible.

Assessment of mobility for research purposes can be made using special apparatus but clinical assessment is usually subjective. It is elicited by exerting pressure on one side of the tooth under examination with an instrument or finger tip, while placing a finger of the other hand on the other side of the tooth and its neighbour which is used as a fixed point so that relative movement can be discerned. Another way of eliciting mobility (although not assessing it) is to place fingers over the facial surfaces of the teeth while the patient grinds the teeth.

The degree of mobility may be graded as follows:

- Grade 1. Just discernible, 0.2–1 mm in a horizontal direction.
- Grade 2. Easily discernible, and over 1 mm labiolingual displacement.
- Grade 3. Well marked labiolingual displacement, mobility of the tooth up and down in an axial direction. There is an element of subjectivity in this grading. No doubt sufficient determination can elicit mobility in perfectly secure teeth!

More refined methods of mobility assessment have been devised. Muhlemann (1954) invented the Periodontometer which measures tooth displacement when a small force was applied to the tooth. More recently, Schulte et al (1992) have produced the Periotest, which is a refinement of the Muhlmann device. Essentially, the Periotest is a horizontal rod which taps the tooth at a known velocity; on impact the tooth is defected, the rod decelerated and the contact time recorded. This ranges between 0.3–2.0ms, being shorter for stable than for mobile teeth.

TOOTH MIGRATION

Movement of a tooth (or teeth) out of its original position in the arch is a common feature of periodontal disease and one which alerts the patient to the problem. Tooth position in health is maintained by a balance of tongue, lip and occlusal forces. Once supporting tissue is lost these forces determine the pattern of tooth migration. The incisors move most frequently in a labial direction but teeth may move in any direction or become extruded (**Fig. 12.4**). Once a tooth migrates, the force on that tooth changes and this may promote further stress and further migration. If an upper incisor migrates labially the lower lip may come to lie lingual to the incisal edge of the tooth and produce further migration.

DISCOMFORT

One of the most important features of chronic periodontitis is the almost total absence of discomfort or pain unless acute inflammation supervenes. This is one of the main distinctions between periodontal and pulp disease. Discomfort or pain on percussion of the tooth indicates some active inflammation of the supporting tissues which is at its most acute in abscess formation when the tooth becomes exquisitely sensitive to touch. Sensitivity to hot and cold is sometimes present when there is gingival recession and root exposure. Indeed one common clinical experience is the appearance of sensitivity, especially to cold, when roots once covered in calculus are cleaned. On occasion, pulp pathology may be a complication of advanced periodontal disease and severe pain may then develop.

ALVEOLAR BONE LOSS

Resorption of alveolar bone and the associated destruction of periodontal ligament is the most important feature of chronic periodontitis, and the one which leads to tooth loss. There is considerable variation in both the form and rate of alveolar bone resorption and in constructing a treatment plan the amount of bone loss, the rate at which resorption is progressing and the pattern of bone loss need to be accurately established. Radiographic examination is an essential part of periodontal diagnosis and with certain limitations, provides evidence of the alveolar bone height, the form of bone destruction, the width of the periodontal ligament space and the density of cancellous trabeculation. Serial radiographs taken over a period of time can provide information about the rate of bone loss. However, radiographic examination without careful clinical examination can be very misleading. A periodontal diagnosis cannot be made from radiographs alone, as there is no way of distinguishing on the radiograph past bone destruction from current bone resorption.

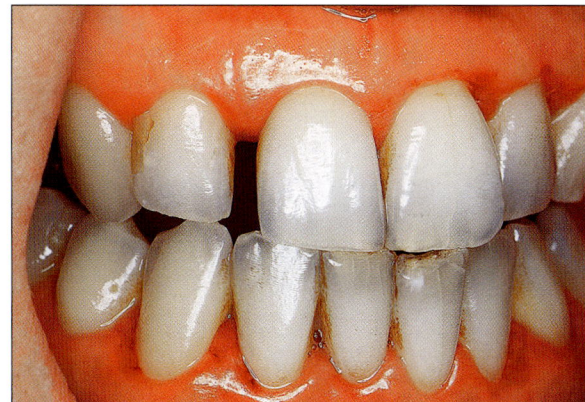

Fig. 12.4 Drifting of the upper incisors which is a feature of advanced chronic periodontitis but may be the first thing to alert some patients to the presence of disease.

Because the images of the facial and lingual plates of bone are largely obscured by the dense image of the tooth, diagnosis depends upon obtaining a clear image of the interdental bone. Careful angulation of the X-ray beam and a standardized routine of exposure and processing the radiographic film is essential.

The first radiographic sign of periodontal destruction is loss of density of the alveolar margin. This is most clearly seen between posterior teeth where in health the broad interdental septum projects a dense and well-defined image of the alveolar margin (**Fig. 12.5**). The image of the narrow interdental septa between anterior teeth is less well defined in health and early pathological changes are less easy to see. With continuing bone resorption the height of the alveolar bone is further reduced (**Fig. 12.6**). Even correctly angulated the radiographs may not disclose the true state of interdental resorption, e.g. an interdental crater between molars can be masked by the images of the facial and lingual walls of the defect.

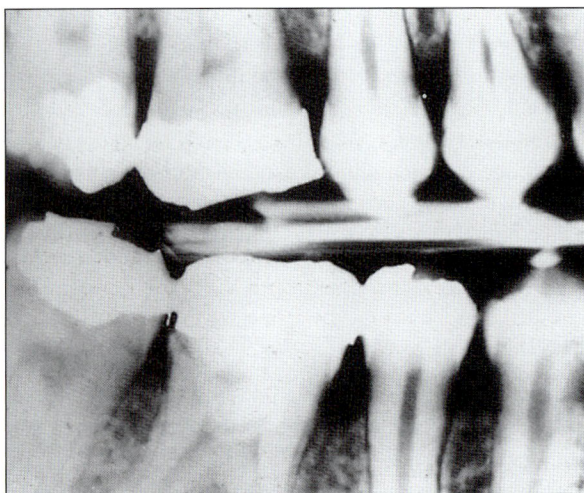

Fig. 12.5 Signs of early marginal bone loss on a bite wing radiograph. Most bone loss is around the upper molars, but note hollowing of the septum between the lower first molar and second premolar, the bite wing film is very useful for revealing early bone loss in posterior segments.

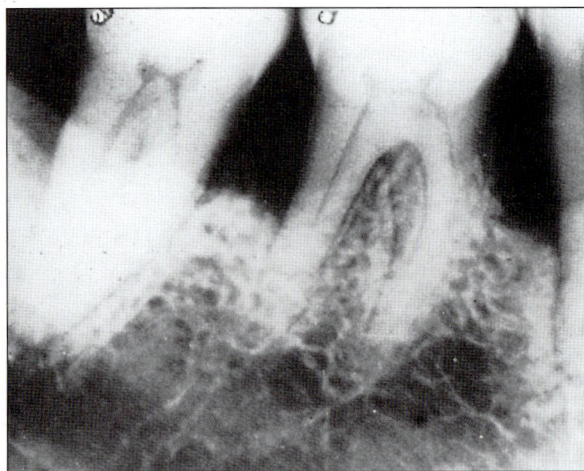

Fig. 12.6 Fairly advanced bone loss in a 46-year-old woman. *Note* irregularity of bone margins with vertical defect distal to the second premolar and second molar.

Bone defects which lie over the facial or lingual aspects of the teeth, e.g. marginal gutters, may be completely obscured and revealed only when flaps are raised at surgery. Moreover, distinguishing between facial and lingual defects may not be possible from radiographic evidence alone.

Two radiographs taken at slightly different angles often reveal defects undetected by one. This is especially true in the diagnosis of furcation defects. These are usually revealed by radiographic examination but the exact form of the defect may not be discernible. The thick palatal root of an upper molar may mask a trifurcation defect. Widening of the periodontal space in the furcation provides evidence of an early lesion. Widening of the periodontal space on one side or all around a tooth frequently indicates excessive occlusal stress. This is sometimes accompanied by widening or funnelling of the coronal aspect of the socket.

All departures from the normal radiographic appearance must be checked against other clinical features, in particular pocket depth and mobility patterns, and if these do not correspond re-examination should be carried out. Clinical and radiographic features taken together should make a reasonable fit which sheds light on both the pathological condition and its aetiology. Thus, where radiographic examination of a mobile tooth reveals that the supporting bone is virtually intact, careful examination of the occlusion is essential. There must always be an identifiable reason for any pathological change. The factors which affect the accuracy of radiographic detection of alveolar bone loss are discussed in Chapter 13.

HALITOSIS AND OFFENSIVE TASTE

The metabolism of many of the oral bacteria, in particular the Gram-negative anaerobic bacteria in saliva, the gingival crevice and plaque, when acting on substrates in the mouth, e.g. food debris and plaque, can produce sulphur-bearing compounds such as hydrogen sulphide and methylmercaptan; these can impart an offensive smell to the mouth and exhaled breath.

An offensive taste and smell frequently accompany periodontal disease, especially when oral hygiene is poor. Acute inflammation, with the production of pus which exudes from pockets on pressure, also causes halitosis. A source of constant surprise is the lack of awareness of many affected individuals and their spouses to the powerful fetor, which like a malignant wind escapes from their mouths when they speak. Lack of sensibility and unconcern about dental health seem to go hand in hand, and as patient cooperation is essential to the success of periodontal treatment, this sensibility, or lack of it, can provide a clue to prognosis.

REFERENCES

Muhlemann HR: Tooth mobility. The measuring method. Initial and secondary tooth mobility, *J Periodontol* 25:22–29, 1954.
Royzman D, Recio L, Badovinac RL, et al: The effect of aspirin intake on bleeding on probing in patients with gingivitis, *J Periodontol* 75:679–684, 2004.
Schulte W, Hoedt B, Lukas D, et al: Periotest for measuring periodontal characteristics – Correlation with periodontal bone loss, *J Periodontal Res* 27:184–190, 1992.

FURTHER READING

Eley BM, Cox SW: Advances in periodontal diagnosis. Part 1. Traditional clinical methods of diagnosis, *Br Dent J* 184:12–16, 1998.

Diagnosis, prognosis and treatment plan

MAKING A DIAGNOSIS

The diagnosis should not be limited to giving a name to the condition. If periodontal disease is to be treated and its recurrence prevented, a diagnosis should include the identification of all aetiological factors, i.e. (1) those factors which predispose to plaque deposition and retention, and (2) those factors, local or systemic, which influence adversely the behaviour of the tissues. It should go without saying that you cannot remove or control factors which have not been identified, yet all too frequently treatment is reduced to the control of signs and symptoms, and inevitably disease recurs.

At the time of the initial examination some attempt should be made to assess the patient's attitude to dental health. Patient cooperation is essential to the success of periodontal treatment and it is this fact which makes the treatment of periodontal disease different from that of caries and other dental diseases when the patient can take a more passive attitude.

PATIENT EXAMINATION

The examination should be methodical and comprehensive and should follow the standard pattern of the classic case history.

Present complaint and its history

A patient with periodontal disease may have no complaint at all and be oblivious to the presence of any disease in the mouth; indeed, the patient may be suspicious of any suggestion that disease is present. The most common complaints are bleeding gums, loose teeth, drifting of the teeth (usually the upper incisors), nasty taste, halitosis, swelling of the gums, discomfort and occasionally acute pain.

Few patients at the initial consultation provide concise and completely relevant information. All too often, the necessary information has to be elicited by abstraction from a long, sometimes rambling, account which must be listened to with patience and close attention. In addition, pertinent questions should be asked:

- Are you in pain?
- Where is the pain?
- Is it a throbbing or dull pain?
- Does the pain keep you awake?
- What brings on the pain – hot, cold, sweet, biting?
- Have you had pain in the past or is this the first time?
- What treatment have you received for pain?
- Do your gums ever bleed?
  - When you brush your teeth?
  - When you eat hard food?
- Did your gums bleed in the past?
- What treatment did you receive?
- Do any of your teeth feel loose?
- Have you always had that space between your front teeth?
- Have you had any swelling in your mouth? Where, when, etc.?

Dental history

- Do you go to the dentist regularly?
- What was the last treatment you received?
- When did you last have a scaling, i.e. cleaning by your dentist?

- Do you have any dentures (false teeth that you can take out) – how long have you had them?
- Have you any false teeth that are fixed in – how long have you had them?

At this stage, questioning about home care can be a waste of time. Answers to such questions as 'How often do you clean your teeth?' are often suspect, as the patient is likely to say what he imagines he is supposed to say, i.e. twice a day, night and morning. Even if this happens to be the truth, it gives no indication of the quality of the performance; only an examination of the mouth provides information about that.

At this time, some idea about habits should be gleaned, e.g. smoking, clenching, night-grinding, biting pencils and so on.

Medical history

Although a medical history may not seem relevant to some patients, it is essential to obtain one for a number of reasons:

1. The patient may be suffering from some condition, e.g. cardiovascular disease, renal disease, etc., which will require special precautions and/or modification of the treatment, and will necessitate communication with the patient's physician.
2. Systemic conditions, e.g. pregnancy, diabetes, will alter the way in which the periodontal tissues behave and may demand medical attention before periodontal treatment can be carried out.
3. The mouth may be the site of some manifestation of a systemic condition, e.g. anaemia, which could affect any periodontal treatment.
4. The patient may be receiving medication, e.g. tricyclic antidepressants for depression, which may conflict with medication involved in the periodontal treatment, e.g. general anaesthetics.

A medical history should record any present illness and medication; any past serious illness and medication, e.g. steroids taken in the recent past, allergies, especially any history of penicillin sensitivity, abnormal bleeding tendencies, in particular excessive bleeding after injury or tooth extraction. The use of a questionnaire may be helpful.

Where some systemic problem exists, communication with the patient's physician is essential.

Patient appraisal

While taking the history, a general appraisal of the patient should be made, and such features as obesity, general posture, pallor, skin rash, heavy breathing, lip posture, should be noted.

Oral examination

The examination of the mouth should be carried out in a methodical and thorough manner; this is the dentist's special area. Halitosis is noted as the mouth is opened, or even earlier when the patient is giving a history. The following areas should be systematically examined:

The oral mucosa

Cheeks, lips, tongue, palate, floor of mouth and vestibules, are examined for ulceration, vesicles, swelling, eroded patches, abnormal colour and white lines or patches. Tooth indentations in the margin of the tongue and interdental keratosis, i.e. a white line in the cheek at the level of the occlusion, often indicates a clenching or grinding habit.

Aphthous ulcers frequently occur in the labial or lingual vestibule or inside the lips. Lichen planus may be seen as fine, interlacing white lines on the cheeks or alveolar mucosa. Vesicles or eroded patches should be fully investigated. A sinus on the alveolar mucosa, with or without the discharge of pus on pressure, indicates the presence of an alveolar abscess.

In the older individual, a squamous-cell carcinoma may appear as a painless swelling, ulcer or eroded white patch in any part of the oral mucosa, but especially in the vestibules. Oral lesions of primary, secondary or tertiary syphilis may appear on the lips, tongue, palate and even the gingivae; widespread candida lesions in a young male could be indicative of HIV infection.

Any departure from the norm must be examined carefully, and if infection or malignant disease is suspected, an examination of the submandibular and cervical lymph nodes will help with a diagnosis. Immediate referral to the physician or appropriate specialist is essential.

Removable appliances

If these are present they should be examined for their fit, design and relationship to any inflammation of the oral mucosa and gingiva.

Oral hygiene

Note presence and position of plaque, supragingival and subgingival calculus. Subgingival calculus can be detected with a probe such as a WHO probe or a Cross calculus probe but may also be seen as a dark blue shadow in the gingival margin. The use of a disclosing agent will help to identify plaque and demonstrate its presence to the patient. Sometimes the location of plaque and calculus points to a predisposing factor, e.g. better oral hygiene on the left side is usually associated with right-handed tooth brushing; interproximal deposits and gingival inflammation may be caused by the overhanging margins of restorations or poor contact relations.

Teeth

Teeth are charted and cavities, restorations and malalignments recorded. Attrition may indicate a grinding habit; abrasion a vigorous and damaging toothbrushing technique.

Gingivae

The gingivae are examined for colour, shape, size and consistency, keeping in mind the picture of health, pink, knife-edged, streamlined and firm, any departure from which could indicate pathology.

Periodontium

The various signs of attachment loss should be looked for, measured and recorded. Periodontal charting should be carried out and should include probing depth and gingival recession measurements on each tooth. In addition, furcation involvement and tooth mobility should be recorded when and where present. Probing depth and recession measurements should be usually made at six points around each tooth. Ideally, true mesial, distal, facial and lingual measurements are required, but this is possible only where teeth are missing, so that unimpeded access to these surfaces is possible. Where proximal teeth are present, measurement is made at the line angles, and on facial and lingual surfaces. Taking six readings on each tooth is ideal but may be very time consuming, and if diagnosis is made at a reasonably early stage in periodontal breakdown, only four measurements made at the mesiobuccal, mesiolingual, distobuccal and distolingual line angles may be sufficient. Where there appears to be furcation involvement of molars, or drifting of incisors, facial and lingual measurements on these teeth are essential.

A pocket-measuring probe must be fine enough to enter a narrow pocket, but must have a blunt end so that the tissue is not perforated. The sharp-ended probe used for the detection of caries should never be used. The pocket-measuring probe should be inserted into the pocket as near parallel to the axis the tooth as possible (**Fig. 13.1**). However, if adjacent teeth are present, parallel placement of the probe at interdental sites will not allow the area under the contact point to be reached and this is the site where the pocket is deepest. Parallel placement will therefore result in a significant underestimation of interproximal pockets. For this reason, it is necessary to slightly angulate the probe beneath the contact area on molar and premolar teeth to reach the base of the deepest interdental pockets (**Fig. 13.1**); the effect of the angulation should be compensated for when recording the measurement. Great care has to be taken to manipulate the probe so that the true depth of the pocket is recorded. Delicate handling of the probe must be employed to negotiate subgingival deposits without impaction against the root surface (**Fig. 13.2**). Vigorous probing is not only painful but likely

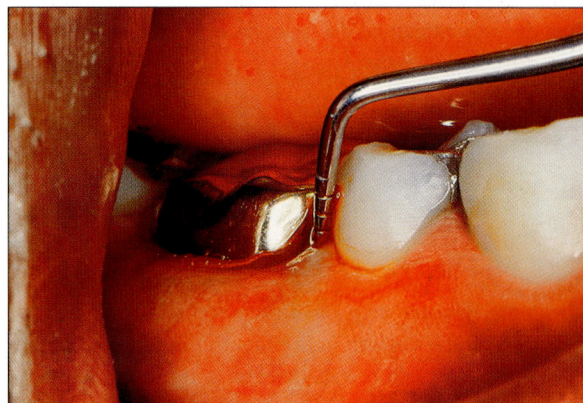

Fig. 13.1 A periodontal probe inserted into the mesiobuccal pocket of the lower right first molar. It has been slightly angled lingually to pass under the contact area to reach the deepest part of the pocket. It is measuring a deep pocket, which would have been missed if the probe had been placed parallel to the tooth surface at the mesiobuccal line angle.

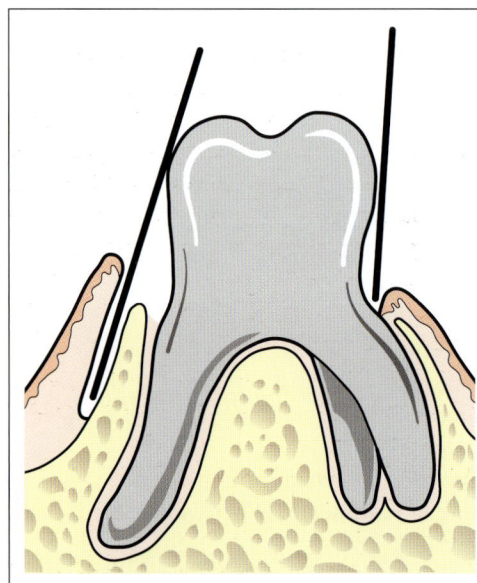

Fig. 13.2 A diagram to show two possible errors in measuring probing depths. The buccally placed probe has passed through the inflamed tissue beyond the base of the pocket and the palatally placed probe has impinged on a bulbous root surface and failed to reach the base of the pocket.

to give an inaccurate reading; even gentle probing of inflamed gingivae can be painful. The problems of pocket measurement can be demonstrated by the fact that pocket measurement after local anaesthesia usually gives greater readings than in the unanaesthetized tissue. If a lot of supragingival calculus is present at the first visit, periodontal charting should be postponed until supragingival scaling has been carried out.

If intrabony pocketing is suspected, in more advanced cases this will usually not be detected by either probing or radiography alone. However, in this situation there is usually lack of agreement between the probing depth measurement and the apparent bone level on the radiograph. In this situation further information may be gained by placing gutta-percha or silver points, which may be calibrated, to the base of the pocket in question during radiographic examination. This will then show the relationship of the pocket to the bone.

In addition to recording pocket depth, it is also important to record gingival recession at all sites where it is present so that the total amount of measured attachment loss can be meaningfully compared with bone levels on radiographs.

It is also important to try to assess the true probing attachment level, i.e. probing depths measured from the amelo-cemental junction (CEJ) or some other fixed point. This would allow more meaningful serial comparisons to be made in order to monitor periodontal progression. Where there is considerable gingival hyperplasia, pocketing may be fairly deep, e.g. 5–7 mm, but attachment loss may be small or nil. Where there has been considerable gingival recession, a shallow pocket may be associated with considerable destruction of the periodontal tissues. Therefore, in order to interpret pocket measurement one must also note:

- The position of the gingival margin on the tooth surface
- The position of the alveolar crest as seen on the radiograph
- The factors affecting the accuracy of periodontal probing.

Radiographic examination

Radiographic examination will demonstrate the position of the alveolar margin and the condition of the alveolar bone. In a child or adolescent, radiographic examination may not be essential but if any doubt exists about the integrity of the alveolar margin, bite wing films of posterior teeth and periapical films of the incisors should provide adequate information. If there is evidence of established bone loss, further radiographic examination can then be undertaken.

In the adult, full mouth examination may be necessary. Vertical bite wing radiographs (**Fig. 13.3A**) are useful for posterior teeth and can be used for teeth with probing depths up to 6 mm; the dentopantomograph (OPT) provides an overall picture, but detail of the alveolar margin is frequently ill defined. Repeat radiographs may be necessary, at intervals (not less than 3 years) determined by patient susceptibility, to show progression. The long-cone paralleling technique provides the most reliable radiographic evidence (**Fig. 13.3B**). The bisecting angle technique is more likely to give a distorted picture of the relationship of the alveolar margin to the CEJ. Rinn bite blocks, film holders and localization devices can be used to ensure that the X-rays pass perpendicular to the teeth and film, preventing any distortion of the bone/teeth relationships. Using these devices can also help to make subsequent radiographs of the same site comparable.

Radiographs may or may not show the presence of intrabony pocketing where the base of the pocket lies within a bone defect (see Ch. 8). Three-walled defects are unlikely to show radiographically due to superimposition of their walls. Two- and one-walled defects are more likely to show up as vertical defects. It may be helpful in situations where an intrabony pocket is suspected to place a radio-opaque marker within the pocket before radiography so that it will appear in the resulting image and mark the base of the pocket in relation to the bone defect (**Fig. 13.4**).

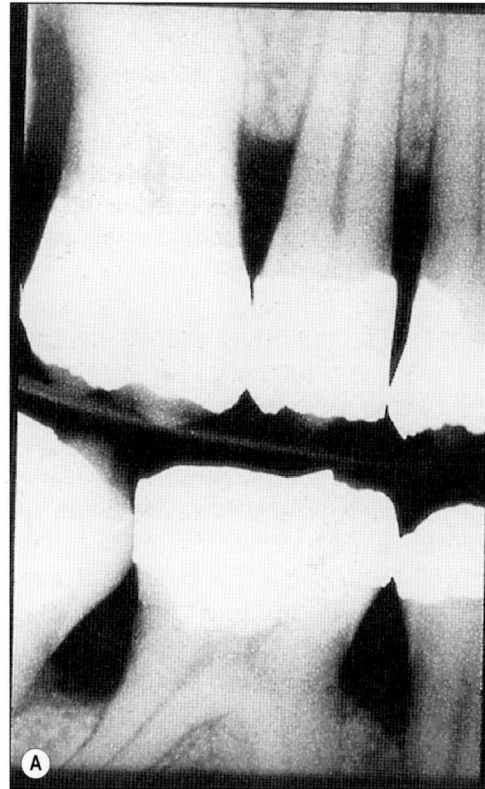

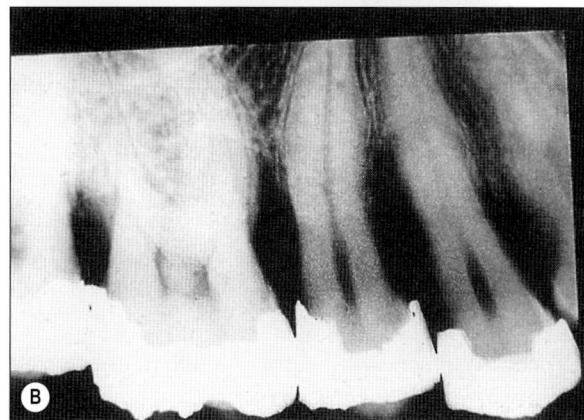

Fig. 13.3 Radiograph taken to show alveolar bone loss. (A) A vertical bite wing radiograph of the right molars and premolars showing horizontal bone loss. (B) A paralleling technique radiograph of upper right molars and premolars showing more advanced horizontal bone loss.

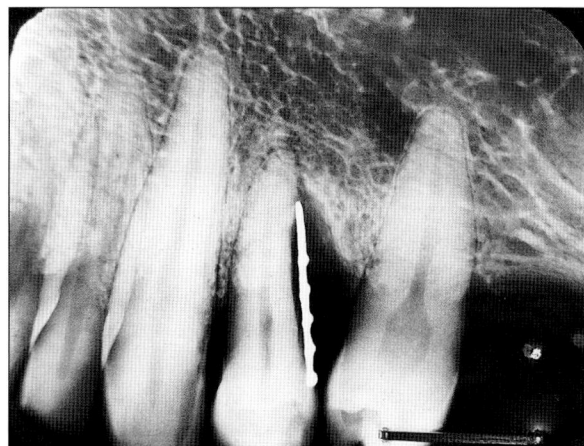

Fig. 13.4 A paralleling technique radiograph of upper right premolars and canine with a radio-opaque (metal) marker within the pocket confirming the presence of an intrabony pocket. The base of the pocket lies within a vertical bony defect distal to upper right first premolar.

Sophisticated techniques such as subtraction radiography and computer-assisted image analysis have been used as research tools to detect small changes in bone mass, but at present these have no place in clinical practice. However, the advent of digital radiography makes the use of such techniques more likely in the future.

It cannot be stressed too strongly that the traditional techniques of clinical radiography can provide a great deal of reliable information, but only if great care is taken in beam angulation, exposure and processing, and in interpretation of the radiographic image.

Occlusion

The examination of occlusion should include:

1. The Angle's classification
2. Overbite and overjet
3. Tooth relation in protrusive and lateral positions and movements
4. Any deviation from the normal path of opening and closure
5. Any temporomandibular joint (TMJ) discomfort of clicking
6. Any spasm in the masticatory muscles
7. Any history of habits, e.g. clenching or grinding the teeth.

The occlusion needs to be examined closely where:

1. Teeth are mobile or sensitive
2. There is discomfort, clicking, deviation of the mandible on opening and closing, or limitation of movement
3. One or more of the masticatory muscles is tender to palpation
4. Radiographs show widening of the periodontal spaces or vertical bone defects, i.e. possible signs of excessive occlusal stress.

ADVANCES IN DIAGNOSTIC TECHNIQUES

The methods described above are suitable for most clinical situations but do suffer from a number of drawbacks. These are:

1. Clinical or radiological measurements of attachment loss are not entirely accurate and if not carried out very carefully, can be misleading. This is particularly the case for periodontal probing but also affects oral radiography
2. Full mouth recording is necessary because of the site specific and episodic nature of much periodontal progression
3. Individual susceptibility to periodontitis, as to all bacterial disease, varies over time and this needs to be determined and taken into account
4. All clinical diagnostic techniques give us retrospective information about past disease and are unable to diagnose disease activity
5. If the periodontal examination is required for periodontal research purposes much more accurate diagnostic techniques are necessary.

All of these issues are discussed below.

FACTORS AFFECTING THE ACCURACY OF PERIODONTAL PROBING

The periodontal probing depth (PPD) is the distance from the gingival margin to the base of the periodontal pocket and it is usually measured at six points around the tooth, i.e. mesial, buccal and distal from the buccal side and mesial, lingual and distal from the lingual side (see Ch. 12). The mesial and distal measurement may not be the same from buccal and lingual sides due to differential bone loss and also because access to them may be better from one side or the other. The amount of gingival recession, i.e. the distance from the cemento-enamel junction (CEJ) to the base of the periodontal pocket should also be measured. These measurements are recorded on to a periodontal chart by the dental nurse during the recording process.

If these measurements are to be related to future serial measurements in order to attempt to monitor disease progression then they must be made very carefully.

In controlled clinical studies, it is necessary to additionally record probing attachment levels (PAL). This is the distance from a fixed, reproducible point and the pocket base. The ideal fixed point is the CEJ if it can be reliably located but alternatives are the occlusal surface or a fixed point on a stent precisely located over the teeth to be recorded.

A periodontal probe must be fine enough to enter a narrow periodontal pocket but must have a blunt end so that it reduces the likelihood of penetration of the tissues at the base of the pocket. Great care must be taken to manipulate the probe to reach the base of the deepest aspect of each pocket without penetrating its base.

A number of factors can affect the accuracy of periodontal probing. These are:

- The size of the probe
- The angulation of the probe
- The contour of the tooth and root surface (**Fig. 13.2**)
- The probing force used (**Fig. 13.2**)
- The inflammatory state of the tissues (**Fig. 13.2**).

A number of studies have shown that periodontal probing often fails to record the true pocket depth (Listgarten et al 1976; Listgarten 1980; van der Velden 1979). These studies have shown a discrepancy between the actual position of the probe and the true base of the pocket in histological sections of block dissections of animal and human cadaver tissue. The size of the probe and its angulation may be controlled but errors resulting from alterations in probing force and the severity of inflammation in the tissues are more difficult to avoid.

With regard to probing force, it has been shown that the force used by different clinicians can vary from 3 to 130 g and may differ by more than 2:1 for the same clinician from one examination to another (Gabathuler & Hassell 1971; Hassell et al 1973). Generally the greater the probing force the greater is the probing depth measured since the probe penetrates deeper into the tissues at the base of the pocket. In order to limit errors due to differences in probing force, pressure sensitive probes have been developed (van der Velden & de Vries 1978; Vitek et al 1979; Polson et al 1980). These enable the dentist to probe with a predetermined force.

If the gingival tissues are inflamed then the marginal tissues may be swollen by oedema or hyperplasia. This alters the position of the gingival margin and produces an element of false pocketing. In addition, in untreated periodontal disease, the connective tissue adjacent to the pocket epithelium is infiltrated with inflammatory fluid and cells and the pocket epithelium is also infiltrated with inflammatory cells and thinned or ulcerated. In this case, these tissues are very easily penetrated by the periodontal probe even with relatively light probing forces and in some instances the probe penetrates as far as the bone margin. This obviously results in an overestimation of the true pocket depth (Polson et al 1980; Armitage et al 1977; Robinson & Vitek 1979). Conversely, when the inflammatory infiltrate decreases following successful treatment and new collagen fibres are laid down in the connective tissue, the dentogingival tissues become more resistant to probing and the tip of the probe usually fails to reach the base of the pocket. Therefore, this often results in an underestimation of the true pocket depth. For these reasons, the difference between probing measurements and the histological 'true' pocket depth may vary by fractions of a millimetre to several millimetres (Listgarten 1980). Thus, manual probing cannot reliably measure changes in PPD of less than 2.5–3 mm (Haffajee & Socransky 1986).

From this discussion it should be realized that the reductions in PPD that follow successful periodontal treatment are produced by the tissue changes outlined above and not by any true gain in connective tissue attachment. In spite of this, these post-treatment reductions in PPD are often reported as a 'gain in clinical attachment', which is very misleading since the changes result from a resolution of inflammation without any true gain in attachment.

THE EPISODIC NATURE OF CHRONIC PERIODONTITIS

A number of longitudinal clinical studies (Socransky et al 1984) have recorded clinical attachment loss at individual sites in different subjects over time periods ranging from 2–5 years. These have revealed that, despite the presence of inflammation, most sites showed no progression during the study period. Instead, attachment loss occurred at only a few sites and even at these sites was interspersed with long periods of stability or quiescence. This type of episodic, site specific attachment loss has given rise to the burst theory of chronic periodontitis (**Fig. 13.5**). It has further been proposed that these bursts might occur randomly throughout an individual's life (random burst) or there may be periods when bursts of periodontal breakdown in many sites are more likely (asynchronous multiple burst).

The implications of the burst theories are that:

■ Gingival inflammation at a site may not indicate that further periodontal breakdown is occurring or that it will occur at a later date
■ Periodontal disease is site specific and may affect different teeth in the same mouth at different rates
■ Full mouth periodontal charting on a regular basis is necessary to identify sites with attachment loss, to determine the pattern and rate of progression and to determine the patient's susceptibility.

■ Individual serial radiographs based on findings in periodontal charting may be needed to confirm disease progression (**Fig. 13.5**) but radiographs must not be repeated without a sound cause and therefore must be based on clinical evidence
■ Each tooth must be considered separately for treatment.

In these studies, only fairly large changes (≥ 3 mm) of clinical attachment level could be reliably measured and smaller changes could not be detected. Therefore, although these studies show clearly that site specific, episodic disease progression does occur they do not preclude other patterns of progression including slow regular progression also occurring. It seems most likely that episodic progression would predominate in susceptible patients with more rapid rates of progression.

SUSCEPTIBLE AND RESISTANT PATIENTS

Periodontal attachment loss has been found to be more marked in some patients than others, even when differences of oral hygiene are taken into account (Löe et al 1978). Studies from a number of different countries have suggested that about 10% of subjects appear to have a high risk of developing destructive periodontal disease and experience severe periodontal destruction with rapid progression and tooth loss (**Fig. 13.6**). About 80% of subjects are susceptible to periodontitis which progresses rather slowly and rarely results in tooth loss. The remaining 10% appear to be relatively resistant to destructive periodontitis (see **Fig. 4.9**, p. 46), despite the continued presence of gingivitis (Löe et al 1978; Page & Schroeder 1986; Papapanou et al 1989). Identification of each patient's individual susceptibility to periodontitis is important since this will determine the type and frequency of treatment that they will require.

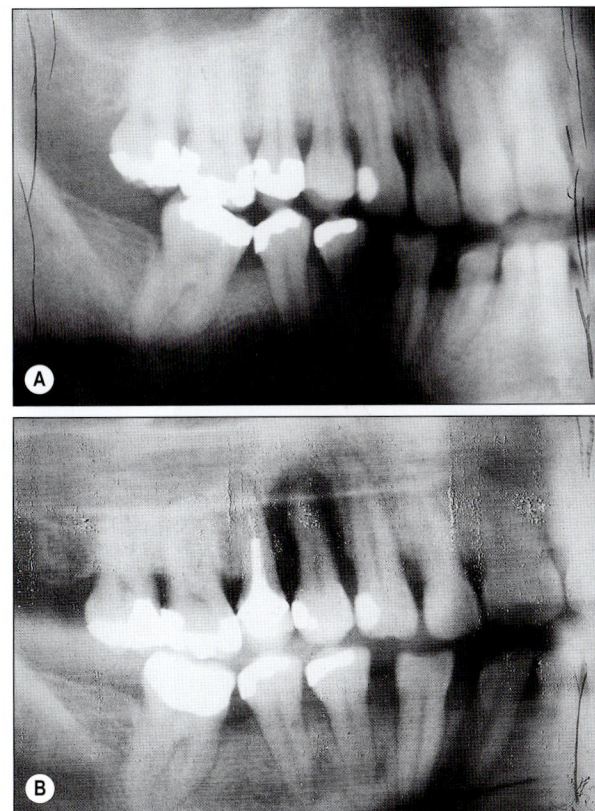

Fig. 13.5 Radiographic evidence of episodic progression of periodontal disease. (A) Part of an orthopantomogram showing molars, premolars, canines and some incisors. Where clearly visible it shows early horizontal bone loss around the upper premolars and canine. The probing depths mesial and distal to the first premolar was 4 mm. (B) An orthopantomogram of the same region taken 8 months later after some restorative and endodontic treatment showing massive bone loss surrounding the upper first premolar. The probing depths mesial and distal to this tooth ranged from 10–12 mm.

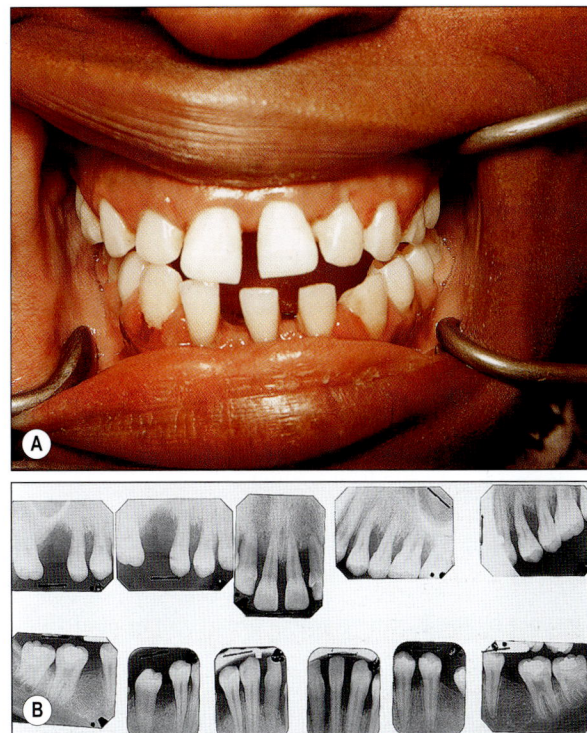

Fig. 13.6 (A) A 15-year-old girl with severe gingival inflammation and advanced periodontitis with drifting of teeth. (B) Radiographs of the same girl showing marked generalized alveolar bone loss. She had already lost a lower incisor due to extreme mobility. Her mother had also lost all her teeth at the same young age, and wore full dentures. No evidence of systemic disease was found; however, all such cases should always be investigated for any underlying systemic cause, such as a leucocyte dysfunction.

ADVANCES IN MEASUREMENT OF PERIODONTAL ATTACHMENT LOSS

The main objective of periodontal diagnosis is to detect changes in periodontal attachment level. The traditional methods of recording this are the use of manual probing with a graduated periodontal probe and radiographic examination. The accuracy of probing is affected by a number of factors including the position and angulation of the probe, the probing pressure and the inflammatory state of the tissues. If probing measurements are to be used sequentially to detect progressive loss of attachment these factors need to be controlled where possible and the measurements need to be made from a fixed reproducible point. This cannot be the gingival margin which can change its position as a result of inflammatory swelling or recession and the ideal reference point is the CEJ. However, the CEJ is difficult to locate precisely because it usually lies subgingivally and it may be obscured by calculus or dental restorations. For these reasons other points such as the occlusal surface or a fixed point on a stent are often used in clinical research studies.

Probing measurements even with those controls are not precisely reproducible between different clinicians even when they standardize their procedures. In addition, replicate measurements of the same site at close time intervals are not always reproducible for the same clinician (Haffajee et al 1983). To overcome these problems in clinical studies they suggested the use of the tolerance method to determine the threshold for confirmed attachment loss based on probing. With this method two replicate measurements of each site are made for each subject and their standard deviation (SD) calculated. The difference between all duplicate measurements for all the test sites within each patient are then used to calculate the patient SD and patient SDs are then averaged to produce a population SD. In a longitudinal clinical study of periodontal attachment loss this method is usually used to confirm measured progressive attachment loss. With this method, for the mean of the second of a pair of attachment level measurements to be considered significantly different from the mean of the first pair then the attachment level change would have to exceed:

- The site threshold which is calculated as 3 site SDs
- The patient threshold which is calculated as 3 patient SDs
- The population threshold which is calculated as 2 population SDs.

The site measurement standard deviation has been calculated as 0.82 mm in the Haffajee studies which makes the subject tolerance 2.46 mm. Thus, using this method any change below 3 mm is considered to be unreliable and this makes it impossible to measure small changes of attachment using manual probing. For this reason, the National Institute for Dental Research (NIDR) of the USA in 1979 requested the development of more sensitive methods (Parakkal 1979). They wanted:

- A precision level of ±0.1 mm and a range of 10 mm
- A constant probing force
- Measurement from a fixed reproducible point
- A guidance system to ensure a reproducible pathway
- A non-invasive procedure
- Digital output of data.

These criteria were met by the Florida research group (Gibbs et al 1988) who developed the Florida probe system. This incorporates:

- Constant probing force
- Precise electronic measurement
- Computer storage of data.

It eliminates errors of visual reading (which becomes more important as you age). It consists of a probe handpiece, a digital readout, a foot switch and a computer interface and computer (Magnusson et al 1988b). It has been found to be significantly superior to manual probing

(Magnusson et al 1988a). Two models have been developed which differ in their fixed reference point. These are the stent and disk models. The probe of the stent model has a 1 mm metal collar that rests on a prepared ledge on a prefabricated vacuoform stent. The disk model has a 11 mm disk which rests on the occlusal surface or incisal edge of the tooth (**Fig. 13.7A**).

The reproducibility of both types of Florida probe has been compared with conventional manual probing (Low et al 1989; Osborn et al 1990). They were both significantly superior to manual probes with a site standard deviation (SD) range of 0.21–0.28 mm. The calculated subject tolerance is 0.63–0.84 mm meaning that changes in attachment of 1 mm can be reliably measured by this method.

The Florida probe can also read probing depths using an interchangeable pocket depth handpiece. This has a collar surrounding the probe which is related to the gingival margin and the distance from this to the base of the pocket is electronically recorded (**Fig. 13.7B**). All of this data along with other readings such as bleeding on probing can be recorded and saved on a disk or printed on to special charts using a suitable compatible printer.

Other electronic probes have been developed and these include:

- The Interprobe (Goodson & Kondon 1988)
  - This has an optical encoder transduction element.
- The Birek probe (Birek et al 1987)
  - This works by constant air pressure and uses the occlusal surface as its reference point. The site SD has been calculated as 0.46 mm and the subject threshold as 1.38 mm.
- The Jeffcoat probe (Jeffcoat et al 1986, 1989)
  - This claims to detect the CEJ automatically and has a calculated site SD of 0.17 mm and a subject threshold of 0.51 mm. This appears to be the lowest subject threshold reported to date.

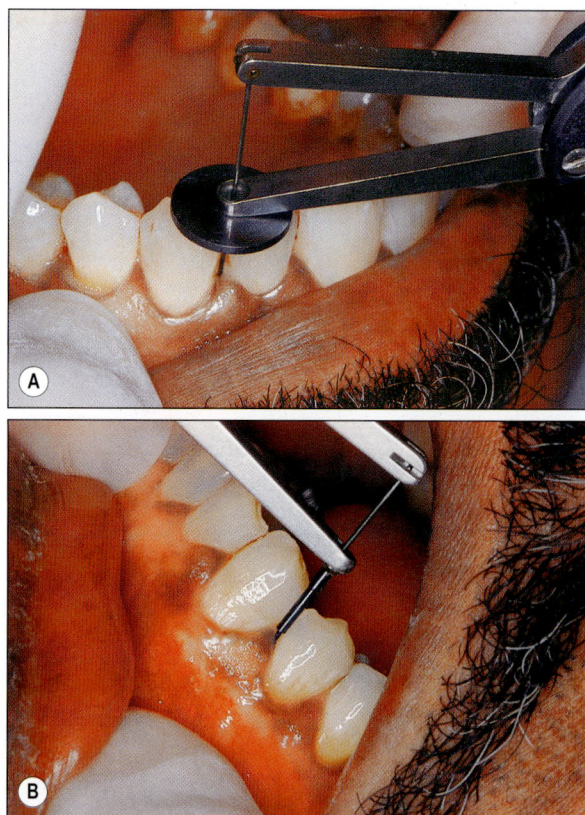

Fig. 13.7 (A) A Florida electronic probe with an attachment level disc on the occlusal surface. (B) A Florida electronic probe with an attachment with a sleeve that is positioned at the gingival margin in question for measuring probing depth.

RADIOGRAPHIC EXAMINATION

Transmission radiography can show the relationship between the alveolar bone margin and the CEJ and changes in the distance from the bone margin to the CEJ, normally 1–2 mm, are indicative of alveolar bone loss. To achieve an accurate display of this distance, the rays must be perpendicular to the tooth and bone surfaces and the tube must also be at the correct antero–posterior angulation. Two types of view can be used in conventional radiography to achieve this:

1. Vertical bite wings (**Fig. 13.3A**)
2. Long cone paralleling views (**Fig. 13.3B**).

To detect serial changes in this relationship further controls are necessary and these involve:

■ A constant film position
■ A constant tube geometry.

A constant film position can be achieved by the use of a stent which can be in the form of an acrylic impression of the occlusal surfaces of the teeth on the bite block of the film holder. A mark can also be made to ensure that the film is always placed in the same position in the holder. By these means the holder is accurately located to the teeth and the film to the holder for each serial radiograph.

A constant tube geometry can be achieved by relating the tube to positioning devices attached to the film holder (Rinn system) or by the use of a cephalostat (Jeffcoat et al 1987).

Bone loss can also be expressed as a percentage of the root length to compensate for errors of foreshortening or elongation.

COMPUTER-AIDED SYSTEMS

Techniques have recently been developed to aid the detection of small serial changes in alveolar bone level. These rely on digitization of the radiographic image to allow computer processing and analysis. Two techniques have been mainly developed for research purpose and these are:

■ Digital subtraction radiology
■ Computer-assisted linear radiography.

However, computer-aided techniques based on the principle of digitization of the image are beginning to be developed for clinical usage and are likely to appear in the near future. These will allow a lower radiation exposure time and also allow the image to be stored in the computer and printed out as many times as required.

Digital subtraction radiology

The best known computer-aided technique is digital subtraction radiology (Webber et al 1982; Gröndahl & Gröndahl 1983; Jeffcoat et al 1987). The purpose of this technique is to subtract all unchanged structures from a pair of serial films and display only the areas of change. For periodontal films, this means subtraction of the teeth, cortical bone and trabecular pattern leaving only bone loss or gain standing out against a neutral grey background.

The digitization process converts the analogue (nearly continuous grey level information) contained in the transmission radiograph to numbers that are proportional to the brightness of the radiograph at a particular location. This is done by taking a picture of the radiograph with a sensitive black and white video camera. The digitizer automatically superimposes a grid over this picture and converts the grey level of the radiograph within each box in the grid to a number ranging from 0 (black) to 255 (white). The fineness of the grid determines the spatial resolution of the digitized image and usually a 512×480 picture element (pixel) grid is used.

This process does not increase the information on the radiograph and in fact decreases it a little. It does, however, put the information in a form that the computer can use so that it can process it in a way in which it will aid the dentist or researcher to detect changes in bone level not visible to the unaided eye from the original radiograph. The computer subtracts all structures present in the first radiograph of the serial pair from those in the second radiograph leaving only bone loss (dark) or bone gain (light). Location of bony change can be more readily seen by superimposing the subtracted image over the original radiograph. Subtracted images can also be colour coded by the computer to increase clarity. Bone loss is usually colour coded red and bone gain green.

If this technique was reliable and accurate it could be useful in assessing the natural history of periodontal disease progression and in longitudinal studies of various types including investigations of potential biomarkers of disease activity or proposed new treatment methods. However, the accuracy of digital subtraction radiography has been questioned by Benn (1990) on the basis of his own measurements using this technique. Subtraction radiography depends critically on the very precise registration of the two sequential radiographs. He created two identical digital images of a single radiograph to test the response of the system to small displacements of 0.1–0.42 mm in the X, Y and XY directions before subtraction. He found that displacements of 0.1–0.14 mm in the Y or XY directions caused 20–25% of crestal pixels to vary by more than ±2.5% of grey range (2.5% is the noise threshold used for this technique). Larger displacements of 0.3–0.42 mm caused 65% of crestal pixels to vary by more than ±2.5% of grey range. Such small displacements would be hard to avoid when using this technique with serial radiographs and so false crestal bone gain or loss could regularly result from these causes. The use of a much higher noise threshold of about ±8% would need to be used to avoid these critical errors.

Computer-assisted linear radiography

Benn (1992) designed a computer-aided method for making linear measurements on serial radiographs using stored regions of interest. In this system, the radiographs are first calibrated and digitized as described above. Under the control of a computer program, regions of interest (ROI) of 7.5 mm × 7.5 mm, sufficient to cover the mesial and distal CEJ to alveolar crest margin regions of adjacent teeth, are chosen. The measuring process involves placing the cursor pixel point on the CEJ and clicking the mouse button which records and marks this position. This is then repeated for the alveolar crest after which the distance is calculated and stored by the computer. The ROI with its marked reference points is also stored. The process is then repeated for the first serial radiograph and the ROI of the first measurement with its marked points is re-displayed close to the area to be measured. This reminds the operator of the chosen reference points reducing the chances of error. The computer automatically calculates the distances, the average distances of the two readings and the difference between the two readings. This process is then repeated for the second serial radiograph initially using prompts for the siting of reference points from the displayed ROI from the first radiograph. When the sites for the second radiograph image have been measured twice the computer automatically calculates the differences between the two films and the confidence value attached to the measured change.

The accuracy and reliability of this system were tested with 28 examiners with minimal training (Benn 1992). They each measured 14 different sites and repeated the process 4 weeks later; 13 out of 14 sites produced an intra-examiner SD threshold of ≤0.15 mm with the ROI method, but 0 out of 14 without. The inter-examiner threshold for 13 out of 14 sites was ≤0.22 mm using the ROI method and 0 out of 14 without. Therefore, this system would appear to be accurate to ≤0.22 mm and would seem to be useful for clinical research.

SPECIAL TESTS

If the severity of the inflammation or the degree of periodontal destruction appears to be out of proportion to the observed aetiological factors, or if general appraisal of the patient suggests that some systemic factor may be operating, then blood and urine examination or other special tests may be required. In such cases it is imperative to communicate with the patient's physician prior to the start of treatment.

MAKING A PROGNOSIS

A prognosis is a prediction of the way in which the tissues are likely to respond to treatment. Before a definitive treatment plan can be formulated, a prognosis must be made. This should allow one to establish not merely what treatment can be carried out but, more importantly, what treatment is justified in the attempt to achieve long-term periodontal stability. Frequently, the patient will ask that such a prediction be made, and the more complicated the treatment the more important making a prognosis becomes. Looking into the future can be a hazardous exercise but a prediction of the way in which the periodontal tissues will behave can be made on the basis of an understanding of the way in which the tissues of that individual have behaved in the past in the face of disease-producing factors.

A number of parameters need to be considered:

1. The extent of periodontal destruction. This is represented by the amount of alveolar bone loss as seen on the radiograph; obviously the greater the amount of bone loss, the poorer the prognosis.
2. The age of the patient. This, together with the extent of periodontal destruction, provides an idea of the rate at which destruction has taken place. The older the individual, the better the prognosis for any given degree of periodontal destruction.
3. The form of the bone loss. The presence of vertical bone defects must mean a less favourable prognosis than where bone loss is horizontal, for several reasons:
    ◆ Because the level of attachment is frequently more apical
    ◆ Because the possibility of fill-in of such defects is uncertain
    ◆ Because the presence of vertical defects may indicate that factors other than plaque-induced inflammation are operating. Furcation involvement can present home care problems, even after satisfactory periodontal treatment, and if the furcation lesion is related to pulp pathology, prognosis is compounded by any defects in endodontic treatment.
4. The possibility of removing aetiological factors. The control of aetiological factors is essential to the achievement of long-term health, but control can only be exercised after these factors have been identified. Without such identification, treatment becomes symptomatic. Careful examination and an understanding of clinical features are essential. It is always necessary to ask: 'Why are these clinical features present?' Patient cooperation is essential for satisfactory plaque control, but is also necessary for the control of predisposing and aggravating aetiological factors, e.g. the replacement of an ill-fitting partial denture. Patient cooperation is more likely to be forthcoming after the patient has been given information about the nature of the problem. Time spent in providing such information and in explaining the rationale behind the treatment plan will improve the chances of achieving a good prognosis.
5. The number, position and form of teeth present. The number of teeth and their position in the arch will determine the occlusal load on each tooth, whether a prosthesis is necessary, and the amount of tooth support for an appliance. In this context, the form of the appliance is extremely important; a removable appliance makes greater demands on the tooth supporting tissues than a fixed appliance.

The symmetrical distribution of the teeth in the arch is likely to provide a better prognosis than where several teeth are placed on one side of the arch. The root base can be a crucial factor in the stability and usefulness of a tooth. An upper molar with widespread roots and therefore a large root base has a much better prognosis than a conical-rooted premolar or incisor with the same amount of bone loss.

6. General health. Although certain conditions do affect the periodontal tissue response, e.g. diabetes, Down's syndrome, agranulocytosis, the general health of the patient does not usually affect the periodontal condition directly, but any debilitation, physical or emotional, can interfere with the patient's oral hygiene regime.
7. The immunological status in relation to plaque bacteria. The individual's response is critical to the development and progress of periodontal destruction, and is the subject of much recent research. As described in Chapter 23, a few young individuals appear to suffer some deficiency in the cell-mediated immune response to plaque antigens which leads to an extremely poor prognosis. It seems likely that other variations in immune response will be identified in the future, and some laboratory tests may be developed which will provide a more objective guide to prognosis than is currently available.

All the factors outlined above must be taken together to provide a periodontal prognosis for that particular individual. This exercise has to be carried out with great care and thought. The assessment of prognosis provides an acid test of the operator's understanding of the biological forces operating in the mouth under examination. Furthermore, the limitations of our understanding of the disease process do handicap our ability to make absolute prognoses.

PERIODONTAL DIAGNOSIS IN GENERAL DENTAL PRACTICE

Since the vast majority of dental patients are treated in dental practices and some stage of periodontal disease affects practically all patients, a minimum standard of basic periodontal examination should be undertaken of all these patients. The following guidelines for this, outlined below, follow those recommended by the British Society of Periodontology (1986) and the Royal College of Surgeons of England, Faculty of Dental Surgery (1997).

BASIC PERIODONTAL EXAMINATION

All patients should be screened for the presence of periodontal diseases as part of their dental examination and the basic periodontal examination (BPE) represents the minimum examination for this purpose. It consists of:

■ A clinical assessment using the Community Periodontal Index of Treatment Needs (CPITN) as detailed in Ch. 10. In older individuals, recession and furcation involvement may be present causing significant attachment to go unrecorded with this system and, for this reason, a modification is recommended. Where the total attachment loss exceeds 7 mm or if a furcation can be probed the sextant is scored by an asterisk (*) rather than the CPITN code.
■ Appropriate supportive dental radiography when indicated by the clinical examination (see below).

The BPE should be performed at the initial dental examination of all new patients and patients with insignificant periodontal disease on the initial visit should be screened again at regular routine dental inspections with a frequency of a least every 12 months. In addition to routine screening, all patients being considered for advanced restorative or orthodontic treatment should be screened.

In view of the evidence for early periodontal breakdown in a few susceptible individuals (Albander et al 1991), screening of children, adolescents and young adults is also advised. Problems arise with false pocketing in children and this must be taken into account by attempting to locate the cemento-enamel junction in sites where pocketing is suspected in these subjects. In patients under 19, only one tooth per sextant needs to be probed and these should be the first molars and the upper left central incisor and the lower right central incisor.

The BPE will need augmentation by detailed periodontal charting (see **Fig. 12.2**) when the screening has revealed significant disease in one or more sextants, i.e. with CPITN codings of 3, 4 or *. This must include:

- Pocket depths (6 points per tooth)
- Recession (6 points per tooth)
- Bleeding on probing
- Mobility
- Furcation involvement.

CPITN (BPE) is not a suitable index to produce a site-related diagnosis which is needed for patients with significant pocketing. It is also not suitable to monitor the response to treatment. In both of these situations full periodontal charting is indicated.

All patients with identifiable disease at screening should be regularly monitored with further CPITN screening if the disease is early, i.e. codes 1, 2 or full periodontal charting in the case of coded 3, 4, *. Results from epidemiological studies show that in the presence of plaque and calculus periodontal disease increases in severity with age. In addition, it has been shown that periodontal disease progresses at different rates in different sites in the mouth and may at individual tooth sites undergo long periods of quiescence or short periods of progression (Lindhe et al 1983; Haffajee et al 1983). Therefore, there is a need to repeat full periodontal charting of patients with initial evidence of periodontitis at regular intervals.

SELECTION CRITERIA FOR PERIODONTAL RADIOGRAPHY

Radiographs should only be taken if their results are likely to affect the patient's treatment and their need should be based on the results of the clinical examination. There is a lack of consensus as to which type of radiograph, i.e. bite wing, site-related periapicals or panoramic tomogram is most appropriate. Osborne and Hemmings (1992) have shown that panoramic radiography is an acceptable alternative to full mouth periapicals on the basis of its diagnostic yield of unsuspected pathology. However, a large proportion of the disease identified by panoramic radiographs does not affect clinical care. Also the accuracy and resolution of panoramic tomograms in detecting the landmarks for assessing bone loss are less than that achievable with properly aligned long cone, paralleling periapicals. For these reasons, there is little to support its use for routine screening of periodontal purposes (Valachovic et al 1986).

Radiographic selection criteria for periodontal disease should take into account the data obtained from a detailed periodontal examination, with particular reference to pocket depths, recession and the overall state of the dentition. The selection criteria below (Table 13.1) are based on those suggested by Hirschmann et al (1994). These are very similar to the recommendations of the Faculty of General Dental Practitioners (UK) (1998, 2004).

Radiographs should not be repeated unless serial periodontal charting indicates significant progression of disease at the site in question.

A recent survey of 800 general dental practitioners (Tugnait et al 2004) on their use of the basic periodontal examination (BPE) and their use and selection of radiographs, found that 91% used BPE for new patients, 56% for all patients and 84% for recall patients. In contrast, their choice of radiographs was not generally in line with the 1998 and 2004 recommendations of the Faculty of General Dental Practitioners (UK).

Table 13.1 *Radiographic selection criteria for periodontal disease*

Disease status	Radiograph
Uniform pocketing <5 mm	Posterior bite wings
Uniform pocketing <5 mm plus ectopic third molars	Panoramic radiograph
Uniform pocketing 5–6 mm plus otherwise sound dentition	Vertical bite wings of molars and premolars plus long cone periapicals of anterior teeth if indicated by pocket depths on these teeth
Irregular pocketing >5 mm or multiple crowned and/or heavily restored teeth or history of endodontic treatment	Full mouth long cone periapicals or panoramic radiograph plus additional long cone periapicals of key sites

If gingival recession is present then these criteria would need adjustment to account for it.

TREATMENT PLAN

The objectives of treatment are:

1. The elimination of disease
2. The restoration of efficient function
3. The production of a satisfactory appearance.

One might also add – a contented patient.

It should be evident from the above list that periodontal treatment is not primarily concerned with the conservation of individual teeth but with the long-term preservation of a healthy dentition. Indeed, there are situations in which individual teeth have to be sacrificed to the greater good. This concept of treating the dentition as a functioning unit is in conflict with the traditional dental teaching, in which the tooth rather than the dentition is the focus of concern.

Because each patient presents an individual problem, one cannot prescribe a rigid pattern of treatment. Treatment is determined not only by the condition defined by the diagnosis but also by the patient's age, general health and their attitudes and aspirations. Nevertheless, it is important that a well-ordered plan of action is designed at the outset, keeping in mind that departures from this plan may be required as treatment proceeds. No treatment, other than emergency treatment, should be started before a plan is established and explained to the patient.

The following outline should provide a guide to treatment management:

1. Emergency treatment
2. Extraction of teeth with poor prognosis
3. Patient information
4. Plaque control and scaling
5. Subgingival scaling and root planing
6. Initial occlusal adjustment
7. Reassessment
8. Surgery
9. Reconstruction
10. Maintenance.

EMERGENCY TREATMENT

The control of pain comes before any other treatment, but to be effective requires accurate diagnosis. An alveolar abscess which is of pulpal origin can be misdiagnosed as a periodontal lesion with consequent errors in treatment and persistence of pain.

Swelling, even without pain, requires immediate attention. Acute infection may require the prescription of antibiotics before further treatment can be carried out, but the use of antibiotics is justified only where pain and infection can be controlled in no other way. A localized and pointing abscess should be treated by incision and drainage rather than with antibiotics.

Large, carious cavities and pulp disease should be treated. Endodontics may be necessary as an emergency measure where there is a pulpitis, apical abscess or a combined periapical-periodontal abscess.

Extremely mobile teeth which seriously interfere with function should be splinted or extracted.

EXTRACTION OF TEETH WITH VERY POOR PROGNOSIS

A decision about extraction should be based not only on the condition of the individual tooth and its supporting tissues but also upon the possible consequences of the extraction. Where periodontal breakdown is advanced, the extraction of weak teeth may create an insoluble prosthetic problem. Such developments need to be anticipated prior to extraction. The provision of removable prostheses may be necessary at this time, and care should be taken with their design, even if temporary.

PATIENT INFORMATION

Some time should be allowed prior to definitive treatment to explain to the patient the nature of the problem and the kind of treatment needed. Where different lines of treatment are available, these options, with their advantages and disadvantages, should be explained. Frequently, decisions have to be made by the patient, and these can be made intelligently only on the basis of information.

PLAQUE CONTROL AND SCALING

Plaque control and scaling are the most important procedures in periodontal treatment. Where the condition is diagnosed and treated at an early stage, they are the only treatments required. They also provide a clue as to patient attitude, dexterity and level of cooperation. Where that level of cooperation is inadequate, any indicated surgical treatment or other complicated treatment will not be justified. This phase of treatment should also include the correction of filling overhangs and the replacement of defective restorations. It is unrealistic and unjust to expect a high level of plaque control where conditions exist which make that impossible; therefore, all plaque retention factors should be corrected at this stage.

SUBGINGIVAL SCALING AND ROOT PLANING

Periodontal pockets require careful subgingival scaling to remove subgingival calculus and root planing to smooth the root surface and remove any necrotic cementum. This is by far the most important procedure in the treatment of chronic periodontitis. If this procedure is carried out successfully it will result in cessation of bleeding on probing and if this sign persists then it is indicative of residual subgingival calculus. The procedure also results in a change in the subgingival flora (see Ch. 15) which itself brings about a resolution of gingival inflammation and a regeneration of junctional epithelium. These changes probably result from changes in the nutritional sources, particularly of protein, brought about by this procedure. They last for about 3 months which is why these procedures need to be repeated 3-monthly.

Subgingival scaling and root planing is a time-consuming procedure which requires appropriate subgingival scalers, freshly sharpened instruments and considerable clinical skill (see Ch. 15).

INITIAL OCCLUSAL ADJUSTMENT

This is necessary for repair of the periodontal lesion and may be carried out alongside plaque control. Gross occlusal disharmonies should be eliminated and temporary splints applied to very mobile teeth. At this stage, any minor tooth movement necessary can be carried out. Such movement should be complete and any retention apparatus should be in place before any surgery is carried out. A bite-guard is provided in cases of definite bruxism.

REASSESSMENT

A reassessment of the periodontal condition should be made at this stage. The tissue response to the treatment already provided may be better than anticipated, so that little or no surgery may be required. Pockets may shrink and mobile teeth become stable after the relatively simple procedures carried out so far. Dramatic stabilization of neighbouring teeth can follow the extraction of an infected tooth.

On the other hand, tissue response or patient cooperation may not be as satisfactory as anticipated and a reappraisal of the case will be needed.

SURGERY

The management of the surgical phase of treatment, when it is required, depends upon the size of the problem and the patient's domestic and work commitments and their physical and emotional status. Not every patient can cope with several surgical procedures under local anaesthesia over an extended period of time. Furthermore, some patients find it difficult to maintain a satisfactory level of plaque control with a surgical wound, sutures and dressings in their mouth. Therefore any necessary surgery should be carried out in as few stages as possible over as short a time as possible. The options available, i.e. local anaesthesia, general anaesthesia or local anaesthesia plus intravenous sedation, should be offered to the patient with explanations of the obvious advantages and disadvantages, so that decisions can be made which meet their individual needs.

The immediate postoperative phase must be closely supervised for the first two postoperative months, after which permanent reconstruction work can be started.

RECONSTRUCTION

This phase should include fine adjustment of the occlusion and the provision of permanent restorative and prosthetic work. In the design of restorations, subgingival preparation should be avoided, except perhaps (minimally) on the labial aspect of upper incisors, where appearance is important. Embrasure spaces, allowing easy interdental cleaning, are essential. A balanced occlusion should be constructed (Ch. 27). Any temporary splints can be removed and the need for permanent splinting can be assessed at this stage (see Ch. 28). If they have not already been made, bite-guards for persistent bruxism can be provided.

MAINTENANCE

Eternal vigilance are the watchwords of successful periodontal treatment and, in that sense, periodontal treatment is never complete. Patients require recall for inspection, oral hygiene monitoring and scaling at 3, 6, 9 or 12-month intervals, depending on their previous disease experience and susceptibility. Individual radiographs may have to be repeated if pocket measurements show that disease is progressing.

One must avoid creating a situation where the patient is totally dependent upon professional care. Some individuals are happy to abdicate responsibility for the state of their mouth to the dentist or hygienist. It is essential to make clear to the patient that in the end the patient must be responsible for his or her own dental health. It is only through a partnership that long-term dental health can be achieved.

REFERENCES

Albander JM, Buischi YA, Barbosa MF: Destructive forms of periodontal disease in adolescents. A 3 year longitudinal study, *J Periodontol* 62:370–376, 1991.

Armitage GC, Svanberg GK, Löe H: Microscopic evaluation of clinical measurements of connective tissue attachment level, *J Clin Periodontol* 4:173–190, 1977.

Benn DK: Limitations of the digital image subtraction technique in assessing alveolar bone crest changes due to misalignment errors during image capture, *Dentomaxillofac Radiol* 19:97–104, 1990.

Benn DK: A computer assisted method for making linear radiographic measurements using stored regions of interest, *J Clin Periodontol* 19:441–448, 1992.

Birek P, McCulloch CH, Hardy V: Gingival attachment level measurements with an automated periodontal probe, *J Clin Periodontol* 14:472–477, 1987.

British Society of Periodontology: Periodontology in general dental practice in the United Kingdom. In Mosedale RF, Floyd PD, Smales FC, editors: *A First Policy Statement*, London, 1986, British Society of Periodontology.

Faculty of General Dental Practitioners UK Royal College of Surgeons (FGDP, UK): *Selection Criteria for Dental Radiography*, London, 1998, FGDP(UK) Royal College of Surgeons.

Faculty of General Dental Practitioners UK Royal College of Surgeons (FGDP, UK): *Selection Criteria for Dental Radiography*, ed 2, London, 2004, FGDP(UK) Royal College of Surgeons.

Gabathuler H, Hassell T: A pressure-sensitive probe, *Helv Odontol Acta* 15:114–117, 1971.

Gibbs CH, Hirschfield JW, Lee JG, et al: Description and clinical evaluation of a new computerized periodontal probe – The Florida Probe, *J Clin Periodontol* 15:137–144, 1988.

Goodson JM, Kondon N: Periodontal pocket depth measurements by fiber optic technology, *J Clin Dent* 1:35–38, 1988.

Gröndah H-G, Gröndahl K: Subtraction radiology for the diagnosis of periodontal bone lesions, *Oral Surg Oral Med Oral Pathol* 55:208–213, 1983.

Haffajee AD, Socransky SS: Attachment level changes in destructive periodontal disease, *J Clin Periodontol* 13:461–472, 1986.

Haffajee AD, Socransky SS, Goodson JM: Comparison of different data analysis for detecting changes in attachment level, *J Clin Periodontol* 10:298–310, 1983.

Hassell TM, Germann MA, Saxer VP: Periodontal probing: investigator discrepancies and correlations between probing force and probing depth, *Helv Odontol Acta* 17:38–42, 1973.

Hirschmann PN, Horner K, Rushton VE: Selection criteria for periodontal radiography, *Br Dent J* 176:324–325, 1994.

Jeffcoat MK, Jeffcoat RL, Jens SC, et al: A new periodontal probe with an automated cement-enamel junction detection, *J Clin Periodontol* 13:276–280, 1986.

Jeffcoat MK, Jeffcoat RL, Captain K, et al: A new periodontal probe with an automated CEJ detection: clinical trials, *J Dent Res* 68:236, 1989.

Jeffcoat MK, Reddy M, Webber RL: Extraoral control of geometry for digital subtraction radiology, *J Periodontal Res* 22:396–402, 1987.

Lindhe J, Haffajee AD, Socransky SS: Progression of periodontal disease in adult subjects in the absence of periodontal therapy, *J Clin Periodontol* 10:433–442, 1983.

Listgarten MA: Periodontal probing: what does it mean? *J Clin Periodontol* 7:165–176, 1980.

Listgarten MA, Mao R, Robinson PJ: Periodontal probing and the relationship of the probe to the periodontal tissues, *J Periodontol* 47:511–513, 1976.

Löe H, Anerud A, Boysen H, et al: The natural history of periodontal disease in Man, *J Periodontol* 49:607–620, 1978.

Low SB, Taylor M, Marks RG, et al: Measuring attachment level with an electronic disk probe, *J Dent Res* 68:359, 1989.

Magnusson I, Fuller WW, Heins PJ, et al: Correlation between electronic and visual readings of pocket depth with a newly developed constant force probe, *J Clin Periodontol* 15:180–184, 1988a.

Magnusson I, Clark WB, Marks RG, et al: Attachment level measurements with a constant force electronic probe, *J Clin Periodontol* 15:185–188, 1988b.

Osborn J, Stoltenberg J, Huso B, et al: Comparison of measurement variability using a standard and constant force probe, *J Periodontol* 61:497–503, 1990.

Osborne GE, Hemmings KW. A survey of disease changes observed on panoramic tomograms of patients attending a periodontal clinic, *Br Dent J* 173:166–168, 1992.

Page RC, Schroeder HE: *Periodontitis in Man and Other Animals*, Basel, 1986, Karger.

Papapanou PN, Wennström JJ, Gröndahl K: A 10 year retrospective study of periodontal disease progression, *J Clin Periodontol* 16:403–411, 1989.

Parakkal PF: Proceedings of the workshop on quantitative evaluation of periodontal diseases by physical measuring techniques, *J Dent Res* 58:547–553, 1979.

Polson AM, Caton JG, Yeaple RN, et al: Histological determination of probe tip penetration into gingival sulcus of humans using an electronic pressure-sensitive probe, *J Clin Periodontol* 7:479–488, 1980.

Robinson PJ, Vitek RM: The relationship between gingival inflammation and resistance to probe penetration, *J Periodontal Res* 14:239–243, 1979.

Royal College of Surgeons of England, Faculty of Dental Surgery: *National Clinical Guidelines. Screening of patients to detect periodontal diseases*, London, 1997, Royal College of Surgeons of England.

Socransky SS, Haffajee AD, Goodson JM, et al: New concepts of destructive periodontal disease, *J Clin Periodontol* 11:21–32, 1984.

Tugnait A, Clerehugh V, Hirschmann PN: Use of basic periodontal examination and radiographs in the assessment of periodontal diseases in general dental practice, *J Dent* 32:17–25, 2004.

Valachovic RW, Douglass CW, Reiskin AB, et al: The use of panoramic radiography in the evaluation of asymptomatic dental patients, *Oral Surg Oral Med Oral Pathol* 61:289–296, 1986.

van der Velden U: Probing force and the relationship of the probe tip to the periodontal tissues, *J Clin Periodontol* 6:106–114, 1979.

van der Velden U, de Vries JH: Introduction of a new periodontal probe: the pressure probe, *J Clin Periodontol* 5:188–197, 1978.

Vitek RM, Robinson PJ, Lautenschlager EP: Development of a force-controlled periodontal instrument, *J Periodontal Res* 14:93–94, 1979.

Webber RL, Ruttimann UE, Gröndahl H-G: X-ray image subtraction as a basis for assessment of periodontal changes, *J Periodontal Res* 17:509–511, 1982.

FURTHER READING

Eley BM, Cox SW: Advances in periodontal diagnosis. 1. Traditional clinical methods of diagnosis, *Br Dent J* 184:12–16, 1998.

Eley BM, Cox SW: Advances in periodontal diagnosis. 2. New clinical methods of diagnosis. *Br Dent J* 184:71–74, 1998.

14 Diagnosis tests of periodontal disease activity

THE RELATIONSHIP OF BACTERIA, SALIVA AND GINGIVAL CREVICULAR FLUID COMPONENTS TO PERIODONTAL DISEASE AND THEIR POSSIBLE USE IN DIAGNOSTIC TESTS

One of the liveliest areas of current periodontal research is concerned with the search for diagnostic tests of periodontal disease activity. These tests have potential relevance to both diagnosis and treatment because current clinical diagnostic methods are not precisely accurate and only allow retrospective diagnosis of attachment loss. To improve on this, however, diagnostic tests would need to be predictive of disease activity rather than just correlate with its occurrence.

Potential biomarkers of disease activity would need to be involved in the disease process in some way and therefore need to undergo extensive and careful basic research investigation before undergoing clinical evaluation. Only when the source, precise nature and the role of the potential marker are known and understood can clinical evaluation be meaningful.

THE PROCESS OF DEVELOPING A PREDICTIVE DIAGNOSTIC TEST

The first consideration is to determine from which source the potential marker should be obtained. Four potential sources are possible:

- Blood or serum
- Saliva.

(Markers from both these sources relate to either the whole patient or the whole mouth.)

- Subgingival plaque sample
- Gingival crevicular fluid (GCF).

(Markers from these sources would relate to the condition of the local periodontal site.) The methods of obtaining these samples are described below.

Periodontal disease progression is site specific and episodic in nature and reflects individual patient susceptibility (see Ch. 13). Since factors in the blood relate to the whole patient they are unlikely to be able to diagnose local site activity. Factors in saliva either come from the salivary glands or the oral flora or from GCF and relate to the whole mouth rather than a local site. They are therefore also very unlikely to be able to help in diagnosing local periodontal activity. At best they could give some information on the patients overall periodontal condition. Therefore factors from subgingival plaque samples or GCF are most likely to give information on local site activity.

Development of a predictive test based on any of the factors discussed in this section requires a combination of basic and applied research over a long time scale and the stages are listed below.

1. Basic research
   - Separation and characterization
   - Investigation of tissue chemistry
   - Investigation of its sources in the periodontal tissue
   - Investigation of its role in the microbiology or pathology of chronic periodontitis

   - Development of a selective and sensitive assay system
   - If GCF samples are to be used then verification is necessary that gingival tissue or bacterial components are the same as those found in GCF.
2. Applied clinical research
   - Ligature induced periodontitis in animals
   - Experimental gingivitis in humans
   - Natural disease process.

Investigations on the natural disease process involve:

- Cross-sectional studies of its relationship to disease severity
- Study of the levels before and after successful periodontal treatment
- Longitudinal studies of its relationship to attachment and bone loss
- Development of simplified test system for chairside use
- Comparison of this simplified system with full laboratory analysis
- Clinical trial using test system.

Each of these stages is detailed below.

BASIC RESEARCH

Separation and characterization

The factor under investigation must first be separated from the complex mixture of substances present in the sampled material. This usually involves a variety of chemical, biochemical, immunochemical or microbiological separation techniques.

Second, the precise nature of the factor must be determined. Tissue factors present in the periodontal tissues or GCF need to be characterized by biochemical or immunocytochemical techniques whilst bacteria need to be speciated by biochemical, immunochemical or genetic techniques.

Third, a number of other factors present in the collection medium may interfere with the detection of the factor under investigation and these interfering factors must be identified and controlled. An example of this might be the presence of natural inhibitors to enzymes under investigation in GCF or blood which may interfere with its detection. Another might be the fastidious growth requirements required by most of the bacteria in subgingival plaque which might interfere with their survival during collection, transport or culture.

Investigation of tissue chemistry

Many factors present in the periodontal tissues pass into GCF in the inflammatory exudate. Before these factors can be assessed their precise biochemical functions in the tissues must be known. For instance, if the factor is an enzyme its normal substrate(s) (i.e. the molecule(s) that the enzyme attacks and cleaves) must be investigated. Its precise mode of action and the precise site(s) of cleavage of the substrate need to be known. Also its requirements for activity, i.e. its pH optimum and the need for co-factors or activators, must be studied. Finally, the normal control mechanisms for the enzyme, e.g. its natural inhibitors need to be investigated.

Investigation of its sources in the periodontal tissue

The precise location of the factor in the periodontal tissues must be studied. For example, the cellular source(s) and precise intracellular location of enzymes in the periodontal tissues need to be determined.

Investigation of its role in the microbiology or pathology of chronic periodontitis

The possible role(s) of the potential marker in periodontal pathology need to be studied. Examples of this would be the association of particular subgingival bacteria with periodontal disease progression and investigations of the ways in which bacterial products could potentially damage the tissues. Another example would be an investigation of the possible role of potential tissue enzyme markers to degrade the various gingival and periodontal tissue components.

Development of a selective and sensitive assay system

The assay system developed to detect a marker must be sensitive, i.e. it must detect the factor in low concentrations in the source material. Also, it must be highly selective, i.e. it should detect the factor in question but should not detect any interfering factors in the source material. An example of this would occur in the detection of enzymes in GCF. A particular substrate used in the assay system might be cleaved by a number of enzymes including the one in question. In this situation the assay system may be made selective by controlling the assay conditions by the inclusion of an appropriate buffer to control the pH, appropriate activators of the enzyme in question and selective inhibitors of the interfering enzymes.

Verification that gingival tissue or bacterial components are the same as those found in gingival crevicular fluid or saliva

If GCF or saliva comprise the source material for the marker then it must first be confirmed that the factor assayed in these sources is the same as that found in the periodontal tissues. This is usually done by careful biochemical investigations of extracts from the periodontal tissues and identical investigations of the factor in GCF or saliva so that their characteristics can be compared.

APPLIED CLINICAL RESEARCH

All of these studies should be blind, i.e. the levels of the marker must be unknown to the clinician carrying out the clinical measurements and vice versa and this must apply until completion of the study. It is also preferable that the clinician carrying out the clinical measurements, usually in duplicate, should be unaware of the measurements recorded at each site. This can be arranged with the use of electronic probes since the values are measured by the computer and displayed on the screen for recording. This screen can be turned away from the clinician and displayed only to the recording dental nurse. Alternatively, they can be stored in the computers memory and printed out later.

Ligature induced periodontitis in animals

Periodontal pockets can be artificially produced in animals, usually dogs, by the placement of silk ligatures into the gingival crevice. The ligatures accumulate plaque and its growth is promoted by giving the animal a soft diet. The ligatures are forced down apically at 2-week intervals for 16–20 weeks. The ligatures detach the junctional epithelium from the tooth and promote inflammation. As a result of this process attachment is rapidly lost and true periodontal pockets form and progressively deepen. Corresponding bone loss also occurs.

The procedure is usually performed on the molars and premolars on one side of the jaw(s) and the other side(s) is/are left alone to serve as the control side(s). Also, the control side is usually given oral hygiene to induce gingival health. The period that the ligatures remain *in situ* is classified as the disease progression phase. After the planned period, usually 16–20 weeks, the ligatures are removed and scaling and root planing are performed to promote the resolution of inflammation. Oral hygiene is also given 3 times/week over the next 8 weeks, which is classified as the disease recovery phase.

This model is usually used for short longitudinal studies spanning the 16–20 weeks of disease progression and the 8 weeks of disease resolution. The levels of the marker are compared at test and control sites both during the disease progression and the disease recovery phases. Pocket depths are measured by manual or electronic probing and bone loss by radiographical techniques. Samples of GCF are collected on strips every 2 weeks before the ligatures are displaced further apically during the disease progression phase and at 2-week intervals in the disease recovery phase.

Experimental gingivitis in humans

Experimental gingivitis is induced in subjects with perfect gingival and periodontal health. These subjects must have no signs of attachment loss and gingival health is enhanced by intensive oral hygiene instruction and any necessary scaling prior to the short experimental period. The point at which full gingival health is obtained serves as the baseline. Gingivitis is then induced over a 10–21 day period by ceasing all oral hygiene procedures and allowing plaque to accumulate. After 10–21 days, oral hygiene procedures are reinstated and the gingivitis resolves over the next 7–10 days. Levels of the marker in GCF is compared at varying time periods from baseline both during the gingivitis promotion phase and the resolution phase.

Experimental gingivitis can also be induced locally by using an acrylic shield to cover the test teeth during oral hygiene procedures. Normal oral hygiene is then carried out with the shield in place which prevents plaque removal in the test (covered) area. The levels of marker can then also be compared at test and control sites during the experimental period.

THE NATURAL DISEASE PROCESS

In these studies, samples of the marker are collected from gingival crevice sites in patients with varying stages of chronic periodontitis.

Cross-sectional studies of marker's relationship to disease severity

Subjects for these studies are usually patients with varying levels of chronic periodontitis ranging from early to advanced chronic periodontitis. They need to have all of their teeth or at least all their functional molar and premolar teeth. GCF or bacterial samples are taken from all the test sites at one time period for each patient, which could be different for any of the other patients.

Levels of the marker (total amounts and concentrations in the case of GCF constituents) are then compared with measurements and indices of disease severity and tested for significance by appropriate statistical tests. The usual measurements of disease severity are probing depth (PD), probing attachment level (PAL) (probing depth from a fixed reference point) and radiographical measurements of bone loss (see Ch. 13). Indices of gingivitis severity, gingival index (GI) (Löe 1967) and gingival bleeding index (GBI) (Barnett et al 1980) and plaque levels, plaque index (Pl.I) (Löe 1967), are also often compared. Since these studies only relate to one point in time of the disease process they can only relate to disease severity at that point in time and give no indication of disease progression. Twenty or more patients are required for these studies for statistical purposes.

Studies of marker levels before and after successful periodontal treatment

These studies usually require patients who have not recently had any periodontal treatment. They need to have varying levels of chronic periodontitis ranging from early to advanced chronic periodontitis. The subjects need to have all or most of their teeth. Samples are taken at baseline before any measurements are made. Then PD and PAL are measured and GI, GBI and Pl.I are scored. The patients then receive a full course of periodontal treatment consisting of oral hygiene instruction and supra- and subgingival scaling and root planing. At 4–8 weeks after the completion of this treatment the samples are taken again and the measurements and indices are repeated.

The levels of the marker (total amounts and concentrations in the case of GCF constituents) are compared before and after treatment and the success of the treatment is measured by similar comparisons of PD, PAL, GI, GBI and Pl.I. All the comparisons are tested for significance by an appropriate statistical test. These studies indicate whether or not the levels of the marker reduce following disease resolution. They do not, however, relate the marker to disease progression which is the function of longitudinal studies.

Longitudinal studies of its relationship to attachment and bone loss

If a potential marker is to be of any use clinically then it must be capable of *predicting* future periodontal attachment loss and this is definitively tested in a carefully constructed longitudinal study of chronic periodontitis patients. In these studies, the level of a marker has to be shown to correlate with confirmed attachment loss not only at the time that loss is recorded but also at a visit before this (i.e. the predictive time).

The number of patients taking part in such a study must be sufficient for meaningful statistical comparisons and is usually between 25 and 75. They need to be carefully chosen with regard to the extent and distribution of their periodontal lesions. They should have all or most of their teeth and a good distribution of moderate/advanced chronic periodontitis lesions. The test teeth are usually the molars and premolars since the disease on these teeth is more likely to progress. The patients should be fit and well and should not be taking any medication, including antibiotics. They should preferably not smoke and the patient group should be balanced for age and sex.

Patients receive standard periodontal treatment, i.e. oral hygiene instruction, supra- and subgingival scaling and root planning, prior to the baseline examination visit. At this visit samples of the marker are first collected from GCF or subgingival plaque and then careful clinical measurements are taken from the chosen sites of the test teeth of probing depth (PD) and attachment level (PAL) from a fixed reproducible point. In addition, gingival and plaque indices are usually scored (Barnett et al 1980; Löe 1967). Also the first set of serial radiographs are usually taken to record the alveolar bone levels. In order for serial radiographs to be comparable, the film to tooth position and tube geometry must be carefully controlled. This will allow meaningful comparisons of serial films (see Ch. 13). Radiographs are usually taken at yearly intervals in a 2-year study.

The patients are then usually monitored every 3 months over the period of the study which can be for anything from 6 months to 2 years. Longer studies give more useful results. At each of these visits, further samples of the marker are taken and the clinical measurements are repeated. The patients are monitored for significant changes in attachment and bone levels and these need to be confirmed to be above the threshold for the method of measurement used.

Assessment of attachment loss

Attachment level change between two points in time is usually assessed retrospectively at the completion of the study by the tolerance method (Haffajee & Socransky 1986). Duplicate measurements of PAL are taken at each time point to calculate examiner error. The standard deviation (SD) of the duplicate measurements at each site, at the first and second time points, are pooled to provide the site SD. The difference between all duplicate measurements for all the test sites within each patient are used to compute the patient SD. Patient SDs are then averaged to produce a population SD. For the mean of the second of a pair of attachment level measurements to be considered significantly different from the mean of the first pair, then the attachment level change needs to exceed:

1. The population threshold which was 2 population SDs
2. The patient threshold which was 3 patient SDs
3. The site threshold which was 3 site SDs.

Measurements of PAL and PD in these studies are usually made with electronic, constant pressure probes (see Ch. 13) which are capable of more reliable measurements. These probes have measurement thresholds of 0.3–0.8 mm compared with 3 mm for manual periodontal probing.

Radiographical measurements

Assessment of progressive bone loss can be made from careful measurements of carefully controlled serial films using conventional radiography (see Ch. 13). A change of 1 mm or more is usually taken as significant. Alternatively, computer-aided systems, such as digital subtraction radiology or computer-assisted linear radiography (see Ch. 13) may be used which are capable of recording smaller changes.

Statistical comparisons

Two types of attachment loss have been identified (Jeffcoat & Reddy 1991) (see also Ch. 8) and these are:

- Rapid, episodic attachment loss (RAL)
- Gradual attachment loss (GAL).

Both types may be identified in longitudinal studies using electronic probes with small measurement thresholds and in this case both types can be compared with the marker. Markers tend to produce better associations with RAL than GAL because of the nature of their temporal patterns.

The levels of the marker must be unknown to the researcher making the attachment level measurements so that the study is blind. Using electronic probes, the attachment level measurements may also be made blind to the clinician since they can be recorded from the computer screen turned away from the clinician making the measurements.

Statistical comparisons are made at the end of the study at both site and patient levels using both total amounts and concentrations of the marker. Site level comparisons can be made between paired attachment loss and non-attachment loss sites. In this case control and test teeth must be of the same type and must have very closely similar baseline clinical measurements. These comparisons are ideal because the sites are paired in the same patient and are independent of patient level influences. The alternative is to pool the attachment loss sites and non-attachment loss sites separately and then to compare them with complex statistical techniques. This situation is fraught with difficulties in trying to compensate for huge numerical imbalances and for patient-related effects (Sterne et al 1990). Because of these factors, they need to use multilayer analyses of variance which are highly complicated. Also, in such a system it is impossible to know the degree of weighting to give to the various patient effects and therefore this can never be precise. For these reasons, comparisons of test and control sites, paired in each patient are to be preferred. The site comparisons must be made at both the time of attachment loss and the predictive time.

Both RAL and GAL sites can be compared in this way but the determination of the predictive time is very difficult with GAL sites because of the long time scale of slow progressive attachment loss. It is probably best to base the statistical comparisons with GAL sites on either the highest value at the GAL site during the study or on its mean level over the whole period of the study. Also a critical value (CV) for diagnostic testing (see below) is much more difficult to assign for GAL sites but could again be based either on an average of the highest values at these sites or an average of their mean levels over the time period of the study. However, it is doubtful if markers are as well suited to the detection of GAL lesions as they may be for RAL lesions.

In addition, the diagnostic efficiency of the marker needs to be tested using 2×2 contingency tables (**Fig. 14.1**). First, a critical value (CV) for the marker has to be determined: one for total amount of the marker and one for its concentration as both need to be tested. They should also be tested at both the attachment loss time and the prediction time. The number of true positive (sites correctly diagnosed as RAL sites by the CV), false positive (sites incorrectly diagnosed as RAL sites by CV), true negative (sites correctly diagnosed as non-attachment loss sites by the CV) and false negative sites (sites incorrectly diagnosed as non-attachment loss sites by the CV) over the course of the study are determined using this value and entered into the 2×2 table. This data is then used to calculate the sensitivity, specificity and positive and negative prediction values as shown in **Figure 14.1**.

All these values should be very high using CVs for both total amount and concentration of the marker and this should be the case at both the attachment loss time and the prediction time for the marker to be clinically useful. However, it is the values at the prediction time which will determine whether or not the marker is capable of predicting periodontal disease activity.

The most important values are the positive and negative prediction values as they determine whether the CV for the marker can correctly distinguish between true RAL sites and true non-attachment loss sites. The positive prediction value represents the percentage of RAL sites correctly identified by the CV of the marker and the negative prediction value the percentage of non-attachment sites correctly identified by the CV of the marker. Both need to be high but the negative prediction value needs to be close to 100% since diagnosing a RAL site as a non-attachment site would result in under-treatment and hence progression of disease at this site. On the other hand misdiagnosing a few non-attachment sites as RAL sites would result in slight over treatment which would not harm the patient.

In addition, patient level comparisons can back up these findings. In this regard, comparisons of the mean levels in attachment loss and non-attachment loss patients give some indication of patient level effects and also give some indication of patient susceptibility.

Development of a simplified test system for chairside use

Potential markers are usually detected by laboratory assays in the clinical studies and these need to be modified to produce an assay system suitable for use in a dental surgery. This involves producing a test kit system which involves no specialized equipment and is easy to read. In this last regard, colour detection systems are usually preferred.

If the sample is collected with a strip (e.g. GCF) it is preferable that this is uncontaminated by reaction chemicals which could be irritant, toxic, carcinogenic or allergenic to the patient. It is important that any chemicals used in the reaction are in clearly and simply labelled plastic containers from which it is easy to dispense the correct amount.

Most enzyme linked immunosorbent assay (ELISA) systems and biochemical and histochemical reactions utilizing simple substrates (see below) are easy to scale down in this way and most commercially available diagnostic kits involve one of these systems. More complicated assay systems are difficult or impossible to scale down and this may preclude some potentially good markers from being used clinically. Some systems using molecular biological techniques such as DNA test kits for putative periodontal pathogens (see below) involve taking a subgingival plaque sample, transferring this to a transport medium and then mailing this to the laboratory for analysis. These are obviously not as convenient as chairside test systems. The details of available commercial kit systems are provided in the relevant parts of this chapter.

Comparison of this system with the laboratory analysis

When the assay system is scaled down to a kit form, it is usually only capable of semi-quantitative analysis and it is necessary to compare the diagnostic accuracy of this system with the full laboratory quantitative analytical system in order to check that the results are closely similar.

Clinical trial

Potential markers which have produced good cross-sectional and longitudinal study results and appear to be capable of predicting periodontal disease activity in research at one centre usually progress to a multicentre trial at several independent centres to see whether their results are comparable. This may either be carried out with the full laboratory quantitative analytical system or the kit form with semi-quantitative analysis. If the results of these trials are good then the diagnostic kit may then be tested in the normal clinical environment with a clinical trial in dental practice.

All of these factors should be taken into account in assessing the potential of a new marker system and should also be used in the assessment of the evidence for the potential markers described below.

THE MAIN CANDIDATES FOR BIOMARKERS

The main candidates in the search for biomarkers have been:

- Bacteria and their products
- Inflammatory and immune products
- Enzymes released from dead cells
- Connective tissue degradation products
- Products of bone resorption.

These will each be considered separately below.

MICROBIOLOGICAL MARKERS

Bacterial plaque plays a primary role in the initiation and progression of periodontal diseases but the composition of the subgingival flora is complex and may vary from patient to patient and site to site. Despite these differences

	Disease present	Disease absent	
Positive test	a True positive	b False positive	Positive predictive value $a/(a + b)$
Negative test	c False negative	d True negative	Negative predictive value $d/(c + d)$
	Sensitivity $a/(a + c)$	Specificity $d/(b + d)$	

Fig. 14.1 Diagnostic testing of critical values of potential markers using 2×2 contingency tables.

and the complex interactions that exist between bacteria and the host, a number of possible pathogens have been suggested on the basis of their association with disease progression, animal pathogenicity and their possession of virulence factors which could damage the tissues (Genco et al 1988; Listgarten 1992; Socransky & Haffajee 1992). The main bacteria are shown below and are more fully discussed in Chapters 2 and 4.

Bacterial associated with periodontal diseases

Porphyromonas gingivalis
Prevotella intermedia
Bacteroides forsythus
Aggregatibacter actinomycetemcomitans
Capnocytophaga ochracea
Eikenella corrodens
Campylobacter (previously *Wolinella*) *recta*
Fusobacterium nucleatum
Treponema denticola

These are commensal bacteria which may be present in the gingival crevice or periodontal pocket, in saliva or on the surface of the oral mucosa. There is no evidence for any one specific pathogen in chronic periodontitis and therefore it may be considered as a non-specific bacterial disease (Theilade 1986). The bacteria listed above tend to be present in higher numbers at active disease sites (Socransky & Haffajee 1992) and in some cases their products are capable of damaging the tissues either directly or indirectly. However, they may also be present in healthy and inactive sites and the composition of all these sites may vary between patients or even in the same patient. Furthermore, the composition of the pocket depends on many factors including the presence of essential nutrients, the redox potential and the effects of the host defence mechanisms and these considerations limit the value of diagnostic tests based on bacteria.

Attempts to relate microbiological data to clinical events are complicated by the technical problems associated with sampling and culturing.

Obtaining a bacterial sample

Samples from the oral mucosa or saliva are obtained with sterile paper points or swabs and then transferred directly into an appropriate anaerobic transport medium. In order to obtain a true sample of subgingival plaque, it is first necessary to remove all traces of supragingival plaque which would otherwise contaminate the sample. The subgingival sample can then be removed either with a fresh, clean and sterile curette or with a sterile paper point. This is then rapidly transferred to the anaerobic transport medium. It is vitally important not to touch any other surface in making this transfer, since this would also contaminate the sample with unwanted bacteria. The wearing of a fresh mask is also necessary for the same reasons.

Virtually all the subgingival bacteria are anaerobic and therefore exposure to the air should be minimal. The anaerobic environment of the transport medium is also necessary for this reason and it should also contain all the necessary nutrients for the particular bacteria in question. The nature of the investigation or test will dictate all the other details.

The relationship of bacteria to periodontal disease progression

A microbiologically based diagnostic system should identify one or more primary pathogens responsible for the disease (Listgarten 1992). It is, however, impossible to determine in a particular patient which bacteria in the subgingival flora are causing periodontal disease and it seems likely that many species may be involved at different stages of the disease. Nevertheless, some bacterial species have been considered by some workers as markers of disease because of their association with sites with progressive attachment loss. However, it must be appreciated that these bacteria are not always present in all such sites and may also be present at stable sites.

Most oral bacteria can be cultured from saliva including the putative periodontal pathogens *A. actinomycetemcomitans*, *P. gingivalis*, *Prevotella intermedia*, *P. nigrescens*, *C. recta*, *E. corrodens*, *F. nucleatum*, *Capnocytophaga* species and spirochaetes (Van Os et al 1986; Frisken et al 1987; Chen et al 1989; Asikainen et al 1991; Muller et al 1997; Von Triol-Linden et al 1995, 1997; Timmerman et al 1998). Their presence and numbers in saliva were shown to reflect their presence and numbers in periodontal pockets in one study (Timmerman et al 1998) but not in another (Muller et al 1997). The numbers of these bacteria in saliva increase with age and are rare in children and healthy young adults and frequent in patients with chronic periodontitis (Matto et al 1996, 1998). In chronic periodontitis patients the numbers of particular bacterial species in saliva have been shown to correlate with clinical parameters of disease severity and to significantly decrease following periodontal treatment (Von Triol-Linden et al 1995). Specific IgA and IgG antibodies are present in saliva to all these bacteria (Nieminen et al 1996).

There is accumulated evidence that the predominant microflora of the periodontal pocket at possible active sites, i.e. those which have shown significant attachment and bone loss within short time intervals, is characterized by the presence of *Porphyromonas gingivalis*, *Prevotella intermedia*, *B. forsythus*, *Peptostreptococcus micros*, *Campylobacter recta*, *F. nucleatum* and *A. actinomycetemcomitans* (Tanner et al 1984; Slots et al 1985, 1986; Dzink et al 1985, 1988; Moore et al 1991). Furthermore, retrospective studies (Slots et al 1986; Bragd et al 1987; Wennström et al 1987; Slots & Listgarten 1988) have suggested that microbiological assays for critical levels of the target bacteria *A. actinomycetemcomitans*, *Porphyromonas gingivalis* and *Prevotella intermedia* at subgingival sites might be of diagnostic value. However, it should be noted that in these studies the samples were taken after breakdown had occurred and although they showed an association between the number of these bacteria and previous attachment loss at the site they were not shown to be predictive of future attachment loss. In another retrospective study (Schmidt et al 1988), a group of 23 untreated and 13 maintenance patients were monitored with the BANA test. They reported selectivity and sensitivity values of 83% for negative and positive tests in the untreated patients. However, the values were much lower on maintained patients and were not diagnostic. Although these studies showed the ability of this test to correctly identify sites pre-defined as healthy or diseased they were not predictive of future periodontal breakdown.

Molecular based methods of detecting individual bacterial species are both very specific and very sensitive (see below). Kawada et al (2004) performed quantitative analyses of *Porphyromonas gingivalis* using the TaqMan real-time PCR system in order to clarify the relationship between the numbers of this organism and periodontal status. They found a significant positive correlation ($p<0.0001$) between the number of *P. gingivalis* and pocket depth and the slope of the regression line indicated that for every 1 mm increase in pocket depth, the number of *P. gingivalis* increased 10-fold. They also found a significant reduction ($p<0.01$) in the numbers of *P. gingivalis* before and after treatment. Their results seem to suggest that the absolute and relative numbers of *P. gingivalis* are closely associated with periodontal status. These techniques may therefore have the potential to clarify this issue.

However, quantitative PCRs represent a field of continuous development, but it is still not the ideal diagnostic to study the subgingival microflora and it is still hampered by the limited information it provides (Sanz et al 2004). Quantitative PCR is still in development; however, the promising early results reported are hampered by the high cost and equipment necessary. Quantitative PCR technology may have a major role in the future as an adjunctive diagnostic tool in both epidemiological and clinical studies in periodontology. However, culture techniques still hold some inherent capabilities, which makes this diagnostic tool the current reference standard in periodontal microbiology.

The numbers of spirochaetes and motile bacteria have been shown to predict future periodontal attachment loss in a 1-year prospective study of patients on maintenance following treatment for periodontitis when no treatment was carried out in the test period (Listgarten & Levin 1981). However, they were not predictive when patients were scaled every 3 months during a 3-year study (Listgarten et al 1986). Furthermore, when *A. actinomycetemcomitans, P. gingivalis* and *Prevotella intermedia* were tested as predictors of future periodontal attachment loss in a similar 3-year study of patients on regular maintenance they were not shown to have any diagnostic potential (Listgarten et al 1991).

Numbers of bacterial species may be determined in a variety of ways (Listgarten 1992) and these include:

Darkground or phase contrast microscopy

The main advantage of these techniques is the ability to count all the bacteria in the sample. The main drawbacks are the inability to speciate microorganisms. However, studies using these techniques have shown that in gingival health there is a scant subgingival flora of cocci and non-motile rods, while in gingivitis there is the appearance of motile rods and spirochaetes and in periodontitis a vast increase in these morphotypes with particularly large numbers of spirochaetes (Listgarten & Levin 1981; Listgarten 1986).

Culture techniques

These techniques are able to analyse the nature of the microorganisms in a sample, since they can be speciated with a variety of laboratory-based methods including selective sub-cultures, biochemical tests, SDS PAGE, gene probes, ribotyping, DNA fingerprinting and cell-wall long chain fatty acid analysis (Genco et al 1986; Greenstein 1988). However, not all bacteria can be readily cultured and the proportional recovery of cultivable species is unlikely to match their proportions in the periodontal pocket. Also, the use of selective media will restrict the species that are able to grow (Mandell & Socransky 1981).

Immunological assays

The use of immunological techniques such as immunofluorescence (Zambon et al 1985b; Zambon et al 1986) or enzyme linked immunosorbent assay, ELISA (Ebersole et al 1984) can detect individual bacterial species. These have proved useful to detect the presence and relative proportions of selected bacterial species. These techniques use specific antibodies which bind to the selected bacterial antigens and are then detected by labelling the primary antibody directly with a fluorescent marker (direct immunofluorescence) (**Fig. 14.2A**) or with a fluorescent secondary antibody (indirect immunofluorescence) (**Fig. 14.2B**). In the ELISA assay

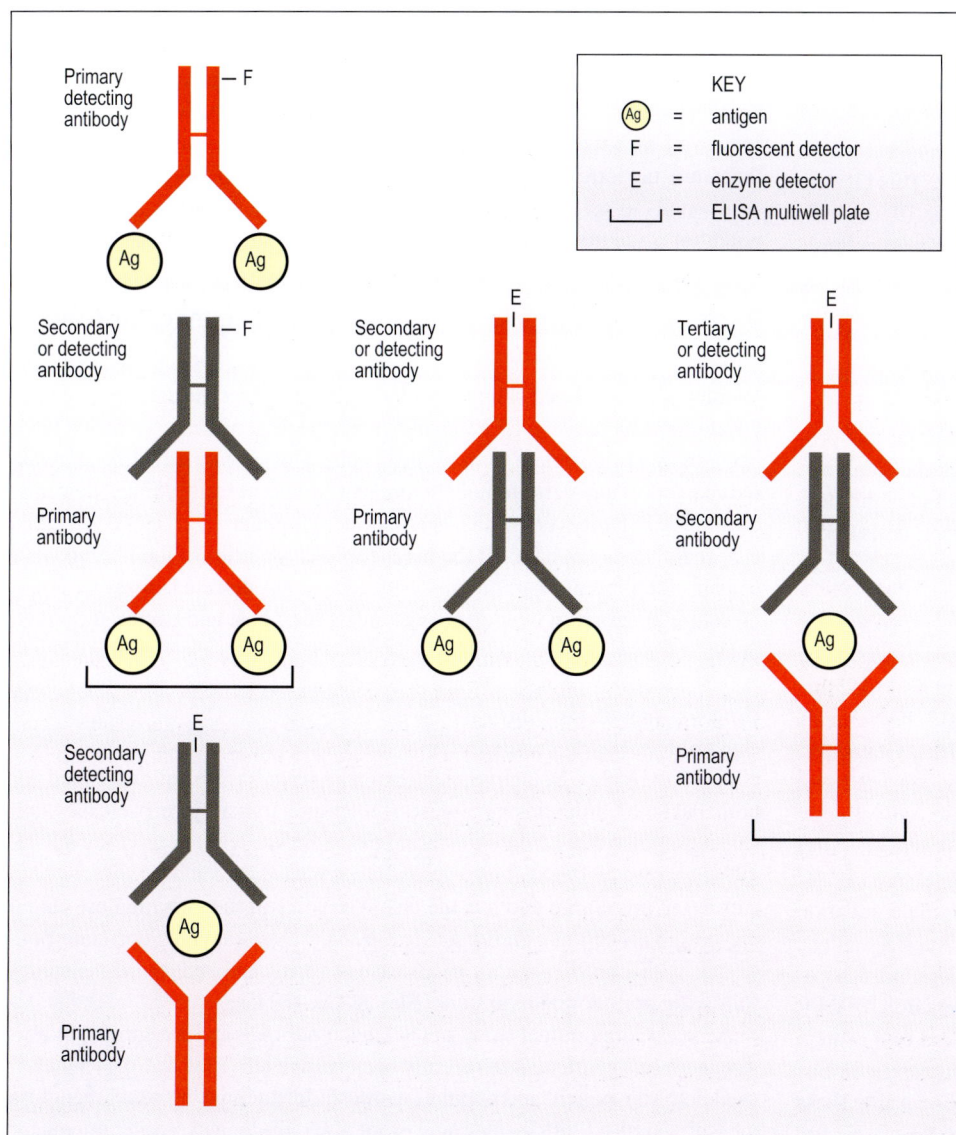

Fig. 14.2 Diagram showing the basis of: (top) direct immunofluorescence, (middle) an enzyme-linked immunosorbent (ELISA) assay (left); indirect ELISA (centre); with third detecting antibody (right) and (bottom) indirect immunofluorescence using a secondary antibody. In ELISA techniques, the detecting antibody is linked to an enzyme, usually horseradish peroxidase or alkaline phosphatase, which catalyses a chain reaction that generates colour.

(Fig. 14.2C), the primary antibody is detected through a colorimetric reaction which is catalysed through an enzyme, either horseradish peroxidase or alkaline phosphatase, linked to the antibody. These techniques are very specific if controls are used to check for non-specific reactions. They can only detect species for which an antibody is available.

DNA probes

DNA probes have been developed to identify nucleotide sequences that are specific for bacteria believed to be of diagnostic significance (Highfield & Dougan 1985), including suspected periodontal pathogens (French et al 1986; Savitt et al 1988; Loesche 1992). These probes can detect as few as 103 cells in a sample and provide information on the presence of selected species in the sample. However, they cannot provide reliable quantitative data and are limited by the availability of probes. They are totally specific and it is possible for a species to be present in large numbers in the sample and not be detected because it was not specifically sought.

A commercial PCR-based method for the detection of periodontopathic species in subgingival plaque samples (MicroDent® test) has been shown to be quicker, easier to use and much more sensitive than culture methods. It employs probes for *Porphyromonas gingivalis, Prevotella intermedia, B. forsythus, A. actinomycetemcomitans* and *T. denticola* (Eick & Pfister 2002).

Enzyme-based assays

BANA assays

Another approach to the detection of selected bacterial species is to look for an enzyme which is unique to one or more of the relevant bacterial species. The plaque sample is exposed to a substrate that can only be hydrolysed by a specific enzyme. An example of this method is the detection of the trypsin-like protease produced mainly by *Porphyromonas gingivalis* and to a much lesser extent by *B. forsythus* and *T. denticola*. This cleaves the benzyl arginine naphthylamide, BANA substrate (Loesche 1986, 1992; Loesche et al 1990). Since some of these species grow poorly in cultures and account for a significant proportion of the protease activity of the subgingival flora, these enzyme assays provide a rapid and inexpensive method of screening samples of these bacteria.

The main drawbacks are a lack of quantitative data and the inability to determine which of the three bacteria are responsible for the enzyme production. In most cases, however, this will be *P. gingivalis* since this produces much more of this protease than the two other bacteria combined (Gazi et al 1994, 1996). Also the BANA system does not include inhibitors of host proteinases which could cleave this substrate and could also contaminate the bacterial sample tested (Cox & Eley 1989).

Quantitative fluorescence polarization

Molecules tagged with a fluorescent label emit fluorescent light in the same polarized plane when excited with plane polarized light provided that the molecule remains stationary throughout the excited state. Instruments (FPM-1TM FP analyser, Jolley Consulting and Research Inc., Grayslake, IL) have been developed to measure this in real-time (Schade et al 1996; Jolley 1996). Labelled proteins have enough mass to rotate only slightly and the emitted light which is measured from them remains polarized. After addition of proteolytic enzymes the millipolarization value (mP) drops with time since the labelled small molecules which result from degradation produce enough kinetic movement to depolarize the light and thus reduce the mP value. A fluorescent moiety 4, 4′ difluoro-5, 7-dimethyl-4-boro-3a, 4a-diaza-s-indacene-3-propionic acid, succinimidyl ester (BODIPY FL C3-SE, Molecular Probes-Inc. – BODIPY®) has been linked to a protein substrate, bovine casein, to produce a suitable fluorescent substrate for this purpose (Schade et al 1996; Jolley 1996) and they have shown that these assays can be carried out in the presence of whole bacteria.

This method has been used to detect *Mycobacterium bovis* extracellular protein (Lin et al 1996) and could be adapted to quantitatively measure proteins or proteases from plaque bacteria.

Volatile sulphur compounds

Volatile sulphur compounds such as hydrogen sulphide, H_2S, methyl mercaptan, CH_3SH, dimethyl sulphide $(CH_3)_2S$ and dimethyl disulphide $(CH_3)_2S_2$ are all toxic by-products of Gram-negative anaerobic bacterial metabolism of sulphur containing amino acids (see Ch. 5). *P. gingivalis, Prevotella intermedia, P. melaninogenica, B. forsythus, T. denticola* and *F. nucleatum* have all been shown to be capable of producing them through their metabolic pathways (Persson et al 1989, 1990c).

A recently developed commercially available instrument, Diamond Probe/Perio 2000 System® (Diamond General Development Corporation, Ann Arbor, USA) has been designed so that it combines the features of a periodontal probe with the detection of volatile sulphur compounds in the periodontal pocket.

It has been found that the levels of volatile sulphur compounds in the periodontal pocket are higher in chronic periodontitis patients than healthy controls (Yaegaki & Sanda 1992a,b). A number of other studies have also indicated that sulphide levels are higher in deeper pockets than shallow ones and decrease when pockets are surgically reduced (Horowitz & Folke 1972; Yaegaki & Sanda 1992a,b). The sulphide readings of the probe have also been shown to relate to clinical parameters of disease severity (Polychronopoulou 1998). However, clinical relevance of these results was hampered by the poor sensitivity of the probe at the low and high ranges of its scale. This resulted in the majority of the readings at both apparently healthy and diseased sites being zero. This sensitivity would need to be improved for this instrument to be suitable for clinical use. Furthermore, there are no longitudinal studies of the relationship of volatile sulphur compounds to periodontal disease progression and therefore its diagnostic potential is unknown.

Bacterial proteases in saliva and gingival crevicular fluid

Saliva

Whole, non-stimulated saliva samples are required for the detection of bacterial enzymes in saliva. The levels of trypsin-like protease in saliva have been shown to correlate with clinical indices of disease severity and also reduce following periodontal treatment (Zambon et al 1985a; Nieminen et al 1993). However, it has been shown (Ingman et al 1993) that this enzyme(s) does not have all the biochemical properties of the *P. gingivalis* trypsin-like protease (gingipain). The enzyme(s) detected in saliva could therefore be either of host origin or a mixture of host and bacterial derived enzymes.

Gingival crevicular fluid

Bacterial proteases are released into the pocket and can be detected in GCF (Cox et al 1989a). Selective biochemical assays have been developed for both bacterial dipeptidylpeptidase (DPP) and trypsin-like proteases and can distinguish them from interfering tissue-derived proteases (Eley & Cox 1994; Gazi et al 1995). The trypsin-like protease detected by this assay is a cysteine proteinase and has the characteristics of the enzyme now called arg-gingipain or arg-gingivain (see Ch. 5). These enzymes correlate positively with clinical indices of disease severity and reduce significantly following periodontal treatment (Eley & Cox 1995a).

A 2-year longitudinal study of GCF bacterial DPP and arg-gingivain/arg-gingipain in 75 patients has recently been completed (Eley & Cox 1996a). It used both site, patient and population thresholds for probing attachment loss measured with a Florida electronic probe and radiological measurements for confirmed progressive attachment loss. All clinical parameters and enzyme levels significantly reduced following basic periodontal treatment prior to baseline. Over the 2 years, there were 124 sites in 49 patients with confirmed attachment loss giving an annual rate of 5.17% of sites. A total of 91 of these sites in 36 patients were rapid episodic attachment loss (RAL) and 33 sites in 22 patients showed gradual progressive attachment loss over a longer time period (GAL). Levels above critical values chosen for both pro teases for total enzyme activities and enzyme concentrations were present at all RAL sites both at the time of attachment loss and 3 months previously (predictive time). They were all significantly higher than values at control sites in the same patients. These levels were also shown to be predictive of attachment loss in diagnostic testing. In this regard, the values for arg-gingivain were somewhat higher overall than those for bacterial DPP. The values for arg-gingivain were 100% (sensitivity) and 99.93% (specificity) for both total enzyme activity and enzyme concentration. The values for bacterial DPP were 100% (sensitivity) and 99.54% (specificity) for total enzyme activity and 100% (sensitivity) and 99.57% (specificity) for enzyme concentration. The differences can be more clearly seen in the positive and negative predictive values calculated in these tests for the two bacterial proteases. The values were 93.81% (positive prediction) and 100% (negative prediction) for arg-gingivain and 60.81% (positive prediction) and 100% (negative prediction) for bacterial DPP.

The mean levels over the 2 years and the highest recorded levels at GAL sites were also above their respective critical values and were statistically significantly higher than those values at control sites in the same patients for both enzymes. In addition, all comparisons of mean patient values in patients with or without attachment loss were highly statistically significant.

Thus, GCF arg-gingivain/arg-gingipain appears to be an excellent predictor and GCF DPP a moderately good predictor of future progressive attachment loss. A test system (see details in following section below) suitable for chairside use has been developed (Cox et al 1990) and has been shown to produce similar results to the laboratory system.

COMMERCIAL DIAGNOSTIC TEST KITS

Diagnostic test kits based on some of these systems have already been marketed. However, most of them were marketed before verifiable evidence of their predictive ability had been shown. They use either paper point or curette bacterial sampling from the pocket and include:

Evalusite (Kodak)

This utilizes enzyme-linked immunosorbent assays (ELISAs) (**Fig. 14.2C**) using antibodies against *Porphyromonas gingivalis*, *Prevotella intermedia* and *A. actinomycetemcomitans* antigens. The reactions are carried out in a simple chairside reaction kit. Subgingival plaque samples are reacted with the antibodies and detection substrate in a multiwell reaction dish.

Omnigene (Omnigene, Inc) and BTD (Biotechnica Diagnostics, Inc)

These are DNA probe systems for a number of subgingival bacteria. A paper point sample of subgingival plaque is placed in the container provided and mailed off to the company for assay. Probes are available for *A. actinomycetemcomitans*, *Porphyromonas gingivalis*, *Prevotella intermedia*, *E. corrodens*, *F. nucleatum*, *C. recta*, *T. denticola* and *T. pectinovorum*.

Perioscan (Oral-B Laboratories)

This is a chairside test kit system which utilizes the BANA (BzArgNA) test for bacterial trypsin-like proteases. These are mainly produced by *Porphyromonas gingivalis* but lesser amounts are also produced by

B. forsythus and *T. denticola*. A subgingival plaque sample is reacted in the kit with the substrate linked to a colour detection system. The system is particularly simple to use.

Diamond Probe/Perio 2000 System®

The Diamond Probe/Perio 2000 System® (Diamond General Development Corporation, Ann Arbor, MI) has been designed so that it combines the features of a periodontal probe with the detection of volatile sulphur compounds in the periodontal pocket. However, since there are no longitudinal studies of the relationship of volatile sulphur compounds to progressive periodontitis its diagnostic potential is unknown.

Potential diagnostic tests worthy of development
Bacterial proteases in gingival crevicular fluid

A test system suitable for chairside use has been developed in conjunction with researchers from Enzyme System Products/Prototek, Dublin, CA (Cox et al 1990) and this can be used to detect the bacterial proteases arg-gingipain/arg-gingivain and DPP in GCF. It is fully described in the section below on hydrolytic and proteolytic host enzymes.

(Note: The commercial firms owning these tests are constantly changing because some of them sell the rights of their products to others. For this reason, the firms cited as owning these tests may not remain accurate over a period of time.)

Advantages and disadvantages of diagnostic tests using bacteria and their products
Advantages

The possible advantages are listed and described below:

- Some appear to be predictive of disease activity in longitudinal studies, e.g. GCF bacterial proteases
- The commercial tests are simple to use
- Results of chairside test kits are available in a short time
- Chairside test kits produce visual results which can be shown to the patient.

All of the markers used in these test systems have been shown to be associated with active sites on a retrospective basis and some, e.g. GCF bacterial proteases appear to be predictive of disease activity in longitudinal studies. The chairside tests are simple to use and their results are available within a relatively short time. They also produce a visual result which can be shown to the patient and related to the site from which they were obtained.

Disadvantages

The main disadvantages are listed and described below:

- Polymicrobial nature of the disease
- Most are not predictive of disease activity
- You need to know which site to sample
- They only detect the bacteria that you look for
- Some need to be sent away to a special laboratory
- Expensive.

Polymicrobial nature of the disease
The subgingival flora is complex and may vary slightly from site to site and patient to patient and no single pathogen is shown to be the cause of chronic periodontitis (see above). The putative periodontal pathogens that have been shown to be associated with progressing sites on a retrospective

basis vary in proportion at both active and stable sites. It is therefore difficult to choose the particular bacterial species to assay as a marker in any particular case.

Predictive ability of bacterial markers

Several putative periodontal pathogens have been shown to be associated with active sites (see above) but none have been shown to be predictive of periodontal disease activity. The BANA test for bacterial trypsin-like activity has been tested for its predictive ability in a clinical setting in a multicentre trial (Loesche et al 1990). It has been shown to correlate well with ELISA test detection of P. gingivalis, B. forsythus and T. denticola but it has relatively poor predictive abilities for periodontal disease activity.

The only bacterial factors that have so far been shown to have good predictive ability (Eley & Cox 1996a) are GCF arg-gingipain/arg-gingivain and bacterial dipeptidyl peptidases (DPPs). In this respect, GCF arg-gingipain/arg-gingivain gave the best results in diagnostic testing (see above). A chair-side diagnostic testing system has been designed for these bacterial enzymes (Cox et al 1990) but this is not yet commercially available.

Which site to sample

It is not possible to sample all the sites in the mouth with any diagnostic test system and therefore the site(s) to be tested have to be preselected. This usually means testing sites which already show clinical signs of previous attachment loss. While these sites are slightly more likely to progress than other sites, the pattern of progression of periodontitis is very irregular and unpredictable. This may make the choice of sites difficult. These comments apply to all markers.

Which bacteria to select as markers

All molecular and antibody detection systems are entirely specific and will therefore only detect the sequence or antigen against which they are directed. Therefore, all DNA probes (Highfield & Dougan 1985; French et al 1986; Savitt et al 1988) and ELISA-based detection systems (Ebersole et al 1984) will only detect the specific bacterial species against which they are directed. You would therefore need to decide which specific bacterial species you wish to detect before deciding on the test system to use. This choice is difficult because there are 12 or more putative periodontal pathogens whose proportions may vary from site to site and from each patient to each patient.

In this regard, the use of bacterial protease markers is less specific. The BANA test (Loesche et al 1990) detects proteases from P. gingivalis, B. forsythus and T. denticola but the majority of this activity comes from P. gingivalis. In respect of GCF bacterial proteases (Gazi et al 1996; Cox & Eley 1989; Cox et al 1992; Eley & Cox 1995, 1996a), these are detected with selective assay systems and thus the situation is a little different. The trypsin-like protease (arg-gingipain) detected in the clinical studies (Eley & Cox 1995, 1996a) is specific for the enzyme from P. gingivalis. In contrast, the bacterial DPPs are produced by P. gingivalis, Prevotella intermedia and Capnocytophaga species and the assay system used detected all of these proteases.

Special laboratory required

Samples for DNA probe (Highfield & Dougan 1985; French et al 1986; Savitt et al 1988) testing of bacterial species have to be sent away to a special laboratory and this has two main disadvantages. First, samples may deteriorate during transit and to minimize this problem the companies offering this service provide transport vessels and media. Second, the result is delayed and is not available to the dentist or patient on the day of the appointment.

Cost

All diagnostic test systems are expensive and in this regard they cannot be used in NHS practice without incurring a financial loss. The cost of the kit and the time involved in taking, reacting and reading the sample would need to be directly added to the patient's bill. The costs are relatively high because you are paying for the development costs of the system, its manufacturing and service costs and the firm's profit. With respect to the relative cost of each system, the DNA probe service is the most expensive and the ELISA and BANA systems the least expensive. These comments apply to all markers.

INFLAMMATORY AND IMMUNE MARKERS

There is no doubt that the bacteria in dental plaque and the subgingival flora are the primary cause of periodontal disease (see Chs 2 and 4). However, these bacteria also trigger inflammatory and immune host responses which, along with the direct effects of the bacteria, cause most of the tissue destruction (Genco 1992). A number of substances are released from inflammatory and immune cells into the tissues and many of these pass into GCF and are thus easily available for analysis (Page 1992; Lamster 1992). Samples of these substances can usually be obtained from paper strip GCF samples.

The substances released by inflammatory and immune cells during the disease process include antibodies (immunoglobulin, Ig), complement proteins, inflammatory mediators such as prostaglandin (PG) and the pro-inflammatory cytokines such as the various interleukins (IL) and tumour necrosis factor (TNF). Those of possible relevance to periodontal pathology are below:

- Immune response
    - Antibody
    - Total IgG and IgG subgroups
    - Complement
- Inflammatory mediators
    - Arachidonic acid derivatives, e.g. PGE_2
    - Cytokines, e.g. IL-1, IL-6.

Sampling of saliva

A whole non-stimulated saliva sample is usually required since it will contain factors from the salivary glands, factors from oral bacteria growing within it and factors from gingival crevicular fluid which flow into it. The sample can usually be spat into a suitable sterile container and then processed according to the requirements of the potential marker of interest.

Sampling of gingival crevicular fluid

GCF is an exudate that can be harvested from the gingival crevice or periodontal pocket using either filter paper strips (**Fig. 14.3**) or micropipette tubes. As the fluid traverses the inflamed tissue, it may pick up enzymes

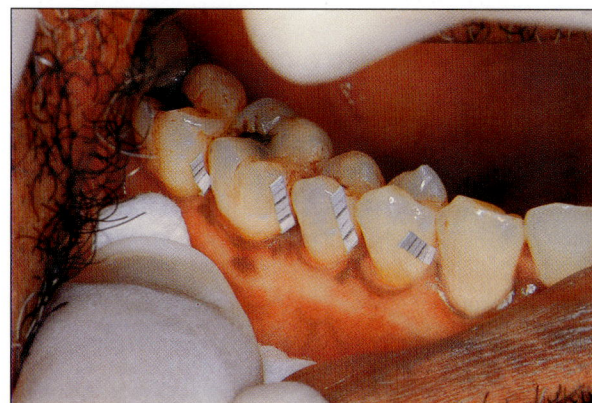

Fig. 14.3 Chromatography paper strips collecting gingival crevicular fluid (GCF) from the mesiobuccal surfaces of the lower right premolars and molars.

and other molecules that participate in the disease process. It can also pick up the products of cell and tissue degradation. Therefore, it offers great potential as a source of factors that may be associated with disease activity.

The exact placement of the sampling device and the collection time are of great importance, since they influence the composition of the GCF collected (Curtis et al 1988; Page 1992). Placement of a sampling device into the crevice or pocket induces a steady flow of exudate, while repeat sampling depletes GCF volume and harvested components per unit of time. Lengthy sampling periods particularly with micropipette tubes will sample mainly inflammatory exudate from vessels rather than the contents of the crevice. The procedure adopted varies for the particular components of interest and its method of analysis but there is general agreement that the method of choice is one which causes the least interference with the site and takes the shortest time to harvest fluid present at the site prior to sampling. Thus, sampling for 30 s or less by the placement of paper strips at the orifice of the site seems to be ideal provided it ensures a sample of sufficient size to analyse with the technique used.

Correlation of host factors with disease

Subgingival temperature

The hyperaemia associated with inflammation increases the local temperature of the part affected and is one of the cardinal signs of inflammation. A device, Periotemp® (Abio Dent, Danvers, MA), has been developed to measure small changes in the sublingual and subgingival temperature. Increased subgingival temperature has been positively correlated with increased pocket depths, decreased attachment levels, clinical parameters of gingival inflammation, higher proportions of putative periodontal pathogens and gingival crevicular fluid enzymes (Haffajee et al 1992a,b,c; Dinsdale et al 1997; Wolff et al 1997). Both the sublingual and subgingival temperatures have also been found to be significantly higher in smokers compared to non-smokers (Dinsdale et al 1997).

One longitudinal study of the relationship between subgingival temperature and progressive attachment loss has been carried out (Haffajee et al 1992a,b,c). A total of 29 chronic periodontitis subjects had clinical parameters and subgingival temperature measured at six sites per tooth every 2 months. Differences between sublingual and subgingival temperatures were also recorded. Attachment loss >2.5 mm occurred at one or more sites at 16 of the 49 subject visits. Elevated mean subgingival temperature was related to subsequent attachment loss particularly in individuals who exhibited more than one progressive site. The odds ratio of a subject exhibiting new attachment loss at one site was 14.5 and at two or more sites was 64.0 if the subject's mean subgingival temperature exceeded 35.5 °C. Subjects with high subgingival temperature and widespread previous attachment loss appeared to be at the greatest risk for new attachment loss. Using diagnostic testing a sensitivity and specificity of 75% and 76%, respectively was found.

Humoral immune response

Patients with various forms of periodontal disease produce antibodies to antigens from periodontopathic bacteria (Lamster 1992; Page 1992). These antibodies can be detected in serum, saliva, gingival tissue and GCF.

Secretory immunoglobulin A (sIgA) is actively secreted into saliva and IgG and M pass into saliva mainly from GCF (Marcotte & Lavoie 1998). Levels of salivary IgG and IgA and specific antibody are very low in healthy patients and there is an increase in salivary IgG in 34% of moderate and 57% of advanced periodontitis patients (Sandholm & Gronblad 1984; Sandholm et al 1987). Specific IgA antibody to *A. actinomycetemcomitans* is present in the saliva of refractory periodontitis patients (Nieminen et al 1993b, 1996). However, the level of this specific antibody

has only been found to be raised in 19% of chronic periodontitis patients (Sandholm et al 1987). In addition, it has been shown that the serum and saliva concentrations of IgG and IgA reduce following periodontal treatment of chronic periodontitis patients probably because of a reduction in the antigenic stimulus (Reiff 1984). This reduction is more pronounced in early periodontitis than in more advanced cases.

In GCF, the total amount of immunoglobulin (Ig) positively correlates with that from adjacent gingival tissue. This shows that both serum and locally produced antibody contributes to that in GCF. The relationship of GCF antibodies to periodontal status has been studied in various ways (Page 1992). These include measuring the total amount of Ig, the relative amounts of IgG subclasses and specific antibody titres to antigens from various periodontal bacteria. These relationships are complex and difficult to interpret.

The total Ig in GCF does not correlate with disease severity or progression and indeed may be lower at progressive sites (Page 1992; Lamster 1992). There has been one report (Reinhardt et al 1989) that compared IgG subclasses in GCF at progressive and stable sites. It found that the concentration of IgG1 and IgG4 subclasses were significantly higher at progressive sites.

Numerous studies (Page 1992; Lamster 1992) have compared specific antibodies titres to antigens from periodontal bacteria with periodontal disease status but these have found no correlation between them. The relationship of specific antibodies in GCF to those in serum is also complex, with some being higher and some lower with considerable variation from patient to patient, site to site, in sequential measurement at the same site.

Thus, specific antibody or total Ig in GCF appears to be of no use in distinguishing between stable and active sites. Furthermore, some evidence suggests that a reduction in specific antibody in serum and consequently GCF in patients with existing disease can place them at risk for further disease progression (Lamster 1992). This relationship has been demonstrated in juvenile periodontitis and acute necrotizing ulcerative gingivitis. Specific antibodies in the gingival tissues and serum are important in modulating the pathology of periodontal diseases but with the present level of knowledge do not appear to offer a means of identifying patients at risk for active disease.

However, some recent research suggests that bacterial specific serum antibody levels and IgG subclass responses may relate to periodontal status. *Porphyromonas gingivalis* has been implicated as a major periodontal pathogen and it has been reported that a positive correlation may exist between IgG levels to *P. gingivalis* and the severity of periodontal disease (Gmür et al 1986; Lopatin & Blackburn 1992; Lamster et al 1998). Antibodies to periodontal bacteria have been reported to vary according to IgG subclass (McArthur & Clark 1993). Furthermore, elevations in *P. gingivalis* specific IgG2, IgG1 and IgG4 in rapidly progressive periodontitis and adult periodontitis have been reported (Kinane et al 1999).

An investigation (Sakai et al 2001) of *P. gingivalis* specific IgG subclasses in adult periodontitis patients and controls has recently been completed. It examined three groups of subjects, 20 treated and maintained adult periodontitis patients, 30 untreated adult periodontitis patients and 19 periodontally healthy patients. The maintained group were seen over 5 years with measurements at both the start and the end of this period. Significantly higher IgG1 levels were seen in both patient groups compared with controls. The untreated group had significantly higher IgG2 responses compared with other groups. The IgG4 levels were significantly higher in the maintained patients compared with the untreated group. Also, a statistically significant correlation between IgG2 levels and changes in bone levels was found in the maintained group. Patients from this group with high IgG2 levels and low IgG4 levels showed greater bone loss than those with low IgG2 and high IgG4, although the mean prevalence of *P. gingivalis* did not differ between the two groups. This work suggests that a persistently high *P. gingivalis* specific IgG2 level after periodontal treatment may be indicative of recurrent or persistent periodontal destruction at the patient level.

Complement

Complement is a battery of nine (or more) related proteins which join together sequentially in an enzyme mediated cascade (**Fig. 14.4**). The major components can be divided into a recognition unit, C1, in the classical pathway, an activation unit, C4, C2, C3, and the membrane unit, C5 through to C9. The complement cascade is initiated by the combination of specific immunoglobulin and the first complement component, C1. It can also be activated by the alternative pathway by other factors such as endotoxin (lipopolysaccharide, LPS) from the cell walls of Gram-negative bacteria. The final product of the cascade is an esterase which damages or lyses the cell walls of bacteria. Two intermediary products of the cascade, C3a and C5a, attach to receptor sites on mast cells and inflammatory cells. They release histamine and other substances from mast cells and prostaglandins from inflammatory cells. These released substances increase vascular permeability. They are also chemotactic for polymorphonuclear neutrophil leucocytes (PMNs). C3a also aids phagocytosis by attaching the antigen to the phagocyte via the C3 receptor on the surface of PMNs, monocytes and macrophages.

Complement proteins are present in GCF from sites with inflammation and the split fragments C3 and Factor B have been detected during experimental gingivitis (Patters et al 1989). However, none of these factors has been associated with disease activity.

Cellular immune response

As periodontal disease is a chronic condition, it is not surprising that activation of the cellular immune mechanism is a feature of periodontal pathology. Neopterin is a well established marker of the immune system and its concentrations in body fluids have been used as an indication of its degree of activation. In this regard, it has been recently shown that neopterin concentrations in saliva significantly correlated with the number of teeth with deep pockets in the mouth. Also when the patients were grouped according to the median number of diseased teeth, the group with 1–20 diseased teeth had significantly higher neopterin concentrations than the group with more than 20 (Vrecko et al 1997).

Cytokines

Cytokines are best described as cell to cell messengers or local hormones. They are all small proteins or peptides which are produced and released by one cell type so that they can link on to a specific receptor on the cell

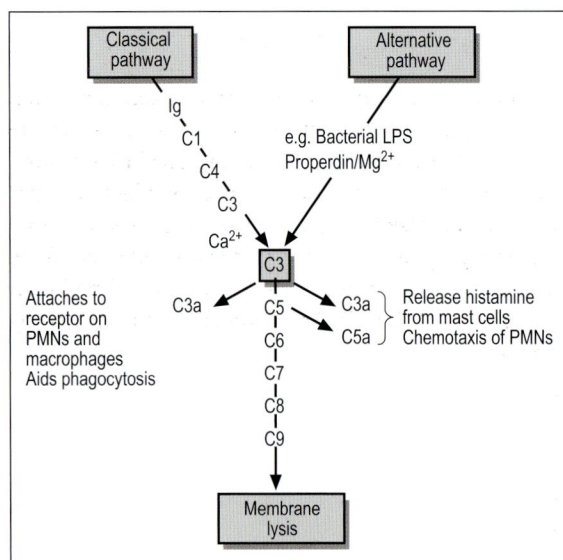

Fig. 14.4 Diagram to show the classical and alternative pathways of the complement cascade.

membrane of another cell(s) of either the same type or another type(s). Attachment to the receptor switches on a particular intracellular messenger system in the cell which leads to a particular function. The best known examples of cytokines are the interleukins (IL) which pass messages between the leucocytes. However, cytokines are involved in the cell to cell communications of most if not all cells in the body and are present in all tissues and body fluids including serum, saliva and GCF. The cell source, target cells and the main action(s) of the common cytokines of relevance to periodontal diseases are shown in Table 3.1.

Saliva

The only potential marker in this class investigated in saliva is platelet activation factor (PAF) which stimulates the activities and production of platelets. Salivary PAF levels have been found to be significantly higher in untreated chronic periodontitis patients compared with controls (Rasch et al 1995; Garito et al 1995). Its levels correlate with clinical indices of disease severity and the extent of disease and also significantly reduce following periodontal treatment.

Gingival crevicular fluid

Interleukin (IL)-1 and tumour necrosis factor alpha (TNF-α) are produced by activated macrophages and other cells and have pro-inflammatory effects of relevance to periodontal pathology which include the stimulation of PGE_2 and collagenase production. Since monoclonal antibodies have been produced for these cytokines they can be measured by ELISA and may therefore have potential for use in a clinical test system.

IL-1α and β are present in inflamed gingiva (Hönig et al 1989). They are also present in GCF from patients with periodontitis with extremely low concentrations at healthy sites (Masada et al 1990). Their levels are reduced following scaling and root planing but did not correlate with probing depth measurements. The amount of IL-1β in GCF also correlated with messenger RNA in adjacent gingival tissue.

TNF-α is also present in GCF but does not correlate with probing depth or gingival inflammation and its total amount was inversely related to tissue inflammation (Rossomando et al 1990).

The levels of IL-1 and IL-6 in refractory periodontitis have also been studied (Reinhardt et al 1993). There were no significant differences in the mean level of IL-1 in refractory or stable patients but refractory sites produced significantly more IL-6.

Lee et al (1995a) measured the levels of IL-1β, IL-2, IL-4, IL-6 and TNF-α in GCF by ELISA assays. Their levels at active and inactive sites in 10 patients with refractory periodontitis were compared in a short 3-month longitudinal study. Active sites were defined as those sites which lost ≥2 mm of attachment, measured with a Florida probe (see Ch. 12), over the 3 months of the study. According to these criteria there were eight active and 12 inactive sites. The active sites had significantly higher levels of IL-2 and IL-6 than the inactive sites at both baseline and the 3-month visit. This suggests that these cytokines might both predict and associate with progressive attachment loss. Also, the levels of IL-1β were significantly higher at active sites at 3 months but not at baseline. They also used subtraction radiology (see Ch. 12) to detect alveolar bone loss over the 3 months and found that sites with bone loss had significantly higher levels of IL-1β and IL-2 than sites with no evidence of bone loss. This suggests that this cytokine might associate with but not predict progressive attachment loss.

However, the level of predictive ability of these cytokines is unclear because the numbers of true and false positive and negative sites were not calculated and were not related in a diagnostic test. This is probably because the small number of active and inactive sites in this study precluded the use of this method of analysis.

The true relationship of these cytokines to periodontal disease activity will only become clearer with another longitudinal study over a longer time period and using greater numbers of chronic periodontitis patients.

IL-8 is secreted by monocytes, macrophages and vascular endothelial cells and mediates chemotaxis and activation of neutrophils (see Ch. 3). Its levels in GCF have been shown (Jin et al 2002) to significantly reduce following periodontal treatment along with corresponding and related reductions in PMN elastase and putative pathogens (P. gingivalis, Prevotella intermedia, A. actinomycetemcomitans, B. forsythus and T. denticola). These are logical relationships, since an absence or reduction of these bacteria would lead to a reduction in the inflammatory stimulus and hence less IL-8 secretion. This would result in less polymorph recruitment, which in turn would lead to less elastase secretion.

Prostaglandins

Prostaglandin E_2 (PGE_2) has pro-inflammatory and immunoregulatory effects and its concentration in gingival tissue is sufficient to elicit significant effects on cell responses and functions (Offenbacher et al 1993). In bone organ culture (see Ch. 5) it stimulates osteoclastic bone resorption. It may thus play a significant role in periodontal pathology.

There is a great deal of evidence which correlates PGE_2 levels in the periodontal tissues and GCF to the severity of periodontal disease. PGE_2 levels are low in health and non-detectable at many sites (Offenbacher et al 1993). In naturally occurring gingivitis, there is a modest rise in GCF PGE_2 levels to about 32 ng/mL and higher (about 53 ng/mL) in experimental gingivitis. Untreated periodontitis patients have significantly higher levels than gingivitis patients.

In one study, following scaling and root planing the periodontitis patients were divided into two groups, those that experienced no further attachment loss and those who experienced one or more sites of 3 mm or more of attachment loss (Offenbacher et al 1986). At this time the group which experienced no further attachment loss in the study period had mean GCF PGE_2 levels which were significantly lower than the group with attachment loss and were similar to those with untreated gingivitis. In contrast, the group which experienced significant attachment loss at one or more sites in the following 6 months had significantly higher mean GCF PGE_2 levels of 113 ng/mL. This observation is the basis of the claim that GCF PGE_2 is predictive for periodontal disease activity (Offenbacher et al 1986).

Levels >66 ng/mL were found to be predictive of further possible loss of attachment and this level was used as a cut off value in a positive and negative screening test. This gave a sensitivity of 0.76, a specificity of 0.96 and an overall predictive value of 0.92–0.95 (Offenbacher et al 1993). This shows that it could be predictive of periodontal disease activity.

DIAGNOSTIC TESTS

Commercial diagnostic tests

A commercial device, Periotemp® (Abio Dent, Danvers, MA), has been developed to measure small changes in the subgingival temperature and positive cross-sectional comparisons with clinical parameters have been found. One longitudinal study of the relationship between subgingival temperature and progressive attachment loss has also been carried out (Haffajee et al 1992a,b,c) and a positive relationship between them has been found.

Potential diagnostic tests worthy of development

Although GCF PGE_2 has considerable potential as a screening test for periodontal activity, strangely no commercial efforts are currently underway to develop one. In this regard, it is now possible to assay GCF PGE_2 with an ELISA assay utilizing a monoclonal rabbit-anti-PGE_2 antibody (Nakashima et al 1994). This technique could be simply modified to develop a diagnostic test system suitable for clinical use.

Cytokines are also assayed using ELISA techniques which could be developed into chairside kits. However, at present the predictive ability of these markers is still in doubt. Thus, the most likely diagnostic marker of the inflammatory and immune factors described above is GCF PGE_2.

Advantages and disadvantages of diagnostic tests using inflammatory mediators

Advantages

The main advantages are:

- Only one, GCF PGE_2 has been shown to be predictive of disease activity in longitudinal studies
- ELISA techniques can be used to detect cytokines and PGE_2 which could be developed into chairside kits which are simple to use
- ELISAs can be read after a short time
- They can be shown to the patient and related to tooth site.

GCF PGE_2 is the best candidate for a marker in this group.

Disadvantages

The main disadvantages are:

- The choice of the most appropriate biomarker may still be difficult at the present state of knowledge
- There is difficulty in determining the sites to sample and when to sample them
- If a moiety is associated with inflammation this may mask its association with destructive disease
- Cost.

The choice of the most appropriate biomarker

Only GCF PGE_2 has been shown to be predictive but IL-2 and IL-6 and possibly IL-1β show promise in this regard. However, in all cases further research is needed to confirm this.

Association of the marker with inflammation

All the inflammatory mediators are associated with gingival inflammation and this association could produce false association with disease activity. It is therefore very important to show that a potential marker has a true association with periodontal disease activity which is independent of any association with gingival inflammation.

HYDROLYTIC ENZYMES OF TISSUE ORIGIN

Inflammation leads to the accumulation of polymorphonuclear neutrophil leucocytes (PMNs), macrophages, lymphocytes and mast cells which are very important in protecting the body against infection. The inflammatory cells contain destructive enzymes within their lysosomes which are normally used to degrade phagocytosed material. These enzymes are however capable of degrading gingival tissue components if released. Such enzymes may be released by inflammatory cells during their function or when they degenerate or die (see Ch. 5). The main enzymes released by these cells are listed below:

- Proteolytic enzymes
  - Collagenases
  - Elastase
  - Cathepsin G
  - Cathepsin B
  - Cathepsin D
  - Dipeptidylpeptidases
  - Tryptase.

- Hydrolytic enzymes
  - Aryl sulphatase
  - β-glucuronidase
  - Alkaline phosphatase
  - Acid phosphatase
  - Myeloperoxidase
  - Lysozyme
  - Lactoferrin.

Collagen degradation is a multistage process (**Fig. 5.3**) and the triple helical region can only be attacked by specific collagenases (MMP1 and 8). The terminal peptides, which contain the sites of intra- and intermolecular cross-links can be attacked by a number of other serine and cysteine proteinases acting in concert (see Chs 1 and 5).

The degradation of collagen is usually preceded by that of the proteoglycans. In proteoglycan degradation (**Fig. 5.4**), protein cleavage occurs first to release the GAGs from the protein core and a number of metallo-, serine and cysteine proteinases can carry out this function. The released GAGs may remain intact or be further degraded by other hydrolytic enzymes.

Thus, all these proteolytic and hydrolytic enzymes can play an important role in periodontal pathology.

Collagenase and related metalloproteinases

Collagenases are part of a family of matrix metalloproteinases (MMPs) which degrade collagen. They are synthesized by macrophages, neutrophils, fibroblasts and keratinocytes and are secreted by these cells as latent enzymes when stimulated by some bacterial products and cytokines. There are two principle types of specific collagenases, MMP-8 found in inflammatory cells such as PMNs and macrophages and MMP-1, found in fibroblasts and other cells (Birkedal-Hansen 1993; Reynolds et al 1994; Reynolds 1996). These cells also produce inhibitors known as tissue inhibitors of metalloproteinases (TIMP) (see Chs 1 and 5).

Latent or pro-collagenases and related enzymes are activated by a number of proteolytic enzymes including tissue plasmin produced from serum plasminogen by plasminogen activator which is secreted by macrophages. They are inactivated by TIMPs and α_2-macroglobulin (Page 1991).

Collagenase-2 (MMP-8), collagenase-1 (MMP-1) and collagenase-3 (MMP-13) activity are present in gingival tissue, saliva and GCF and can be assayed biochemically with collagen substrates (Sorsa et al 1990) and immuno-detected using monoclonal (Chen et al 2000; Hanemaaijer et al 1997) or polyclonal antibodies with the ELISA technique (Ingman et al 1996; Matsuki et al 1996) or Western blotting (Kiili et al 2002). MMP-1 (collagenase-1), MMP-8 (collagenase-2), MMP-2 (Gelatinase- A) and MMP-9 (Gelatinase- B) (see Ch. 1 and Table 1.1) are present in both GCF and saliva (Sorsa et al 1990; Ingman et al 1994; Makela et al 1994; Westerlund et al 1996) and in both situations MMP-8 and MMP-9 predominate as they are produced by PMNs. In addition, the MMP-8 present in both situations in untreated chronic periodontitis patients has been found to be predominantly in the active form whilst that present in healthy or treated chronic periodontitis patients is mainly in the inactive or latent form (Uitto et al 1990; Hayakawa et al 1994).

Emingil et al (2006) carried out a study of gingival crevicular fluid matrix metalloproteinase-25 and -26 levels in periodontal diseases. It demonstrated the presence of soluble or shed forms of MMP-25 and MMP-26 in GCF of patients with different periodontal diseases. Increased levels and activation of MMP-25 and MMP-26 in GCF were associated with an enhanced severity of periodontal inflammation, and suggested that these MMPs could participate in the progression of periodontal diseases.

Tüter et al (2005) evaluated the effects of basic periodontal treatment on GCF levels of matrix metalloproteinase (MMP)-3 and tissue inhibitors of metalloproteinase (TIMP)-1. They showed that the clinical improvements were accompanied by a reduction in MMP-3 and an increasing in TIMP-1 GCF levels.

Saliva

Salivary levels of MMP-8 and 9 are significantly higher in untreated chronic periodontitis patients than healthy controls (Hayakawa et al 1994; Ingman et al 1996; Matsuki et al 1996; Makela et al 1994). Levels of MMP-8 also correlate with indices of disease severity (Sorsa et al 1994) and levels of MMP-8, 2, 9 significantly decrease following periodontal treatment (Uitto et al 1990; Hayakawa et al 1994; Makela et al 1994). In addition, TIMP-1 is significantly lower in untreated chronic periodontitis patients than healthy controls (Hayakawa et al 1994; Matsuki et al 1996).

By contrast, in localized juvenile periodontitis (LJP) salivary MMP-1 predominates but the levels of collagenase present in this condition are significantly less than in either untreated or treated chronic periodontitis or healthy patients (Ingman et al 1993). In addition, the levels of TIMP-1 are significantly increased in LJP cases, compared with that in either healthy or chronic periodontitis patents.

There are no longitudinal studies of salivary MMPs because salivary samples relate to the whole oral cavity and unable to give information on site related periodontal disease progression.

Gingival crevicular fluid

The 80, 75 and 60 kDa bands corresponding to the prepro-, pro- and active forms of collagenase-2 (MMP-8) have been detected by Western blotting in GCF (Kiili et al 2002). The 43 and 38 kDa bands of the active fibroblast type MMP-8 and the 60 kDa pro- and the 40 kDa active form of collagenase-3 (MMP-13) were also detected. In addition, a small amount of the >100 kDa form representing enzyme-inhibitor complex was also found. The percentage of the total absorbance of the MMP-8 and -13 bands correlated significantly with gingival and bleeding indices (Kiili et al 2002).

The level of GCF collagenase in naturally occurring and experimental gingivitis was assayed and the amounts correlated with the severity of inflammation (Kowashi et al 1979; Overall & Sodek 1987). Collagenase levels also correlated with the amount of attachment loss in ligature-induced periodontitis in dogs and latent enzyme predominated at healthy and gingivitis sites (Kryshalskyi et al 1986; Kryshalskyi & Sodek 1987).

In human periodontitis, GCF collagenase activity has been shown to increase with increasing severity of gingival inflammation and increasing pocket depth and alveolar bone loss (Villela et al 1987; Larivee et al 1986; Overall & Sodek 1987; Golub et al 1976; Häkkarainen et al 1988). Total enzyme and active enzyme levels are significantly higher and enzyme inhibitor levels are lower at diseased sites compared with healthy or treated sites (Larivee et al 1986).

It has also been shown that the predominating collagenase in GCF is MMP-8 mainly from PMNs and that GCF levels of MMP-8 and 9 are significantly higher in untreated chronic periodontitis patients than healthy controls (Sorsa et al 1990; Ingman et al 1996; Westerlund et al 1996; Makela et al 1994). Furthermore, it has been shown that the relationship between MMPs and LJP is the same in GCF and saliva (Ingman et al 1993).

Chen et al (2000) showed that total MMP-8 and MMP-8 concentration reduced significantly following periodontal treatment. This was also confirmed by Figueredo et al (2004). In addition, Chen et al (2000) showed that this enzyme demonstrated more significant correlations with clinical parameters with further decreases after successful periodontal treatment than either elastase or cathepsin B. This might reflect more effective complexing of this enzyme with inhibitors as the periodontal condition improves and this contention is supported by the finding in this study that the amount of the inhibitor α_2-macroglobulin also decreased significantly following treatment.

The same research group has developed immunological assay systems that can detect different MMPs (Kiili et al 2002) and has recently developed a two epitome monoclonal system for MMP-8 (Chen et al 2000; Hanemaaijer et al 1997). This latter system has also been developed as a chairside test system for GCF samples (Mäntylä et al 2003). This system has been shown to compare closely with the laboratory system and has been used in a small cross-sectional and a before and after treatment study using 11 periodontitis, 10 gingivitis and eight healthy subjects. They found that the median concentrations of MMP-8 were statistically significantly higher in periodontitis subjects than gingivitis subjects which were higher than healthy subjects. The levels at diseased sites and in diseased patients significantly reduced following treatment. Using a threshold of 1 mg/L the chairside test provided a sensitivity of 83% and specificity of 96%. This system is thus able to differentiate periodontitis from gingivitis and monitor the treatment of periodontitis (Mäntylä et al 2003).

A longitudinal study of GCF collagenase levels and periodontal attachment loss has been carried out by Lee et al (1995b). This study measured the relative amounts of active and latent collagenase relative to GCF by functional assays in a 12-month longitudinal cohort study. Comparisons were made between 14 subjects with inflammation and a previous history of progressive attachment loss (progressive periodontitis: group 1), 27 subjects with inflammation and previous attachment loss but now clinical stable (stable periodontitis: group 2) and 17 subjects with inflammation and no attachment loss (gingivitis: group 3).

Subjects with progressive and stable periodontitis (groups 1 and 2) were given basic periodontal treatment and were then monitored 3 months later. All subjects were then monitored monthly for attachment loss with a constant pressure probe and a threshold of 2 mm was used for confirmed attachment loss. GCF samples were taken from six specific sample teeth in each subject and from other teeth that lost attachment of 2 mm or more. Subjects in group 1 were rejected from the study if they did not lose attachment after 1 year and further subjects were recruited until 14 had lost attachment. The samples were all analysed at the end of the study so that all attachment loss sites were included. Inhibitors and blocking antibodies were used to determine the cellular source of GCF collagenase and this was found to be PMNs.

There were 14 sites which lost attachment in excess of the tolerance level; one in each of the chosen patients in group 1. Active collagenase activity was pooled from the six sites per subject for the group comparisons and this was significantly higher in group 1 subjects compared with groups 2 and 3. In contrast, latent collagenase was 2-fold higher in group 2 than group 1.

There was a wide variation in active collagenase levels at sites with progressive attachment loss and in these sites there was a significant increase with time. However, there were sharp elevations in active enzyme level at the time of attachment loss in only eight out of the 14 sites which lost attachment. Furthermore, as seven sites which lost attachment did not show these elevations, although it was not calculated in this study, the diagnostic sensitivity and specificity values for active collagenase as a predictor of attachment loss would have been low. In spite of the apparent poor predictive qualities of these enzymes measured in this way, one commercial test kit has been developed (see below).

Many of the earlier studies described above relating collagenases to periodontal disease severity or activity have used biochemical assays with collagen substrates. They generally assumed that they were measuring neutrophil collagenases but it is now known that this assay probably reflected the combined action of several collagenolytic enzymes including collagenases 1, 2, 3 (MMP-1, -8, -13), gelatinases A and B (MMP-2, -9), membrane-type-1-MMP (MT-1-MMP, MMP-14) and bacterial collagenases in GCF. Now that ELISA assays have been developed for many individual MMPs, it is possible to assay for them individually. It has been shown by using these techniques that the inflammatory cell MMP (MMP-8) relates

positively to indices of periodontal severity and significantly decreased following treatment (Mäntylä et al 2003). It is therefore possible that MMP-8 might give better results in a longitudinal study to those given by a mixture of enzymes in previous studies using biochemical assays.

In this regard, there has been a short 3-month longitudinal study of GCF MMP-8 using 20 chronic periodontitis patients with sampling of four sites of each before and after treatment and after the 3-month maintenance treatment (Kinane et al 2003). It showed significant reductions in MMP-8 concentrations following treatment ($p<0.005$). However, the difference between baseline and post-maintenance levels was highly significant ($p<0.001$) for both absolute amounts and concentrations. Mäntylä et al (2006) monitored the periodontal disease status in smokers and non-smokers using a gingival crevicular fluid matrix metalloproteinase-8-specific chair-side test. They found that at sites of periodontal disease progression, the distribution of MMP-8 concentrations was broader than in stable sites, indicating a tendency for elevated concentrations in patients with periodontal disease. The mean MMP-8 concentrations in smokers were lower than in non-smokers, but in smokers' and non-smokers' sites with progressive disease, MMP-8 concentrations were similar. Sites with exceptionally elevated MMP-8 concentrations were clustered in smokers who also showed a poor response to scaling and root planing (SRP). In these sites, the MMP-8 concentration did not decrease with scaling and root planing (SRP) and these sites were easily identified by the MMP-8 test. They concluded that persistently elevated GCF MMP-8 concentrations may indicate sites at risk, as well as patients with poor response to conventional periodontal treatment.

Pozo et al (2005) analysed the metalloproteinases (MMPs) and tissue inhibitors of metalloproteinases (TIMPs) in gingival crevicular fluid from periodontitis-affected patients and compared them with clinical parameters. They found significant correlations between the severity of the periodontal disease and the actual MMP activity, the active form of MMP-8 and the low level of both TIMP-1 and TIMP-2.

Cysteine proteinases

Cathepsins B, L and H are a family of intracellular cysteine proteinases which can degrade extracellular components including collagen (Dickinson 2002). They act at acid pH and are primarily involved in intracellular degradation but are also active extracellularly when released during inflammation. They are also particularly active during bone resorption (see Ch. 5). They are produced principally by fibroblasts, macrophages (Kennett et al 1994a) and osteoclasts (Vaes 1988). Ultrastructural studies have also shown cathepsin B localized within lysosomes and associated with the surface membrane of macrophages (Kennett et al 1997b). In addition, cathepsin B was seen on the surface of collagen fibrils in the adjacent connective tissue to these cells and this suggests that it could play a role in connective tissue degradation. Cysteine proteinases are inhibited by α_2-macroglobulin and the tissue inhibitors known as cystatins (Eley & Cox 1991). Fibroblasts and some macrophages in human gingiva contain α_2-macroglobulin (Kennett et al 1994a) and the active cysteine proteinase activity in gingival tissue and GCF is a balance between enzyme and inhibitors.

Saliva

There are no studies on cysteine proteinase potential markers because there is a high level of cystatin (tissue inhibitors of cysteine proteinases) in saliva which is sufficient to inhibit the activities of this group of enzymes in this situation.

Gingival crevicular fluid

Cathepsins B and L are present in gingival tissue and GCF (Cox & Eley 1989a; Eley & Cox 1991) as are also their inhibitors (Eley & Cox 1991). GCF levels of cathepsins B and L significantly correlate with increasing gingival inflammation, probing depth, probing attachment level and bone loss (Eley & Cox 1992b,c). In addition, levels of cathepsins B and L significantly decrease following periodontal treatment (Cox & Eley 1992; Eley & Cox 1992d). Zero or very low levels are present at healthy sites, low levels at gingivitis sites and high levels at periodontitis sites (Eley & Cox 1993).

To date (early 2009) there has been only one longitudinal study of GCF cathepsin B activity and periodontal attachment loss (Eley & Cox 1996b). This was a 2-year study of 75 patients using both site, patient and population thresholds for probing attachment loss measured with a Florida electronic probe and radiological measurements to determine confirmed progressive attachment loss. All clinical parameters and enzyme levels were significantly reduced following basic periodontal treatment prior to baseline.

Over the 2 years there were 121 sites in 49 patients with confirmed attachment loss giving an annual rate of 5.04% of sites. A total of 90 of these sites in 37 patients were rapid episodic attachment loss (RAL) and 31 sites in 21 patients showed gradual progressive attachment loss over a longer time period (GAL). Levels above critical values chosen for total cathepsin B activity and enzyme concentration were present at all RAL sites, both at the time of attachment loss and 3 months previously (predictive time). They were all significantly higher than control sites in the same patients.

These levels were also shown to be predictive of attachment loss in diagnostic testing. There were values of 100% (sensitivity) and 99.83% (specificity) for total enzyme activity and 100% (sensitivity) and 99.75% (specificity) for enzyme concentration. In addition, there were values of 86.53% (positive prediction) and 100% (negative prediction) for total enzyme activity and 81.08% (positive prediction) and 100% (negative prediction) for enzyme concentration.

The mean levels over the 2 years and the highest recorded values at GAL sites were also both above their respective critical values and were statistically significantly higher than those values at control sites in the same patients. In addition, all comparisons of mean patient values in patients with or without attachment loss were statistically significant.

Thus, GCF cathepsin B appears to be a good predictor of future progressive attachment loss. A test system suitable for chairside use has been developed (Cox et al 1990) and has been shown to produce similar results to the laboratory system (see below).

Aspartate proteinases

Cathepsin D is found in gingival tissue and GCF and GCF levels have been shown to correlate significantly with increasing gingival inflammation, probing depth, probing attachment level and bone loss (Ishikawa et al 1972). No longitudinal studies have been carried out relating this proteinase to periodontal attachment loss.

Serine proteinases

Elastase

Elastase in gingival tissue is produced by neutrophil polymorphonuclear leucocytes (PMNs) and is held in the cell in an inactive form probably bound with an inhibitor (Kennett et al 1995). It is inhibited in the tissues by α_1-proteinase inhibitor (α_1 PI), α_2-macroglobulin (α_2-M), secretory leucocyte protease inhibitor (SLPI) and skin antileukoproteinase (SKALP). α_2-M is found in many fibroblasts and also some macrophages which may also contain α_1 PI (Kennett et al 1995). SLPI is found in saliva (Wahl et al 1997; Cox et al 2003) and mast cells (Westin et al 1999) and SKALP in oral and other epithelial cells (Cox et al 2001, 2003).

Active elastase can only occasionally be detected in gingival tissue biochemically (Eley & Cox 1990) or histochemically (Kennett et al 1995) and is probably only detectable in an active state where there is an enzyme-inhibitor

imbalance and this is usually seen either adjacent to junctional epithelium where PMNs are migrating into the crevice or in granulation tissue at the advancing front of the lesion (Kennett et al 1995).

Elastase is able to degrade proteoglycans and can also activate latent collagenase (Eley & Cox 1990). Collagenases are unable to degrade collagen until the terminal peptide region of the molecule which contains intermolecular cross-links is first cleaved. This can also be carried out by elastase. It may thus have an important role in periodontal pathology.

Elastase is present in both saliva and GCF and can be biochemically assayed from these sources. In this regard, Cox et al (2006) found that proteases and inhibitors in GCF and saliva were better related to elastase activity in these fluids than the clinical variables and concluded that SLPI may be an important inhibitor of elastase activity in the periodontium.

Saliva

Salivary elastase levels are very low in periodontally healthy patients and zero in edentulous patients (Pederson et al 1995). The mean elastase level rose significantly in successive patient groups from gingivitis to early periodontitis to moderate periodontitis to advanced periodontitis. Its levels also correlated with indices of disease severity and with the number of deep pockets present (Uitto et al 1996). Some 85% of patients with one deep (≥ 6 mm) periodontal pocket had elevated levels of salivary elastase. Levels also decreased significantly following periodontal treatment (Nieminen et al 1993). Importantly, salivary elastase levels are not a good indicator for gingivitis, as only 45% of these patients had detectable elastase in their saliva (Uitto et al 1996). In addition, its levels did not significantly rise during the progression of experimental gingivitis. Finally, salivary elastase levels are much lower in untreated localized juvenile periodontitis than in untreated chronic periodontitis and in fact are little different from control levels in healthy patients (Ingman et al 1993).

Gingival crevicular fluid

GCF elastase levels significantly correlate with increasing gingival inflammation, probing depth, probing attachment level and bone loss (Eley & Cox 1992b,c) and its level also significantly reduces following periodontal treatment (Cox & Eley 1992; Eley & Cox 1992d). Zero or very low levels are present at healthy sites, low to moderate levels at gingivitis sites and very high levels at periodontitis sites (Eley & Cox 1993).

Takashi et al (2005) evaluated the potential of gingival crevicular fluid assays as a screening methodology for periodontal disease activity including haemoglobin, albumin, transferrin, α-1-antitrypsin, fibronectin, IgA, IgG, IgM, lactoferrin, myeloperoxidase and neutrophil elastase, all conducted at a commercial laboratory. They used a very small study group of 27 subjects. This cross-sectional study suggested a potential for the combination of IgA and neutrophil elastase.

A 6-month longitudinal study using a test kit system for elastase measurements has been reported (Palcanis et al 1992). This study used small thresholds of probing attachment loss of 0.4, 0.6 and 1 mm measured with a Florida probe (see Ch. 13) and bone loss detected by subtraction radiology (see Ch. 13) to determine when attachment loss occurred. It showed significant differences of total elastase activity at baseline in progressive and non-progressive sites assessed 2–6 months later.

Results from a 2-year longitudinal study of 75 patients using both a higher threshold and radiological examination to determine confirmed progressive attachment loss (Eley & Cox 1996c) showed similar and better results. All clinical parameters and enzyme levels were significantly reduced following basic periodontal treatment prior to baseline. Over the 2 years, there were 119 sites in 48 patients with confirmed attachment loss giving an annual rate of 4.96% of sites. A total of 89 of these sites in 36 patients were rapid episodic attachment loss (RAL) and 30 sites in 21 patients showed gradual progressive attachment loss (GAL) over a long time period.

Levels above critical values chosen for total elastase activity and enzyme concentration were present at all RAL sites both at the time of attachment loss and 3 months previously (predictive time). They were all significantly higher than values at control sites in the same patients. These levels were also shown to be predictive of attachment loss in diagnostic testing. There were values of 100% (sensitivity) and 99.95% (specificity) for total enzyme activity and 100% (sensitivity) and 99.91% (specificity) for enzyme concentration. In addition, there were values of 95.70% (positive prediction) and 100% (negative prediction) for total enzyme activity and 68.46% (positive prediction) and 100% (negative prediction) for enzyme concentration.

Also the means levels over the 2 years and the highest recorded values at GAL sites were both above their respective critical values and were statistically significantly higher than those values at control sites in the same patients. In addition, all comparisons of mean patient values in patients with or without attachment loss were highly statistically significant.

In addition, the levels of GCF elastase have also been compared at healthy, gingivitis and histologically confirmed attachment loss sites in beagle dogs with ligature-induced periodontitis (Renvert et al 1998). At the attachment loss sites, maximum histological attachment loss was found to coincide with the period of maximum GCF elastase activity and there was significant correlation between the two during the first 7 days of ligature placement. In contrast, the healthy and gingivitis sites had minimal levels of enzyme activity throughout the study period.

Thus, GCF elastase appears to be a good predictor of future progressive attachment loss. A test system suitable for chairside use has been developed (Cox et al 1990) and has been shown to produce similar results to the laboratory system. A commercial system based on the same biochemistry has also been developed (Palcanis et al 1992).

Tryptase

Tryptase activity is present in large amounts in gingival tissue and in small amounts in GCF when measured biochemically (Eley & Cox 1990; Cox & Eley 1989a,b,c) and it has been localized to gingival mast cells (Kennett et al 1993). In the mast cell granules it is stabilized as an active tetramer by association with heparin and is released by these cells on degranulation.

Tryptase can cleave the third component of complement and can activate latent collagenase. It can stimulate the release of collagenase from gingival fibroblasts and in inflamed gingival tissues mast cell degranulation occurs in areas of connective tissue breakdown.

In dogs, an inhibitor of mast cell degranulation has been shown to significantly reduce the rate of alveolar bone loss (Jeffcoat et al 1985). Thus, tryptase could be involved in the pathogenesis of periodontitis.

In humans, GCF tryptase activity correlates with clinical parameters of disease severity including probing attachment and bone loss (Eley & Cox 1992b,c) and significantly reduces following periodontal treatment (Cox & Eley 1992; Eley & Cox 1992d). Zero to very low levels are present at healthy sites, low levels at gingivitis sites and moderately high levels at periodontitis sites (Eley & Cox 1993). The test system for chairside use (Cox et al 1990) described in the previous section could be used with this enzyme.

Dipeptidylpeptidase (DPPs)

DPP II which is active at acid pH and DPP IV which is active at alkaline pH are present in gingival tissue and GCF (Cox & Eley 1989; Cox et al 1992).

Within gingival tissue DPP II is a lysosomal enzyme present in fibroblasts (Kennett et al 1994b, 1996). In GCF smears it is also present in macrophages (Cox et al 1995; Kennett et al 1997a). This may suggest that

this enzyme within macrophages is in an inactive form in gingival tissue, but in an active form in migrated cells in GCF.

DPP IV is a lysosomal enzyme present in macrophages, T-lymphocytes and fibroblasts (Kennett et al 1994b, 1996). Using immunogold localization with electron microscopy, DPP IV was present on the surface membrane of T-lymphocytes, macrophages and fibroblasts (Kennett et al, unpublished data).

GCF DPP II and IV need to be distinguished from bacterial DPPs and selective assays have been developed for this purpose (Cox et al 1989a; Eley & Cox 1995a). They are able to cleave glycol prolyl residues and may play a role in collagen degradation after the action of other enzymes.

Both tissue DPP II and IV correlate with clinical parameters of disease severity and significantly reduce following periodontal treatment (Eley & Cox 1992a,b,c,d; Cox & Eley 1992). Zero or very low levels are present at healthy sites, low levels at gingivitis sites and high levels at periodontitis sites (Eley & Cox 1993).

A 2-year longitudinal study of both GCF DPP II and DPP IV in 75 patients has recently been completed (Eley & Cox 1995b). It used both site, patient and population thresholds for probing attachment loss measured with a Florida electronic probe and radiological measurement to determine confirmed progressive attachment loss. All clinical parameters and enzyme levels significantly reduced following basic periodontal treatment prior to baseline.

Over the 2 years, there were 120 sites in 49 patients with confirmed attachment loss giving an annual rate of 5.0% of sites. Some 88 of these sites in 35 patients were rapid episodic attachment loss (RAL) sites and 32 sites in 20 patients showed gradual progressive attachment loss (GAL) over a longer time period.

Levels above critical values chosen for both DPP II and DPP IV (total enzyme activities and enzyme concentrations) were present at all RAL sites both at the time of attachment loss and 3 months previously (predictive time). They were all significantly higher than controls sites in the same patients.

These levels were also shown to be predictive of attachment loss in diagnostic testing. These values were 100% (sensitivity) and 99.58% (specificity) for total enzyme activities; 100% (sensitivity) and 99.34% (specificity) for enzyme concentrations in respect of DPP II; 100% (sensitivity) and 99.48% (specificity) for total enzyme activities and 100% (sensitivity) and 99.17% (specificity) in respect of DPP IV. In addition, there were values of 70.96% (positive prediction) and 100% (negative prediction) for total enzyme activity; 60.68% (positive prediction) and 100% (negative prediction) for enzyme concentration in respect of DPP II; 66.17% (positive prediction) and 100% (negative prediction) for total enzyme activity and 55% (positive prediction) and 100% (negative prediction) for enzyme concentration in respect of DPP IV.

The mean levels over the 2 years and the highest recorded values at GAL sites for both proteases were also above their respective critical values and were statistically significantly higher than those values at control sites in the same patients. In addition, all comparisons of mean patient values in patients with or without attachment loss were highly statistically significant.

Thus, both GCF DPP II and DPP IV appear to be good predictors of future progressive attachment loss. A test system suitable for chairside use has been developed (Cox et al 1990) and has been shown to produce similar results to the laboratory system.

Protease inhibitors

The two main endogenous protease inhibitors, α_1-proteinase inhibitor (α_1 PI) and α_2-macroglobulin (α_2-M), are present in serum, saliva and GCF (Sandholm 1986; Roa et al 1995). The levels of α_1 PI in saliva and GCF do not significantly vary in healthy and periodontally diseased patients.

On the other hand, the levels of α_2-M are significantly higher in chronic periodontitis patients compared with gingivitis patients and the levels in gingivitis patients are significantly higher compared with healthy patients (Pederson et al 1995). α_2-M is found in many fibroblasts and also some macrophages which may also contain α_1 PI (Kennett et al 1995). Two further elastase inhibitors are present in gingival tissue, secretory leucocyte protease inhibitor (SLPI) from saliva and mast cells (Wahl et al 1997; Cox et al 2003; Westin et al 1999) and skin antileukoproteinase (SKALP) from epithelial cells (Cox et al 2001, 2003).

The GCF levels of α_1 PI and SLPI have been compared before and after periodontal treatment of 21 chronic periodontitis patients by ELISA (Nakamura-Minami et al 2003). A significant reduction in the α_1 PI levels were found 4 weeks after treatment. In the 2 weeks following treatment the SLPI level rose and then did not change up to 4 weeks after treatment. At baseline, α_1 PI levels were significantly higher at bleeding compared with non-bleeding sites.

Cystatins are tissue derived inhibitors of cysteine proteinases. Cystatin C is produced by many cells and tissues and has a general distribution, while cystatins S, SA, SN and D are produced by glandular acinar cells and are mainly found in glandular secretions including saliva. Cystatin A is produced by inflammatory cells and is the main cystatin in GCF. Saliva contains cystatins S, SA, SN and D produced by the salivary glands, cystatin C from other cells and possibly cystatin A from GCF. GCF contains cystatin A from inflammatory cells and sometimes lesser amounts of cystatin C from other cells.

Total salivary cystatins were found to be significantly higher in chronic periodontitis patients compared with gingivitis patients and periodontally healthy patients (Henskens et al 1993a). However, the levels of protein and albumin followed the same pattern, so it is possible that the changes were due to differences in the salivary flow rate. However, it has also been found that the levels of cystatin C were also higher in chronic periodontitis patients compared with healthy patients (Henskens et al 1993b). It has also been found that saliva from healthy patients contains mainly cystatin S, while that from chronic periodontitis patients contains both S and C (Henskens et al 1994, 1996a). It has also been shown that salivary total cystatins and cystatin C in chronic periodontitis patients were reduced significantly following periodontal treatment (Henskens et al 1996b).

The levels of cystatins in GCF is significantly lower than in saliva (Blankenvoorde et al 1997). Also cystatins S and SN and C could not be detected in GCF but cystatin A was found in every GCF sample analysed and was also found in saliva. Cystatin A in saliva could either come from GCF or migrating inflammatory cells.

β-glucuronidase and arylsulphatase

Extensive studies have been carried out on β-glucuronidase and arylsulphatase and this work is reviewed in Lamster (1992) and Page (1992). Both of these enzymes are lysosomal and are found in PMNs. β-glucuronidase is an acid hydrolase which is considered to be a marker for primary granule release by these cells.

In cross-sectional studies both these enzymes in GCF have been shown to have statistically significant correlations with gingival inflammation, pocket depth and alveolar bone loss. The levels of these enzymes are also higher in diseased relative to healthy sites and their levels drop following periodontal treatment (Lamster 1992).

During a 4-week period of experimental gingivitis, the level of these enzymes increased for the first 3 weeks and then levelled off or dropped. The level of both enzymes increased with increasing pocket depths and β-glucuronidase was also positively associated with spirochaetes *Porphyromonas gingivalis*, *Prevotella intermedia* and lactose-negative black pigmenting bacteria in the subgingival flora and was negatively associated with cocci (Lamster 1992).

A 6-month longitudinal study, where GCF β-glucuronidase activity was related to disease activity defined as loss of attachment of 2.0 mm or more over that period, has been reported (Lamster et al 1988). Those sites which showed the highest β-glucuronidase activity at baseline and again at 3 months had the highest association with loss of attachment. Critical values at these sites had a sensitivity and specificity of 89% in diagnostic testing.

In a further study (Lamster et al 1991), 59 patients were similarly followed for 1 year and it was shown that persistently elevated β-glucuronidase levels were associated with disease activity that could be predicted from 3–6 months in advance. In this study, critical values of β-glucuronidase had a sensitivity of 92% and a selectivity of 86%, respectively in diagnostic testing. All of these results were related to total β-glucuronidase activity per 30 s sample and not to enzyme concentration.

The association with disease activity has been confirmed in a multicentre trial in which 140 patients were followed for 6 months and this showed a total predictive value as high as 90% (Lamster 1992). This has so far only been reported in oral presentations published as abstracts and reported in Lamster (1992). However, the baseline data for this study has been reported in full (Lamster et al 1994). Thus, total β-glucuronidase activity per 30 s sample appears to be a good predictor of future attachment loss.

A diagnostic kit based on GCF β-glucuronidase is being commercially developed by Abbott Laboratories, North Chicago, IL.

Alkaline phosphatase

Alkaline phosphatase is thought to play a role in bone metabolism and is found in PMNs. A cross-sectional study of GCF alkaline phosphatase in periodontitis patients showed that it positively and significantly correlated with pocket depth but not with bone loss (Ishikawa & Cimasoni 1970) and is found at higher levels at diseased than healthy sites (Chapple et al 1994). A longitudinal study (Binder et al 1987) which related GCF levels to periodontal attachment loss of >2 mm showed that active sites yielded 20 times the activity in serum and were significantly associated with periodontal disease activity. However, when the data was calculated in terms of false positives and negatives using the most favourable cut-off point, 73% of active sites were identified, although 36% of the inactive sites were included. This would seem to indicate that its predictive value is low.

Acid phosphatase

Acid phosphatase is present in inflammatory cells and has been detected in GCF (Binder et al 1987). Levels, however do not correlate with measurements of either disease severity or activity.

Myeloperoxidase, lysozyme and lactoferrin

Myeloperoxidase, lysozyme and lactoferrin are found in PMNs and can be detected in saliva and GCF.

Myeloperoxidase

Myeloperoxidase (MPO) is a potent antibacterial enzyme produced by PMNs. Salivary MPO levels are significantly higher in untreated chronic periodontitis patients compared with healthy control subjects and their levels significantly reduce following periodontal treatment (Over et al 1993; Guven et al 1996; Suomalainen et al 1996). GCF MPO levels are higher at periodontitis sites than control sites and the levels decrease significantly following periodontal treatment. However, MPO activity was not found to correlate with clinical indices of disease severity (Smith et al 1986; Cao & Smith 1989).

The choice of the most appropriate biomarker

Of the potential markers described here, cathepsin B, elastase, dipeptidyl peptidase II and IV and β-glucuronidase have been shown in longitudinal studies to be predictive of periodontal disease progression. Collagenase, tryptase, alkaline phosphatase, arylsulphatase and myeloperoxidase have been shown in cross-sectional studies, and in some cases longitudinal studies, to be associated with disease severity and activity. However, they are not predictive in disease activity which is the basic requirement of a diagnostic test. Acid phosphatase, lysozyme and lactoferrin at present do not appear to be associated with either disease activity or severity.

Association of the marker with inflammation

All enzymes released from inflammatory cells are likely to be associated with gingival inflammation. Since gingival inflammation is often present in the absence of disease activity (i.e. progressive periodontal attachment loss), this association with inflammation could produce false association with disease activity. It is therefore very important to show that a potential marker has a true association with periodontal disease activity which is independent of and stronger than any association it may have with gingival inflammation. This is most clearly shown in comparisons of true and false positive and negative sites in respect of confirmed attachment loss which are used to compute the sensitivity, specificity and positive and negative predictive values quoted in the sections on each marker.

Biological control mechanisms

All diagnostic tests should reflect an understanding of the role played by biological control mechanisms in determining the levels of the test substance. For instance, protease levels in gingival tissue are determined partly by a balance between the enzyme and its natural inhibitors. Serine proteinases like elastase are inhibited by α_1-proteinase inhibitor, α_2-macroglobulin, SLPI and SKALP. Cysteine proteases are inhibited by α_2-macroglobulin and cystatins. The level of enzyme in the tissues and to some extent GCF must therefore depend upon the enzyme inhibitor balance. In addition, the level of inflammatory cell proteinases in GCF also depends on release from inflammatory cells that have migrated into the crevice.

ENZYMES RELEASED BY DEAD CELLS (CYTOSOLIC ENZYMES)

Enzymes released from dead cells (cytosolic enzymes) include:

- Aspartate amino transferase (AST)
- Lactate dehydrogenase (LDH).

Aspartate amino transferase (AST) and lactate dehydrogenase (LDH) are soluble cytoplasmic enzymes which are confined to the cell cytoplasm but are released by dead or dying cells. Since cell death is an integral and essential component of periodontal tissue destruction they should be released during this process and should pass with the inflammatory exudate into GCF.

Aspartate amino transferase

Levels of AST in serum and cerebrospinal fluid have been used for a number of years in medicine as an indicator of tissue necrosis and cell death. In dogs, GCF AST levels have been shown to increase during the development of ligature induced experimental periodontitis (Chambers et al 1984). In human experimental gingivitis, levels in GCF samples harvested during the development and resolution of the condition were significantly associated with gingival inflammation (Persson et al 1990a). In a cross-sectional study, GCF AST was shown to correlate with clinical indices of disease severity (Imrey et al 1991).

In longitudinal studies, GCF AST levels have been related to confirmed attachment loss (Persson et al 1990b; Chambers et al 1991). Elevated GCF AST levels were strongly associated with disease active sites in contrast to disease inactive sites and active sites contained 725 units of AFC more than inactive sites. Sites with severe inflammation also yielded more AST than less inflamed sites. However, there is no evidence to indicate that GCF AST levels are predictive of disease activity because the positive correlations were made at the time of attachment loss rather than before it.

A multicentre trial was performed using a dichotomous colorimetric test which becomes positive when 800 units or more of GCF AST are present. Samples were taken before and after periodontal treatment and showed that levels were reduced below the detection limit following treatment (Page 1992).

Lactate dehydrogenase (LDH)

LDH has been correlated with probing depth and other clinical indices of disease severity in cross-sectional studies. It has also been related to periodontal disease activity in a longitudinal study. However, in both cases, the level of correlation was less than for β-glucuronidase which was included in the same studies (Lamster et al 1988).

Sampling gingival crevicular fluid for these components

Samples of GCF for the detection of both LDH and AST can be collected on conventional paper strips left *in situ* for 30 s.

Degradation products of degenerating cells

Epithelial cells produce the protein keratin and this forms the cornified layer on the surface of stratified squamous epithelia. Keratin may be released into the environment of these cells when they turnover rapidly, are damaged or degenerate. This discarded keratin has been detected in saliva and GCF (McLaughlin et al 1996). In chronic periodontitis patients, the keratin concentrations in GCF were found to be significantly greater at sites exhibiting gingivitis or periodontitis than at healthy sites but no differences were detected between gingivitis and periodontitis sites. No differences were also seen for these groupings in the salivary levels of keratin. The presence of keratin in GCF may reflect damage to the pocket epithelium which occurs in these conditions. However, since this product is unable to distinguish between gingivitis and periodontitis in a cross-sectional study, it has no potential as a marker for periodontal disease activity.

COMMERCIAL TEST KIT

The only commercial test kit based on factors released from tissue degradation is that based on GCF AST (Persson et al 1995).

Periogard AST in gingival crevicular fluid

The (Colgate) test kit uses paper point GCF samples and colorimetric detection. The test kit consists of a tray with two test wells for each tooth and appropriate reagents for conducting the test. The strip containing the GCF sample is placed into an appropriate test well and two drops of one reagent (10 mM Tris HCl with 0.067% Triton X-100, pH 6.0) are added. At the same time, positive and negative control wells are prepared using the strips provided. Two drops of a solution provided (260 mM L-aspartic acid, 33 mM 2-oxogluteric acid, 4.3 mM disodium EDTA, 1.6% polyvinylpyrrolidone, 0.067% Triton X-100, 2.7 mM sorbic acid in 100 mM Tris HCl, pH 6.0) are added to the wells and allowed to incubate at room temperature. After 9 min incubation the substrate/detection solution (1 mg Fast red RC diazotized salt in 1% methanol, 0.067% Triton X-100, in 230 mM Tris HCl, pH 8.0) is mixed and two drops are added at 10 min; 5 min later, the

test results can be read by eye by comparing the test well colour with the colour of the positive control. A colour of greater intensity over that of the negative control is scored as positive and one of lesser or equal intensity as a negative result. The test is designed to be positive at ≥800 mIU AST activity and negative at values below 800 mIU.

(Note: The commercial firms owning these tests are constantly changing because some of them sell the rights of their products to others. Therefore, the firms cited as owning these tests may not remain accurate in the future.)

Advantages and disadvantages of diagnostic tests using cytosolic enzymes

Advantages

The possible advantages are:

- Both of these potential markers associate with disease activity but do not predict it
- Tests can be devised which are simple to use
- They can be read after relatively short periods
- They can be shown to patients and related to tooth site affected.

Disadvantages

The main disadvantages are:

- The choice of the most appropriate biomarker is difficult at the present state of knowledge
- There is difficulty in determining the sites to sample and when to sample them
- Cost.

The choice of the most appropriate biomarker

Neither AST or any of the other markers in this section have been shown to be predictive for disease activity in human chronic periodontitis.

MARKERS OF CONNECTIVE TISSUE DEGRADATION

During its passage through the inflamed tissue, GCF could pick up normal components of the extracellular matrix or tissue degradation products released during the destructive process. The components that could be involved in this process are listed below:

- Connective tissue
  - Collagens I, III, V
  - Proteoglycans
  - Hyaluronan
  - Fibronectin.
- Basement membrane
  - Collagen IV
  - Laminin.

The detection of the breakdown products of these macromolecules could be indicative of tissue breakdown. These include:

Component	Breakdown product
Collagen	Hydroxyproline
	Collagen cross-links
	N-propeptide
Proteoglycan	Glycosaminoglycans (GAGs)
GAGs	Heparan sulphate
	Chondroitin-4-sulphate
	Chondroitin-6-sulphate

Fibronectin

Fibronectin, a normal component of serum and the connective tissue matrix, is present in GCF and more intact molecules are present in samples from healthy and treated sites than from diseased sites (Talonpoika et al 1989; Lopatin et al 1989). In addition, the number of intact molecules increased following treatment of the diseased sites. There are no longitudinal studies of this molecule.

Hydroxyproline-containing peptides

Hydroxyproline-containing peptides are released during collagen degradation. They have been shown to be present in GCF harvested from dogs during the development of experimental periodontitis (Svanberg 1987). However, the relationship of this peptide to human destructive periodontitis has not been studied to date.

Glycosaminoglycans

The extracellular ground substance of connective tissues contains a series of hexuronate-containing heteropolysaccharides termed glycosaminoglycans (GAGs) which are linked to a specific core protein to form high molecular weight aggregates called proteoglycans. The connective tissue breakdown which occurs during periodontitis includes proteoglycan degradation and this process involves proteolytic enzymes which release GAGs from the protein core. The GAGs may then pass into GCF via the inflammatory exudate where they have been detected (Embery et al 1982).

The GAGs in GCF from individual sites of defined clinical conditions have been investigated with cellulose-acetate electrophoresis (Embery et al 1982; Last et al 1985). The non-sulphated GAG, hyaluronic acid, was present in all samples and was the only major GAG found in chronic gingivitis patients. An additional sulphated GAG, identified by enzyme digestion as chondroitin-4-sulphate, was detected in GCF from sites with untreated advanced periodontitis. Initial GCF samples from early periodontitis and juvenile periodontitis also contained this GAG. This GAG was, however, not detected after periodontal treatment of these sites with subgingival scaling, pocket reduction surgery or daily irrigation of the pockets with a chlorhexidine solution.

Sulphated GAGs were also detected in GCF samples from around teeth undergoing orthodontic movement, teeth subject to occlusal trauma and from samples of healing tooth-extraction wounds. Thus, the presence of sulphated GAGs in GCF appears to correlate on a cross-sectional basis with those clinical conditions in which degradation changes are occurring in the deeper periodontal tissues (Last et al 1985). For this reason, the electrophoretic profile or the presence of chondroitin-4-sulphate in GCF may be a method for indicating active periodontal disease.

So far, no longitudinal studies have been carried out to relate GCF GAGs to periodontal disease activity. Also, unfortunately, it may be difficult to design a diagnostic test based on these techniques. This is first, because a large sample of GCF is required to detect GAGs and this necessitates collection with a micropipette for 15 min and second, because cellulose-acetate electrophoresis and enzyme digestion are used for their detection and identification.

Proteoglycan degradation products

The degradation products (unsaturated disaccharide isomers) of enzymic degradation of chondroitin sulphate have been shown to be present in whole saliva (Okazaki et al 1996). This group has shown that the salivary levels of these products are significantly higher in untreated chronic periodontitis patients than healthy control subjects.

Antioxidant activity and capacity

Inflammatory cells produce reactive oxygen species (ROS) within their phagolysosomes and these may spill over into the tissues during phagocytosis or when they degenerate. This may cause bystander tissue damage around these cells. ROS have a great capacity to damage cells and tissues and are scavenged for within the tissues by antioxidants.

The antioxidant capacity of saliva has been investigated in healthy and chronic periodontitis patients (Moore et al 1994). The major aqueous antioxidant component of whole saliva was found to be uric acid with lesser contributions from ascorbic acid and albumin. Using biochemical methods, the antioxidant capacity of the saliva was not found to be compromised in chronic periodontitis patients and this was attributed to increased salivary flow and antioxidant flow from GCF.

An enhanced chemiluminescent assay can be used to measure the total antioxidant (AO) capacity of serum, saliva and GCF (Chapple et al 1997). In saliva and GCF an AO response was found which was not present in the serum of the same patients. This group investigated the peripheral (serum) and local (saliva) AO capacities of chronic periodontitis and healthy patients. There were no differences in the serum AO capacities but the salivary total AO concentrations were significantly lower in the chronic periodontitis group compared with the healthy group. Thus the saliva of chronic periodontitis patients may have a reduced AO capacity which could result from increased ROS production by inflammatory cells. The enhanced chemiluminescent assay provides a rapid and simple method of measuring the total antioxidant defence in small volumes of biological fluid and hence could have diagnostic use. However, much more work on its relationship to the progression of periodontal disease needs to be done before this could be properly assessed.

Sampling gingival crevicular fluid for these components

GCF for the detection of fibronectin and hydroxyproline-containing peptides can be collected on paper strips. However, the detection of GAGs in GCF requires a large volume of fluid produced over long collection times of around 15 min using micropipettes. This is impractical in the clinical situation and can also significantly affect GCF composition over that which is produced by short collection times. The longer collection time will collect fluid which mostly consists of continuously stimulated inflammatory exudate rather than the residual fluid which additionally contains components from the local environment.

Methods of isolation and detection

The biochemical techniques used to isolate and detect some of these components are difficult to modify for chairside use. These methods are listed below:

- Hydroxyproline high pressure liquid chromatography (HPLC), ion exchange chromatography
- Collagen cross-links HPLC
- GAGs cellulose acetate extraction and staining.

Problems with the possible clinical use of tissue degradation products

- Most involve complex and expensive techniques to isolate and detect.
- If present in GCF they usually require long collection times using a micropipette to obtain sufficient quantities to analyse.
- Long GCF collection times affect its composition.
- The normal cycle of synthesis and degradation of connective tissue and bone needs to be considered.
- Most are not suitable for chairside use because it is difficult to develop a simplified detection system.

BONE RESORPTION

Bone specific proteins

Several bone morphogenic proteins are involved in bone mineralization and some connective tissue proteins also play an important role in this process (Bowers et al 1989). Some of those given below have been considered as possible markers of bone resorption and hence periodontal disease activity. These proteins are:

- Osteonectin
- Bone phosphoprotein (*N*-propeptide)
- Osteocalcin
- Telopeptides of type I collagen
- Collagen I
- Proteoglycans.

Osteonectin and bone phosphoprotein (N-propeptide)

Osteonectin is a normal component of bone matrix which is thought to play an important role in the initial phase of mineralization (Termine et al 1981). Bone phosphoprotein, which is an amino propeptide extension (*N*-propeptide) of the α-1 chains of type I collagen, appears to be involved in the attachment of connective tissue cells to the substratum (Bowers et al 1989).

Both of these proteins have been detected in GCF from patients with periodontitis (Bowers et al 1989). In addition, the total amount of both GCF osteonectin and bone phosphoprotein have been shown to increase in line with the site probing depth (Bowers et al 1989). They therefore may be associated with periodontal disease severity. However, no longitudinal studies of these proteins have been reported.

Osteocalcin

Osteocalcin is a 5.4 kDa calcium binding protein of bone and is the most abundant non-collagenous protein of the mineralized tissues (Lian et al 1988). It contains three residues of a specialized calcium binding amino acid known as γ-carboxyglutamic acid and this allows specific changes that promote hydroxyapatite binding and subsequent accumulation of bone (Hauschka et al 1975). Osteocalcin also chemotactically attracts osteoclast progenitor cells and blood monocytes (Glowacki & Lian 1987; Mundy & Proser 1987). In addition, it is stimulated by vitamin D3 (Price & Baukol 1980) producing concentrations that inhibit collagen synthesis in osteoblasts, promote bone resorption (Calalis & Lian 1988) and stimulate the differentiation of progenitor cells capable of bone resorption (Lian et al 1985). Furthermore, elevated levels of osteocalcin are found in the blood during periods of rapid bone turnover such as osteoporosis and fracture repair (Yasuruma et al 1987; Slovik et al 1984). For all these reasons osteocalcin has been suggested as a possible marker for bone resorption and hence periodontal disease progression.

Two cross-sectional studies of the relationship of GCF osteocalcin levels to periodontal disease severity have been published. The first of these studied 19 patients, five with chronic gingivitis and 14 with chronic periodontitis, at their initial visits (Kunimatsu et al 1993). Insignificant amounts of osteocalcin were found in gingivitis patients, whereas in periodontitis patients higher levels of osteocalcin were found which significantly correlated with the clinical parameters. The levels were highest at the sites with marked inflammation and the results suggested that GCF osteocalcin levels reflected the degree of inflammation at the sampled sites. The second study (Nakashima et al 1994) investigated 17 patients and compared the GCF osteocalcin levels at healthy, gingivitis and periodontitis sites. They found that osteocalcin was present at both healthy and diseased sites and the mean concentrations in GCF were more than 10 times greater

than normal serum levels. They also found that the total amounts of GCF osteocalcin at diseased sites were significantly higher than those at healthy or gingivitis sites. In addition, the total amounts of GCF osteocalcin significantly correlated with clinical parameters. However, when the GCF osteocalcin concentrations were compared they correlated with GI but not with PD.

There have been no human longitudinal studies relating GCF osteocalcin levels to periodontal disease activity but recently there has been one study relating these levels to the progression of ligature induced experimental periodontitis in beagle dogs (Giannobile et al 1995). A total of 36 experimental sites and 36 control sites were examined longitudinally at 2-week intervals over 6 months. The GCF osteocalcin was measured by radioimmunoassays. Standardized radiographs were taken at 2-weekly intervals to measure the linear loss of alveolar bone and the percentage bone loss at each 2-week interval was calculated using a previously described method (Jeffcoat & Williams 1984). Also, active bone loss was monitored monthly by assessing the uptake of a bone-seeking radioactive technetium compound (99m-Tc-MDP) using a previously described nuclear medicine technique (Jeffcoat et al 1987).

GCF osteocalcin levels increased significantly after 2 weeks following the initiation of the disease and this increase preceded significant increases in the bone-seeking radiopharmaceutical uptake (BSRU) by 2 weeks and the radiographical evidence of bone loss by 4 weeks. The BSRU was significantly elevated at experimental as compared with control sites at 4 weeks and 8 weeks post-disease initiation. GCF osteocalcin levels peaked at 8 and 10 weeks following ligature placement at levels nearly 10-fold greater than those at contralateral control sites. Following the removal of the ligatures, the GCF osteocalcin levels dropped precipitously approaching control levels.

The diagnostic ratios of GCF osteocalcin concentration predicting active bone loss were calculated and were 56% (sensitivity), 78% (specificity), 87% (positive prediction) and 34% (negative prediction). This indicates that GCF osteocalcin may serve as a predictor of active bone loss in experimental periodontitis but the low figure for negative prediction means that it would fail to predict a significant number of truly active sites. If this were translated to a clinical situation it would mean that these sites would not be treated.

Osteocalcin can be assayed using polyclonal or monoclonal antibodies by an enzyme-linked immunosorbent assay (ELISA) or a radioimmune assay. An ELISA technique could be simplified and developed for use in a diagnostic test suitable for dental practice.

Cross-linked carboxyterminal telopeptide of type I collagen

The pyridinoline cross-linked carboxyterminal telopeptide of type I collagen (CTP) is a 12–20 kDa fragment of bone type I collagen (**Fig. 14.7**) released by digestion with trypsin or bacterial collagenase (Risteli et al 1993). Type I collagen makes up about 90% of the organic matrix of bone. During synthesis of bone collagen pyridinoline cross-links are formed between the telopeptide regions of an α_1 collagen molecule and the helical region of another such molecule. This increases the mechanical stability of the structure.

CTP has recently been shown to correlate with bone turnover in myxoedema, thyrotoxicosis, primary hyperparathyroidism and postmenopausal

osteoporosis (Eriksen et al 1993). Elevated CTP has also been shown to coincide with the bone resorptive rate (Eriksen et al 1993; Hassager et al 1994).

CTP has been detected in GCF (Giannobile et al 1995; Talonpoika and Hämäläinen 1994), in periodontitis patients (Talonpoika and Hämäläinen 1994) and in experimental periodontitis in dogs (Giannobile et al 1995).

There has been one recent cross-sectional study of GCF CTP in humans (Talonpoika and Hämäläinen 1994). This was a study of 20 patients who were divided into a periodontitis-affected group (13 subjects) and a periodontitis-free group (7 subjects). GCF was collected from 126 sites in all these patients. Four subjects from the periodontitis-affected group received periodontal treatment and GCF samples were additionally collected 2, 5, 10, 20 and 40 days after treatment. GCF CTP was determined by a radioimmunological method. Significantly higher GCF CTP concentrations were found in the periodontitis-affected group compared with the periodontitis-free group and the GCF levels were 100 times higher than serum reference levels. Significant positive correlations were found between the total amount of GCF CTP per site and pocket depth, radiological bone loss, papillary bleeding index and plaque index.

Periodontal treatment reduced the GCF CTP concentrations to levels found in healthy subjects. However, there were large variations in the amounts of GCF CTP found in individual patients and at individual sites within each patient. In this regard, some CTP levels below the detection limit were found in deep pockets and some high levels were found in periodontitis-free individuals. Thus, it is possible that GCF CTP levels reflect local type I collagen degradation in the periodontal tissues which may or may not be reflected in the clinical parameters found at the site sampled.

There have been no human longitudinal studies relating GCF CTP levels to periodontal disease activity but recently there has been one relating these levels to the progression of ligature induced experimental periodontitis in beagle dogs (Giannobile et al 1995). This had the same study design as the one described above for osteocalcin and the experimental details are the same. GCF CTP was detected by radioimmunoassays. The GCF CTP levels increased significantly after 2 weeks following the initiation of the disease. This increase preceded significant increases in the bone-seeking radiopharmaceutical uptake (BSRU) by 2 weeks and the radiographical evidence of bone loss by 4 weeks. The BSRU was significantly elevated at experimental as compared with control sites at 4 and 8 weeks post-disease initiation. GCF CTP levels remained elevated throughout the entire disease progression phase.

The GCF CTP levels dropped precipitously following the removal of the ligatures and approached control levels. The diagnostic ratios of GCF CTP in predicting active bone loss were calculated at all time periods and these were 95% (sensitivity), 81% (specificity), 87% (positive prediction) and 91% (negative prediction). These values were all considerably better than those for GCF osteocalcin and indicate that GCF CTP relate positively to indices of active alveolar bone loss in experimental periodontitis and may serve as markers for future alveolar bone loss. However, its clinical use will depend on the results of human longitudinal studies.

Sampling gingival crevicular fluid for these components

The detection of osteonectin requires the use of nitrocellulose strips as it cannot be recovered from conventional strips (Bowers et al 1989). In contrast, GCF samples for the detection of osteocalcin and CTP (Giannobile et al 1995)

Fig. 14.7 A diagram showing the pyridinoline cross-linked carboxyl telopeptide of type I collagen (CTP). This is found at the carboxyterminal end of bone type 1 collagen.

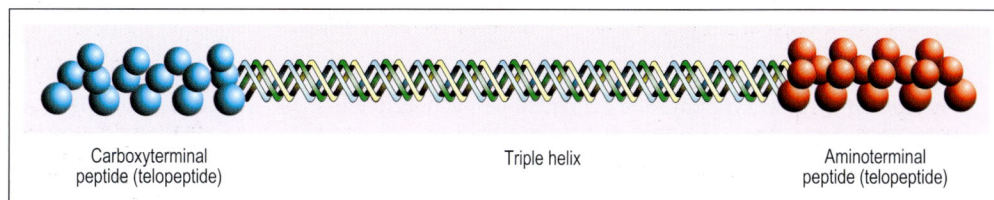

Carboxyterminal peptide (telopeptide)   Triple helix   Aminoterminal peptide (telopeptide)

were collected on conventional paper strips left *in situ* for 30 s. However, in some studies of osteocalcin and CTP multiple strip collection was used using two in succession for 1 min at the same site (Nakashima et al 1994) or three strips together at the same site for very short periods of collection (Talonpoika and Hämäläinen 1994). Clearly, some standardization of collection technique is required if the data from such studies is to be compared.

Development of diagnostic tests

Most of the potential markers in this group could easily be adapted into test kits as their detection involves the use of specific polyclonal or monoclonal antibodies. In this regard, the techniques of osteocalcin utilizes either ELISA (Kunimatsu et al 1993; Nakashima et al 1994) or radioimmunoassays (Giannobile et al 1995); those for CTP utilize radioimmunoassays (Giannobile et al 1995; Talonpoika and Hämäläinen 1994) and those for osteonectin and *N*-propeptide utilize ELISA (Bowers et al 1989).

Advantages and disadvantages of diagnostic tests using markers of bone resorption

Advantages

- Some of these potential markers associate with disease activity but do not predict it
- Simple to use
- Can be read after relatively short periods
- Can be shown to patients and related to tooth site affected.

GCF CTP levels appear to predict active bone loss in experimental periodontitis in dogs but have yet to be tested in a longitudinal study in humans.

Disadvantages

- The choice of the most appropriate biomarker is difficult at the present state of knowledge
- There is difficulty in determining the sites to sample and when to sample them
- Cost.

The choice of the most appropriate biomarker

None of markers in this section have been shown in human longitudinal studies of chronic periodontitis to predict disease activity. Osteocalcin and CTP seem to relate to alveolar bone resorption and may thus have potential as markers on the basis of cross-sectional human studies and studies on experimental periodontitis in dogs.

CLINICAL USES OF A PREDICTIVE DIAGNOSTIC TEST

If a reliable predictive test were developed, it could predict future periodontal activity and thus enable site specific treatment to be given before irreversible damage had occurred. For this to be the case, the marker must have been shown in human longitudinal studies to have highly statistically significant correlations with confirmed attachment loss, both at the predictive and the attachment loss periods. It should also have very high positive and negative predictive values in diagnostic testing using 2×2 contingency tables. Multicentre studies are also desirable. Only markers with these credentials should be used in clinical practice for the reasons listed below:

- To prevent destructive disease
- To prevent progression of disease
- To identify high risk patients
- To target treatment to specific sites
- To monitor the effects of periodontal treatment.

A periodontal diagnostic test could only help to prevent destructive disease if such a test was predictive of impending attachment loss at healthy gingival sites. If this were the case, it would only be possible to achieve this goal if all the sites in the mouth were tested regularly. Even if this were possible, disease progression could occur at any time between each test appointment and therefore could easily be missed.

It is also of no use using a marker which correlates with gingival inflammation because although this precedes attachment loss, it can be present for long periods without resulting in attachment loss. In addition, in some sites and some patient's mouths it may never result in attachment loss. Furthermore, gingival inflammation is easy to detect clinically and can easily be reversed with good plaque control and scaling, providing no plaque retentive factors such as poor restorations are present.

Finally, since no attachment loss has occurred in the healthy patient, we have no idea of their susceptibility to periodontal disease, as we cannot relate the amount of attachment loss to their age. It is therefore not possible to determine how frequently to test the patient or indeed which sites in the mouth to test. If a test were ever used for this purpose it would probably be best to test the most common tooth sites to show attachment loss such as mesially and distally to the first molars.

A predictive periodontal diagnostic test could be used to prevent progression of periodontal disease if tooth sites with previous attachment loss were regularly tested. However, it would still be possible for progression to occur between test visits, although this is less likely if these patients are on effective 3-monthly maintenance visits.

Some diagnostic tests may be capable of identifying high risk patients by using mean values of the marker for the mouth from several sites. For this to be the case, a long duration longitudinal study must have shown highly statistically greater mean values for the marker in attachment loss patients (i.e. those which showed progressive attachment loss during the study) compared with non-attachment loss patients (i.e. those patents which did not show attachment loss during the study).

If a predictive test correctly identified a site with impending attachment loss, it could target treatment to that site and thus should prevent the attachment loss from occurring. A test could also help to monitor periodontal treatment as its level should reduce if the treatment is successful. However, as periodontal disease is site specific and its progression may be episodic it is difficult to determine which sites to test or when to test them. This will therefore always be a problem demanding sound clinical judgement.

REFERENCES

Asikainen S, Alaluusua S, Saxen L: Recovery of Actinobacillus actinomycetemcomitans from teeth, tongue and saliva, *J Periodontol* 62:203–206, 1991.
Barnett ML, Ciancio SG, Mather ML: The modified papillary bleeding index: comparison with gingival index during the resolution of gingivitis, *J Prev Dent* 6:135–138, 1980.
Binder TA, Goodson JM, Socransky SS: Gingival fluid levels of acid and alkaline phosphatase levels, *J Periodontal Res* 22:14–19, 1987.
Birkedal-Hansen H: Role of matrix metalloproteinases in human periodontal diseases, *J Periodontol* 64:474–484, 1993.
Blankenvoorde MF, Henskens YM, Van der Weijden GA, et al: Cystatin A in gingival crevicular fluid of periodontal patients, *J Periodontal Res* 32:533–538, 1997.
Bowers MR, Fisher LW, Termine JD, et al: Connective tissue-associated proteins in crevicular fluid: Potential markers for periodontal diseases, *J Periodontol* 60:448–451, 1989.
Bragd L, Dahlén G, Wikström M, et al: The capability of Actinobacillus actinomycetemcomitans, Bacteroides gingivalis and Bacteroides intermedius to indicate progressive periodontitis, *J Clin Periodontol* 14:95–99, 1987.
Calalis E, Lian JB: 1, 25 dihydroxyvitamin D3 effects on collagen and DNA synthesis in periosteum and periosteum-free calvaria, *Bone* 6:457–460, 1988.
Cao CF, Smith QT: Crevicular fluid myeloperoxidase at healthy, gingivitis and periodontitis sites, *J Clin Periodontol* 16:17–20, 1989.
Chambers DA, Crawford JM, Mukherjee S, et al: Aspartate aminotransferase increases in crevicular fluid during experimental periodontitis in beagle dogs, *J Periodontol* 55:526–530, 1984.
Chambers DA, Imrey PB, Cohen RL, et al: A longitudinal study of aspartate aminotransferase in human gingival crevicular fluid, *J Periodontal Res* 26:65–74, 1991.

Chapple IL, Glenwright HD, Matthews JB, et al: Site-specific alkaline phosphatase levels in gingival crevicular fluid in health and gingivitis: cross-sectional studies, *J Clin Periodontol* 24:146–152, 1994.

Chapple IL, Mason GI, Garner I, et al: Enhanced chemiluminescent assay for measuring the antioxidant capacity of serum, saliva and crevicular fluid, *Ann Clin Biochem* 34:412–421, 1997.

Chen CK, Dunford RG, Reynolds HS, et al: Eikenella corrodens in the human oral cavity, *J Periodontol* 60:611–616, 1989.

Chen H-Y, Cox SW, Eley BM, et al: Matrix metalloproteinase-8 levels and elastase activities in gingival crevicular fluid from chronic adult periodontitis patients, *J Clin Periodontol* 27:366–369, 2000.

Cox SW, Cho K, Eley BM, et al: A simple, combined fluorogenic and chromogenic method for the assay of proteases in gingival crevicular fluid, *J Periodontal Res* 25:164–171, 1990.

Cox SW, Eley BM: The detection of cathepsin B- and L-, elastase-, tryptase-, trypsin- and dipeptidyl peptidase IV-like activities in gingival crevicular fluid from gingivitis and periodontitis patients using peptidyl derivatives of 7-amino-4-trifluomethylcoumarin, *J Periodontal Res* 24:353–361, 1989a.

Cox SW, Eley BM: Identification of a tryptase-like enzyme in extracts of inflamed human gingiva by effector and gel-filtration studies, *Arch Oral Biol* 34:219–221, 1989b.

Cox SW, Eley BM: Tryptase-like activity in crevicular fluid from gingivitis and periodontitis patients, *J Periodontal Res* 24:41–44, 1989c.

Cox SW, Eley BM: Cathepsin B/L-, elastase-, tryptase-, trypsin- and dipeptidyl peptidase IV-like activities in gingival crevicular fluid: a comparison of levels before and after basic periodontal treatment of chronic periodontitis patients, *J Clin Periodontol* 19:333–339, 1992.

Cox SW, Gazi MI, Eley BM: Dipeptidyl peptidase II- and IV- like activities in gingival tissue and crevicular fluid from human periodontitis lesions, *Arch Oral Biol* 37:167–173, 1992.

Cox SW, Kennett CN, Eley BM: Evaluation of the cellular contribution to protease activities in gingival crevicular fluid, *J Dent Res* 75:846, 1995, Abstract 193.

Cox SW, Eley BM, Proctor GB, et al: Elastase inhibitors from gingival homogenates, gingival epithelial cells and saliva, *J Dent Res* 80:1153, 2001.

Cox SW, Eley BM, Carpenter GH, et al: Skin antileukoproteinase in gingival tissue homogenates and epithelial cell media, *J Dent Res* 82:C-511, 2003, Abstract 282.

Cox SW, Rodriguez Gonzalez EM, Booth V, et al: Secretory leukocyte protease inhibitor and its potential interactions with elastase and cathepsin B in gingival crevicular fluid and saliva from patients with chronic periodontitis, *J Periodontal Res* 41:477–485, 2006.

Curtis MA, Griffiths GS, Price SJ, et al: The total protein concentration of gingival crevicular fluid; variation with sampling time and gingival inflammation, *J Clin Periodontol* 15:628–632, 1988.

Dickinson DP: Cysteine peptidases of mammals: their biological roles and potential effects in the oral cavity and other tissues in health and disease, *Crit Rev Oral Biol Med* 13:238–275, 2002.

Dinsdale CRJ, Rawlinson A, Walsh TF: Subgingival temperature in smokers and non smokers, *J Clin Periodontol* 24:761–766, 1997.

Dzink JL, Haffajee AD, Socransky SS: The predominant cultivable microbiota of active and inactive lesions of destructive periodontal diseases, *J Clin Periodontol* 15:316–323, 1988.

Dzink JL, Tanner ARC, Haffajee AD, et al: Gram negative species associated with active destructive periodontal lesions, *J Clin Periodontol* 12:648–659, 1985.

Ebersole JL, Frey DE, Taubman MA, et al: Serological identification on oral Bacteroides sp. By enzyme-linked immunosorbent assay, *J Clin Microbiol* 19:639–644, 1984.

Eick S, Pfister W: Comparison of a microbial cultivation and a commercial PCR based method for the detection of periodontopathogenic species in subgingival plaque samples, *J Clin Periodontol* 29:638–644, 2002.

Eley BM, Cox SW: A biochemical study of serine proteinase activities at local gingivitis sites in human chronic periodontitis, *Arch Oral Biol* 35:23–27, 1990.

Eley BM, Cox SW: Cathepsin B and L-like activities at local gingival sites of chronic periodontitis patients, *J Clin Periodontol* 18:499–504, 1991.

Eley BM, Cox SW: Crevicular fluid dipeptidyl peptidase activities before and after periodontal treatment, *J Dent Res* 71:622, 1992a.

Eley BM, Cox SW: Cathepsin B/L-, elastase-, tryptase-, trypsin- and dipeptidyl peptidase IV-like activities in gingival crevicular fluid: correlation with clinical parameters in untreated chronic periodontitis patients, *J Periodontal Res* 27:62–69, 1992b.

Eley BM, Cox SW: Correlation of gingival crevicular fluid proteases with clinical and radiological parameters of periodontal attachment loss, *J Dent* 20:90–99, 1992c.

Eley BM, Cox SW: Cathepsin B/L-, elastase-, tryptase-, trypsin- and dipeptidyl peptidase IV-like activities in gingival crevicular fluid: a comparison of levels before and after periodontal surgery in chronic periodontitis patients, *J Periodontol* 63:412–417, 1992d.

Eley BM, Cox SW: Gingival crevicular fluid inflammatory cell proteases at healthy, gingivitis and periodontitis sites, *J Dent Res* 72:705, 1993.

Eley BM, Cox SW: Bacterial proteases before and after periodontal treatment, *J Dent Res* 73:799, 1994, Abstract.

Eley BM, Cox SW: Bacterial proteases in gingival crevicular fluid before and after periodontal treatment, *Br Dent J* 178:133–139, 1995a.

Eley BM, Cox SW: Correlation between gingival crevicular fluid dipeptidyl peptidase II and IV activity and periodontal attachment loss, A 2-year longitudinal study in chronic periodontitis patients. *Oral Dis* 1:201–213, 1995b.

Eley BM, Cox SW: Correlation between gingivain/gingipain and bacterial dipeptidyl peptidase in gingival crevicular fluid and periodontal attachment loss in chronic periodontitis patients. A 2-year longitudinal study, *J Periodontol* 67:703–716, 1996a.

Eley BM, Cox SW: The relationship between gingival crevicular fluid cathepsin B activity and periodontal attachment loss in chronic periodontitis patients. A 2-year longitudinal study, *J Periodontal Res* 31:381–392, 1996b.

Eley BM, Cox SW: A 2-year longitudinal study of elastase in gingival crevicular fluid and periodontal attachment loss, *J Clin Periodontol* 23:681–692, 1996c.

Embery G, Oliver WM, Stanbury JB, et al: The electrophoretic detection of acid glycosaminoglycans in human gingival sulcus fluid, *Arch Oral Biol* 27:177–179, 1982.

Emingil G, Kuula H, Sorsa T, et al: Gingival crevicular fluid matrix metalloproteinase-25 and -26 levels in periodontal disease, *J Periodontol* 77:664–671, 2006.

Eriksen EF, Charles P, Melsen F, et al: Serum markers of type I collagen formation and degradation in metabolic bone disease: correlation with bone histomorphometry, *J Bone Miner Res* 8:127–132, 1993.

Figueredo CMS, Areas A, Miranda LA, et al: The short-term effectiveness of non-surgical treatment in reducing protease activity in gingival crevicular fluid from chronic periodontitis patients, *J Clin Periodontol* 31:615–619, 2004.

French CK, Savitt ED, Simon SL, et al: DNA probe detection of periodontal pathogens, *Oral Microbiol Immunol* 1:58–62, 1986.

Friedman SA, Mandel ID, Herrera MS: Lysozyme and lactoferrin quantifications in the crevicular fluid, *J Periodontol* 54:347–350, 1983.

Frisken KW, Tagg JR, Laws AJ: Suspected periodontopathic microorganisms and their oral habitats in young children, *Oral Microbiol Immunol* 2:60–64, 1987.

Garito ML, Prihoda TJ, McManus LM: Salivary PAF levels correlate with the severity of periodontal inflammation, *J Dent Res* 74:1048–1056, 1995.

Gazi MI, Cox SW, Clark DT, et al: Cathepsin B, tryptase and Porphyromonas gingivalis trypsin-like protease in gingival crevicular fluid, *J Dent Res* 73:799, 1994.

Gazi MI, Cox SW, Clark DT, et al: Comparison of host tissue and bacterial dipeptidylpeptidases in human gingival crevicular fluid by analytical isoelectric focusing, *Arch Oral Biol* 40:731–736, 1995.

Gazi MI, Cox SW, Clark DT, et al: A comparison of cysteine and serine proteinases in human gingival crevicular fluid with host tissue, saliva and bacterial enzymes by analytical isoelectric focusing, *Arch Oral Biol* 41:393–400, 1996.

Genco RC, Zambon JJ, Christersson LA: Use and interpretation of microbiological assays in periodontal diseases, *Oral Microbiol Immunol* 1:73–79, 1986.

Genco RC, Zambon JJ, Christersson LA: The origin of periodontal infections, *Adv Dent Res* 2:245–259, 1988.

Genco RJ: Host responses in periodontal diseases: Current concepts, *J Periodontol* 63:338–355, 1992.

Giannobile WV, Lynch SE, Denmark RG, et al: Crevicular fluid osteocalcin and pyridinoline cross-linked carboxyterminal telopeptide of type I collagen (ICTP) as markers of rapid bone turnover in periodontitis. A pilot study in beagle dogs, *J Clin Periodontol* 22:903–910, 1995.

Glowacki J, Lian JB: Impaired recruitment by osteoclast progenitors by osteocalcin deficient bone implants, *Cellular Differentiation* 21:247–254, 1987.

Gmür R, Hrodek K, Saxer UP, et al: Double-blind analysis of relation between adult periodontitis and systemic host responses to suspected periodontal pathogens, *Infect Immun* 52:768–776, 1986.

Golub LM, Siegel K, Ramamurthy NS, et al: Some characteristics of collagenase activity in gingival crevicular fluid and its relationship to gingival disease in humans, *J Dent Res* 55:1049–1057, 1976.

Greenstein G: Microbiological assessments to enhance periodontal disease diagnosis, *J Periodontol* 59:508–515, 1988.

Guven Y, Satman I, Dinccag N, et al: Salivary peroxidase activity in whole saliva of patients with insulin-dependent (type 1) diabetes mellitus, *J Clin Periodontol* 23:879–881, 1996.

Haffajee AD, Socransky SS: Attachment level changes in destructive periodontal disease, *J Clin Periodontol* 13:461–472, 1986.

Haffajee AD, Socransky SS, Goodson JM: Subgingival temperature. I. Relation to baseline clinical parameters, *J Clin Periodontol* 19:401–408, 1992a.

Haffajee AD, Socransky SS, Goodson JM: Subgingival temperature. II. Relation to future attachment loss, *J Clin Periodontol* 19:409–416, 1992b.

Haffajee AD, Socransky SS, Goodson JM: Subgingival temperature. III. Relation to microbial counts, *J Clin Periodontol* 19:417–422, 1992c.

Häkkarainen K, Uitto V-J, Ainamo J: Collagenase activity and protein content of sulcular fluid after scaling and occlusal adjustment of teeth with deep periodontal pockets, *J Periodontal Res* 23:204–210, 1988.

Hanemaaijer R, Sorsa T, Konttinen YT, et al: Matrix metalloproteinase-8 is expressed in rheumatoid synovial fibroblasts and endothelial cells. Regulation by tumor necrosis factor-alpha and doxycycline, *J Biol Chem* 272:31504–31509, 1997.

Hassager C, Jensen LT, Pødenphant J, et al: The carboxyterminal pyridinoline cross-linked telopeptide of type I collagen in serum as a marker of bone resorption: the effect of nandrolone decanoate and hormone replacement therapy, *Calcif Tissue Int* 54:30–33, 1994.

Hauschka PV, Lian JB, Gallop PM: Direct identification of the calcium-binding amino acid gamma-carboxyglutamic acid in mineralized tissue, *Proceedings of the Royal Academy of Science USA* 72:3925, 1975.

Hayakawa H, Yamashita K, Ohwaki K, et al: Collagenase activity and tissue inhibitor of metalloproteinases-1 (TIMP-1) content in human whole saliva from clinically healthy and periodontally diseased subjects, *J Periodontal Res* 29:305–308, 1994.

Henskens YM, van der Velden U, Veerman EC, et al: Protein, albumin and cystatin concentrations in saliva of healthy subjects and of patients with gingivitis or periodontitis, *J Periodontal Res* 28:43–48, 1993a.

Henskens YM, van der Velden U, Veerman EC, et al: Cystatin C levels of whole saliva are increased in periodontal patients, *Ann N Y Acad Sci* 694:280–282, 1993b.

Henskens YM, Veerman EC, Mantel MS, et al: Cystatins S and C in human whole saliva in glandular salivas in periodontal health and disease, *J Dent Res* 73: 1606–1614, 1994.

Henskens YM, van den Keijbus PA, Veerman EC, et al: Protein composition of whole and parotid saliva in healthy and periodontitis subjects, *J Periodontal Res* 31: 57–65, 1996a.

Henskens YM, van der Weijden GA, van den Keijbus PA, et al: Effects of periodontal treatment on the protein composition of whole and parotid saliva, *J Periodontol* 67:205–212, 1996b.

Highfield PE, Dougan G: DNA probes for microbial diagnosis, *Med Lab Sci* 42: 352–360, 1985.

Hönig C, Rordorf-Adam C, Siegmund C, et al: Increased interleukin beta (IL-1b)-concentration in gingival tissue from periodontitis patients, *J Periodontal Res* 24: 362–367, 1989.

Horowitz A, Folke EA: Hydrogen sulphide and periodontal disease, *Periodontal Abstr* 2:59–62, 1972.

Imrey PB, Crawford JM, Cohen RL, et al: A cross-sectional analysis of aspartate aminotransferase in human gingival crevicular fluid, *J Periodontal Res* 26:75–84, 1991.

Ingman T, Sorsa T, Konttinen YT, et al: Salivary collagenase, elastase- and trypsin-like proteases as biochemical markers of periodontal tissue destruction in adult and localized juvenile periodontitis, *Oral Microbiol Immunol* 8:298–305, 1993.

Ingman T, Sorsa T, Lindy O, et al: Multiple forms of gelatinases/type IV collagenases in saliva and gingival crevicular fluid of periodontitis patients, *J Clin Periodontol* 21:26–31, 1994.

Ingman T, Tervahartiala T, Ding Y, et al: Matrix metalloproteinases and their inhibitors in gingival crevicular fluid and saliva of periodontitis patients, *J Clin Periodontol* 23:1127–1132, 1996.

Ishikawa I, Cimasoni G, Ahmad-Zadeh C: Possible role of lysosomal enzymes in the pathogenesis of periodontitis. A study of cathepsin D in human gingival fluid, *Arch Oral Biol* 17:111–117, 1972.

Ishikawa I, Cimasoni G: Alkaline phosphatase in human gingival fluid and its relationship to periodontitis, *Arch Oral Biol* 15:1401–1404, 1970.

Jeffcoat MK, Reddy MS: Progression of probing attachment loss in adult periodontitis, *J Periodontol* 62:185–189, 1991.

Jeffcoat MK, Williams RC: Relationships between linear and area measurements of bone levels utilising a simple computerised technique, *J Periodontal Res* 19:191–198, 1984.

Jeffcoat MK, Williams RC, Johnson HG, et al: Treatment of periodontal disease in beagles with lodoxamide ethyl, an inhibitor of mast cell release, *J Periodontal Res* 20:532–541, 1985.

Jeffcoat MK, Williams RC, Caplan ML, et al: Nuclear medicine techniques for the detection of active alveolar bone loss, *Adv Dent Res* 1:80–84, 1987.

Jin LJ, Leung WK, Corbet EF, et al: Relationship of changes in interleukin-8 levels and granulocyte elastase activity in gingival crevicular fluid to subgingival periodontopathogens following non-surgical periodontal therapy in subjects with chronic periodontitis, *J Clin Periodontol* 29:604–614, 2002.

Jolley ME: Fluorescence polarization assays for the detection of proteases and their inhibitors, *Journal of Biomedical Screening* 1:33–38, 1996.

Kawada M, Yoshida A, Suzuki N, et al: Prevalence of Porphyromonas gingivalis in relation to periodontal status assessed by real-time PCR, *Oral Microbiol Immunol* 19:289–292, 2004.

Kennett CN, Cox SW, Eley BM, et al: Comparative histochemical and biochemical studies of mast cell tryptase in human gingiva, *J Periodontol* 64:870–877, 1993.

Kennett CN, Cox SW, Eley BM: Comparative histochemical, biochemical and immunocytochemical studies of cathepsin B in human gingiva, *J Periodontal Res* 29:203–213, 1994a.

Kennett CN, Cox SW, Eley BM: Histochemical, immunocytochemical and biochemical studies of dipeptidyl peptidases in human gingival tissue, *J Dent Res* 74:845, 1994b, Abstract 192.

Kennett CN, Cox SW, Eley BM: Localisation of active and inactive elastase, alpha-1-proteinase inhibitor and alpha-2-macroglobulin in human gingiva, *J Dent Res* 74: 667–674, 1995.

Kennett CN, Cox SW, Eley BM: The histochemical and immunocytochemical localisation of dipeptidylpeptidase II and IV in human gingiva, *J Periodontol* 67:846–852, 1996.

Kennett CN, Cox SW, Eley BM: Investigations into the cellular contribution of host tissue protease activity in gingival crevicular fluid, *J Clin Periodontol* 24:424–431, 1997a.

Kennett CN, Cox SW, Eley BM: Ultrastructural localisation of cathepsin B in gingival tissue from chronic periodontitis patients, *Histochem J* 29:727–734, 1997b.

Kiili M, Cox SW, Chen HY, et al: Collagenase-2 (MMP-8) and collagenase-3 (MMP-13) in adult periodontitis: molecular forms and levels in gingival crevicular fluid and immunolocalisation in gingival tissue, *J Clin Periodontol* 29:224–232, 2002.

Kinane DF, Mooney J, Ebersole JL: Humoral immune response to Actinobacillus actinomycetemcomitans and Porphyromonas gingivalis in periodontal disease, *Periodontol 2000* 20:289–340, 1999.

Kinane DF, Darby IB, Said S, et al: Changes in gingival crevicular fluid matrix metalloproteinase-8 levels during periodontal treatment and maintenance, *J Periodontal Res* 38:400–404, 2003.

Kowashi Y, Jaccard F, Cimasoni G: Increase of free collagenase and neutral protease activities in the gingival crevice during experimental gingivitis in Man, *Arch Oral Biol* 34:645–650, 1979.

Kryshalskyi E, Sodek J: Nature of collagenolytic enzyme and inhibitor activity in gingival crevicular fluid from healthy and inflamed periodontal tissues of beagle dogs, *J Periodontal Res* 22:264–269, 1987.

Kryshalskyi E, Sodek J, Ferrier JM: Correlation of collagenolytic enzymes and inhibitors in gingival crevicular fluid with clinical and microscopic changes in experimental periodontitis in the dog, *Arch Oral Biol* 31:21–31, 1986.

Kunimatsu K, Mataki S, Tanaka H, et al: A cross-sectional study of osteocalcin levels in gingival crevicular fluid from periodontitis patients, *J Periodontol* 64:865–869, 1993.

Lamster IB: The host response in gingival crevicular fluid: potential applications in periodontitis clinical trials, *J Periodontol* 63:1117–1123, 1992.

Lamster IB, Holmes LG, Gross KBW, et al: The relationship of β-glucuronidase activity in crevicular fluid to clinical parameters of periodontal disease. Findings from a multicenter study, *J Clin Periodontol* 21:118–127, 1994.

Lamster IB, Oshrain RL, Harper DS, et al: Enzyme activity in crevicular fluid for detection and prediction of clinical attachment loss in patients with chronic adult periodontitis, *J Periodontol* 59:516–523, 1988.

Lamster IB, Oshrain RL, Celenti RS, et al: Indicators of the acute inflammatory and humoral immune responses in gingival crevicular fluid: relationship to active periodontal disease, *J Periodontal Res* 26:261–263, 1991.

Lamster IB, Kaluszhner-Shapira I, HerrerAbreu M, et al: Serum IgG responses to Actinobacillus actinomycetemcomitans and Porphyromonas gingivalis: implications for periodontal diagnosis, *J Clin Periodontol* 25:510–516, 1998.

Larivee L, Sodek J, Ferrier JM: Collagenase and collagenase inhibitor activity in crevicular fluid of patients receiving treatment for localised juvenile periodontitis, *J Periodontal Res* 21:702–715, 1986.

Last KS, Stanbury JB, Embery G: Glycosaminoglycans in human gingival crevicular fluid as indicators of active periodontal disease, *Arch Oral Biol* 30:275–281, 1985.

Lee H-J, Kang IK, Chung CP, et al: The subgingival microflora and gingival crevicular fluid cytokines in refractory periodontitis, *J Clin Periodontol* 22:885–890, 1995a.

Lee W, Aitken S, Sodek J, et al: Evidence of a direct relationship between neutrophil collagenase activity and periodontal tissue destruction in vivo: role of active enzyme in human periodontitis, *J Periodontal Res* 30:23–33, 1995b.

Lian JB, Gundberg CM: Osteocalcin: biochemical considerations and clinical applications, *Clin Orthop Relat Res* 226:267–291, 1988.

Lian JB, Couttes MC, Canalis E: Studies of the hormone regulation of osteocalcin synthesis in cultured fetal rat calvaria, *J Biol Chem* 260:8706, 1985.

Lin M, Sugden EA, Jolley ME, et al: Modification of the Mycobacterium bovis extracellular protein MPB70 with fluoroscein for rapid detection of specific serum antibodies by fluorescence polarization, *Clinical and Diagnostic Immunology* 3:438–443, 1996.

Listgarten MA: Direct microscopy of periodontal pathogens, *Oral Microbiol Immunol* 1:31–36, 1986.

Listgarten MA: Microbial testing in the diagnosis of periodontal disease, *J Periodontol* 63:332–337, 1992.

Listgarten MA, Levin S: Positive correlation between proportions of subgingival spirochaetes and motile bacteria and susceptibility of human subjects to periodontal deterioration, *J Clin Periodontol* 8:122–138, 1981.

Listgarten MA, Schifter CC, Sulivan P, et al: Failure of a microbial assay to reliably predict disease recurrence in a treated periodontitis population receiving regularly scheduled prophylaxes, *J Clin Periodontol* 13:768–773, 1986.

Listgarten MA, Slots J, Nowotny AH, et al: Incidence of periodontitis recurrence in treated patients with and without cultivable Actinobacillus actinomycetemcomitans, Porphyromonas gingivalis and Prevotella intermedia: a prospective study, *J Periodontol* 62:377–386, 1991.

Löe H: The gingival index, the plaque index and the retention index systems, *J Periodontol* 38:610–616, 1967.

Loesche WJ: The identification of bacteria associated with periodontal disease and dental caries by enzymatic methods, *Oral Microbiol Immunol* 1:65–70, 1986.

Loesche WJ: DNA probe and enzyme analysis in periodontal diagnosis, *J Periodontol* 63:1102–1109, 1992.

Loesche WJ, Bretz W, Lopatin D, et al: Multi-center clinical evaluation of a chairside method for detecting certain periodontopathic bacteria in periodontal disease, *J Periodontol* 61:189–196, 1990.

Lopatin DE, Caffessee ER, Bye FL, et al: Concentrations of fibronectin in the sera and crevicular fluid in various stages of periodontal disease, *J Clin Periodontol* 16: 359–364, 1989.

Lopatin DE, Blackburn E: Avidity and titre of immunoglobulin G subclasses to Porphyromonas gingivalis in adult periodontitis patients, *Oral Microbiol Immunol* 7:332–337, 1992.

Makela M, Salo T, Uitto VJ, et al: Matrix metalloproteinases (MMP-2 and MMP-9) of the oral cavity: cellular origin and relationship to periodontal status, *J Dent Res* 73: 1397–1406, 1994.

Mandell RL, Socransky SS: Selective medium for Actinobacillus actinomycetem-comitans and the incidence of the organism in juvenile periodontitis, *J Periodontol* 52: 593–598, 1981.

Mäntylä P, Stenman M, et al: Gingival crevicular fluid collagenase-2 (MMP-8) test stick for chairside monitoring of periodontitis, *J Periodontal Res* 38:436–439, 2003.

Mäntylä P, Stenman M, Kinane D, et al: Monitoring periodontal disease status in smokers and nonsmokers using a gingival crevicular fluid matrix metalloproteinase-8-specific chair-side test, *J Periodontal Res* 41:503–512, 2006.

Marcotte H, Lavoie MC: Oral microbial ecology and the role of salivary immunoglobulin A, *Microbiol Mol Biol Rev* 62:71–109, 1998.

Markkanen H, Syrjanen SM, Alakuijala P: Salivary IgA, lysozyme and beta 2-microglobulin in periodontal disease, *Scand J Dent Res* 94:115–120, 1986.

Masada MP, Persson R, Kenney JL, et al: Measurement of interleukin-1a and 1b in gingival crevicular fluid: implications for the pathogenesis of periodontal disease, *J Periodontal Res* 25:156–163, 1990.

Matsuki H, Fujimoto N, Iwata K, et al: A one-step sandwich enzyme immunoassay (EIA) system for human matrix metalloproteinase 8 (neutrophil collagenase) using monoclonal antibodies, *Clinica Chimica Acta* 31(244), 129–143, 1996.

Matto J, Saarela M, Von Triol-Linden B, et al: Similarity of salivary and subgingival Prevotella intermedia and Prevotella nigrescens isolates by arbitrarily primed polymerase chain reaction, *Oral Microbiol Immunol* 11:395–401, 1996.

Matto J, Saarela M, Alaluusua S, et al: Detection of Porphyromonas gingivalis from saliva by PCR using a simple sample processing method, *J Clin Microbiol* 36:157–160, 1998.

McArthur WP, Clark WB: Specific antibodies and their potential role in periodontal diseases, *J Periodontol* 64:807–818, 1993.

McLaughlin WS, Kirkham J, Kowalik MJ, et al: Human gingival crevicular fluid keratin at healthy, chronic gingivitis and chronic adult periodontitis sites, *J Clin Periodontol* 23:331–335, 1996.

Moore S, Calder KA, Miller NJ, et al: Antioxidant activity of saliva and periodontal disease, *Free Radic Res* 21:417–425, 1994.

Moore WEC, Moore LH, Ranney RR: The microflora of periodontal sites showing active destruction progression, *J Clin Periodontol* 18:729–739, 1991.

Muller HP, Heinecke A, Borneff M, et al: Microbial ecology of Actinobacillus actinomycetemcomitans, Eikenella corrodens and Capnocytophaga spp. In adult periodontitis, *J Periodontal Res* 32:530–542, 1997.

Mundy GR, Proser JW: Chemical activity of the gamma-carboxyglutamic acid-containing protein in bone, *Calcif Tissue Int* 40:57, 1987.

Nakamura-Minami M, Furuichi Y, Ishikawa K, et al: Changes in α1-protease inhibitor and secretory leukocyte protease inhibitor levels in gingival crevicular fluid before and after non-surgical periodontal treatment, *Oral Dis* 9:249–254, 2003.

Nakashima K, Roehrich N, Cimasoni G: Osteocalcin, prostaglandin E2 and alkaline phosphate in gingival crevicular fluid: their relations to periodontal status, *J Clin Periodontol* 21:327–333, 1994.

Nieminen A, Nordlund L, Uitto VJ: The effect of treatment on the activity of salivary proteases and glycosidases in adults with advanced periodontitis, *J Periodontol* 64:297–301, 1993a.

Nieminen A, Kari K, Saxen L: Specific antibodies against Actinobacillus actinomycetemcomitans in serum and saliva of patients with advanced periodontitis, *Scand J Dent Res* 101:196–201, 1993b.

Nieminen A, Asikainen S, Tokko H, et al: Value of some laboratory and clinical measurements in the treatment plan for advanced periodontitis, *J Clin Periodontol* 23:572–581, 1996.

Offenbacher S, Heasman PA, Collins JG: Modulation of host PGE$_2$ secretion as a determinant of periodontal disease expression, *J Periodontol* 64:432–444, 1993.

Offenbacher S, Odle BM, Van Dyke TE: The use of crevicular fluid prostaglandin E$_2$ levels as a predictor of periodontal attachment loss, *J Periodontal Res* 21:101–112, 1986.

Okazaki J, Kamada A, Gonda Y, et al: High-performance liquid chromatography analysis of chondroitin sulphate isomers in human whole saliva in a variety of clinical conditions, *Oral Dis* 2:224–227, 1996.

Over C, Yamalik N, Yavuzyilmaz E, et al: Myeloperoxidase activity in peripheral blood neutrophils, crevicular fluid and whole saliva of patients with periodontal disease, *J Nihon Univ Sch Dent* 35:235–240, 1993.

Overall CM, Sodek J: Initial characterisation of a neutral metalloproteinase, active on 3/4-collagen fragments, synthesised by ROS 17/2.8 osteoblastic cells, periodontal fibroblasts, and identified in gingival crevicular fluid, *J Dent Res* 66:1271–1282, 1987.

Page RC: The role of inflammatory mediators in the pathogenesis of periodontal disease, *J Periodontal Res* 26:230–242, 1991.

Page RC: Host response tests for diagnosing periodontal diseases, *J Periodontol* 63:356–366, 1992.

Palcanis KG, Larjava IK, Wells BR, et al: Elastase as an indicator of periodontal disease progression, *J Periodontol* 63:237–274, 1992.

Patters MR, Niekrash CE, Lang NP: Assessment of complement cleavage in gingival fluid during experimental gingivitis, *J Clin Periodontol* 16:33–37, 1989.

Pederson ED, Stanke SR, Whitener SJ, et al: Salivary levels of alpha-2-macrogobulin, alpha-1-antitrypsin, C-reactive protein, cathepsin G and elastase in humans with and without destructive periodontal disease, *Arch Oral Biol* 40:1151–1155, 1995.

Persson GR, De Rouen TA, Page RC: Relationship between levels of aspartate aminotransferase in gingival crevicular fluid and gingival inflammation, *J Periodontal Res* 25:17–24, 1990a.

Persson GR, De Rouen TA, Page RC: Relationship between gingival crevicular fluid levels of aspartate aminotransferase and active tissue destruction in treated chronic periodontitis patients, *J Periodontal Res* 25:81–87, 1990b.

Persson S, Claesson R, Carlsson J: The capacity of the subgingival microbiota to produce volatile sulphur compounds in human serum, *Oral Microbiol Immunol* 4:169–172, 1989.

Persson S, Edlund MB, Claesson R, et al: The formation of H$_2$S and CH$_3$SH by oral bacteria, *Oral Microbiol Immunol* 5:195–201, 1990c.

Persson GR, Alves ME, Chambers DA, et al: A multicenter clinical trial of periogard in distinguishing between diseased and healthy sites, I, Study design, methodology and therapeutic outcome, *J Clin Periodontol* 22:794–808, 1995.

Pinducciu G, Micheletti L, Piras V, et al: Periodontal disease, oral microbial flora and salivary antibacterial factors in diabetes mellitus type 1 patients, *Eur J Epidemiol* 12:631–636, 1996.

Polychronopoulou T: *A study of a probe to measure volatile sulphides and clinical parameters in periodontal health and disease*. M. Dent. Sci. Thesis, 1998, University of Liverpool.

Pozo P, Valenzuela MA, Melej C, et al: Longitudinal analysis of metalloproteinases, tissue inhibitors of metalloproteinases and clinical parameters in gingival crevicular fluid from periodontitis-affected patients, *J Periodontal Res* 40:199–207, 2005.

Price PA, Baukol SA: 1, 25(OH)$_2$D$_3$ increases the synthesis of the vitamin K dependent protein by osteosarcoma cells, *J Biol Chem* 255:1160–1163, 1980.

Rasch MS, Mealey BL, Woodard DS, et al: The effect of initial therapy on salivary platelet activating factor levels in chronic adult periodontitis, *J Periodontol* 66:613–623, 1995.

Reiff RL: Serum and salivary IgG and IgA response to initial preparation therapy, *J Periodontol* 55:299–305, 1984.

Reinhardt RA, McDonald TL, Bolton RW, et al: IgG subclasses in gingival crevicular fluid from active versus stable periodontal sites, *J Periodontol* 60:44–50, 1989.

Reinhardt RA, Masada MP, Kaldahl WB, et al: Gingival fluid IL-1 and IL-6 levels in refractory periodontitis, *J Clin Periodontol* 20:225–231, 1993.

Renvert S, Wikström M, Mugrabi M, et al: Association of crevicular fluid elastase-like activity with histologically-confirmed attachment loss in ligature-induced periodontitis in beagle dogs, *J Clin Periodontol* 25:368–374, 1998.

Reynolds JJ: Collagenases and tissue inhibitors of metalloproteinases; a functional balance in tissue degradation, *Oral Dis* 2:70–76, 1996.

Reynolds JJ, Hembry RM, Meikle MC: Connective tissue degradation in health and periodontal disease and the role of matrix metalloproteinases and their natural inhibitors, *Adv Dent Res* 8:312–319, 1994.

Risteli J, Elomaa I, Neimi S, et al: Radioimmunoassay for the pyridinoline cross-linked carboxyterminal peptide of type I collagen: a new serum marker of bone collagen degradation, *Clin Chem* 39:635–640, 1993.

Roa RN, Balamuralikrishnan K, Vasantkumar A, et al: A study of antitrypsin and macroglobulin levels in serum and saliva of patients with gingivitis, *Indian J Dent Res* 6:41–46, 1995.

Rossomando EF, Kennedy JE, Hadjimichael J: Tumor necrosis factor alpha in gingival crevicular fluid as a possible indicator of periodontal disease in humans, *Arch Oral Biol* 35:431–434, 1990.

Sakai Y, Shimauchi H, Ito H- O, et al: Porphyromonas gingivalis specific IgG subclass antibody levels as immunological risk indicators of periodontal bone loss, *J Clin Periodontol* 28:853–859, 2001.

Sandholm L: Proteases and their inhibitors in chronic inflammatory periodontal disease, *J Clin Periodontol* 13:19–26, 1986.

Sandholm L, Gronblad E: Salivary immunoglobulins in patients with juvenile periodontitis and their healthy siblings, *J Periodontol* 55:9–12, 1984.

Sandholm L, Tolo K, Olsen I: Salivary IgG, a parameter of periodontal disease activity? High responder to Actinobacillus actinomycetemcomitans Y4 in juvenile and adult periodontitis, *J Clin Periodontol* 14:289–294, 1987.

Sanz M, Lau L, Herrera D, et al: Methods of detection of Actinobacillus actinomycetemcomitans, Porphyromonas gingivalis and Tannerella forsythensis in periodontal microbiology, with special emphasis on advanced molecular techniques: a review, *J Clin Periodontol* 31:1034–1047, 2004.

Savitt ED, Strzemoko MN, Vaccaro KK, et al: Comparison of cultural methods and DNA probe analysis for the detection of A. actinomycetemcomitans, P. gingivalis, and B. intermedius in subgingival plaque samples, *J Periodontol* 59:431–438, 1988.

Schade SZ, Jolley ME, Sarauer BJ, et al: BODIPY-alpha-casein, a pH-independent protein substrate for protease assays using fluorescence polarization, *Anal Biochem* 243:1–7, 1996.

Schmidt EF, Bretz WA, Hutchinson RA, et al: Correlation of the hydrolysis of benzoyl-arginine-naphthylamide (BANA) by plaque with clinical parameters and subgingival levels of spirochaetes in periodontal patients, *J Dent Res* 67:1505–1509, 1988.

Slots J, Emrich LJ, Genco R: Relationship between some subgingival bacteria and periodontal pocket depth and gain or loss of attachment after treatment of adult periodontitis, *J Clin Periodontol* 12:540–552, 1985.

Slots J, Bragd L, Wikström M, et al: The occurrence of Actinobacillus actinomycetemcomitans, Bacteroides gingivalis and Bacteroides intermedius in destructive periodontal disease in adults, *J Clin Periodontol* 13:570–577, 1986.

Slots J, Listgarten MA: Bacteroides gingivalis, Bacteroides intermedius and Actinobacillus actinomycetemcomitans in human periodontal diseases, *J Clin Periodontol* 15:85–93, 1988.

Slovik M, Gundberg CM, Neer RM, et al: Clinical evaluation of bone turnover by serum osteocalcin measurements, *J Clin Endocrinol Metab* 59:228–230, 1984.

Smith QT, Hinrichs JE, Melnyk RS: Gingival crevicular fluid myeloperoxidase at periodontitis sites, *J Periodontal Res* 21:45–55, 1986.

Socransky SS, Haffajee AD: The bacterial etiology of destructive periodontal disease: current concepts, *J Periodontol* 63:322–337, 1992.

Sorsa T, Suomalainen K, Uitto J: The role of gingival crevicular fluid and salivary interstitial collagenases in human periodontal disease, *Arch Oral Biol* 35:193S–196S, 1990.

Sorsa T, Ding Y, Salo T, et al: Effects of tetracyclines on neutrophil, gingival and salivary collagenases. A functional and western-blot assessment with special reference to their cellular sources in periodontal diseases, *Ann N Y Acad Sci* 732:112–131, 1994.

Sterne JAC, Curtis MA, Gillett IR, et al: Statistical models for data from periodontal research, *J Clin Periodontol* 17:129–137, 1990.

Suomalainen K, Saxen L, Vilja P, et al: Peroxidases, lactoferrin and lysozyme in peripheral blood neutrophils, gingival crevicular fluid and whole saliva of patients with localized juvenile periodontitis, *Oral Dis* 2:129–134, 1996.

Svanberg GK: Hydroxyproline determination in serum and gingival crevicular fluid, *J Periodontal Res* 22:133–138, 1987.

Takashi H, Ryoichi M, Yukiko S, et al: Relationship between periodontal disease status and combination of biochemical assays of gingival crevicular fluid, *J Periodontal Res* 40:331–338, 2005.

Talonpoika JT, Heino J, Larjava H, et al: Gingival crevicular fluid fibronectin degradation in periodontal health and disease, *Scand J Dent Res* 97:415–421, 1989.

Talonpoika JT, Hämäläinen MM: Type I collagen carboxyterminal telopeptide in human gingival crevicular fluid in different clinical conditions and after periodontal treatment, *J Clin Periodontol* 21:320–326, 1994.

Tanner ARC, Socransky SS, Goodson JM: Microbiota of periodontal pockets losing alveolar crestal bone, *J Periodontal Res* 19:279–291, 1984.

Termine JD, Kleinmann HK, Whitson SW, et al: Osteonectin, a bone-specific protein linking mineral to collagen, *Cell* 26:99–105, 1981.

Theilade E: The non-specific theory in microbial etiology of inflammatory periodontal diseases, *J Clin Periodontol* 13:905–911, 1986.

Timmerman MF, Van der Weijden GA, Armand S, et al: Untreated periodontal disease in Indonesian adolescents: clinical and microbiological baseline data, *J Clin Periodontol* 25:215–224, 1998.

Tüter G, Bülent K, Serdar M, et al: Effects of phase I periodontal treatment on gingival crevicular fluid levels of matrix metalloproteinase-3 and tissue inhibitor of metalloproteinase-1, *J Clin Periodontol* 32:1011–1015, 2005.

Uitto VJ, Suomalainen K, Sorsa T: Salivary collagenase. Origin, characteristics and relationship to periodontal health, *J Periodontal Res* 25:135–142, 1990.

Uitto VJ, Nieminen A, Coil J, et al: Oral fluid elastase as an indicator of periodontal health, *J Clin Periodontol* 23:30–60, 1996.

Vaes G: Cellular biology and biochemical mechanism of bone resorption, *Clin Orthop Relat Res* 231:239–271, 1988.

Van Os JH, de Jong MH, Van der Hoeven H: Growth of supragingival plaque organisms in enrichment cultures in saliva, *J Dent Res* 65:836, 1986.

Villela B, Cogan RB, Bartolucci AA, et al: Collagenolytic activity in crevicular fluid from patients with chronic adult periodontitis, localised juvenile periodontitis and gingivitis, and from healthy control subjects, *J Periodontal Res* 22:381–389, 1987.

Von Triol-Linden B, Torkko H, Alaluusua S, et al: Salivary levels of suspected periodontal pathogens in relation to periodontal status and treatment, *J Dent Res* 74:1789–1795, 1995.

Von Triol-Linden B, Alaluusua S, Wolf J, et al: Periodontitis patient and the spouse: periodontal bacteria before and after treatment, *J Clin Periodontol* 24:893–899, 1997.

Vrecko K, Staedtler P, Mischak I, et al: Periodontitis and concentrations of the cellular immune activation marker neopterin in saliva and urine, *Clin Chim Acta* 268:31–40, 1997.

Wahl SM, McNeely TB, Janoff EN, et al: Secretory leukocyte protease inhibitor (SLPI) in mucosal fluids inhibits HIV-1, *Oral Dis* 3:i564–i569, 1997.

Wennström JL, Dahlén G, Swensson J, et al: Actinobacillus actinomycetemcomitans, Bacteroides gingivalis and Bacteroides intermedius: Predictors of attachment loss? *Oral Microbiol Immunol* 2:158–163, 1987.

Westerlund U, Ingman T, Lukinmaa PL, et al: Human neutrophil gelatinase and associated lipocalin in adult and localized juvenile periodontitis, *J Dent Res* 75:1553–1563, 1996.

Westin U, Polling A, Ljungkrantz I, et al: Identification of SLPI (secretory leukocyte protease inhibitor) in human mast cells using immunohistochemistry and in situ hybridisation, *Biol Chem* 380:489–493, 1999.

Wolff LF, Koller NJ, Smith QT, et al: Subgingival temperature relation to gingival crevicular fluid enzymes, cytokines and subgingival plaque organisms, *J Clin Periodontol* 24:900–906, 1997.

Yaegaki K, Sanda K: Biochemical and clinical factors influencing oral malodour in periodontal patients, *J Periodontol* 63:783–789, 1992a.

Yaegaki K, Sanda K: Volatile sulfur compounds in mouth air from clinically healthy subjects and patients with periodontal disease, *J Periodontal Res* 27:233–238, 1992b.

Yamalik N, Ozer N, Caglayan F, et al: Determination of pseudocholinesterase activity in gingival crevicular fluid, saliva and serum from patients with juvenile periodontitis and rapidly progressive periodontitis, *J Dent Res* 69:87–89, 1990.

Yamalik N, Ozer N, Caglayan F, et al: The effect of periodontal therapy on salivary pseudocholinesterase activity, *J Dent Res* 70:988–990, 1991.

Yasuruma S, Aloia J, Yeh J, et al: Serum osteocalcin and total body calcium in normal, pre- and postmenopausal women and postmenopausal osteoporotic patients, *J Clin Endocrinol Metab* 64:681, 1987.

Zambon JJ, Nakamura N, Slots J: Effect of periodontal therapy on salivary enzyme activity, *J Periodontal Res* 20:652–659, 1985a.

Zambon JJ, Reynolds HS, Chen P, et al: Rapid detection of periodontal pathogens in subgingival plaque. Comparison of indirect immunofluorescence microscopy with bacterial cultures for detection of Bacteroides gingivalis, *J Periodontol* 56:32–40, 1985b.

Zambon JJ, Bochacki V, Genco RJ: Immunological assays for putative periodontal pathogens, *Oral Microbiol Immunol* 1:39–44, 1986.

FURTHER READING

Eley BM, Cox SW: Advances in periodontal diagnosis. 3. Assessing potential markers of periodontal disease activity, *Br Dent J* 184:109–113, 1998.

Eley BM, Cox SW: Advances in periodontal diagnosis. 4. Potential microbial markers, *Br Dent J* 184:161–166, 1998.

Eley BM, Cox SW: Advances in periodontal diagnosis. 5. Potential inflammatory and immune markers, *Br Dent J* 184:220–223, 1998.

Eley BM, Cox SW: Advances in periodontal diagnosis. 6. Proteolytic and hydrolytic enzymes of inflammatory cell origin, *Br Dent J* 184:268–271, 1998.

Eley BM, Cox SW: Advances in periodontal diagnosis. 7. Proteolytic and hydrolytic enzymes link with periodontitis, *Br Dent J* 184:323–328, 1998.

Eley BM, Cox SW: Advances in periodontal diagnosis. 8. Commercial diagnostic test kits based on GCF proteolytic and hydrolytic enzyme levels, *Br Dent J* 184:373–376, 1998.

Eley BM, Cox SW: Advances in periodontal diagnosis. 9. Markers of cell death and tissue degradation, *Br Dent J* 184:427–430, 1998.

Eley BM, Cox SW: Advances in periodontal diagnosis. 10. Markers of bone resorption, *Br Dent J* 184:489–492, 1998.

15 Basic treatment of chronic gingivitis and periodontitis

The basic treatment of periodontal disease is best divided into the treatment of chronic gingivitis and chronic periodontitis. The treatment of gingivitis mainly centres around plaque control and is relatively simple. The treatment of periodontitis involves the meticulous debridement of the root surface within the periodontal pocket and requires much skill and considerable time.

CHRONIC GINGIVITIS

Treatment has three components which are carried out concurrently:

1. Instruction in home care
2. Removal of plaque and calculus by scaling
3. Correction of plaque-retention factors.

These three exercises are interdependent. The removal of plaque and calculus cannot be completed without the correction of plaque-retention factors and rendering the mouth plaque free provides no benefit if no effort is made to prevent the recurrence of plaque deposition or to ensure its swift removal after deposition.

In some patients, especially the young, calcified deposits may be negligible and the treatment of gingival inflammation is largely a matter of plaque control (Ch. 11). Where calcified deposits are present, scaling may be needed and when deposits are heavy it may not be possible to remove all deposits in one appointment. Furthermore, resolution of gingival inflammation, especially when longstanding, may take a number of weeks. These facts must be explained to the patient. It is essential to establish a partnership of effort to restore gingival health (**Fig. 15.1**).

INSTRUCTION IN HOME CARE

Patients bear the major responsibility for their own dental health, particularly when disease is present. The presence of disease indicates (1) past neglect and (2) vulnerability to disease, which needs to be explained to the patient.

The organization of treatment needs to be very carefully planned but it is impossible to prescribe a general timetable which could apply to every patient and each individual requires a personal schedule. It is also necessary to make it clear that gingival health will not be achieved overnight and that treatment is likely to take several months. Depending on the severity of the gingival inflammation, the state of oral hygiene, the presence of aggravating factors and the patient's perceived concern, a series of appointments can be made. Some instruction in home care must be given on the first visit when scaling is started.

Where oral hygiene is poor, subsequent appointments may need to be made at weekly intervals especially where there is subgingival calculus. The proportion of time spent on scaling and oral hygiene instruction must vary with individual needs but in most cases, the earlier appointments are largely given over to scaling and as the patient feels and sees the improvement in gingival health which this brings about, his home care efforts can be stimulated. The patient is always advised to bring his toothbrush with him and visits can be started by using a disclosing agent and encouraging the patient to 'get the stain off'. At this time difficult areas are defined and modifications to his technique devised. Encouragement is always helpful, criticism rarely; a positive approach is essential to patient cooperation.

Treatment should continue until both oral hygiene and gingival condition are satisfactory. Recall appointments are then made at suitable intervals dictated by the patient's condition.

SCALING

This is the removal of all tooth deposits, supragingival calculus, subgingival calculus, plaque and stains. It must be carried out thoroughly; inflammation persists if all tooth deposits are not removed. Scaling technique can be learned only by constant practice but a number of conditions are essential to an effective technique:

1. The operation must be undertaken methodically, working around the mouth and around each tooth in an orderly manner.
2. The correct instrument should be used, i.e. one which fits well against the tooth surface to be cleaned. A fairly large bladed instrument can be used to remove supragingival calculus; a much smaller one is necessary for the removal of subgingival calculus.
3. Each stroke of the instrument should be deliberate and effective. It is very easy to scratch around ineffectively or to use the instrument so that it actually damages the tooth surface (**Fig. 15.2**). A firm finger

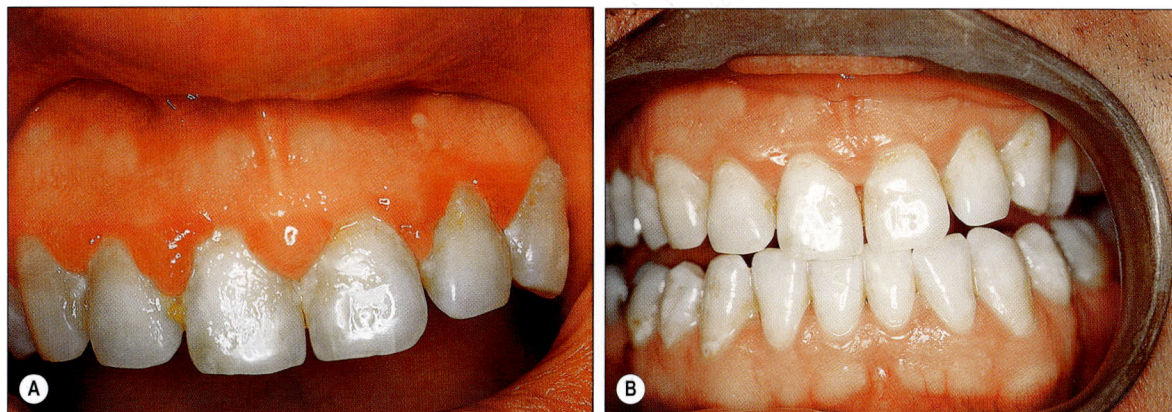

Fig. 15.1 (A) Gingival inflammation associated with poor oral hygiene prior to treatment. (B) The gingival condition after instruction in home care and scaling over a course of 8 weeks. It shows resolution of the condition to complete gingival health.

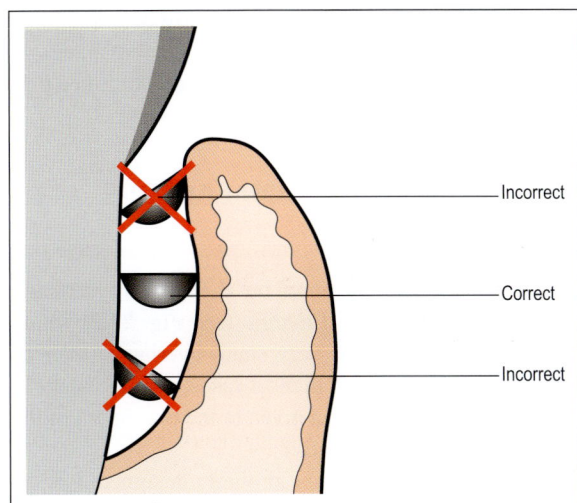

Fig. 15.2 Diagram to show the angulation of a curette blade against the tooth surface. Incorrect positioning may make the use of the instrument ineffective or damaging.

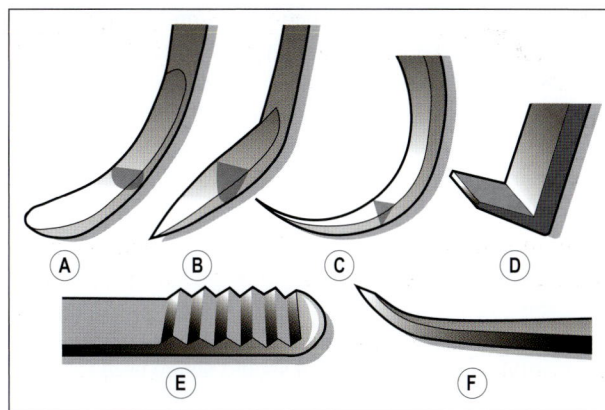

Fig. 15.3 Diagram to show the blades of various scaling instruments: (A) curette, (B) Jaquette scaler, (C) sickle, (D) hoe, (E) file (much enlarged), (F) chisel.

rest on the teeth is essential for controlled use of the instrument. The movement of the instrument can be divided into two phases:

- The exploratory stroke in which the apical limit of deposits is defined. In the removal of subgingival calculus this is a blind procedure and one carried out entirely by tactile sensation. The exploratory stroke must be gentle but deliberate so that the tissue, hard or soft, is not damaged.
- The working stroke which removes the deposits. In this action the instrument blade is pressed against the tooth surface and brought deliberately and slowly in a coronal direction bringing the deposits with it.

4. The tooth surface should be rendered clean and smooth. The surface can be examined with a suitable instrument, e.g. the Cross calculus probe, to detect any residual deposits. Sometimes the gingival margin can be retracted and the subgingival tooth surface visualized by blowing warm air gently into the gingival crevice.

Scaling instruments

Hand instruments

A large number of instruments are available and each operator will choose those which he or she finds most effective. The names of the instruments describe the design of the instrument and their mode of action: curettes, hoes, files, sickles and chisels. The instruments have three parts: a handle, a shank and blade. The handle needs to fit into the hand so that it is stable and cannot slip under pressure. The shank of the instrument varies in length and angulation so that all tooth surfaces are accessible to the blade, thus a short shank may be used in shallow pockets and a long shank in deep pockets and for interproximal sites at the back of the mouth. The blade has one or more edges designed to remove deposits from the tooth surface or soft tissue from the crevicular face of the gingiva. The edges of the blade must be kept sharp if the instrument is to be effective.

Curettes (Fig. 15.3A) – have a double-edged, spoon-shaped blade which is curved to conform to the tooth surface. Most surfaces can be reached with a pair (left and right) of curettes. Because of the small size and shape of the blade it can be inserted under the gingival margin. The most common types of curette are the McCall, Younger-Goode, Universal and Gracey. These instruments are mostly used for subgingival scaling and are described in more detail in the section on the treatment of chronic periodontitis.

Jaquette scalers (Fig. 15.3B) – the blade of this instrument is triangular in cross-section and it has two cutting edges. It is available in different sizes; the large blade is used for superficial scaling, the smaller blade for subgingival scaling. It comes in a set of three with differently angulated shanks for use in different parts of the mouth.

Sickle scalers (Fig. 15.3C) – these have a sickle-shaped blade which is triangular in cross-section so that there are two cutting edges. The blade may also be curved in a lateral plane so that it fits against the tooth surface. They are available in several sizes, the larger ones being used for superficial scaling.

Hoes (Fig. 15.3D) – as the name implies, are hoe-shaped instruments which are available as a set of four, each shank angulated differently so that all tooth surfaces may be reached. In use, the blade is inserted lightly under the gingival margin keeping the shank parallel to the axis of the tooth; the blade is then pressed against the tooth surface apical to the deposits of calculus and pulled in a coronal direction detaching the calculus. These are mainly used for subgingival scaling (see below).

Files (Fig. 15.3E) – these are indeed files which because of their very small dimensions can be inserted extremely easily into the gingival crevice or pocket. They are used like hoes.

Chisels (Fig. 15.3F) (watch-spring or push scaler) – these scalers are designed for the removal of interproximal deposits in the front of the mouth.

The ultrasonic scaler

Ultrasonic vibrations, i.e. above the range of normal hearing (above 20 000 Hz), can be used to remove tooth deposits. The ultrasonic scaler unit comprises an ultrasonic generator and a water supply. The instrument tip is vibrated between 25 000 and 42 000 Hz and this action fragments deposits on the tooth surfaces against which it is placed. Special tips are used under a cooling water spray as the vibration creates heat. The water spray also has a detergent effect which helps cleaning.

Several tips are available and these include a chisel-shaped tip, a beaver-tail tip, a universal tip, shaped mid-way between a sickle and a curette, and a periodontal probe-shaped tip. The chisel shaped tip is used to remove supramarginal ledges of calculus on anterior teeth and is placed against the proximal tooth surface and is used with a horizontal push stroke. The beaver-tail tip is used to remove very heavy supragingival calculus deposits and a horizontal stroke is used on proximal surfaces and vertical strokes on buccal and lingual surfaces. The universal tip is the most commonly used to remove heavy submarginal deposits and can be used supra- and subgingivally. It is used with vertical strokes on proximal surfaces and oblique strokes on buccal and lingual surfaces. The periodontal probe-shaped tip is used for subgingival scaling and is particularly useful in furcation areas. An oblique stroke is used in all situations.

The instrument is applied to the tooth or root surface with soft stroking movements. Unlike a hand instrument, in using the ultrasonic scaler there is no tactile sensation in the operator's fingers, therefore it is essential to avoid excessive pressure.

The ultrasonic scaler can also be used to remove tooth stains and cement. It must be used with great care against ceramics. It can also discolour composite restorations as the metal tip can be abraded by the composite so that metal particles become incorporated in its surface. Some patients find ultrasonic scaling painful and in these cases it should not be used.

Its main advantages are that it removes heavy calculus and stain with less operator fatigue and less soft tissue trauma. In addition, fragments of calculus and other debris are flushed out by the water spray. However, it is more difficult to carry out definitive subgingival calculus removal with this instrument because of the lack of tactile sensation. It is also possible to produce surface irregularities of root cementum and dentine or even enamel if the tip is used incorrectly. Also, continuous contact with a surface or insufficient water coolant may result in heat build up giving rise to pulpal sensitivity.

It is best to use the ultrasonic instrument to remove supragingival and the more superficial subgingival deposits and then to complete the scaling with hand instruments. It can also be used effectively for repeat scaling of periodontal pockets at maintenance visits, provided that all subgingival calculus deposits have been removed previously by hand instruments at the first treatment visits. Special tips are available for subgingival scaling.

It can also be used to remove stains such as those from tobacco, tea, coffee or chlorhexidine, to remove cement and orthodontic bonding materials and even with heavy inserts to reduce or remove amalgam overhangs.

A chlorhexidine mouthwash given for 2 min before ultrasonic scaling reduces the number of salivary bacteria which are sprayed on to the operator from the aerosol produced during its use. It is also essential to wear a mask, and protective glasses are used to reduce operator exposure through this aerosol.

The ultrasonic scaler should *not* be used in patients with:

- A pacemaker since electromagnetic sound waves from the ultrasonic unit may interfere with the electronic function of the pacemaker
- Contagious diseases such as hepatitis, HIV infection, tuberculosis, throat and respiratory infections since the microorganisms are spread in the aerosol from the instrument
- Uncontrolled diabetes
- Debilitating diseases or chronic nutritional deficiencies
- Desquamative gingivitis
- Deep, pus-producing pockets
- Undergoing prolonged antibiotic or steroid therapy.

The ultrasonic scaler should also not be used adjacent to:

- Composite resin fillings since the vibrations may cause marginal leakage and loss of retention
- Porcelain inlays or crowns since the vibrations can cause porcelain margins to fracture.

Ultrasonic scalers are not well tolerated by children and patients with exposed, sensitive root surfaces. Finally, ultrasonic scalers may detect leaky fillings by stimulating pain and painful sites should be investigated for this possibility.

Tooth polishing

Rough surfaces become sites of plaque and calculus deposition, therefore the tooth surface must be made smooth as well as free of calculus, plaque and stain. After scaling any residual plaque and stain should be removed using rotating cup-shaped brushes or rubber cups and a small amount of abrasive polishing paste. The brush should be rotated slowly and applied intermittently to the tooth surface to avoid overheating. An advantage of the rubber cup is that it can be taken below the gingival margin. Linen polishing strips can be used to polish interproximal tooth surfaces.

CORRECTION OF PLAQUE-RETENTION FACTORS

Faulty restorations

Restorations may be rough and badly contoured but the most frequent and important fault is the overhanging cervical margin (see **Fig. 27.3**) which collects plaque and prevents its removal. Very small overhangs may be removed using polishing burrs or strips but in most cases, it is necessary to replace the restoration, with careful attention given to the placement of the matrix band and the use of interdental wedges.

Marginal ridges and contact points must be properly designed. Undercontoured restorations should be replaced. Any caries under the margin of the restoration must be identified and a new restoration placed. Where possible, the margins of restorations should be placed coronal to the gingival margin (see Ch. 30).

Subgingival margins and particularly overhanging margins on posterior or anterior crowns (see **Fig. 30.2**) produce the worst problems and necessitate replacement of the offending restoration.

Faulty appliances

Removable prosthetic or orthodontic appliances may irritate the tissues in several ways (see Ch. 4). They can compress or rub the gingiva directly or act to retain plaque against the gingiva. A removable partial denture should be designed so that as far as possible it is tooth borne and gingiva free. Where contact with the gingiva is unavoidable the fit should be good and pressure on the tissue should be avoided. The model should never be carved to produce lines of pressure, nor should relief areas be provided in an attempt to avoid pressure, as these provoke gingival hyperplasia which fills the relief chamber. Appliances must be kept scrupulously clean and not worn at night.

Fixed appliances must be designed so that they do not promote plaque stagnation or impede plaque removal. Fixed orthodontic appliances can present a difficult problem for the young patient to keep clean and the patient must be taught how to look after the appliance without at the same time damaging it. Fortunately young tissues recover quickly when the appliance is removed and thorough oral hygiene measures instituted.

The modern revival of tribal customs in the form of body piercings when intraoral can cause direct gingival trauma when applied intraorally. The most common offender in this respect is the tongue stud.

Crowns and bridges

The margins of crowns and bridge abutments should fit precisely, without marginal excess or deficiency. The margins should also be accessible for cleaning. Faulty crowns and bridges associated with periodontal problems usually need replacing. In constructing these restorations certain rules should be followed (see Ch. 30):

1. Restoration margins should be supragingival except on the labial face of upper incisors where cosmetic considerations dictate that the crown margin should be just hidden.
2. The provision of adequate embrasure spaces is imperative. The design of pontics is particularly important and the ridge-lap pontic should be avoided where possible and bullet-shaped pontics or sanitary pontics should be used for posterior bridges. The pontics of anterior bridges usually need to slightly overlap the ridge labially for aesthetic reasons. These pontics can be made cleanable by sloping

the ridge surface of the pontic so that it lies above the ridge palatally or lingually and by keeping a sufficient embrasure space to allow the passage of floss via a threader or the use of superfloss.

3. Over contouring crowns should be avoided.

Lack of lip-seal

Although not a plaque-retention factor, lack of lip-seal does seem to render the exposed gingiva more vulnerable to plaque irritation. Once upon a time, the oral screen was prescribed to wear during sleep, the theory being that it would seal the mouth, prevent evaporation of saliva and dehydration of the tissues. Smearing the gingiva with petroleum jelly was a popular practice and even Sellotaping the lips was recommended! None of these measures was aimed at the cause of the problem, the plaque. Patients with lack of lip-seal need to have their particular vulnerability carefully explained so that they can cooperate intelligently. With a clean mouth the patient can breathe through any available orifice without jeopardizing gingival health.

Tooth malalignment

Frequently orthodontic treatment is carried out to correct tooth malalignment which appears to be associated with gingival inflammation. A large proportion of this effort is wasted because the patient's home care is inadequate to clean even well-aligned teeth. On the other hand, some patients' efforts are effective enough to clean malaligned teeth and therefore do not need orthodontic treatment. Such treatment is justified where the patient is obviously trying to control plaque deposition and fails only in areas of malalignment.

Gingivoplasty

Gingival swelling creates gingival or 'false' pockets. When hyperplastic gingivitis has been present for a relatively short time, the main component of the swelling is inflammation and given adequate scaling the inflammation resolves and the swelling reduces. In the case of longstanding irritation there is a great deal of fibrous tissue formation which does not resolve on scaling. The pocket persists and plaque re-deposits so that inflammation is maintained. If pocketing and gingival enlargement persist after repeated scaling and assiduous patient effort over a period of several months, surgical re-shaping of the gingiva, i.e. gingivoplasty, is indicated. It may also be needed after recurrent episodes of acute ulcerative gingivitis where tissue destruction has resulted in the saucer-shaped gingival defects characteristic of this disease.

Gingivoplasty is a gingivectomy with the limited aim of improving gingival contour, i.e. producing a streamlined contour with a knife-edged and scalloped margin and interdental sluice-ways (**Fig. 15.4**). Details of the technique are given in Chapter 19.

CHRONIC PERIODONTITIS

Although chronic gingivitis may remain contained for many years, in many people failure to control the inflammation will eventually lead to periodontitis. The susceptibility to periodontitis is variable and its rate of progression varies from one person to another and from one tooth to another. Traditionally chronic periodontitis has been thought to advance slowly and progressively but a number of longitudinal clinical studies of untreated chronic periodontitis have produced results that are inconsistent with this view (Goodson et al 1982; Socransky et al 1984). They suggest that the disease progresses by short and recurrent bursts of activity, probably of acute inflammation at specific sites, which are followed by long but variable periods of remission. Many tooth sites within an

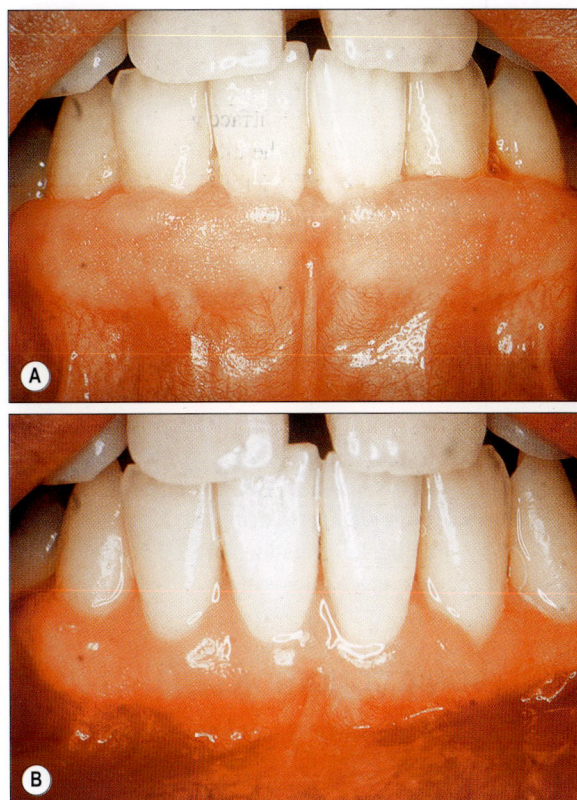

Fig. 15.4 (A) Gingival hyperplasia and deformity which failed to resolve following a prolonged period of scaling and home care. (B) Gingival condition following surgical reshaping, i.e. gingivoplasty.

affected individual may remain free of destructive periodontal activity and indeed some patients remain free from destructive periodontal disease throughout their lives. It is also suggested that destructive periodontal disease activity may occur more frequently during certain periods of an individual's life.

At the time of an examination, many periodontal pockets may be inactive, so that periodontal examination will reveal evidence of past disease rather than present activity. Since there are currently no certain means either to diagnose current activity or to predict when disease activity will occur, the only way to be sure that periodontal disease is actually progressing is to keep it under careful longitudinal observation. This method, however, has the obvious disadvantage that further periods of destruction will have to occur before they can be detected and treated. Therefore it is important to treat all periodontal pockets when they are first detected, and to aim at the removal of all soft and hard deposits from the root surface, to create conditions which allow the patient to perform efficient plaque control, and to eliminate all factors which would prevent the patient from maintaining that plaque control. Controlling dental plaque and supra- and subgingival scaling and root planing are often referred to as cause-related therapy since these measures are directly aimed at controlling the factors causing the condition. The principle stages of this treatment are:

- Treatment of any acute condition
- Patient motivation (see Ch. 11)
- Demonstration of oral hygiene techniques (see Ch. 11)
- Anti-smoking advice
- Supragingival scaling (see above)
- Removal of any plaque-retention factors (see above)
- Subgingival scaling and root planing (root surface debridement)
- Occlusal adjustment if appropriate (see Ch. 27)
- Monitoring response to therapy.

The objectives of this treatment are:

1. The resolution of the disease process
2. The creation of conditions that will mitigate against recurrence of disease.

TREATMENT OF ACUTE CONDITIONS

Acute conditions associated with chronic periodontitis should be treated without delay. The treatment of an acute lateral periodontal abscess and acute ulcerative gingivitis is described in Chapters 22 and 24.

In addition, a careful watch should be kept for sites of active disease which should be treated immediately. Patients may complain of local symptoms at these sites, such as discomfort, itching or gingival bleeding, and they will usually show signs of acute inflammation with redness, swelling and bleeding on probing. These sites should be treated by immediate, careful subgingival scaling and root planing under local anaesthesia. The pocket can be washed out by subgingival irrigation with a 0.2% chlorhexidine solution using a blunt needle and a 5 mL syringe.

TREATMENT OF CHRONIC CONDITIONS

Subgingival scaling and root planing

All patients, other than those with acute problems, should first receive thorough supragingival scaling, as this will reduce gingivitis and bleeding. It is also important to have a full pocket chart before starting subgingival scaling.

Subgingival scaling is the most conservative method of pocket reduction and, where pocketing is shallow, it is the only treatment required. However, when pockets deepen to 5 mm or more, additional measures are required. The commonest of these is *root planing* which seeks to remove embedded calculus, necrotic cementum and to smooth the root surface. This is an integral part of the subgingival scaling procedure in these situations.

Subgingival calculus is hard and tenaciously adherent to the root surface and CEJ and is difficult to remove. It is firmly attached to the root because the calcification process involves filamentous bacteria which may themselves penetrate into the surface cementum. Surface irregularities, such as the small pits previously occupied by Sharpey's fibres, are penetrated by apatite crystals firmly locking the calculus to the root surface. It can be particularly adherent in areas with difficult access such as furcations between multirooted teeth and in grooves and concavities on the root surface.

The object of *root planing (root surface debridement)* is to remove necrotic cementum and embedded calculus and to smooth the root surface. It is also concerned with the removal of cementum infiltrated with toxic material of bacterial origin such as endotoxin (LPS). However, recently it has been found that this material is only loosely associated with the root surface (Moore et al 1986) and can be removed by hand or ultrasonic scaling without the need for cementum removal. This indicates that the aim of scaling and root planing should be to produce a smooth, deposit-free root surface with the minimal removal of cementum.

Effects of subgingival scaling and root planing

Subgingival scaling and root planing significantly alter the bacterial composition of the pocket. Dark ground microscopy techniques show that this treatment results in a marked decrease in the number of motile rods and spirochaetes and a corresponding increase in cocci (Listgarten et al 1978). The time taken for bacterial re-population to occur is variable, ranging from 1 to 6 months (Listgarten et al 1978; Mousques et al 1980). Cultural studies have also shown significant reductions in the numbers of obligate anaerobes and black pigmented *Bacteroides* species (Walsh et al 1986). These prolonged reductions in the numbers of Gram-negative anaerobic bacteria

and spirochaetes probably result from changes in the pocket environment, brought about by subgingival scaling, which makes it less favourable for the growth of these fastidious bacteria. It may reduce the nutritive sources for the proteolytic subgingival bacteria by reducing inflammation and thus gingival crevicular fluid (GCF) flow and by removing subgingival calculus, which probably soaks up inflammatory exudate and slowly releases it to the adjacent bacteria. The rate of decolonization is affected by the standard of oral hygiene since a re-growth of supragingival plaque will favour selective decolonization of the pocket (Magnusson et al 1984).

Recently, some studies using light microscopy, scanning electron microscopy and bacterial culture have shown that some bacteria may invade cementum and radicular dentine within periodontal pockets (Adriaens et al 1984; 1987; 1988a,b; Giuliana et al 1997). These studies have even suggested that the dentinal tubules may act as reservoirs of putative periodontal pathogens (Ch. 5). These findings suggest that radicular dentine could act as a bacterial reservoir from which periodontal pathogens can recolonize treated periodontal pockets and could thus contribute to the recurrence of disease. Root planing could reduce this potential source of decolonization. However, some studies indicate that these bacteria may penetrate into the dentine tubules (Giuliana et al 1997), which is well beyond the capacity of root planing for access.

Scaling and root planing are effective at reducing gingival inflammation and pocket depth. When combined with good oral hygiene and regular maintenance these effects can be prolonged over several years (Pihlstrom et al 1983; Ramfjord et al 1987; Badersten et al 1987). These studies indicate that these measures alone can be effective in treating and maintaining patients with moderate and even advanced chronic periodontitis but it must be remembered that treatment is very time consuming and demanding, particularly in patients with deep pocketing, and requires frequent maintenance visits. In the studies quoted above, the time taken for scaling and root planing ranged from 5 to 8 h and the patients were recalled for maintenance treatment every 2–4 months. Relapses did occur in some patients despite these measures. Obviously the patient's susceptibility to periodontal disease is a factor but it is also becoming clear that it is very difficult to remove all calculus deposits from deep pockets by 'blind' subgingival scaling. Several studies have shown that some calculus frequently remains after careful subgingival scaling and the incidence increases with increasing pocket depths (Rabbani et al 1981; Eaton et al 1985). This is less common following surgical exposure by flap procedures (Caffesse et al 1986).

Subgingival scaling and root planing are indicated for periodontal pockets of 4 mm or more and if necessary, should be carried out under local anaesthesia. Although ultrasonic scalers are equally effective as hand scaling in removing calculus and root associated products, they have more limited access to deep pockets and fail to give the operator tactile information. They are therefore less capable of definitive subgingival calculus removal.

The techniques of subgingival scaling and root planing

The main hand instruments used for scaling and root planing are *hoes* and *curettes* and it is essential that these instruments are sharp. The cutting edges of these instruments become blunted after use during a single treatment session and therefore they need to be sharpened before they are next used.

Hoes are used to remove resistant deposits of calculus but care should be taken to avoid excessive pressure or incorrect positioning of the instrument, as this may groove the root surface (**Fig. 15.5A**). The hoe should be gently manipulated to the base of the pocket and then carefully manoeuvred to engage the deepest edge of the calculus deposit. It is then positively planed in a coronal direction with its cutting edge being maintained in contact with the root surface to remove the deposit. A firm finger rest and a finger pull movement are necessary to accomplish this movement.

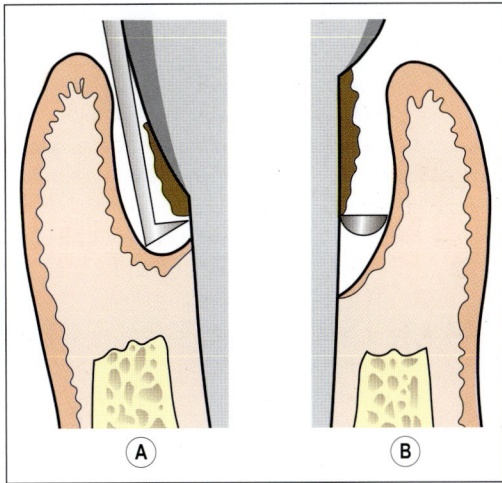

Fig. 15.5 Diagram to show the use of instruments and their correct placement in subgingival scaling: (A) a hoe is used to remove resistant deposits, (B) a curette is used to remove fine deposits and to root plane.

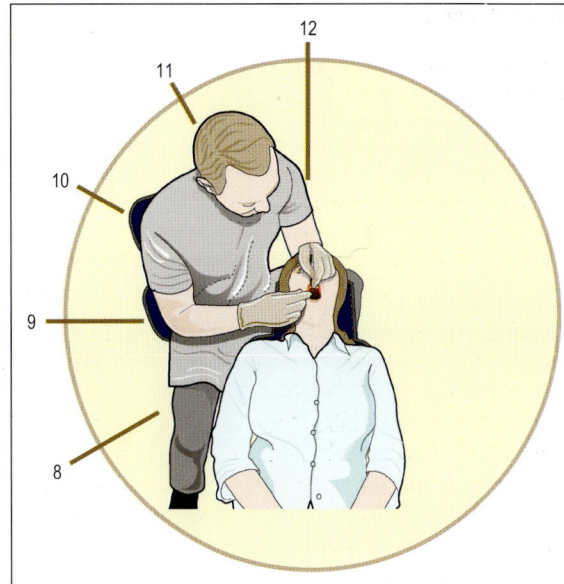

Fig. 15.6 Operator positions for scaling procedures related to a 12-hour clock. This system is used in the text to describe these positions.

Curettes are used to remove residual fine deposits of calculus and to plane and smooth the root surface (**Fig. 15.5B**). They are carefully manipulated to the base of the pocket to engage the deepest edge of the deposit and are then planed upwards in contact with the root surface using a finger movement. In many situations, it is easier to use curettes for the whole process of scaling and root planing. If the intention is to avoid trauma to the soft tissue, single-sided curettes such as the *Gracey curettes* can be used. These are particularly good instruments for finishing and smoothing the root surface and for repeat subgingival scaling procedures at maintenance visits. Subgingival scaling and root planing may be painful due either to sensitivity of the soft tissues or the root surface and these procedures are best carried out under local analgesia.

The patient may also experience some discomfort following root planing and it may be wise to advise the use of a chlorhexidine mouthwash to supplement oral hygiene for 1 or 2 days. Healing will take place over several days and will be aided by meticulous oral hygiene.

The first requirements in deciding on the instruments and technique to use are a detailed knowledge of the root anatomy of individual teeth and their precise probing depths. This is of particular importance when furcation involvement is present on molar or premolar teeth. The details of the essential factors in subgingival scaling technique are described below.

Operator and patient positions

The patient and operator position is of great importance and with low-seated dentistry, the patient's head is placed in the lap of the operator with the light directed into the mouth from a position vertically above it so that it is not impeded by the operator in any position round the patient. The operator can then rotate around the patient to gain access to particular tooth surfaces and these positions can be related to the face of a clock projected over the face of the subject with 12 o'clock above the midpoint of the top of the head and 6 o'clock below the midpoint of the chin (**Fig. 15.6**). This is very clearly described in Nield and Houseman (1988) for both right and left handed operators.

Using this system, the following positions are adopted assuming a right handed operator:

Mandibular teeth
- The buccal surfaces of the right mandibular molars and premolars and lingual surfaces of left mandibular molars and premolars (**Fig. 15.7A**):
  - Operator in 9 o'clock position to the right side of the patient, looking down into mouth. The patient's head is straight ahead with the chin inclined down. The patient's head is turned slightly away from operator when required.

- The buccal surfaces of the left mandibular molars and premolars and lingual surfaces of left mandibular molars and premolars (**Fig. 15.7B**):
  - Operator in either the 9 o'clock or the 11 o'clock position to the right side of the patient, looking down into mouth. The patient's head is turned towards operator with chin inclined down.

The mandibular incisors, facial aspects
- For tooth surfaces towards operator (**Fig. 15.7C**):
  - Operator in 8 o'clock position on right side of patient. The patient's head is straight ahead with chin inclined down.
- For tooth surfaces away from operator (**Fig. 15.7D**):
  - Operator in 12 o'clock position behind the patient. The patient's head is straight ahead with chin inclined down.

The mandibular incisors, lingual aspects
- For tooth surfaces towards operator (**Fig. 15.7E**):
  - Operator in 8 o'clock position on right side of patient. The patient's head is straight ahead with chin inclined down.
- For tooth surfaces away from operator (**Fig. 15.7F**):
  - Operator in 12 o'clock position behind the patient. The patient's head is straight ahead with chin inclined down.

Maxillary teeth
- The buccal surfaces of right maxillary molars and premolars and lingual aspects of left maxillary molars and premolars (**Fig. 15.8A**):
  - Operator in the 9 o'clock position to the right side of the patient with the patient's head straight or slightly turned away from operator for buccal surfaces and always turned away for the lingual surfaces with the patient's chin inclined up.
- The buccal surfaces of left maxillary molars and premolars and lingual aspects of right maxillary molars and premolars (**Fig. 15.8B**):
  - Operator in either the 9 o'clock or the 11 o'clock position to the right side. The patient's head is turned toward operator for both buccal and lingual aspects with chin inclined up.

The mandibular incisors facial aspects
- For tooth surfaces towards operator (**Fig. 15.8C**):
  - Operator should be in the 8 o'clock position to the right of the patient. The patient's head is straight ahead with chin inclined up.
- For tooth surfaces away from operator (**Fig. 15.8D**):
  - Operator should be in the 12 o'clock position behind the patient. The patient's head is straight ahead with chin inclined up.

Fig. 15.7 (A) Head position for buccal surfaces of right mandibular molars and premolars and lingual surfaces of the left mandibular molars and premolars. (B) Head position for buccal surface of left mandibular molars and premolars and lingual surfaces of right mandibular molars and premolars. (C) Head position for facial aspects of the mandibular incisors, right surfaces. (D) Head position for facial aspects of the mandibular incisors, left surfaces. (E) Head position for lingual aspects of the mandibular incisors, right surfaces using a mirror. (F) Head position for lingual aspects of the mandibular incisors, left surfaces using a mirror.

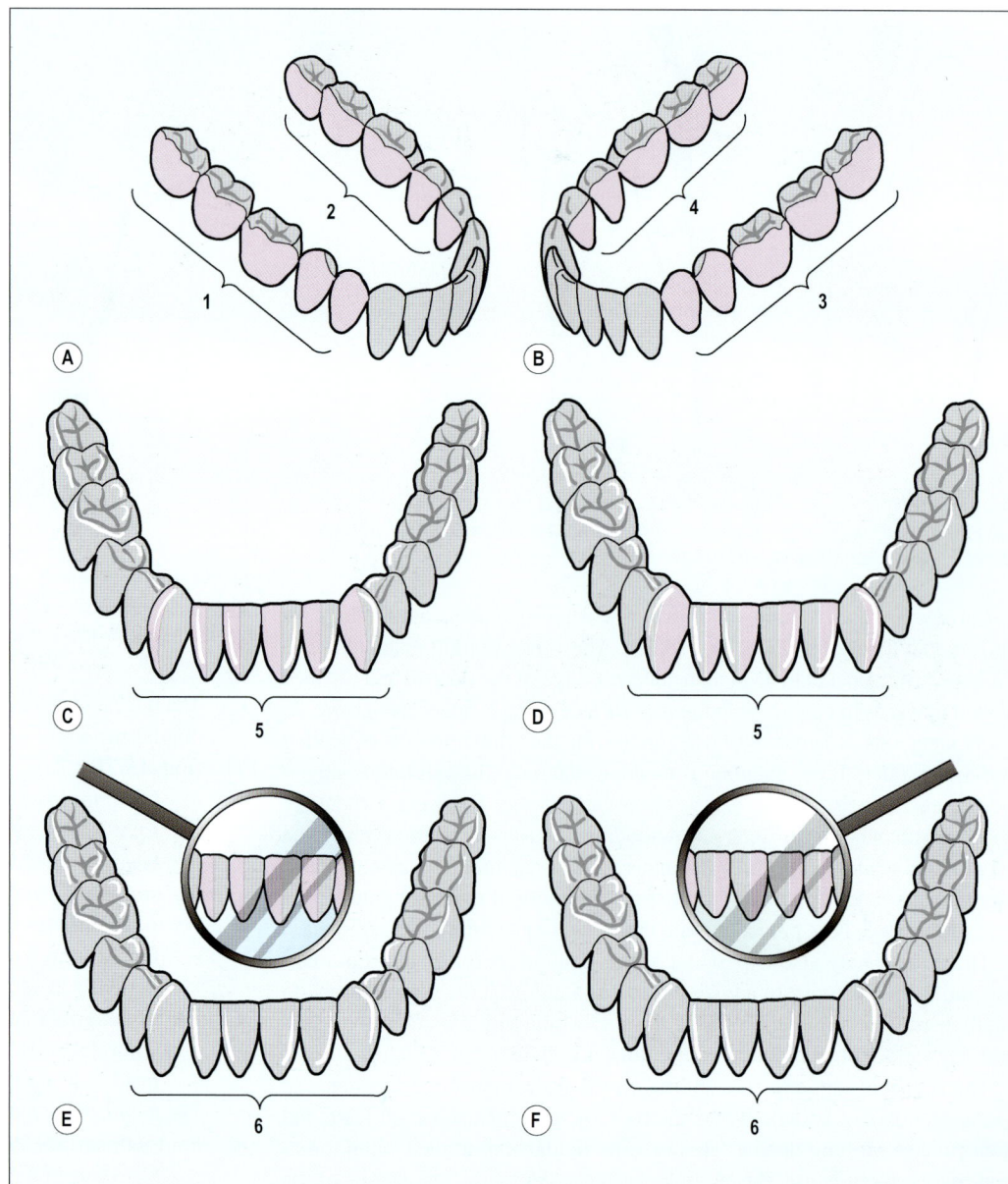

The mandibular incisors lingual aspects
- For tooth surfaces towards operator (**Fig. 15.8E**):
  - Operator should be in the 8 o'clock position to the right of the patient. The patient's head is straight ahead with chin inclined up.
- For tooth surfaces away from operator (**Fig. 15.8F**):
  - Operator should be in the 12 o'clock position behind the patient. The patient's head is straight ahead with chin inclined up.

These positions relate to right-handed operators and would need to be reversed for left-handed operators. Full details can be found in Nield and Houseman (1988, pp 17–59).

The parts of a subgingival scaler

A subgingival scaling instrument consists of a *handle* with a variety of designs to aid gripping, a *shank* extending from the handle to the working end and the *working end* itself (**Fig. 15.9**). These scalers are mostly double-ended with a pair of complimentary shanks and working ends per handle. These may be permanently attached to the handle or may screw into it and thus be replaceable. The *shank* may be straight as in most anterior scalers or angled or curved as in posterior scalers to aid access to these teeth. They may be flexible as in Gracey curettes to increase tactile sense or rigid or semi-rigid in most other scalers to increase strength. The *working end* consists of a smooth rounded *back* which joins two *lateral surfaces* which meet the *face* at the *cutting edges* (**Fig. 15.10A**). The *tip* end of the face is known as the *toe*, the middle as the *middle* and the back end as the *heel* sections (**Fig. 15.10B**). The tip may be pointed as in the sickle scaler or rounded in curettes. The working end usually has two functional cutting edges as in universal curettes but may only have one as in hoes or one functional one as in Gracey curettes. The cutting edge(s) must be kept sharp by regular sharpening i.e. either after or before each use. Full details can be found in Nield and Houseman (1988, pp 179–196).

Instrument grasp

Scalers are invariably held by a *modified pen grasp* (**Fig. 15.11**). The tips of *thumb* and *index finger* hold the scaler and these fingers should be opposite one another near the junction of the handle and shank towards the working end of the instrument in double-ended scalers. The handle should rest against the hand somewhere between your thumb and the area behind the second knuckle of your index finger. When you are working on mandibular teeth, the handle usually rests against the index finger and working on maxillary teeth the handle usually rests closer to the thumb.

The *middle finger* rests lightly on the shank and is used to feel the shank's vibration when the instrument's working surface is moving over the root surface. The pad of this finger contacts the instrument and helps to guide the instrument. Another portion of its pad rests against the ring finger.

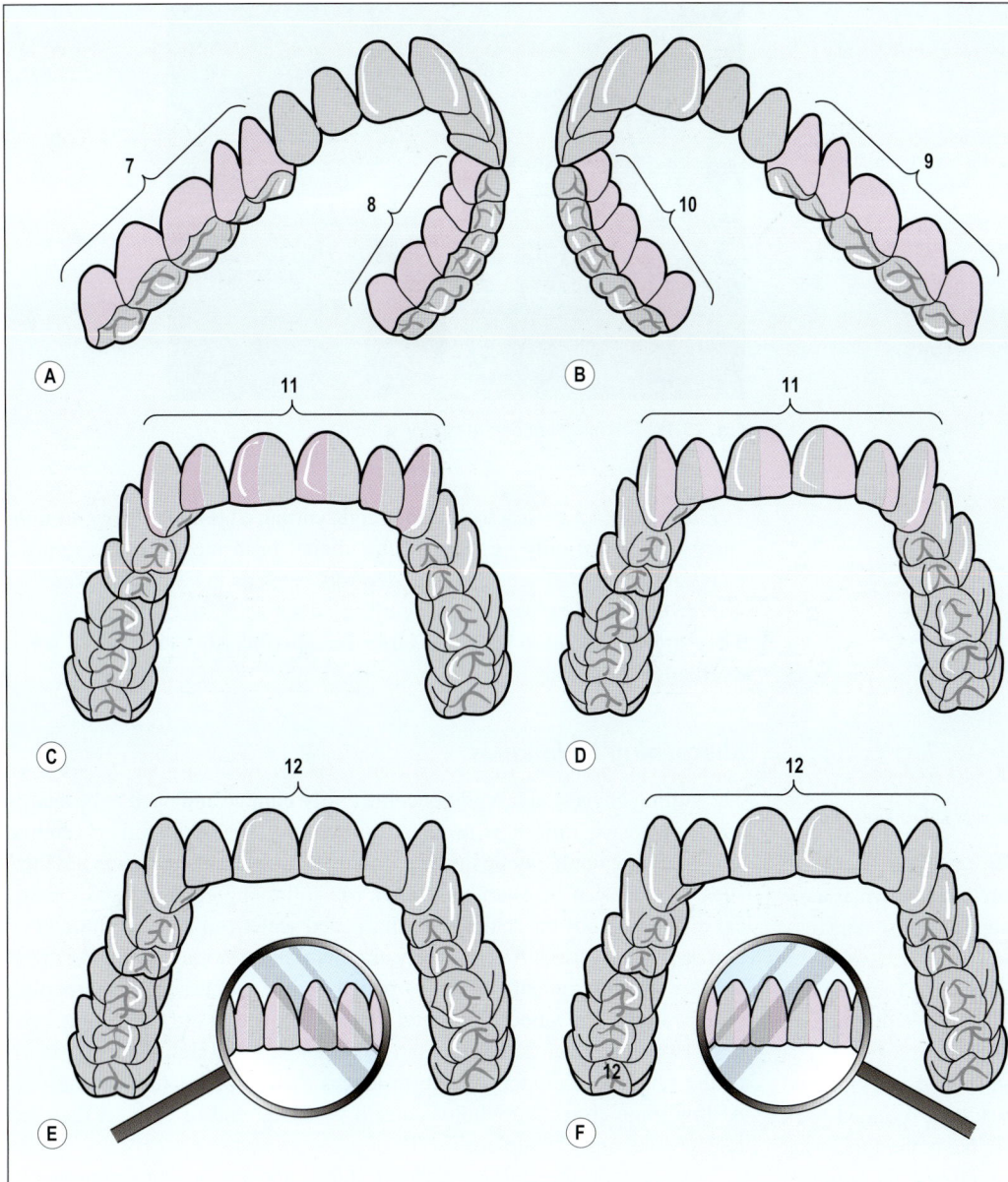

Fig. 15.8 (A) Head position for buccal surfaces of right maxillary molars and premolars and palatal surfaces of the left maxillary molars and premolars. (B) Head position for buccal surface of left maxillary molars and premolars and palatal surfaces of right maxillary molars and premolars. (C) Head position for facial aspects of the maxillary incisors, right surfaces. (D) Head position for facial aspects of the maxillary incisors, left surfaces. (E) Head position for palatal aspects of the maxillary incisors, right surfaces using a mirror. (F) Head position for palatal aspects of the maxillary incisors, left surfaces using a mirror.

The *ring finger* contacts the patient's tooth to stabilize the hand in the patient's mouth. Your hand and the instrument are balanced on this finger. The *little finger* has no function and is held comfortably away.

The *index* and *middle* fingers are bent and the *thumb* held straight or slightly curved while the *ring* finger is held straight with the knuckles locked so that it balances the hand. A dental mirror may be held in the other hand when appropriate. The fingers of the other hand or the mirror may be used to deflect the lips, cheek or tongue when necessary.

Full details can be found in Nield and Houseman (1988, pp 67–164).

Instrument insertion

The face of the scaler is placed flat against the tooth surface with the toe-third of the instrument in contact with the tooth (**Fig. 15.14A**). The working end is then slid under the gingival margin and moved to the base of the pocket (**Figs. 15.12, 15.14B**). In this position, the soft tissue wall of the pocket will only come in contact with the rounded back of the scaler and thus will not be traumatized. It must be ensured that the working end has passed over the calculus deposit so that the cutting edge can be subsequently positioned below its apical margin. When this position is reached, the instrument must be turned to bring the cutting edge into contact with the root surface at the correct working angulation. This is usually at an angle of 70–80° to the root surface (**Figs. 15.13, 15.14C**).

Instrument activation

Using this grasp, the scaler may rock using wrist rotation for lateral movement, rotated by an action similar to turning a door knob for rotating curved movement or moved up (apico-coronally) by a digital pulling movement over the root surface. The latter is the most frequent scaling movement for most subgingival scaling procedures. With this technique it is inserted below the calculus deposit and its sharp cutting edge is applied to the root surface (see above). The working tip is then planed over the root surface by an upward pull of the thumb and index finger, guided by the middle finger and stabilized against the teeth by the ring finger (**Fig. 15.14**).

Working end design

The design of the main scalers has already been described and the following description is confined to the working ends of the instruments and their uses.

Most working ends have a smooth back surface and a face. The face and the lateral surface in curettes, sickle scalers and Jaquettes meet to form a cutting edge running along the full length of the face. There may be one or two cutting edges depending on the design of the instrument. The cutting edge must be kept sharp for the instrument to function efficiently and this is accomplished by grinding the lateral surface(s) and face with sharpening

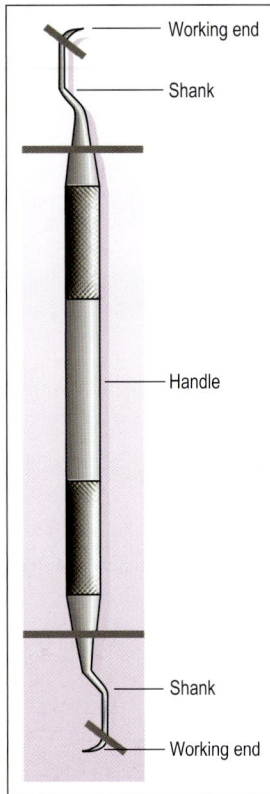

Fig. 15.9 The parts of a subgingival scaler (curette): handle; shank; working end.

stones (see above). The rounded working end of a curette is known as a toe and that of a sickle or Jaquette as a tip. Both curettes and sickle scalers may have either straight or curved cutting edges.

Sickle or *Jaquette* scalers have two cutting edges and are triangular in cross-section. They are strong instruments mainly suited to supragingival scaling and the removal of heavy calculus deposits.

Curettes usually have two cutting edges, a spoon-shaped working end and the cutting edges meet in a rounded toe. They have a rounded back and are semicircular in cross-section. *Gracey curettes* have one functional cutting edge, the lower, and are designed to avoid trauma to the gingival tissue adjacent to the root surface. *Curettes* are the main scalers for subgingival scaling.

Periodontal hoes have one cutting edge at a 99–100° angle to the shank. They can be used to remove heavy subgingival deposits but must be used with care to avoid grooving the root surface. These scalers can only be used with a digital pull movement in an apico-coronal direction.

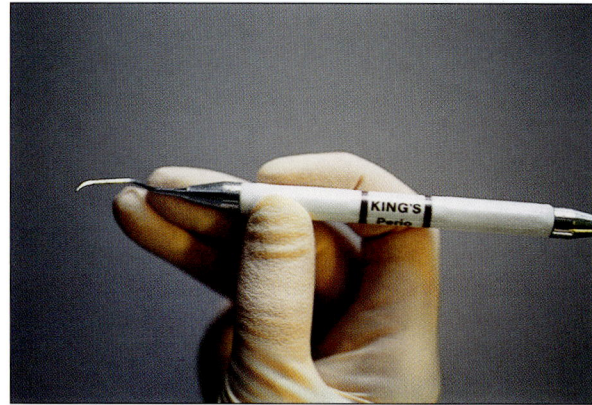

Fig. 15.11 The modified pen grasp for scaling.

Push scalers or chisels have one straight cutting edge and a heavy, straight shank. They can only be used with a digital push movement to remove heavy interproximal supragingival deposits between the lower incisors.

Periodontal files have many cutting edges at 90–105° to the shank. They are mainly used to crush large calculus deposits or remove some overhanging margins.

Sharpening techniques

The cutting edge(s) of a scaler become easily blunted and need to be sharpened after each time it is used. A dull cutting edge will fail to remove subgingival calculus deposits and could result in damage to the soft tissues. Scalers can be sharpened after use following cleaning and chemical disinfection of the scaler. The sharpened scaler can then be autoclaved before it is next used. Alternatively, the sharpening stone may be sterilized to allow the instruments to be sharpened before use. Frequent sharpening will minimize the amount of metal that is removed in the sharpening process. However, over time, successive sharpenings will thin the working tip of the scaler to an extent which produces danger of fracture during use. At this stage either the whole scaler or working end or ends, if they are replaceable, must be replaced.

The design of the working end will dictate the sharpening technique. In this respect, cutting edges may be straight or curved and this must be preserved in the sharpening process.

To sharpen a scaler, one needs a properly prepared *sharpening stone*, a *stable flat working surface* and a *plastic testing stick*. If the stone is of natural material then it should be lubricated on both sides with a few drops of oil. If it is synthetic, then it should be lubricated on both sides, with water.

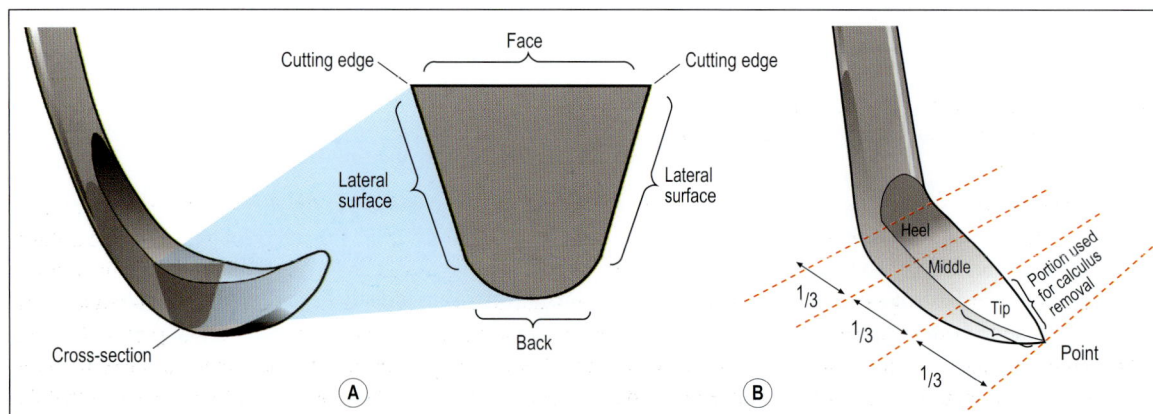

Fig. 15.10 The parts of the working end of a scaler: (A) showing the cutting surfaces, face, back and lateral surfaces; (B) showing the heel, middle, tip and point.

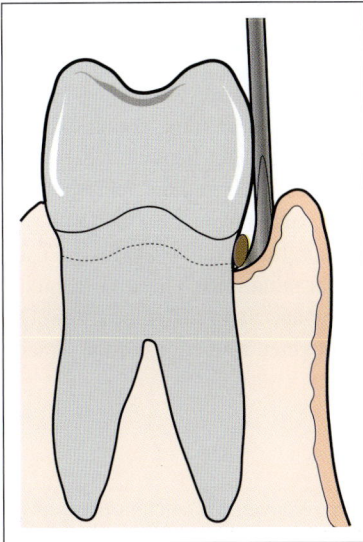

Fig. 15.12 Diagram showing instrument insertion into the pocket.

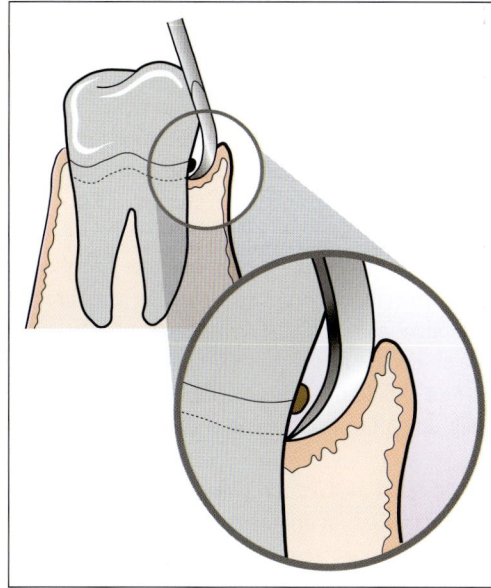

Fig. 15.13 Diagram showing scaler working end positioned for scaling stroke.

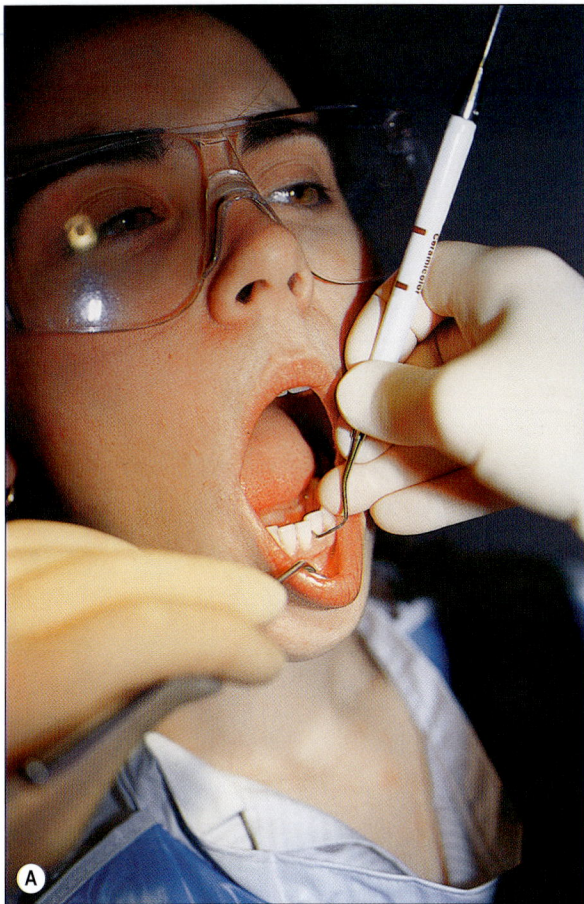

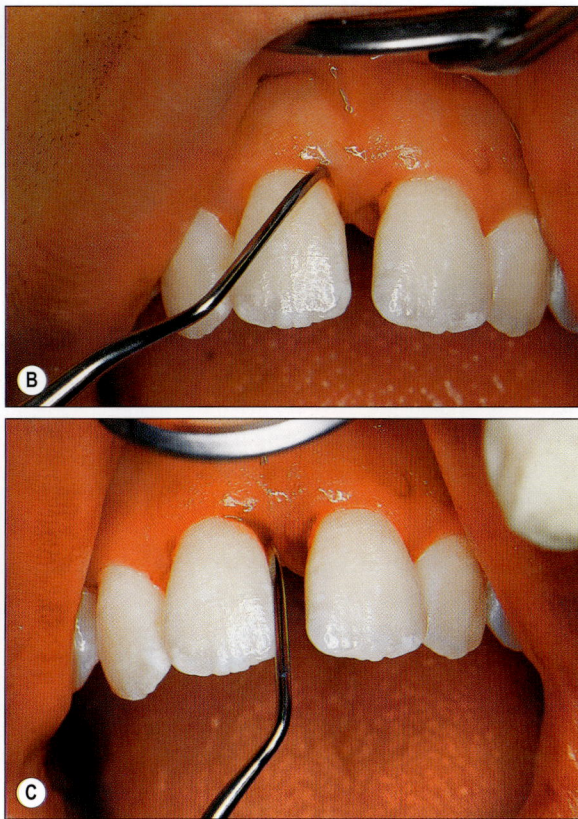

Fig. 15.14 The positioning of a subgingival scaling instrument (curette) ready for subgingival scaling: (A) scaler applied to tooth surface with steadying finger on adjacent teeth; (B) curette introduced into pocket; (C) cutting edge positioned for scaling stroke.

Look carefully at the instrument to see whether it has straight or curved cutting edges; whether it ends in a rounded or pointed toe and whether it has a rounded back. Divide the face into heel, middle and toe sections since all three cannot be sharpened together because: (a) the entire edge may not be dull since the anterior two-thirds is most frequently used and (b) the instrument may have curved cutting edges. Sharpen each of these three sections in turn, starting at the heel. The extent of sharpening needed for any one of these sections depends on the state of their edges. The sharpening stone will be placed on the *lateral surface* so that it is in contact with the cutting edge of each section to be sharpened.

The grasp of the instrument is important in sharpening procedures because it maintains control of the instrument during the sharpening process and holds it at the correct angulation. First, grasp the instrument in a palm grip in your left hand if you are right-handed and in your right hand if you are left-handed. The instrument's handle should lie in your palm between the fingers and thumb with the fingers and thumb wrapped around. Second, make a fulcrum on the edge of the stable working table with the inner edge of your hand so that the *terminal shank* of the scaler is perpendicular to the work surface with the *toe* pointing directly towards you. The instrument should remain in this position throughout the sharpening procedure. Third, grip the stone in between the tips of the fingers of the other hand, confining your grasp to the lower half of the stone. Fourth, place the stone against the working end of the instrument, lying against the *lateral surface* to be sharpened and establish a 90° angle between the *face* and the *stone*. Fifth, close this angle to 70°–80° by moving the stone closer to the lateral surface. The stone is now in the correct position to sharpen your instrument. With the stone correctly positioned in contact with the *heel* section, sharpen this portion with rhythmic up and down strokes, always ending on a downward stroke. When the heel section is sharp, proceed to the *middle* section and then the *toe* section up to the point or rounded end of the toe using the same procedure. Sixth, when this is complete, swing the stone around to contact the opposite cutting edge using the surface of the stone closest to your hand. Then use the same procedure to sharpen the three sections of this surface. In this procedure the *face* should not be touched because abrasion of this surface would quickly thin down the working tip and could result in its fracture during use.

Note that some instruments, such as *Gracey curettes*, have only one functional cutting edge and in this situation only this edge should be sharpened. When sharpening a curette also use semicircular strokes around the back to bend in and smooth the junction with this surface.

Finally, using the plastic test stick, test the entire length of both cutting edges remembering that the cutting edge should be at an 80° angle to the surface of the test stick.

The technique for sharpening periodontal *hoes* or *files* is obviously different. First, place the instrument horizontally on the table and hold it there firmly with your left hand (right hand if left-handed). Second, for a *hoe*, place the edge of the stone, held in your other hand, into the V-shaped groove adjacent to the single cutting edge, so that its adjacent flat surface lies on the wall ending at the cutting edge. Third, sharpen this surface by moving the stone back and forth. For a *file*, repeat this process in each groove of the instrument.

Full details can be found in Nield and Houseman (1988, pp 471–482).

Subgingival calculus removal

Any of the three strokes described, i.e. lateral, rotation and digital pull may be used using curettes. Each separate stroke should progress around the tooth root in a systematic manner to cover the whole area of root within the pocket. One way of doing this is to divide the root surface into contiguous zones which are instrumented sequentially. The curette must be sharp to function and needs to be re-sharpened after each use.

A subgingival scaler can be used both as a scaler and a calculus explorer. The working tip is first moved to the base of the pocket in the first zone and moved upward against the root until calculus is detected. It is then activated to remove the deposit. It is then replaced to the base of the pocket in the same position and used as a calculus explorer to detect if any residual deposits are present. This is continued until this part of the root is smooth. The process then moves to the next zone of the root and continues until the whole circumference of the root is smooth. It then proceeds to the next tooth until the planned area of subgingival scaling is completed.

Calculus removal in different areas of the mouth

Anterior teeth – Supragingival calculus can be removed by the use of sickle, Jaquette 1 and push scalers (see above). The push scaler is used for heavy interdental calculus around the lower incisors and the others for all other situations. The ultrasonic scaler can also be used.

Subgingival scaling is carried out with curettes and hoes. Hoes are used for heavy deposits in accessible areas. Anterior curettes can be of either the universal or Gracey type (see below). The universal anterior curette has a straight shank and a working end with two, parallel, straight cutting edges. The back is rounded and semicircular in cross-section. There are four Gracey curettes suitable for anterior teeth, Gracey 1, 2, 3 and 4, each with a straight shank one functional straight cutting edge (see below).

Posterior teeth (molars and premolars) – Supragingival calculus can be removed by the use of sickle, Jaquette 2 and 3 and large spoon excavator (see above). The sickle and excavator are used for heavy buccal to the molars' calculus and the Jaquette 2 and 3, with their angled shanks, for all other deposits in particular those in interproximal areas.

Subgingival scaling is carried out with curettes and hoes. Hoes are used for heavy deposits and curettes for all other situations. These instruments have angled and or curved shanks to allow access to different areas. The curettes may be of the universal type with two cutting edges or the Gracey type with only one functional cutting edge.

Gracey curettes

Gracey curettes were specifically designed to remove light calculus deposits on root surfaces within the periodontal pocket. They have special design features to carry out this function. First, since the working end must reach around the tooth into a deep periodontal pocket, these curettes have very long, curved functional shanks. Second, as these deposits are located within a periodontal pocket and cannot be seen, these curettes have flexible shanks to allow the operator to feel the calculus. Third, they have a working end design that allows these curettes to be inserted to the base of the pocket without traumatizing the delicate periodontal tissues lining the pocket. The working ends are tilted so that one cutting edge will be at the correct angle to the root surface, while the opposite edge is angled away from the soft tissue wall of the pocket (**Fig. 15.15**). Finally, the shanks and working ends of these curettes are designed to adapt to specific surfaces of individual teeth. Thus, Gracey 13 and 14 curettes will adapt to mesial surfaces and 11 and 12 to mesial surfaces of posterior teeth.

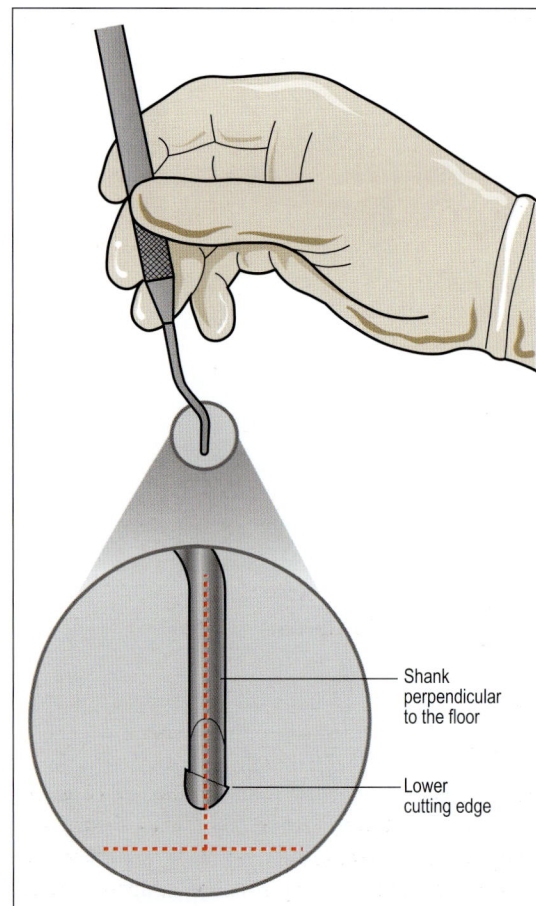

Shank perpendicular to the floor

Lower cutting edge

Fig. 15.15 Diagram illustrating the working end of a Gracey scaler showing the angled cutting edge.

The working end of a Gracey curette has two curved cutting edges that meet to form a rounded toe and has a rounded back which is semicircular in cross-section. The working end is tilted in relation to the terminal shank making one cutting edge lower than the other. This allows insertion into the pocket without trauma from the opposite edge. The lower functional edge then is placed at the correct angle to the root. Only the lower cutting edge is used for scaling and *only* this edge should be sharpened. Each Gracey curette is area specific and this means that correct adaptation to difficult areas can be achieved. However, several instruments are required to scale the whole mouth. These instruments have long functional shanks with multiple shank bends and this design allows easy access to areas within deep pockets.

The flexibility of the shanks of Gracey curettes is ideal for the detection and removal of fine deposits but makes the instruments unsuitable for the removal of heavy deposits which is usually carried out with universal curettes which have shorter rigid shanks. There are, however, situations with heavy subgingival deposits where access is impossible with universal curettes and for these modified Gracey curettes with rigid shanks have been manufactured. These rigid shank Gracey curettes should not be used for definitive scaling and root planing because this design results in limited transfer of tactile sensation to the operator which in root planing could result in excessive removal of root surface.

Choosing the correct instrument – The area-specific curettes are combined in pairs to make double-ended instruments as follows:

Gracey 1–2	Gracey 11–12
Gracey 3–4	Gracey 11–14
Gracey 5–6	Gracey 12–13
Gracey 7–8	Gracey 13–14
Gracey 9–10	

A reasonable selection of these instruments suitable for most areas of the mouth would be one double-ended anterior and several double-ended posterior Gracey (G) curettes, e.g. G 1–2, G 11–14, G 12–13.

The correct Gracey curette for different areas of the mouth are listed below:

Area of use	Gracey curette
Anteriors (incisors and canines)	Gracey 1
	Gracey 2
	Gracey 3
	Gracey 4
Anteriors and premolars	Gracey 5
	Gracey 6
Buccal and lingual surfaces of molars	Gracey 7
	Gracey 8
	Gracey 9
	Gracey 10
Buccal, lingual and mesial surfaces of molars	Gracey 11
	Gracey 12
Distal surfaces of molars	Gracey 13
	Gracey 14

In using these instruments, great care must be taken in selecting the correct instrument, in determining the lower cutting edge of the instrument and placing the cutting edge at the correct angle to the tooth. If the correct curette is selected, these criteria can be met by placing the shank nearest to the working end parallel to the tooth with the cutting edge against the tooth surface. This principle works \for buccal, lingual, mesial and distal surfaces alike.

Insertion of a Gracey curette into the pocket – On *proximal surfaces* a finger rest is established and the correct cutting edge is placed against the proximal surface. Next the instrument handle is raised or lowered so that the whole working end *face* is in contact with the tooth surface, i.e. a zero face to tooth angulation. The working end is next slid along the tooth surface in an apical direction until the base of the pocket is reached. The finger rest is maintained while the instrument handle is adjusted so that the shank nearest to the working end is parallel to the proximal surface being instrumented. This places the lower cutting end at the correct angulation to the root surface.

On *buccal* or *lingual* surfaces a finger rest is established and the correct lower cutting edge is placed against the tooth surface. The handle is then raised or lowered so that the *toe* of the working end is pointing directly into the pocket. The working end is then slid into the pocket until it reaches its base. The handle is then raised or lowered until the shank nearest to the working end is parallel to the tooth surface to be instrumented which places the cutting edge at the correct angulation to start the working stroke.

Instrumentation – When instrumenting *anterior teeth* subgingivally using G 1–2, it is usual to start on the midline of the labial surface with the toe pointing towards the proximal surface and then to instrument across the root and on to the mesial surface. Then the working end of the double-ended instrument is changed and positioned at the midline with the toe pointing distally so the rest of the labial surface and the distal aspect is instrumented. This is then repeated for all the teeth and the process repeated for the lingual surfaces. A combination of vertical and lateral working strokes can be used.

On *posterior teeth* it is usual to use vertical working strokes on proximal surfaces and mainly oblique working strokes on buccal and lingual surfaces. When instrumenting *posterior teeth* subgingivally using G 11–14 or G 12–13, it is usual to begin near the distobuccal or distolingual line angle and work across the root surface and on to the distal surface. The end is then changed and is positioned with the toe at this line angle pointing mesially. The rest of the buccal (or lingual) surface is then instrumented working on to the mesial surface. Overlapping strokes are used to avoid missing any area of the root. Each tooth is instrumented in order, completing one surface (buccal or lingual) before passing to the next one.

Universal curettes

Universal curettes have paired, mirror image working ends and two cutting edges per working end. Both cutting edges can be used for scaling and both must be sharpened. The shank next to the working end is set perpendicular to the working end face. These instruments can be used to scale subgingivally in all areas of the mouth.

These instruments have curved, semi-rigid shanks and are therefore suitable for removal of moderately heavy or fine deposits of subgingival calculus. Each working end has two parallel, straight cutting edges which meet to form a rounded toe. They have rounded backs which are semi-circular in cross-section. Each universal curette has extensive applications throughout the mouth. The shanks of anterior universal curettes are straight whilst those designed for posterior teeth are curved or angled.

Choosing the correct instrument

In order to determine the correct instrument to use, first choose either an anterior (straight shank) or posterior (curved or angled shank) instrument. The correct working tip for posterior teeth is then determined as follows. First hold the selected curette in the standard finger grip and establish a finger rest. Then place the working end on the buccal surface of the first lower right premolar with shank nearest to the working end approximately parallel to the tooth's long axis and resting on the tooth with the tip of the toe pointing towards the front of the mouth. The handle should be directed out of the mouth and held as parallel as possible to the long axis of the tooth. If the shiny instrument face and both cutting edges are pointing inwards towards the tooth, then this is the right end to use. If they are pointing outwards, then the working end at the other end of the double-ended instrument is the correct one to use. The same working tip will be appropriate for the lingual surfaces of these teeth and both cutting edges are used for one aspect of the sextant. The same system can be applied to the other upper or lower posterior sextants.

The correct working tip for anterior teeth is determined as follows. First choose an anterior curette and hold the instrument in the standard finger grip to establish a finger rest. Place the working end of the instrument on the labial surface of a maxillary central incisor with the tip pointing in the direction in which you are working. The handle should be parallel to the long axis of the tooth. If the tip is directed distally and the face and cutting edges are turned inwards towards the tooth surface, then this is the correct end to use for surfaces facing away from you. If they turn away from the surface then change to the other end of the instrument. Lingual areas can be tested in the same way. One working end of the anterior universal curette is used for surfaces turned away from you and the other for surfaces turned towards you in the same sextant.

Insertion of curette into the pocket – For *proximal surfaces* first establish a finger rest and place the correct working end against the proximal surface with the face against the surface. Then align the handle so it is parallel to the occlusal surface of posterior teeth of the incisal edge of anterior teeth. The entire working end face should now be in contact with the tooth surface. Next, slide the working end along the side of the tooth and beneath the gingival margin and down to the base of the pocket. For *buccal or lingual surfaces* place the appropriate working end on the buccal or lingual surface where you want to insert the instrument. Then, raise or lower the instrument handle until the toe of the working end is pointing towards the gingival margin with the face flush with the tooth surface. Finally, slide the working end under the gingival margin and down to the base of the periodontal pocket.

Instrumentation – When instrumenting *anterior teeth* subgingivally using the appropriate working end of an anterior universal curette, the same sequence is used as has been previously described for Gracey curettes. When the curette reaches the base of the pocket it is turned so that the appropriate cutting edge is at the correct angle with the root and the active working stroke is commenced. A combination of vertical and lateral working strokes can be used. One working end will be used to scale the surfaces facing away from you and the other for surfaces facing towards you.

For *posterior teeth* first choose one working end of the appropriate posterior universal curette. When the curette reaches the base of the pocket it is turned so that the appropriate cutting edge is at the correct angle with the root and the active working stroke is commenced. On posterior teeth it is usual to use vertical working strokes on proximal surfaces and mainly oblique working strokes on buccal and lingual surfaces. For lower teeth start at the distal line angle of the lower right last molar and scale towards the distal proximal surface. Then scale from this point towards the mesial proximal surface and repeat this sequence on all the teeth in the sextant. One working end is used for all these surfaces but one cutting edge is used on the distal sequence and the other cutting edge on the mesial sequence. This process is repeated on the lingual aspects of this sextant and then for the other mandibular and maxillary posterior sextants. In all cases, overlapping strokes are used to avoid missing any deposits. Full details can be found in Nield and Houseman (1988, pp 201–304).

Root planing (root surface debridement)

This technique is used to remove surface irregularities encountered after subgingival calculus removal and necrotic cementum.

Roughness caused by instrumentation

Firm scaling strokes used to remove subgingival calculus also remove a small amount of cementum resulting in some notching of the root surface. Careful root planing needs to be carried out to smooth the root surface.

Necrotic cementum – Cementum exposed by the apical migration of the junctional epithelium is altered by exposure to subgingival plaque within the pocket. It may become hypermineralized, demineralized (root caries) or necrotic. Also bacterial products may become superficially absorbed into its surface. For the tissues to heal following scaling altered or necrotic cementum needs to be removed by root planing.

Embedded calculus – Some residual embedded calculus often remains following subgingival scaling and is removed by root planing.

Procedure

This procedure is required for all root surfaces exposed by periodontal disease within periodontal pockets. All subgingival scaling procedures should have been completed before this procedure is carried out.

Root planing is carried out with the appropriate Gracey curettes. These curettes must be freshly sharpened. A standard modified pen grip is used with appropriate finger rest and light shaving pressures rather than a cutting action is used which can only be obtained with the flexible shanks of the Gracey curettes. The optimum angle to the root surface of between 60 and 70° is necessary and is obtained with the correct placement of the appropriate Gracey curettes. The strokes should be long and made in various directions, e.g. vertical, oblique and circumferential and numerous strokes, often 20–40 are needed to complete one surface. An efficient sequence similar to that for subgingival scaling needs to be carried out to cover all the teeth requiring this procedure. A good knowledge of root anatomy is necessary for this procedure.

This procedure is considerably more difficult because the root surface cannot be seen. In this regard, Geisinger et al (2007) showed that the use of the fibreoptic periodontal endoscope to visualize the subgingival structures resulted in a statistically significant overall improvement in calculus removal during SRP, which was most evident in deeper probing depths. However, Michaud et al (2007) studied the use of a dental endoscope as an aid to subgingival calculus removal on multirooted teeth and found that although there was 1.16% less residual calculus at test versus control sites, there were no statistically significant differences in residual calculus between groups at deeper probing depths or at sites with deep furcation invasions.

TISSUE RESPONSE TO SCALING AND ROOT PLANING

The tissue response to even perfect scaling is variable. There are several possible consequences:

1. The pocket wall may shrink completely. This is most likely to happen when the pocket is fairly shallow and the inflammatory element in the pocket wall dominates over the fibrous tissue component. This is usually the case in young people where the walls of pockets as deep as 6 mm may shrink completely (**Fig. 15.16A**).
2. With resolution of inflammation the collagen bundles of the gingival fibre system are reformed so that the gingival cuff contracts against the tooth surface and the crevicular epithelium heals to form a long epithelial attachment which may become adherent to the tooth surface by hemidesmosomes. Thus, a wide gingival cuff is formed which is not supported by bone (**Fig. 15.16B**). The integrity of this cuff depends on the length of the adherence, its strength, the strength of the collagen bundles of the gingival fibres and the level of oral hygiene. If plaque-induced inflammation recurs the cuff collapses readily.

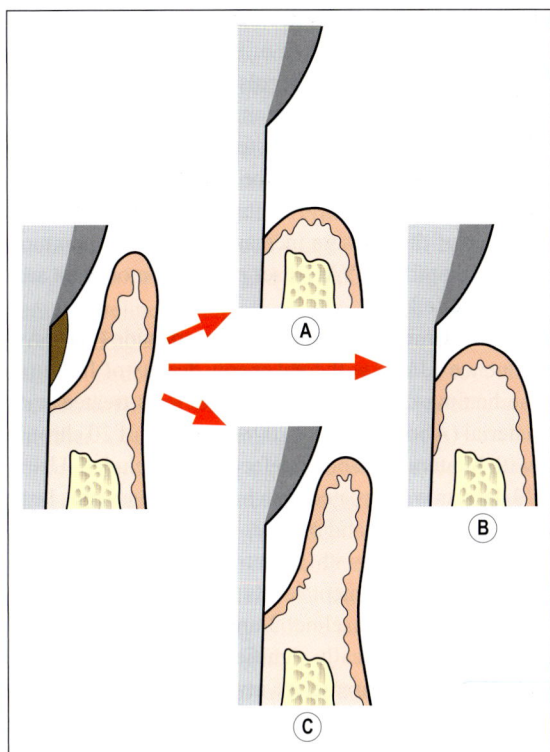

Fig. 15.16 Diagram to show some possible tissue changes that may follow scaling: (A) complete shrinkage of the pocket with resolution of inflammation; (B) reformation of gingival fibres plus some shrinkage of the pocket wall to form wide gingival cuff with long junctional epithelium; (C) little shrinkage of the pocket wall and pocket remains patent. The tissue changes following scaling frequently represent a combination of these possibilities.

3. Little shrinkage of the pocket wall may take place and the pocket may remain patent. This occurs most commonly when the pocket is deep and its wall is composed predominantly of fibrous tissue (**Fig. 15.16C**).
4. Frequently, the gingival response represents a combination of these possibilities.
5. There is a significant alteration in the bacterial composition of the pocket with a marked decrease in the number of motile rods, Gram-negative anaerobes and spirochaetes and a corresponding increase in cocci for periods of about 3 months. This brings about the resolution of inflammation, healing and formation of a long junctional epithelium and maintains it for the duration of the bacterial changes, i.e. for approximately 3 months.

Effects of smoking on periodontal treatment

There is a strong relationship between smoking and periodontal disease severity and progression (see Ch. 4) and therefore one would expect smokers to respond poorly to periodontal therapy and to require more treatment. This has been shown to be the case (Goultschin et al 1990). Smoking also appears to adversely alter the tissue response to various forms of periodontal treatment and the clinical reductions in probing depth achieved by scaling and root planing have been shown to be significantly less in smokers than in non-smokers (Preber and Bergström 1986; Ah et al 1994; Newman et al 1994; Grossi et al 1997). However, one study showed that smoking had no influence on the nature of bacterial flora before or after treatment (Preber et al 1995), while another (Grossi et al 1997) showed that smokers had lesser reductions in *Porphyromonas gingivalis* and *Bacteroides forsythus* than non-smokers in response to periodontal therapy. Thus, its effects on the bacterial flora are unclear.

In addition to these cross-sectional studies, there have now been some longitudinal studies on this subject. Machtei et al (1998) considered the change in attachment and bone levels 1 year after basic treatment.

Non-smokers had a relatively stable bone height whilst smokers exhibited an annualized rate of bone loss of 1.17 mm. This difference in long-term response between smokers and non-smokers was confirmed in a 5-year follow-up study (Boström et al 1998).

Two studies (MacFarlane et al 1992; Woolf et al 1994) found that about 90% of the patients who fail to respond to treatment were smokers. A more recent study (Colombo et al 1998) found that only 25% of refractory cases were current smokers but that another 40% were former smokers. However, Boström et al (1998) found that many former smokers return to their addiction and other authors (Gonzalez et al 1996) found the self-reporting status of former smokers unreliable.

Although smokers will also benefit from treatment, albeit to a lesser degree, treatment failures tend to predominate among smokers (Kinane & Radvar 1997). This group also found that the response to mechanical therapy was particularly poor for smokers in deep pockets. There is also evidence that stopping smoking benefits the periodontal condition and past smokers seem to respond in a similar way to non-smokers to periodontal therapy (Kaldahl et al 1996; Grossi et al 1997). All smoking patients should be informed of these associations and should be actively discouraged from smoking.

The use of ultrasonic or piezoelectric scalers for subgingival root debridement

Ultrasonic or piezoelectric scalers may be effectively used for subgingival root debridement if suitably small and correctly shaped tips are available for use which can gain access to the subgingival root surface in the clinical situation. There are indeed some studies which show that they can produce a significantly smoother root surface than hand instruments (Kawashima et al 2007).

Effects of laser radiation to the periodontal pocket

Irradiation of the periodontal pocket with the laser such as the infrared (Er) YAG laser has a bactericidal effect and has the ability to remove plaque and calculus with the effect limited to a very thin layer of the surface (Ishikawa et al 2004). It is also effective for implant maintenance. In addition, it also possesses suitable characteristics for oral soft and hard tissue ablation and has recently been applied for effective elimination of granulation tissue, gingival melanin pigmentation and gingival discolouration. Contouring and cutting of bone can be achieved with minimal damage and faster healing.

There have been some initial studies on the effects of subgingival laser radiation on the bacterial flora of the periodontal pocket and the clinical condition. One of these (Schwartz et al 2003) investigated the effects of an Er:YAG laser at 160 mJ/pulse and 10 Hz compared with subgingival scaling and root planing in a 2-year follow-up split-mouth study. It found no statistical differences between them in terms of changes in clinical attachment level or the darkfield microscopy bacterial flora and this suggested that laser irradiation could be of possible clinical use. However, another study (Folwaczny et al 2003) investigated the histological effects of the same laser on the root surfaces of teeth in cadaver skulls by scanning electron microscopy. It found that the laser radiation produced surface and sub-surface structural changes in the cementum and underlying dentine probably as the result of thermal damage. This could therefore affect the clinical usefulness of this type of laser in this regard.

Another study (Eberhard et al 2003) compared the efficacy of subgingival calculus removal by either mechanical debridement (SRP) or the Er:YAG laser. The mesial and distal surfaces of 30 periodontally involved and untreated single-rooted teeth, planned for extraction, were divided into test and control sites. Subgingival plaque samples were taken before and after the treatments and evaluated by culture and DNA probe analysis. The morphology of the extracted teeth was evaluated by digitized planimetry and scanning electron-microscopy. Following laser irradiation, $68.4 \pm 14.04\%$ of the root surface was free of calculus in contrast to

tend to deteriorate after 3 months if periodontal pockets remain, since they cannot be reached by the patient's oral hygiene procedures. Therefore, if successful pocket elimination periodontal surgery is not carried out, maintenance subgingival scaling will be necessary every 3 months to produce a suitable bacterial flora to maintain periodontal stability. There is evidence that even with good treatment of periodontal disease, the disease will return and progress unless an effective maintenance programme is established and carried out.

Maintenance involves:

- Regular monitoring of the periodontal status by regular periodontal charting
- Further radiographs when indicated by clinical evidence of progression
- Regular checks on oral hygiene
- Simple scaling when necessary
- Regular subgingival scaling of all residual periodontal pockets every 3 months. These are usually sites with probing depths of 5 mm or more. This is by far the most important procedure since it is responsible for maintaining a 'healthy' subgingival bacterial flora
- Treatment of recurrent periodontitis by appropriate means.

If effective subgingival scaling and root planing were carried out 3 months ago, then no new subgingival calculus deposits are likely but some residual fine deposits which remain even after these procedures could be present. The residual pockets are best scaled with Gracey curettes which are suited to the detection and removal of fine calculus deposits. If no residual deposits are detected then fine gently planing strokes with these instruments can be used. Alternatively, if suitable fine subgingival curette-shaped tip or probe-shaped tip inserts are available for an ultrasonic scaler, then this instrument can be used for this purpose. It is also necessary to have the water spray outlet for the ultrasonic scaler incorporated into the tip so that the coolant water is carried down into the pocket. The tip should be passed to the base of each pocket and carried over all the root surfaces of the involved teeth.

EVIDENCE FOR THE BENEFICIAL EFFECT OF MAINTENANCE CARE

All the available evidence indicates that the maintenance of periodontal stability following a course of periodontal treatment depends on regular maintenance visits.

Lövdal et al (1961) monitored 1428 subjects aged 20–40 years in an industrial company over 5 years following basic periodontal treatment. They were seen 2–4 times per year for maintenance treatment. There was a 60% improvement in their gingival condition and tooth loss was reduced by 50%.

Suomi et al (1971) monitored loss of attachment in young patients with gingivitis and early periodontitis. After periodontal treatment, one group received maintenance treatment every 3 months and the other (control group) received no further treatment. The plaque and gingivitis levels were significantly lower in the maintained group and the clinically measured loss of attachment per surface over the test period was 0.08 mm compared with 0.30 mm in the control group.

Ramfjord et al (1973) carried out longitudinal clinical studies of the effect of maintenance on 104 patients, 13–64 years of age, with advanced periodontitis. They were seen every 3 months for maintenance treatment over a 7-year period. This group recorded a low annual loss of attachment of 0.04 mm per tooth in these patients over this period. Better results were also found in those patients who maintained excellent plaque control compared with those with consistently poor oral hygiene (Knowles et al 1979; Ramfjord et al 1982).

Nyman et al (1975) investigated 20 patients with advanced periodontitis who were treated with periodontal treatment including periodontal surgery. They were divided into test and control groups and the test group received professional cleaning and oral hygiene instruction every 2 weeks for 2 years while the control group was recalled for scaling every 6 months but no efforts were made to maintain good oral hygiene. They found that the test group lost no further attachment over the 2 years while the control group lost an average of 2 mm of attachment over the same time period.

Axelsson and Lindhe (1978, 1981a) investigated a test group of 375 patients aged 20–71 years and a similar control group over 3 years. The test group was given comprehensive maintenance treatment every 2 months for the first 2 years and 3-monthly during the last year. The control group was seen annually by their dentists for traditional dental care. The test group had probing depth reductions of about 0.5 mm and little or no attachment loss, while the control group had probing depth increases of about 0.5 mm and lost significant attachment averaging between 0.17 and 0.3 mm per tooth surface.

Axelsson and Lindhe (1981b) also showed the value of maintenance treatment for patients treated for advanced periodontitis. They examined the patients before treatment, 2 months after the last surgical procedure, and after 3 and 6 years. A total of 52 patients were given maintenance treatment every 2 months for the first 2 years and every 3 months for the last 4 years. The remaining 25 were sent back to their referring dentists with instructions for future care. The maintained group had low plaque scores and showed no loss of attachment over the whole time period. In contrast, the non-recalled group showed increasing plaque scores and gingivitis and signs of recurrent periodontitis. In the maintained group, 99% of teeth either improved or lost less than 1 mm of attachment compared with 45% of the non-recall group, while the other 55% of teeth in this group had lost between 2 and 5 mm of attachment by the 6-year visit.

All the above studies were carried out in controlled conditions in dental schools but their results are also supported by reviews of patients treated and maintained for up to 50 years in various dental practices (Oliver 1969; Ross 1971; Hirschfeld & Wasserman 1978). The patients studied had all been referred to specialist periodontal practices, and the majority of cases had advanced disease. In all three studies, the average loss of teeth per year was dramatically reduced so that fewer teeth were lost per patient than in the general population. One of the studies (Hirschfeld & Wasserman 1978) reported the loss of teeth in 600 patients who had been maintained from 15–53 years. Over the entire observation period, the average loss was 1.8 per individual. Half the patients lost no teeth, 199 patients lost 1–3 teeth while 25 patients (4.2% of total group) lost 13.3 teeth per individual. This last group was aptly described as the downhill group and probably was comprised of the patients most highly susceptible to periodontal breakdown.

A systematic review of maintenance care in chronic periodontitis patients (Heasman et al 2002) compared those studies including only supragingival scaling with those including subgingival scaling. It found a significantly higher amount of clinical attachment level gain in those including subgingival scaling. This supports both the use of maintenance treatment and the inclusion, when necessary, of subgingival scaling in the treatment of chronic periodontitis patients.

Fujise et al (2006) investigated the occurrence of microbial recolonization during early periodontal maintenance. They found that severe periodontitis sites before active periodontal treatment seemed to place them at risk of *P. gingivalis* recolonization in the early maintenance period, and felt that this microbial restoration could be a cause of recurrent periodontitis.

Thus these studies clearly show the effectiveness of long-term maintenance treatment for periodontal patients but also show a variation of response in some individuals. Taken as a whole, all these studies clearly show the great importance of regular and careful maintenance treatment for periodontal patients in maintaining periodontal stability. They also clearly show that failure to carry out effective maintenance treatment nearly always leads to periodontal breakdown and progression irrespective of the type and quality of the original treatment.

PERIODONTAL TREATMENT IN GENERAL DENTAL PRACTICE

Since the vast majority of dental patients are treated in dental practices and some stage of periodontal disease affects practically all patients, a minimum standard of basic periodontal treatment should be undertaken in all these patients. Guidelines for this have been published by the British Society of Periodontology (1986) and the Royal College of Surgeons of England, Faculty of Dental Surgery (1997). The appropriate basic periodontal treatment for general dental practice should include:

- Patient motivation
- Oral hygiene instruction
- Anti-smoking advice
- Supragingival scaling
- Removal of plaque-retention factors
- Subgingival scaling and root planing
- Monitoring response to therapy
- Possible use of adjunctive antimicrobial agents.

All of these have been described above. However, patients requiring more complex treatment are best referred for specialist care in either hospital periodontal departments or specialist periodontal practices.

The biggest drawback to effective periodontal treatment is the time it takes. The restrictions of National Health Service (NHS) dentistry also make the provision of adequate treatment for periodontitis very difficult and where appropriate treatment is allowed by the schedule, it is not rewarded with fees which adequately cover the time necessary to carry it out under the present remuneration system. Treatment of periodontitis is therefore much more suited to private dental practice. In spite of this, periodontal diagnosis and treatment has always had a recognized place in general dental practice (Smales 1993).

However, recently, the quality and appropriateness of the management of periodontal diseases in the general dental services have been questioned. The Green paper on the future of NHS dentistry questioned whether the 14.6 million scale and polishes done in 1993/4 at a cost of £108 million were all essential on clinical grounds (Her Majesty's Stationery Office 1994). The Scottish Dental Practice Board (1995) showed that in Scotland, while 1.3 million scales and polishes were carried out in the year 1994/5, only 2000 courses of multi-visit periodontal treatment were provided. This disparity between simple and complex treatment contrasts with the published data on the epidemiology of the severity of periodontal disease in this region which shows that 15% of patients aged 35–44 years have advanced bone loss (Jenkins & Kinane 1989).

The NHS fee structure has been cited as a major factor in limiting the provision of periodontal treatment in NHS general dental practice (Butterworth & Sheiham 1991) and this in turn could diminish the diagnostic and treatment skills of many general dental practitioners. This view has been supported by a recent study to identify factors influencing the provision of periodontal care in dental practice (Chestnutt & Kinane 1997). This survey analysed the returns to the Scottish Practice Board and data from 375 completed questionnaires from Scottish dental practitioners. It confirmed that the majority of periodontal treatment consisted of a simple scale and polish, with multi-visit periodontal treatment comprising less than 0.2% of all non-surgical periodontal treatment claimed from the Board. While the majority of survey respondents were confident in their ability to diagnose periodontal disease only 40% were confident in treating it. Patient related factors, such as difficulty in motivation and lack of compliance, were seen in this and other studies (Nevins 1996; Noaves et al 1996) as a major hindrance to disease management. Time factors and the low level of fees were also cited as major obstacles to NHS periodontal treatment by more than 50% of respondents.

While about half of the respondents claimed that they would use the Community Periodontal Index of Treatment Needs (CPITN) or its derivative, the Basic Periodontal Examination (BPE) as a screening system on new patients, only 22% of respondents stated that they would probe all adults as part of their routine examination. As periodontal disease only gives rise to symptoms at an advanced stage and earlier signs, such as bleeding on brushing, are so common as to be ignored by a majority of patients (Lang & Corbet 1995), periodontal probing is essential to accurate periodontal diagnosis.

About half of the survey respondents (Chestnutt & Kinane 1997) employed a hygienist in their practice. A similar percentage claimed to undertake complex periodontal treatment and these were mostly dentists employing a hygienist and attending postgraduate courses. Only 89 of these dentists claimed to do this work themselves and 107 referred these cases to their hygienist. In this regard, it has been clearly shown that practices employing hygienists provide a more periodontally-orientated mix of services (Brown 1996). Furthermore, practitioners attending postgraduate courses most frequently request periodontal courses above all others (Davis & Pitts 1994; Chestnutt & Kinane 1997).

The discrepancy between the number of NHS claims for multi-visit subgingival scaling (0.2%) and the number of survey respondents claiming that they carried out this procedure (54%) suggest that most of these procedures were carried out under private rather than NHS contract. Private treatment for this procedure is encouraged by the low NHS fee, the need for prior approval and the fact that most NHS patients will be paying the full fee for the NHS procedure anyway.

Some 89% of respondents (Chestnutt & Kinane 1997) claimed to refer complex cases for specialist periodontal treatment but only 4% of these did so once a month or more. It is now accepted that while gingivitis is extremely prevalent, periodontitis has a more skewed distribution with advanced disease affecting relatively few 'high risk' individuals (Jenkins & Kinane 1989). Such patients may require specialist periodontal care.

However, many patients are becoming more informed about the nature of periodontal disease and as they also become more litigation conscious, failure to provide adequate diagnosis and treatment of these conditions may render a practitioner liable to claims of malpractice (Killila 1993). In addition, a recent report from a leading medical protection society (Dental Protection 1996) has claimed that over the last few years, it has recorded a steady increase in the number of complaints and claims that relate to the failure to identify, record and appropriately treat periodontal disease.

While fiscal arrangements are no impediment to adequate periodontal care in private dental practice, either under a fee or insurance system, they are a major obstacle to its provision in NHS practice. The results of the surveys quoted above indicate that there must be considerable doubts as to whether current arrangements for periodontal diagnosis and treatment are satisfactory in NHS general dental practice. Clearly there is an urgent need to develop evidence-based clinical guidelines and adequate fiscal arrangements to facilitate periodontal care under the NHS. While all patients would benefit from oral hygiene instruction and simple scaling, greater emphasis needs to be placed on the appropriate treatment of early to moderate periodontitis. There is also a need to identify high risk patients and to refer them for specialist periodontal care.

Referral for specialist treatment

The following categories of patients may be referred for specialist care:

1. Patients with good compliance who have residual active periodontitis after basic treatment and might benefit from more complex treatment like periodontal surgery. Patients with inadequate plaque control should not be referred until they can demonstrate motivation to improve this situation.
2. When a diagnosis of early onset periodontitis such as rapidly progressive periodontitis, juvenile periodontitis or prepubertal periodontitis is suspected.

3. Patients where complex treatment planning is required, e.g. combined periodontal and endodontic lesions; combined periodontal and orthodontic treatment; planning of fixed prosthodontics and implants for periodontal cases.
4. Patients with medical conditions predisposing to gingival or periodontal disease or periodontal disease progression, e.g.
   - Organ transplant patients
   - Patients taking anti-convulsive drugs
   - Diabetic patients
   - Patients with immunosuppression
   - Patients with renal disease.
5. Patients at special risk of complication from dental treatment, e.g.
   - Patients on anticoagulant therapy
   - Patients at risk for bacterial endocarditis
   - Patients with immunosuppression.

INFECTION CONTROL IN PERIODONTAL TREATMENT

Good cross-infection control procedures are necessary for all dental procedures and are particularly important in periodontal treatment. These procedures are well set out in a BDA Advice sheet (BDA Advisory Service 1996) and therefore will only be summarized here.

Most periodontal procedures such as subgingival scaling result in bleeding and therefore blood contamination of instruments, the dental unit and the operator and his/her staff is a major problem and for these reasons, cross-infection control measures are particularly important. Potentially infectious patients such as those carrying viruses such as hepatitis B/C or HIV are a particular risk in these situations. However, these risks should be covered by universal cross-infection control measures, since an accurate history of these conditions is often not given or unavailable.

UNIVERSAL PROCEDURES

A thorough medical history should be obtained at the first visit and then regularly updated. Patients should not be refused treatment on medical grounds since it is unethical to do so, and also illogical since many undiagnosed carriers of infectious disease pass undetected through practices or clinics every day. All information provided by the patient must be treated with complete confidentiality.

Equipment

The design of a surgery must allow easy cleaning of all surfaces and adequate ventilation. All equipment must be designed to allow cleaning and disinfection of all surfaces in the operative area and all water lines should be appropriately treated. Foot rather than hand chair controls are to be preferred as this cuts down on contamination. All surfaces likely to be contaminated during treatment must be cleaned and disinfected between patients and covered with a removable barrier, such as cling film, during the treatment session.

The water from dental units contains more bacteria than tap water (Martin 1987; Smith et al 2002). This is mainly due to water stagnation in the plastic tube delivery system in modern dental units. Whereas the copper pipes of general water system release copper ions which are bactericidal, plastic tubes are neutral but encourage biofilm development. These biofilms contain mainly species of bacteria and fungi present in the source water. The regular use of chemical disinfections is not effective in preventing bacterial contamination of the water from dental units because the bacteria are protected within the biofilm from their effect (Martin 1987; Smith et al 2002). The bacteria found in plastic tube biofilms can include potentially pathogenic species such as *Legionella* (Atlas et al 1995).

For these reasons dental units should be flushed for a significant time before use each day. As a consequence, sterile fluids should be used as irrigants for surgical procedures particularly for immunosuppressed patients. One study (Fulford et al 2004) investigated the dental unit waterlines of 25 units in eight general practices. A total of 57 samples were taken from the triple syringe, the air rotor and the source water supply. Half of these water samples were found to exceed the ADA and BDA recommended total viable counts of microorganisms.

Various means of decontaminating biofilms in dental unit tubing have been tried and Wirthlin et al (2004) have compared the effectiveness of an alkaline peroxide product, a freshly mixed chlorine dioxide product and a buffer-stabilized chlorine dioxide product with flushing and drying as the control. They found that the chlorine dioxide waterline cleaners were the most effective decontaminants compared with the control ($p=0.001$) and the alkaline cleaner ($p=0.001$).

Instruments

All stainless steel instruments should be first cleaned to remove blood and debris and then autoclaved. The appropriate time and temperature must be adhered to for autoclaving, i.e. 134–138°C for at least 3 min and longer times for lesser temperatures. If a hot air oven is used for any instruments, then a time of 120 min at 160°C must be used.

Pre-sterilized disposables should be used for syringe needles and surgical blades. Equipment which is difficult to clean such as aspirator tips, saliva ejector tips and three-in-one air/water tips are also available as disposable items.

Operator

Single use disposable gloves should be used for all clinical procedures and these should be sterile for surgical procedures. Operators should wear appropriate clinical clothing, eye protection and masks. The latter two items are particularly important when using instruments that create an aerosol, such as ultrasonic scaling.

Staff

All staff must be fully trained in cross-infection control procedures.

Immunization

It is imperative that all staff are immunized against the common preventable infections, such as hepatitis B, poliomyelitis, rubella, pertussis, diphtheria, tetanus and tuberculosis. All clinical personnel must provide evidence of effective hepatitis B vaccination.

REFERENCES

Aboelsaad NS, Soory M, Gadalla LM, et al: *Effect of soft laser and bioactive glass on bone regeneration in the treatment of infra-bony defects (a clinical study)*, 2008a, Lasers in Medical Science [Epub ahead of print].

AboElsaad NS, Soory M, Gadalla LM, et al: *Effect of soft laser and bioactive glass on bone regeneration in the treatment of bone defects (an experimental study)*, 2008b, Lasers in Medical Science [Epub ahead of print].

Adriaens PA, Claeys GW, De Boever JA: Colonization of human dentin by a mixed flora of oral bacteria in vitro, *Caries Res* 18:160, 1984.

Adriaens PA, Loesche WJ, De Boever JA: Bacteriology of the flora present in the roots of periodontally diseased teeth, *J Dent Res* 66:338, 1987.

Adriaens PA, De Boever JA, Loesche WJ: Bacterial invasion in root cementum and radicular dentin of periodontally diseased teeth in humans, *J Periodontol* 59:222–230, 1988a.

Adriaens PA, Edwards CA, De Boever JA, et al: Ultrastructural observations on bacterial invasion in cementum and radicular dentin of periodontally diseased human teeth, *J Periodontol* 59:493–503, 1988b.

Ah MKB, Johnson GK, Kaldahl WB, et al: The effect of smoking on the response to periodontal therapy, *J Clin Periodontol* 21:91–97, 1994.

Ambrosini P, Miller N, Briançon S, et al: Clinical and microbiological evaluation of the effectiveness of the Nd:Yap laser for the initial treatment of adult periodontitis. A randomized controlled study, *J Clin Periodontol* 32:670–676, 2005.

Atlas RM, Williams JF, Huntington MK: Legionella contamination of dental unit waters, *Appl Environ Microbiol* 61:1208–1213, 1995.

Axelsson P, Lindhe J: The effect of controlled oral hygiene procedures on caries and periodontal disease in adults, *J Clin Periodontol* 5:133–151, 1978.

Axelsson P, Lindhe J: The effect of controlled oral hygiene procedures on caries and periodontal disease in adults. Results after 6 years, *J Clin Periodontol* 8:239–248, 1981a.

Axelsson P, Lindhe J: The significance of maintenance care in the treatment of periodontal disease, *J Clin Periodontol* 8:281–295, 1981b.

Badersten A, Nilveus R, Egelberg J: 4 year observations of basic periodontal therapy, *J Clin Periodontol* 14:438–444, 1987.

Boström L, Linder LE, Bergström J: Influence of smoking on the outcome of periodontal surgery. A 5-year follow-up, *J Clin Periodontol* 25:194–201, 1998a.

British Society of Periodontology: Periodontology in general dental practice in the United Kingdom. In Mosedale RF, Floyd PD, Smales FC, editors: *A First Policy Statement*, London, 1986, British Society of Periodontology.

British Dental Association Advisory Service: *Infection Control in Dentistry*, London, 1996, British Dental Association, Advice Sheet 12.

Brown LF: A comparison of patients attending practices employing or not employing dental hygienists, *Aust Dent J* 41:47–52, 1996.

Butterworth M, Sheiham A: Changes in the Community Periodontal Index of treatment needs (CPITN) after periodontal treatment in general dental practice, *Br Dent J* 171:363–366, 1991.

Caffesse RG, Sweeney PL, Smith BA: Scaling and root planing with and without periodontal flap surgery, *J Clin Periodontol* 13:205–211, 1986.

Chestnutt IG, Kinane DF: Factors influencing the diagnosis and management of periodontal disease by general dental practitioners, *Br Dent J* 183:319–324, 1997.

Cobb CM: Lasers in periodontics: a review of the literature, *J Periodontol* 77:545–564, 2006.

Colombo AF, Eftimiadi C, Haffajee AD, et al: Serum IgG2 level, Gm(23) allotype and FcgammaRIIa and FcgammaRIIIb receptors in refractory periodontal disease, *J Clin Periodontol* 25:465–474, 1998.

Crespi R, Barone A, Covani U: Er:YAG laser scaling of diseased root surfaces: a histologic study, *J Periodontol* 77:218–222, 2006.

Davis MN, Pitts NB: Topics for general practitioner continuing education: survey of Scottish views, *Eur J Prosthodont* 1:23–25, 1994.

Dental Protection: Dentolegal aspects of periodontal disease, *Dental Protection, Dental News* 17:3–4, 1996.

Eaton KA, Kieser JB, Davies RM: The removal of root surface deposits, *J Clin Periodontol* 12:141–152, 1985.

Eberhard J, Ehlers H, Falk W, et al: Efficacy of subgingival calculus removal with Er:YAG laser compared to mechanical debridement: an in situ study, *J Clin Periodontol* 30:511–518, 2003.

Folwaczny M, Benner K-U, Flasskamp B, et al: Effects of 2.94 μm Er:YAG laser radiation on root surfaces treated in situ: a histological study, *J Periodontol* 74: 360–365, 2003.

Fujise O, Miura M, Hamachi T, et al: Risk of Porphyromonas gingivalis recolonization during the early period of periodontal maintenance in initially severe periodontitis sites, *J Periodontol* 77:1333–1339, 2006.

Fukui M, Yoshioka M, Satomura K, et al: Specific-wavelength visible light irradiation inhibits bacterial growth of Porphyromonas gingivalis, *J Periodontal Res* 43:174–178, 2008.

Fulford MR, Walker JT, Martin MV, et al: Total viable counts, ATP, and endotoxin levels as potential markers of microbial contamination of dental unit water systems, *Br Dent J* 196:157–159, 2004.

Geisinger ML, Mealey BL, Schoolfield J, et al: The effectiveness of subgingival scaling and root planing: an evaluation of therapy with and without the use of the periodontal endoscope, *J Periodontol* 78:22–28, 2007.

Giuliana G, Ammatuna P, Pizzo G, et al: Occurrence of invading bacteria in radicular dentin of periodontally diseased teeth: microbiological findings, *J Clin Periodontol* 24:478–485, 1997.

Gonzalez YM, De-Nardin A, Grossi SG, et al: Serum cotinine levels, smoking and periodontal attachment loss, *J Dent Res* 75:796–802, 1996.

Goodson JR, Turner ACR, Haffajee AD, et al: Patterns of progression and regression of advanced destructive periodontal disease, *J Clin Periodontol* 9:472–481, 1982.

Goultschin J, Sgan Cohen HD, Donchin M, et al: Association of smoking with periodontal treatment needs, *J Periodontol* 61:364–367, 1990.

Grossi SG, Zambon J, Machtei EE, et al: Effects of smoking and smoking cessation on healing following mechanical periodontal therapy, *J Am Dent Assoc* 128:599–607, 1997.

Heasman PA, McCraken GI, Steen N: Supportive periodontal care: the effect of periodic subgingival debridement with supragingival prophylaxis with respect to clinical outcomes, *J Clin Periodontol* 29:S163–S172, 2002.

Her Majesty's Stationery Office: *Improving NHS Dentistry*, London, 1994, Her Majesty's Stationery Office.

Hill RW, Ramfjord SP, Morrison EC, et al: Four types of periodontal treatment compared over 2 years, *J Periodontol* 52:655–667, 1981.

Hirschfeld L, Wasserman B: A long-term survey of tooth loss in 600 treated periodontal patients, *J Periodontol* 49:225–237, 1978.

Ishikawa I, Aoki A, Takasaki AA: Potential applications of Erbium:YAG laser in periodontics, *J Periodontal Res* 39:275–285, 2004.

Jenkins WM, Kinane DF: The 'high risk' group in periodontitis, *Br Dent J* 167:189–171, 1989.

Kaldahl WB, Johnson GK, Patil KD, et al: Levels of cigarette consumption and response to periodontal therapy, *J Periodontol* 67:675–681, 1996.

Kawashima H, Sato S, Kishida M, et al: A comparison of root surface instrumentation using two piezoelectric ultrasonic scalers and a hand scaler in vivo, *J Periodontal Res* 42:90–95, 2007.

Kinane DF, Radvar M: The effect of smoking on mechanical and antimicrobial periodontal therapy, *J Periodontol* 68:467–472, 1997.

Killila BA: Dental profession liability issues, *J Indian Dent Assoc* 72:22–24, 1993.

Knowles JW, Burgett FG, Nissle RR, et al: Results of periodontal treatment related to pocket depth and attachment level. Eight years, *J Periodontol* 50:225–233, 1979.

Lang NP, Corbet EF: Periodontal diagnosis in daily practice, *Int Dent J* 45:3–15, 1995.

Listgarten MA, Lindhe J, Hellden L: Effects of tetracycline and/or scaling on human periodontal disease. Clinical microbiological and histological observations, *J Clin Periodontol* 5:246–271, 1978.

Lövdal A, Arno A, Schei O, et al: Combined effect of subgingival scaling and controlled oral hygiene on the incidence of gingivitis, *Acta Odontol Scand* 19:537–555, 1961.

Magnusson I, Lindhe J, Yoneyama T, et al: Recolonisation of the subgingival microbiota following scaling in deep pockets, *J Clin Periodontol* 11:193–207, 1984.

MacFarlane GD, Herzberg MC, Wolff LF, et al: Refractory periodontitis associated with abnormal polymorphonuclear leucocyte phagocytosis and cigarette smoking, *J Periodontol* 63:908–913, 1992.

Machtei EE, Hausmann E, Schmidt M, et al: Radiographic and clinical responses to periodontal therapy, *J Periodontol* 69:590–595, 1998.

Martin MV: The significance of bacterial contamination of dental unit water supplies, *Br Dent J* 163:152–154, 1987.

Michaud RM, Schoolfield J, Mellonig JT, et al: The efficacy of subgingival calculus removal with endoscopy – aided scaling and root planing: A study on multirooted teeth, *J Periodontol* 78:2238–2245, 2007.

Miyazaki A, Yamaguchi T, Nishikata J, et al: Effects of Nd:YAG and CO_2 laser treatment and ultrasonic scaling on periodontal pockets of chronic periodontitis patients, *J Periodontol* 74:175–180, 2003.

Moore J, Wilson M, Kieser JB: The distribution of bacterial lipopolysaccharide (endotoxin) in relation to periodontally involved root surfaces, *J Clin Periodontol* 13:748–751, 1986.

Mousques T, Listgarten MA, Phillips RW: Effect of scaling and root planing on the composition of the human subgingival microbial flora, *J Periodontal Res* 15:144–151, 1980.

Nevins M: Long-term periodontal maintenance in private practice, *J Clin Periodontol* 23:273–277, 1996.

Newman MG, Kornman KS, Holzman S: Association of clinical risk factors with treatment outcomes, *J Periodontol* 65:489–497, 1994.

Nield JS, Houseman GA: In *Fundamentals of Dental Hygiene Instrumentation*, Philadelphia 1988, Lea and Febiger, pp 17–482.

Noaves AB, Noaves AB Jr, Moares N, et al: Compliance with supportive periodontal therapy, *J Periodontol* 67:213–216, 1996.

Nyman S, Rosling B, Lindhe J: Effect of professional tooth cleaning on healing after periodontal surgery, *J Clin Periodontol* 2:80–86, 1975.

Oliver RC: Tooth loss with and without periodontal therapy, *Dent Abstr* 17:8–9, 1969.

Papapanou PN, Sedaghatfar MH, Demmer RT, et al: Periodontal therapy alters gene expression of peripheral blood monocytes, *J Clin Periodontol* 34:736–747, 2007.

Pihlstrom BL, McHugh RB, Oliphant TH, et al: Comparison of surgical and non surgical treatment of periodontal disease. A review of current studies and additional results after 6.5 years, *J Clin Periodontol* 10:524–541, 1983.

Pourzarandian A, Watanabe H, Ruwanpura SMPM, et al: Er:YAG laser irradiation increases prostaglandin E2 production via the induction of cyclooxygenase-2 mRNA in human gingival fibroblasts, *J Periodontal Res* 40:182–186, 2005.

Preber H, Bergström J: The effect of non-surgical treatment on periodontal pockets in smokers and non-smokers, *J Clin Periodontol* 13:319–323, 1986.

Preber H, Linder L, Bergström J: Periodontal healing and the periopathogenic microflora in smokers and non-smokers, *J Clin Periodontol* 22:946–952, 1995.

Rabbani GM, Ash MM, Caffesse RG: The effectiveness of subgingival root planing in calculus removal, *J Periodontol* 52:119–123, 1981.

Ramfjord SP, Knowles JW, Nissle RR, et al: Longitudinal study of periodontal therapy, *J Periodontol* 44:66–77, 1973.

Ramfjord SP, Morrison EC, Burgett FG, et al: Oral hygiene and maintenance of periodontal support, *J Periodontol* 53:26–30, 1982.

Ramfjord SP, Caffesse RG, Morrison EC, et al: 4 modalities of periodontal treatment compared over 5 years, *J Clin Periodontol* 14:445–452, 1987.

Ross IF: The results of treatment. A long term study of one hundred and eighty patients, *Parodontologie* 25:125–134, 1971.

Royal College of Surgeons of England, Faculty of Dental Surgery: *National Clinical Guidelines. Screening of patients to detect periodontal diseases*, London, 1997, Royal College of Surgeons of England.

Scottish Dental Practice Board: *Annual Report 1994/5*, Edinburgh, 1995, Scottish Dental Practice Board.

Schwartz F, Sculean A, Berakdar M, et al: Periodontal treatment with an Er:YAG laser or scaling and root planing. A 2-year follow-up split mouth study, *J Periodontol* 74:590–596, 2003.

Sculean A, Schwarz F, Berakdar M, et al: Periodontal treatment with an Er:YAG laser compared to ultrasonic instrumentation: a pilot study, *J Periodontol* 75:966–973, 2004.

Smales FC: Periodontology in general dental practice, *Int Dent J* 43:193–199, 1993.

Smith AJ, McHugh S, McCormick L, et al: A cross sectional study of water quantity from dental unit water lines in dental practices in the West of Scotland, *Br Dent J* 193:645–648, 2002.

Socransky SS, Haffajee AD, Goodson JM, et al: New concepts of destructive periodontal disease, *J Clin Periodontol* 11:21–32, 1984.

Stambaugh RV, Dragoo M, Smith DM, et al: The limits of subgingival curettage, *Journal of Periodontal Restorative Dentistry* 1:31–41, 1981.

Suomi JD, Greene JC, Vermillion JR, et al: The effect of controlled oral hygiene procedures on the progression of periodontal disease in adults: results after third and final year, *J Periodontol* 42:152–160, 1971.

Teughels W, Newman MG, Coucke W, et al: Guiding periodontal pocket recolonisation: a proof of concept, *J Dent Res* 86:1078–1082, 2002.

Theodoro LH, Haypek P, Bachmann L, et al: Effect of ER:YAG and diode laser irradiation on the root surface: morphological and thermal analysis, *J Periodontol* 74:838–843, 2003.

Tunkel J, Heinecke A, Flemmig TF: A systematic review of the efficiency of machine-driven and manual subgingival debridement in the treatment of chronic periodontitis, *J Clin Periodontol* 29:S72–S81, 2002.

Van der Weijden GA, Timmerman MF: A systematic review on the clinical efficiency of subgingival debridement in the treatment of chronic periodontitis, *J Clin Periodontol* 29:S55–S71, 2002.

Walsh MM, Buchanan SA, Hoover CI, et al: Clinical and microbiological effects of single dose metronidazole on scaling and root planing in treatment of adult periodontitis, *J Clin Periodontol* 13:151–157, 1986.

Westfelt E, Nyman S, Socransky SS, et al: Significance of frequency of professional tooth cleaning for healing following periodontal surgery, *J Clin Periodontol* 10:148–156, 1983.

Wirthlin MR, Marshall GW, Rowland RW: Formation and decontamination of biofilms in dental waterlines, *J Periodontol* 74:1595–1609, 2004.

Woolf L, Dahlen G, Aeppli D: Bacteria as risk markers for periodontitis, *J Periodontol* 65:498–510, 1994.

Wylam JM, Mealey BL, Mills MP, et al: The clinical effectiveness of open versus closed scaling and root planing on multi-rooted teeth, *J Periodontol* 64:243–253, 1993.

FURTHER READING

Nield JS, Houseman GA: In *Fundamentals of Dental Hygiene Instrumentation*, Philadelphia 1988, Lea and Febiger, Operator positions, pp 17–58; Scaling techniques, pp 67–324; Sharpening techniques, pp 471–482.

The use of antiseptics, enzymes and oxygenating agents as adjuncts in supragingival plaque control

16

Antimicrobials used in periodontal treatment can be divided into two main groups:

1. Agents directed against supragingival plaque development
2. Agents directed against subgingival bacteria.

Antimicrobial and anti-plaque agents used to inhibit bacterial plaque formation and thus to prevent or resolve chronic gingivitis can only affect supragingival plaque. They should be clearly distinguished from agents directed against subgingival plaque and therefore used to treat chronic periodontitis which will be considered in Chapter 17.

SUPRAGINGIVAL PLAQUE CONTROL

A number of chemotherapeutic agents have been studied to control supragingival plaque. These agents can be divided into enzymes, bisbiguanide antiseptics, quaternary ammonium antiseptics, phenolic antiseptics, other antiseptics, oxygenating agents, metal ions and natural products (Addy 1986) and are shown in Table 16.1 and discussed below.

Throughout this chapter, the terms 'plaque inhibitory', 'anti-plaque' and 'anti-gingivitis' have been used according to the clarification of terminology suggested by the European Federation of Periodontology at its second workshop. This defines a plaque inhibitory effect as one reducing plaque to levels insufficient to prevent the development of gingivitis; an anti-plaque effect as one which produces a prolonged and profound reduction in plaque sufficient to prevent the development of gingivitis; and anti-gingivitis, as an anti-inflammatory effect on the gingival health not necessarily mediated through an effect on plaque.

ENZYMES

Two approaches to plaque control with enzymes have been tried:

1. Studies of enzymes interfering with bacterial attachment, including dextranases and proteolytic enzymes. The results of these have been promising in animal studies but inconclusive in humans (Addy 1986).
2. Potentiation of host defences, which involves potentiation of salivary antibacterial activity using the enzymes amyloglucosidase and glucose oxidase to produce hydrogen peroxide from dietary fermentable carbohydrates. This in turn converts thiocyanate to hypothiocyanate in the presence of salivary lactoperoxidase, which then acts as a bacterial inhibitor by interfering with cell metabolism. There is *in vitro* evidence for this process but such activity in the mouth has not yet been demonstrated. Clinical studies of the use of this system as a mouthwash and a toothpaste (Zendium) have given conflicting results.

ANTISEPTICS

Bisbiguanide antiseptics

Several bisbiguanide antiseptics possess anti-plaque activity, including chlorhexidine, alexidine and octenidine (Addy 1986). Chlorhexidine gluconate, however, is the most studied bisbiguanide and is the one on which there is most information on toxicology.

These antiseptics are able to kill a wide range of microorganisms by damaging the cell wall. The anti-plaque properties of chlorhexidine are unsurpassed by other agents and it has much greater effects than other antiseptics of similar or greater antibacterial activity. This appears to be due to the adsorption of the dicationic chlorhexidine molecule on to oral surfaces and its release at bacteriostatic levels for prolonged periods.

Chlorhexidine

The digluconate of chlorhexidine (1:6-Di 4′-chlorophenyl-diguanido-hexane) is a synthetic antimicrobial drug which has been widely used as a broad spectrum antiseptic in clinical and veterinary medicine since 1953. It has been available in Europe for over 25 years and has been successfully used in the dental field over that period. As an antimicrobial agent, chlorhexidine is effective *in vitro* against both Gram-positive and Gram-negative bacteria (Davies et al 1954; Hennessy 1973; Emilson 1977), yeasts and fungi (Budtz-Jorgensen & Löe 1972) and facultative aerobes and anaerobes (Davies et al 1954). Its antibacterial action is due to an increase in cellular membrane permeability followed by coagulation of the cytoplasmic macromolecules (Hennessy 1977). It has also been shown that chlorhexidine can reduce the adherence of *Porphyromonas gingivalis* to epithelial cells (Grenier 1996). This effect is probably due

Table 16.1 *Chemical supragingival plaque control*

Enzymes	Bisbiguanides	Quaternary ammonium compounds	Phenolic compounds
Protease	Chlorhexidine	Cetylphyridinium chloride	Thymol
Lipase	Alexidine	Benzalkonium chloride	4-Hexylresorcinol
Nuclease	Octenidine		2-Phenylphenol
Dextranase			Eucalyptol
Mutanase			Listerine
Glucose oxidase			
Amyloglucosidase			

Fluorides	Metal ions	Oxygenating agents	Other antiseptics
Sodium fluoride	Copper	Peroxide	Iodine
Sodium monofluorophos-phate	Tin		Povidone iodine
Stannous fluoride	Zinc		Chloramine-T
Amine fluoride			Sodium hypochlorite
			Hexetidine
			Triclosan
			Salifluor
			Delmopinol

Reproduced from the Journal of Clinical Periodontology (1986) by kind permission of Dr M. Addy and the Editor.

227

to the binding of chlorhexidine to the bacterial outer membrane and it therefore could have similar effects on the adherence of other plaque bacteria.

Plaque and subgingival bacteria grow in a biofilm (see Chs 2, 17) and this structure reduces the effectiveness of chemotherapeutic agents. Noiri et al (2003) investigated the effects of chlorhexidine on *P. gingivalis* in artificial biofilms in an intraoral device. *P. gingivalis* biofilms were prepared on hydroxyapatite discs. At baseline and 24, 72 and 144 h after perfusion of chlorhexidine, two discs from each device were used to assess its antimicrobial effects by adenosine triphosphate (ATP) bioluminescence and its morphological changes by scanning electron microscopy (SEM). Close relationships in the results were found between both methods. A significant decrease in ATP content was found between the chlorhexidine-treated and control groups ($p<0.001$). The extracellular matrix structure and *P. gingivalis* cellular structure were altered in the presence of chlorhexidine. Thus, chlorhexidine was effective at reducing the viability of *P. gingivalis* biofilms.

It has been shown that an 0.2% chlorhexidine gluconate mouthrinse will prevent the development of experimental gingivitis after the withdrawal of oral hygiene procedures (Hull 1980; Addy 1986). It has thus been shown to be an effective anti-plaque and anti-gingivitis agent. However, when used as an adjunct to normal oral hygiene measures, variable results are achieved, suggesting that chlorhexidine is more effective in preventing plaque accumulation on a clean tooth surface than in reducing preexisting plaque deposits. It is thus able to inhibit plaque formation in a clean mouth but will not significantly reduce plaque in an untreated mouth. For these reasons chlorhexidine mouthwash should never be given to patients before the necessary periodontal treatment has been carried out and then should only be used for the specific reasons set out below.

Substantivity of chlorhexidine

The ability of drugs to adsorb on to and bind to soft and hard tissues is known as substantivity and this property was first described for chlorhexidine in the 1970s (Rölla et al 1971; Bonesvoll et al 1974; Bonesvoll & Gjermo 1978). Substantivity is influenced by the concentration of the medication, its pH and temperature and the length of time of contact of the solution with the oral structures (Bonesvoll et al 1974). This property of chlorhexidine was associated with its ability to maintain effective concentrations for prolonged periods of time (Gjermo et al 1974; Bonesvoll & Gjermo 1978) and this prolongation of its action made it especially suitable for the inhibition of plaque formation.

Safety of chlorhexidine

The safety of an antimicrobial agent is tested in animal studies prior to its clinical use and then all side effects are carefully investigated in human studies.

Animal experiments with radiolabelled chlorhexidine have shown that the primary route of excretion is through the faeces. There is minimal metabolic cleavage and no evidence of formation of carcinogenic substances has been reported (Winrow 1973). Chlorhexidine is poorly absorbed by the gastrointestinal tract and it therefore displays very low toxicity (oral LD50 is 1800 mg/kg and the intravenous LD50 is 22 mg/kg). No tetragenic alterations have been found following long-term use (Faulkes 1973).

The most common side-effect of chlorhexidine is the formation of extrinsic stain on the teeth and tongue following its use as a mouthwash (Addy 1986).

Clinical usage

There are now quite a few commercially available chlorhexidine mouthwashes in the UK and the rest of Europe. Those in the UK, such as Corsodyl, contain 0.2% chlorhexidine and recommend a 10 mL volume per rinse. The chlorhexidine mouthwash available in the USA, Peridex, contains 0.12% chlorhexidine and recommends a 15 mL volume per rinse. The factor governing the effectiveness of these mouthwashes is the dose of chlorhexidine delivered and 10 mL of 0.2% solution delivers 20 mg and 15 mL of 0.12% solution delivers

18 mg (Binney et al 1995). Since both of these amounts are similar and above the therapeutic dose, either of the formulations is equally effective.

Zanatta et al (2007) carried out a randomized, controlled clinical trial on the effect of 0.12% chlorhexidine gluconate rinsing on previously plaque-free and plaque-covered surfaces. They found that the mouthrinse had little anti-plaque and anti-gingivitis effect on previously plaque-covered surfaces. These results confirm the diminished effect of this mouthwash on structured biofilm and reinforce the necessity of biofilm disruption before the initiation of a chlorhexidine mouthrinse.

Chlorhexidine and fluoride have valuable preventive roles in dental disease and there is also evidence that in caries prevention they may act together to provide additional benefits. For this reason, combined chlorhexidine and fluoride have been investigated. One study (Jenkins et al 1993a) used an 0.12% chlorhexidine and 100 ppm fluoride mouthrinse in combination with toothbrushing in a randomized, double-blind parallel design involving 99 subjects over 6 weeks. The anti-plaque effects were the same as with a conventional chlorhexidine mouthwash. Similar results were seen in a study using an 0.05% sodium fluoride and 0.05% chlorhexidine mouthwash (Joyston-Bechal & Hernaman 1993).

It is more difficult to incorporate chlorhexidine into toothpastes and gels because of the binding of chlorhexidine to components in the toothpaste. This reduces its activity by decreasing the number of active cationic sites (Addy et al 1989). However, some formulations have been achieved which avoid this problem. In comparing the effect of potential plaque inhibitory ingredients in toothpastes, the plaque inhibitory effects of the other ingredients need to be taken into account. In this regard, it has been shown that commercial toothpastes containing various formulations of fluoride all reduce the rate of plaque regrowth compared with water in a 4-day study (Binney et al 1996).

More recently, toothpastes have been formulated to ensure a high availability of the contained antiseptic. A 1% chlorhexidine toothpaste of this type has been formulated and has been investigated in a 19-day, randomized double-blind, placebo-controlled, crossover experimental gingivitis clinical trial (Jenkins et al 1993b). The toothpastes were used as slurries, which were rinsed around the mouth twice per day for 1 min during the experimental period. Plaque and gingivitis scores were highly significantly reduced and stain scores were significantly increased in the active toothpaste period with respect to those in the placebo period. Thus, this particular formulation of chlorhexidine toothpaste does seem to provide a sufficient dose of chlorhexidine for a similar clinical effect to that seen with chlorhexidine mouthrinsing.

Chlorhexidine has also been incorporated into a sugar-free chewing gum (Fertin A/S, Vejle, Denmark) and in this form, the chlorhexidine molecule remains unbound. The chewing gum contains 20 mg of chlorhexidine diacetate and this has been compared with the effects of a 0.2% chlorhexidine mouthwash and a placebo gum in a clinical study (Smith et al 1996). A total of 151 subjects were divided into three groups, one using the chlorhexidine gum, one using 0.2% chlorhexidine mouthwash and one a placebo gum, and were tested for their anti-plaque effects after 4 and 8 weeks. The subjects using the gum chewed two pieces twice per day for 10 min and the mouthwash subjects rinsed twice per day for 1 min. There were significant and similar anti-plaque effects of the chlorhexidine gum and mouthwash and this was not seen with the placebo gum. Tooth staining was seen both with the chlorhexidine gum and mouthwash but the intensity and extent of staining was less with the gum.

In a similar study, the use of chlorhexidine gum has also been found to reduce plaque levels significantly more than the use of xylitol and sorbitol gums and also the subjects' regular plaque control routines (Tellefsen et al 1996). Therefore, the use of chlorhexidine gum could be a good method of using chlorhexidine in longer-term users (see below).

Side-effects of chlorhexidine usage

Although chlorhexidine is not toxic, it has an unpleasant taste, alters taste sensation and produces brown staining on the teeth which is difficult to remove (**Fig. 16.1**). This can also affect the mucous membranes and the

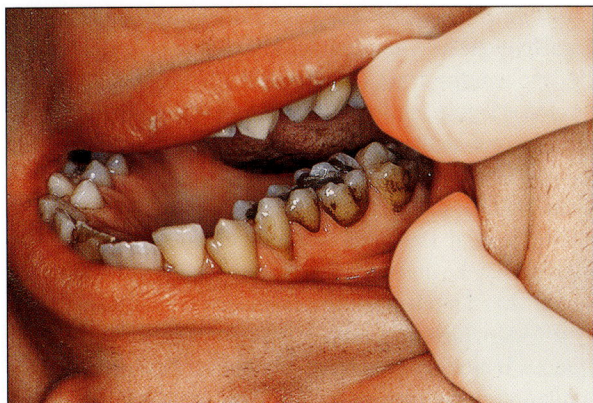

Fig. 16.1 Chlorhexidine tooth staining after 3 weeks of twice daily rinsing.

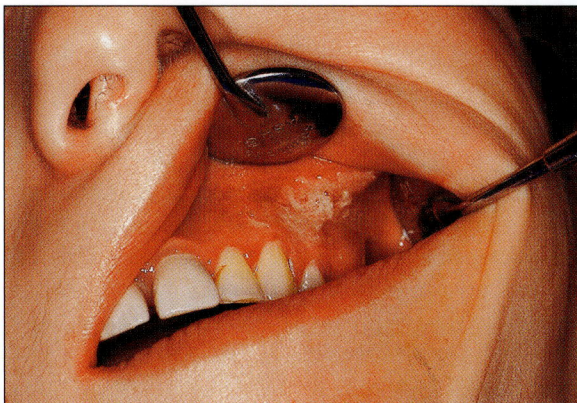

Fig. 16.2 Buccal mucosal ulceration occurring 1 week after twice daily rinsing with chlorhexidine mouthwash following periodontal surgery.

tongue and may be related to the precipitation of chromogenic dietary factors on to the teeth and mucous membranes. It is probable that one cationic group attaches chlorhexidine to the tooth or mucosal surface, whilst the other cationic group produces the bactericidal effect of damaging the bacterial cell wall. However, this cationic group can also attach dietary factors, such as gallic acid derivatives (polyphenols) found in food and many beverages including tea and coffee and tannins from wines, to the molecule and hence to the tooth surface. Chlorhexidine does also encourage supragingival calculus formation and the resulting calcified and stained areas adhere strongly to the tooth (or restoration) surface and are difficult to remove.

There is also individual variation between subjects in the amount of stain which forms following the use of cationic antiseptic mouthwashes such as chlorhexidine. In this regard a recent *in vitro* study (Sheen et al 2001a) has shown that individual saliva samples from different subjects support different rates of staining in a standardized model of cationic mouthwash staining on Perspex specimens. Although the mechanism behind these differences is currently unknown this may be one of the reasons for this variation in staining.

The stained areas are resistant to polishing and can only be removed by scaling and in this regard ultrasonic scaling is the most effective method. They also tend to stain the margins and surfaces of composite and glass ionomer restorations and these stains are particularly resistant to removal by scaling. Scaling procedures are also liable to damage the surface of these restorations and therefore reduce their effective life.

It is important to advise patients using chlorhexidine mouthwash to avoid the intake of tea, coffee and red wine for the duration of its use. One should also severely restrict its use in patients with visible anterior composite and glass ionomer restorations.

It is also worth stating that chlorhexidine formulations which do not stain are ineffective in inhibiting plaque. This is because the second cationic group of the molecule has reacted with something in the formulation and thus is unavailable for either a beneficial bactericidal effect or the unwanted staining effect. This has been clearly shown in a comparison of a number of commercial chlorhexidine mouthwashes which differed in their content of binding additives. Those which effectively bound-up the chlorhexidine did not produce staining but also lacked a significant antiplaque effect (Addy & Wade 1995; Harper et al 1995). Mouthwashes with this reduced effect include, at the time of writing, the French Eludril. The formula of British Eludril has now been changed to prevent the binding of chlorhexidine and as a result this product is now effective and causes tooth staining like the other effective products. However, at the time of writing, the formula of the French product has not been changed and hence it remains ineffective and does not cause staining (Addy, personal communication).

In an effort to reduce staining, anti-adhesive molecules have also been combined with chlorhexidine in experimental mouthwashes. These combined mouthwashes have no effect on 4-day plaque regrowth and do not cause increased tea staining almost certainly for the same reasons stated above (Moran et al 1995; Addy et al 1995).

Other much rarer side-effects of chlorhexidine mouthwash are mucosal erosion (**Fig. 16.2**) and parotid swelling (Addy 1986).

For these reasons, the prolonged use of chlorhexidine should be avoided in normal periodontal patients. It is useful for short periods (up to 2 weeks) when oral hygiene may be difficult or impossible, such as during acute oral infections or following periodontal surgery. It may occasionally be used as an adjunct to mechanical oral hygiene in initial periodontal treatment, when the gingivae may be sore after subgingival scaling. Mouthwashing should be limited to 2–3 days, after which normal brushing and flossing must be resumed.

Chlorhexidine mouthwash may also be used during periods of intermaxillary fixation following the treatment of fractures or skeletal surgery when effective oral hygiene is not possible lingually and interdentally. During this period, the patient should also be seen regularly for professional cleaning by a dentist or hygienist to limit staining.

More prolonged use of chlorhexidine may be justified in physically and mentally handicapped patients, in medically compromised patients predisposed to oral infections and as an adjunct to oral hygiene in fixed orthodontic appliance wearers. All of these patients should also be seen for regular professional cleaning. In many of these special cases, the mouthwash or gel will be used over a prolonged period and severe staining will be a problem. This can be minimized by using concomitant toothbrushing and by avoiding the intake of certain foods and drinks such as tea and coffee (see above).

With increasing pocket depth, subgingival plaque becomes inaccessible to both oral hygiene procedures and anti-plaque mouthrinses. In this regard it has been shown that mouthwashes do not penetrate into the gingival crevice or periodontal pocket (Flotra et al 1972; Flotra 1973). Therefore, antibacterial mouthrinses, toothpastes and gum have no place in the treatment or control of periodontitis.

It is also doubtful if antibacterial mouthrinses have any place in treating existing gingivitis, since in this situation there will be an established subgingival flora within the gingival (false) pocket and the mouthwash would not reach this vital area. Therefore, it is inappropriate to use any antiseptic mouthwash in the treatment of either gingivitis or periodontitis unless effective subgingival scaling has first been carried out. In this regard it is also worth noting that while chlorhexidine, because of its good substantivity, is effective in preventing plaque formation on a clean surface and thus the development of gingivitis, it is much less effective in penetrating a thick layer of established plaque in an untreated diseased situation.

Quaternary ammonium compounds

Quaternary ammonium compounds such as cetylpyridinium chloride (CPC) have moderate plaque inhibitory activity (Lobene et al 1977; Ciancio 1986). Although they have greater initial oral retention and equivalent antibacterial activity to chlorhexidine, they are less effective in inhibiting plaque and preventing gingivitis. One reason for this may be that these compounds are rapidly desorbed from the oral mucosa (Holbeche et al 1975; Bonesvoll & Gjermo 1978; Roberts & Addy 1981). It has also been found that the antibacterial properties of these compounds are considerably reduced once adsorbed on to a surface and this may be related to the monocationic nature of these compounds. The cationic groups of each molecule bind to receptors on the mucosa producing the mucosal retention but because of the monocationic nature of these molecules this process leaves few unattached sites available for its antibacterial function.

A CPC pre-brushing mouthrinse used as an adjunct to mechanical oral hygiene has not been found to have a beneficial effect on plaque accumulation (Moran & Addy 1991). With regard to conventional use, Jenkins et al (1994) compared the plaque-inhibitory potential of 0.05% and 0.1% CPC, 0.05% chlorhexidine and control mouthrinses used twice daily during a 4-day period of non-brushing. The 0.1% CPC-rinse had the lowest plaque scores, being approximately 26% lower than the control rinse and 7% lower than the 0.05% chlorhexidine rinse. The 0.05% CPC and chlorhexidine mouthwashes were very similar in their effects. The relatively poor effect of the 0.05% chlorhexidine and CPC mouthwashes is undoubtedly due to the low concentration in these formulations yielding too low a total dose for the expected effect. Also, the short duration of this study makes it impossible to detect an anti-plaque effect on gingivitis which would be expected from a normal chlorhexidine mouthrinse. It does, however, show that the CPC 0.1% mouthwash did produce a limited but statistically significant reduction in plaque growth.

A slow release system containing CPC has been tried to increase the retention time for CPC in the mouth (Vandekerchhove et al 1995). The plaque inhibitory effects over 18 days of this device was compared with that of a CPC mouthrinse, CPC lozenges (Cepacol®) and a chlorhexidine mouthrinse (Peridex®). As expected, the chlorhexidine mouthrinse (Peridex®) had the most profound effects on plaque and gingivitis and these were not approached by the other formulations. However, there were also no differences between any of the CPC formulations which showed that the slow release system had no effect on the efficacy of CPC. All the CPC formulations and Peridex produced tooth staining and this was worst with the CPC lozenges.

All cationic antiseptics including chlorhexidine and CPC are adversely affected by toothbrushing with toothpaste. A recent study (Sheen et al 2001b) has shown that toothpaste used before and particularly after mouthrinsing significantly reduced both tooth staining and the plaque inhibitory effects of both these agents. This suggests that these antiseptics should only be used a considerable time (2–3 h) after toothbrushing. In addition, this evidence puts into question some of the home-use studies on such agents.

Phenolic antiseptics

Phenols, either alone or in combination, have been used in mouthrinses or lozenges for a considerable time. When used at high concentrations relative to other compounds they have been shown to reduce plaque accumulation (Gomer et al 1972; Lusk et al 1974; Fornell et al 1975). Listerine® is an essential oil/phenolic mouthwash which has been shown to have moderate plaque inhibitory effects and some anti-gingivitis effects in a number of short- and long-term home use studies (Lamster et al 1983; Gordon et al 1985; De Paula et al 1989). On the basis of these studies it has been accepted by the American Dental Association to be an aid to home oral hygiene measures.

The effects of Listerine® on 4-day plaque regrowth during abstinence from mechanical oral hygiene has been compared with those from chlorhexidine and anti-adhesive mouthwashes (Moran et al 1995). An 0.2% chlorhexidine mouthrinse was significantly more effective than Listerine which was in turn more effective than the anti-adhesive mouthwashes alone or in combination with chlorhexidine, which it inactivates (see above). It was, however found to be slightly more effective than triclosan mouthwash in plaque inhibition (Moran et al 1997). Its anti-inflammatory effects shown in the home-use studies may be due to its antioxidative activity (Firatli et al 1994). Thus, Listerine® has a moderate effect on plaque regrowth and some anti-inflammatory effects which may reduce the severity of gingivitis. Its lack of profound plaque inhibitory effects is probably because, unlike chlorhexidine, it has poor oral retention.

Hexetidine

Hexetidine has some plaque inhibitory activity but this is low in comparison with chlorhexidine (Bergenholz & Hanstrom 1974; Roberts & Addy 1981; Harper et al 1995; Addy & Wade 1995). Its substantivity (oral retention) is between 1 and 3 h (Harper et al 1995) which accounts for the reported plaque inhibitory effects of Oraldene® the UK product (Roberts & Addy 1981). However, one study which investigated its adjunctive effect on aphthous ulcer patients did not show any added benefit over mechanical oral hygiene (Chadwick et al 1991). It can cause oral ulceration at concentrations >0.1% (Bergenholz & Hanstrom 1974). It has also been shown that combining zinc with hexetidine improves its plaque inhibiting activities probably by acting synergistically with it (Giersten et al 1987).

Povidone iodine

Povidone iodine appears to have no significant anti-plaque activity when used as a 1% mouthwash (Addy et al 1977) and the absorption of significant levels of iodine may make this compound unsatisfactory for prolonged use in the oral cavity (Fergerson et al 1978). Also, it could cause a problem of iodine sensitivity in sensitized individuals.

Triclosan

Triclosan, a trichlora-2′-hydroxydiphenyl ether, is a non-ionic antiseptic which lacks the staining effects of cationic agents. It has been used recently in a number of the commercial toothpastes and mouthwashes and produces moderate plaque inhibitory effects when used as a mouthwash in combination with zinc (Moran et al 1992a; Schaeken et al 1994). In one study (Moran et al 1992a) the combination mouthwash produced inhibition of plaque regrowth during a 4-day period with abstinence from mechanical oral hygiene but this study raised doubts as to the individual contribution of triclosan to this effect. The use of a combination of zinc and triclosan arose from the concept that agents with different modes of action might have synergistic or additive effects but the separate and combined effect of triclosan have been investigated and these are described below.

The effects of zinc/triclosan and chlorhexidine mouthwashes were compared in a 3-week clinical trial (Schaeken et al 1994) where abstinence from brushing was produced by wearing an acrylic tooth shield over the test area of the mouth during brushing. Two experimental mouthwashes containing 0.4% zinc sulphate and 0.15% triclosan were compared with 0.12% chlorhexidine (positive control) and placebo (negative control) mouthwashes. The two experimental mouthwashes differed only in their ethanol and humectant content. The mouthwashes were used twice daily after brushing for 3 weeks. In the negative control subjects the plaque and gingival bleeding scores rose above their pre-study levels. In the subjects using the first zinc/triclosan mouthwash these levels were significantly lower than the control levels but the change was not significant for the second zinc/triclosan mouthwash. The first zinc/triclosan mouthwash had higher concentrations of ethanol and humectant which probably improved the effect by increasing the solubilization of triclosan which has a low solubility in water. As expected the plaque and gingivitis scores were the lowest in the subjects using chlorhexidine mouthwash.

The effects of these same two experimental zinc/triclosan mouthwashes were compared with a non-active control mouthwash over 28 weeks (Schaeken et al 1996). The subjects were divided into three groups and each was given one of the three mouthwashes which they used twice per day after brushing. Assessments were made of the clinical status and levels of salivary *Streptococcus mutans*. At 4-week plaque and calculus scores all groups were low compared with baseline but thereafter they progressively increased. Plaque and gingival bleeding scores were significantly lower in subjects using the experimental mouthwashes than those using the control mouthwash. Calculus scores were also significantly lower at 28 weeks for the subjects using the second experimental mouthwash. No significant changes in salivary *S. mutans* numbers were seen. The only adverse effect seen was some tooth staining.

Another crossover study (Ramberg et al 1996) compared the effect of 0.06% triclosan, 0.12% chlorhexidine and placebo mouthwashes on *de novo* plaque formation over 18 days at healthy and inflamed gingival sites of 10 volunteers. No significant differences in the gingivitis scores were found between the three mouthwashes but both active mouthwashes produced significant reductions of plaque formation compared with the control mouthwash. These reductions were significantly greater for the chlorhexidine compared with the triclosan mouthwash. They also found that more plaque formed at inflamed sites than healthy sites regardless of which mouthwash was used.

While triclosan itself has little or no substantivity, there is evidence that its oral retention can be increased by its combination with copolymers of methoxyethylene and maleic acid (Gantrex®, ISP Corp) (Deasy et al 1991; Lobene et al 1992). Furthermore, there is also evidence from two short-term (Deasy et al 1991; Lobene et al 1992) and two longer-term trials (Worthington et al 1993; Ayad et al 1995) conforming to the Council on Therapeutics, American Dental Association (1986) Guidelines that the combination of 0.03% triclosan with Gantrex® used as a pre-brushing rinse can produce significant adjunctive effects to mechanical oral hygiene in further reducing plaque levels and gingivitis.

Moreover, there is evidence that triclosan may also act as an anti-inflammatory agent in mouthrinses and toothpastes (Kjaerheim et al 1996). In this way, it has been shown to reduce the inflammatory reaction to sodium lauryl sulphate on the gingiva (Waaler et al 1994) and skin, and the skin reaction to nickel hypersensitivity (Barkvoll & Rölla 1995). In addition, it has been shown to reduce histamine induced dermal inflammation and reduce the severity and healing period of aphthous ulceration (Skaare et al 1996). The mechanism of this property has been investigated *in vitro* (Gaffar et al 1995) and it has been shown to inhibit both cyclo-oxygenase and lipoxygenase, thus reducing the synthesis of prostaglandins and leukotrienes.

This issue is further complicated by the fact that the anti-inflammatory and antibacterial properties of triclosan combinations are affected by the nature of the solvents in the formulation (Jenkins et al 1991; Kjaerheim et al 1994a,b; Skaare et al 1997).

Thus, triclosan mouthwashes reduce plaque accumulation but to a much lesser extent than chlorhexidine. However, the extent of their plaque inhibitory effects seems to be dependent both upon the presence of co-polymers in the formulation to increase the oral retention of triclosan and upon triclosan's anti-inflammatory and hence anti-gingivitis effect. The anti-inflammatory effect of triclosan depends upon its ability to penetrate into the gingival tissues and this is in turn dependent upon the nature of the solvent(s) in the mouthwash formulation.

Triclosan has also been added to a number of experimental and commercial toothpastes with and without zinc and it appears to produce moderate inhibition of plaque formation (Saxton 1986; Jenkins et al 1989a). These and other studies have shown that zinc citrate and triclosan toothpastes (Saxton 1986; Jenkins et al 1989a; Saxton et al 1987; Saxton & Van der Ouderaa 1989; Svatun et al 1987, 1989, 1990; Stephen et al 1990) and triclosan/copolymer (Stephen et al 1990; Cubells et al 1991; Cummins 1992; Deasy et al 1992) have produced greater reductions of plaque and gingivitis than brushing alone. However, one study has shown that it has plaque inhibitory effects which are little different from other detergent based commercial toothpastes regardless of whether it is present with or without zinc (Jenkins et al 1989b).

The effects of a triclosan dentifrice on the microbial composition of supragingival plaque over 6 months has also been studied (Walker et al 1994). Both test and placebo dentifrice produced significant reductions in the total bacterial counts and a non-significant reduction in the anaerobic count. Neither dentifrice resulted in detrimental shifts in the microbial composition of the flora nor in the emergence of periodontal or opportunistic pathogens. There was also no difference in the proportion of the flora resistant to triclosan regardless of whether the triclosan or placebo toothpaste was used. Thus, the extended use of a 0.3% triclosan/0.2% copolymer toothpaste appears to be safe to use and does not seem to disrupt the normal oral flora.

In another study (Renvert & Birkhed 1995) the effects of three commercial triclosan toothpastes, Colgate Paradent (triclosan/copolymer), Pepsodent Gum Health (triclosan/zinc citrate), Dentosal Friskt Tandkött (triclosan/pyrophosphate), and a placebo toothpaste on plaque, gingivitis and the salivary microflora were compared over 6 months in 112 subjects. Colgate Paradent reduced plaque scores by 36% and Pepsodent Gum Health by 6% and there were increased scores of 5% for Dentosal Friskt Tandkött and 2% for the placebo. Gingival bleeding scores reduced in all groups with no significant differences between them. There was an increase in the number of streptococci over time with Dentosal, Pepsodent and placebo but not Colgate toothpastes. This would seem to indicate that only the triclosan/copolymer formulation significantly reduced plaque levels with respect to the control during this period of normal usage.

Another study (Binney et al 1995) also compared the effects of a commercially available triclosan/copolymer toothpaste, a sodium fluoride containing toothpaste, a chlorhexidine rinse (positive control) and saline rinse (negative control) on 4-day plaque regrowth. The toothpastes were made into a slurry for rinsing around the mouth so that the compounding effect of mechanical brushing was avoided. Chlorhexidine was significantly more effective than all the other agents tested and both toothpastes were significantly better than the saline rinse. There was no significant difference between the two toothpaste rinses.

These studies show that triclosan toothpaste offers only moderate plaque inhibiting properties when compared with conventional toothpaste. However, they have also been shown to reduce gingival inflammation better than mechanical brushing alone when used in addition to normal brushing (Saxton 1986; Jenkins et al 1989a; Saxton et al 1987; Saxton & Van der Ouderaa 1989; Svatun et al 1987, 1989, 1990; Stephen et al 1990; Cubells et al 1991; Cummins 1992; Deasy et al 1992) and this may be associated with triclosan's anti-inflammatory properties. However, these effects are much less profound when triclosan toothpastes are used as slurries to mitigate against the confounding effects of mechanical plaque removal and in this form they are no more effective than a conventional toothpaste without triclosan or any other antimicrobial agent (Binney et al 1995; Jenkins et al 1989).

Oxybenzone

Oxybenzone, or benzophenone-3, is a monomethyloxylated derivative of 2-hydroxybenzophenone and has been used in sunscreens and cosmetics for many years (Jannesson et al 2004). It also occurs naturally in flower pigments and has been approved safe by The Cosmetic Review Expert Panel for topical use. It is a phenolic compound similar in structure to triclosan (see above). It has been tested *in vitro* for its ability to inhibit prostaglandin E_2 (PGE_2) from cultured human embryo mesenchymal cells in a similar way to triclosan (Jannesson et al 2004). It was also evaluated *in vivo* in the form of an oxybenzone-containing dentifrice. A 6-week clinical trial was carried out of its effects on plaque and gingivitis levels in 66 gingivitis subjects. A dose-dependent inhibition of PGE_2 was found in the cultured mesenchymal cells following oxybenzone exposure. In the clinical trial, a 25% reduction in the gingival index was observed in the oxybenzone group compared with a 2% reduction in the placebo group ($p<0.001$). Plaque levels were reduced in both groups with no significant differences between them. This indicates that the use of an oxybenzone-containing dentifrice may reduce gingivitis.

Delmopinol

Several substituted amine alcohols such as Octapinol hydrochloride have been shown to inhibit plaque accumulation (Attström et al 1983; Brecx et al 1987). Further studies have been carried out on the related morpholino-ethanol derivative, delmopinol hydrochloride. Both *in vitro* (Simonsson et al 1991a) and *in vivo* studies (Collaert et al 1992) show that it inhibits plaque growth and reduces gingivitis. One study suggested that delmopinol has only limited substantivity in comparison to chlorhexidine and inhibited salivary bacteria for only 30 min as compared with several hours for chlorhexidine (Moran et al 1992b). However, the substantivity test used in this study was designed for antibacterial agents that act directly on bacteria and thus reduce their numbers. Since delmopinol is not a true antibacterial agent in this sense and has virtually no inhibitory concentration it may not be correct to test its substantivity in this way.

A suggested mode of action for the plaque inhibiting effects of delmopinol is interference with plaque matrix formation and reduction of bacterial adherence (Simonsson et al 1991b). In this regard, it has been shown that delmopinol interferes with the synthesis of extracellular matrix and in particular dextrans (Steinberg et al 1992). It has also been shown to inhibit the growth of dextran-producing streptococci (Elworthy et al 1995). These two mechanisms may produce loosely adherent plaque that is more easily removed by mechanical cleaning procedures (Rundegren et al 1992). It would therefore seem more suitable for a pre-brush mouthrinse.

A trial of 0.1% and 0.2% delmopinol hydrochloride mouthrinses as adjuncts to normal oral hygiene has been carried out (Claydon et al 1996). This was a 6-month home-use, placebo-controlled, double-blind, randomized study and was structured to conform with the ADA Council of Dental Therapeutics guidelines. The 450 healthy subjects were either given one of the delmopinol mouthrinses or a placebo mouthrinse to use for 1 min twice a day after brushing. At baseline and at 3 and 6 months, they were scored for plaque, gingivitis, tooth stain and supragingival calculus and plaque was collected for microbiological analysis. The oral mucosa was also examined and they were questioned about adverse reactions. At the start and end of the trial a full medical examination, including haematological and biochemical tests, was carried out. A few adverse signs and symptoms were reported and these included transitory numbness of the tongue, tooth and tongue staining, taste disturbance and rarely mucosal soreness and erosion. All these local side-effects were less commonly reported at 6 months compared with 3 months and only six subjects withdrew from the study because of adverse events. No systemic effects attributable to the agent were observed and no shifts in haematological and biochemical parameters occurred. Both test groups showed significant decreases in plaque, gingivitis and calculus scores with few differences between them but there were some significant differences in plaque scores

in favour of 0.2% delmopinol. Tooth staining was increased in the delmopinol groups but not calculus. The reductions in gingivitis seen in this study suggests that delmopinol may have an anti-inflammatory and hence an anti-gingivitis effect. In addition, the reductions in both plaque and gingivitis also suggest that it may be a true anti-plaque agent.

The microbiological effects of the above study were investigated on plaque collected at 12, 24 and 36 weeks (Elworthy et al 1995). There were no consistent effects on the microscopical or total counts. However, there was a significant reduction in the proportion of dextran-producing streptococci in the active compared with the control group throughout treatment. There was no colonization by *Candida* or major shift in bacterial composition in the active group nor was there any decrease in susceptibility to delmopinol. Thus, delmopinol seems to mediate its anti-plaque effect without causing a major shift in bacterial populations apart from the reduction in dextran-producing streptococci.

The effectiveness of 0.2% delmopinol and 0.2% chlorhexidine mouthwashes have also been compared in a 4-week, double-blind, randomized, placebo-controlled clinical study of 57 patients with gingivitis (Halse et al 1995). The patients all received professional cleaning before baseline and were either given delmopinol, chlorhexidine or placebo mouthwashes to use 10 mL twice/day after brushing. The plaque index and plaque wet weight were used to score plaque and gingival fluid flow and bleeding on probing to score gingivitis. With respect to plaque, both chlorhexidine and delmopinol significantly reduced scores relative to the placebo and there were no significant differences between the effects of chlorhexidine and delmopinol. In respect of gingivitis, there were no significant differences between the effects of delmopinol, chlorhexidine and placebo mouthrinses. The same adverse effects as were described above were reported for both active mouthwashes. A transient anaesthetic effect on the oral mucosa was more commonly reported in the delmopinol group while chlorhexidine produced more tooth and tongue staining than delmopinol.

This same group (Halse et al 1998a) compared the use of 0.2% delmopinol, 0.2% chlorhexidine and placebo mouthwashes over 6 months in 149 patients. It showed that both active mouthwashes significantly reduced the levels of plaque and gingivitis over this period. The chlorhexidine mouthwash produced somewhat greater reductions in plaque but in terms of gingivitis there was no difference in the effects of both active mouthwashes. This study shows a much better effect of delmopinol on gingivitis over this longer period than its effect in the short term (Halse et al 1995) and this study also supports the previous findings of another group (Claydon et al 1996).

A further study by the same group (Halse et al 1998b) on 68 of these patients showed that neither mouthwash produced an undesirable shift in the bacterial flora in saliva or dental plaque. There were slight reductions in the total cultivated counts in both areas but no changes in bacterial proportions and no increase in the growth of staphylococci, enteric bacteria or yeasts. Furthermore, there was no change in the MIC values for individual bacterial species in subjects using the 0.2% delmopinol mouthwash over this time period, which indicates that no adaptation to this agent had taken place. Finally, neither delmopinol nor chlorhexidine showed any residual effects on the plaque bacteria by the end of treatment. Thus, the use of delmopinol seemed to be accompanied by a composition of the plaque and salivary flora associated with healthy conditions in the oral cavity.

Another study compared the plaque inhibitory effects of 0.1%, 0.2% delmopinol mouthwashes and a placebo mouthwash in 'slow' and 'rapid' plaque formers (Zee et al 1997). It confirmed the beneficial effects of both delmopinol mouthwashes versus the placebo but found no differences in its effect on slow or rapid plaque formers.

Therefore, it would seem that delmopinol is well-tolerated and may produce a true anti-plaque effect. It thus holds promise as a useful agent for mouthwashes and possibly toothpastes.

Salifluor

Salifluor is a salicylamide (5*N*-octanoyl-3'-trifluoromethylsalicylanide) which has both antibacterial and anti-inflammatory properties (Genco 1994). The possibility that 5-alkyl-salicylanides like salifluor may have a plaque inhibitory effect was suggested by Coburn et al (1981) from *in vitro* studies. Recently, a combination of salifluor and polyvinylmethylether/malic acid (OVM/MA) have been investigated *in vitro* (Nabi et al 1996) and the combination was shown to enhance the uptake of salifluor on saliva-coated hydroxyapatite discs and to reduce plaque growth in an artificial mouth.

Three related double-blind, randomized, crossover clinical trials into the effect of mouthrinses containing salifluor on plaque and gingivitis have been carried out (Furuichi et al 1996). In each study, 10 medically and dentally healthy dental students were used and the effects of 0.08%, 0.12% and 0.2% salifluor, 0.12% chlorhexidine and control mouthwashes were compared with a washout period between each. In the first study, they found that the salifluor mouthrinses were significantly more effective than control rinses and equally effective as 0.12% chlorhexidine in retarding 4-day plaque growth. In the second study oral hygiene was stopped for 2 weeks to induce gingivitis and then the teeth were professionally cleaned. Plaque was then allowed to form again for a further 4 days during which time either the control, the 0.12% salifluor or 0.12% chlorhexidine mouthwash, was used. The results showed that mouthwashes containing 0.12% salifluor and 0.12% chlorhexidine inhibited plaque formation to the same extent as both inflamed and non-inflamed sites but the effects of both mouthrinses were less at inflamed compared with non-inflamed sites. In the third study, oral hygiene was stopped for 2 weeks and during this time one of the 3 mouthrinses was used. Clinical measurements and plaque samples for dark ground microscopy were taken at baseline and days 4, 7 and 14. The sequence was repeated for each mouthwash with a washout period between each. There was no difference between 0.12% salifluor and 0.12% chlorhexidine mouthwashes in their ability to retard *de novo* plaque formation and the development of gingivitis during the 14-day period. The microbial examination showed that in the control group the percentage of cocci decreased and the percentage of filaments, fusiformis and spirochaetes increased while in the salifluor and chlorhexidine groups no distinct changes occurred in the composition of the supragingival plaque.

These studies demonstrate the potential of salifluor as an effective antiplaque agent. However, the mechanisms behind the anti-microbial and anti-inflammatory properties of salifluor are not yet properly understood. Therefore, the clinical use of salifluor should be further studied in the longer term to include a detailed evaluation of possible side-effects before it can be released for routine clinical use.

METAL IONS

A number of metal ions have been studied for their effects on plaque and zinc, copper and tin have been shown to possess plaque inhibitory activity. Both copper and tin suffer from the local side effect of staining. Some fluoride compounds such as stannous fluoride and amine fluorides also have plaque inhibitory effects but not as a result of the fluoride ion itself but rather due to the effect of stannous ion or surface-active amine portion of the molecule.

Studies on the effect of metal ions on plaque accumulation have been contradictory (Addy 1986) and factors like concentration and frequency of use may explain the differences. Of further interest is the apparent additive or synergistic effect of the combination of zinc and other metal ions with other antiseptics (Waaler & Rölla 1980). This effect has been noted with zinc combined with hexetidine (Giersten et al 1987), triclosan (Schaeken et al 1996) and sanguinarine (Southard et al 1987).

Little is known of the mechanisms by which metal ions exert their effects. It has been suggested that zinc may assist the inhibition of glycolysis by

sanguinarine (Southard et al 1987) which could in turn limit plaque formation. It has also been reported to improve the bactericidal activities of sanguinarine against certain oral organisms and to enhance the efficiency of other antiseptics such as triclosan and hexetidine in inhibiting plaque. It has also been noted (Ingram et al 1992) that zinc is retained by dental plaque and inhibits its regrowth without disrupting the oral ecology.

Acidified sodium chlorite

Acidified sodium chlorite is a potent broad spectrum antimicrobial agent formed from the combination of a solution of sodium chlorite and protic acid. It forms a semi-stable solution of acidified chlorite (chlorous acid) which has been shown to be strongly antibactericidal to transient aerobic bacteria. It may thus inhibit early plaque formation and has been shown to have an equivalent plaque inhibitory effect to chlorhexidine (Yates et al 1997). However, this agent has a pH of 2.9 which is erosive to enamel (Pontefract et al 2001) and this precludes the use of this agent in a mouthwash or toothpaste.

Cetyl dimethicone copolymer

A commercial denture cleaner containing cetyl dimethicone co-polymer has been produced and one group has investigated its effectiveness (Sheen & Harrison 2000). This silicone polymer appears to be able to inhibit the formation of plaque and stain on the surface of acrylic dentures. Soaking the denture daily in this solution reduced plaque growth by up to 51% in comparison with a water control. This could be a useful aid to denture hygiene and be particularly useful for partial dentures adjacent to natural teeth.

NATURAL PRODUCTS

Studies on the plant extract sanguinarine chloride have shown that it produces moderate reductions in plaque and gingivitis. The zinc present in the formulations could be partly responsible for the effect.

Sanguinarine

Chemically, sanguinarine is a benzophenanthridine alkaloid derived from the alcoholic extraction of powdered rhizomes of the bloodroot plant, *Sanguinaria canadensis*, which grows in Central and South America and Canada. After precipitation and purification of the alcohol extract an orange powder containing 30–35% sanguinarine is obtained. Sanguinarine contains the chemically reactive iminium ion, which is probably responsible for its activity. It appears to be retained in plaque for several hours after use and is poorly absorbed from the gastrointestinal tract. Several clinical studies have been carried out into its effects (Grenby et al 1995).

A sanguinarine mouthrinse and toothpaste regime given for 6 months during orthodontic treatment reduced plaque by 57%, gingival inflammation by 60% and bleeding on probing by 45% compared with figures of 27%, 21% and 30% for the placebo control group (Hannah et al 1989). Another study of sanguinarine mouthrinse and toothpaste (Kopczyk et al 1991) carried out under the ADA guidelines in 120 subjects showed 13–17% lower plaque scores and 16–18% less gingival inflammation compared with a placebo group after a 6-month treatment period.

Reviews on antimicrobial mouthrinses including sanguinarine (Mandel 1988; Overholser 1988) conclude that short-term studies on sanguinarine have shown variable but significant plaque inhibitory effects but no effect on gingivitis. On the other hand, two studies of sanguinarine toothpastes, used alone without the mouthwash, have shown no detectable plaque inhibitory or anti-inflammatory effects (Schonfeld et al 1986; Mallatt et al 1989).

In respect of its possible modes of action, it has been shown that sanguinarine at a concentration of 16 μg/mL completely inhibited 98% of microbial isolates from human dental plaque (Dzink & Socransky 1985) and that sanguinarine and zinc act synergistically in suppressing the growth of various oral strains of streptococci and actinomyces (Eisenberg et al 1991).

Some studies have compared the activity of sanguinarine with other antimicrobial antiseptics. A small group of 14 healthy volunteers were used in an experimental gingivitis study and subjects used either a sanguinarine-zinc (Veadent) or a chlorhexidine mouthwash (Moran et al 1988). This showed that the chlorhexidine mouthwash was significantly more effective than sanguinarine-zinc in inhibiting plaque formation and the development of gingivitis. The effects of various mouthwashes on 21 patients with gingivitis were examined by Wennström and Lindhe (1986) and this study showed that both chlorhexidine and sanguinarine mouthwashes produced significant plaque inhibition compared with a non-active placebo but only chlorhexidine reduced gingivitis. Sigrist et al (1986) compared the effectiveness of sanguinarine-zinc (Veadent®), chlorhexidine and essential oil/phenolic (Listerine) mouthwashes with a placebo mouthwash in an experimental gingivitis study over 21 days. All these active mouthwashes significantly inhibited plaque accumulation with respect to the placebo but only chlorhexidine was effective in preventing the development of gingivitis. In a further placebo-controlled study in the USA, the effectiveness of sanguinarine-zinc (Veadent®), chlorhexidine and essential oil/phenolic (Listerine) mouthwashes were again compared with a placebo mouthwash, this time in a 6-month study (Grossman et al 1989). Again all the active mouthwashes significantly reduced plaque scores compared with the placebo but only chlorhexidine was able to significantly reduce gingivitis.

It is doubtful to what extent zinc contributes to the plaque inhibitory properties of sanguinarine-zinc mouthwashes. The interaction of zinc and sanguinarine has been investigated in some detail by Southard et al (1987) and they concluded that the effect on plaque was more determined by sanguinarine concentration than by the presence or absence of zinc. However, the addition of zinc did produce a slight enhancement of its effects.

In conclusion, sanguinarine appears to be an effective plaque inhibitory agent but is less effective in this regard than chlorhexidine. Also, unlike chlorhexidine, it is not able to prevent the development of gingivitis. Furthermore, the mouthwash is a much more effective plaque inhibitory agent than the toothpaste which may be devoid of activity. This may be due to the binding of other components in the toothpaste to the chemically reactive site of the sanguinarine molecule.

Propolis

Propolis (Murray et al 1997) is a naturally occurring bee product used by bees to seal openings in their hives. It mainly consists of wax and plant extracts and contains flavones, flavanones and flavonols. It has been used in homeopathic remedies as an antiseptic, anti-inflammatory, antimycotic and bacteriostatic agent and because of these properties it has been suggested as a constituent of a plaque inhibitory mouthwash.

A double-blind, parallel clinical study of the effectiveness of a propolis mouthwash has been carried out with negative and positive controls (Murray et al 1997). This showed that it had a very low level of clinical effectiveness and was not significantly better in inhibiting de novo plaque growth than the negative control. It does not therefore appear to have any use as a mouthwash.

Garlic (*Allium sativum*)

Garlic (*Allium sativum*) has long been known to have antibacterial, antifungal and antiviral properties but there is little information on its effects against oral bacterial species particularly putative periodontal pathogens or their enzymes. Bakri and Douglas (2005) tested the ability of filter sterilized, aqueous extract of garlic to inhibit the growth of a range of oral species and to inhibit the trypsin-like and total protease activity of *Porphyromonas gingivalis*. They found that the garlic extract inhibited the growth and killed most of the organisms tested. Time-kill curves for *S. mutans* and *P. gingivalis*, showed that killing of the latter started almost immediately, whereas there was a delay before *S. mutans* was killed. The garlic extract also inhibited the trypsin-like and total protease activity of *P. gingivalis* by 92.7% and 94.88%, respectively. These data indicate that garlic extract inhibits the growth of oral pathogens and certain proteases and so may have therapeutic value in inhibiting bacteria associated with chronic periodontitis.

OXYGENATING AGENTS

Oxygenating agents such as hydrogen peroxide and buffered sodium peroxyborate and peroxycarbonate in mouthrinses have a beneficial effect on acute ulcerative gingivitis, probably by inhibiting anaerobic bacteria. As obligate anaerobes are important in the development of gingivitis and periodontitis these effects could be useful. The information relating to the value of these agents in suppressing supragingival plaque formation is limited although some retardation of plaque growth has been noted with the use of oxygenating mouthwashes (Wennström & Lindhe 1979). In view of the importance of obligate anaerobic bacteria in the development of gingivitis and periodontitis these compounds deserve further investigation (Addy 1986).

THE POSSIBLE USES OF ANTISEPTIC MOUTHWASHES

The main uses of antibacterial mouthwashes are as follows:

1. To replace mechanical toothbrushing when this is not possible in the following situations:
   - After oral or periodontal surgery and during the healing period
   - After intermaxillary fixation used to treat jaw fractures or following cosmetic jaw surgery
   - With acute oral mucosal or gingival infections when pain and soreness prevents mechanical oral hygiene
   - For mentally or physically handicapped patients who are unable to brush their teeth themselves. However, these patients may also not be able to use a mouthwash so that swabbing the gingival margins by a care worker may be the only option. This may not necessarily be easier for the care worker to carry out than brushing. The long-term use of effective agents has the major disadvantage of causing tooth staining.

2. As an adjunct to normal mechanical oral hygiene in situations where this may be compromised by discomfort or inadequacies:
   - Following subgingival scaling and root planing when the gingiva may be sore for a few days. The use of a mouthwash is usually only necessary for about 3 days in this situation
   - Following scaling when there is cervical hypersensitivity due to exposed root surface. Its use needs to be combined with measures to treat the hypersensitivity since the duration for the use of the mouthwash should usually not exceed 2 weeks to avoid tooth staining. However, patients vary considerably in the amount of staining they experience and some may have staining within a few days and others show little after 1 month's use
   - Following scaling in situations where the patients oral hygiene remains inadequate. The inadequacy needs to be remedied quickly since the duration of mouthwash use should not exceed 2 weeks in order to avoid staining. It would be better to have a suitable antibacterial agent which does not cause significant staining in a toothpaste or pre-brush rinse, such as triclosan, for this purpose in view of the above restriction.

Anti-plaque mouthwashes have no place in the treatment of existing perio-dontal disease, either gingivitis or periodontitis, since they cannot either reach the subgingival environment or penetrate thick layers of established plaque (see above).

All effective antibacterial, anti-gingivitis mouthwashes (bisguanides) cause staining (**Fig. 16.1**) and this severely limits their use (see above). They should therefore only be used for short periods (up to 2 weeks) in professionally cleaned mouths to prevent the development of gingivitis when oral hygiene may be difficult or impossible (see above).

All patients using antibacterial mouthwashes for short periods should be told to avoid drinking tea, coffee and red wine in order to minimize the tooth staining. Such mouthwashes should generally not be used for smokers since they would cause major tooth staining in this situation.

While many of the agents discussed above have significant plaque inhibitory activity when compared with an inactive placebo the extent of this varies amongst different agents and different formulations, e.g. mouthwash and toothpaste. Many of the more effective agents share the side-effect of producing tooth staining which may limit their longer term use. Only one group of agents that are in general use, the bisguanides of which chlorhexidine is the most effective, produce true anti-plaque activity and thus are able to prevent the development of an experimental gingivitis. This is because they combine substantivity (oral retentiveness) with antibacterial activity and thus remain active in the mouth for long periods after their use.

Effective anti-plaque agents must have these combined properties to work. The bisguanides are therefore the only group of mouthwashes with therapeutic efficiency and all the others are normally compared against this yardstick. All other agents have only plaque inhibitory effects and thus are not therapeutically effective and can at best be used as adjunctives to mechanical cleaning measures such as toothbrushing.

Two other experimental agents, delmopinol and salifluor, also hold promise in this regard and both of these have anti-inflammatory and hence anti-gingivitis effects in addition to plaque inhibitory effects.

Assessing manufacturers claims about mouthwashes

The degree of effectiveness of a commercial mouthwash is vary variable and depends on the composition of both the active and various additional agents within the mouthwash. Their characteristics are best assessed under the following headings:

- Substantivity to the oral surface
- Range of antibacterial activity against the various plaque bacteria
- Possible anti-inflammatory effect
- Acceptable taste
- Ability to promote fresh mouth sensation.

They can be grouped into three categories on the basis of these properties:

Group A

These are mouthwashes with good substantivity and antibacterial spectrum and thus have both anti-gingivitis and anti-plaque effects. The only agents with these properties are the bisguanides, the best of which is chlorhexidine. These can be used to replace mechanical cleaning methods for short periods when this is not possible. The main drawback of the bisguanides is staining which is strongly linked to their substantivity. It precludes their prolonged use. Commercial chlorhexidine mouthwashes which do not produce staining are inactive usually because the active chlorhexidine molecules have been bound to another constituent of the mouthwash.

Two other agents, salifluor and delmopinol, either achieve or come close to achieving these properties but probably by rather different mechanisms to chlorhexidine.

Group B

These are agents with little or no substantivity but with a good antibacterial spectrum. Therefore, they have plaque inhibitory effects but lack true anti-plaque effects. They thus cannot be used to replace toothbrushing but can be used as adjunctives to mechanical cleaning. They include cetyl pyridinium chloride, the essential oil/phenolic mouthwash, Listerine®, and triclosan. In the case of triclosan additional constituents such as zinc citrate or a copolymer can enhance it anti-plaque effects possibly in the case of the latter by increasing its retention time in the mouth when used as a constituent in mouthwashes or toothpastes.

Group C

These are antiseptic mouthwashes that have been shown to have antibacterial effects *in vitro* but in clinical studies have been shown to have either varying plaque inhibitory effects from moderate to low or no statistical difference from the negative control. These include hexetidine (Oraldene®), povidone iodine, oxygenating agents and the natural product sanguinarine (Veadent®) which is a benzophenanthridine alkaloid. These would have limited or no adjunctive effects when combined with mechanical cleaning and therefore can not be recommended for this purpose.

SUBGINGIVAL PLAQUE CONTROL

As periodontal disease is caused by bacteria the use of antibacterial agents would appear to be reasonable in its treatment. However, for their use to be effective certain conditions need to be fulfilled:

1. They should be effective against the bacteria involved in the lesion
2. They should reach the site of infection in sufficient concentration for an adequate length of time
3. Their efficiency should outweigh all contraindications, e.g. side-effects
4. They should not be used in situations where other conventional means of treatment are equally effective.

These agents can be taken systemically or applied locally into the periodontal pocket. Agents taken systemically must reach the periodontal pocket in a sufficient concentration to be inhibitory to the subgingival bacteria whilst agents applied locally must also remain in a sufficient concentration for an adequate length of time.

Agents used systemically are always antibiotics whilst those applied locally into the periodontal pocket can be either antibiotics or antiseptics.

ANTISEPTIC AGENTS FOR SUBGINGIVAL PLAQUE CONTROL

The association of bacteria with periodontal disease has given rise to considerable interest in the development and use of non-antibiotic antimicrobial agents for its management. These have to be applied locally into the periodontal pocket in slow release agents. Interest has mainly centred on their use as adjunctives to scaling and root planing.

The gingival crevice or periodontal pocket is not reached by chemical agents in mouthwashes or toothpastes, which have their effect purely on supragingival plaque. This is the main reason that such mouthwashes have no place in the treatment of established gingivitis or periodontitis. More recently local drug delivery systems have been developed to carry antibiotics into the pocket area and some of these have been used to deliver antiseptics.

REFERENCES

Addy M: Chlorhexidine compared with other locally delivered antimicrobials, *J Clin Periodontol* 13:957–964, 1986.

Addy M, Griffiths C, Isaac R: The effect of povidone iodine on plaque and salivary bacteria. A double-blind crossover trial, *J Periodontol* 48:730–732, 1977.

Addy M, Rawle L, Handley R, et al: The development and *in vitro* evaluation of acrylic strips and dialysis tubing for local drug delivery, *J Periodontol* 53:693–699, 1982.

Addy M, Jenkins S, Newcombe R: Studies of the effect of toothpaste rinses on plaque regrowth. (1) Influence of surfactants on chlorhexidine efficiency, *J Clin Periodontol* 16:380–384, 1989.

Addy M, Wade W: An approach to efficacy screening of mouthrinses: studies on a group of French products (I) Staining and antimicrobial properties in vitro, *J Clin Periodontol* 22:717–722, 1995.

Addy M, Moran J, Newcombe R, et al: The comparative tea staining of phenolic, chlorhexidine and anti-adhesive mouthrinses, *J Clin Periodontol* 22:923–928, 1995.

Attström R, Matsson L, Edwardsson S, et al: The effect of Octapinol on dentogingival plaque and development of gingivitis. III. Short-term studies in humans, *J Periodontal Res* 14:445–451, 1983.

Ayad F, Berta R: Effects on plaque and gingivitis of a triclosan/copolymer pre-brush rinse: a six month study in Canada, *J Can Dent Assoc* 61:53–56, 1995.

Bakri IM, Douglas CWI: Inhibitory effect of garlic extract on oral bacteria. *Arch Oral Biol* 50:645–651, 2005.

Barkvoll P, Rölla G: Triclosan protects the skin against dermatitis caused by sodium lauryl sulphate exposure, *J Clin Periodontol* 21:717–719, 1994.

Barkvoll P, Rölla G: Triclosan reduces the clinical symptoms of the allergic patch reaction (APR) elicited with 1% nickel sulphate in sensitized patients, *J Clin Periodontol* 22:485–487, 1995.

Bergenholz A, Hanstrom L: The plaque inhibiting effect of hexedine (Oraldene) mouthwash compared with that of chlorhexidine, *Community Dent Oral Epidemiol* 2:70–74, 1974.

Binney A, Addy M, McKeown S, et al: The effect of a commercially available triclosan-containing toothpaste compared with a sodium-fluoride-containing toothpaste and a chlorhexidine rinse on 4-day plaque regrowth, *J Clin Periodontol* 22:830–834, 1995.

Binney A, Addy M, McKeown S, et al: The choice of controls in toothpaste studies. The effect of a number of commercially available toothpastes compared with water on 4-day plaque regrowth, *J Clin Periodontol* 23:456–459, 1996.

Bonesvoll P, Gjermo P: A comparison between chlorhexidine and some quaternary ammonium compounds with regard to retention, salivary concentration and plaque inhibitory effect in the human mouth after mouthrinses, *Arch Oral Biol* 23:289–294, 1978.

Bonesvoll P, Lökken P, Rölla G: Influence of concentration, time, temperature and pH on the retention of chlorhexidine in the human oral cavity after mouthrinses, *Arch Oral Biol* 19:1025–1029, 1974.

Brecx M, Theilade J, Attstrom R, et al: The effect of chlorhexidine and Octapinol on early dental plaque formation. A light and electron microscopic study, *J Periodontal Res* 22:290–295, 1987.

Budtz-Jorgensen J, Löe H: Chlorhexidine as a denture disinfectant in the treatment of denture stomatitis, *Scand J Dent Res* 80:457–464, 1972.

Chadwick B, Addy M, Walker DM: Hexedine mouthwash in the management of minor aphthous ulceration and as an adjunct to oral hygiene, *Br Dent J* 171:83–87, 1991.

Claydon N, Hunter L, Moran J, et al: A 6-month home usage of 0.1% and 0.2% delmopinol mouthwashes. I. Effect on plaque, gingivitis, supragingival calculus and tooth staining, *J Clin Periodontol* 23:220–228, 1996.

Coburn RA, Batista AJ, Evans RT, et al: Potential salicylamide antiplaque agents. In vitro antibacterial activity against Actinomyces viscosus, *J Med Chem* 24:1245–1249, 1981.

Collaert B, Attstrom R, DeBrune N, et al: The effect of delmopinol rinsing on dental plaque formation and gingivitis healing, *J Clin Periodontol* 19:274–280, 1992.

Cosyn J, Wyn I: A systematic review on the effects of the chlorhexidine chip when used as an adjunct to scaling and root planing in the treatment of chronic periodontitis, *J Periodontol* 77:257–264, 2006.

Council on Therapeutics, American Dental Association: Guidelines for acceptance of chemotherapeutic products for the control of plaque and gingivitis, *J Am Dent Assoc* 112:529–532, 1986.

Cubells AB, Dalmau LB, Petrone ME, et al: The effect of a triclosan/copolymer/fluoride dentifrice on plaque formation and gingivitis: a six months clinical study, *J Clin Dent* 2:63–69, 1991.

Cummins D: Mechanisms of actions of clinically proven antiplaque agents. In Embery G, Rölla G, editors: *Clinical and Biological Aspects of Dentifrices*, Oxford, 1992, Oxford University Press, pp 205–228.

Davies G, Francis J, Martin A, et al: 1: 6Di-4′-chlorophenyl-diguanidohexane, Laboratory investigation into a new antibacterial agent of high potency, *Br J Pharmacol* 9: 192–196, 1954.

De Paula LG, Overholser CD, Meiller TF, et al: Chemotherapeutic inhibition of supragingival dental plaque and gingivitis development, *J Clin Periodontol* 16: 311–315, 1989.

Deasy MJ, Battista G, Rustogi KN, et al: Antiplaque efficacy of a triclosan/copolymer prebrush rinse: a plaque prevention clinical study, *Am J Dent* 5:91–94, 1991.

Deasy MJ, Singh SM, Rustogi KN, et al: Effect of a dentifrice containing triclosan and a copolymer on plaque formation and gingivitis, *Clin Prev Dent* 13:12–19, 1992.

Dzink JJ, Socransky SS: Comparative in vitro activity of sanguinarine against microbial isolates, *Antimicrob Agents Chemother* 27:663–665, 1985.

Eisenberg AD, Young DA, Fan-Hse J, et al: Interactions of sanguinarine and zinc on oral streptococci and Actinomyces species, *Caries Res* 25:185–190, 1991.

Elworthy AJ, Edgar R, Moran J, et al: A 6-month home usage of 0.1% and 0.2% delmopinol mouthwashes. II. Effects on plaque microflora, *J Clin Periodontol* 22: 527–532, 1995.

Emilson C: Susceptibility of various microorganisms to chlorhexidine, *Scand J Dent Res* 85:255–265, 1977.

Faulkes E: Some toxicological observations of chlorhexidine, *J Periodontal Res* 12(Suppl):131–148, 1973.

Fergerson MM, Geddes DAM, Wray D: The effect of povidone iodine mouthwash on thyroid function and plaque accumulation, *Br Dent J* 148:14–16, 1978.

Firatli E, Unal T, Onan U, et al: Antioxidative activities of some chemotherapeutics: a possible mechanism of reducing inflammation, *J Clin Periodontol* 21:680–683, 1994.

Fletcher JM, Wilson M: The effectiveness of a redox agent, methylene blue, on the survival of Porphyromonas gingivalis in vitro, *Curr Microbiol* 26:85–90, 1993.

Flotra L: Different modes of chlorhexidine application and related side effects, *J Periodontal Res* 12:S41–S44, 1973.

Flotra L, Gjermo P, Rölla G, et al: A 4-month study of the effect of chlorhexidine mouthrinses on 50 soldiers, *Scand J Dent Res* 80:10–17, 1972.

Fornell J, Sundin Y, Lindhe J: Effect of Listerine on dental plaque and gingivitis, *Scand J Dent Res* 83:18–25, 1975.

Friedman MA, Golomb G: New sustained dosage form of chlorhexidine for dental use. I. Development and kinetics of release, *J Periodontal Res* 17:323–328, 1982.

Furuichi Y, Ramberg P, Lindhe J, et al: Some effects of mouthrinses containing salifluor on de novo plaque formation and developing gingivitis, *J Clin Periodontol* 23: 795–802, 1996.

Gaffar A, Scherl D, Affitto J, et al: The effect of triclosan on the mediators of gingival inflammation, *J Clin Periodontol* 22:480–484, 1995.

Genco RJ: Pharmaceuticals and periodontal diseases, *J Am Dent Assoc* 125:11S–19S, 1994.

Gibson MT, Mangat D, Gagliano G, et al: Evaluation of the efficiency of a redox agent in the treatment of chronic periodontitis, *J Clin Periodontol* 21:690–700, 1994.

Giersten E, Svatun B, Saxton A: Plaque inhibition by hexedine and zinc, *Scand J Dent Res* 95:49–54, 1987.

Gjermo P, Bonesvoll P, Rölla G: Relationship between plaque inhibiting effect and the retention of chlorhexidine in the oral cavity, *Arch Oral Biol* 19:1031–1034, 1974.

Gomer RM, Hobroyd SV, Fedi PF, et al: The effects of oral rinses on the accumulation of dental plaque, *J Am Society Prev Dent* 2:12–14, 1972.

Gordon JM, Lamster IB, Sieger MC: Efficacy of Listerine antiseptic in inhibiting the development of plaque and gingivitis, *J Clin Periodontol* 12:697–704, 1985.

Grenby TH: The use of sanguinarine mouthwashes and toothpastes compared with some other antimicrobial agents, *Br Dent J* 178:254–258, 1995.

Grenier D: Effect of chlorhexidine on the adherence properties of Porphyromonas gingivalis, *J Clin Periodontol* 23:140–142, 1996.

Grossman E, Meckel AH, Issacs RL, et al: A clinical comparison of antimicrobial mouthrinses: effects of chlorhexidine, phenolics and sanguinarine on dental plaque and gingivitis, *J Periodontol* 60:435–440, 1989.

Halse JC, Ainamo J, Etemadzadeh H, et al: Plaque formation and gingivitis after mouthrinsing with 0.2% delmopinol hydrochloride, 0.2% chlorhexidine digluconate and placebo for 4 weeks following initial professional tooth cleaning, *J Clin Periodontol* 22:533–539, 1995.

Halse JC, Attström R, Edwardsson S, et al: 6-month use of 0.2% delmopinol hydrochloride in comparison with 0.2% chlorhexidine digluconate and placebo. I. Effect on plaque formation and gingivitis, *J Clin Periodontol* 25:746–753, 1998a.

Halse JC, Edwardsson S, Rundegren J, et al: 6-month use of 0.2% delmopinol hydrochloride in comparison with 0.2% chlorhexidine digluconate and placebo. II. Effect on plaque and salivary microflora, *J Clin Periodontol* 25:841–849, 1998b.

Hannah JJ, Johnson JD, Kuftinee MM: Long-term evaluation of toothpaste and oral rinse containing sanguinaria extract in controlling plaque and gingival inflammation and sulcular bleeding during orthodontic treatment, *Am J Orthod Maxillofac Orthop* 96:199–207, 1989.

Harper PR, Milsom S, Wade W, et al: An approach to efficacy screening of mouthrinses: studies on a group of French products (I) Inhibition of salivary bacteria and plaque in vivo, *J Clin Periodontol* 22:723–727, 1995.

Heasman PA, Soskolne A, Smart G, et al: Subgingival administration of Perio Chips in patients with chronic periodontitis, *J Dent Res* 74:481, 1995.

Hennessy T: Some antibacterial properties of chlorhexidine, *J Periodontal Res* 8(Suppl):61–67, 1973.

Hennessy T: Antibacterial properties of Hibitane, *J Clin Periodontol* 4:36–48, 1977.

Holbeche JD, Ruljancich MK, Reade P: A clinical trial of cetylpyridinium chloride mouthwash, *Aust Dent J* 20:397–404, 1975.

Hull P: Chemical inhibition of plaque, *J Clin Periodontol* 7:431–442, 1980.

Ingram GS, Horay CP, Stead WJ: Interaction of zinc with dental mineral, *Caries Res* 26:248–253, 1992.

Jannesson L, Birked D, Scheri D, et al: Effect of oxybenzone on PGE2-production in vitro and on plaque and gingivitis in vivo, *J Clin Periodontol* 31:91–94, 2004.

Jeffcoat MK, Bray KS, Ciancio SG, et al: Adjunctive use of a subgingival controlled-release chlorhexidine chip reduces probing depth and improves attachment level compared with scaling and root planing alone, *J Periodontol* 69:989–997, 1998.

Jeffcoat MK, Palcanis KG, Weatherford TW, et al: Use of a biodegradable chlorhexidine chip in the treatment of adult periodontitis: Clinical and radiographic findings, *J Periodontol* 71:256–262, 2000.

Jenkins S, Addy M, Newcombe R: Toothpastes containing 0.3% and 0.5% triclosan. I. effects on 4-day plaque regrowth, *Am J Dent* 2:211–214, 1989a.

Jenkins S, Addy M, Newcombe R: Studies of the effect of toothpaste rinses on plaque regrowth. II. Triclosan with and without zinc citrate formulations, *J Clin Periodontol* 16:385–387, 1989b.

Jenkins S, Addy M, Newcombe R: Triclosan and sodium lauryl sulphate mouthrinses, II. effects on 4-day plaque regrowth, *J Clin Periodontol* 18:145–148, 1991.

Jenkins S, Addy M, Newcombe R: Evaluation of a mouthrinse containing chlorhexidine and fluoride as an adjunct to oral hygiene, *J Clin Periodontol* 20:20–25, 1993a.

Jenkins S, Addy M, Newcombe R: The effects of a chlorhexidine toothpaste on the development of plaque, gingivitis and tooth staining, *J Clin Periodontol* 20:59–62, 1993b.

Jenkins S, Addy M, Newcombe R: A comparison of cetylpyridinium chloride, triclosan and chlorhexidine mouthrinse formulations for the effect on plaque regrowth, *J Clin Periodontol* 21:441–444, 1994.

Joyston-Bechal S, Smales FC, Duckworth R: Effect of metronidazole on chronic periodontal disease in subjects using a topically applied chlorhexidine gel, *J Clin Periodontol* 11:53–62, 1984.

Joyston-Bechal S, Hernaman N: The effect of a mouthrinse containing chlorhexidine and fluoride on plaque and gingival bleeding, *J Clin Periodontol* 20:49–53, 1993.

Kaner D, Bernimoulin J-P, Hopfenmüller W, et al: Controlled-delivery chlorhexidine chip versus amoxicillin/metronidazole as adjunctive antimicrobial therapy for generalized aggressive periodontitis: a randomized controlled clinical trial, *J Clin Periodontol* 34:880–891, 2007.

Kenney EB, Ash M: Oxidation-reduction potential of developing plaque, periodontal pocketing and gingival sulci, *J Periodontol* 40:630–633, 1969.

Killoy WJ: The use of locally-delivered chlorhexidine in the treatment of periodontitis. Clinical results, *J Clin Periodontol* 25:953–958, 1998.

Kjaerheim V, Waaler SM, Rölla G: Organic solvents and oils as vehicles for triclosan mouthrinses: a clinical study, *Scand J Dent Res* 102:306–308, 1994a.

Kjaerheim V, Waaler SM, Rölla G: Significance of choice of solvents for the clinical effect of triclosan-containing mouthrinses, *Scand J Dent Res* 102:202–205, 1994b.

Kjaerheim V, Skaare A, Barkvoll P, et al: Antiplaque-, antibacterial- and anti-inflammatory properties of triclosan mouthrinses in combination with zinc citrate or polyvinylmethylether maleic acid (PVA-MA) copolymer, *Eur J Oral Sci* 104:529–534, 1996.

Kopczyk RA, Abrams H, Brown AT, et al: Clinical and microscopical effects of sanguinaria-containing mouthrinse and dentifrice with and without fluoride during 6 months of use, *J Periodontol* 62:617–622, 1991.

Lamster IB, Alfano MC, Sieger MC, et al: The effect of Listerine antiseptic on reduction of existing plaque and gingivitis, *Clin Prev Dent* 5:12–15, 1983.

Lerner E, Barak M, Landau I, et al: Chlorhexidine release profile from a Perio Chip – in vitro and in vivo studies, *J Dent Res* 75:431, 1996.

Lobene RR, Lobene S, Soparker PM: The effect of cetylpyridinium chloride mouthrinse on plaque and gingivitis, *J Dent Res* 56:595, 1977.

Lobene RR, Singh SS, Garcia L, et al: Clinical efficacy of a triclosan/copolymer pre-brush rinse: a plaque removal study, *J Clin Dent* 3:54–58, 1992.

Lusk SS, Bowers GM, Tow HD, et al: Effects of an oral rinse on experimental gingivitis, plaque formation and formed plaque, *J Am Society Prev Dent* 4:31–37, 1974.

Mallatt ME, Beiswanger BB, Drook CA, et al: Clinical effect of a sanguinaria dentifrice on plaque and gingivitis in adults, *J Periodontol* 60:91–95, 1989.

Mandel ID: Chemotherapeutic agents for controlling plaque and gingivitis, *J Clin Periodontol* 15:488–498, 1988.

Moran J, Addy M: The effects of a cetylpyridinium chloride prebrushing rinse as an adjunct to oral hygiene and gingival health, *J Periodontol* 62:562–564, 1991.

Moran J, Addy M, Newcombe R: A clinical trial to assess the efficacy of sanguinarine-zinc mouthrinse (Veadent) compared with a chlorhexidine mouthwash, *J Clin Periodontol* 15:612–616, 1988.

Moran J, Addy M, Roberts S: The comparison of a natural product, triclosan and chlorhexidine mouthwashes on 4-day plaque regrowth, *J Clin Periodontol* 19:578–582, 1992a.

Moran J, Addy M, Wade WG, et al: A comparison of delmopinol and chlorhexidine on plaque regrowth over a 4-day period and salivary bacterial counts, *J Clin Periodontol* 19:749–753, 1992b.

Moran J, Addy M, Newcombe R, et al: The comparative effects of phenolic, chlorhexidine and anti-adhesive mouthrinses, *J Clin Periodontol* 22:929–934, 1995.

Moran J, Addy M, Newcombe R: A 4-day plaque regrowth study comparing an essential oil mouthrinse with a triclosan mouthrinse, *J Clin Periodontol* 24:636–639, 1997.

Murray MC, Worthington HV, Blinkhorn HS: A study to investigate the effect of a propolis-containing mouthrinse on the inhibition of de novo plaque formation, *J Clin Periodontol* 24:796–798, 1997.

Nabi N, Kashuba B, Lucchesi S, et al: In vitro and in vivo studies of salifluor/PVM/MA copolymer/NaF combination as an antiplaque agent, *J Clin Periodontol* 23:1084–1092, 1996.

Noiri Y, Okami Y, Takahashi Y, et al: Effects of chlorhexidine, minocycline, and metronidazole on Porphyromonas gingivalis strain 381 in biofilms, *J Periodontol* 74:1647–1651, 2003.

Overholser CD: Longitudinal clinical studies with antimicrobial mouthrinses, *J Clin Periodontol* 15:517–519, 1988.

Polson AM, Stoller NH, Hanes PJ, et al: 2 multi-centre trials assessing the clinical efficacy of 5% sanguinarine in a biodegradable drug delivery system, *J Clin Periodontol* 23:782–788, 1996.

Pontefract H, Hughes J, Kemp K, et al: The erosive effects of some mouthrinses on enamel. A study in situ, *J Clin Periodontol* 28:319–324, 2001.

Ramberg P, Furuichi Y, Volpe AR, et al: The effects of antimicrobial mouthrinses on de novo plaque formation at sites with healthy and inflamed gingiva, *J Clin Periodontol* 23:7–11, 1996.

Renvert S, Birkhed D: Comparison between 3 triclosan dentifrices on plaque, gingivitis and salivary microflora, *J Clin Periodontol* 22:63–70, 1995.

Roberts WR, Addy M: Comparison of the in vivo and in vitro antibacterial properties of antiseptic mouthrinses containing chlorhexidine, alexidine, cetylpyridinium chloride and hexedine, *J Clin Periodontol* 8:295–310, 1981.

Rölla G, Löe H, Schiöt C: Retention of chlorhexidine in the human oral cavity, *Arch Oral Biol* 16:1109–1116, 1971.

Rosling BG, Slots J, Webber RL, et al: Microbiological and clinical effects of topical subgingival antimicrobial treatment on human periodontal disease, *J Clin Periodontol* 10:487–514, 1983.

Rundegren J, Simonsson T, Petersson L, et al: Effect of delmopinol on cohesion of glucan-containing plaque formed by Streptococcus mutans in a flow system, *Scand Dent J* 71:1792–1796, 1992.

Saxton CA: The effects of a dentifrice containing zinc citrate and 2.2.4'-hydroxydiphenol, *J Periodontol* 57:555–562, 1986.

Saxton CA, Van der Ouderaa F: The effect of a dentifrice containing zinc citrate and triclosan on developing gingivitis, *J Periodontal Res* 24:75–80, 1989.

Saxton CA, Lane RM, van der Ouderaa F: The effects of a toothpaste containing a zinc salt and a non-cationic antimicrobial agent on plaque and gingivitis, *J Clin Periodontol* 14:144–148, 1987.

Schaeken MJM, van der Hoeven JS, Saxton CA, et al: The effect of mouthrinses containing zinc and triclosan on plaque accumulation and development of gingivitis in a 3-week clinical test, *J Clin Periodontol* 21:360–364, 1994.

Schaeken MJM, van der Hoeven JS, Saxton CA, et al: The effect of mouthrinses containing zinc and triclosan on plaque accumulation, development of gingivitis and formation of calculus in a 28 week clinical test, *J Clin Periodontol* 23:465–470, 1996.

Schonfeld SE, Farnoush A, Wilson SG: In vivo antiplaque activity of a sanguinarine-containing dentifrice in comparison with conventional toothpastes, *J Periodontal Res* 21:298–303, 1986.

Sheen S, Harrison A: Assessment of plaque prevention on dentures using an experimental cleaner, *J Prosthet Dent* 84:594–601, 2000.

Sheen S, Banfield N, Addy M: The propensity of individual saliva to cause extrinsic staining in vitro – a developmental method, *J Dent* 29:99–102, 2001a.

Sheen S, Owers R, Addy M: The effect of toothpaste on the propensity of chlorhexidine and cetyl Pyridium chloride to produce staining in vitro: a possible predictor study, *J Clin Periodontol* 28:46–51, 2001b.

Sigrist BE, Gusberti FA, Brecz MC, et al: Efficacy of supervised rinsing with chlorhexidine gluconate in comparison to phenolic and plant alkaloid compounds, *J Periodontal Res* 21(Suppl):60–73, 1986.

Simonsson T, Bondesson H, Rundegren J, et al: Effect of delmopinol on in vitro dental plaque formation, bacterial acid production and the number of microorganisms in human saliva, *Oral Microbiol Immunol* 6:305–309, 1991a.

Simonsson T, Arnebrant T, Peterson L: The delmopinol on the salivary pellicles, the wettable tooth surfaces in vivo and bacterial cell surfaces in vitro, *Biofouling* 3:251–260, 1991b.

Skaare AB, Herlofson BB, Barkvoll P: Mouthrinses containing triclosan reduce the incidence of recurrent aphthous ulcers (RAU), *J Periodontol* 23:778–781, 1996.

Skaare AB, Kjaerheim V, Barkvoll P, et al: Does the nature of the solvent affect the anti-inflammatory capacity of triclosan, *J Clin Periodontol* 24:124–128, 1997.

Smith AJ, Moran J, Dangler LV, et al: The efficacy of an antigingivitis chewing gum, *J Clin Periodontol* 23:19–23, 1996.

Soskolne A, Golomb G, Friedman M, et al: New sustained release dosage form of chlorhexidine for dental use. II. Use in periodontal therapy, *J Periodontal Res* 18:330–336, 1983.

Soskolne A, Heasman PA, Smart G, et al: European multi-centre study: sustained local delivery of chlorhexidine as an adjunct to scaling and root planing in the treatment of periodontal diseases, *J Periodontol* 68:32–38, 1997.

Soskolne A, Proskin HM, Stabholz A: Probing depth changes following 2-years of periodontal maintenance therapy including adjunctive controlled release of chlorhexidine, *J Periodontol* 74:420–427, 2003.

Southard GL, Parsons LG, Thomas LG, et al: The relationship of sanguinaria extract concentration and zinc ion to plaque and gingivitis, *J Clin Periodontol* 14:315–319, 1987.

Stabholz A, Sela MN, Friedman M, et al: Clinical and microbiological effects of sustained release chlorhexidine in periodontal pockets, *J Clin Periodontol* 13:783–788, 1986.

Steinberg D, Beeman D, Bowen WH: The effect of delmopinol on glucosyl transferase absorbed to saliva-coated hydroxyapatite, *Arch Oral Biol* 37:33–38, 1992.

Stephen KW, Saxton CA, Jones CL, et al: Control of gingivitis and calculus by a dentifrice containing a zinc salt and triclosan, *J Periodontol* 61:674–679, 1990.

Svatun B, Saxton CA, van der Ouderaa F, et al: The influence of a dentifrice containing a zinc salt and a non-cationic antimicrobial agent on the maintenance of gingival health, *J Clin Periodontol* 14:457–461, 1987.

Svatun B, Saxton CA, Rölla G, et al: One year study of the efficacy of a dentifrice containing a zinc citrate and triclosan to maintain gingival health, *Scand J Dent Res* 97:242–246, 1989.

Svatun B, Saxton CA, Rölla G: Six month study of the effect of a dentifrice containing a zinc citrate and triclosan on plaque, gingival health and calculus, *Scand J Dent Res* 98:301–304, 1990.

Tellefsen G, Larsen G, Kaligithi K, et al: Use of chlorhexidine chewing gum significantly reduces dental plaque formation compared to similar xylitol and sorbitol products, *J Periodontol* 67:181–183, 1996.

Vandekerchhove BNA, Van Steenberge D, Tricio J, et al: Efficacy on supragingival plaque control of cetylpyridinium chloride in a slow-release dosage form, *J Clin Periodontol* 22:824–829, 1995.

Waaler SM, Rölla G: Plaque inhibition effect of combinations of chlorhexidine with metal ions zinc and tin, *Acta Odontol Scand* 38:213–217, 1980.

Waaler SM, Rölla G, Skjörland KK, et al: Effects of oral rinsing with triclosan and sodium lauryl sulfate on dental plaque formation: a pilot study, *Scand J Dent Res* 101:192–195, 1994.

Walker CB, Borden LC, Zambon JJ, et al: The effects of a 0.3% triclosan-containing dentifrice on the microbial composition of supragingival plaque, *J Clin Periodontol* 21:334–341, 1994.

Wennström J, Lindhe J: The effect of hydrogen peroxide on developing plaque and gingivitis in man, *J Clin Periodontol* 6:115–130, 1979.

Wennström J, Lindhe J: The effect of mouthrinses on parameters characterising human periodontal disease, *J Clin Periodontol* 13:86–93, 1986.

Wilson M, Gibson M, Strahan JD, et al: A preliminary evaluation of the use of a redox agent in the treatment of periodontal disease, *J Periodontal Res* 27:522–527, 1992.

Winrow M: Metabolic studies with radiolabelled chlorhexidine in animals and man, *J Periodontal Res* 12(Suppl):45–48, 1973.

Worthington HV, Davies RM, Blinkhorn AS, et al: A six-month clinical study of the effect of a pre-brush rinse on plaque removal and gingivitis, *Br Dent J* 75:322–326, 1993.

Yates R, Moran J, Addy M, et al: The comparative effect of acidified sodium chlorite and chlorhexidine mouthrinse on plaque regrowth and salivary bacterial counts, *J Clin Periodontol* 24:603–609, 1997.

Zee K-Y, Rundegen J, Attström R: Effect of delmopinol hydrochloride mouthrinse on plaque formation and gingivitis in 'rapid' and 'slow' plaque formers, *J Clin Periodontol* 24:486–491, 1997.

Zanatta FB, Antoniazzi RP, Rösing CA: The effect of 0.12% chlorhexidine gluconate rinsing on previously plaque-free and plaque-covered surfaces: a randomized, controlled clinical trial, *J Periodontol* 78:2127–2134, 2007.

ANTIBIOTICS AND PERIODONTAL TREATMENT

Until recently, there has been a justifiable reserve in the dental profession regarding the use of antibiotics to treat periodontal disease. However, in the past few years, interest in the use of antibiotics for this purpose has increased and many clinical trials of their use have been published.

Several criteria must be met before the use of antibiotics can be justified. These are:

- That the nature of the bacterial flora associated with periodontal disease must be amenable to control by antibiotics
- Antibiotics must be shown either to be superior in controlling the disease than traditional clinical treatment or to act as useful adjunctives to it
- Antibiotics used must be free from adverse side effects and from the induction of hypersensitivity or bacterial resistance
- They must achieve effective concentrations in the periodontal pocket where the causative bacteria reside.

The antibiotics most commonly used in the treatment of periodontal patients are:

- Penicillins
- Tetracyclines
- Metronidazole
- Erythromycin
- Clindamycin
- Vancomycin
- Gentamicin.

CLASSIFICATION OF ANTIBIOTICS

Antibiotics are classified according to their structures (Mandel & Petri 1996a,b; Chambers & Sande 1996a,b; Sande et al 1996; Tracey & Webster 1996) into:

- Beta-lactams – Those which contain a β-lactam ring nucleus and these include the penicillins, cephalosporins and cephalomycins
- Aminoglycosides – These are either derived from various species of the *Streptomyces* fungi and end in mycin, e.g. streptomycin and tobramycin or from *Micromonospora purpura*, which is not a fungus and hence end in 'micin', e.g. gentamicin and semi-synthetic drugs such as amikacin
- Sulphonamides – The names of this group contain 'sulpha' or 'sulfa'
- Tetracyclines – These all have a four-ringed structure and their names end in 'cycline'
- Azoles – These all contain an azole ring and their names end in 'azole', e.g. metronidazole
- Quinolones – These are all structurally related to nalidixic acid and most end in 'oxacin', e.g. ciprofloxacin
- Macrolides, e.g. erythromycin
- Others – structurally unrelated to any of these groups. They include chloramphenicol, clindamycin (a lincinoid) and vancomycin.

NATURAL PRODUCTION OF ANTIBIOTIC BY BACTERIA OR FUNGI

Antibiotics are medically useful not only due to their effects on bacteria but also because they do not have similar effects on human cells which are sufficiently different from bacterial cells to escape destruction (Chamber & Sande 1996; Laurence et al 1997).

People tend to think of antibiotics as a human invention but this is far from the truth. Ever since the British biologist, Alexander Fleming discovered in 1928 the antimicrobial activity of a substance released from the *Penicillium* fungus, the substance which was aptly called penicillin, people have realized that bacteria and fungi can manufacture powerful antibiotics. Thus, antibiotics are manufactured by the very classes of organisms they aim to destroy.

Scientists are still not clear why these organisms manufacture antibiotics. One theory is that they are designed to inhibit other competing species of the bacteria trying to inhabit a new environment but this seems inconsistent with certain features of antibiotics. In this regard, one would expect an organism in search of a new environment to lack the resources to make complex antibiotics and therefore for them to be simple compounds (Amábile-Cuevas et al 1995). This is not the case and antibiotics are complex molecules which require a good deal of energy for their manufacture. Furthermore, they are produced by organisms in a stationary stage of their life cycle, which seems incompatible with competition in a new environment.

On the other hand, other workers (Davies 1990) have proposed that antibiotics are vestiges of ancient metabolic systems, dating back to some of the very first organisms on Earth. Many antibiotics bind to cellular structures and could have facilitated the synthesis of biological molecules such as peptides or stimulated other metabolic pathways. As biochemistry evolved, it is likely that these ancient binding molecules were replaced by enzymes, which proved much more efficient. However, the ancient binding molecules may have persisted in bacteria and fungi and now function as antibiotics.

THE STRUCTURE AND ORIGINS OF ANTIBIOTICS

A variety of techniques have been used to determine the chemical structure of naturally produced antibiotics and the detailed structure of most of these is now known.

Penicillin – (Laurence et al 1997; Mandel & Petri 1996b) originates from the *Penicillium* fungus but since the structure of its nucleus was determined many new penicillins have been synthesized. This has vastly increased the antibacterial range of these antibiotics and increased their adsorptions from a variety of routes. This has been achieved by adding appropriate side chains to the β-lactam nucleus (**Fig. 17.1**). Cephalosporins also contain the β-lactam nucleus and individual cephalosporins are based on changes in two side chains (**Fig. 17.2**).

Tetracycline – (Laurence et al 1997; Chambers & Sande 1996b) is produced by species of *Streptomyces*. It has a four-ringed parent structure (**Fig. 17.3**) and a family of tetracyclines have been produced by altering side chains.

Metronidazole – (Laurence et al 1997; Tracey & Webster 1996) is a benzimidazole (**Fig. 17.4**) which was synthesized for use as an anthelminthic agent. Its action against anaerobic bacteria was discovered as a result of its administration to a patient with a trichomonal vaginitis who was also suffering from oral acute necrotizing ulcerative gingivitis (ANUG) (Shinn 1962; Shinn et al 1965). It was found to bring about a swift resolution of the ANUG. It has been shown to be active against most strictly anaerobic bacteria.

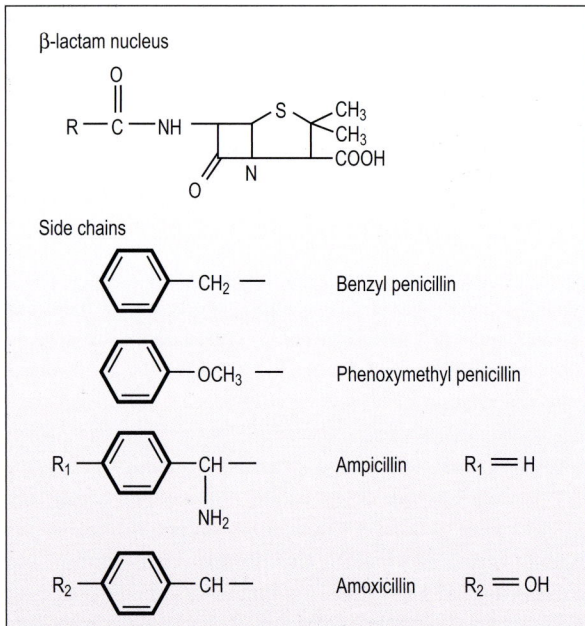

Fig. 17.1 The chemical structure of the β-lactam nucleus and the side chains of penicillins in common use.

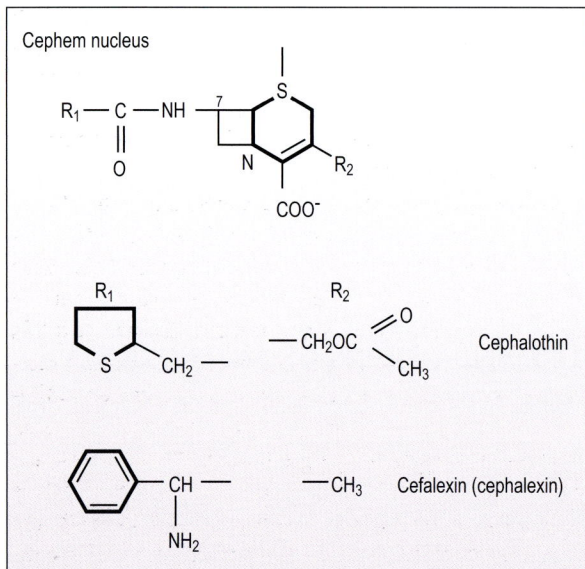

Fig. 17.2 The chemical structure of the cephalosporins: the Cephem nucleus and two common side chains.

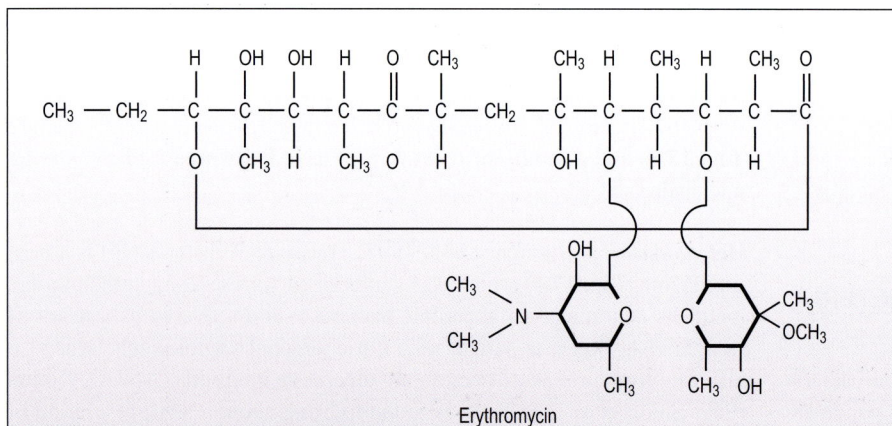

Fig. 17.3 The chemical structure of the tetracyclines.

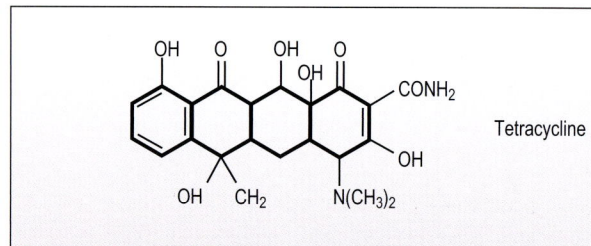

Fig. 17.4 The chemical structure of metronidazole.

Erythromycin – (Laurence et al 1997; Sande et al 1996) is a macrolide antibiotic with a complex structure (**Fig. 17.5**) produced by species of *Streptomyces*.

Clindamycin – (Laurence et al 1997; Sande et al 1996) is produced by the soil bacterium, *Bacillus fragilis*. Its structure is shown in **Figure 17.6**.

Gentamicin – (Laurence et al 1997; Sande et al 1996) is an aminoglycoside antibiotic (**Fig. 17.7**) produced by *M. purpura*.

Vancomycin – (Laurence et al 1997; Sande et al 1996) is a complex tricyclic glycopeptide (**Fig. 17.8**) and its structure has only recently been chemically determined. It is produced by a species of *Streptomyces*.

MODE OF ACTION OF ANTIBIOTICS

The precise chemical mode of action varies from one antibiotic to another. Antibiotics are either bactericidal, i.e. they kill sensitive bacteria, or bacteriostatic, i.e. they inhibit multiplication of sensitive bacteria and permit the normal host defences to destroy the microorganisms (Amábile-Cuevas et al 1995; Neu 1991). Bactericidal antibiotics are usually the first choice in treating infections but in general, provided that an adequate concentration of the antibiotic is achieved at the site of infection and the host defences are normal, there is little difference in the

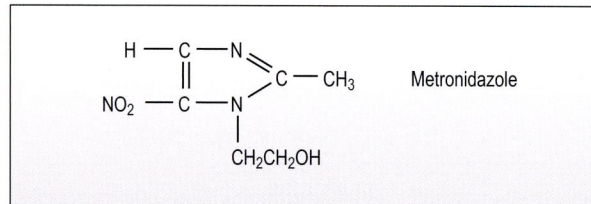

Fig. 17.5 The chemical structure of erythromycin.

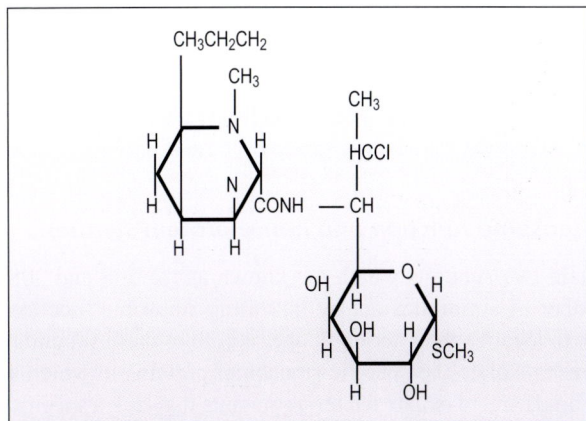

Fig. 17.6 The chemical structure of clindamycin.

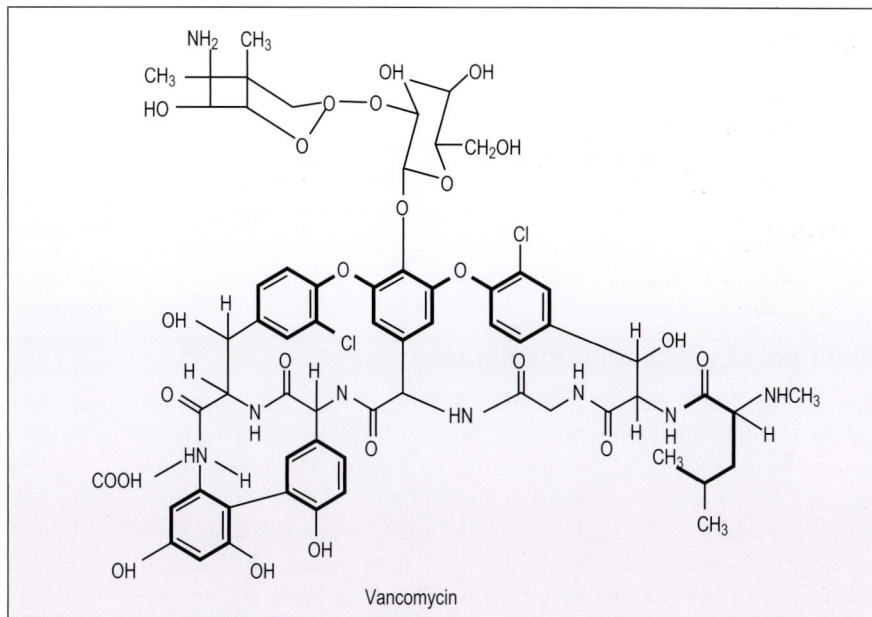

Fig. 17.8 The chemical structure of vancomycin.

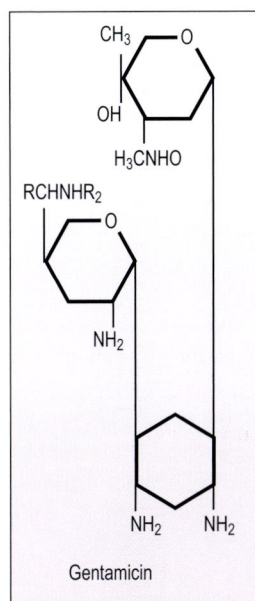

Gentamicin

Fig. 17.7 The chemical structure of gentamicin.

for antibiotics attacking the cell wall is the peptidoglycan layer. This layer is essential for the survival of the bacteria in hypotonic environments and loss of this layer destroys the rigidity of the cell wall and results in death.

Peptidoglycan synthesis occurs in three stages. The first stage takes place in the cytoplasm and involves the synthesis of low molecular weight precursors and fosfomycins and cycloserine inhibit enzymes involved in this process.

The second stage is catalysed by membrane bound enzymes and bacitracin interacts with a critical step in this process.

The third stage involves polymerization of the subunits and the attachment of the nascent peptidoglycan to the cell wall. β-lactam antibiotics inhibit the final enzymes in this process and these enzymes have been termed the penicillin binding proteins. These enzymes are different in Gram-positive and Gram-negative species and these differences explain differences in the antibacterial spectra of different β-lactam antibiotics. The penicillin binding protein to which a particular β-lactam antibiotic binds affects the morphogenic response of the bacterium to the agent. Binding to one protein-binding protein results in rapid lysis because the cell wall bulges and the bacterium bursts. Binding to another which is involved in forming the septum between dividing cells results in the failure of this function so that the bacteria continue to grow into long filaments, which eventually die. Mecillinam (an amidino penicillin) does not bind to the penicillin-binding proteins of Gram-positive bacteria and thus does

effectiveness of both types. Penicillin and metronidazole are examples of bactericidal antibiotics and tetracycline and erythromycin examples of bacteriostatic ones. However, some antibiotics such as erythromycin may be bacteriostatic at lower concentrations and bactericidal at higher ones.

The antibiotics used in treatment of infections act by one of the following mechanisms (Amábile-Cuevas et al 1995; Neu 1991):

- Inhibition of cell wall synthesis
- Inhibition of cytoplasmic membrane function
- Inhibition of nucleic acid synthesis
- Inhibition of ribosomal function and hence protein synthesis
- Inhibition of folate metabolism.

These are illustrated in **Figure 17.9**.

Inhibitors of cell wall synthesis

Gram-positive bacterial cell walls contain peptidoglycan and teichoic or teichuronic acid and the bacterium may be surrounded by a protein or polysaccharide envelope. Gram-negative bacterial cell walls contain peptidoglycan, lipopolysaccharide, lipoprotein, phospholipid and protein. The critical site

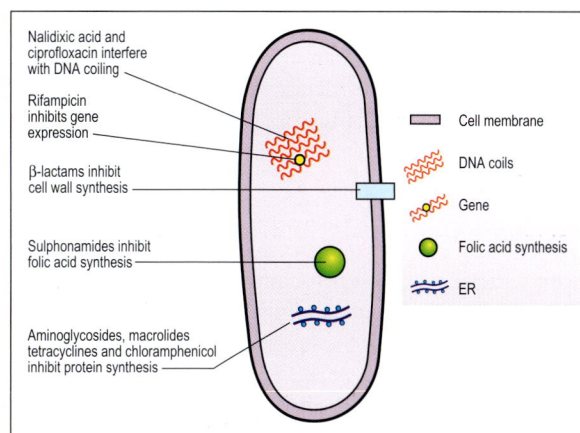

Fig. 17.9 The various mechanisms of action of different classes of antibiotics.

not affect these bacteria. Similarly, aztreonam (a monobactam) only binds to Gram-negative penicillin-binding proteins and does not inhibit Gram-positive or anaerobic species.

Vancomycin interferes with cell wall synthesis by combining with substrates essential for cell wall formation. Because it is a high-molecular weight polypeptide it cannot cross the cytoplasmic membrane or pass through the complex outer cell wall of Gram-negative bacteria. It binds to the terminus of the growing peptidoglycan molecule and prevents the interaction of muramidases with the glycan chain.

Inhibitors of cytoplasmic membrane function

Cytoplasmic membranes are composed of protein, lipid and lipoprotein and act as a diffusion barrier for water, nutrients and ions and a transport system. The membranes are composed of a lipid matrix with globular proteins distributed to penetrate through the lipid bilayer. Agents that cause disorganization of these membranes can be divided into cationic, anionic and neutral agents. Polymyxins B and E are octapeptides which inhibit Gram-negative bacteria that have negatively charged lipids at their surface. They probably displace Mg^{2+} and Ca^{2+} from the negatively charged phosphate groups on the membrane lipids since the activity of the polymyxins is antagonized by Mg^{2+} and Ca^{2+}. They thus disrupt membrane permeability so the contents leak out and the cell dies. The polymyxins cannot be used systemically since they bind to various body tissue ligands and are thus potent toxins for the kidney and nervous system in particular. Gramicidins also affect membrane function by producing aqueous pores in the membranes. They can also only be used topically.

Inhibition of nucleic acid synthesis

Antimicrobial agents can interfere with nucleic acid synthesis at several different levels including:

- Inhibiting nucleic acid synthesis
- Inhibiting nucleic acid conversion
- Preventing DNA functioning as a proper template
- Interfering with polymerases involved in the replication and transcription of DNA.

Interference with nucleotide synthesis

The antiviral and antifungal agents using this mechanism are described in Chapter 24.

Inhibition of DNA-directed DNA polymerase

Rifamycins inhibit DNA-directed DNA polymerase. Polypeptide chains in RNA polymerase attach to a factor that confirms specificity for the recognition of promoter sites that initiate the transcription of DNA. Rifampicin binds strongly to a subunit of RNA polymerase and interferes specifically with the initiation process. It has no effect once the polymerization has begun.

Inhibition of DNA replication

DNA gyrase unwinds the negative supercoiling in the closed-circular duplex DNA of bacteria and is essential for the replication of circular chromosomes. It is also involved with the breakage and reunion of DNA strands. It consists of two components, A and B, with the A subunit more abundant. Quinolones such as nalidixic acid bind to the A component of Gram-negative bacteria and inhibit its action. The newer fluorinated quinolones, ciprofloxacin and norfloxacin also bind to the DNA gyrase of both Gram-positive and negative bacteria.

Nitroimidazoles, such as metronidazole inhibit anaerobic bacteria and protozoa. The nitro group of the nitrosohydroxyl amino moiety is reduced by an electron transfer protein in anaerobic bacteria. The reduced drug causes strand breaks in the DNA. Mammalian cells are unharmed because they lack the enzymes to reduce the nitro group of these agents.

Inhibition of ribosome function and hence protein synthesis

Ribosomes contain two subunits which are known as the 50S and 30S subunits. A number of antibiotics act by inhibiting ribosome function and it is possible to localize their action to one or both of these subunits. It is also possible to isolate the specific ribosomal proteins to which a particular agent binds and to isolate bacterial mutants that lack a specific ribosomal protein and therefore show resistance to that antibiotic.

Aminoglycosides are composed of complex sugars connected in glycosidic linkages. Different members of this group differ both in the molecular nucleus, which can be streptidine or 2-deoxystreptidine and in the aminohexoses linked to the nucleus. The activity of these agents is dependent on the free NH_4 and OH groups by which they bind to specific ribosomal proteins. Streptomycin, which contains the streptidine nucleus, binds to a specific S12 protein in the 30S subunit and causes the ribosome to misread the genetic code. The other aminoglycosides, gentamicin, tobramycin and amikacin, are all 2-deoxystreptidine derivatives and bind not only the specific S12 protein in the 30S subunit but also the L6 protein of the 50S subunit. This latter binding is important in terms of the resistance of bacteria to the aminoglycosides. It is probable that the aminoglycosides can also combine with other binding sites on the 30S subunit and thus kill bacteria by inducing the formation of aberrant, non-functioning complexes as well as by causing misreading. Spectinomycin is an aminocyclitol antibiotic, used in the treatment of penicillin-resistant gonorrhoea and is closely related to the aminoglycosides. It binds to a different protein on the 30S subunit and is bacteriostatic rather than bactericidal.

The other agents which bind to proteins of the 30S subunit are the tetracyclines. They appear to inhibit the binding of aminoacyl-tRNA into its site on the bacterial ribosome. The binding is short lived rather than permanent so that these agents are bacteriostatic. However, they inhibit a wide range of bacteria, *Chlamydiae* and mycoplasmas.

There are three important groups of antibiotics that inhibit the 50S ribosomal subunit: chloramphenicol, the macrolides and the lincinoids. Chloramphenicol inhibits peptide bond formation by binding to a peptidyltransferase enzyme on the 50S subunit and is a bacteriostatic agent that inhibits both Gram-negative and positive bacteria. Macrolides are large lactone ring compounds that bind to the 50S subunit and probably impair the peptidyltransferase reaction or translocation or both. The most important macrolide is erythromycin which inhibits Gram-positive bacteria and a few Gram-negative species such as *Haemophilus, Mycoplasma, Chlamydia* and *Legionella*. Lincinoids, such as clindamycin, have similar sites of action. The macrolides and lincinoids are usually bacteriostatic inhibiting only the formation of new peptide chains.

Inhibition of folate metabolism

Both the sulphonamides and trimethoprim interfere with the folate metabolism in the bacterial cell by competitively blocking the biosynthesis of tetrafolate, which acts as a carrier of one carbon fragment. This is necessary for the ultimate synthesis of DNA, RNA and bacterial wall proteins. Unlike mammals, bacteria and protozoan parasites lack the transport system to take up preformed folic acid from their environment. Most of these organisms must synthesize folates, although some are capable of using exogenous thymidine, circumventing the need for folate metabolism.

Sulphonamides competitively block the conversion of pteridine and p-aminobenzoic acid (PABA) to dihydrofolic acid by the enzyme pteridine synthetase. Sulphonamides have a greater affinity than PABA for pteridine synthetase. Trimethoprim has a very high affinity for bacterial dihydrofolate reductase (10 000 to 100 000 times higher than for the mammalian enzyme). When bound to this enzyme it inhibits the synthesis of tetrafolate.

DRAWBACKS TO THE USE OF ANTIBIOTICS IN PERIODONTAL TREATMENT

The over-use and frequent misuse of antibiotics in medicine, dentistry, veterinary practice, farming and food production has severely reduced the clinical effectiveness of commonly used antibiotics in one of five ways.

The possible drawbacks to the use of antibiotics are:

- Gastrointestinal disturbances
- Possible toxic effects
- Alterations in commensal flora
- Hypersensitivity
- The development of bacterial resistance to antimicrobials.

Gastrointestinal disturbances

All antibiotics can potentially cause gastrointestinal (GI) disturbances either by direct irritative effects or by causing alterations in the gut commensal flora (Neu 1991; Green & Harris 1993; Chambers et al 1996; Laurence et al 1997). The broad spectrum agents are more likely than narrow spectrum agents to severely affect the gut flora. By suppressing the growth of susceptible gut organisms they can also cause an overgrowth of naturally resistant organisms and in this way an overgrowth of *Clostridium difficile* can occur. This bacteria produces a toxin that damages the gut mucosa resulting in diarrhoea and even in severe cases pseudomembranous colitis. Mild GI disturbances can occur with all broad spectrum antibiotics, moderate ones with the macrolides, particularly erythromycin and clindamycin when they are prescribed for longer periods. The agents which are better absorbed from the GI tract such as amoxicillin cause less GI disturbance than those more poorly absorbed such as ampicillin. The newer macrolide analogues, azithromycin, clarithromycin and roxithromycin appear to cause less GI disturbance than erythromycin (Standing Medical Advisory Committee, SMAC 1999a).

Toxic effects

Toxic effects vary from agent to agent and from patient to patient (Neu 1991; Green & Harris 1993; Chambers et al 1996; Bull 1997). They may also depend on the dosage used, the plasma level and the duration of the course of treatment. They include renal and liver damage, nerve damage, blood dyscrasias, platelet damage and haemolytic anaemia. They are best considered separately for each antibiotic group and only those used in dentistry will be described.

Penicillins

Generally well-tolerated and adverse effects limited to GI effects described above and hypersensitivity reactions described below.

Cephalosporins

Early members of this group were mildly nephrotoxic but the later ones are not. Hypoprothrombinaemia with resulting haemorrhage reported with one agent only in this group, latamoxef.

Macrolides

Main adverse effects are GI disturbance and possible hypersensitivity described in other sections.

Tetracyclines

These agents deposit in developing bones and teeth. Therefore, these antibiotics should not be prescribed during pregnancy or to children under the age of 12 as this will result in irreversible internal tooth staining.

Nitroimidazoles

Metronidazole can cause gastric disturbance and also resembles the anti-alcohol drug, Antabuse. Patients taking metronidazole should therefore refrain from consuming alcoholic drinks since this would produce marked nausea. Metronidazole can also produce some central nervous disturbance in some patients leading to dizziness, headache and epileptiform seizures and also peripheral neuropathy.

Glycopeptides

Vancomycin can cause renal damage and this relates to the dose, plasma level and duration of the course of treatment.

Alterations in commensal flora

The administration of an antibiotic will result both in an effect against the pathogenic agent and also against all members of the commensal flora of the mouth, nose and intestines which are also susceptible to it (Neu 1991; Green & Harris 1993; Chambers et al 1996). This may then result in the overgrowth of those members of the commensal flora which are resistant to it. These effects on the commensal flora occur with all antibiotics but are most profound with broad spectrum agents. The effects are also greater the longer the duration of the treatment.

These effects can result in the overgrowth of *Candida* in the mouth, oral pharynx or vagina and overgrowth of certain intestinal commensals such as *Clostridium difficile* resulting in diarrhoea or colitis.

Hypersensitivity

Hypersensitivity to antibiotics can be mediated by a number of different immunological mechanisms including immediate types I, II, III and delayed type IV hypersensitivity (Riott 1997). The immune system can recognize components or degradation products of antibiotics which act as haptens. These reactions occur more frequently in subjects genetically predisposed to hypersensitivity such as those who suffer from hay fever, eczema and asthma and both the numbers of these subjects and the number of patients hypersensitive to antibiotics is increasing.

The descriptions and reports of hypersensitivity to antibiotics are rarely if ever grouped into these types but are rather based on the signs and symptoms produced by them. Those reported in the literature can be divided into:

1. Angioneurotic oedema, urticaria and anaphylactic shock
2. Red-man syndrome
3. Maculopapular rashes (**Fig. 17.10**)
4. Serum sickness-like syndromes
5. Drug fever
6. Erythema multiforme/Steven–Johnson syndrome
7. Adverse skin reactions in patients with lymphoid diseases.

Angioneurotic oedema, urticaria and anaphylactic shock

This is mediated by type I hypersensitivity and can take the form angioneurotic oedema, urticaria or anaphylactic shock with each exposure to the antigen giving a more severe reaction. These reactions are reported (Bull 1997; Sher 1983) to occur in <0.05% of penicillin treated patients, although penicillin reactions accounts for most drug-related anaphylactic

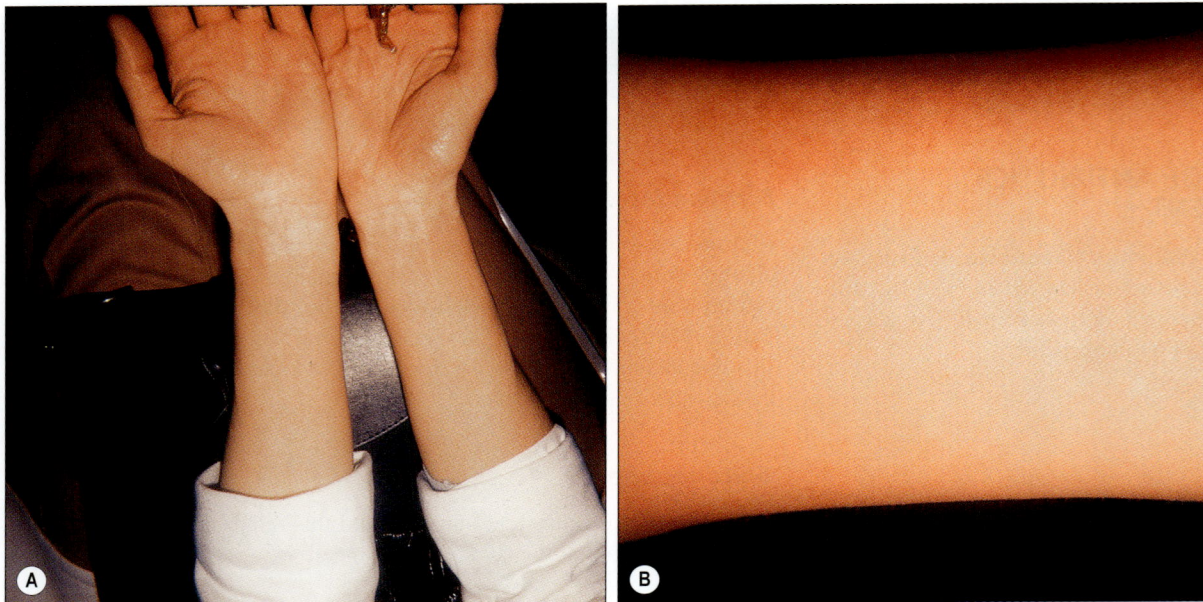

Fig. 17.10 (A) Macular rash on forearm due to erythromycin hypersensitivity; (B) the same close up.

episodes. Full anaphylactic shock only occurs in <2 per 100 000 treatments. The reactions occur in most cases to penicillin degradation products including penicilloyl derivatives. A history of penicillin hypersensitivity precludes the further use of any penicillin derivative. However, the public perception of penicillin hypersensitivity appears to be greater than its absolute incidence. In a recent investigation (Surtees et al 1991) of 132 patients with alleged penicillin hypersensitivity only four patients had a positive radioallergosorbent test (RAST) and the 128 patients who were negative were re-challenged with oral penicillin without ill effects.

These reactions may also occur with other antibiotics including cephalosporins (Bull 1997; Meyer 1985) and quinolones (Bull 1997; Paton & Reeves 1991).

Red-man syndrome

This appears to be mediated by type I mechanisms. The red-man syndrome (Bull 1997; Wallace et al 1991) gets its name from the redness of the skin seen in this condition and is caused by hypersensitivity to vancomycin. The reaction produces flushing, itching, dyspnoea, chest pain and hypotension and can progress to full anaphylactic shock.

Maculopapular rashes

These reactions can be caused by hypersensitivity to β-lactams and sulphonamides and less frequently by other antimicrobials (Bull 1997; Collaborative Study Group 1973). They are particularly common reactions to ampicillin with an incidence of 7% but occur less frequently with other penicillins. It appears to be mainly mediated by type III mechanisms involving IgG and IgM antibodies. The serum levels of IgM antibodies are raised in this condition (Bull 1997; Levine 1996). It also occurs in 1–2% of patients given parenteral cephalosporins (Bull 1997; Meyer 1985). In addition 10% of patients who have previously developed a penicillin rash will also produce one if exposed to cephalosporins (Bull 1997; Dash 1975). Rashes also occur in about 3% of patients given co-trimoxazole (Bull 1997; Jick 1982) and these reactions can range from maculopapular rashes to Steven Johnson syndrome (see below). Rashes are rare with macrolides but can occur as a reaction to clindamycin (Bull 1997; Geddes et al 1970).

Serum sickness-like syndromes

This occurs as a result of type III mechanisms where there is an excess of antigen and this results in the formation of antigen-antibody complexes. The increased vascular permeability allows these complexes to be deposited in different parts of the vascular bed, particularly in the glomeruli of the kidneys. The condition is characterized by fever, swollen lymph nodes, a generalized urticarial rash and painful swollen joints. It is also associated with low serum complement and transient albuminuria (Riott 1997). These reactions can occur to β-lactams, particularly cefaclor and to sulphonamides and rarely fluoroquinolones (Bull 1997; Platt et al 1988). There were 638 reports of this reaction to cefaclor, 51 to co-trimoxazole, 28 to cefalexin (cephalexin) and 10 to amoxicillin in a study published in 1988 (Platt et al 1988).

Drug fever

This produces raised body temperature, malaise and mental confusion. It may be produced in a similar way to the serum sickness-like syndrome described above but this is far from clear. It occurs as a reaction to long acting sulphonamides but can also occur with β-lactams and other agents particularly after prolonged therapy (Bull 1997). There appears to be a particularly high incidence of this condition in high dosage treatment with ureidopenicillins when 32% of patients treated in this way in a recent study (Lang et al 1991) were affected.

Erythema multiforme/Steven–Johnson syndrome

In the 1960s, 30% of the cases of severe erythema multiforme were caused by long acting sulphonamides (Bull 1997; Rallison et al 1961) and this condition had a mortality of 25%. Similar reactions have been produced, albeit at a lower incidence with co-trimoxazole and these have resulted in 14 deaths (Bull 1997; Ball 1986). These reactions have also been occasionally seen with penicillins, cephalosporins and other antimicrobial agents (Bull 1997). The immunological basis of this reaction is undoubtedly delayed type IV hypersensitivity.

Adverse skin reactions in patients with lymphoid diseases

An increased number of skin reactions identical to those seen in hypersensitivity to antibiotics have been reported in patients with lymphoid disorders taking these antibiotics. They have been observed in patients with

Epstein–Barr virus infection (glandular fever), cytomegalovirus infections and chronic lymphatic leukaemia taking ampicillin (Bull 1997; Pullen et al 1967). A similar reaction has been reported in response to amoxicillin in patients with HIV infection and AIDS (Bull 1997; Battegay et al 1989). The commonest reaction of this type, however, seems to be to co-trimoxazole given to AIDS patients to treat *Pneumocystis carinii* pneumonia and the reaction seems to be effected by the use of corticosteroids (Bull 1997; Caumes et al 1994). Thus, it would seem that a variety of lymphoid disorders increase the rate of hypersensitivity reactions to some penicillins and sulphonamides.

The development of bacterial resistance to antimicrobials

The over-use and frequent misuse of antibiotics in medicine, dentistry, veterinary practice, farming and food production has severely reduced the clinical effectiveness of commonly used antibiotics in one of two ways (Neu 1991; Green & Harris 1993; Chambers et al 1996):

1. The antibiotic either kills or suppresses the bacteria sensitive to it but does not affect those strains which are naturally resistant to it. This favours the growth of these resistant strains which then increase in number. Further exposure to the same antibiotic, particularly a short time after it was last prescribed, progressively increases the number of resistant strains.
2. Bacteria resistant to a particular antibiotic possess gene(s) coding for factor(s) producing this resistance and may pass copies of them to other bacteria in structures known as plasmids and transposons (see below). The recipient bacteria could be of the same or closely related species or in some cases different species. This process of gene transfer in plasmids and transposons may represent a primitive form of sexual reproduction. In this way the genes concerned with antibiotic resistance can be passed from the resistant bacteria to other bacteria in the subject. The resistant bacteria can then spread to many other subjects by common means of transmission either producing antibiotic resistant infections in the recipient subjects or passive carriage of the resistant strains in the commensal flora of their skin, nose or throat.

THE BACTERIAL GENOME

Bacteria, like all other organisms, encode their genetic information in DNA and replication of this DNA is essential to the inheritance of these traits in future generations (Holmes & Joblin 1991). Gene expression involves transcription of the DNA into messenger RNA and translation of the RNA sequence into an amino acid sequence and thus a protein product.

The main bacterial chromosome is a circular structure that functions as a self-replicating genetic element (replicon) (Holmes & Joblin 1991). Extra chromosomal genetic elements such as plasmids and bacteriophages (viruses which infect bacteria) are separate, circular non-essential replicons which often contain genes coding for virulence factors and bacterial resistance.

MUTATIONS

Mutations are heritable changes in the genome due either to irreparable damage to the gene or mistakes in the replication process (Holmes & Joblin 1991). The mutation rate in bacteria is determined by the accuracy of DNA replication, the occurrence of damage (e.g. UV light, ionizing radiation, mutagenic chemicals, viruses) and the effectiveness of DNA repair mechanisms. Therefore, mutations can occur spontaneously but are rare in individual bacteria. However, mutations are inheritable and may spread to other unaffected bacteria by several mechanisms.

Mutations can be classified on the basis of the changes in the DNA (Holmes & Joblin 1991). Some are limited to short sections of DNA, e.g. nucleotide substitution, micro-deletion, micro-insertion whereas others involve larger regions of DNA and include deletions or insertions or re-arrangements of sections. If the mutation produces no functional or structural change they are known as silent mutations, if they result in the substitution of one amino acid they are known as missense mutations and if they result in failure to produce a protein product they are known as nonsense mutations.

EXCHANGE OF GENETIC MATERIAL BY BACTERIA

Normal bacterial reproduction is asexual and involves replication of DNA and binary fission. However, genetic material can also be passed to another bacteria by sexual processes (Holmes & Joblin 1991). This is important for the long-term success of the species because it increases the chances for rare, independent mutations to spread to other bacteria and be subject to the processes of natural selection. Sexual exchange of DNA between bacteria enables the genome to evolve much more rapidly than by mutation alone.

The sexual processes in bacteria involve the transfer of genetic information from a donor to recipient and result in either the substitution of donor alleles for recipient alleles or addition of donor alleles to the recipient (Holmes & Joblin 1991). The sexual processes involved are:

- Transformation
- Transduction
- Conjunction
- Transposition.

Transformation

When a bacteria lyses it releases fragments of its DNA into the external environment. It has been shown that segments of this released DNA can be taken up by recipient bacteria (Holmes & Joblin 1991). If the donor and recipient bacteria are closely enough related then recombination occurs between the transforming segment of donor DNA and the recipient bacterial chromosome. To be active in transformation the DNA molecules must consist of at least 500 nucleotides. This process was first discovered in *Streptococcus pneumoniae* and was later shown to occur in *Haemophilus, Neisseria, Bacillus* and *Staphylococcal* species (Standing Medical Advisory Committee, SMAC 1999b).

Transduction

Bacteriophage viruses can function as vectors to introduce DNA from donor bacteria. In some bacteriophages, known as generalized transducing phages, a small section of the viral DNA produced during lytic growth is aberrant and comes to contain random fragments of the bacterial genome instead of phage DNA (Holmes & Joblin 1991; Berg & Howe 1989; Calender 1988; Miller et al 1989). When such a phage infects other bacteria it will carry these donor genes into the recipient genome along with the viral genes. In this situation either abortive transduction or complete transduction may occur. In abortive transduction the donor genes fail to undergo homologous recombination with the recipient genome whereas in complete transduction the donor genes are recombinated into the recipient genome. Complete transduction results in a stable recombinant genome that can express the donor genes and pass them on to future generations.

Conjunction

In conjunction (Holmes & Joblin 1991; Berg & Howe 1989; Calender 1988; Miller et al 1989; Amábile-Cuevas et al 1995; Di Vita & Mekalanos 1989; Kohara et al 1987; Neidhardt et al 1987) there is direct contact between donor and recipient bacteria and this leads to the formation of a cytoplasmic bridge between them which allows the transfer of part or all of the genome from donor to recipient (**Fig. 17.11**).

This process has been closely studied in *Escherichia coli* (Holmes & Joblin 1991; Kohara et al 1987; Neidhardt et al 1987) and the process appears to be broadly similar in other Gram-negative bacteria. Donor ability is determined by the presence of specific conjunctive plasmids known as fertility (F)

Fig. 17.11 The process of transfer of antibiotic resistance genes between bacteria (conjunction): (A) two plasmids with different resistance genes; (B) transfer of resistance gene from one plasmid to another in the same bacterial cell by transposition or integration; (C) a bacterial cell containing a multiple resistance gene plasmid; (D) transfer of the genes from one multiple resistance gene plasmid to another across a conjunctive bridge; (E) donor and recipient bacterial cell after this process.

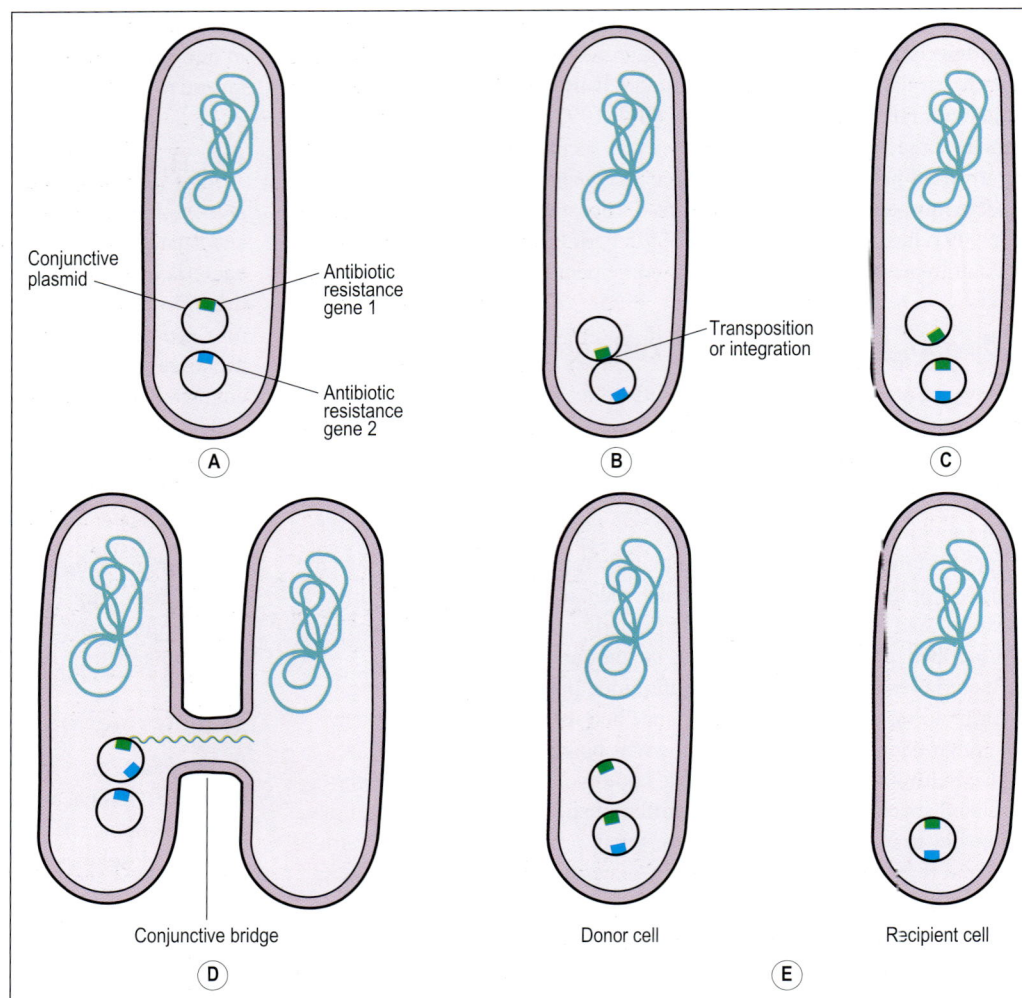

plasmids. Strains of *E. coli* with this plasmid are known as F+ strains and function as donors and strains which lack it are known as F− strains and act as recipients. The conjunctive function genes on the F plasmid are a cluster of genes which code for pili, known as F pili and the synthesis and transfer of DNA during mating and the suppression of the ability of the F+ donor to act as a recipient. Each F+ donor has three F pili that bind to a specific outer membrane protein (the ompA protein) on the recipient F− bacteria and this initiates the mating. A cytoplasmic bridge is then formed and one strand of F plasmid DNA is transferred from donor to recipient, beginning and ending at a unique origin and termination. This strand is then converted in the recipient bacteria into a circular, double stranded DNA F plasmid. The donor bacteria then synthesizes a new strand to replace the one donated. Both bacteria now become F+ donor strains and can therefore spread this plasmid among other genetically similar bacteria. The F plasmid may remain as an extra chromosomal plasmid or become integrated into the main chromosome (homologous recombination).

Whilst Gram-negative bacteria use pili to initiate mating, Gram-positive bacteria do not (Holmes & Joblin 1991). However, instead donor Gram-positive bacteria produce adhesins that cause them to aggregate with recipient bacteria and this process initiates mating.

Some species of both Gram-negative and -positive bacteria possess bacterial resistance genes and these genes are nearly always contained on plasmids (**Fig. 17.11A**). These resistance genes can be transferred from one plasmid to another in the same bacterial cell and in this way, a single plasmid can collect a number of different resistance genes (**Fig. 17.11B, C**). Examples of these bacteria are those which are naturally resistant to an antibiotic and these include those bacteria that actually produce antibiotic molecules. Other bacteria have acquired these genes from other resistant bacteria by the sexual

processes described above and below. The plasmids containing these resistance genes are known as resistance (R) plasmids. It has been shown that the R+ plasmid can function in a similar way to F+ plasmid since they can code for factors in the mating process like the formation of pili or adhesin molecules and the formation of an intracytoplasmic bridge (**Fig. 17.11D, E**). They can also transfer R-plasmid DNA in a similar way to F plasmids. Also once transferred the donor strand can integrate into the genome by a process of homologous recombination. The recombination process involves breaking and joining parental DNA molecules to form hybrid recombinant molecules either in a new plasmid or in the main chromosome.

In a similar way to F-plasmids, R+ donors convert R− recipients to become future R+ donors and hence the transferred genes can become widely spread in the bacterial population (Holmes & Joblin 1991).

Transposition

Transposons are segments of DNA that can move from one site in a DNA molecule to another target site in the same or a different DNA molecule (Holmes & Joblin 1991; Kingsman et al 1998). This transposition process is independent of generalized recombination. Because of these unique properties transposons are extremely important elements in widely dispersing newly acquired genes and they can:

- Cause mutations
- Mediate genomic rearrangements
- Function as portable regions of genetic homology
- Contribute to the dissemination of their contained genes within bacterial populations.

The insertion of a transposon can often interrupt the linear sequence of a gene and inactivate it. Also, transposons are important in causing deletions, duplications and inversions of DNA segments as well as fusions between self replicating elements (replicons). However, transposons themselves are not self replicating elements and must become integrated into other replicons to be stably maintained in the bacterial genome.

Most transposons share a number of common features (Holmes & Joblin 1991; Kingsman et al 1998). Each encodes the functions necessary for transposition including encoding for a transposase enzyme that interacts with specific sequences at the ends of the transposon section. During transposition, a short sequence of DNA is duplicated and the transposon is inserted between the directly repeated target sequences. The length of this short duplication varies with each transposon. The process involves cleavage of DNA at the target site and is followed by synthesis of new complimentary strand corresponding to the region between the cleavage sites.

If excision of the transposon from the donor site is followed by its insertion into a target site the process is known as non-replicative transposition whereas if the transposon is first replicated at the donor site and a copy inserted at the target site it is called replicative transposition (Holmes & Joblin 1991; Kingsman et al 1998). Most bacterial transposons can be divided into three classes:

1. Insertion sequences and composite transposons
2. TnA family
3. Mutator bacteriophages.

Insertion sequences and composite transposons

Insertion sequences only code for the functions needed for transposition. They are short and vary from 750–1500 nucleotide pairs.

Composite transposons vary in length from 2000–40000 nucleotide pairs. They contain insertion sequences at each end and other genes coding for other varied functions between them. These can include genes for the production of adherence antigens, toxins and other virulence factors or genes that code for various forms of bacterial resistance. Examples of these latter genes are the Tn5 and Tn10 genes which determine kanamycin and tetracycline resistance respectively.

TnA family

These transposons all have larger terminal repeats than composite transposons. Their terminal insertion sequences encode for the functional enzymes, transposase and resolvase. These transposons include members (Tn3 and Tn1000) which encode ampicillin resistance and are found on the R plasmid. The TnA family has a place in medical history since it was responsible for the spread of high level resistance to ampicillin to *Haemophilus influenzae* and *Neisseria gonorrhoeae* during the 1970s and severely limited the use of this antibiotic in treating infections by these bacteria. It resulted in the dissemination of ampicillin resistance genes from the Enterobacteriaceae to plasmids in *Haemophilus* and *Neisseria* species.

Mutator phages

These are transposons which are contained in a specialized group of bacteriophages. In these phages the entire phage genome functions as a transposon and replication of the phage occurs by replication transposition. When the phages infect bacteria prophage integration can occur at many different sites with the bacterial chromosome and therefore this process often causes mutations (hence the name mutator phage). These phages have probably been very important in spreading bacterial resistance genes into

plasmids that were initially devoid of them. They also function in spreading numerous different resistance genes into bacteria resulting in the formation of multiple resistance R-plasmids. This is supported by the fact that some multiple-antibiotic-resistance plasmids have individual transposons with several resistance genes while others have multiple resistance gene containing transposons at several sites and still others contain complex hybrid resistance transposons formed by integration of one transposon into another. Thus, step-wise acquisition of resistance genes in this way can lead to the formation of complex transposons that encode multiple resistance determinants.

The extensive therapeutic use of antibiotics by the medical, dental and veterinary professions and their incorporation into animal feed as 'growth promoters' has provided huge selective advantages for bacteria with R-plasmids (Holmes & Joblin 1991). In this situation transformation, transduction, conjugation and transposition provide the means for the wide dissemination of R-plasmids both within and between bacterial species. After an R-plasmid, carrying a transposon is introduced into a new bacterial host, the transposons and its contained resistance genes can jump from the plasmid into the main chromosome. This guarantees the stability of these resistance genes in the new bacterium since it is not necessary for them to undergo homologous recombination to achieve this. This favours the spread of resistance genes between different bacterial species. It also ensures the new genes are associated with transposons, which in turn assures the easy future spread of these genes between species.

MECHANISMS OF RESISTANCE

The mechanisms of bacterial resistance which are either present in naturally resistant bacteria, produced by mutations or acquired from other bacteria by the methods described above are shown below (Neu 1991; Amábile-Cuevas et al 1995; Standing Medical Advisory Committee, SMAC 1999b):

- Increasing destruction of the antimicrobial agent
- Reducing drug uptake
- Increasing drug excretion
- Altering the antimicrobial agent's target so that it is no longer bound by the drug
- Activating an alternative metabolic pathway that by-passes the target.

These are shown in Table 17.1 and illustrated in **Figure 17.12**. Only those agents used in dental treatment or antibiotic prophylaxis will be detailed.

Table 17.1 *The mechanisms of actions of antibiotics*

Antibiotic	Resistance mechanism
β-lactams, Aminoglycosides, Chloramphenicol, Erythromycin, Tetracycline	Chemically modified by enzymes
Erythromycin, Tetracycline	Actively removed from cell
Erythromycin	Enzymatic modification of target
β-lactams, Fusidic acid	Proteins bind to and sequester antibiotics within target cell
Sulphonamides, Trimethoprim	Synthesis of enzymes insensitive to the action of the drug

Fig. 17.12 The mechanisms by which bacteria gain resistance to antibiotics. Bacteria develop a variety of mechanisms to combat the effects of antibiotics. Some bacteria produce enzymes that can dismantle antibiotic molecules and this is responsible for resistance to the β-lactams, aminoglycosides and chloramphenicol. These enzymes may be secreted and thus attack the antibiotic outside the cell before they enter it, or may attack the antibiotic within the cell if they have already passed through the surface membrane. Other bacteria produce cellular pumps, which remove the antibiotics from the cell as soon as they enter it. This mechanism is responsible for resistance to tetracyclines and erythromycin. Another mechanism is the modification of the bacterial metabolic enzyme affected by the antibiotic so that the antibiotic will no longer bind to it. Thus, the bacterial enzyme may continue to function normally. This mechanism may produce resistance to sulphonamides and trimethoprim. In a similar way, other bacteria alter the target molecule affected by the antibiotic so that it can no longer key into its receptor site on the molecule. This mechanism may produce resistance to tetracyclines and erythromycin.

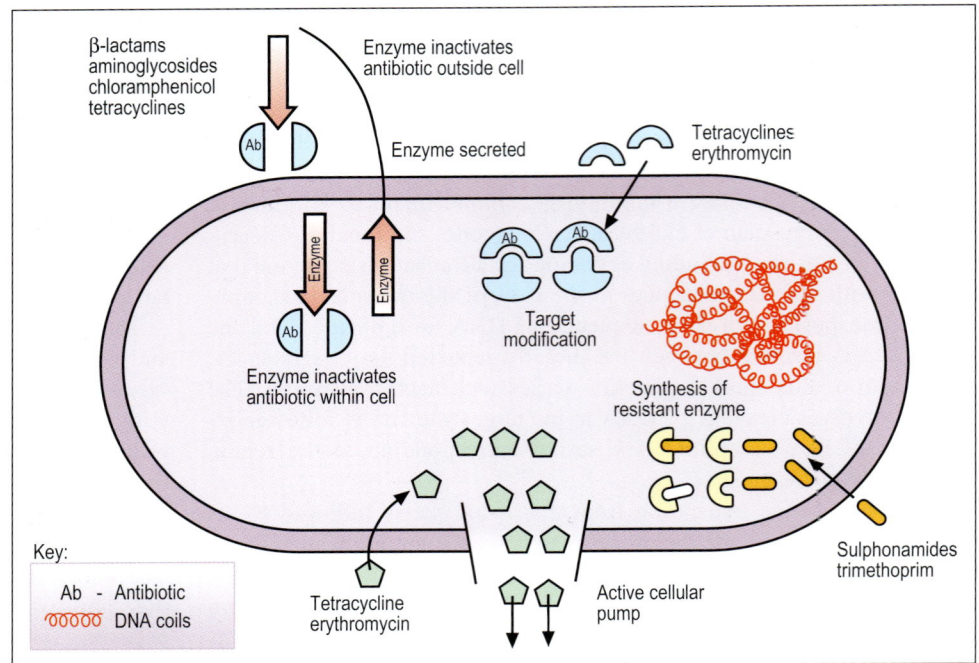

Increasing destruction of the antimicrobial agent

β-Lactamase resistance

This is probably the best known mechanism of resistance and the resistance of *E. coli* to penicillin by this mechanism was first recognized in 1940 (Neu 1991; Standing Medical Advisory Committee, SMAC 1999b). Also in the 1940s the acquired resistance of *staphylococci* to this antibiotic was also shown to be due to a penicillinase. These enzymes can attack all β-lactam antibiotics, i.e. penicillins, cephalosporins, carbapenems and monobactams. They are widely distributed in nature and may be classified according to the compound they destroy, i.e. penicillinases, cephalosporinases, etc. The main action of these enzymes is to alter the β-lactam nucleus. This mechanism can be circumvented by the use of a β-lactamase inhibitor such as clavulanic acid and this is used in the combination of amoxicillin with clavulanic acid in Augmentin® (Farmer & Reading 1982; Todd & Benfield 1990).

In Gram-positive species, β-lactamases are primarily exo-enzymes that are excreted into the milieu around the bacteria whereas in both aerobic and anaerobic Gram-negative bacteria they are contained in the periplasmic space where they effectively protect the penicillin binding proteins. In both groups, they may either be chromosomal or plasmid mediated or constitutive or inducible.

Virtually all hospital isolates of *Staphylococcus aureus* and epidermidis produce β-lactamases as do up to 80% of the community acquired isolates. Resistance of staphylococci to penicillins was initially overcome with the anti-staphylococcal penicillins and cephalosporins. However, this has led to these bacteria both producing more and different β-lactamases so that they can destroy these new penicillins and cephalosporins. They can also develop other mechanisms of resistance. In 1974 *H. influenza* was shown to posses plasmid-mediated β-lactamase and this is now present in over 35% of the strains of this bacteria. The TnA transposon has become more widespread and the resistance of *Haemophilus* and *Neisseria* seems to be increasing year on year. The *Haemophilus* β-lactamase is structurally the same enzyme as that found in *E. coli*, *Salmonella*, *Shigella* species and *N. gonorrhoeae*. It has been called the TEM enzyme after the initials of a Greek girl from whom the *E. coli* strain containing a plasmid β-lactamase was first isolated. The most common plasmid-mediated β-lactamase is TEM-1 and this accounts for up to 80% of plasmid related

β-lactamase resistance worldwide. New plasmid-related β-lactamases that can hydrolyse compounds such as inomethoxy cephalosporin, which is not destroyed by other plasmid-related β-lactamases, have recently appeared and are likely to increase in frequency in the future. These new enzymes have a different amino acid sequence which permits binding to the cephalosporin and its subsequent breakdown.

Chromosomal, constitutively produced β-lactamases are produced by many *Enterobacter*, *Citrobacter*, *Proteus*, *Pseudomonas* and *Klebsiella* species as well as many anaerobic species (Neu 1991; Standing Medical Advisory Committee, SMAC 1999b). β-lactamases produced by these bacteria vary in their ability to degrade the various classes of β-lactam antimicrobials. However, β-lactamase activity is only one component of the β-lactam resistance of Gram-negative bacteria since this derives from a combination of decreased drug entry, β-lactamase stability and the affinity of the compounds for the penicillin-binding proteins.

Handal et al (2004) carried out a study to assess the extent of β-lactamase-producing bacteria in the periodontal pocket. They obtained subgingival plaque samples from 25 patients with refractory marginal periodontitis in the USA. β-Lactamase-positive isolates were characterized using commercial diagnostic kits and partial sequencing of the 16S rRNA gene. The susceptibilities to different antimicrobial agents were tested and, in addition, the isolates were screened for the presence of extended spectrum β-lactamases (ESBLs). β-Lactamase-producing bacteria were detected in 18 (72%) patients. The most prominent β-lactamase-producing organisms belonged to the anaerobic genus *Prevotella*. Other enzyme-producing anaerobic strains were *Fusobacterium nucleatum*, *Propionibacterium acnes* and *Peptostreptococcus* sp. Facultative bacteria, such as *Burkholderia* spp., *Ralstonia pickettii*, *Capnocytophaga* spp., *Bacillus* spp., *Staphylococcus* spp. and *Neisseria* sp., were also detected among the enzyme-producers. Minimum inhibitory concentrations (MICs) of ampicillin and amoxicillin were in the range 1.5–256 µg/mL and 4–256 µg/mL, respectively, for the isolates of the *Prevotella* species. All *Prevotella* isolates were susceptible to amoxicillin/clavulanate and metronidazole, but they showed variable resistance to tetracyclines. Two of the *Prevotella* isolates had high MICs of cefotaxime and ceftazidime. ESBL activity was not detected in any of the β-lactamase-producing isolates by the Etest method. Thus, this study demonstrated a wide variety of β-lactamase-producing bacteria that may play a role in refractory periodontal disease.

Reducing drug uptake

Tetracycline resistance

This form of resistance is due to a decrease in the level of accumulation of the drug probably both as a result of decreased uptake and increased efflux (Neu 1991; Standing Medical Advisory Committee, SMAC 1999b). Resistant bacteria bind less tetracycline and pump out any that does accumulate by an energy-dependent process.

Tetracycline resistance is very common in both Gram-positive and negative bacterial species and in most cases is plasmid-related and inducible. However, in some bacteria types like *Proteus* it is chromosomal.

Plasmid genes for tetracycline resistance have been found in enteric bacteria and the most common of these, TetB, is present in *H. influenzae*. Tetracycline resistance in *Staphylococcus aureus* is due to genes present on small multicopy plasmids and these genes are also present in non-conjunctive plasmids in *Streptococcus faecalis*. However, they are found on the main chromosome of group *B. streptococci*, oral *Streptococci* and *Clostridia* spp., such as *C. difficile*.

Plasmid resistance to tetracyclines can be partially overcome by modifying the tetracycline nucleus and minocycline and doxycycline will inhibit some tetracycline resistant streptococci and some *Staphylococcus aureus* strains. However, this has not overcome the resistance of the members of the Enterobacteriaceae, particularly *Pseudomonas* and *Bacteroides* ssp.

Tetracycline resistance is a major concern because it is located near the insertion sites of the plasmids and these plasmids readily acquire other genetic information to enlarge the spectrum of resistance. The widespread use of tetracyclines in animal feeds is probably a major factor in the extensive, worldwide resistance in members of the Enterobacteriaceae, particularly enteric species like Salmonella, to tetracyclines and many other antimicrobial drugs. Not only can tetracycline resistance move among members of the Enterobacteriaceae on plasmids but plasmids mediating tetracycline resistance have also moved between *S. aureus, S. epidermidis, S. pyogenes, S. pneumoniae* and *S. faecalis*.

Aminoglycoside resistance

In the most important form of this resistance the drug is inactivated outside the bacterial cell and this also results in poor uptake of the drug (Neu 1991). Other forms of resistance, such as altered binding sites on the 30S ribosome, are much less common.

In the Enterobacteriaceae and *Pseudomonas* spp. the aminoglycosides pass through porin channels in the periplasmic space designed to admit cationic molecules. They are then actively translocated across the cell membrane by an energy-dependent proton-motive force and once into the cytoplasm they bind to some ribosomes located just below the membrane, only binding to ribosomes actively engaged in protein synthesis. All aminoglycosides have free amino and hydroxyl groups that are essential to their binding to the ribosomal proteins and bacteria resistant to aminoglycosides contain in their periplasmic space enzymes that phosphorylate or acetylate these essential groups. The modified aminoglycosides do not bind well to the ribosomes.

Aminoglycoside-modifying enzymes have been found in Gram-positive species such as *Staphylococcus aureus, Streptococcus faecalis, S. pyogenes* and *S. pneumoniae* and Gram-negative species such as the Enterobacteriaceae and *P. aeruginosa* (Neu 1991). Many of the genes for these enzymes are carried on transposons.

Anaerobic bacteria such as *Bacteroides* species are resistant to aminoglycosides because they lack an oxygen-dependent transport system to move the drug across the cytoplasmic membrane.

Although most of the resistance of *Staphylococcus aureus* to aminoglycosides is due to modifying enzymes some small colony variants of staphylococci also show resistance probably due to a defect in adenylate cyclase or cyclic adenosine 5′-monophosphate (cAMP)-binding proteins.

This prevents the transport of aminoglycosides into the cytoplasm. Also some members of the Enterobacteriaceae and *P. aeruginosa* may be resistant to aminoglycosides due to alteration of porin channels. These bacteria do not take up any of the drug but unlike other resistant bacteria they lack aminoglycoside-inactivating enzymes.

Increasing drug excretion

Some resistant bacteria allow antibiotics like tetracycline or the macrolides to enter the bacteria cell but have developed molecular pumps which pump the drug out again by an energy-dependent process (Amábile-Cuevas et al 1995; Standing Medical Advisory Committee, SMAC 1999b). Altering the antimicrobial agent's target so that it is no longer bound by the drug.

β-Lactams

Altered penicillin-binding proteins which bind β-lactams poorly has explained a number of cases of bacterial resistance to penicillins and cephalosporins (Neu 1991; Standing Medical Advisory Committee, SMAC 1999b). It is responsible for *Streptococcus pneumoniae* resistance to penicillin G and *Staphylococcus aureus* resistance to β-lactamase-stable penicillins (meticillin-resistant strains). Also meticillin-resistant *S. aureus* (MRSA) strains are resistant to all penicillins, cephalosporins and carbapens by the same mechanism.

The resistance of group D streptococci to beta-lactam antibiotics appears to be the result of lower affinity of the penicillin binding proteins for penicillin. In addition, resistance of *Neisseria gonorrhoeae* to penicillin is also due to a diminished affinity of this target (Neu 1991; Standing Medical Advisory Committee, SMAC 1999b).

Macrolides and lincomycins

The resistance to macrolides and lincomycins is due to methylation of the two adenine nucleotides in the 23S component of 50S RNA. The methylated RNA binds these drugs much less well than unmethylated RNA (Neu 1991; Standing Medical Advisory Committee, SMAC 1999b). The gene responsible for the enzyme causing this resistance is present on plasmids and transposons. These genes can therefore spread between species. The induction of resistance varies between species but in most Gram-positive bacteria such as Staphylococci and Streptococci erythromycin is a more effective inducer of resistance than clindamycin. Activating an alternative metabolic pathway that by-passes the target.

β-lactams

Whilst no bacteria appear to have synthesized a new type of cell wall resistant to β-lactams, some streptococci lack the hydrolytic enzymes required for forming new cell wall and therefore β-lactamases do not lyse these bacteria (Neu 1991; Standing Medical Advisory Committee, SMAC 1999b). This change converts a bactericidal antibody into a bacteriostatic agent.

SIGNIFICANCE OF BACTERIAL PLAQUES (BIOFILMS)

Interactions between bacteria allow them to associate together in close proximity in colonies and plaques and in these relationships they are not affected by antibiotics as readily (Amábile-Cuevas et al 1995). Bacteria can produce a biofilm on a variety of surfaces where they become protected from the effects of heat, ultraviolet light, viruses and antibiotics. These films can form on the tooth surface, catheters, implants, dental units and tubing, endotracheal tubes, contact lenses and silicone surfaces. Bacteria living in multi-species biofilms including dental plaque live in a special microniche where nutrients are provided by neighbouring cells and diffusion. It has been shown that all forms of resistance to antibiotics can rapidly increase in these films. Probably, the close contact in the biofilm of a great diversity of bacterial species greatly increases the chances of plasmid and transposon exchange. These factors are very pertinent to some of the current usages of antibiotics in dentistry such as their local application into the periodontal pocket.

There are two principle forms of dental biofilms, i.e. supragingival or dental plaque and the subgingival bacterial flora (see Ch. 2). Some of the bacteria in dental plaque are related to dental caries and all of them are related to the onset of chronic gingivitis. Many of the bacteria in the subgingival flora are related to the onset and progression of chronic periodontitis and it is in this latter situation where antibiotics are occasionally used.

The large numbers of different bacteria within the periodontal pocket exist as interdependent microcolonies on the root surface, pocket epithelial lining and the pocket space itself. These represent highly organized biofilms (Finegold 1989). The usually quoted minimum bactericidal concentrations (MBC) or minimum inhibitory concentrations (MIC) for antibiotics relate to independent bacterial growth (planktonic conditions) and not to their growth in biofilms (Amábile-Cuevas et al 1995). As the target for the *in vivo* concentration of an antibiotic is often taken as its *in vitro* concentration inhibiting or killing 90% of tested isolates (MBC90 or MIC90), the decreased susceptibility of bacteria in a biofilm needs to be taken into account. In this respect, there is no direct evidence on which to base an estimate of the MICs or MBCs of periodontal pathogens growing in their organized biofilms. However, estimates from other biofilm infections indicate that the necessary MICs and MBCs are at least 50 times higher than those for bacteria grown under planktonic conditions (Anwar et al 1992; Brown & Gilbert 1993; Vorachit et al 1993).

A recent study (Wright et al 1997) compared the MIC values for the effect of metronidazole on *Porphyromonas gingivalis* grown under planktonic conditions and as a biofilm on the surface of hydroxyapatite. Growth on the biofilm was still active after exposure to 20 μg/mL of metronidazole which is 160 times the MIC for the planktonic growth of this bacteria. This bacteria present in a biofilm would therefore be resistant to the concentrations of metronidazole found in tissues following systemic administration. Another study (Larsen 2002) produced *P. gingivalis* biofilms in anaerobic chambers and compared them with normal planktonic cultures of the bacterium with respect to antibiotic susceptibility. They were exposed to varying therapeutic concentrations of metronidazole, amoxicillin and doxycycline. It was found that the MICs for the biofilms in respect of the three antimicrobials were at least twice that of planktonic cultures and MBCs were at least eight times higher and in the case of doxycycline they were up to 64 times higher.

Noiri et al (2003) investigated the effects of minocycline and metronidazole on *P. gingivalis* in artificial biofilms in an intraoral device. *P. gingivalis* biofilms were prepared on hydroxyapatite discs. At baseline and 24, 72 and 144 h after perfusion of minocycline or metronidazole two discs from each device were used to assess its antimicrobial effects by adenosine triphosphate (ADP) bioluminescence and its morphological changes by scanning electron microscopy (SEM). Minocycline caused a decrease ($p<0.05$) in the ADP content and some morphological change in *P. gingivalis* structure. However these effects were much less than those produced by chlorhexidine (see Ch. 16). Furthermore, metronidazole showed no significant effect against *P. gingivalis* biofilms. This shows how well the biofilm structure can protect against the effects of these antimicrobial agents on bacteria.

The relationship between antibiotic use and bacterial resistance

The evidence that the extensive use of antibiotics in medical, dental and veterinary practice and in animal meat production and horticulture whether appropriate or not causes resistance is overwhelming, although mostly circumstantial (Standing Medical Advisory Committee, SMAC 1999c). This is as follows:

First, there is no evidence of acquired resistance prior to the antimicrobial era (Hughes & Datta 1983). Second, the introduction of new antimicrobial agents has been followed repeatedly with the emergence of resistance (Fish et al 1995; Livermore 1992). The timescale has varied, mainly reflecting the complexity of the evolutionary process required for resistance, but the pattern is consistent. The relationship between use and resistance is most obvious when it is mutational as this may be selected during therapy causing clinical failure (Chow et al 1991). Third, subjects receiving antimicrobial treatment tend to develop a resistant commensal flora. If they subsequently develop a further infection, caused by an opportunistic pathogen from within their own bacterial flora, it is much more likely to be resistant than in patients who have not received prior treatment (Chow et al 1991; McGowen & Gerding 1996; Muder et al 1997; Shlaes et al 1997). Fourth, resistance is greatest where the use of antimicrobials is heaviest and this applies at both national and clinical unit level. This is clearly shown by the higher levels of resistance in intensive care units compared with general hospital wards or outpatient clinics (Chow et al 1991; Muder et al 1997; Huovinen et al 1997; Manian et al 1996; Parry et al 1989).

While exposure to antibiotics is the major factor in selecting bacterial resistance it should also be remembered that plasmids also confer resistance to topical disinfectants including chlorhexidine, quaternary ammonium compounds, triclosan and other phenolic compounds widely used in dentistry. Furthermore, the excessive and unnecessary use of disinfectants may serve to conserve plasmids that also determine antimicrobial resistance (Standing Medical Advisory Committee, SMAC 1999c).

The extent of the bacterial resistance problem

The overuse and inappropriate use of antibiotics and the spread of resistance genes by plasmid transfer (see above) has resulted in the development of bacterial infections resistant to one or more prescribed antibiotics. Bacterial resistance is accumulating worldwide and although the UK has a better situation in this respect than many other countries, the trends here are for progressively more resistance to develop (Standing Medical Advisory Committee, SMAC 1999d). At this point in time, the worst problem in this regard is with the meticillin-resistant *S. aureus* (MRSA). However, other major problems include those with *Streptococcus pneumoniae*, *enterococci* and many Gram-negative opportunists, *Salmonellae*, *Neisseria gonorrhoeae* and *Mycobacterium tuberculosis*. Furthermore, resistance is also now emerging in a number of clinically important fungi and viruses as well.

Staphylococcus aureus is a classical wound pathogen and can cause either superficial or deep seated infections (Standing Medical Advisory Committee, SMAC 1999d). It is also carried as a skin commensal by about 30% of the population and this proportion is dramatically higher in medical or dental staff who are regularly in contact with infected patients or other carriers. This property coupled with its strong ability to develop multiple resistances to important antimicrobials makes this bacteria a highly successful and adaptable pathogen.

When penicillin was first introduced in 1944, over 95% of *S. aureus* isolates were strongly susceptible to it. Since then progressive resistance had developed first to penicillin, then to the new penicillins (meticillin and flucloxacillin), gentamicin and tetracyclines leaving *S. aureus* only consistently susceptible to the glycopeptides, vancomycin and teicoplanin (Standing Medical Advisory Committee, SMAC 1999d). From 1998 intermediate resistance to vancomycin and teicoplanin were first reported (Hiramatsu et al 1997; Smith 1997; Ploy et al 1998) and these vancomycin-intermediate *S. aureus* (VISA) infections are resistant to all currently available antimicrobial agents and their number is increasing.

The use of topical mupirocin was introduced to attempt to reduce the carriage rate of staff and *S. aureus* isolates were at first universally susceptible to it. However, both low and high level forms of resistance to this agent are emerging and increasing in number (Eltringham 1997; Kavi 1987; Maples et al 1995).

MRSA infection is primarily a problem of hospital cross-infection (Department of Health and Social Security 1998) and tends to be spread when patients move from ward to ward, hospital to hospital or hospital to nursing home. Effective control has been achieved in the Netherlands and Scandinavia by identification and treatment of carriers, isolation or cohorting of those with MRSA infection and very strict hygiene policies within hospitals (Standing Medical Advisory Committee, SMAC 1999d).

The percentage of MRSA infections in the UK increased from 1.5% in 1989–91–13.2% in 1995, 21.1% in 1996 and 31.7% in 1997. Similar trends in resistance to erythromycin, gentamicin and ciprofloxacin were recorded over the same time period (Speller et al 1997; Johnson & James 1997; Standing Medical Advisory Committee, SMAC 1999d).

The incidence of MRSA varies in different parts of the world (Standing Medical Advisory Committee, SMAC 1999d; Speller et al 1997; Johnson & James 1997). It is lowest in those countries with very strict infection control policies and highest in those with liberal policies. In 1997, the percentage incidence of MRSA was <1% in Scandinavia and Holland, 28% in the USA, 32% in the UK, 40% in Belgium and 70% in Japan and Korea.

Enterococci are gut commensals (gut flora) which when introduced to other areas of the body can cause infections in immunocompromised patients (Standing Medical Advisory Committee, SMAC 1999d). These infections are a particular problem in renal dialysis and bone marrow transplant units where they may cause wound and urinary tract infections, septicaemia and endocarditis.

Enterococci are intrinsically resistant to quinolones and cephalosporins and readily gain resistance to other antibiotics such as penicillins, tetracyclines, macrolides, chloramphenicol and trimethoprim leaving only glycopeptides for their treatment (Neu 1991; Paton & Reeves 1991). However, a high level aminoglycoside resistance has now emerged and spread and many of the glycopeptide-resistant enterococci (GRE), particularly *Enterococcus faecium*, are resistant to all available antibiotics (Standing Medical Advisory Committee, SMAC 1999d; Woodford et al 1995). Glycopeptide-resistance spread by transferable plasmids which have the potential to transfer it into more pathogenic species (Noble & Howell 1995).

Reports of GRE infection in the UK rose from two in 1987 to 57 in 1996 (Standing Medical Advisory Committee, SMAC 1999d; Woodford et al 1995). In 1996, GRE infection was first reported in Sweden, Australia, Germany, Italy and Canada. In the USA, the percentage of States with hospitals reporting GRE infections increased from 27% in 1989–93 to 44% in 1994–95 (Archibald et al 1997).

Streptococcus pneumoniae is most important cause of lobar pneumonia which may also lead to bacteraemia and is also a frequent cause of otitis media and bacterial meningitis (Standing Medical Advisory Committee, SMAC 1999d).

S. pneumoniae was exquisitely susceptible to penicillin (Standing Medical Advisory Committee, SMAC 1999d) but low-level penicillin resistance was first reported in the late 1960s and by the late 1970s high level resistance had began to appear (Standing Medical Advisory Committee, SMAC 1999d; McCracken 1995).

From 1990–1995 (Laurichesse et al 1996) the rates of resistance to penicillin increased from 1.5 to 3.9% and to erythromycin from 2.8–5.1% (Laurichesse et al 1996). Penicillin resistant strains are more likely to be cross resistant to other antimicrobials and 36% of penicillin-resistant *S. pneumoniae* tested by the PHLS antibiotic reference Unit between 1993 and 1995 were resistant to erythromycin and many were also resistant to tetracycline and chloramphenicol (Goldstein & Acar 1996). The rates of resistance are even higher in other countries and by 1992 rates of 20% were reported in France, 25% in Romania, 44.3% in Spain and 57.8% in Hungary (Standing Medical Advisory Committee, SMAC 1999d; Applebaum 1992). In Iceland, rates rose from <1% in 1988 to 20% in 1993 by the import of resistant *S. pneumoniae* strains by returning holiday-makers and their dissemination to child care facilities (Soares et al 1992). Similar dissemination of these resistant species has occurred in the USA (Standing Medical Advisory Committee, SMAC 1999d; Applebaum 1992).

Many Gram-negative rods act as opportunistic pathogens in hospitals, particularly among immunocompromised patients and may infect virtually any site. In the community at large, the commonest bacteria to cause urinary tract infections is *Escherichia coli* as the result of passage from the gut (Standing Medical Advisory Committee, SMAC 1999d).

These bacteria develop resistance to penicillins, tetracyclines, chloramphenicol, aminoglycosides, trimethoprim and many cephalosporins usually by transferable plasmids. However, resistance to quinolones, some cephalosporins and carbapenems occurs by chromosomal mutation (Standing Medical Advisory Committee, SMAC 1999d; Livermore 1995; Livermore & Yuan 1996). In the UK the rates of resistance to commonly used antibiotics remained low and between 1989 and 1997 these antibiotics retained good activity against the major species. However, over this period, the level resistance of *E. coli*, *Klebsiella* spp. and *Enterobacter* spp. to ampicillin and trimethoprim rose markedly (Standing Medical Advisory Committee, SMAC 1999d). Similar rates of resistance have been reported in other countries (Standing Medical Advisory Committee, SMAC 1999d).

Several bacterial species are important in food poisoning and most of these infections are acquired from animals. Bacterial resistance to antimicrobials is acquired within the food animal before transmission to man via the food chain (Standing Medical Advisory Committee, SMAC 1999d).

These infections are most commonly caused by *Salmonella enteritidis*, *S. typhimurium*, *S. virchow* and *S. hadar* (Standing Medical Advisory Committee, SMAC 1999d). Resistance to antibiotics in these bacteria is mainly due to the use of a variety of antimicrobials in food animals for growth promotion. The resistant bacteria then infect humans via the food chain. Most resistance is concentrated in *S. typhimurium* and from 1964–1968 there were epidemics of multi-resistant *S. typhimurium* in bovines and humans in the UK. As a result the Swann Committee recommended that certain antimicrobials should only be available on prescription for veterinary use and should not be used for growth promotion (Anon 1969) and legislation followed. From 1970 to 1975 these infections in cattle were rare and only about 8% of salmonellae from cattle and 3% from humans were multi-resistant (Rowe & Threlfall 1984). However, from 1975 to the mid-1980s there was a substantial upsurge in the incidence of multi-resistant *S. typhimurium* from food animals, particular bovines and an increase in multi-resistant isolates from humans (Threlfall et al 1978). A feature of this period was sequential acquisition of plasmids and transposons coding for resistance to multiple antibacterial agents. This followed the introduction as therapeutic agent in calf husbandry of new antibacterial agents, notably apramycin, a gentamicin analogue (Threlfall et al 1985; 1986). By the end of 1990, 60% of *Salmonella* isolates from cattle were multi-resistant (Threlfall et al 1993).

From 1991 to 1996 there was a further substantial increase in multi-resistance of *S. enteritidis, S. typhimurium, S. virchow* and *S. hadar* (Standing Medical Advisory Committee, SMAC 1999d) and these species accounted for 89% non-typhoid salmonellae referred to the PHLS (Ridley et al 1996). The most resistant species was *S. typhimurium* and 80% of isolates from humans received in 1996 were multi-resistant (Public Health Laboratory Service 1998). This strain is now established in poultry, sheep and pigs and has also been isolated from many human foods. This strain is also increasingly resistant to sulphonamides, trimethoprim and ciprofloxacin (Threlfall et al 1996). Multiple resistant *S. virchow* infections are mainly seen in patients with recent foreign travel (Threlfall et al 1992).

Campylobacter coli and *C. jejuni* can cause severe food poisoning (Standing Medical Advisory Committee, SMAC 1999d). Macrolides and ciprofloxacin are the commonly used antimicrobials for these infections and emerging resistance is a particular concern particularly in patients infected abroad (Gaunt & Piddock 1996). However, the incidence of ciprofloxacin-resistant *Campylobacter* isolates in Oxfordshire rose from 3% in 1991 to 7% in 1995 and half of the patients gave no history of recent foreign travel. The main cause appeared to be increasing quinolone use in poultry farming (Bowler et al 1996). Ciprofloxacin-resistant *C. jejuni* isolates have been recovered from retail carcasses UK-bred and imported chickens (Gaunt & Piddock 1996). Between 1982 and 1989 the incidence of ciprofloxacin-resistant *Campylobacter* spp. isolated from chickens in the Netherlands rose from 0% to 14% and this was paralleled by an increase in humans from 0% to 11%. This increase followed the extensive use of enrofloxacin, a ciprofloxacin analogue, by the poultry industry (Endz et al 1991).

In 1997 in the UK all isolates tested by the PHLS were found to be resistant to trimethoprim and 89% were also resistant to one or more other antimicrobials. Rising rates of resistance to colimycin, tetracyclines and ciprofloxacin were also found (Standing Medical Advisory Committee, SMAC 1999d).

Neisseria gonorrhoeae causes gonorrhoea and has progressively developed total resistance to sulphonamides and ever increasing levels of resistance to penicillin.

Gonococci show great heterogeneity and a remarkable ability to acquire DNA from other gonococci and related species (Cambell 1944; Dees & Colston 1937; O'Rourke & Stevens 1993). This permits rapid evolution of resistance in this species. Sulphonamides were invariably effective against gonorrhoea at its introduction in 1937 (Cambell 1944), but were almost invariably found to be ineffective by 1944 (Dees & Colston 1937).

The development of penicillin resistance was slower but progressive and led to the prescription of ever-increasing doses of penicillins, so that the maximum possible single dose of amoxicillin (3.5 g) is now administered to patients with gonorrhoea in the UK, together with an excretion-blocking agent (probenecid) (Standing Medical Advisory Committee, SMAC 1999d). It is also associated with moderate cross-resistance to other unrelated antibiotics, especially tetracycline and erythromycin. In the developing world, such resistance is very frequently seen.

Plasmid-mediated ability to produce β-lactamases (penicillinase producing *N. gonorrhoeae*, PPNG) was first detected in 1974 in gonococci from the Far East and from West Africa (Cambell 1944; Ashford et al 1976; Phillips 1976). Following its introduction PPNG soon spread worldwide. Initially the plasmids were restricted to a few phenotypes, but they then disseminated gradually. The incidence of PPNG in the developing world has risen to 50% of all *N. gonorrhoeae* isolates.

N. gonorrhoeae with plasmid-mediated tetracycline resistance were first reported in 1987 (Hook et al 1987; Lind 1990). They remain uncommon in the UK but isolates from travellers indicate higher prevalences elsewhere (Fontanals et al 1989).

Ciprofloxacin is very effective against penicillin-resistant isolates and is now used for this purpose in the UK. However, it too is used elsewhere and this is resulting in a gradual increase in MICs for UK isolates and in a slow increase in the proportion of frankly resistant strains.

In the developing world the situation is far worse, with very high levels of resistance engendered by lack of alternative antibacterial agents and misuse of available drugs (Standing Medical Advisory Committee, SMAC 1999d; Botha 1985).

N. meningitidis is the major cause of bacterial meningitis (Standing Medical Advisory Committee, SMAC 1999d). This species is quite closely related to *N. gonorrhoeae*, but fortunately is less adept at acquiring resistance.

N. meningitidis isolates highly resistant to benzylpenicillin have not yet been identified in England and Wales, but have been reported in patients from South Africa (Hughes & Datta 1983) and more recently from Spain (Fontanals et al 1989). Isolates with reduced penicillin susceptibility occur in the UK and since 1984 the proportion of UK isolates with reduced penicillin susceptibility has increased from <1%, in 1985/6 to nearly 14% in 1995/6. Rifampicin is the most widely used prophylactic agent for contacts of meningococcal cases (Standing Medical Advisory Committee, SMAC 1999d). Resistance has never exceeded 0.4% in any given year. Most of the resistant isolates are from those who have received recent rifampicin

chemoprophylaxis, an observation that accords with the ability of rifampicin to select mutational resistance and highlights the need to use chemoprophylaxis in a targeted fashion and sparingly.

Tuberculosis (TB) remains the commonest bacterial cause of death from any single infectious agent in adults worldwide, with an estimated 8 million new cases and 3 million deaths annually, mostly in the developing world (Standing Medical Advisory Committee, SMAC 1999d). A steady decline in clinical cases in the developed world and some parts of the developing world, ceased or reversed in the mid-1980s.

Unusually among bacterial infections, *Mycobacterium tuberculosis* infections require treatment with combinations of three or four agents for at least 6 months. Monotherapy leads rapidly to resistance, by selecting spontaneous mutants. Even with combination therapy, resistance emerges when there is non-compliance by the patient, incorrect dosage by the physician or malabsorption.

The greatest treatment problem relates to individuals with multi-resistant TB isolates (Standing Medical Advisory Committee, SMAC 1999d) and mortality in these cases is very high.

A review was carried out of *M. tuberculosis* isolates submitted to the PHLS from residents of England and Wales between 1982 and 1991 (Warburton et al 1993). Overall, 6.1% of the first isolates from newly diagnosed patients were resistant to isoniazid and 0.6% were multi-drug resistant. Isoniazid resistance rates (with or without resistance to other drugs) were 4.6% in 1993, 5.4% in 1994 and 5.5% in 1995. Multi-drug resistance rose from 0.6%, in 1993 to 1.2% in 1994 and 1995.

The reported resistance rates in *M. tuberculosis* were higher in the USA, where a 1993–96 survey estimated that 8.4% of isolates were initially resistant to isoniazid and 2.2% were multidrug resistant (Moore et al 1997).

FUTURE PROSPECTS FOR ANTIMICROBIAL RESISTANCE

The current literature shows that existing resistances have spread and it is likely that new types will evolve. The past decade has revealed new genetic mechanisms of resistance such as mosaic gene information (Spratt 1994) and integrins (Hall et al 1991) that facilitate the evolution and spread of bacterial antimicrobial resistance. The decade has also shown that multidrug efflux pumps are important resistance mechanisms which have been previously underestimated (Nikaido 1996). More fundamentally, the rate of evolution has run more swiftly than would be predicted from known genetic processes. This implies the existence of other genetic processes that we do not yet understand. A controversial proposal that bacteria undergo favourable mutations under selection pressure may be relevant in this context (Cairns et al 1988). Such a mechanism would accelerate the evolution of resistance.

Several key developments seem likely from the present evidence. First, it seems inevitable that vancomycin-intermediate MRSA (VISA) will spread. During the few months that the Standing Medical Advisory Committee, SMAC's Subgroup on Antimicrobial Resistance has been in existence, VISA have been encountered in the USA and France, as well as in Japan, where they were first reported (Hiramatsu et al 1997; Smith 1997; Ploy et al 1998). Furthermore it has been shown that gene exchange can occur between enterococci and staphylococci and it is likely that the VanA system of resistance in enterococci will spread to MRSA, resulting in the acquisition of high-level glycopeptide resistance. Spread of VanA to *S. pneumoniae* and other α-haemolytic streptococci is also possible. This could occur in the same way that other enterococcal and staphylococcal genes transfer to these species (Schaberg & Zervos 1986). The consequences would be severe since glycopeptides are the drugs of last resort against β-lactam-resistant α-haemolytic streptococci in endocarditis and against β-lactam-resistant *S. pneumoniae* in meningitis.

Second, current data show that Gram-negative bacteria susceptible to only one or two antibacterial agents are common and are likely to spread. Often, the last drugs to retain activity are the carbapenems, imipenem and meropenem. Carbapenem resistance is now found increasingly in *Acinetobacter* spp. worldwide (Afzal-Shah & Livermore 1998). Furthermore, plasmid-mediated carbapenems (carbapenem-destroying enzymes) have emerged in enterobacteria and *Pseudomonas* spp. in Japan (Livermore 1997). These enzymes give complete resistance to all β-lactam antimicrobials. These enzymes have a flexible structure, with a large active site, implying that it will be extremely difficult to redesign β-lactams that evade hydrolysis. During the 6 months following the establishment of the SMAC Sub-group, the PHLS Antibiotic Reference Unit has received *Pseudomonas aeruginosa* isolates from England with a carbapenemase and with complete antimicrobial cross-resistance (Standing Medical Advisory Committee, SMAC 1999d).

Third, quinolones have retained good activity against many Gram-negative rods resistant to other antibacterial agents and, until 1997, such resistance that did occur always proved to be mutational rather than plasmid-associated. However, in 1997, an *E. coli* isolate was described in Spain with transferable quinolone resistance (Martinez-Martinez 1997) and this seems likely to spread.

Other resistances to be feared in the future are those in species that have so far remained remarkably susceptible. Obvious risks are penicillin resistance in *N. meningitidis* and *S. pyogenes*. Resistance in *N. meningitidis* follows the same evolutionary course as in *N. gonorrhoeae*, albeit more slowly and there is every reason to suppose that substantive penicillin resistance will ultimately emerge. Penicillin resistance in *S. pyogenes* is remarkable for its continued absence. This was the most feared of hospital wound pathogens and has remained exquisitely sensitive to penicillin since the 1940s. Nevertheless, gene exchange occurs between *S. pyogenes* and staphylococci (Schaberg & Zervos 1986) and there is a risk that β-lactamase production may spread from the latter to the former. It seem obvious that bacterial, fungal and viral evolution has not finished yet (Standing Medical Advisory Committee, SMAC 1999d).

CONTROL OF THE USE OF ANTIBIOTICS

If inappropriate and excessive use of antibiotics on the scale of today were to continue then it is likely that the majority of serious bacterial infections will become resistant to all the antibiotics available today. It is also extremely unlikely that new antibiotics would appear at a fast enough rate to solve these problems and even if they did it would be very likely that bacteria would develop insensitivity to these new antibiotics in turn by the same mechanisms.

It is therefore extremely important that antibiotics are only prescribed when correctly indicated for infections known to be sensitive to the antibiotic in question. They should never be prescribed as blanket cover for the imprecise diagnosis of an infection or for conditions that can be equally or better treated by other means. It is also vitally important that all other unnecessary uses of antibiotics, such as additives to farm animal feed, are totally eliminated.

In respect of periodontal disease it is pertinent that no single pathogen is involved in its aetiology so that no precise antibiotic treatment to eliminate a single pathogen can be used. At the best, therefore, antibiotics used in periodontal treatment will suppress some of the bacteria in the subgingival flora for a variable period after which they will grow back, since they are all members of the indigenous flora. This change in the subgingival flora can be equally or better achieved by subgingival scaling (see Ch. 15 and below) which has been shown in some studies to be effective for longer periods. Therefore, antibiotics can never be primary agents in treating periodontal diseases and should only be used for the few situations where

for one reason or another conventional treatment fails to be effective, even when it is efficiently carried out and repeated. These situations will be described below.

POSSIBLE PERIODONTAL USES OF ANTIMICROBIALS

The antimicrobials most commonly used as adjunctives in the treatment of chronic periodontitis are tetracyclines and metronidazole. Both of these antibiotics are broad spectrum agents aimed at many different bacteria within the periodontal pocket rather than a single pathogen. For this reason the rationale for their use has to be questioned. In addition, tetracyclines and an amoxicillin/metronidazole combination have been suggested to treat juvenile periodontitis (see Ch. 23). An acute periodontal abscess may occasionally require antibiotics (see Ch. 22) and metronidazole is the agent of choice in treating acute necrotizing ulcerative gingivitis (see Ch. 25). Finally, amoxicillin, erythromycin, clindamycin, vancomycin and gentamicin all have a place in the prophylaxis of transient bacteraemia in susceptible patients (see Ch. 18). The factors involved in the possible use of antibiotics are considered in detail below.

THE NATURE OF PERIODONTAL INFECTIONS

Although the primary cause of inflammatory periodontal disease is bacterial, no single causative pathogen has been found (Ch. 4). Thus, chronic periodontitis seems best regarded as a non-specific bacterial disease caused by a local imbalance in the local indigenous bacterial population (Theilade 1986). However, the bacteria in the subgingival plaque are the primary aetiological agent in periodontitis (Tonetti 1994), which also results from the sequelae of quantitative and qualitative changes in both the subgingival microflora and the inflammatory response to its presence (Loesche 1976). Certain indigenous bacteria may play a more important role in the disease process because they possess virulence factors that may enable them to damage host defences or degrade host tissues. However, there is no evidence that eradication of suspected pathogens of chronic periodontitis without the suppression of other members of the flora is effective in treating chronic periodontitis. If, as seems to be the case, all the suspected pathogens are members of the normal oral flora their permanent eradication by antibiotics will not be possible because they will reestablish themselves after treatment.

However, it is known that transient shifts in the subgingival bacterial flora can be produced both by scaling and root planing (see Ch. 15) and the systemic administration or local application of some antibiotics. A number of studies have been carried out into the most promising antibiotics, tetracycline and metronidazole and these will be described below along with the few advantages and many disadvantages for using them.

There is a much stronger case for using appropriate antibiotics to treat acute necrotizing ulcerative gingivitis (Ch. 25) and the early stages of juvenile periodontitis (Ch. 23) as they appear to be associated with selective growth of a much narrower range of bacteria.

However, because of the possibility of inducing bacterial resistance and antibiotic hypersensitivity (see below) by over prescription of antibiotics, these drugs should never be prescribed if other means of treatment are possible.

THE SPECTRUM OF ANTIBIOTICS

The spectrum of action of antibiotics varies considerably and depends on their mode of action. It is obviously necessary for the antibiotic of choice to be strongly active against the causative bacteria of the disease. An example of this affecting the choice of an antibiotic for periodontal purposes is in the use of metronidazole, which is strongly active against strictly anaerobic bacteria but is only weakly active against facultative, capnophilic aerobes such as *Eikenella corrodens*, *Capnocytophaga* spp. and *Aggregatibacter actinomycetemcomitans*. Generally antibiotics with a lower potential for sensitization and bacterial resistance (see below) should be preferred for treating periodontal diseases.

Antibiotics are primarily used for treating specific exogenous bacterial infections where the infection can be treated with a narrow spectrum antibiotic specifically directed against the foreign pathogen. During treatment the susceptible pathogens and any indigenous bacteria sensitive to the antibiotic will be either killed (bactericidal antibiotic) or stopped from multiplying (bacteriostatic antibiotic). Bacteriostatic antibiotics depend upon the host defence mechanisms to rid the body of the suppressed pathogens. The success of the treatment depends on which bacteria regrow after the treatment is stopped. If the indigenous bacteria regrow rapidly after treatment they will prevent the reestablishment of the pathogens (van Palenstein Helderman 1986).

If different antibiotics are combined in a treatment regime then the ones with differing modes of action are likely to be additive in most cases. However, the combination of tetracycline and penicillin is contraindicated since the former antagonizes the latter.

THE SITE OF ACTION OF ANTIBIOTICS FOR PERIODONTAL TREATMENT

The site of action for an antimicrobial agent treating periodontal disease is the periodontal pocket and it is essential that it should achieve a high concentration at this site (van Palenstein Helderman 1986).

Antibiotics for treating periodontal disease can be administered either systemically or locally. The local method seems better for achieving high local concentrations of the drug but this method should not be used with antibiotics such as penicillin that carry a high risk of sensitization. The inaccessibility of the pocket is a problem in this regard and cannot be reached by antimicrobials in mouthrinses, ointments, toothpastes or chewing gum. This problem can be overcome by subgingival irrigation but daily irrigation is not practical since it is patient dependent. To avoid this problem, slow release devices have been developed that can be inserted by the dentist into the pocket, extending down to its base. These currently include hollow and monolithic fibres (Goodson et al 1979, 1983) and acrylic strips (Addy 1986) and slow release gels (Norling et al 1992).

Systemically administered antibiotics can also reach the pocket in gingival crevicular fluid, which is an exudate. This has been shown to occur with tetracyclines (Gordon et al 1981), clindamycin (Walker et al 1981a), metronidazole (Notten et al 1982) and amoxicillin and an amoxicillin/clavulanic acid combination (Augmentin®) (Tenenbaum et al 1997). Tetracycline and its derivatives achieve higher concentrations in crevicular fluid than in serum, possibly by binding to calcium-containing substances (Baker et al 1983). The antibiotic concentrations in crevicular fluid, achieved using either the systemic route or local delivery systems, are higher than those necessary to inhibit the sensitive bacteria *in vitro* (van Palenstein Helderman 1986) but it must be remembered that we are dealing with a biofilm where higher concentrations are needed.

CLINICAL TRIALS OF ANTIBIOTICS IN THE TREATMENT OF CHRONIC PERIODONTITIS

A number of clinical trials of the use of antibiotics for the treatment of chronic periodontitis have been carried out. They have used antibiotics either as the sole treatment, or in combination with scaling and root planing and in both cases have compared the results obtained with scaling and root planing alone. All of these have involved the use of either a tetracycline or metronidazole.

Local application can produce a much higher concentration in the pocket with a much lower total dose and very low systemic levels. However, local application does not affect the reservoirs of bacteria at other sites in the mouth and only maintains bactericidal levels for about 24 h. It is also much more expensive.

FACTORS AFFECTING LOCAL DELIVERY OF ANTIMICROBIAL AGENTS INTO THE PERIODONTAL POCKET

A pharmacological agent must reach its site of action and be maintained there at a sufficient concentration for a sufficient time for an effect to occur and these three criteria affect the local delivery of agents to the periodontal pocket.

Site of action

The targets for locally delivered pharmacological agents include bacteria residing in the periodontal pocket and bacteria possibly invading the junctional epithelium and adjacent connective tissue or the exposed root cementum or dentine (Saglie et al 1982, 1988; Adriaens et al 1988). Most methods of local delivery, including irrigating solutions, place the agent down to the base of the pocket (Pitcher et al 1980). However, it should be recognized that gaining access to the pocket does not necessarily mean gaining access to target bacteria. Extracellular components of the bacterial biofilm may impair diffusion or inactivate a significant proportion of the applied active agent and thus may protect biofilm bacteria from the action of an antimicrobial agent. In addition, it may prevent the agent from diffusing into the soft tissue wall or exposed root surface.

Concentration

To be effective against target bacteria, the antimicrobial agent should reach the site of action at a concentration higher than its minimal efficacious concentration. Definition of the desired concentration range is a key aspect in maximizing therapeutic efficiency of an agent and minimizing its expected side-effects.

The first approximation of the desired concentration of antimicrobials comes from *in vitro* experiments looking at the susceptibility of the target bacteria to different concentrations of the drug in terms of its effects on growth inhibition (MIC) and bacterial killing (MBC). The *in vivo* concentration of an antimicrobial is usually based on the *in vitro* concentration of that agent which inhibits or kills 90% of the target bacteria in culture (MIC90 and MBC90). It must, however, be realized that these *in vitro* concentrations are determined with the bacteria growing in culture under planktonic conditions whereas the bacteria in the subgingival flora are residing in an organized biofilm. In these situations the real therapeutic concentration is likely to be at least 50 times higher than the *in vitro* MIC90 or MBC90 (Anwar et al 1992; Brown & Gilbert 1993; Vorachit et al 1993). However, it is also true that sub-MIC concentrations of antibiotics can also modulate bacterial metabolism and impair production of virulence and colonization factors and may thus make bacteria more susceptible to the effects of the immune system (Hansberger 1992).

It is necessary to adjust the therapeutic dose to take account of side-effects of the drug which are also associated with the local concentration. The pharmacological effect of any drug, including antibiotics, is characterized by a certain therapeutic range which is the range of concentrations above the minimal effective concentration and below the concentration that produces substantial toxicity or side-effects. The most important concentration dependent side-effect of local delivery of antimicrobials is the overgrowth of non-susceptible microorganisms and these effects occur at both ends of the concentration spectrum. After exposure to marginally effective concentrations, resistant bacteria may repopulate the whole ecological niche, while after exposure to highly effective concentrations, overgrowth of intrinsically non-susceptible microorganisms including yeasts is more likely to occur.

Time

Once a drug reaches the site of action in an effective concentration, it must remain at the site for long enough for its pharmacological effect to occur. Different classes of antibiotics inhibit or kill infecting bacteria by different mechanisms, e.g. interference with cell wall growth, inhibition of protein synthesis or inhibition of DNA synthesis. Antibiotics using these different specific mechanisms have been shown to require different durations of exposure to effective concentrations. Therefore, the duration of antimicrobial levels of the drug may therefore be of critical importance in the case of some antibiotics.

Moreover, these assumptions are based on *in vitro* experiments and should be considered further when the target bacteria are not living in planktonic conditions such as in the periodontal pocket. In this respect metronidazole requires rapidly proliferating bacteria to work effectively. However, in organized biofilms most of the bacteria display a very slow growth rate and this may seriously limit the effectiveness of many antibiotics (Evans et al 1990; Ashby et al 1994).

An inflammatory infiltrate, gingival crevicular fluid (GCF), constantly flows into the periodontal pocket. It has been estimated that the fluid present in a 5 mm periodontal pocket is replaced about 40 times/h (Goodson 1989) and such a high clearance is the result of a low volume and high flow rate (Binder et al 1987). Therefore, it is apparent that following subgingival placement of a drug, it will be rapidly removed from the pocket according to an exponential decay equation (Benet et al 1996).

The expected half time of elimination of a subgingivally placed pharmacological agent (i.e. the time necessary to reduce its concentration by half) is about 1 min. This is in good agreement with experimental observations of about 1.5 min obtained following subgingival irrigation with 1% ofloxacin solution (Higashi et al 1990) or the subgingival placement of fluorescein gel (Oosterwaal et al 1990).

This high rate of clearance of a drug placed into the periodontal pocket represents the major obstacle in attempting to maintain antimicrobial action following subgingival irrigation or placement of non-binding substances. Therefore longer antimicrobial action requires systems to establish drug reservoirs which are able to release active medication in sufficient quantities to counteract the expected continuous loss over time effected by the flow of GCF.

The effects of antibiotics as the sole agent

Short-term use of systemic or local tetracycline and metronidazole produce a marked reduction in Gram-negative anaerobes and spirochaetes and improvements in the clinical condition, i.e. reduction in probing pocket depth (PPD) and bleeding on probing (BOP). Similar results have been shown with the local delivery of tetracycline in hollow or solid fibres (Goodson et al 1979, 1983; Lindhe et al 1979) or metronidazole in acrylic strips (Addy 1986). Re-establishment of the pocket flora after antibiotic treatments occurs between 8 and 12 weeks (Lindhe et al 1979).

These studies show that, whilst marked reductions in the number of subgingival bacteria can be achieved with these antibiotics, these are often less than can be achieved by scaling and root planing and tend to persist for shorter periods.

The effects of antibiotics as adjunctives to scaling and root planing

Since it is impossible to remove the whole pocket flora by scaling and root planing, the use of antibiotics as adjunctives to these procedures might enhance their effects. To test this possibility a number of studies have been carried out to compare the combined effects of antibiotics and scaling and root planing with the effects of scaling and root planing alone (Listgarten et al 1978; Lindhe et al 1979, 1983). In both groups the changes in the flora were maintained for up to 25 weeks.

Ehmke et al (2005) showed that over the 24-month period, a single course of the administered adjunctive antimicrobial therapy led to a relative risk reduction of 62% for attachment loss at deep sites. However, with the exception of *A. actinomycetemcomitans*, it failed to induce long-term changes in the prevalence profiles of oral colonization.

Systemic use

Human clinical trials of systemic treatment with tetracycline in combination with scaling and root planing have not shown any more benefit over scaling and root planing alone (Listgarten et al 1978). On the other hand, there are other studies using systemic metronidazole as an adjunctive which show more marked and prolonged improvements in the clinical condition (Loesche et al 1985, 1991; Joyston-Bechal et al 1984, 1986; Söder et al 1990). However, all these improvements had disappeared 3 years after treatment (Joyston-Bechal et al 1986).

Loesche and his co-workers have carried out three double-blind clinical trials of systemic metronidazole in the treatment of periodontal disease and have observed each time a significant clinical improvement in the group receiving metronidazole (Loesche et al 1985, 1991, 1992). In these patients there was a significant rapid decline or disappearance of spirochaetes. Systemic metronidazole as an adjunctive to scaling was also found significantly to reduce the need for periodontal surgery (Loesche et al 1992). However, a few patients in the metronidazole groups appeared to be non-responsive to the drug. In another study (Loesche et al 1993), the compliance in taking the drug was investigated by measuring the reduction in spirochaetes and it was found that only 10 patients out of 18 in the study were compliant in regularly taking the drug. These 10 patients experienced a significantly greater clinical benefit than the eight non-compliant patients.

A systematic review of the adjunctive systemic use of antibiotics compared with subgingival scaling and root surface debridement alone has been reported (Herrera et al 2002). Out of 158 retrieved publications, only 25 passed their inclusion criteria as randomized, controlled clinical trials of 6 months or more duration. Only limited meta-analysis was possible. This process excluded the publications on all antibiotics except those on metronidazole, amoxicillin/metronidazole combination and the macrolide, spiramycin. It showed that systemic spiramycin had a slight adjunctive effect ($p=0.014$) on probing pocket depth (PPD) reduction but not on gain in clinical attachment level (CAL). Systemic amoxicillin/metronidazole combination had a slight adjunctive effect ($p=0.001$) on CAL gain but not PPD reduction. Furthermore, these effects were only found in patients with deep PPDs (>6 mm). The effects of systemic, adjunctive metronidazole on these parameters were not statistically significant. Thus the evidence of clinically relevant beneficial adjunctive effects of systemic antibiotics in the treatment of periodontal disease is weak and is outweighed by their other disadvantages.

Local delivery

The effect of local tetracycline and metronidazole with local administration or slow release devices as an adjunctive to scaling and root planing has also been studied. Similar changes were seen with and without the adjunctives and thus no additional benefit appeared to accrue (Lindhe et al 1979, 1983; Addy 1986).

Further studies (Norling et al 1992) on local delivery of tetracycline and metronidazole have been carried out more recently following the incorporation of these antibiotics into biodegradable slow-release gels (**Figs 17.13, 17.14**). Studies of the release characteristics from these gels have shown that both the 2% minocycline (Dentomycin®) gel (Satomi et al 1987) and the 25% metronidazole (Elyzol®) gel (Stoltze 1992) produced levels above the MIC for suspected pathogens for 12–24 h after treatment. It has also been shown that the systemic absorption, including that from swallowed excess gel, was less than that absorbed from one 200 mg metronidazole tablet taken orally (Stoltze & Stellfeld 1992).

Further human studies with these agents for 2% minocycline gel (Van Steenberge et al 1993; Vandekerckhove et al 1998), locally-delivered 10% doxycycline hyclate (Drisko 1998; Wennström et al 2001), 25% metronidazole gel (Klinge et al 1992a; Ainamo et al 1992; Pedrazzoli would have to treat nine sites to gain an additional 0.3 mm of probing depth reduction. Another similar study (Paquette et al 2003) reported that the adjunctive use of minocycline microspheres in smokers with chronic periodontitis showed a significantly greater reduction (*p* >0.05) in probing depth after 9 months in the test group compared with the control. However, the mean difference between 1.19 mm compared with 0.90 mm would not be of any clinical significance and would be much less than variations in probing between the clinicians used in this study and also the effect of smoking.

An 18-month, randomized, double-blind, parallel, comparative study of locally applied minocycline (Timmerman et al 1996) was carried out in 20 healthy patients with moderate to severe periodontitis. The adjunctive effect of either active or placebo gel and scaling and root planing was compared with regard to clinical and microbiological effects. The active or placebo gel was applied at baseline, 2-weeks, 1, 3, 6, 9 and 12 months. Over the 18-month period no differences were observed between test and control sites with regard to probing depth or probing attachment level. Over a 15-month period there were significant reductions in the numbers of putative periodontal pathogens in all the treated sites but there were no significant differences between test and placebo sites. *Candida albicans* and Enterobacteriaceae were only detected in small numbers at each time interval in a limited number of patients and no changes in their proportions or prevalence were seen in any of these patients during the study. Thus, this group of patients responded favourably to scaling and root planing and did not benefit from the adjunctive use of minocycline gel. This study clearly shows that locally applied antibiotics do not have a place in the routine treatment of chronic periodontitis.

Greenstein (2006) reviewed the controlled clinical trials on local antibiotic delivery and found that several local drug delivery systems employed as mono therapies improved periodontal health but their results were not statistically significantly different over those attained with scaling and root planing (SRP) alone. In contrast, many local drug delivery devices when used as adjuncts to SRP provided a statistically significant enhancement of parameters commonly used to monitor periodontal status. However, mean improvements with respect to probing depth reduction or gain of clinical attachment were often limited to tenths of millimetres which is of no clinical significance. There was also conflicting data with respect to the ability of local drug delivery to enhance results of SRP at deep probing sites.

Local delivery using slow release fibre

Two types of fibre system have been investigated for carriage of tetracycline for local delivery into the periodontal pocket. These are:

1. Drug filled hollow fibres (Goodson et al 1979)
2. Ethylene vinyl acetate copolymer (EVA) fibres (Goodson et al 1985).

Monolithic fibres of EVA with a diameter of 0.5 mm containing 25% tetracycline have been used in a number of clinical trials and were marked under the trade name of Actisite®.

It has been found that these fibres placed into the periodontal pocket maintained an average of 1590 μg/mL (0.16%) of tetracycline over 10 days (Tonetti et al 1990). This concentration is above that necessary to inhibit growth of the susceptible bacterial species (Walker et al 1981b).

The fibres are used to fill the periodontal pocket under treatment. The end of the fibre is first applied with a flat plastic instrument into the deepest part of the pocket and then successive layers are then packed in wrapping the fibre around the tooth so that all the subgingival areas are filled. A floss threader can be used to pass the fibre between the teeth. When the packing process is complete excess fibre is cut off with scissors and the fibre is retained by applying a thin layer of cyanoacrylate adhesive to the tooth and top layers of the fibre at the gingival margin. The time taken to apply

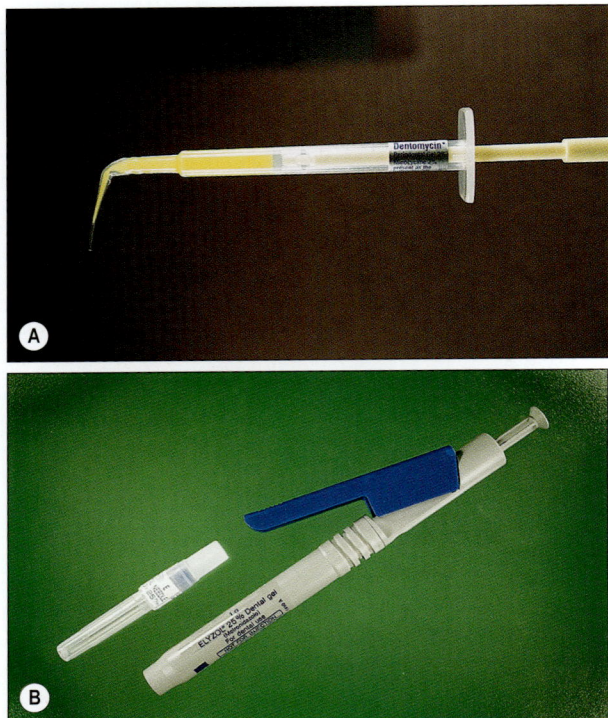

Fig. 17.13 Local delivery systems for antibiotic slow release gels: (A) the delivery system for 2% minocycline (Dentomycin®); (B) the delivery system for 25% metronidazole (Elyzol®)

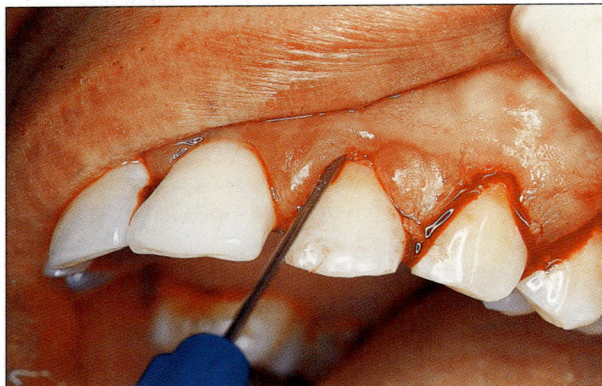

Fig. 17.14 Metronidazole (Elyzol®) being delivered into a periodontal pocket.

et al 1992; Magnusson 1998) and a single application of 5% metronidazole in a collagen slow release device (Hitzig et al 1997) produced similar findings to those already reported. Similar results were found using 25% metronidazole gel in experimental periodontitis in dogs (Klinge et al 1992b). Similar results have been achieved with topical irrigation with tetracycline-HCl solution (100 mg/mL) and this might in part be due to absorption of the compound on to root dentine and its subsequent release (Christersson et al 1993). Irrigation for long periods (5 min) is, however, necessary to achieve release of therapeutic concentrations of active antibiotic.

Similar results have been achieved with microencapsulated spheres of minocycline in a controlled clinical trial (Williams et al 2001a). A 9-month multicentre, controlled trial of 748 subjects (Williams et al 2001b) has been carried out comparing subgingival scaling alone with subgingival scaling with unfilled microspheres and subgingival scaling with minocycline microspheres. It found a significant reduction in mean probing depths in all groups after treatment and a significantly greater, albeit very slight, reduction in the minocycline group. The difference was of no clinical significance and the figures indicate that one the fibre varies from 5 to 15 min per tooth depending on the pocket depth and position of the tooth. The fibre is left in the pocket for about 10 days after which the fibre is removed with a scaler or tweezers. When the fibre is removed the pocket is dilated and the root surface within the pocket can be clearly seen. This may reveal any residual calculus which may have been left on the tooth following the preceding subgingival scaling procedures. This can be more easily seen and removed at this stage. The tissues then readapt to this clean root surface during the subsequent healing period.

EVA fibres containing 25% tetracycline (EVA-TC fibres) have been subject to a number of laboratory and clinical studies.

Tonetti et al (1990) investigated their delivery characteristics and compared them with subgingival irrigation. They found that following subgingival irrigation of 1% and 10% tetracycline solutions into the periodontal pocket the gingival crevicular fluid (GCF) concentration decayed exponentially with half times of 4.2 and 12.2 h, respectively. In contrast, EVA-TC fibres packed into the pocket and left *in situ* for 10 days maintained a constant GCF concentration of 1590 μg/mL over the 10 days. After removal of the fibres the tetracycline concentration decreased exponentially with a half time of 4.5 h.

The serum concentration resulting from EVA-TC fibre placement has been studied by Rapley et al (1992). They placed the fibres in eight deep pockets of four adult chronic periodontitis patients for 10 days and took plasma samples at baseline, 1 h, 3 h, 3 days and 10 days. The maximum tetracycline local dose averaged 105 mg with a range of 91–126 mg. This produced no detectable serum level >0.1 μg/mL. Thus, local EVA-TC fibre placement appears to result in insignificant systemic uptake of tetracycline.

The tissue concentration of tetracycline following EVA-TC fibre placement into periodontal pockets was studied in 10 chronic periodontitis patients (Ciancio et al 1992). It evaluated the tetracycline concentration in the gingival tissue adjacent to the fibre-treated periodontal pockets. Either placebo fibre or EVA-TC fibre were randomly assigned to two non-adjacent pockets in each subject and fibres left *in situ* for 8 days after which the fibres were removed and periodontal surgery, allowing a biopsy of one interdental papilla from each of the two test sites in each quadrant, was performed. One biopsy was analysed for tetracycline concentration by high performance liquid chromatography (HPLC) and the second was examined by light and ultraviolet (UV) fluorescence microscopy to determine the localization of residual tetracycline and intensity of inflammatory cell infiltrates in the adjacent periodontal tissues. They found a mean tissue tetracycline concentration of 64.4 ng/mg which corresponds to 43 μg of tetracycline. The levels at placebo sites were below the detection limit of the HPLC system. Also, tetracycline fluorescence was seen in the soft tissue wall at depths ranging from 1 to 20 μm. Therefore, some tetracycline from the EVA-TC fibre placed in the periodontal pocket may pass through the damaged pocket epithelium into the adjacent periodontal tissue.

Morrison et al (1992) studied the effect on the root surface within the pocket from a 10 day exposure to EVA-TC fibre placement. Eight patients with four teeth with terminal periodontitis which required extraction were selected for treatment. The teeth of each patient were randomly assigned to one of four treatment groups, i.e. no treatment control, scaling and root planing only, EVA-TC fibre only and EVA-TC fibre plus scaling and root planing. The root surfaces were examined by fluorescent light microscopy (FLM), scanning electron microscopy (SEM) and energy dispersive spectroscopy (EDS). SEM revealed a visible reduction in the subgingival plaque on the root surfaces in the EVA-TC fibre and fibre plus scaling groups in comparison to the control group. In contrast, the scaling and root planing group showed randomly distributed areas of residual subgingival plaque and calculus. EDS analysis of large crystals adhering to the root surfaces of EVA-TC fibre and fibre plus scaling teeth revealed high chloride peaks which were suggestive of residual tetracycline. These crystals were not present in the other groups.

FLM examination of EVA-TC fibre and fibre plus scaling teeth showed a superficial penetration of tetracycline into the root surface to a depth of about 10 μm. Thus, EVA-TC fibre treatment appears to be effective over 10 days in clearing subgingival plaque from the root surface and also appears to result in some absorption of tetracycline into the root surface.

One of the main drawbacks to local antibiotic therapy is the possible development of bacterial resistance (see above). For this reason antibiotic resistance of the subgingival microbiota following EVA-TC fibre treatment has been studied using three approaches (Goodson & Tanner 1992). First, they assessed the ability of the subgingival microbiota to grow on media containing tetracycline. High percentages of tetracycline-resistant bacteria appeared at EVA-TC fibre treated sites and within the saliva 1 week after treatment as compared with pretreatment levels. However, by 1 month post-treatment the number had returned to levels comparable to those at pretreatment. In a second approach they took subgingival isolates following treatment and grew them on media without antibiotics. They then took selected isolates and determined their Gram-stain and cell morphology characteristics. It showed that the subgingival sites became colonized with Gram-positive cocci during the same time period in which the increase in the number of tetracycline-resistant bacteria developed. Since most Gram-positive cocci are intrinsically resistant to tetracycline this may account for the transient increase in tetracycline-resistant bacteria seen following EVA-TC fibre treatment. In a third approach the antibiotic-resistance of subgingival Gram-negative bacteria was determined before and after EVA-TC fibre treatment. The predominant cultivable microbiota of nine sites from three subjects were isolated immediately before and 6 months after EVA-TC fibre treatment. Gram-negative rods were characterized and tested for sensitivity to tetracycline (minimum inhibitory concentration (MIC) 1–128 μg/mL), penicillin at 80 μg/mL and erythromycin at 8 μg/mL. None of the Gram-negative rods were resistant to tetracycline either before or after treatment. Before treatment 98% were susceptible to tetracycline at 1–2 μg/mL and after treatment 88% were susceptible. The percentage of Gram-negative rods showing intermediate sensitivity (MIC 4–8 μg/mL) changed from 2% before treatment to 5.2% after treatment. In no case was penicillin or erythromycin resistance associated with increased resistance to tetracycline.

This study appears to show that no significant bacterial resistance develops following EVA-TC fibre therapy. This could result from thee reasons. First, there is a high concentration of tetracycline in the pocket throughout the 10 day application which is vastly in excess of the MIC (Tonetti et al 1990). This would inhibit virtually all the susceptible bacteria at this site. It could also inhibit bacteria on the root surface as tetracycline appears to absorb into this surface following EVA-TC fibre treatment (Morrison et al 1992). Second, tetracycline from EVA-TC fibre treatment does find its way into the adjacent gingival tissues and may thus inhibit any susceptible bacteria at this site (Ciancio et al 1992). Third, tetracycline does not appear to become systemically absorbed to any significant level from the local site (Rapley et al 1992) and may not stimulate resistance at other sites.

However, this study does not take account of three important factors (see above). First, tetracycline is bacteriostatic rather than bactericidal and its affects on the susceptible bacteria are less prolonged and may thus allow the long term development of resistance. Second, some strains of bacteria from species normally susceptible to an antibiotic are naturally resistant. Thus, inhibition of susceptible strains will select for these resistant strains and allow them to multiply. Third, and most importantly, antibiotic-resistant bacteria can transfer antibiotic-resistance genes to non-resistant bacteria in plasmids and this can involve bacteria of the same or different species (see above). Since there is a significant reservoir of natural or acquired tetracycline-resistant bacteria in all periodontal pockets and gingival crevices and these bacteria are in very close relationship with each other in this environment, there is a very real possibility of tetracycline resistance developing as a result of local tetracycline treatment.

This equally applies to all other antibiotics used locally or systemically in periodontal treatment. Therefore, one should always be very cautious in using antibiotics and should only consider using them for periodontal treatment when repeated conventional treatment is not effective.

In addition, there have been other single site studies (Heijl et al 1991) and multicentre studies (Goodson et al 1991a,b,c; Newman et al 1994) which have compared the effects of EVA-fibres or placebo-fibres with or without additional subgingival scaling and root planing. The multicentre studies involved large numbers of subjects (107–113) and were well designed. They all showed that EVA-fibres alone produce similar but lesser clinical and microbiological changes to scaling and root planing alone and that these effects were enhanced when their use was combined with scaling and root planing. Furthermore, they all found no statistical difference between the microbiological changes produced between adjunctive EVA-fibre placement and scaling and root planing alone. In terms of clinical effects both multicentre studies showed slightly enhanced effects from the use of adjunctive EVA-fibre compared with scaling and root planing alone and these benefits appeared to last up to 6 months. However, the clinical relevance of this must be in doubt since there were no differences in the microbiological changes and it is these changes which are responsible for producing and maintaining the clinical improvements. Overall, these results indicate that EVA-TC fibre therapy has no place in the routine management of periodontal disease but might enhance the effectiveness of subgingival scaling and root planing at localized recurrent periodontitis sites which fail to respond to repeated mechanical therapy.

The effect of EVA-TC fibre treatment on recurrent lesions has been also investigated in a private periodontal practice situation (Corsair 1994). This was a long-term study of 31 patients who produced recurrent, refractory lesions during maintenance care. Patients were evaluated 1, 3, 6, 12 and 24 months after the use of EVA-TC fibre. These treated sites showed probing depth reductions, apparent clinical attachment gains and reductions in bleeding on probing which were maintained for up to 24 months. Although there were no controls in this study it did show that a combination of EVA-TC fibre treatment and scaling was effective in sites previously refractory to conventional treatment in a private practice situation.

Although all of these clinical studies, which have been recently reviewed by Tonetti (1998), show that EVA-TC fibre treatment is effective they do not show that it is significantly better than subgingival scaling and root planing in most situations. Therefore, one should always be very cautious in using antibiotics and should only consider using them for periodontal treatment when repeated conventional treatment is not effective at a local site.

Thus, some studies do and some do not show a statistically significant adjunctive benefit of locally delivered antimicrobials (Killoy 2002). There has also been a recent meta-analysis of 29 suitable studies of local tetracycline used alone or as an adjunct with scaling and root planing or the use of a placebo (Pavia et al 2003). Local use of tetracycline alone did not perform better than scaling and root planing, whereas it did perform better than a placebo. Adjunctive tetracycline did produce small but significantly better reductions in probing depth compared with scaling and root planing alone. However, they were not large enough to be clinically significant. Furthermore, this must be also gauged against the adverse effects of the widespread use of tetracyclines.

There has also been a further systematic review of studies of one or more local agents as adjunctives to subgingival scaling (Bonito et al 2005). The most positive results occurred for tetracycline, minocycline and metronidazole but the marginal improvements in PPD and CAL were a fraction of the improvement from subgingival scaling alone. Thus, such improvements, even if statistically significant, are not clinically meaningful.

Therefore, the use of adjunctive tetracycline or other antibiotics should only be considered if basic treatment of a tooth site fails to give clinical benefit when retreated at least twice. Also, it is difficult to choose between the various agents and delivery systems so it usually comes down to a choice of the method which works best for the clinician and individual patient. In general terms because of the significant risks of bacterial resistance to antibiotics it may be better to choose an antiseptic based system like the Perio Chip® (see Ch. 16) in preference to the antibiotic-based systems.

DEVELOPMENT OF BACTERIAL RESISTANCE OF PERIODONTAL BACTERIA TO ANTIBIOTICS USED IN PERIODONTAL THERAPY

The use of systemic antibiotics can easily produce bacterial resistance by the methods described above and this is particularly the case if:

- Doses of the same antibiotic are repeated within relatively short time periods
- Inappropriate antibiotics are prescribed
- Sub-optimal doses of antibiotic are given
- The prescribed regime is not adhered to by the patient.

Furthermore, oral administration of antibiotics also open the possibility of the development of resistance in members of the gastrointestinal bacterial flora. Finally, the appropriateness of the use of antibiotic therapy for chronic periodontitis could be questioned in view of the non-specific nature of the bacterial causation of that disease.

Local application may reduce the risk of systemic side-effects, as the dose absorbed is minimized. Also, the chances of the development of resistance in the gastrointestinal flora are reduced as little of the drug reaches this area. In this respect, the use of excessive amounts of antibiotic gel should be avoided as any that spills over into the mouth will be swallowed.

In the oral cavity, however, local application of antibiotic may pose an increased risk of the development and selection of resistant bacterial strains within the pocket flora possibly causing further deterioration or recurrence of periodontal disease (Larsen & Fiehn 1997). Resistance may also be produced as a result of sub-inhibitory antibiotic concentrations developing in the periodontal pocket due to rapid wash out of the antibiotic from this site. Growth of bacteria at sub-inhibitory concentrations of antibiotic facilitates the development of resistance and the emergence of a high proportion of resistant bacteria in periodontal pockets after the long-term low-dose administration of tetracycline has been shown (Kornman & Karl 1982; Williams et al 1979).

Local delivery of antibiotics to periodontal pockets produces very high concentrations initially but as the antibiotic is constantly washed out from the pocket this is quickly succeeded by sub-inhibitory concentrations, which may well facilitate the development of bacterial resistance. A recent study (Larsen & Fiehn 1997) investigated the possible development of resistance in suspected periodontal pathogens after exposure to sub-inhibitory concentrations of the two most commonly used antibiotics for local application in the treatment of periodontal disease, minocycline and metronidazole. The minimum inhibitory concentration (MIC) of 18 reference strains and 12 clinical isolates was determined. Subsequently, all strains with a MIC of $<8\,\mu g/mL$ were exposed to serial passage on plates containing sub-inhibitory and gradually increasing concentrations of these antibiotics, until growth was inhibited. Initially most strains were inhibited at $\geq 0.25\,\mu g/mL$ of minocycline and $0.5\,\mu g/mL$ of metronidazole, although *A. actinomycetemcomitans* was resistant to metronidazole. After growth at sub-inhibitory concentrations, eight strains survived 1–2 times and 11 strains survived 8–32 times their initial MIC of metronidazole. With respect to minocycline *A. actinomycetemcomitans* survived 8–64 times their initial MIC while all other strains survived 1–8 times their MIC. Thus, significant resistance to these antibiotics was shown to develop in suspected periodontal pathogens and this could easily occur following their local application. Furthermore, widespread appearance of tetracycline resistance in medically important bacteria has limited the use of this antibiotic in the treatment of medical infections (Speer et al 1992).

In the oral cavity, tetracycline resistance has also been shown to correlate to prior administration of this antibiotic and while resistance was only seen in 1–7% of isolates in patients not treated with antibiotics, it was seen in over 20% of isolates following tetracycline treatment (Fiehn & Westergaard 1990; Olsvik et al 1995; Walker et al 1983). In some studies of systemic administration (Fiehn & Westergaard 1990; Hawley et al 1980; Heimdahl & Nord 1983) the percentage of resistant organisms has been shown to return to baseline levels after 3 months.

Studies of local application of tetracyclines (Goodson & Tanner 1992; Larsen 1991; O'Connor et al 1990; Preus et al 1995) have shown a similar pattern possibly because of the initial very high concentration of antibiotic for the first 48 h. However, it cannot be excluded that resistance may increase further upon repeated exposure to sub-inhibitory concentrations by the frequent use of subgingival antibiotics in maintenance patients and this could lead to resistance levels in periodontopathic bacteria with clinical implications.

Common to all these studies was, however, the maintenance of high inhibitory concentrations in the periodontal pocket for 1–3 weeks. In the older studies (Kornman & Karl 1982; Williams et al 1979) resistance was determined after systemic administration of low, sub-inhibitory doses of tetracyclines over long periods and these recorded resistance in up to 77% of isolates and one (Kornman & Karl 1982) showed that 26% of isolates were still resistant 6–24 months after discontinuation of this antibiotic.

Rodrigues et al (2004) evaluated longitudinally the tetracycline resistance patterns of the subgingival microbiota of periodontitis subjects treated with systemic or local tetracycline therapy plus scaling and root planing (SRP). A total of 30 chronic periodontitis patients were randomly assigned to three groups: SRP plus 500 mg of systemic tetracycline twice/day for 14 days; SRP alone and SRP plus tetracycline fibres (Actsite®) at four selected sites for 10 days. Subgingival plaque samples were obtained from four sites with probing pocket depths (PPD) ≥6 mm in each patient at baseline, 1 week, 3, 6 and 12 months post-therapy. The percentage of resistant microorganisms was determined and the isolates identified by DNA probes and the checkerboard method. The percentage of resistant microorganisms increased significantly at 1 week in the tetracycline groups, but dropped to baseline levels over time. The SRP plus Actsite® group presented the lowest proportions of resistant species at 6 and 12 months. No significant changes were observed in the SRP group. The predominant tetracycline-resistant species included *Streptococcus* spp., *Veillonella parvula*, *Peptostreptococcus micros*, *Prevotella intermedia*, *Gemella morbillorum* and *A. actinomycetemcomitans* (Aa). A high percentage of sites with resistant Aa, *Porphyromonas gingivalis* and *Tannerella forsythensis* was observed in all groups at baseline. However *T. forsythensis* was not detected in any group and *P. gingivalis* was not present in the SRP plus Actsite® group at 1 year post-therapy. Aa was still frequently detected in all groups after therapy. However, the greatest reduction was observed in the SRP plus Actsite® group. Thus, local or systemically administered tetracycline results in selection of subgingival species probably from those intrinsically resistant to this drug. Although the percentage of sites harbouring periodontal pathogens resistant to tetracycline were quite elevated in this population, both therapies were effective in reducing their prevalence over time. However, resistance from this small pool could very easily pass from species to species by a variety of methods in the close relationships of dental plaques.

Resistance to metronidazole is less common in spite of the fact that it has been used extensively (Edwards 1993; Garcia-Rodriguez et al 1995). The development of metronidazole resistance has not been studied following its systemic use in periodontal patients but one study of its local application (Pedrazzoli et al 1992) reported no increase in resistance 6 months after therapy.

However, in other parts of the body resistance to metronidazole has been described in *Bacteroides* species and in *Helicobacter pylori* causing active gastritis and peptic ulcers (Banatavala et al 1994; Edwards 1993;

Noache et al 1994; Sprott et al 1983). *H. pylori* resistance has been shown to develop during antibiotic treatment (Goodwin et al 1988; Hirschl et al 1988) and the prevalence of resistance is associated with previous intake of metronidazole (Banatavala et al 1994). In *Bacteroides* species, resistance to metronidazole has been shown to be transferable by several mechanisms (Garcia-Rodriguez et al 1995). Furthermore, in a group of patients *H. pylori* gastric infection, pretreatment metronidazole-susceptible isolates were shown to be genetically identical to post treatment metronidazole-resistant isolates and this suggests that resistance had developed in the existing flora (Rautelin et al 1994).

These *in vivo* studies complement *in vitro* studies on the development of metronidazole resistance in *H. pylori*. These studies exposed the bacteria to serial passage on plates containing sub-inhibitory concentrations of metronidazole and found increased resistance in up to 75% of the strains (Haas et al 1990; van Zwet et al 1994). Furthermore, in the majority of isolates the acquired resistance was stable (van Zwet et al 1994). This is in agreement with the study of Larsen and Fiehn (1997) which showed that metronidazole resistance of 32 times their initial MIC developed in suspected periodontal pathogens including *P. gingivalis, P. anaerobius, Prevotella intermedia* and *Fusobacterium nucleatum*.

Thus, it has been shown that bacterial resistance to metronidazole can develop in previously susceptible bacteria including putative periodontal pathogens. Therefore, the use of this antibiotic should be restricted to situations where it is absolutely necessary.

Studies of the effects of a single course of either amoxicillin, metronidazole or doxycycline (Feres et al 1999, 2001, 2002) on the susceptibilities of subgingival bacteria showed that the numbers of resistant bacteria increased in the first weeks after therapy but returned to baseline levels 90 days after therapy. This shows good recovery after single therapy episodes but the results would probably have been greater and much more prolonged after repeated antibiotic administrations.

Another study (Sanai et al 2002) of 150 children of 8–11 showed that 31% of them already harboured putative periodontal pathogens including *Porphyromonas gingivalis, Prevotella intermedia* and *P. nigrescens* in their mouths and that two-thirds of the isolates from these subjects carried the erm (F), erythromycin resistance and tet (Q), tetracycline resistance genes. Thus many of the commensal bacteria acquired by children from contact with adults already carry antibiotic resistance genes.

Lakhssassi et al (2005) studied the antibiotic susceptibilities of *P. gingivalis, Prevotella intermedia, T. forsythia, F. nucleatum* and *Peptostreptococcus micros* to 10 commonly used antibiotics. It was found to vary according to bacterial species and antimicrobial molecules. The variability seemed to be greater with older molecules (penicillin G, tetracycline, erythromycin) than with more recent ones (amoxicillin, amoxicillin/clavulanate, ampicillin and doxycycline), which showed more stable results. *Prevotella intermedia* appeared to be the bacteria most resistant to penicillins and showed the highest coefficient of variation.

van Winkelhoff et al (2005) compared the antimicrobial susceptibility profiles of five periodontal bacteria isolated from periodontitis patients in Spain and in the Netherlands. Subgingival plaque samples from adult patients with periodontitis were collected and cultured on selective and non-selective plates. *A. actinomycetemcomitans, Porphyromonas gingivalis, Prevotella intermedia, F. nucleatum* and *Macromonas micros* were isolated and used for minimal inhibitory concentration tests using the Epsilometer (Etest) technique. Eight different antibiotics were tested on all bacterial isolates. MIC50 and MIC90 values for each antibiotic and each species were determined and the percentage of resistant strains was calculated. Significantly higher MIC values were noted in Spanish strains of *F. nucleatum* for penicillin and ciprofloxacin, of *P. intermedia* for penicillin, amoxicillin and tetracycline, of *M. micros* for tetracycline, amoxicillin and azithromycin and of *Porphyromonas gingivalis* for tetracycline and ciprofloxacin. Based on breakpoint concentrations, a higher number of resistant strains in Spain were found in *F. nucleatum* for penicillin, amoxicillin and metronidazole, in *Prevotella intermedia* for tetracycline and amoxicillin and in *A. actinomycetemcomitans* for amoxicillin and azithromycin. Resistance of *Porphyromonas gingivalis* strains was not observed for any of the antibiotics tested both in Spain and the Netherlands. This showed that differences exist in the susceptibility profiles of periodontal pathogens isolated from periodontitis patients in Spain and in the Netherlands. This implicates that antibiotic susceptibility testing is necessary to determine efficacy of antimicrobial agents. Also, clinical studies with antibiotics should take these differences into account. The information from the present study indicates that it may not be possible to develop uniform protocols for usage of antibiotics in the treatment of severe periodontitis in the European Union.

All these studies show the importance of:

■ Limiting the use of antibiotics to situations when it is absolutely necessary
■ Avoiding the repeat use of the same antibiotic within 3 months of its previous administration
■ Achieving high inhibitory concentrations at the treatment site (the periodontal pocket) for the whole duration of the treatment whether using systemic or local administration.

THE NON-ANTIBIOTIC PROPERTIES OF TETRACYCLINES

Tetracyclines (TCs) have been found to inhibit host-derived collagenases and some other matrix metalloproteinases (MMPs) by a mechanism independent of the well known antimicrobial activity of these drugs (Golub et al 1983, 1984, 1985, 1987, 1991, 1992; Rifkin et al 1993; Ryan et al 1996). The first discovery that tetracyclines can inhibit host-derived MMPs by a mechanism independent of their antimicrobial properties was made in germ-free rats with experimentally induced diabetes, a model of excess collagenase activity (Golub et al 1983).

Available antimicrobial TCs with these properties are minocycline, doxycycline and tetracycline itself. Recently, however, Golub and co-workers (Golub et al 1987, 1991, 1992; Rifkin et al 1993; Yu et al 1993) have synthesized 10 different analogues of the tetracycline molecule which are known as chemically modified tetracyclines (CMTs) and all of these totally lack antimicrobial properties. In spite of this, nine of them exhibited strong collagenase inhibition properties. The CMT that lost its anticollagenase activity was CMT-5 and this was the pyrazole analogue, in which the carbon-11 carbonyl oxygen and carbon-12 hydroxy groups were replaced by nitrogen atoms. This eliminated the important Zn^{2+} and Ca^{2+} binding site in the tetracycline molecule, which is active at physiological pH.

The mechanism proposed to explain these anticollagenase properties concerned the Zn^{2+} and Ca^{2+} binding properties of the TC molecule and explained the ability of TCs to inhibit already active collagenase or gelatinase in the extracellular matrix. It is supported by several pieces of recent evidence. First, adding excess Zn^{2+} or Ca^{2+} ions eliminates this property (Golub et al 1983; Yu et al 1991). Second, collagenase now appears to contain secondary Zn^{2+} and Ca^{2+} ions outside the catalytic domain of the enzyme, in addition to those within this domain. These secondary ions help to maintain the conformity and catalytic activity of the enzyme (Lovejoy et al 1994). The proposed mechanism suggested that TCs interacted with these secondary metal ions in particular Zn^{2+} (Golub et al 1991). Third, the mechanism of this action is not associated with fragmentation of the MMP molecule and the results of *in vitro* experiments suggest a non-competitive action of these drugs (Sorsa et al 1994). Thus, these findings suggest that TCs other than CMT-5 may bind secondary Zn^{2+} and to a lesser extent Ca^{2+} in collagenase, thus altering the conformity of the enzyme molecule and blocking its catalytic activity.

TCs have been found to inhibit collagenases from a number of cell and tissue sources including PMNs, macrophages, osteoblasts, osteoclasts, chondrocytes and tumour cells and rat skin and gingiva and human gingiva (Golub et al 1991; Rifkin et al 1993). Recent studies show that different tissues and cells vary in their susceptibility to TC collagenase inhibition and members of the TC family vary in regard to their collagenase inhibitory activity. In respect of the first point, collagenase and other MMPs from PMNs (MMP-8,9) are highly sensitive to TC inhibition whilst those from fibroblasts (MMP-1,2) are relatively resistant (Ingman et al 1993). With regard to the second point, the semi-synthetic TCs, doxycycline and minocycline and the CMTs, are more potent for this action than tetracycline itself (Rifkin et al 1993; Ryan et al 1996).

TCs and CMTs have also been found to inhibit bone resorption at concentrations within the normal therapeutic dose range of these drugs (Rifkin et al 1993). They appear to reduce the degradation of osteoid by inhibition of osteoblast collagenase. They also appear to increase bone formation by increasing alkaline phosphatase and collagen synthesis by these cells. They appear to decrease bone resorption by elevating osteoclast intracellular calcium levels, decreasing the osteoclast ruffled border, decreasing osteoclast acid production, decreasing osteoclast secretion of cysteine proteinases (cathepsins B and L) and inhibiting osteoclast MMPs.

In animal model studies, three different models have been studied (Rifkin et al 1993). First, the effect of TCs was studied on the excessive alveolar bone loss seen in surgically de-salivated rats and it was found to reduce the bone loss in these animals compared to controls untreated with TCs. Second, its effect on accelerated periodontal disease in diabetic rats was studied. Severe disease was produced by inducing accelerated plaque formation and this was then exacerbated by making the animals diabetic by the administration of streptozotocin. Daily tetracycline or CMT-1 administration reduced the excessive collagenase activity in their gingival tissue and reduced the severity of the disease. Interestingly, while tetracycline induced the emergence of tetracycline resistant bacteria in their oral cavities, the use of CMT-1 did not have this unwanted effect. Third, their effects on gnotobiotic rats monoinfected with *P. gingivalis* were studied (Rifkin et al 1993; Golub et al 1994). The infected animals showed marked gingival inflammation and bone loss compared with non-infected controls. Daily administration of either CMT-1, with no antimicrobial properties and doxycycline, with antimicrobial properties, for 8 weeks at normal therapeutic dosage resulted in significant reductions in both gingival inflammation and alveolar bone loss and also significantly reduced gingival tissue collagenase concentration.

Finally, it has been found that CMT-1 administration can normalize the collagen metabolism in diabetic rats which otherwise exhibit severe collagen depletion in the skin and gingiva (Yu et al 1993).

In human studies, TCs, given in normal therapeutic doses, have been shown to reduce collagenase, in particular MMP-8, activity in gingival tissue, gingival crevicular fluid (GCF) and saliva (Golub et al 1985, 1991; Rifkin et al 1993; Sorsa et al 1994). The majority of gingival tissue extracellular collagenase and GCF collagenase activity comes from inflammatory cells rather than fibroblasts and it is that form of MMP activity that is most susceptible to TCs. In addition, it has been found that a 3-week course of regular dose doxycycline reduced periodontal attachment loss in refractory periodontitis patients 7 months after stopping the treatment (Lee et al 1991). It has also been found that doxycycline inhibited both PMN produced MMPs in gingival tissue and also bacterial collagenase produced by *P. gingivalis* (Golub et al 1995).

The type of periodontal disease being potentially treated is important since the type of predominating MMP in gingival tissue, GCF and saliva varies (Ingman et al 1993). In adult chronic periodontitis the PMN-derived MMPs (MMP-8, 9) predominate which are highly sensitive to inhibition with TCs and CMTs while in localized juvenile periodontitis, the fibroblast-derived MMP-1 predominates, albeit at low levels and this is relatively resistant to these drugs. In this regard, it has been shown that MMP-8 was inhibited *in vitro* by doses of TCs of 75 μM/L, while MMP-1 was relatively insensitive to 100 μM/L (Ingman et al 1993; Sorsa et al 1994). MMP-1 was however inhibited by doses of 600 μM/L. It would therefore appear that adult chronic periodontitis is more likely to be effectively treated by the anti-collagenase effects of TCs than localized juvenile periodontitis.

Thus, it would appear that CMTs lacking antimicrobial effects and hence the unwanted effects of inducing bacterial resistance, might have a therapeutic role in the treatment of adult chronic periodontitis in the future. Their proven abilities to both inhibit inflammatory cell MMPs and favourably modify bone metabolism would seem to be of major significance in this regard.

Recently, a 20 mg capsule of doxycycline hyclate (Periostat®) has been approved by the United States of America Food and Drug Administration for adjunctive use in the treatment of adult periodontitis and may be prescribed twice daily. The mechanism of action postulated is its suppression of collagenase activity, particularly MMP-8 from PMNs (Ciancio 2002). Although this drug is one of the tetracycline family of antimicrobial agents and at higher dosage does have an antimicrobial effect, it is postulated not to have this effect at this low dosage. However, one study (Walker 2000) has shown that this regime does significantly decrease the number of spirochaetes and motile rods and increase the number of coccoid bacteria suggesting that it does have some antimicrobial action in the longer term. It is therefore possible that it could stimulate, if used over a prolonged time, the development of bacterial resistance to tetracycline. Therefore it would seem preferable to use a non-antimicrobial chemically modified form of tetracycline (CMT) for this purpose such as CMT 1–4, 6–10 (Golub et al 1987, 1991, 1992; Rifkin et al 1993; Yu et al 1993) rather than doxycycline. One clinical study (Caton et al 2000) reported the results of a 9-month clinical trial of Periostat® as an adjunctive to scaling and root planing (SRP) compared to a placebo plus SRP in 190 adult periodontitis patients. It showed that the test group had a statistically significantly greater numbers of treated sites which attained clinically significant reductions in probing depths (≥2 mm) and gains in clinical attachment level (≥3 mm) than the control group. This result needs to be confirmed by further independent studies.

The effect of low dose doxycycline as an adjunct to replaced flap surgery in patients with advanced periodontitis has been investigated (Gapski et al 2004). A total of 24 subjects were enrolled into a 12-month, randomized, placebo-controlled, double-masked trial and clinical and microbiological data were recorded in response to 6 months therapy of either placebo capsules plus replaced flap surgery or low-dose (20 mg) doxycycline plus replaced flap surgery. Data were recorded at baseline and 3, 6, 9 and 12 months after surgery. Patients treated with adjunctive low dose doxycycline had greater reductions in probing depths and greater gains in clinical attachment level than the placebo group with a low level of statistical significance ($p<0.05$). There were no significant differences in microbiological data between the two groups suggesting that the low dose doxycycline did not produce any significant shifts in the microbiota. A further multicentre trial shows similar results (Preshaw et al 2004) as does another similar, double-masked, randomized, placebo-controlled, study (Lee et al 2004). Thus this shows a small adjunctive benefit of this regime with both basic and surgical treatment. However, the small benefits may not justify its use due to possible effects of this regime on bacterial resistance stated below.

Four studies summarized in one report (Ciancio 2000) sought to assess whether long-term therapy with twice daily Periostat® changed the antibiotic susceptibly of the oral flora of periodontal patients. They appeared to show that the MIC levels remained the same in the test and control groups at 18 and 24 months of the 2-year studies. Another study by the same research group (Walker et al 2000) also appeared to show that long-term twice daily Periostat® had no effects on the composition of the faecal or vaginal microflora in the test group compared with a control group.

Payne et al (2007) investigated the efficacy of 2-year continuous sub-antimicrobial dose doxycycline on alveolar bone in post-menopausal osteopenic, oestrogen-deficient women undergoing periodontal maintenance in a 2-year double-blind, placebo-controlled, randomized clinical trial. However, in these women with periodontitis sub-antimicrobial dose doxycycline did not differ overall from placebo and thus was of no benefit.

Soory (2008) in a review for non-antimicrobial actions of tetracyclines in combating oxidative stress in periodontal and metabolic disease showed that tetracyclines had diverse mechanisms of overcoming oxidative stress and enhancing matrix synthesis.

While these studies seem to indicate that this regime had no effects on bacterial resistance to tetracyclines it is difficult to know whether this will remain true in the future particularly if its use increases. Furthermore, its apparent clinical benefits need to be confirmed by other independent studies.

POSSIBLE INDICATIONS FOR ANTIBIOTIC USE IN PERIODONTAL TREATMENT

It seems from current available evidence that although systemic administration and local application of tetracycline and metronidazole can produce similar clinical and bacteriological effects to scaling and root planing they appear to offer no significant advantages and used on their own are generally inferior to scaling and root planing (see above). There are also compelling reasons for avoiding antibiotics in situations where other treatments are equally effective because of the risks of developing bacterial resistance to their effects (see above). It should also be realized that the concentrations of antibiotic needed to kill or inhibit the growth of bacteria within a biofilm such as dental or subgingival plaque is 50–200 times higher than that for bacteria growing planktonically (Anwar et al 1992; Brown & Gilbert 1993; Vorachit et al 1993; Wright et al 1997). This almost certainly means that bacteria in this situation are likely to be resistant to the concentrations of antibiotic likely to present in the periodontal pocket following systemic administration of an antibiotic. However, the use of the adjunctive antibiotic gels or fibres occasionally may be advantageous in a few situations (Goodson 1994). These are:

- Deep pockets with very difficult access for scaling and root planing
- Deep pocket sites in refractory or rapidly progressive periodontitis
- Pockets exuding pus.

They should, however, only be considered for use if these sites persistently fail to respond to repeated scaling and root planing. In this situation several studies have indicated that 1% metronidazole gel, 1% chlorhexidine gel and tetracycline-loaded fibres produced short-term resolution of persistent refractory pocket sites (Perinetti et al 2004; Aimetti et al 2004). However, when tested for their ability to inhibit *P. gingivalis* within an artificial biofilm *in vitro* (see above) only chlorhexidine inhibited it strongly and tetracycline and metronidazole had only weak effects (Noiri et al 2003). Moreover, antimicrobials cannot be repeated so may only delay a recurrent problem.

Strategy for the use of adjunctive local antimicrobials

1. Subgingival antimicrobials should never be used alone since mechanical disruption of the biofilm is necessary to achieve their penetration to the active sites (Tonetti 1998). Furthermore, even the best delivery systems with the best pharmacokinetic profiles and effecting substantial depression of subgingival microbiota, are unable to completely disinfect a periodontal pocket. They should therefore only be used as adjunctive to scaling and root planing.
2. Since, the changes in the bacterial flora by antimicrobials are similar in amount and duration to that produced by scaling and root planing they should only be considered for use in pockets that are refractory to repeated use of this procedure.

Ciancio SG: Systemic medications: clinical significance in periodontics, *J Clin Periodontol* 29(Suppl 2):17–21, 2002.

Ciancio SG, Cobb CM, Leung M: Tissue concentration and localisation of tetracycline following site-specific therapy, *J Periodontol* 63:849–853, 1992.

Collaborative Study Group: Prospective study of the ampicillin rash, *Br Med J* 1:7–9, 1973.

Corsair A: Long-term effect of tetracycline fibres on recurrent lesions in periodontal maintenance patients, *Periodontal Clin Investig* 16:8–13, 1994.

Dash CH: Penicillin allergy and cephalosporins, *J Antimicrob Chemother* 1(Suppl): 107–118, 1975.

Davies J: What are antibiotics? Archaic functions for modern activities, *Mol Microbiol* 4:1227–1232, 1990.

Dees J, Colston J: Use of sulphonamide in gonococcal infections: a preliminary report, *J Am Med Assoc* 108:1855–1858, 1937.

Department of Health and Social Security: *Guidance on the control of infection in hospitals prepared by the joint DHSS/PHLS Hospital Infection Working Group ('The Cooke Report')*, London, 1998, DHSS.

Di Vita VJ, Mekalanos JJ: Genetic control of bacterial virulence, *Am Rev Genet* 23:455–482, 1989.

Drisko CH: The use of locally-delivered doxycycline in the treatment of periodontitis. Clinical results, *J Clin Periodontol* 25:947–952, 1998.

Edwards DI: Nitroimidazole drugs – action and resistance mechanisms. II. Mechanisms of resistance, *J Antimicrob Chemother* 31:201–210, 1993.

Ehmke B, Moter A, Beikler T, et al: Adjunctive antimicrobial therapy of periodontitis: long-term effects on disease progression and oral colonization, *J Periodontol* 76:749–759, 2005.

Eltringham I: Mupirocin resistance and methicillin-resistant Staphylococcus aureus (MRSA), *J Hosp Infect* 35:1–8, 1997.

Endz HP, Ruijs GJ, van Klingeren B, et al: Quinolone resistance in Campylobacter isolated from man and poultry following the introduction of fluoroquinolones in veterinary medicine, *J Antimicrob Chemother* 27:199–208, 1991.

Evans D, Allison D, Brown M, et al: Effect of growth rate on resistance of Gram-negative biofilms to cetrimide, *J Antimicrob Chemother* 26:473–478, 1990.

Farmer T, Reading C: Beta-lactamases of Brauhamella catarrhalis and their inhibition by clavulanic acid, *Antimicrob Agents Chemother* 21:506–508, 1982.

Feres M, Haffajee AD, Gonclaves C, et al: Systemic doxycycline administration in the treatment of periodontal infections. II. effect on antibiotic resistance of subgingival species, *J Clin Periodontol* 26:784–792, 1999.

Feres M, Haffajee AD, Allard KA, et al: Change in subgingival microbial profiles in adult periodontitis subjects receiving either systemically administered amoxicillin or metronidazole, *J Clin Periodontol* 28:597–609, 2001.

Feres M, Haffajee AD, Allard KA, et al: Antibiotic resistance of subgingival species during and after antibiotic therapy, *J Clin Periodontol* 29:724–735, 2002.

Fiehn N-E, Westergaard J: Doxycycline-resistant bacteria in periodontally diseased individuals after systemic doxycycline therapy and in healthy individuals, *Oral Microbiol Immunol* 5:219–222, 1990.

Finegold SM: Classification and taxonomy of anaerobes. In Finegold SM, George WL, editors: *Anaerobic Infections in Humans*, San Diego, 1989, Academic Press, pp 23–26.

Fish DN, Piscitelli SC, Danziger LH: Development of resistance during antimicrobial therapy: a review of antibiotic classes and patient characteristics in 173 studies, *Pharmacotherapy* 15:279–291, 1995.

Fontanals D, Pineda V, Pons I, et al: Penicillin-resistant beta-lactamase producing Neisseria meningitidis in Spain, *Eur J Clin Microbiol Infect Dis* 8:90–91, 1989.

Gapski R, Barr JL, Sarment DP, et al: Effect of systemic matrix metalloproteinase inhibition on periodontal wound repair: a proof of concept trial, *J Periodontol* 75: 441–452, 2004.

Garcia-Rodriguez JA, Garcia-Sánchez JE, Munoz-Bellido JL: Antimicrobial resistance in anaerobic bacteria: current situation, *Anaerobe* 1:69–80, 1995.

Gaunt PN, Piddock LJV: Ciprofoxacin resistant Campylobacter spp. in humans; an epidemiological and laboratory study, *J Antimicrob Chemother* 37:747–757, 1996.

Geddes AM, Bridgwater FAJ, Williams DN, et al: Clinical and bacteriological studies with clindamycin, *Br Med J* 2:703–704, 1970.

Gill Y, Scully C: British oral and maxillofacial surgeons' views on the aetiology and management of acute pericoronitis, *Br J Oral Maxillofac Surg* 29:180–182, 1991.

Goldstein FW, Acar JF: Antimicrobial resistance among lower respiratory tract isolates of Streptococcus pneumoniae: results of a 1992–1993 Western Europe and USA collaborative surveillance study. The Alexander Project Collaborative Group, *J Antimicrob Chemother* 38(Suppl A):71–84, 1996.

Golub LM, Lee HM, Lehrer G, et al: Minocycline reduces gingival collagenolytic activity during diabetes: preliminary observations and a proposed new mechanism, *J Periodontal Res* 21:18, 516–526, 1983.

Golub LM, Ramamurthy NS, McNamara TF, et al: Tetracyclines inhibit tissue collagenase activity: a new mechanism in the treatment of periodontal disease, *J Periodontal Res* 19:651–655, 1984.

Golub LM, Wolff M, Lee HM, et al: Further evidence that tetracyclines inhibit collagenase activity in human crevicular fluid and from other mammalian sources, *J Periodontal Res* 20:12–23, 1985.

Golub LM, McNamara TF, D'Angelo G, et al: A non-antimicrobial chemically-modified tetracycline inhibits mammalian collagenase activity, *J Dent Res* 66:1310–1314, 1987.

Golub LM, Ramamurthy NS, McNamara TF: Tetracyclines inhibit connective tissue breakdown: new therapeutic implications for an old family of drugs, *Crit Rev Oral Biol Med* 2:297–322, 1991.

Golub LM, Suomalainen K, Sorsa T: Host modulation with tetracyclines and their chemically modified analogues, *Curr Sci Curr Opin Dent* 2:80–90, 1992.

Golub LM, Evans RT, McNamara TF, et al: A non-antimicrobial tetracycline inhibits gingival matrix metalloproteinases and bone loss in Porphyromonas gingivalis-induced periodontitis in rats, *Ann N Y Acad Sci* 732:96–111, 1994.

Golub LM, Sorsa T, Lee H-M, et al: Doxycycline inhibits neutrophil (PMN)-type matrix metalloproteinases in adult periodontitis gingiva, *J Clin Periodontol* 22:100–109, 1995.

Goodson JM: Pharmacokinetics principles controlling efficacy of oral therapy, *J Dent Res* 68:1625–1632, 1989.

Goodson JM: Antimicrobial strategies or treatment of periodontal disease, *Periodontol 2000* 5:142–168, 1994.

Goodson JM, Tanner A: Antibiotic resistance of the subgingival microflora following local tetracycline treatment, *Oral Microbiol Immunol* 7:113–117, 1992.

Goodson JM, Haffajee AD, Socransky SS: Periodontal therapy by local delivery of tetracycline, *J Clin Periodontol* 6:83–92, 1979.

Goodson JM, Holborow D, Dunn R, et al: Monolithic tetracycline containing fibres for control delivery to periodontal pockets, *J Periodontol* 54:575–579, 1983.

Goodson JM, Hogan PE, Dunham SL: Clinical responses following periodontal treatment by local drug delivery, *J Periodontol* 56:81–87, 1985.

Goodson JM, Ugini MA, Kent RL, et al: Multicenter evaluation of tetracycline fibre therapy: I, experimental design, methods and baseline data, *J Periodontal Res* 26:361–370, 1991a.

Goodson JM, Ugini MA, Kent RL, et al: Multicenter evaluation of tetracycline fibre therapy: II. Clinical response, *J Periodontal Res* 26:371–379, 1991b.

Goodson JM, Tanner A, McArdle S, et al: Multicenter evaluation of tetracycline fibre therapy: III. microbiological response, *J Periodontal Res* 26:440–451, 1991c.

Goodwin CS, Marshall BJ, Blincow ED, et al: Prevention of nitroimidazole resistance in Campylobacter pylori by coadministration of colloidal bismuth subcitrate: clinical and in vitro studies, *J Clin Pathol* 41:207–210, 1988.

Gordon JM, Walker CB, Murphy JC, et al: Tetracycline levels achievable in gingival crevice fluid and in vitro effect on subgingival organisms. Part 1. Concentrations in crevicular fluid after repeated doses, *J Periodontol* 52:609–612, 1981.

Green RJ, Harris ND: Infections and antimicrobial therapy. In *Pathology and Therapeutics for Pharmacists. A Basis for Clinical Pharmacy Practice*, London, 1993, Chapman and Hall, Ch. 12, pp 548–581.

Greenstein G: Local drug delivery in the treatment of periodontal diseases: assessing the clinical significance of the results, *J Periodontol* 77:565–578, 2006.

Haas CE, Nix DE, Schentag JJ: *In vitro* selection of resistant Heliobacter pylori, *Antimicrob Agents Chemother* 34:1637–1641, 1990.

Haffajee AD, Uzel NG, Arguello EI, et al: Clinical and microbiological changes associated with the use of combined antimicrobial therapies to treat 'refractory' periodontitis, *J Clin Periodontol* 31:869–877, 2004.

Hall RM, Brookes DE, Stokes HW: Site-specific insertion of genes into integrins: role of the 59-base element and determination of the recombination cross-over point, *Mol Microbiol* 5:1941–1959, 1991.

Handal T, Olsen I, Walker CB, et al: Beta-lactamase production and antimicrobial susceptibility of subgingival bacteria from refractory periodontitis, *Oral Microbiol Immunol* 19:303–308, 2004.

Hansberger H: Pharmacodynamic effects of antibiotics. Studies on bacterial morphology, initial killing, post-antibiotics effect and effective regrown time, *Scand J Infect Dis* 81(Suppl):1–52, 1992.

Hawley RJ, Lee LN, LeBlanc DJ: Effects of tetracycline on the streptococcal flora of periodontal pockets, *Antimicrob Agents Chemother* 17:372–378, 1980.

Heijl L, Dahlen G, Sundin Y, et al: A 4-quadrant comparative study of periodontal treatment using tetracycline-containing drug delivery fibres and scaling, *J Clin Periodontol* 18:111–116, 1991.

Heimdahl A, Nord CE: Influence of doxycycline on the normal oral flora and colonisation of the oral cavity and colon, *Scand J Infect Dis* 15:293–302, 1983.

Herrera D, Roldán S, Sanz M: The periodontal abscess: a review, *J Clin Periodontol* 27:377–386, 2000.

Herrera D, Roldán S, González I, Sanz M: The periodontal abscess. I. Clinical and microbiological findings, *J Clin Periodontol* 27:387–394, 2000a.

Herrera D, Roldán S, O'Connor A, Sanz M: The periodontal abscess. II. Microbiological efficiency of 2 systemic antibiotic regimens, *J Clin Periodontol* 27:387–394, 2000b.

Herrera D, Sanz M, Jepsen S, et al: A systematic review on the effect of systemic antimicrobials as an adjunct to scaling and root planning in periodontitis patients, *J Clin Periodontol* 29(Suppl 3):136–159, 2002.

Higashi K, Morisaki K, Hayashi S, et al: Local ofloxacin delivery using a controlled-release insert (PT-01) in the human periodontal pocket, *J Periodontal Res* 25:1–5, 1990.

Hiramatsu K, Hanaka H, Ino T, et al: Methicillin-resistant Staphylococcus aureus clinical strain with reduced vancomycin susceptibility, *J Antimicrob Chemother* 40:135–136, 1997.

Hirschl AM, Hentschel E, Schütze K, et al: The efficiency of antimicrobial treatment of Campylobacter pylori-associated gastritis and duodenal ulcer, *Scand J Gastroenterol* 23:76–81, 1988.

Hitzig C, Fosse T, Charbit Y, et al: Effects of combined topical metronidazole and mechanical treatment on the subgingival flora of deep periodontal pockets in cuspids and bicuspids, *J Periodontol* 68:613–617, 1997.

Holmes RK, Joblin MC: Genetics. In Baron S, editor: *Medical Microbiology*, ed 3, 1991, New York, 1991, Churchill Livingstone, Ch. 5, pp 91–122.

Hook EWD, Judson FN, Handsfield HH, et al: Auxotype/serovar diversity and antimicrobial resistance of Neisseria gonorrhoeae in two mid-sized American cities, *Sex Transm Dis* 14:141–146, 1987.

Hughes VM, Datta N: Conjunctive plasmids in bacteria of the pre-antibiotic era, *Nature* 302:725–726, 1983.

Huovinen P, Seppala H, Kataja J, et al: The relationship between erythromycin consumption and antibiotic resistance in Finland. Finnish Study Group for Antimicrobial Resistance, *Ciba Found Symp* 207:36–41, 1997.

Ingman T, Sorsa T, Konttinen YT, et al: Salivary collagenase, elastase- and trypsin-like proteases as biochemical markers of periodontal tissue destruction in adult and localized juvenile periodontitis, *Oral Microbiol Immunol* 8:298–305, 1993.

Jick H: Adverse reactions to trimethoprim-sulfamethoxazole in hospitalized patients, *Rev Infect Dis* 4:426–428, 1982.

Johnson AP, James D: Continuing increase in invasive methicillin-resistant Staphylococcus aureus infections, *Lancet* 350:1710, 1997.

Joyston-Bechal S, Smales FC, Duckworth R: Effect of metronidazole on chronic periodontal disease in subjects using a topically applied chlorhexidine gel, *J Clin Periodontol* 11:53–62, 1984.

Joyston-Bechal S, Smales FC, Duckworth R: A follow-up study 3 years after metronidazole therapy for chronic periodontal disease, *J Clin Periodontol* 13:944–949, 1986.

Kavi J: Mupirocin-resistant Staphylococcus aureus, *Lancet* 2:1472–1473, 1987.

Killoy WJ: The clinical significance of local chemotherapies, *J Clin Periodontol* 29(Suppl):22–29, 2002.

Kingsman AJ, Charter KF, Kingsman SM: *Transposition 43rd Symposium for Society for General Microbiology*, Cambridge, 1998, Cambridge University Press.

Klinge B, Kuvatanasuhati J, Attström R, et al: The effect of topical metronidazole therapy on experimentally-induced periodontitis in the beagle dog, *J Clin Periodontol* 19:702–707, 1992a.

Klinge B, Attström R, Karring T, et al: Three regimes of topical metronidazole therapy compared with subgingival scaling on periodontal pathology in adults, *J Clin Periodontol* 19:708–714, 1992b.

Kohara Y, Adiyama K, Isona K: The physical map of the whole E. coli chromosome: application of a new strategy for rapid analysis and sorting of a large genome, *Cell* 50:495–508, 1987.

Kornman KS: Controlled-release local delivery antimicrobials in periodontics: prospects for the future, *J Periodontol* 64:782–791, 1993.

Kornman KS, Karl EH: The effect of long-term, low-dose tetracycline therapy on the subgingival microflora in refractory adult periodontitis, *J Periodontol* 53:604–610, 1982.

Lakhssassi CN, Elhajoui N, Lodter J, et al: Antimicrobial susceptibility variation of 50 anaerobic periopathogens in aggressive periodontitis: an interindividual variability study, *Oral Microbiol Immunol* 20:244–252, 2005.

Lang R, Lishner M, Ravid M: Adverse reaction to prolonged treatment with high dosage carbenicillin and ureidopenicillins, *Rev Infect Dis* 13:68–72, 1991.

Larsen T: Occurrence of doxycycline-resistant bacteria in the oral cavity after local administration of doxycycline in patients with periodontal disease, *Scand J Infect Dis* 23:89–95, 1991.

Larsen T, Fiehn, NE: Development of resistance to metronidazole and minocycline *in vitro*, *J Clin Periodontol* 24:254–259, 1997.

Larsen T: Susceptibility of Porphyromonas gingivalis biofilms to amoxicillin, doxycycline and metronidazole, *Oral Microbiol Immunol* 17:267–271, 2002.

Laurence DE, Bennett DN, Brown MJ: Infection and inflammation. In *Clinical Pharmacology*, ed 8, New York, 1997, Churchill Livingstone. Section 3. Chs. 11–14, pp 187–248.

Laurichesse H, Grimaud O, Waight P: Pneumococcal bacteria and meningitis in England and Wales 1993–1995, *Commun Dis Public Health* 1:22–27, 1996.

Lee W, Aitken S, Kulkarni G, et al: Collagenase activity in recurrent periodontitis: relationship to disease progression and doxycycline therapy, *J Periodontal Res* 26:479–485, 1991.

Lee J-Y, Lee Y-M, Shin S-Y, et al: Effect of subantimicrobial dose doxycycline as an effective adjunct to scaling and root planing, *J Periodontol* 75:1500–1508, 2004.

Levine BB: Penicillin allergy and the heterogeneous immune response to benzylpenicillin, *J Clin Investig 1996* 45:1898–1906, 1996.

Lewis MA, MacFarlane TW, McGowan DA: A microbiological and clinical review of the acute dentoalveolar abscess, *Br J Oral Maxillofac Surg* 28:359–366, 1990.

Lind I: Epidemiology of antibiotic-resistant Neisseria gonorrhoeae in industrialised and developing countries, *Scand J Infect Dis Suppl* 169:77–82, 1990.

Lindhe J, Heijl L, Goodson JM, et al: Local tetracycline delivery using hollow fibre devices in periodontal therapy, *J Clin Periodontol* 6:141–149, 1979.

Lindhe J, Liljenberg B, Adielson B, et al: Use of metronidazole as a probe in the study of human periodontal disease, *J Clin Periodontol* 10:100–111, 1983.

Listgarten MA, Lindhe J, Helldén L: Effect of tetracycline and/or scaling in human periodontal disease, *J Clin Periodontol* 5:246–271, 1978.

Livermore DM: Beta-lactamases in clinical and laboratory resistance, *Clin Infect Dis* 15:824–839, 1992.

Livermore DM: Beta-lactamases in laboratory and clinical resistance, *Clin Microbiol Rev* 8:557–584, 1995.

Livermore DM: Acquired carbapenemases, *J Antimicrob Chemother* 39:673–676, 1997.

Livermore DM, Yuan M: Antibiotic resistance and production of extended-spectrum-beta-lactamases among Klebsiella spp from intensive care units in Europe, *J Antimicrob Chemother* 38:409–427, 1996.

Loesche WJ: Chemotherapy of dental plaque infections, *Oral Science Review* 9:65–107, 1976.

Loesche WJ, Syed SA, Morrison EC, et al: Metronidazole in periodontitis. I. Clinical and bacteriological results after 15 to 30 weeks, *J Periodontol* 55:325–335, 1985.

Loesche WJ, Schmidt E, Smith BA, et al: Effects of metronidazole on periodontal treatment needs, *J Periodontol* 62:247–257, 1991.

Loesche WJ, Giordano JR, Hujoel PP, et al: Metronidazole in periodontitis: Reduced needs for surgery, *J Clin Periodontol* 19:103–112, 1992.

Loesche WJ, Grossman N, Giordano JR: Metronidazole in periodontitis. IV. The effect of patient compliance on treatment parameters, *J Clin Periodontol* 20:96–104, 1993.

Lovejoy B, Cleasby A, Hassell A, et al: Structure of the catalytic domain of fibroblast collagenase complexed with an inhibitor, *Sci* 263:375–377, 1994.

Magnusson I: The use of locally-delivered metronidazole in the treatment of periodontitis. Clinical results, *J Clin Periodontol* 25:959–963, 1998.

Mandell GL, Petri WA: Antimicrobial agents: sulphonamides, trimethoprim-sulfamethoxazole, quinolones and agents: for urinary tract infections. In Goodman-Gilman A, Hardman JG, Limbird LE, Molinoff PB, Ruddon RE, editors: *Goodman & Gilman's the pharmacological basis of therapeutics*, ed 9, Section IX, Chemotherapy of microbial disease, New York, 1996a, McGraw-Hill, Ch. 44, pp. 1057–1072.

Mandell GL, Petri WA: Antimicrobial agents: penicillins, cephalosporins and other beta-lactam antibiotics. In Goodman-Gilman A, Hardman JG, Limbird LE, Molinoff PB, Ruddon RE, editors: *Goodman & Gilman's the pharmacological basis of therapeutics*, ed 9, Section IX, Chemotherapy of microbial disease, 1996b, New York, McGraw-Hill, Ch. 45, pp. 1073–1102.

Mandell RC, Tripodi LS, Savitt E, et al: The effect of treatment on Actinobacillus actinomycetemcomitans in localized juvenile periodontitis, *J Periodontol* 57:94–99, 1986.

Manian FA, Meyer L, Jenne J, et al: Loss of antimicrobial susceptibility in aerobic gram-negative bacilli repeatedly isolated from patients in intensive care units, *Infect Control Hosp Epidemiol* 17:222–226, 1996.

Maples RR, Speller DC, Cookson BD: Prevalence of Mupirocin resistance in Staphylococcus aureus, *J Hosp Infect* 29:153–155, 1995.

Martin MV, Longman LP, Hill JB, et al: Acute dentoalveolar infections: an investigation of the duration of antibiotic therapy, *Br Dent J* 183:135–137, 1997.

Martinez-Martinez L: ICAAC Abstract LB-20. In *ICAAC 1997*, Washington DC, 1997, American Society for Microbiology, p. 12.

McCracken GH Jr.: Emergence of resistant Streptococcus pneumoniae: a problem in pediatrics, *Pediatr Infect Dis J* 14:211–215, 1995.

McGowen JE Jr., Gerding DN: Does antibiotic restriction prevent resistance? *New Horiz* 4:370–376, 1996.

Meyer BK: Comparative toxicities of the 3rd generation cephalosporins, *Am J Med* 79(Suppl 12):96–103, 1985.

Miller JF, Mekalananos JJ, Falkow S: Coordinate regulation and sensory transduction in the control of bacterial virulence, *Sci* 243:916–922, 1989.

Mombelli A, Lehmann B, Tonetti M, et al: Clinical response to local delivery tetracycline in relation to overall and local periodontal conditions, *J Clin Periodontol* 24:470–477, 1997.

Moore M, Onorato IM, McCray E, et al: Trends in drug-resistant tuberculosis in the United States, 1993–1996, *J Am Med Assoc* 278:833–837, 1997.

Morrison SL, Cobb CM, Kazakos G, et al: Root surface characteristics associated with subgingival placement of monolithic tetracycline-impregnated fibres, *J Periodontol* 63:137–143, 1992.

Muder RR, Brennen C, Drenning SD, et al: Multiple resistant gram-negative bacilli in a long-term care facility; a case control study of patient risk factors and prior antibiotic use, *Infect Control Hosp Epidemiol* 18:809–813, 1997.

Neidhardt FC, Ingraham JL, Low KB: *Escherichia coli, Salmonella typhimurium: Cellular and Molecular Biology*, Washington DC, 1987, American Society for Microbiology.

Neu HC: Antimicrobial chemotherapy. In Baron S, Jennings PM, editors: *Medical Microbiology*, ed 3, New York, 1991, Churchill Livingstone, Ch. 11, pp 179–201.

Newman MG, Kornman KS, Doherty FM: A 6-months multi-center evaluation of adjunctive tetracycline fibre therapy in conjunction with scaling and root planing in maintenance patients: clinical results, *J Periodontol* 65:685–691, 1994.

Nikaido H: Multidrug efflux pumps of gram-negative bacteria, *J Bacteriol* 178:5853–5859, 1996.

Noache LA, Langenberg WL, Bertola MA, et al: Impact of metronidazole resistance on the eradication of Helicobacter pylori, *Scand J Infect Dis* 26:321–327, 1994.

Noble WC, Howell SA: Labile antibiotic resistance in Staphylococcus aureus, *J Hosp Infect* 31:135–141, 1995.

Noiri Y, Okami Y, Narimatsu M, et al: Effects of chlorhexidine, minocycline and metronidazole on Porphyromonas gingivalis strain 381 in biofilms, *J Periodontol* 74:1647–1651, 2003.

Norling T, Lading P, Engström S, et al: Formulation of a drug delivery system based on a mixture of monoglycerides and triglycerides for use in the treatment of periodontal disease, *J Clin Periodontol* 19:687–692, 1992.

Notten F, Koek-van Oosten A, Mikx F: Capillary agar diffusion assay for measuring metronidazole in human gingival crevicular fluid, *Antimicrob Agents Chemother* 21:836–837, 1982.

O'Connor BC, Newman HN, Wilson M: Susceptibility and resistance of plaque bacteria to minocycline, *J Periodontol* 61:228–233, 1990.

O'Rourke M, Stevens E: Genetic structure of Neisseria gonorrhoeae populations: a non-clonal pathogen, *J Genetic Microbiol* 139:2603–2611, 1993.

Olsvik B, Hansen BF, Tenover F, et al: Tetracycline resistant microorganisms recovered from patients with refractory periodontal disease, *J Clin Periodontol* 22:391–396, 1995.

Oosterwaal P, Mikx F, Reggli H: Clearance of a topical applied fluorescein gel from periodontal pockets, *J Clin Periodontol* 17:613–615, 1990.

Paquette D, Oringer R, Lessem J, et al: Locally delivered minocycline microspheres for treatment of periodontitis in smokers, *J Clin Periodontol* 30:787–794, 2003.

Parry MF, Panzer KB, Yukna ME: Quinolone resistance: Susceptibility data from a 300-bed community hospital, *Am J Med* 87(5A):12S–16S, 1989.

Paton DH, Reeves DS: Clinical features and management of adverse effects of the quinolone antibacterials, *Drug Saf* 6:8–27, 1991.

Pavia M, Nobile CGA, Angelillo IF: Meta-analysis of local tetracycline in treating chronic periodontitis, *J Periodontol* 74:916–932, 2003.

Payne JB, Stoner JA, Nummikoski PV, et al: Subantimicrobial dose doxycycline effects on alveolar bone loss in post-menopausal women, *J Clin Periodontol* 34:776–787, 2007.

Pedrazzoli V, Kilian M, Karring T: Comparative clinical and microbiological effects of topical subgingival application of metronidazole 25% dental gel and scaling in the treatment of adult periodontitis, *J Clin Periodontol* 19:715–722, 1992.

Perinetti G, Paolantonio M, Cordella C, et al: Clinical and microbiological effects of subgingival administration of two active gels on persistent pockets of chronic periodontitis patients, *J Clin Periodontol* 31:282–285, 2004.

Phillips I: Beta-lactamase-producing, penicillin-resistant gonococcus, *Lancet* 2:656–657, 1976.

Pitcher G, Newman H, Strahan J: Access to subgingival plaque by disclosing agents using mouthwashes and direct irrigation, *J Clin Periodontol* 7:300–302, 1980.

Platt R, Dreis MW, Kennedy DL, et al: Serum sickness-like reactions to amoxicillin, cefaclor, cephalexin and trimethoprim-sulfamethoxazole, *J Infect Dis* 158:474–477, 1988.

Ploy MC, Grelaud C, Martin C, et al: First clinical isolate of vancomycin-intermediate Staphylococcus aureus in a French hospital, *Lancet* 351:1212, 1998.

Preshaw PM, Hefti AF, Novak MJ, et al: Subantimicrobial dose doxycycline enhances the efficacy of scaling and root planing in chronic periodontitis: A multicenter trial, *J Periodontol* 75:1068–1076, 2004.

Preus HR, Lassen J, Aass A, et al: Bacterial resistance following subgingival and systemic administration of minocycline, *J Clin Periodontol* 22:380–384, 1995.

Public Health Laboratory Service: *Submission to the House of Lords Inquiry*, London, 1998, House of Lords.

Pullen H, Wright N, Murdock J, et al: Hypersensitivity reactions to antibacterial drugs in infectious mononucleosis, *Lancet* 2:1176, 1967.

Rallison ML, O'Brien J, Good RA: Severe reaction to long acting sulphonamides, *Paediatr* 28:908–917, 1961.

Rapley JW, Cobb CM, Killoy WJ, et al: Serum levels of tetracycline during treatment with tetracycline-containing fibres, *J Periodontol* 62:817–820, 1992.

Rautelin H, Tee W, Seppälä K, et al: Ribotyping patterns and emergence of metronidazole resistance in paired clinical samples of Helicobacter pylori, *J Antimicrob Chemother* 32:1079–1082, 1994.

Ridley AM, Punia P, Ward LR, et al: Plasmid characterization and pulsed-field electrophoretic analysis demonstrate that ampicillin-resistant strains of Salmonella enteritidis phage type 6a are derived from Salm. enteritidis phage type 4, *J Appl Bacteriol* 81:613–618, 1996.

Rifkin BR, Vernillo AT, Golub LM: Blocking periodontal disease progression by inhibiting tissue destructive enzymes: a potential role of tetracyclines and their chemically modified analogues, *J Periodontol* 64:819–827, 1993.

Riott IM: Hypersensitivity. In *Riott's essential immunology*, ed 9, Oxford, 1997, Blackwell Science, Ch. 16, pp 328–352.

Rodrigues RMJ, Gonçalves C, Souto R, et al: Antibiotic resistance profile of the subgingival microbiota following systemic or local tetracycline therapy, *J Clin Periodontol* 31:420–427, 2004.

Ross BC, Czajkowski L, Vandenberg KL, et al: Characterization of two outer membrane protein antigens of Porphyromonas gingivalis that are protective in a murine lesion model, *Oral Microbiol Immunol* 19:6–15, 2004.

Rowe B, Threlfall EJ: Drug resistance in Gram-negative aerobic bacteria, *Br Med Bull* 40:68–76, 1984.

Ryan ME, Ramamurthy S, Golub LM: Matrix metalloproteinases and their inhibition in periodontal treatment, *Curr Opin in Periodontol* 3:85–96, 1996.

Saglie R, Newman M, Carranza F, et al: Bacterial invasion of gingiva in advanced periodontitis in humans, *J Periodontol* 53:217–222, 1982.

Saglie R, Pertuiset J, Rezende M, et al: In situ correlation immuno-identification of mononuclear cells and invasive bacteria in diseased gingiva, *J Periodontol* 59:688–696, 1988.

Sanai Y, Persson GR, Starr JR, et al: Presence and antibiotic resistance of Porphyromonas gingivalis, Prevotella intermedia and Prevotella nigrescens in children, *J Clin Periodontol* 29:929–934, 2002.

Sande MA, Chambers HF, Kupusnik-Uner JE: Antimicrobial agents: Tetracyclines, chloramphenicol, erythromycin and miscellaneous antibacterial agents. In Goodman-Gilman A, Hardman JG, Limbird LE, Molinoff PB, Ruddon RE, editors: *Goodman & Gilman's the Pharmacological Basis of Therapeutics*, ed 9, Section IX, Chemotherapy of microbial disease, New York, 1996, McGraw – Hill, Ch. 47, pp 1123–1154.

Satomi A, Vraguchi R, Ishikawa I, et al: Minocycline hydrochloride concentration in periodontal pockets after administration of LS-007, *J Assoc Periodontol* 29:937–943, 1987.

Schaberg DR, Zervos MJ: Intergeneric and interspecies gene exchange in gram-positive cocci, *Antimicrob Agents Chemother* 30:817–822, 1986.

Sher TH: Penicillin hypersensitivity, *Rev Pediatr Clin North Am* 30:161–176, 1983.

Shinn DL: Metronidazole in acute ulcerative gingivitis, *Lancet* 1:1191, 1962.

Shinn DL, Squires S, McFadzean JA: The treatment of Vincent's disease with metronidazole, *Dent Pract* 15:275–280, 1965.

Shlaes DM, Gerding DN, John JF Jr, et al: Society for Healthcare Epidemiology of America and Infectious Diseases Society of America. Joint Committee on the Prevention of Antimicrobial Resistance: guidelines for the prevention of antimicrobial resistance in hospitals, *Clin Infect Dis* 25:584–599, 1997.

Slots J, Rosling B: Suppression of periodontopathic microflora in localized juvenile periodontitis by systemic tetracycline, *J Clin Periodontol* 10:465–486, 1983.

SMAC, Standing Medical Advisory Committee, Subgroup on Antimicrobial Resistance: In *The path of least resistance*, Ch. 4, Antimicrobial agents, London, 1999a, Department of Health, pp 17–19.

SMAC, Standing Medical Advisory Committee, Subgroup on Antimicrobial Resistance: In *The path of least resistance*, Ch. 5, Basis of resistance, London, 1999b, Department of Health, pp 20–23.

SMAC, Standing Medical Advisory Committee, Subgroup on Antimicrobial Resistance: In *The path of least resistance*, Ch. 6, Does the use of antimicrobial agents cause resistance? London, 1999c, Department of Health, pp 24.

SMAC, Standing Medical Advisory Committee, Subgroup on Antimicrobial Resistance: In *The path of least resistance*, Ch.10, Current resistance problems in the UK and worldwide, London, 1999d, Department of Health, pp 33–54.

Smith TC: ICAAC Abstract LB-16. In *ICAAC*, Washington DC, 1997, American Society for Microbiology, pp 11.

Soares S, Kristinsson KG, Musser JM, et al: Evidence for the introduction of a multi-resistant clone of serotype 6B Streptococcus pneumoniae form Spain into Iceland in the late 1980s, *J Infect Dis* 168:158–163, 1992.

Söder PÖ, Frithiof L, Wikner S, et al: The effect of systemic metronidazole after non-surgical treatment in moderate and advanced periodontitis in young adults, *J Periodontol* 61:281–288, 1990.

Soory M: A role for non-antimicrobial actions of tetracyclines in combating oxidative stress in periodontal and metabolic diseases, *The Open Dentistry Journal* 2:5–12, 2008.

Sorsa T, Ding Y, Salo T, et al: Effects of tetracyclines on neutrophil, gingival and salivary collagenases. A functional and western-blot assessment with special reference to their cellular sources in periodontal diseases, *Ann N Y Acad Sci* 732:112–131, 1994.

Speer BS, Shoemaker NB, Salyers AA: Bacterial resistance to tetracycline: mechanisms, transfer and clinical significance, *Clin Microbiol Rev* 5:387–399, 1992.

Speller DCE, Johnson AP, James D, et al: Resistance to methicillin and other antibiotics in Staphylococcus aureus from blood and cerebrospinal fluid, England and Wales, 1989–1995, *Lancet* 350:323–325, 1997.

Spratt BG: Resistance to antibiotics mediated by target alterations, *Science* 264:388–393, 1994.

Sprott MS, Ingham HR, Hickman JE, et al: Metronidazole resistant anaerobes, *Lancet* 8335:1230, 1983.

Stoltze K, Stellfeld M: Systemic absorption of metronidazole after application of a 25% metronidazole dental gel, *J Clin Periodontol* 19:693–697, 1992.

Stoltze K: Concentration of metronidazole in periodontal pockets after application of a 25% metronidazole dental gel, *J Clin Periodontol* 19:698–701, 1992.

Surtees SJ, Stockton MG, Gietzen TW: Allergy to penicillin: fact or fiction, *Br Med J* 302:1051–1052, 1991.

Tenenbaum H, Jehl F, Gallion C, et al: Amoxicillin and clavulanic acid concentrations in gingival crevicular fluid, *J Clin Periodontol* 24:804–807, 1997.

Theilade E: The non-specific theory in microbial etiology of inflammatory periodontal diseases, *J Clin Periodontol* 13:905–911, 1986.

Threlfall EJ, Ward LR, Rowe B: Spread of multiresistant strains of Salmonella typhimurium phage types 204 and 193 in Britain, *Br Med J* 2:997, 1978.

Threlfall EJ, Rowe B, Fergerson JL, et al: Increasing incidence of resistance to gentamicin and related aminoglycosides in Salmonella typhimurium phage type 204c in England, Wales and Scotland, *Vet Rec* 117:355–357, 1985.

Threlfall EJ, Rowe B, Fergerson JL, et al: Characterization of plasmids conferring resistance to gentamicin and apramycin in strains of Salmonella typhimurium phage types 204c isolated in Britain, *J Hyg* 97:419–426, 1986.

Threlfall EJ, Hall ML, Rowe B: Salmonella bacteraemia in England and Wales, 1981–1990, *J Clin Pathol* 45:34–36, 1992.

Threlfall EJ, Ward LR, Rowe B: A comparison of multiple drug resistance in salmonellas from humans and food animals in England and Wales, 1981 and 1990, *Epidemiol Infect* 111:189–197, 1993.

Threlfall EJ, Frost JA, Ward L, et al: Increasing spectrum of resistance in multiresistant Salmonella typhimurium, *Lancet* 347:1053–1054, 1996.

Timmerman MF, van der Weijden GA, van Steenbergen TJM, et al: Evaluation of the long-term efficacy and safety of locally-applied minocycline in adult periodontitis patients, *J Clin Periodontol* 23:707–716, 1996.

Todd PA, Benfield P: Amoxycillin/clavulanic acid. An update of its antibacterial activity, pharmokinetic properties and therapeutic use, *Drugs* 39:264–307, 1990.

Tonetti MS: Etiology and pathogenesis. In Lang NP, Karring T, editors: *Proceedings of the 1st European Workshop on Periodontology*, Berlin, Germany, 1994, Quintessence Publishing, pp 54–89.

Tonetti MS: Local delivery of tetracycline: from concept to clinical application, *J Clin Periodontol* 25:969–977, 1998.

Tonetti MS, Cugini MA, Goodson JM: Zero-order delivery with periodontal placement of tetracycline-loaded ethylene vinyl acetate fibres, *J Periodontal Res* 25:243–249, 1990.

Tonetti MS, Mombelli A, Lehmann B, et al: Impact of oral ecology on the recolonisation of locally treated pockets, *J Dent Res* 74:481, Abstract 642, 1995.

Tracey JW, Webster LT: Trypanosomiasis, Leishmaniasis, Amebiasis, Giardiasis, Trichomoniasis and other protozoal infections. In Goodman-Gilman A, Hardman JG, Limbird LE, Molinoff PB, Ruddon RE, editors: *Goodman & Gilman's the Pharmacological Basis of Therapeutics*, ed 9, Section IX, Chemotherapy of microbial disease, New York, 1996, McGraw-Hill, Ch. 41, pp 987–1008.

Vandekerckhove BN, Quirynen M, van Steenberghe D: The use of locally-delivered minocycline in the treatment of chronic periodontitis. A review of the literature, *J Clin Periodontol* 25:964–968, 1998.

van Palenstein Helderman WH: Is antibiotic therapy justified in the treatment of human chronic inflammatory periodontal disease? *J Clin Periodontol* 13:932–938, 1986.

Van Steenberge D, Bercy P, Hohl J, et al: Subgingival minocycline hydrochloride ointment in moderate to severe chronic adult periodontitis: randomised, double-blind, vehicle-controlled, multi-centre study, *J Periodontol* 64:637–644, 1993.

van Winkelhoff AJ, Rodenberg AJ, Goené RJ, et al: Metronidazole plus amoxicillin in the treatment of Actinobacillus actinomycetemcomitans associated periodontitis, *J Clin Periodontol* 16:128–131, 1989.

van Winkelhoff AJ, Herrera D, Oteo A, et al: Antimicrobial profiles of periodontal pathogens isolated from periodontitis patients in the Netherlands and Spain, *J Clin Periodontol* 32:893–898, 2005.

van Zwet AA, Thijs JC, Schievink-de Vries W, et al: In vitro studies on stability and development of metronidazole resistance in Helicobacter pylori, *Antimicrob Agents Chemother* 38:360–362, 1994.

Vorachit M, Lam K, Jayanetra P, et al: Resistance of Pseudomonas pseudomallei growing on a biofilm on silastic discs to ceftazidime and co-trimoxazole, *Antimicrob Agents Chemother* 37:2000–2002, 1993.

Wade AB, Blake GC, Mirza KB: Effectiveness of metronidazole in treating the acute phase of ulcerative gingivitis, *Dent Pract* 16:440–443, 1966.

Wallace MR, Mascola JR, Oldfield EC: The red man syndrome: incidence, aetiology and prophylaxis, *J Infect Dis* 164:1108–1185, 1991.

Walker CB, Gordon JM, Cornwall HA, et al: Gingival crevicular fluid levels of clindamycin compared with its minimal inhibitory concentrations for periodontal bacteria, *Antimicrob Agents Chemother* 19:867–871, 1981a.

Walker CB, Gordon JM, McQulkin SJ, et al: Tetracycline: levels achievable in gingival crevice fluid and *in vitro* effect on subgingival organisms. Part II Susceptibilities of periodontal bacteria, *J Periodontol* 52:613–616, 1981b.

Walker CB, Gordon JM, Socransky SS: Antibiotic sensitivity testing of subgingival plaque samples, *J Clin Periodontol* 10:422–432, 1983.

Walker C, Nango S, Lennon J, et al: Effect of sub-antimicrobial dose doxycycline (SDD) on the intestinal and vaginal flora, *J Dent Res* 79(Special Issue):608 Abstract 3718, 2000.

Warburton AR, Jenkins PA, Waight PA, et al: Drug resistance in initial isolates of Mycobacterium tuberculosis in England and Wales, 1982–1991, *Commun Dis Rep CDR Rev* 3:R175–R179, 1993.

Wennström JL, Newman HN, Griffiths GS, et al: Utilisation of locally delivered doxycycline in non-surgical treatment of chronic periodontitis. A comparative multicenter trial of two treatment approaches, *J Clin Periodontol* 28:753–761, 2001.

Williams BL, Østerberg SK, Jørgensen J: Subgingival microflora of periodontal patients on tetracycline therapy, *J Clin Periodontol* 6:210–221, 1979.

Williams RC, Paquette D, Offenbacher S, et al: Treatment of periodontitis by local administration of a micro-encapsulated antibiotic: a controlled trial, *J Periodontol* 72:753–761, 2001a.

Williams RC, Paquette D, Offenbacher S, et al: Treatment of periodontitis by local administration of minocycline microspheres, a controlled trial, *J Periodontol* 72:1535–1544, 2001b.

Woodford N, Johnson AP, Morrison D, et al: Current perspectives on glycopeptide resistance, *Clin Microbiol Rev* 8:585–615, 1995.

Wright TL, Ellen RP, Lacriox JM, et al: Effects of metronidazole on Porphyromonas gingivalis biofilms, *J Periodontal Res* 32:473–477, 1997.

Yu L, Smith G, Hasty K, et al: Doxycycline inhibits type XI collagenolytic activity of extracts from human osteoarthritic cartilage and of gelatinase, *J Rheumatol* 18:1450–1452, 1991.

Yu Z, Ramamurthy NS, Leung M, et al: Chemically-modified tetracycline normalizes collagen metabolism in diabetic rats: a dose response study, *J Periodontal Res* 28:420–428, 1993.

Antibiotic prophylaxis for susceptible patients undergoing periodontal treatment

ANTIBIOTIC PROPHYLAXIS

Please note that current (2009) legislation in the UK means that this procedure is no longer necessary.

RATIONALE

Microorganisms may settle on the endocardium damaged or rendered defective by acquired or congenital heart disease and may cause infective endocarditis. It was therefore accepted that antibiotic prophylaxis should be administered whenever susceptible patients were exposed to bacteraemia (British Society for Antimicrobial Chemotherapy (BSAC) 1982). Bacteraemia may arise from certain dental procedures, operations on the upper respiratory tract such as tonsillectomy and adenoidectomy and genitourinary and gastrointestinal tract instrumentation or operation (BSAC 1982; Elliott 1939; Durack 1979). Although bacteraemia may follow these procedures, the likelihood of infective endocarditis resulting seemed to vary considerably and with many procedures the risk was insignificant.

In Britain the introduction of antibiotic prophylaxis was not followed by a decline in the incidence of infective endocarditis (Office of Population Census and Survey 1980). In the 1920s, when virtually every patient who contracted infective endocarditis died, the Registrar General registered about 1000 deaths annually in England and Wales. Currently, the mortality from this condition is about 30% and in 1979, the Office of Population Census and Surveys reported 280 deaths suggesting an annual incidence rate similar to the 1920s.

Although there is no clear evidence in humans for the protective effect of antibiotic prophylaxis for dental procedures (Cawson 1981) and fewer than 15% of patients with infective endocarditis give a history of relevant dental treatment in the preceding 3 months (Cherubin & Neu 1971; Cates & Christie 1951), the British Society for Antimicrobial Chemotherapy still believed that the circumstantial evidence was strong enough to warrant advising antibiotic prophylaxis (BSAC 1982).

SUSCEPTIBLE PATIENTS

Possible susceptible patients may be in three possible categories:

- Patients with a susceptible heart condition
- Patients with prosthetic joint replacements
- Immunosuppressed patients.

Patients with a susceptible heart condition

These patients can be further divided into three further categories of high, moderate and negligible risks and these are summarized in Table 18.1.

High risk

Patients in this category have a higher risk than the other categories for contracting infective endocarditis either with or without exposure to a treatment induced bacteraemia and also have a higher level of mortality following this infection (Dajani et al 1997a,b; Steckelberg & Wilson 1993; Saiman et al 1993). The conditions in this category are:

- Prosthetic heart valves including both bioprosthetic and homograft valves
- Previous history of infective endocarditis
- Complex cyanotic congenital heart disease (e.g. single ventricle states, transposition of great arteries and Fallot's tetralogy)
- Surgically constructed systemic – pulmonary shunts or conduits.

Full antibiotic prophylaxis usually with additional cover is recommended for this group.

Moderate risk

Patients in this category have a lesser risk of contracting infective endocarditis than the high risk group but a higher risk than the general population with no known risks (Dajani et al 1997a,b; Steckelberg & Wilson 1993; Saiman et al 1993; Gersony et al 1993). They comprise the following categories:

- Most other congenital cardiac malformations other than those above or below
- Acquired valvular dysfunction, e.g. Rheumatic heart disease
- Hypertrophic cardiomyopathy
- Mitral valve prolapse with valvular regurgitation and/or thickened leaflets.

Table 18.1 *Conditions which require or do not require antibiotic prophylaxis to protect from the risks from transient bacteraemia*

Conditions at risk and requiring antibiotic cover	Conditions not at risk
Ventricular septal defect (ASD)	Angina
Primum atrial septal defect (ASD)	Myocardial infarction
ASD repaired with prosthetic patch	Ventricular aneurysm
Post valvotomy	Innocent systolic murmur
Pulmonary stenosis	Ligated ductus arteriosus
Patent ductus arteriosus	ASD – unrepaired or repaired without patch
Coarctation of the aorta	Coronary artery bypass graft
Complex cyanotic heart disease (e.g. single ventricular states, transposition of great arteries and Fallot's tetralogy)[a]	Rheumatic fever without history and evidence of valvular disease[b]
Surgically constructed systemic– pulmonary shunts or conduits[a]	Hip or knee prosthesis
Bicuspid aortic valve	Permanent pacemaker
Murmurs of doubtful origin[b]	
Acquired valvular disfunction, e.g. rheumatic heart disease	
Mitral valve prolapse with valvular regurgitation and/or thickened leaflets[b]	
Hypertrophic cardiomyopathy[b]	
AV malformation or fistula	
History of infective endocarditis[a]	
Prosthetic valve replacement including both bioprosthetic and homograft valves[a]	

[a]High risk.
[b]Need cardiac examination to confirm.

The congenital heart conditions in this group comprise the uncorrected patent ductus arteriosus, ventricular septal defect, primum atrium septal defect, coarctation of the aorta and bicuspid aortic valve. The acquired conditions include valvular defects or dysfunction either as a result of rheumatic heart disease, collagen vascular disease or hypertrophic cardiomyopathy.

Mitral valve prolapse (MVP) is a common condition and the need for prophylaxis for this condition is controversial as only a small percentage of MVP patients develop complications at any age (Prabha and O'Rourke 1997; Boudoulas & Wooley 1995; Carabello 1993). MVP represents a spectrum of vascular changes and clinical behaviour. In addition, dehydration and tachycardia are common causes of intermittent MVP (Dajani et al 1997a). Abnormal motion of normal mitral valves can be detected by an echocardiogram and is seen in a proportion of normal adults and adolescents. The high prevalence of such motion in young adults indicates that MVP is often an abnormality of volume status, adrenergic state or growth phase and not of valve structure or function.

When MVP occurs without leaking and no Doppler-demonstrated regurgitation, the risk of endocarditis following exposure to a bacteraemia is no greater than that in the normal population (Saiman et al 1993; Prabha and O'Rourke 1997; Carabello 1993) and antibiotic prophylaxis is not needed. However, patients with prolapsing and leaking mitral valves, evidenced by the audible clicks and murmurs of mitral regurgitation are recommended to receive antibiotic prophylaxis (Carabello 1993; Devereux et al 1986, 1994; Danchin et al 1989; MacMahon et al 1987; Marks et al 1989; Zuppiroli et al 1995; Wooley et al 1991; Morelas et al 1992; Weissman et al 1994; Nishimura et al 1985; McKinsey et al 1987; Devereux et al 1989; Stoddard et al 1995; Awadallah et al 1991; Cheitlin et al 1997; La Porte et al 1999; Waldman et al 1997; Little 1997).

MVP also occurs with myxomatous degeneration of the mitral valve and this condition has a spectrum of manifestations (Skiest & Coykendall 1995; Wooley et al 1991). The mitral valves in these conditions appear thickened on the echocardiogram due to accumulation of proteoglycan deposits and the amount of thickening is variable and may increase with age. Patients with myxomatous mitral valve degeneration with regurgitation are recommended for antibiotic prophylaxis (Marks et al 1989; Nishimura et al 1985; McKinsey et al 1987). These are more commonly older men which have an increased risk of developing infective endocarditis (Devereux et al 1986; MacMahon et al 1987; Marks et al 1989; Devereux et al 1989; Stoddard et al 1995).

The vast majority of children with chest pain or fatigue do not have any form of heart disease but careful evaluation is nevertheless required in children who have isolated clinical findings such as a non-injection systolic click, since this may be an indicator of important mitral valve abnormality requiring antibiotic prophylaxis (Awadallah et al 1991). In some reports, MVP has emerged as an important underlying diagnosis associated with infective endocarditis in the paediatric group (Saiman et al 1993; Awadallah et al 1991).

A clinical approach (Cheitlin et al 1997) to the determination of the need for antibiotic prophylaxis in patients with MVP is shown in **Figure 18.1**.

Negligible risks

Although infective endocarditis may develop in any individual including those with no underlying cardiac defect, the negligible risk category includes those cardiac conditions in which the risk of development of endocarditis is not higher than that of the general population (Dajani et al 1997a). Whereas in paediatric patients innocent heart murmurs may be clearly defined by auscultation, in the adult population other procedures such as echocardiogram may be necessary to confirm that the murmur is innocent. Individuals with innocent murmurs have structurally normal hearts and do not require antibiotic prophylaxis.

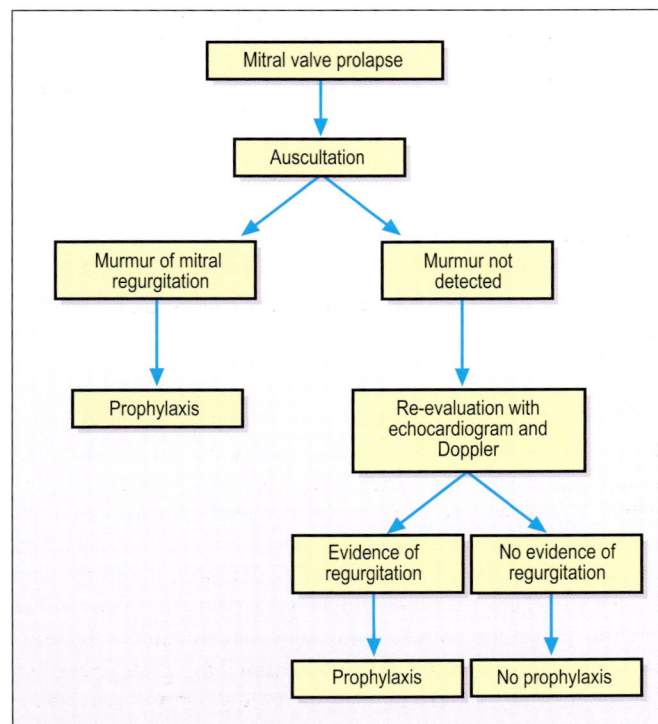

Fig. 18.1 A scheme for assessment of mitral valve prolapse with regard to the need for antibiotic prophylaxis.

The identification of subjects in this category involves a considerable degree of cooperation between the medical and dental practitioner. Clearly the dentist alone can only try to identify at risk patients by taking a careful medical history, asking about the precise nature of any heart disease and of any history of rheumatic fever or cardiac surgery.

A history of rheumatic fever alone is not a reason for antibiotic prophylaxis since these patients may or may not have rheumatic valvular disease. The value of a history alone is limited since the dentist cannot carry out the appropriate physical examination of the patient to confirm the findings. Furthermore, the patient's history of past events such as rheumatic fever may be vague and misleading. Also the patient may be unaware of the presence of certain susceptible cardiac defects, which produce no symptoms, such as bicuspid aortic valves, or may even seek to conceal them. If there is any reason to suspect a susceptible cardiac lesion it is best for the dentist to contact the patient's medical practitioner for further information or in previously undiagnosed cases, arrange through the doctor for an examination by a cardiologist.

Patients with prosthetic joint replacements

Dental procedures leading to bacteraemia have been implicated as possible causes of a few cases of late infections of prosthetic hip and knee arthroplasties (La Porte et al 1999; Waldman et al 1997; Little 1997; Skiest & Coykendall 1995). However, the number of these is very small and the time pattern of these late infections does not seem to associate with that which one would expect if they were related to dental bacteraemias. Thus, the role of antibiotic prophylaxis in patients with prosthetic joints who require dental treatment is highly controversial (Sandhu et al 1997).

La Porte et al (1999) investigated 2973 patients with total hip arthroplasties found 52 patients with late joint infections, three of which seemed to be associated with extensive dental procedures because of the nature of the bacteria infecting the joint. However, one of these patients had diabetes and another had rheumatoid arthritis both of which are known to predispose the patient to infection. The conclusion of the study was that only patients with predisposing systemic disease should receive antibiotic prophylaxis for relevant dental procedures.

A similar study (Waldman et al 1997) of total knee arthroplasties examined the records of 3490 cases treated at one centre between 1982 and 1983. They identified 62 cases of late infections with seven cases apparently related to extensive dental procedures. They also investigated a further 12 cases of late infections referred from other centres, two of which were apparently associated to extensive dental procedures. Of these nine patients, eight received no cover but one had received standard recommended antibiotic cover. However, five of these nine cases had systemic risk factors predisposing them to infection.

Surveys of dentists and orthopaedic surgeons in the UK and USA between 1994 and 1995 (Jaspers & Little 1985; Shrout et al 1994) found that both groups recommended cover for prosthetic joint replacement patients undergoing relevant dental treatment. However, opinions on this matter now seem to have changed. A review of cases of prosthetic joint infections concluded that most of these were due to wound contamination at the time of surgery and only a few due to haematogenous spread from a distant infective site (Devereux et al 1994). An extensive review of the related literature by this group failed to associate prosthetic joint infections with transient bacteraemias from dental procedures.

Several studies have described systemic factors predisposing to infection to be involved in most of the cases of joint infection with any apparent association to dental procedures (La Porte et al 1999; Waldman et al 1997; Little 1997). However, most evidence seems to relate these late infections to wound contamination or spread from other areas of infection and to be unrelated to dental procedures (Little 1997).

Based on these findings both the American Dental Association and the American Association of Orthopaedic Surgeons recommend cover only for patients with systemic factors predisposing to infection undergoing extensive dental procedures related to bacteraemia (Anonymous 1997).

The situation in the UK is similar. A Working Party of the British Society of Antimicrobial Chemotherapy recently suggested that there was no evidence to support the use of antibiotic prophylaxis in these patients (Sandhu et al 1997; Grant & Hoddinott 1992; Mason et al 1992). However, it has also been suggested that not all patients with prosthetic joints present a similar risk and that certain patients may require cover (Sandhu et al 1997; Mason et al 1992; Tyne & Ferguson 1991; Field & Martin 1991). These patients include those with rheumatoid arthritis, diabetes mellitus and immunosuppression, those on steroids and possibly those with re-operated hips.

This poses the question of who is in the best position to assess the need in these cases. Another study examined how closely the recommendations of the British Society for Antimicrobial Chemotherapy (BSAC) were being followed by British maxillofacial and orthopaedic surgeons (Jaspers & Little 1985). It also looked at differences between maxillofacial and orthopaedic surgeons in the management of these patients. This showed that 77.7% of the orthopaedic surgeons recommended the use of antibiotic cover for dental treatment while only 29% of maxillofacial surgeons did so. There were also differences in the antibiotic of choice between these groups. Most of the maxillofacial surgeons recommended either amoxicillin or clindamycin while the majority of orthopaedic surgeons recommended the use of a cephalosporin, in spite of the fact that this is not the most efficacious antibiotic against oral streptococci which are the most likely infecting bacteria in these cases.

Thus, this matter is far from resolved. It would seem most appropriate for dental surgeons to follow the guidelines of the BSAC in not giving cover in most cases. In the case of the special risk groups described above they should consult with the patient's orthopaedic surgeon. However, they should make sure that if cover is recommended that the appropriate regime is given.

In this regard the latest advice of the British Society for Antimicrobial Chemotherapy (La Porte et al 1999; Sandhu et al 1997; Anonymous 1997; Grant & Hoddinott 1992; Mason et al 1992) is that patients with prosthetic joint implants (including total hip and knee replacements) do not require antibiotic prophylaxis for dental treatment. The Working Party considers that it is unacceptable to expose patients to the adverse effects of antibiotics when there is no evidence that such prophylaxis is of any benefit, but those who develop any concurrent infection need prompt treatment with antibiotics to which the infecting microorganisms are sensitive. The Working Party also commented that joint infections rarely follow dental procedures and are even more rarely caused by oral streptococci.

Immunosuppressed patients

Immunosuppressed patients are more susceptible to infections and may need antibiotic treatment when they are exposed to infection. These patients may include those with rheumatoid arthritis or diabetes mellitus, those on steroids, those with immunosuppression due to radiotherapy, those on immunosuppressive drugs or those with immunosuppressive infections (Walter 1997). Each case should be considered separately on its individual merits and the decision needs to be taken by the physician in charge of the patient's treatment.

Septicaemia is a cause of death in haematopoietic stem cell transplantation (HSCT) and extraction of teeth with advanced periodontitis has been advocated before HSCI to prevent septicaemia in myeloablated hosts. However, a study (Akintoye et al 2002) found no relationship between radiographic periodontal status and septicaemia or mortality for 100 days after transplantation (see Ch. 6).

The advice of the British Society for Antimicrobial Chemotherapy (BSAC 1982; Little 1997; Grant & Hoddinott 1992) is that patients who are immunosuppressed, including transplant patients and patients with indwelling intraperitoneal catheters do not require antibiotic cover for dental treatment provided that there is no other indication for prophylaxis. The Working Party has commented that there is little evidence that dental treatment is followed by infection in immunosuppressed and immunocompromised patients nor is there any evidence that dental treatment is followed by infection in patients with indwelling intraperitoneal catheters.

DENTAL CAUSES OF TRANSIENT BACTERAEMIA

It has long been known that bacteraemia can arise from oral and dental sepsis and following tooth extraction (Okell & Elliott 1935; Sale 1938). Furthermore, transient bacteraemia from oral sources may occur in the absence of dental procedures when there is poor oral hygiene, periodontal disease or periapical infection and is stimulated by normal functions such as eating, chewing and toothbrushing. The incidence is directly proportional to the degree of gingival inflammation and infection (Eley 1983a; Binder et al 1984; Pallasch & Slots 1991, 1996; Forner et al 2006). Individuals at risk should establish and maintain the best oral health possible to reduce this continuous source of potential bacteraemias (Guntheroth 1984; Kay 1986; Eley 1983b; Roberts et al 1997; 1998a,b). Possible causes of transient bacteraemias are shown in Table 18.2 and described in detail below.

TOOTH EXTRACTION AND ORAL AND PERIODONTAL SURGERY

Bacteraemia and in some cases infective endocarditis has long been shown to be occasionally produced by tooth extraction (Okell & Elliott 1935; Sale 1938). Three cases of bacterial endocarditis have been shown to occur in a study in children with congenital heart disease following dental extraction, despite the administration preoperatively of appropriate antibiotics (O'Sullivan et al 1996).

Table 18.2 *Conditions and procedures which can produce a transient bacteraemia*

Chewing, toothbrushing and flossing in the presence of gingival inflammation

Spread from local areas of infections

Oral surgical procedures including tooth extraction

Intraligamental local anaesthetic injection

Reimplantation of avulsed teeth

Dental implant placement

Periodontal probing

Polishing of teeth and implants when gingival bleeding expected

Supragingival scaling which traumatized the gingivae

Subgingival scaling and root planing

Subgingival placement of antimicrobial fibres or strips (if ever indicated in these patients)

Periodontal surgery

Restorative procedures which involve trauma to the gingival margin or crevice

Endodontic instrumentation when there is a danger of going through the apex

Endodontic (apical) surgery

Initial placement of orthodontic bands but not brackets

It has also been shown that the frequency and severity of the bacteraemia relates to the nature and extent of the surgical procedure. The prevalence and intensity of bacteraemia of dental origin were examined in 207 children undergoing dental surgery (Roberts et al 1998b). They were divided into four groups: a baseline group with no surgical intervention (group I), a single tooth extraction group (group II), a multiple tooth extractions group (group III), and mucoperiosteal flap elevation group (group IV). Bacterial cultures were positive in 11% of group I at the time of testing, 43% of group II, 54% of group III, and 43% of group IV. When organisms were isolated, the intensity of bacteraemia ranged from 1 to 3400 colony forming units per millilitre (cfu/mL).

Another study (Rajasuo et al 2004) investigated the bacteraemia caused by surgical removal of partially erupted mandibular third molars. Bacterial samples were taken pre-operatively from the pericoronal pocket of these teeth and post operatively from the extraction socket from 16 young adults. Blood samples were taken from the antecubital vein up to 30 min after surgery. Some 88% of the subjects had detectable bacteraemia, 50% 1 min after the incision, and 44% immediately after tooth removal. The respective percentages at 10, 15 and 30 min were 44%, 25% and 13%. The blood cultures contained 31 species (74% anaerobes), with 3.9±2.6 species isolated per subject. Most prevalent were the anaerobes *Prevotella*, *Eubacterium* and *Peptostreptococcus* spp. and the aerobes viridans-group streptococci and *Streptococcus milleri* group. Any species found in the blood of a subject was also isolated from the mouth and 93% of pericoronal pockets and 43% of extraction sockets. Surgical dental extraction clearly causes bacteraemia of a high frequency and is relatively long lasting.

PERIODONTAL TREATMENT

Severe prosthetic valve-related endocarditis has been shown to occur following simple scaling (Doerffel et al 1997). Gingival trauma will occur in all forms of scaling but will be much greater following subgingival scaling in patients with periodontitis. The resulting bacteraemia has also been found to be more frequent and greater following subgingival scaling (Pallasch & Slots 1991, 1996). Bacteraemia has even been shown to follow tooth polishing in a few cases in one study (Roberts et al 1997).

Kinane et al (2005) carried out a single blind parallel study of 2 weeks duration in 30 volunteers with untreated periodontal disease. A periodontal probing depth chart was carried out followed by a baseline blood sample. A further blood sample was collected 2 weeks later. Full-mouth ultrasonic scaling was then performed and a final blood sample taken. Blood samples were analysed for bacteraemia using conventional microbiological culture and polymerase chain reaction (PCR) using universal bacterial primers that target the 16S ribosomal RNA gene of the vast majority of bacteria. Using culture methods, the incidence of bacteraemias was as follows: following ultrasonic scaling (13%), periodontal probing (20%) and toothbrushing (3%). PCR analysis revealed bacteraemia incidences following ultrasonic scaling, periodontal probing and toothbrushing of 23%, 16% and 13%, respectively. These findings suggest that detectable dental bacteraemias induced by periodontal procedures are at a lower level than previously reported.

Lafaurie et al (2007) evaluated the frequency of periodontopathic and other subgingival anaerobic and facultative bacteria in the bloodstream following scaling and root planing (SRP). 42 patients with severe generalized chronic periodontitis (GChP) and generalized aggressive periodontitis (GAgP) were included in the study. A total of 80.9% of the patients presented positive cultures after SRP and it occurred more frequently immediately after treatment; however, 19% of the patients still had microorganisms in the bloodstream 30 min after the procedure. The periodontopathic microorganisms more frequently identified were *Porphyromonas gingivalis* and *Macromonas micros*, *Campylobacter* spp., *Eikenella corrodens*, *Tannerella forsythensis*, *Fusobacterium* spp. and *Prevotella intermedia* were isolated less often. *Actinomyces* spp. were also found frequently during bacteraemia after SRP. Thus, SRP induced bacteraemia associated with anaerobic bacteria, especially in patients with periodontal disease.

ORAL HYGIENE PROCEDURES

Oral hygiene procedures such as toothbrushing, flossing and the use of interproximal brushes are necessary to achieve and maintain periodontal health. However, they can also stimulate transient bacteraemias particularly in the presence of gingival inflammation and periodontal disease (Pallasch & Slots 1991; Guntheroth 1984). In a study (Roberts et al 1997) of 735 anaesthetized children aged 2–16 years in which blood samples for cultures were obtained 30 s after each of 13 dental operative procedures, it was shown that a bacteraemia was produced at baseline (no procedure) on 9.4% occasions. In comparison, toothbrushing alone caused a bacteraemia on 38.5% of occasions. Bacteraemia has also been shown to occur following the use of air polishing (Hunter et al 1989) or an oral irrigator in subjects with gingivitis or periodontitis (Romans & App 1971; Felix et al 1971).

PERIODONTAL EXAMINATION

Bacteraemia of oral origin may result from periodontal probing. A study by Daly et al (1997) investigated 30 healthy adult patients with untreated periodontitis by taking blood samples for culture before and after periodontal probing. A positive bacteraemia was recorded for three of the patients prior to probing. Following probing, 13 patients (43%) exhibited bacteraemia of oral origin. *Viridans streptococci* were the most common isolates (45%). Patients at risk of developing infective endocarditis with radiographic evidence of periodontitis should have periodontal probing carried immediately prior to periodontal treatment when this is to be carried out under antibiotic prophylaxis in order to avoid repeated doses of antibiotic prophylaxis.

LOCAL ANAESTHESIA

It has been shown (Roberts et al 1998a) that the administration of local anaesthetic injections may produce transient bacteraemia but that the frequency was much greater with some forms than others. 143 children, aged

1 year 11 months to 19 years 4 months, undergoing general anaesthesia had blood samples taken after local anaesthesia. The injection methods were buccal infiltration, conventional intraligamental, and a modified intraligamental. A subgroup of 50 had blood taken before any dentogingival manipulative procedures to provide a baseline level of bacteraemia. The percentage prevalence of bacteraemia was baseline level 8%, buccal infiltration analgesia 16%, modified intraligamental analgesia 50% and conventional intraligamental analgesia 97%. The intraligamental techniques had statistically significantly greater percentage prevalence of bacteraemia compared with baseline and other methods. This may have implications for the use of intraligamental local anaesthesia in dental treatment and this technique would seem to be contraindicated in patients at risk of infective endocarditis.

RESTORATIVE PROCEDURES

Bacteraemia can follow restorative procedures that traumatize the gingival tissues. The frequency and severity relates to the extent of the trauma. A study (Roberts et al 1997, 1998a) investigated the frequency of bacteraemia following 13 dental operative procedures in 735 anaesthetized children aged 2–16 years. Four procedures used in conservative dentistry caused bacteraemias significantly more often than the baseline value of 9.4%. These were polishing teeth 24.5%, intraligamental injection 96.6%, rubber dam placement 29.4%, and matrix band with wedge placement 32.1%. The organisms isolated were typical of odontogenic bacteraemias in that 50% of the isolates were identified as varieties of *Viridans streptococci*. Recently, a very low frequency of bacteraemia (11%), using PCR bacterial identification, was found following conventional root canal therapy (Savarrioa et al 2005).

WHICH DENTAL PROCEDURES WARRANT ANTIBIOTIC PROPHYLAXIS?

It is clearly not practical or sensible to cover all these possible sources of bacteraemia with antibiotic prophylaxis. The latest suggestions (Dajani et al 1997a) are to give cover when it is necessary for the following:

- Dental extractions
- Oral and *Periodontal S*urgery
- Scaling – particularly subgingival scaling
- Periodontal probing
- Dental implant placement
- Reimplantation of avulsed teeth
- Endodontic instrumentation when there is a risk of going through apex
- Endodontic (apical) surgery
- Initial placement of orthodontic bands but not brackets
- Intraligamental local anaesthetic injection
- Polishing of teeth and implants but only where gingival bleeding is expected
- Subgingival placement of antimicrobial fibres or strips (if ever indicated in these patients).

Cover is not needed for (Dajani et al 1997a):

- Restorative dentistry (operative and prosthodontic)[a]
- Careful use of retraction cord[b]
- All local anaesthesia except intraligamental
- Intracanal root canal treatment (i.e. not beyond the root apex)
- Post placement and build-up
- Placement of rubber dam
- Placement of removable prosthetic and orthodontic appliances.

[a]Restoration of caries and missing teeth.
[b]Clinical judgement needed as prophylaxis required if procedure causes bleeding.

RECOMMENDATIONS FOR ANTIBIOTIC PROPHYLAXIS

A number of factors influence the choice of antimicrobial agents such as bactericidal activity against the potential pathogens, relative toxicity, preferred route of administration, the nature of the cardiac abnormality and the history of drug allergy (BSAC 1982). The recommendations of the BSAC (1982) differed slightly in detail from those of their American counterpart (American Heart Association 1977). These differences were partly because of poor patient compliance to the American regimes which is reported to be 15% (Brookes 1980).

It has also been shown in some studies that the application of an antiseptic to the gingival margin or the use of a chlorhexidine mouthwash immediately prior to a procedure may reduce the severity of the bacteraemia (Jones et al 1970).

Most patients that require antibiotic prophylaxis are likely to be seen in general dental practice and in this situation an oral administration is preferred and much more likely to be complied with (Dajani et al 1997a). Many organisms may cause infective endocarditis but the viridans group of streptococci are by far the commonest cause. For these reasons the penicillins are the mainstay of agents used for prophylaxis. In this regard the broader spectrum amoxicillin is now preferred to penicillin V principally because of its significantly better absorption from oral administration and its ability to maintain high blood levels for the necessary period (Shanson et al 1978; Shanson et al 1980).

On this basis, the recommendations of the BSAC (1982) were to use oral amoxicillin 3 grams (g) orally, 1 h pre-operation. Children under 10 would receive one-half and those under 5 one-quarter of the adult dose. These doses were administered at the surgery under direct supervision. Patients allergic to penicillin were recommended to receive erythromycin stearate 1.5 g orally 1–2 h preoperative and 0.5 g 6 h later. The proportional reductions for children were the same as those for penicillins. This modified regime was recommended because erythromycin is less bactericidal than amoxicillin and has a less predictable absorption. This advice has recently been modified (see below).

It has also been shown that patients who had recently received penicillins were liable to harbour bacteria resistant to these drugs (Garod & Waterworth 1962; Spencer et al 1970). In these circumstances it seems better to use an alternative drug such as clindamycin or erythromycin.

For patients receiving general anaesthesia (GA) when oral administration is contraindicated the recommended regime was 1 g amoxicillin by intramuscular (i.m.) injection, followed by 0.5 g, 6 h later. The proportional reductions for children were the same as those above. At this time, it was also recommended to give this injection in 2.5 mL of 1% lidocaine (lignocaine) hydrochloride to reduce the pain of injection. This advice has been recently withdrawn (see below) (Littler et al 1997).

For patients in the high risk category, it was recommended to additionally administer gentamicin 120 mg i.m. either 1 h pre-operation for subjects treated under local anaesthesia (LA) or in those being treated under GA immediately before induction. Children should receive 2 mg gentamicin/kg body weight. Gentamicin is not particularly active against streptococci but gentamicin has been shown to act synergistically with penicillins in this respect (Watt 1978).

Patients who are allergic to penicillin or who have received it in the previous month and were undergoing GA were recommended to receive vancomycin as an alternative. Vancomycin alone has been used successfully in treating streptococcal infections including enterococci. However, a combination of vancomycin and gentamicin has been shown to be more reliably bactericidal in this respect (Watankunakorn & Bakie 1973; Shanson & Nomnyak 1982). They thus recommended that for GA patients that 1 g vancomycin be given by slow intravenous (i.v.) infusion over 30 min followed by 120 mg gentamicin i.v. Children should be given vancomycin 20 mg and gentamicin 2 mg/kg body weight. A related drug teicoplanin can also be used as an alternative to vancomycin since it can be given at or 15 min prior to induction. The recommended dose is 400 mg i.v. for adults with child doses of 6 mg/kg .

Roberts and Holzel (2002) have retrospectively investigated the efficiency of i.v. antibiotic regimes for children with severe congenital heart defects undergoing comprehensive dental treatment under GA. The antibiotics were administered i.v. immediately before the treatment and blood samples for culture were taken at the completion of the treatment. The overall percentage of positive cultures was 16% and was not significantly different for children given either i.v. ampicillin or i.v. amikacin and teicoplanin (16.7% vs 22.2%). Thus, in these children the bacteraemia associated with dental treatment was reduced by these antibiotics but still occurred in 16% of cases. However, amikacin and teicoplanin appear to be an effective alternative regimen in children that are allergic to penicillins or who have received them in the previous month.

The only changes proposed by the recent British Working Party (Littler et al 1997) was to cease to recommend giving i.m. amoxicillin in lidocaine (lignocaine) hydrochloride. This was because the revised data sheet on amoxicillin warned that it may now precipitate due to insolubility in this mixture because it was manufactured with marginally higher concentrations of amoxicillin to meet stringent legal requirements. They also report that there was international consensus on the use of amoxicillin.

American authorities (Dajani et al 1994) recommended the oral dose of amoxicillin as 2 g rather than 3 g. There is little difference in efficiency of the two doses initially but the 3 g dose has been shown to produce a higher serum level after 10–12 h (BSAC 1982; Littler et al 1997). The main reason for the difference was that the 3 g sachet of amoxicillin that was available in the UK was not available in the USA and therefore not available for their studies on optimum dose (Dajani et al 1994). In the UK, the 2 g dose was originally proposed in 1978 (BSAC 1982) but was replaced by the 3 g sachet when it became available which was then shown to have a better pharmacodynamic profile and patient acceptability (BSAC 1982; Littner et al 1986).

The only subsequent changes in the recommendations for cover have centred around the use of erythromycin as an alternative to amoxicillin when this was contraindicated. In this regard clindamycin, azithromycin and clarithromycin have been suggested as better alternatives (Pelletier et al 1975; Glauser & Francioli 1982; Dall et al 1990; Hall et al 1996; Vermot et al 1996; Rouse et al 1997).

Carmona et al (2007) analysed the efficacy of antibiotic prophylaxis in the prevention of bacteraemia following dental manipulations and in the prevention of bacterial endocarditis, reviewing both animal models and human studies. They noted that antibiotic prophylaxis guidelines remained consensus-based, and that there was scientific evidence of the efficacy of amoxicillin in the prevention of bacteraemia following dental procedures. However, the results reported did not confirm the efficacy of other recommended antibiotics. The majority of studies on experimental models of bacterial endocarditis have verified the efficacy of antibiotics administered after the induction of bacteraemia, confirming the efficacy of antibiotic prophylaxis in later stages in the development of bacterial endocarditis. However there was no scientific evidence that prophylaxis with penicillin was effective in reducing bacterial endocarditis secondary to dental procedures in patients considered to be 'at risk'.

Azithromycin has replaced clindamycin oral suspension for prophylaxis in children (Addy & Martin 2004). It was also recommended by the American Heart Association for prophylaxis in adults. The available evidence from animal models supported the efficiency of this drug as a prophylactic agent against oral streptococci and its pharmacological properties seem to make it a promising therapeutic adjunct in the management of odontological infections (Addy & Martin 2004). At present, there are only a small number of studies on the effectiveness of this relatively new drug. Further studies comparing this compound with other commonly used antibiotics would be of benefit in assessing its relative value.

In this regard, earlier work using the rabbit experimental aortic valve endocarditis model (Pelletier et al 1975) showed that at that time penicillin G and streptomycin in combination were the only agents in single dosage which could prevent the development of endocarditis stimulated by the inoculation of *V. streptococci*. It also showed that multiple doses of phenoxymethyl penicillin (penicillin V) or cefazolin alone or with streptomycin over 48 h also prevented its development. However, erythromycin uniformly failed to protect animals from bacterial endocarditis but showed greater prophylactic efficacy only when a low inoculum of streptococci was used.

Another study using the rat experimental aortic valve endocarditis model stimulated by inoculation of either *Streptococcus sanguis*, *S. intermedius* or *S. mitior* compared the effects of erythromycin, clindamycin and doxycycline as prophylactic agents (Glauser & Francioli 1982). Significant protection was achieved with all three antibiotics, but only clindamycin was fully effective against all three species at doses that simulated serum levels achievable in humans after oral administration. Endocarditis was prevented by antibiotic concentrations in serum far below minimal bactericidal concentrations for these streptococci. Furthermore, serum concentrations at the time of bacterial challenge were not bactericidal. Therefore, it was concluded that single doses of non-bactericidal antibiotics apparently prevented endocarditis in rats by mechanisms other than bacterial killing.

Members of the *Viridans* streptococcal group produce glycocalyx on their surface and it has been shown that abundant glycocalyx production by these bacteria in the rabbit model of endocarditis is associated with delayed antimicrobial sterilization. Furthermore, enzymatic digestion of the glycocalyx with dextranase has been shown to enhance antibiotic activity (Dall et al 1990).

The effect of clindamycin given three times daily was studied in rabbits with experimental aortic valve endocarditis caused by high glycocalyx-producing *V. streptococci* (Dall et al 1990). This revealed that animals receiving clindamycin had smaller vegetations which were sterilized more quickly than those in control animals or animals receiving penicillin or dextranase alone. Penicillin plus dextranase treatment allowed greater bacterial killing than penicillin alone but did not differ significantly from clindamycin treatment. In addition, electron micrographs revealed markedly less cell-adherent glycocalyx on bacteria grown *in vitro* in the presence of clindamycin than those grown with penicillin or neither. Therefore, it is hypothesized that clindamycin inhibits glycocalyx production *in vivo*, allowing better antimicrobial penetration in the infected cardiac vegetation.

In a human study (Hall et al 1996), erythromycin and clindamycin were compared for antibiotic prophylaxis. A total of 38 healthy patients were randomized to receive either erythromycin (1 g) or clindamycin (0.6 g) orally 1.5 h prior to dental extraction. Blood samples for microbiological investigation were collected before, during and 10 min after surgery. The incidence of bacteraemia with *V. streptococci* was 79% in the erythromycin group and 74% in the clindamycin group with no statistical difference between them in the incidence or magnitude of the bacteraemia with *V. streptococci* or anaerobic bacteria. A total of 96 aerobic and 133 anaerobic strains recovered from the blood samples were tested for their susceptibility to erythromycin and clindamycin as well as to penicillin V and ampicillin. The antimicrobials were found to be highly active against the majority of bacteria except for some *enterococci*, *staphylococci* and *Veillonella*. It was hypothesized that protection from endocarditis by prophylaxis with either erythromycin or clindamycin must be due to elimination of bacteria at later stage in the development of the disease, rather than by elimination of bacteria from blood during the short period of postoperative bacteraemia.

Clarithromycin has been also compared with clindamycin for single-dose prophylaxis of streptococcal endocarditis in rats (Vermot et al 1996). Achieving serum levels mimicking those in humans, the two antibiotics prevented endocarditis in animals challenged with both small and large amounts of bacterial inocula. Clarithromycin was marginally superior to clindamycin against small amounts of inocula and it was concluded that clarithromycin could be also considered for endocarditis chemoprophylaxis in humans.

In another study (Rouse et al 1997) the efficacy of azithromycin or clarithromycin was compared to that of amoxicillin, clindamycin, or erythromycin for the prevention of *Viridans* group streptococcal experimental endocarditis in rabbits. Animals with catheter-induced aortic valve vegetations were given either no antibiotics or two doses of each antibiotic. Antibiotics were administered 30 min before and 5.5 h after intravenous infusion of 5×10^5 CFU of *S. milleri*. At 48 h after the bacterial inoculation, the rabbits were killed and aortic valve vegetations were aseptically removed and cultured for bacteria. Infective endocarditis occurred in 88% of untreated animals, 1% of animals receiving amoxicillin, 9% of animals receiving erythromycin, 0% of animals receiving clindamycin, 2.5% of animals receiving clarithromycin, and 1% of animals receiving azithromycin. All five regimens were more significantly effective than no prophylaxis. Erythromycin was less effective than amoxicillin or clindamycin. Azithromycin or clarithromycin was as effective as amoxicillin, clindamycin, or erythromycin for the prevention of *Viridans* group streptococcus experimental endocarditis in this model.

It has also been shown that 600 mg of clindamycin i.v. given to 31 patients was able to penetrate to most tissues including muscle, bone, mucosa and skin between 15 min and 8 h after administration (Mueller et al 1999). It was demonstrated that clindamycin concentrations above the MIC90 of those pathogens most likely to cause oral wound contamination were reached in all the tissues investigated. Already 15 min after administration, tissue concentrations above the MIC90 were reached and were still detectable in the last samples taken between 4 and 8 h after the last clindamycin administration. This shows that from the pharmacokinetic point of view, clindamycin is suitable for antibiotic prophylaxis.

Finally, it has also been shown that clindamycin has a much lower ability to produce hypersensitivity reactions than previously claimed (Mazur et al 1999). In 3896 clindamycin administrations between 1995 and 1997, 14 (0.47%) adverse reactions were reported and seven of these were compounded by the co-administration of other agents. Thus, its potential to stimulate hypersensitivity appears low.

Thus, clindamycin, azithromycin and clarithromycin appear to be better agents than erythromycin for use as alternatives to amoxicillin in prophylaxis both when given orally or parenterally.

Earlier recommendations of the Working Party for antibiotic prophylaxis are shown in **Figure 18.2** for procedures under local analgesia and in **Figure 18.3** for those procedures under general anaesthesia. The necessary percentage reductions of doses for children on the basis of age and weight are shown in Table 18.3.

MANAGEMENT OF CASES REQUIRING ANTIBIOTIC COVER

In addition, the prophylactic use of antibiotics should be reduced to the minimum by sensible management (Eley 1983a). Patients which give a history of rheumatic fever should be sent to a cardiologist for cardiac investigations to see whether the patient has actually suffered from rheumatic heart disease. When such patients were investigated in this way, many were found to have no cardiac disease and thus did not need prophylactic antibiotic cover. An examination by a cardiologist should also be arranged for apparently healthy patients reporting cardiac murmurs if the exact status is not already known and available from their general medical practitioner.

If antibiotic prophylaxis is required for patients at risk from a transient bacteraemia then treatment producing a bacteraemia should be organized in the minimum number of visits and at least 6 weeks should elapse before antibiotic administration is repeated.

IS ANTIBIOTIC PROPHYLAXIS STILL JUSTIFIED FOR ALL RISK GROUPS

Prophylactic antibiotics are given to patients at risk from infective endocarditis on the premise that certain dental procedures cause bacteraemia and infective endocarditis carries a high morbidity and mortality (Durack 1995, 1998). In this regard it has been shown that prophylactic antibiotics can prevent induced infective endocarditis in experimental animals (Moreillon et al 1986; Malinverni et al 1987; Dajani et al 1997a,b) and on these grounds it was widely recommended for this purpose in humans (Durack 1995; Dajani et al 1997a,b). Compliance with these regimes is less than perfect (van der Meer et al 1992a) and apparent failures far from rare (Durack et al 1983). Moreover, the recommended procedures were so entrenched that failure to give medication could have generated malpractice claims (Martin et al 1997). However, neither the effectiveness of prophylaxis in humans nor its cost-effectiveness have been proven and probably never will be (Durack 1995). In addition, the foundation of this practice has been seriously questioned (Guntheroth 1984; Clemens & Ransohoff 1984; Bor & Himmelstein 1984; Pallasch 1989; van der Meer et al 1992b,c; Wahl 1994; Roberts 1999; Epstein 1999).

Fig. 18.2 Antibiotic regimens for patients at risk from transient bacteraemia when treated under local analgesia.

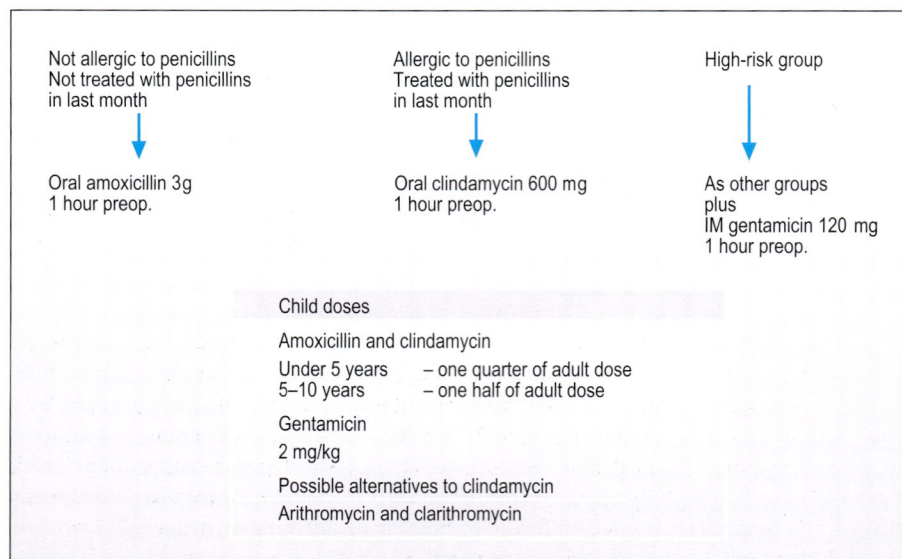

Not allergic to penicillins Not treated with penicillins in last month	Allergic to penicillins Treated with penicillins in last month	High-risk group
Oral amoxicillin 3g 1 hour preop.	Oral clindamycin 600 mg 1 hour preop.	As other groups plus IM gentamicin 120 mg 1 hour preop.

Child doses

Amoxicillin and clindamycin

| Under 5 years | – one quarter of adult dose |
| 5–10 years | – one half of adult dose |

Gentamicin

2 mg/kg

Possible alternatives to clindamycin

Arithromycin and clarithromycin

Not allergic to penicillins
Not treated with penicillins
in last month

IV amoxicillin 1 g
at induction plus
oral amoxicillin 500 mg
6 hours later

or

IV amoxicillin 3 g
4 hours prehinduction
plus
oral amoxicillin 3 g
as soon as possible
after recovery

or

Oral amoxicillin 3 g
plus
oral probenecid 1g
4 hours preop.

Child doses

Amoxicillin and clindamycin

Under 5 years — one quarter of adult dose
5–10 years — one half of adult dose

Gentamicin
2 mg/kg

Vancomycin
20 mg/kg

Teicoplanin
6 mg/kg

Allergic to penicillins
treated with penicillins
in last month

IV vancomycin 1 g
over at least 100 mins plus
IV gentamicin 120 mg
at induction

or

IV teicoplanin 400 mg
plus
IV gentamicin 120 mg
at induction

or

IV clindamycin 300 mg
over at least 10 mins
plus
at induction
oral clindamycin 300 mg

High-risk group

IV amoxicillin 1 g
plus
IV gentamicin 120 mg

or

If allergic to penicillin
or
treated with penicillin
in last month

either

IV vancomycin 1 g
over at least 100 minutes
plus
IV gentamicin 120 mg
at induction

or

IV teicoplanin 400 mg
plus
IV gentamicin 120 mg
at induction

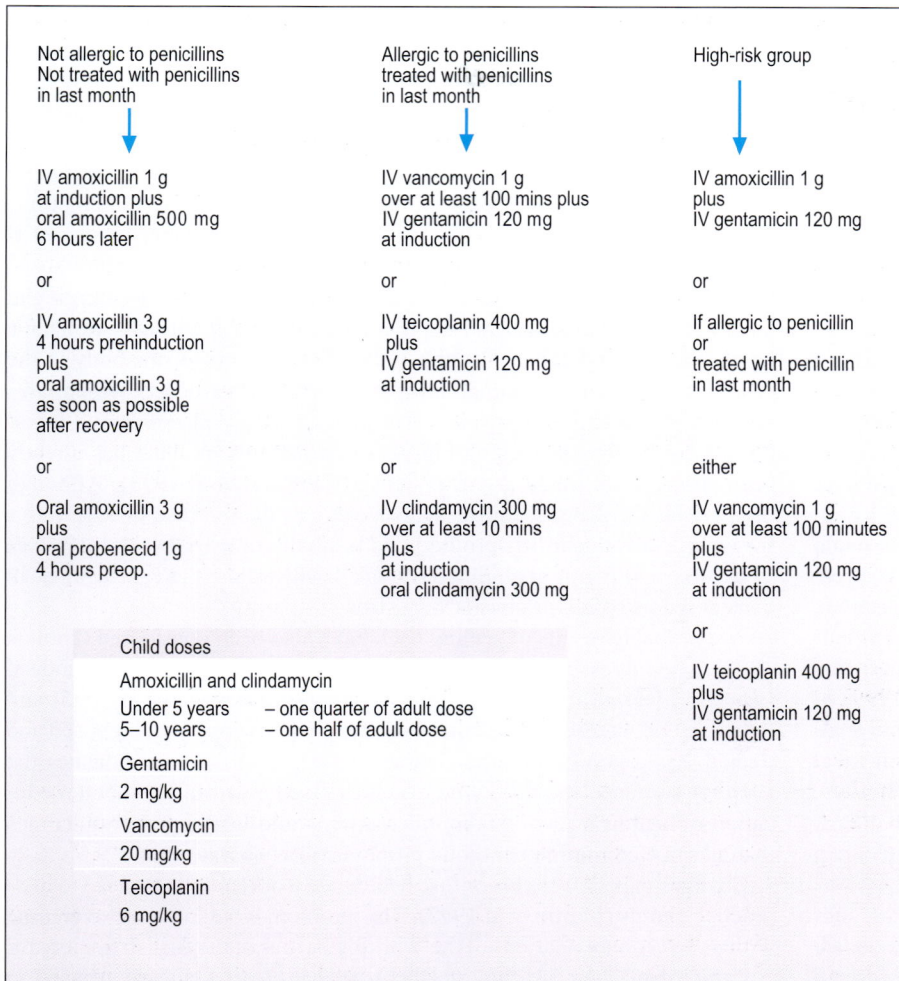

Fig. 18.3 Antibiotic regimens for patients at risk from transient bacteraemia when treated under general anaesthesia.

Table 18.3 *The percentage of the adult dose for children*

Age	Ideal bodyweight		Height		Body surface	Percentage of adult dose
	(kg)	**(lb)**	**(mm)**	**(inches)**		
Children						
Newborn	3.4	7.5	500	20	0.23	12.5
1 month	4.2	9.0	550	22	0.26	14.5
3 months	5.6	12	590	23	0.32	18
6 months	7.7	17	670	26	0.40	22
1 year	10	22	760	30	0.47	25
3 years	14	31	940	37	0.62	33
5 years	18	40	1080	42	0.73	40
7 years	23	51	1200	47	0.88	50
12 years	37	81	1480	58	1.25	75
Adult						
Male	68	150	1727	68	1.8	100
Female	56	123	1626	64	1.6	100

A case control study (Strom et al 1998) compared 273 cases of infective endocarditis, 104 (38%) of whom knew of a previous heart condition with a control group and showed no link between infective endocarditis and dental procedures. The incubation period before the onset of symptoms when endocarditis follows dental treatment is usually short (Stortebaum et al 1997) and in the study above (Strom et al 1998) the risk of infective endocarditis was no higher in the first month after dental treatment than after 2–3 months. This is consistent with a lack of a link between them.

This, of course does not prove that dental treatment never results in infective endocarditis as it has been shown that it occasionally does (Okell & Elliot 1935; Sale 1938; Stortebaum et al 1997; Droz et al 1997). Furthermore, appropriate antibiotic prophylaxis does not always protect against infective endocarditis since a report has been published on two patients with known congenital heart disease in whom endocarditis developed after dental extractions, despite the appropriate administration of the recommended antibiotics (O'Sullivan et al 1996). The Strom et al (1998) study does however indicate that this event is too rare to justify antibiotic prophylaxis for all cases at risk. It also supports the results of previous case control studies in the Netherlands and France (van der Meer et al 1992b,c; Lacassin et al 1995).

In contrast to the irrelevance of dental treatment, Strom et al (1998) emphasized the importance of the nature of the underlying cardiac valvular abnormality and the risk factors of prosthetic valves and a history of previous infective endocarditis since these factors produced high odds ratios in their statistical analysis. In this study (Strom et al 1998) no particular type of dental treatment, not even dental extractions, was linked to infective endocarditis. However, dental extractions were prominent in case reports of infective endocarditis after dental treatment (Okell & Elliot 1935; Sale 1938; O'Sullivan et al 1996; Droz et al 1997; Doerffel et al 1997). Furthermore, dental extractions were more prone than any other procedure to produce bacteraemia (Okell & Elliot 1935; Roberts et al 1998b). In this regard, Strom et al (1998) reported that only six out of 273 patients with infective endocarditis had had dental extractions within 2 months compared with none of the controls. These figures were much too small to produce statistical significance, but they did indicate the real possibility of a type II statistical error with regard to extractions (Durack 1998). This possibility was crucial but did not detract from the main findings of the study.

Thus, in summary, four major case control studies (van der Meer et al 1992a,b; Strom et al 1998; Lacassin et al 1995) and several outcome analyses and commentaries (Guntheroth 1984; Clemens & Ransohoff et al 1984; Bor & Himmelstein 1984; Pallasch 1989; Wahl 1994; Roberts 1999, Epstein 1999) have presented substantial grounds on which to challenge the value of the practice of administering antibiotic before dental treatment to prevent infective endocarditis (Durack 1998).

In a commentary on the study by Strom et al (1998), Durack (1998) suggested that the time had come to scale back on antibiotic prophylaxis. He felt that the list of dental procedures requiring prophylaxis should be downgraded to only dental extractions and gingival surgery including implant placement and the cardiac conditions requiring cover were limited to prosthetic heart valves including both bioprosthetic and homograft valves, previous history of infective endocarditis, complex cyanotic congenital heart disease (e.g. single ventricle states, transposition of great arteries and Fallot's tetralogy) and surgically constructed systemic – pulmonary shunts or conduits. This corresponded with the cardiac conditions classified in the high risk category. He recommended that when any of these conditions were present, prophylaxis followed the recommendations of the British Society for Antimicrobial Chemotherapy (BSAC 1982; Littler et al 1997) or the American Heart Association (Dajani et al 1997a,b) depending on their place of work.

In these proposals (Durack 1998) mitral valve prolapse (MVP) was not included in the conditions requiring cover in spite of the fact that a significant proportion of infective endocarditis cases did occur in patients with MVP. This is because the number of patients with MVP was large and the risk incurred by any individual MVP patient, including those with echocardiographic and Doppler confirmation of regurgitation, was much lower than that for a patient with a prosthetic heart valve or a previous episode of infective endocarditis or both (Strom et al 1998). Furthermore the prognosis of *Viridans* streptococcal infective endocarditis was very good following appropriate antibiotic treatment (Durack 1998).

The changes recommended by Durack (1998) would have eliminated most of the prophylactic antibiotic doses given to dental patients and resulted in several important benefits. Decreased use of antibiotics would have resulted in fewer side-effects such as hypersensitivity reactions and gastrointestinal upsets. In this regard three times more people die from anaphylaxis due to antibiotics than die from endocarditis (Clemens & Ransohoff 1984; Bor & Himmelstein 1984). It would also result in considerably more convenience for patients and less work for health care workers. The resultant financial gain would be refocused on high risk procedures and patients. Evidence (van der Meer et al 1992b,c; Strom et al 1998; Lacassin et al 1995) showed that with this policy it was possible to retain 80% of any putative benefits from current antibiotic prophylaxis for less than 20% of the cost.

Selection for antibiotic resistance is probably the strongest argument for this change. *V. streptococci* are traditionally susceptible to penicillins but they have been shown to be starting to develop resistance (Doern et al 1996, 2001). Because they are feeble pathogens in normal, healthy hosts, this sea change has not achieved the notoriety of the resistance emerging in pneumococci, enterococci and staphylococci. However, this may well have its own dark significance (Durack 1998). The entrance of the body to the oropharynx shelters a standing army of *Viridans streptococci* which have not only the potential to accept resistance genes via plasmids and transposons from passing bacteria but also to donate them. This has already been shown to occur with pneumococci (Dowson et al 1993). Although the magnitude of the selective pressure due to the overuse of antibiotics for infective endocarditis prophylaxis is small compared with their uses in treatment it is not negligible (Durack 1998). Thus, the case against ill considered use of antibiotics is very strong.

The probable results of scaling back have also been considered (Durack 1998). The increase in infective endocarditis would be very small indeed (van der Meer et al 1992b,c; Strom et al 1998; Lacassin et al 1995) and infective endocarditis after dental treatment, when promptly diagnosed and treated, has a good prognosis (Durack 1998). Best practice indicates the need for vigilance and follow-up to achieve the best results and better education of healthcare workers in this matter would lead to better outcomes than unselected routine antibiotic prophylaxis as operates now.

Changes in policy could confuse healthcare workers and also lead to malpractice claims (Martin et al 1997). This problem would only be overcome with new recommendations of the Working Parties of the British Society for Antimicrobial Chemotherapy and the American Heart Association based on these new findings and conditions. Malpractice claims would then be minimized by emphasizing that antibiotics are not generally required except for a subgroup of high risk patients. Clinical judgement would always need to be used in these situations (Dajani et al 1997a).

Children were excluded from the case control studies (van der Meer et al 1992b,c; Strom et al 1998; Lacassin et al 1995) and the problems of the patterns of major congenital heart disease and surgery were not addressed. However, it was generally accepted that most of the severe cases in this category were included in the high risk group and thus should always receive antibiotic prophylaxis.

There have been nine changes in the American recommendations for antibiotic prophylaxis over the years (Durack 1998) and several others in Britain and Europe. At first, these recommendations were steered by paediatric cardiologists who were experts on rheumatic fever. Later influences came from infective disease specialists which resulted in more extensive use. There then followed enthusiasm for parenteral regimes fuelled by the publication of many studies which showed parenteral antibiotics to be most effective in preventing experimental animal endocarditis caused by bacteraemia (Durack 1995; Moreillon et al 1986; Malinverni et al 1987). These were then modulated by the emergence of effective and convenient oral regimes (BSAC 1982; Shanson et al 1978; Shanson et al 1980; Littler et al 1997; Shanson & Nomnyak 1982; Dajani et al 1997b). The emphasis changed again with further evidence from the epidemiological and outcome studies (van der Meer et al 1992b,c; Strom et al 1998; Lacassin et al 1995).

It would seem most sensible to stay with the current Working Party recommendations in response to pressure from recent findings which protect against malpractice claims. We should also attempt to raise the level of oral and particularly periodontal health in all the risk groups since this would reduce and possibly eliminate the bacteraemias that result from normal function, i.e. chewing, toothbrushing and flossing when the gingival margin is inflamed. These normal procedures may well result in greater overall exposures to bacteraemia than treatment procedures (Durack 1998). Furthermore, good overall oral health should remove the need for extractions and other forms of minor oral surgery which constitute the greatest dental treatment risk to these patients.

Latterly, recommendations of the British Cardiac Society and the Royal College of Physicians (2004) on the dental aspects of endocarditis prophylaxis differed significantly from previous international consensus guidance, reported above. It recommended its additional use for a range of restorative procedures including placement of rubber dam, matrix band use, wedging and retraction cord placement and the use of i.v. antibiotics for high risk cases. This flies in the face of recent scientific research and the wealth of evidence showing the effectiveness of oral administration, reported above. These all suggested that current regimes were unnecessarily stringent (Dajani et al 1997a; Seymour et al 2000). It would also result in a wholly undesirable increase in antibiotic use and an associated increase in complications such as hypersensitivity and bacterial resistance. Furthermore, there was no evidence associating restorative procedures with endocarditis.

Following these reports, there has now been new guidelines from a new report of the British Society for Antimicrobial Chemotherapy (BSAC), which brings the findings of all these new reports together (Gould et al 2006). A summary of this is set out below.

A BSAC group of experts spent a lot of time in again reviewing the evidence for possible risk of endocarditis following certain dental procedures. This time they concluded that there was no evidence that these procedures increased the risk for infective endocarditis. They therefore recommended that the current practice of giving antibiotic prophylaxis to patients with medium and low risks for infective endocarditis should be stopped and only be continued for those in the high risk group. The main reasons given were the lack of any supporting evidence that dental treatment can lead to infective endocarditis and the increasing worry that the administration of antibiotics may lead to other serious complications such as anaphylaxis or antibiotic resistance. This new report should now serve as the basis for the use of antibiotic prophylaxis by all dental practitioners and dental groups. However, this report was sent (May 2007) to the National Institute for Clinical Excellence (NICE) and their report and decision were awaited at the end of this year. In 2008, a clinical practice guideline on prophylaxis against infective endocarditis was being developed for use in the NHS in England, Wales and Northern Ireland. Registered stakeholders for the prophylaxis against infective endocarditis (IE) guidelines were invited to comment on the provisional recommendations via the NICE website.

In 2008 NICE reported and recommended the following:

■ Antibiotic prophylaxis against IE was not required for patients at risk for IE undergoing dental treatment
■ Patients must maintain a high standard of oral hygiene
■ They should receive a chlorhexidine mouthwash prior to treatment
■ Patients in the higher risk group for IE should receive antibiotic prophylaxis. These include
  ◆ acquired valvular stenosis or regurgitation
  ◆ valve replacement
  ◆ congenital heart disease including surgically corrected defects but excluding isolated atrial septal defect and corrected ductus arteriosis.

Thus these recommendations were very similar to those outlined previously in this chapter.

Although current legislation in the UK (2009) states that no antibiotic cover is required prior to dental procedures.

MAINTENANCE OF GOOD DENTAL HEALTH

Transient bacteraemia may also arise from normal functional activity and tooth cleaning when gingivitis or periodontitis is present (Pallasch & Slots 1991, 2000; Roberts et al 1997; Roberts 1999) and is best prevented by the maintenance of dental health and the prevention and early treatment of periodontal diseases. A good preventive programme in these patients from an early age should help to prevent dental caries and chronic periodontitis and thus obviate the need for dental extractions, subgingival scaling and other surgery requiring prophylactic antibiotics in most patients (Eley 1983b). Good oral hygiene should also prevent gingivitis which can lead to transient bacteraemia. Appropriate periodontal and restorative care must be made available to these patients and all teeth retained in these patients' mouths should be periodontally stable.

REFERENCES

Addy LD, Martin MV: Azithromycin and dentistry – a useful agent? *Br Dent J* 197: 141–143, 2004.

Akintoye SO, Brennan MT, Graber CJ, et al: A retrospective investigation of advanced periodontal disease as a risk factor for septicaemia in hematopoietic stem cell and bone marrow transplant recipients, *Oral Surg Oral Med Oral Pathol Oral Radiol Endod* 94:581–608, 2002.

American Heart Association: Committee on Prevention of Rheumatic Fever and Bacterial Endocarditis. Prevention of bacterial endocarditis, *Circulation* 56: 139A–143A, 1977.

Anonymous: Advisory statement. Antibiotic prophylaxis for dental patients with total joint replacements. American Dental Association; American Academy of Orthopaedic Surgeons, *J Am Dent Assoc* 128:1004–1008, 1997.

Awadallah SM, Kavey REW, Byrum CJ, et al: The changing patterns of infective endocarditis in childhood, *Am J Cardiol* 68:90–94, 1991.

Binder IB, Naiderof IJ, Garvey GJ: Bacterial endocarditis: a consideration for physicians and dentists, *J Am Dent Assoc* 109:415–420, 1984.

Bor DH, Himmelstein DU: Endocarditis prophylaxis for patients with mitral valve prolapse. A quantitative analysis, *Am J Med* 76:711–717, 1984.

Boudoulas H, Wooley CF: Mitral valve prolapse. In Emmanauilides GC, Reimenschneider TA, Allen HD, Gutegsell HP, editors: *Moss and Adam's Heart Disease in Infants, Children and Adolescents Including Fetus and Young Adult*, ed 5, Baltimore, MD, 1995, Williams and Wilkins, pp 1063–1086.

British Cardiac Society and the Royal College of Physicians: *Dental aspects of endocarditis prophylaxis: new recommendations from the British Cardiac Society Guidelines and the Royal College of Physicians Clinical Effectiveness and Evaluation Unit*. Online. Available: www.rceng.ac.uk. 2004.

Brookes SL: Compliance with AHA guidelines for prevention of bacterial endocarditis, *J Am Med Assoc* 101:41–43, 1980.

BSAC: The antibiotic prophylaxis of infective endocarditis. Report of a working party of the British Society for Antimicrobial Chemotherapy, *Lancet* 2:1323–1326, 1982.

Carabello BA: Mitral valve prolapse, *Curr Probl Cardiol* 7:423–478, 1993.

Carmona T, Dios DP, Scully C: Efficacy of antibiotic prophylactic regimens for the prevention of bacterial endocarditis of oral origin, *J Dent Res* 86:1142–1159, 2007.

Cates JE, Christie RV: Subacute bacterial endocarditis: a review of 442 patients treated at 4 centres appointed by Penicillin Trials Committee of Medical Research Committee, *Q J Med* 20:93–130, 1951.

Cawson RA: Infective endocarditis as a complication of dental treatment, *Br Dent J* 151:409–414, 1981.

Cheitlin MD, Alpert JS, Armstrong WF, et al: American College of Cardiologists/ American Heart Association guidelines for the clinical application of echocardiography: a report of the American College of Cardiologists/American Heart Association task force on Practical Guidelines (Committee on Clinical Applications of Echocardiography), *Circulation* 95:1686–1744, 1997.

Cherubin CE, Neu HE: Infective endocarditis at the Presbyterian Hospital in New York City from 1938–1967, *Am J Med* 51:83–96, 1971.

Clemens JD, Ransohoff DF: A quantitative assessment of pre-dental antibiotic prophylaxis with mitral valve prolapse, *J Chronic Dis* 37:531–544, 1984.

Dajani AS, Bawden RE, Berry MC: Oral amoxicillin prophylaxis for endocarditis: what is the optimum dose? *Clinical Infective Disease* 18:157–160, 1994.

Dajani AS, Taubert KA, Wilson W, et al: Prevention of bacterial endocarditis. Recommendation by the American Heart Association, *J Am Med Assoc* 277: 1794–1801, 1997a.

Dajani AS, Taubert KA, Wilson W, et al: Prevention of bacterial endocarditis. Recommendations by the American Heart Association, *Circulation* 96:358–366, 1997b.

Dall L, Keilhofner M, Herndon B, et al: Clindamycin effect on glycocalyx production in experimental viridans streptococcal endocarditis, *J Infect Dis* 161: 1221–1224, 1990.

Daly C, Mitchell D, Grossberg D, et al: Bacteraemia caused by periodontal probing, *Aust Dent J* 42:77–80, 1997.

Danchin N, Briancon S, Mathieu P, et al: Mitral valve prolapse as a risk factor for infective endocarditis, *Lancet* 1:743–745, 1989.

Devereux RD, Hawkins I, Kramer-Fox R, et al: Complications of mitral valve prolapse; disproportionate occurrence in men and older patients, *Am J Med* 81:751–758, 1986.

Devereux RB, Kramer-Fox R, Kligfield P: Mitral valve prolapse: causes, clinical manifestations and management, *Ann Intern Med* 111:305–317, 1989.

Devereux RB, Frary CJ, Kramer-Fox R, et al: Cost effectiveness of infective endocarditis prophylaxis for mitral valve prolapse with or without mitral regurgitation murmur, *Am J Cardiol* 74:1024–1029, 1994.

Doerffel W, Fietze I, Baumann G, et al: Severe prosthetic valve-related endocarditis following dental scaling: a case report, *Quintessence Int* 28:271–274, 1997.

Doern GV, Brueggemann A, Holley HP Jr., et al: Antimicrobial resistance of Streptococcus pneumoniae recovered from outpatients in the United States during the winter months of 1994 to 1995: results of a 30-center national surveillance study, *Antimicrob Agents Chemother* 40:1208–1213, 1996.

Doern GV, Heilmann KP, Huynh HK, et al: Antimicrobial resistance among clinical isolates of Streptococcus pneumoniae in the United States during 1999–2000, including a comparison of resistance rates since 1994–1995, *Antimicrob Agents Chemother* 45:1721–1729, 2001.

Dowson CG, Coffey TJ, Kell C, et al: Evolution of penicillin resistance in Streptococcus pneumoniae: the role of Streptococcus mitis in the formation of low affinity PBP2B in S. Pneumoniae, *Mol Microbiol* 9:635–643, 1993.

Droz D, Koch L, Lenain A, et al: Bacterial endocarditis: results of a survey in a children's hospital in France, *Br Dent J* 183:101–105, 1997.

Durack DT: Prophylaxis of endocarditis. In Mandell GI, Douglas RG, Bennett JE, editors: *Principles and Practice of Infectious Diseases,* New York, 1979, John Wiley, pp 701–710.

Durack DT: Prevention of infective endocarditis, *N Engl J Med* 332:38–44, 1995.

Durack DT: Antibiotics for prevention of endocarditis during dentistry: time to scale back? *Ann Intern Med* 129:829–831, 1998.

Durack DT, Kaplan EL, Bisno AL: Apparent failures of endocarditis prophylaxis. Analysis of 52 cases submitted to the national registry, *JAMA* 250:2318–2355, 1983.

Eley BM: Infective endocarditis: a dentist's view. 1. Aetiology and dental treatment, *Cardiology in Practice* 1:35–38, 1983a.

Eley BM: Infective endocarditis: a dentist's view. 2. Prevention, *Cardiology in Practice* 1:16–19, 1983b.

Elliott SD: Bacteraemia following tonsillectomy, *Lancet* 2:589–592, 1939.

Epstein JB: Infective endocarditis and dentistry: outcome-based research, *J Can Dent Assoc (Tor)* 65:95–96, 1999.

Felix JE, Rosen S, App GR: Detection of bacteremia after use of oral irrigation device on subjects with periodontitis, *J Periodontol* 42:785–787, 1971.

Field EA, Martin MV: Prophylactic antibiotics for patients with artificial joints undergoing oral and dental surgery: necessary or not? *British Journal of Maxillofacial Surgery* 29:341–346, 1991.

Forner L, Larsen T, Kilian M, et al: Incidence of bacteremia after chewing, tooth brushing and scaling in individuals with periodontal inflammation, *J Clin Periodontol* 33:401–407, 2006.

Garod LP, Waterworth PM: The risks of extraction during penicillin treatment, *Br Heart J* 39:46, 1962.

Gersony WM, Hayes CT, Driscoll DJ, et al: Bacterial endocarditis in patients with aortic stenosis, pulmonary stenosis or ventricle septal defect, *Circulation* 87(Suppl 1):121–126, 1993.

Glauser MP, Francioli P: Successful prophylaxis against experimental streptococcal endocarditis with bacteriostatic antibiotics, *J Infect Dis* 146:806–810, 1982.

Gould FK, Elliott TSJ, Foweraker J, et al: Guidelines for prevention of endocarditis: report of the Working Party of the British Society for Antimicrobial Chemotherapy, *J Antimicrob Chemother* 57:1035–1042, 2006.

Grant A, Hoddinott C: Joint replacement, dental surgery, and antibiotic prophylaxis, *Br Med J* 304:959, 1992.

Guntheroth WG: How important are dental procedures as a cause of endocarditis, *Am J Cardiol* 54:797–801, 1984.

Hall G, Nord CE, Heimdahl A: Elimination of bacteraemia after dental extraction: comparison of erythromycin and clindamycin for prophylaxis of infective endocarditis, *J Antimicrob Chemother* 37:783–795, 1996.

Hunter KD, Hollborrow DW, Kardos TB, et al: Bacteremia and tissue damage following air polishing, *Br Dent J* 167:275–277, 1989.

Jaspers MT, Little JW: Prophylactic antibiotic coverage in patients with total arthroplasty: current practice, *J Am Dent Assoc* 111:943–948, 1985.

Jones JC, Catchen JL, Goldberg JR, et al: Control of the bacteraemia associated with the extraction of teeth, *Oral Surg Oral Med Oral Pathol* 30:453–459, 1970.

Kay D: Prophylaxis for infective endocarditis; an update, *Ann Intern Med* 104:419–423, 1986.

Kinane DF, Riggio MP, Katie F, et al: Bacteraemia following periodontal procedures, *J Clin Periodontol* 32:708–713, 2005.

Lacassin F, Hoen B, Leport C, et al: Procedures associated with infective endocarditis in adults. A case control study, *Eur Heart J* 16:1968–1974, 1995.

Lafaurie GI, Mayorga-Fayad I, Torres MF, et al: Periodontopathic microorganisms in peripheric blood after scaling and root planing , *J Clin Periodontol* 34:873–887, 2007.

La Porte DM, Waldman BJ, Mont MA, et al: Infections associated with dental procedures in total hip arthroplasty, *J Bone Joint Surg* 81:56–59, 1999.

Little JW: Patients with prosthetic joints: are they at risk when receiving invasive dental procedures? *Spec Care Dentis* 17:153–160, 1997.

Littler WA, McGowen DA, Shanson DC: Changes in recommendations about prophylaxis for prevention of endocarditis, *Lancet* 350:1100, 1997.

Littner MM, Kaffe T, Tamse A, et al: A new concept on chemoprophylaxis of bacterial endocarditis resulting from dental treatment, *Oral Surg Oral Med Oral Pathol* 61:338–342, 1986.

MacMahon SW, Roberts JK, Kramer-Fox R, et al: Mitral valve prolapse and infective endocarditis, *Am Heart J* 113:1291–1298, 1987.

Malinverni R, Francioli PB, Glauser MP: Comparison of single and multiple doses of prophylactic antibiotics in experimental streptococcal endocarditis, *Circulation* 76:378–382, 1987.

Marks AR, Choong CY, Sanfilippo AJ, et al: Identification of high-risk and low-risk subgroups of patients with mitral valve prolapse, *N Engl J Med* 320:1031–1036, 1989.

Martin MV, Butterworth ML, Longman LP: Infective endocarditis and the dental practitioner: a review of 53 cases involving litigation, *Br Dent J* 182:465–468, 1997.

Mason JC, Dollery CT, So A, et al: An infected prosthetic hip – is there a role for antibiotic prophylaxis? *Br Med J* 305:300–302, 1992.

Mazur N, Greenberger PA, Regalado J: Clindamycin hypersensitivity appears to be rare, *Ann Allergy Asthma Immunol* 82:443–445, 1999.

McKinsey RS, Ratts TE, Bisno AL: Underlying cardiac lesions in adults with infective endocarditis, *Am J Med* 82:681–688, 1987.

Moreillon P, Francioli P, Overhalse D, et al: Mechanisms of successful amoxicillin prophylaxis of experimental endocarditis due to Streptococcus intermedius, *J Infect Dis* 154:801–807, 1986.

Morelas AR, Romanelli R, Boucek RJ, et al: Myxoid heart disease, an assessment of extravascular cardiac pathology in severe mitral valve prolapse, *Hum Pathol* 23:129–137, 1992.

Mueller SC, Henkel KO, Neumann J, et al: Preoperative antibiotic prophylaxis in maxillofacial surgery: penetration of clindamycin into various tissues, *J Craniomaxillofac Surg* 27:172–176, 1999.

Nishimura RA, McGoon MD, Shub C, et al: Echocardiographically documented mitral valve prolapse, *N Engl J Med* 313:1305–1309, 1985.

O'Sullivan J, Anderson J, Bain H: Infective endocarditis in children following dental extraction and appropriate antibiotic prophylaxis, *Br Dent J* 181:64–65, 1996.

Office of Population Census and Survey: *Mortality Statistics for 1979*, London, 1980, HM Stationery Office.

Okell CC, Elliott SD: Bacteraemia and oral sepsis with special reference to subacute endocarditis, *Lancet* 2:868–872, 1935.

Pallasch TJ: A critical appraisal of antibiotic prophylaxis, *Int Dent J* 39:183–896, 1989.

Pallasch TJ, Slots J: Antibiotic prophylaxis for medical-risk patients, *J Periodontol* 62:227–231, 1991.

Pallasch TJ, Slots J: 1996 Antibiotic prophylaxis and medically compromised patients, *Periodontology* 10:107–138, 2000.

Pelletier LL Jr, Durack DT, Petersdorf RG: Chemotherapy of experimental streptococcal endocarditis. IV. Further observations on prophylaxis, *J Clin Invest* 56:319–330, 1975.

Prabha SD, O'Rourke RA: Mitral valve prolapse. In Rahimtoola SA, editor: *Atlas of Heart Diseases: Valvular Heart Disease*, Vol. XI, St Louis, MO, 1997, Mosby Year Books, pp 1–10.

Rajasuo A, Perkki K, Nyfors S, et al: Bacteremia following surgical dental extraction with emphasis on anaerobic strains, *J Dent Res* 83:171–174, 2004.

Roberts GJ: Dentists are innocent: 'Everyday' bacteraemia is the real culprit: a review and assessment of the evidence that dental surgical procedures are a principal cause of bacterial endocarditis in children, *Pediatr Cardiol* 20:317–325, 1999.

Roberts GJ, Holzel HS, Sury MR, et al: Dental bacteremia in children, *Pediatr Cardiol* 18:24–27, 1997.

Roberts GJ, Watts R, Longhurst P, Gardner P: Bacteremia of dental origin and antimicrobial sensitivity following oral surgical procedures in children, *Pediatr Dent* 20:28–36, 1998a.

Roberts GJ, Simmons NB, Longhurst P, et al: Bacteraemia following local anaesthetic injections in children, *Br Dent J* 185:295–298, 1998b.

Roberts GJ, Holzel HS: Intravenous antibiotic regimes and prophylaxis of odontogenic bacteraemia, *Br Dent J* 193:525–527, 2002.

Romans AR, App GR: Bacteremia, a result from oral irrigation in subjects with gingivitis, *J Periodontol* 42:757–760, 1971.

Rouse MS, Steckelberg JM, Brandt CM, et al: Efficacy of azithromycin or clarithromycin for prophylaxis of viridans group streptococcus experimental endocarditis, *Antimicrob Agents Chemother* 41:1673–1676, 1997.

Saiman L, Prince A, Gersony WM: Pediatric infective endocarditis in the modern era, *J Pediatr* 122:847–853, 1993.

Sale L: Some tragic results following extraction of teeth, *J Am Dent Assoc* 26:1647–1651, 1938.

Sandhu SS, Lowry JC, Reuben SF, et al: Who decides on the need for antibiotic prophylaxis in patients with major arthroplasties requiring dental treatment: is it a joint responsibility? *Ann R Coll Surg Engl* 79:143–147, 1997.

Savarrioa L, Mackenzie D, Riggioa M, et al: Detection of bacteraemias during non-surgical root canal treatment, *J Dent* 33:293–303, 2005.

Seymour RA, Lowry R, Whitworth JM, et al: Infective endocarditis, dentistry and antibiotic prophylaxis: a time to rethink, *Br Dent J* 189:610–616, 2000.

Shanson DC, Cannon P, Wells M: Amoxicillin compared to penicillin V for the prophylaxis of dental bacteraemia, *J Antimicrob Chemother* 4:431–436, 1978.

Shanson DC, Ashford RFU, Sing LJ: High dose amoxicillin for preventing endocarditis, *Br Med J* 280:446, 1980.

Shanson DC, Namnyak S: Viridans streptococci with reduced bactericidal susceptibility to erythromycin, rifampicin, vancomycin and aminoglycosides. Current chemotherapy and immunotherapy. In Peri P, Grassi CC, editors: *Proceedings of the 12th International Congress of Chemotherapy, Florence, Italy, 19–24th July 1981,* Washington DC, 1982, American Society for Microbiology, pp 311–313.

Shrout MK, Scarbrough F, Powell BJ: Dental care and the prosthetic joint patient: a survey of orthopedic surgeons and general dentists, *J Am Dent Assoc* 125:429–436, 1994.

Skiest DJ, Coykendall AL: Prosthetic hip infection related to a dental procedure despite antibiotic prophylaxis, *Oral Surg Oral Med Oral Pathol Oral Radiol Endod* 79:661–663, 1995.

Spencer WM, Thornesbury C, Moody MD, et al: Rheumatic fever chemoprophylaxis and penicillin resistant gingival organisms, *Ann Intern Med* 73:683–687, 1970.

Steckelberg JM, Wilson WR: Risks for infective endocarditis. Infective disease, *Clin North Am* 7:9–19, 1993.

Stoddard MF, Prince CR, Dillon S, et al: Exercise-induced mitral regurgitation is a predictor of morbid events in subjects with mitral valve prolapse, *Am J Cardiol* 25:693–699, 1995.

Stortebaum M, Durack D, Beeson P: The 'incubation period' of subacute bacterial endocarditis, *Yale Journal of Biological Medicine* 50:49–58, 1997.

Strom BL, Abrutyn E, Berlin JA, et al: Dental and cardiac risk factors for infective endocarditis. A population-based, case-control study, *Ann Intern Med* 129:761–769, 1998.

Tyne GM, Ferguson JW: Antibiotic prophylaxis in patients during dental treatment in patients with prosthetic joints, *J Bone Joint Surg* 73:191–194, 1991.

van der Meer JT, Van Wijk W, Thompson J, et al: Awareness of the need and actual use of prophylaxis: lack of patient compliance in prevention of bacterial endocarditis, *J Antimicrob Chemother* 29:187–194, 1992a.

van der Meer JT, Thompson J, Valkenburg HA, et al: Epidemiology of bacterial endocarditis in The Netherlands. II. Antecedent procedures and use of prophylaxis, *Arch Intern Med* 152:1869–1873, 1992b.

van der Meer JT, Van Wijk W, Thompson J, et al: Efficiency of antibiotic prophylaxis for prevention of native valve endocarditis, *Lancet* 339:135–139, 1992c.

Vermot D, Entenza JM, Vouillamoz J, et al: Efficacy of clarithromycin versus that of clindamycin for single-dose prophylaxis of experimental streptococcal endocarditis, *Antimicrob Agents Chemother* 40:809–811, 1996.

Wahl MJ: Myths of dentally induced endocarditis, *Arch Intern Med* 154:137–144, 1994.

Waldman BJ, Mont MA, Hungerford DS: Total knee arthroplasty infections associated with dental procedures, *Clin Orthop Relat Res* 343:164–172, 1997.

Walter H: Antibiotic prophylaxis in the dental surgery, *Dent Update* 24:271–277, 1997.

Watankunakorn C, Bakie C: Synergism of vancomycin–gentamicin and vancomycin–streptomycin against enterococci, *J Antimicrob Agents Chemother* 4:120–124, 1973.

Watt B: Streptococcal endocarditis: a penicillin alone or a penicillin with an aminoglycoside? *J Antimicrob Chemother* 4:107–109, 1978.

Weissman J, Pini R, Roman MT, et al: In vivo mitral valve morphology and motion in mitral valve prolapse, *Am J Cardiol* 73:1080–1088, 1994.

Wooley CF, Baker PB, Kolibash AT, et al: The floppy, myxomatous mitral valve, mitral valve prolapse and mitral regurgitation, *Prog Cardiovasc Dis* 33:397–433, 1991.

Zuppiroli A, Rinaldi M, Kramer-Fox R, et al: Natural history of mitral valve prolapse, *Am J Cardiol* 75:1028–1032, 1995.

INTRODUCTION

As described in Chapter 15, there are limitations to what can be achieved by subgingival scaling and root planing. Increased probing depths, and the presence of defective restorations especially overhanging margins, limit what can be accomplished by this 'blind' procedure. It has been claimed that a pocket depth of about 5 mm represents the limit for efficient debridement, but there is much debate about this.

Many studies have compared the results of surgical (open) and non-surgical (closed) procedures (among them, Hill et al 1981; Brayer et al 1989; Wylam et al 1993). The Wylam study is especially interesting as it compared the clinical effectiveness of the open and closed techniques on multi-rooted teeth and demonstrated heavy residual deposits in furcations after both procedures; better results were obtained on external root surfaces using the open procedures. These workers state that hand instrumentation alone is inadequate for debridement in furcations, and they suggest that ultrasonic instrumentation or rotating burrs are necessary. Kaldahl et al (1993) have reviewed over 20 longitudinal studies that compared the results of surgical and non-surgical treatment, and they conclude that:

1. Both surgical and non-surgical procedures produce improvement in clinical parameters, i.e. gingival inflammation and bleeding, and reduction in pocket depth
2. Surgical procedures produced greater short-term reduction in probing depth, but long-term results were mixed
3. A comparison of those surgical procedures that did not include manipulation of alveolar bone with those that included bone resection, showed mixed results.

A more recent clinical trial (Serino et al 2001) was designed to determine the initial outcome of non-surgical and surgical access treatment in subjects with advanced periodontal disease and the incidence of recurrent disease during 12 years of maintenance following active therapy. The 64 subjects in the trial had generalized gingival inflammation and a minimum of 12 teeth with deep pockets of ≥6 mm and with ≥6 mm of alveolar bone loss. They were randomly assigned to two treatment groups, surgical (SU) and non-surgical (SRP). The subjects in the SU group received surgical access therapy, while in SRP group non-surgical treatment was provided. This was followed by a maintenance care programme with meticulous supportive periodontal therapy 3–4 times per year. If a subject exhibited marked disease progression between annual examinations he/she was exited from the study and given additional treatment. The study found that surgical therapy was more effective than non-surgical scaling and root planing in reducing the overall mean probing pocket depth and in reducing deep pockets. Furthermore, more SRP-treated subjects exhibited signs of advanced disease progression in the 1–3 year period following active therapy than SU-treated subjects. Thus, in subjects with advanced periodontal disease, surgical therapy provided better short and long-term periodontal pocket reduction and led to fewer subjects requiring additional adjunctive therapy.

A recent systematic review of the effect of surgical therapy compared with subgingival debridement in the treatment of chronic periodontitis has been reported (Heitz-Mayfield et al 2002). Out of 589 abstracts retrieved, they found only six randomized, controlled trials of 12 months' duration which met their inclusion criteria and were suitable for meta-analysis. They showed that, in areas of deep pocketing (>6 mm), surgical therapy resulted in 0.6 mm more probing depth (PPD) reduction and 0.2 mm more clinical attachment level (CAL) gain than subgingival debridement. In areas of moderate pocketing (4–6 mm) subgingival debridement resulted in 0.4 mm more CAL gain and 0.4 mm less PPD reduction than surgical therapy. In areas of shallow pocketing (1–3 mm), both procedures resulted in CAL loss but this loss was 0.5 mm less for subgingival debridement. Thus both subgingival debridement and surgical therapy are effective methods for the treatment of chronic periodontitis in terms of CAL gain and reduction in gingival inflammation. However, surgical therapy in deep pocket areas resulted in more PPD reduction and CAL gain.

Thus there is a measure of agreement that surgical treatment is more effective in cases of more advanced periodontal disease.

One must conclude from the results of these studies that much rests on:

1. The appropriateness of the technique used to the pathological situation. This highlights the crucial nature of precise diagnosis and the identification of all the factors involved in the production of the lesion
2. The competence of the operator in executing different procedures
3. The production of a tissue anatomy which facilitates the patient's home care efforts; this remains central to long-term success regardless of operator invention.

The type of surgical treatment necessary depends upon the form of the lesion, which can be described as:

1. Simple or suprabony, in which all the walls of the lesion are in soft tissue and are uncomplicated by mucogingival problems
2. Intrabony lesions where the base of the pocket is apical to the bone margin and therefore one or more of the pocket walls are bounded by bone
3. Pockets complicated by mucogingival problems such as high muscle attachments or the absence of attached gingiva.

The most difficult lesions to treat are those intrabony defects associated with mucogingival problems and furcation involvement.

CONTRAINDICATIONS TO SURGERY

These may be oral or systemic.

1. Patients of advanced age where teeth may last for life without resorting to radical treatment. Procedures indicated in someone of 60 may not be justified in someone of 70.
2. The presence of systemic disease, such as severe cardiovascular disease, malignancy, kidney and liver disease, blood diseases and bleeding disorders, uncontrolled diabetes, etc. Consultation with the patient's physician is essential.
3. Where thorough subgingival scaling and conscientious home care will remove or control the lesion.
4. Where patient motivation is obviously inadequate.
5. In the presence of acute infection.
6. Where the postoperative appearance would be so poor as to cause patient distress.
7. Where the prognosis is so poor that tooth loss is inevitable.

Some situations may require delay or special preoperative attention. An inadequately controlled diabetic patient will need to be stabilized. Surgery in the pregnant patient is best delayed until after parturition, except where acute lesions develop.

Patients with a history of valvular disease, open heart surgery and congenital heart defects must have preoperative antibiotic cover (see Ch. 18). Patients on various drugs, anticoagulants, steroids and antidepressants require special attention as directed by their physician. A thorough medical history is always essential.

SMOKING AND PERIODONTAL SURGICAL TREATMENT

Smoking is known to adversely affect all forms of periodontal treatment (see Chs 4, 15) and this is particularly important in surgical treatment. In longitudinal studies of groups of smokers and non-smokers who had undergone periodontal surgery (Preber & Bergström 1990; Ah et al 1994), smokers exhibited greater post-treatment probing depths and less gain in clinical attachment levels than non-smokers. Smokers also show much worse long-term responses to periodontal surgery than non-smokers (Boström et al 1998). A recent controlled study of the effect of smoking on flap surgery healing (Scabbia et al 2001) had similar findings.

All periodontal patients, and particularly potential surgery patients, should be actively discouraged from smoking.

PREPARATION FOR SURGERY

Patients should have completed basic treatment and reassessment and have good oral hygiene before being considered for surgery. They must be provided with information about what surgery can achieve in their case, about prognosis, limitations or complications and the problems of the postoperative period.

Information also must be provided about the available anaesthesia and analgesia. The most common method of organization of the surgery is to carry this out in stages on sections of the mouth, either a segment or quadrant at one time, under local anaesthesia in the dental chair. Where full-mouth surgery is required this will involve the patient in several procedures over many weeks. Alternatively, full-mouth surgery can be carried out under general anaesthesia in hospital. As full-mouth surgery can be an extremely lengthy procedure, involving a long general anaesthetic and postoperative care, an overnight stay in hospital is recommended. A third option, where several surgical stages are to be avoided, is to carry out surgery under local anaesthesia plus intravenous sedation. Whichever of the alternatives is used depends on patient preference, their emotional state and their work and domestic commitments. Comprehensive information and discussion are essential to meet the patient's needs.

PERIODONTAL SURGICAL TECHNIQU

The aims of periodontal surgery are:

1. To arrest the progress of periodontal disease and p
2. To attempt to produce regeneration of tissue dest

Thus, the various surgical techniques may also be divided into these same two groups. These are:

1. Those that are limited to eliminating disease and producing conditions which obviate against its recurrence. These can be further divided into two subgroups:
   a. Procedures aimed at pocket elimination or reduction:
      – Gingivectomy
      – Inverse bevel gingivectomy
      – Apical reposition flap.
   b. Procedure to expose the root surface for open scaling and root planing:
      – Replaced flap (Modified Widman flap). This procedure should produce a long junctional epithelium.
2. Those that eliminate disease and also aim to produce regeneration of periodontal tissue which has been destroyed by disease, and thereby produce increased attachment level:
   a. Guided tissue regeneration (GTR)
   b. Bone grafting.

In this context it is important to distinguish two forms of healing:

1. The adherence of a long junctional epithelium to the root surface so that clinical probing depth may be reduced
2. The formation of new connective tissue attachment consisting of periodontal ligament fibres embedded into bone and cementum.

These end-results are illustrated in **Figure 19.1**.

Simple suprabony pockets can be treated by any of these procedures, choosing whichever is most appropriate. Compound intrabony pockets require access by means of a flap procedure and their treatment is discussed in Chapter 20. Mucogingival problems associated with periodontal pockets which extend close to or beyond the mucogingival junction must be treated by an apically repositioned flap in order to increase the zone of attached gingiva.

PROCEDURES FOR POCKET ELIMINATION

GINGIVECTOMY

Gingivectomy is the complete removal of the soft-tissue wall of the pocket.

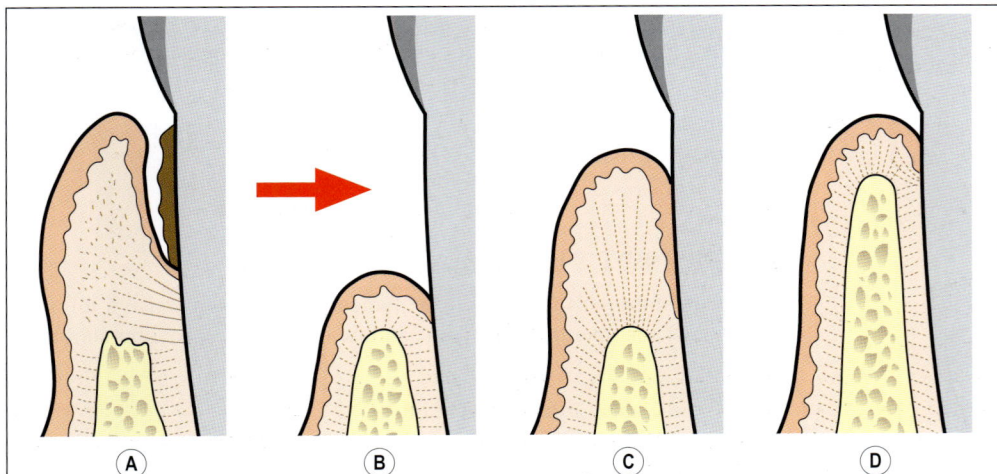

Fig. 19.1 (A) Periodontal lesion; (B) the result of radical elimination of the lesion; (C) the result of a replaced flap with a long junctional epithelium; (D) regeneration of bone and fibrous attachment.

Indications for gingivectomy

1. The presence of suprabony pockets >5 mm which persist despite repeated subgingival scaling and root planing and conscientious home care, and where gingivectomy would leave an adequate zone of attached gingiva
2. The presence of persistent gingival swelling where 'real' pocketing may be shallow but there is considerable gingival enlargement and deformity. If the gingival tissue is fibrous, gingivectomy may be the treatment most likely to produce a satisfactory result
3. The presence of furcation involvement (without associated bone defects) where there is a wide zone of attached gingiva
4. A gingival abscess, i.e. an abscess contained entirely by soft tissue
5. A pericoronal flap.

Gingivectomy is a radical procedure which has been largely replaced by more conservative flap techniques. However, it remains the treatment of choice where recontouring of deformed tissue is needed particularly for hyperplastic gingival tissues (**Fig. 19.3A**), and where access and a precise and predictable anatomy are required to facilitate restorative treatment.

The procedure is given in detail as it provides a model for other surgical procedures.

Procedure

Pocket marking For complete removal of the pocket wall, the apical limit of the pocket must be identified and marked using either pocket marking forceps (**Fig. 19.2**) or a periodontal probe. A series of such markings on both facial and lingual gingivae provides a guide for gingivectomy incision.

The gingivectomy incision The incision can be made with several knives: e.g. Swann-Morton Nos 12 or 15 on a conventional scalpel handle; the Blake knife which uses disposable blades; special gingivectomy knives, such as the Kirkland, Orban or Goldman–Fox knives which have to be sharpened. The choice of knife is entirely personal but where possible the use of disposable blades is to be recommended.

The incision must be made apical to the markings, i.e. apical to the base of the pocket, and at an angle of 45° so that the blade completely perforates the gingiva to the base of the pocket (**Fig. 19.2**). A continuous incision (not

an interrupted scalloped incision) which follows the base of the pockets is made. The correct incision will both remove the pocket wall and produce a streamlined tissue contour; if the incision is too flat the postoperative contour will be unsatisfactory. The most common fault is to incise in a coronal position so that the base of the pocket wall is retained with the possibility of disease recurrence. Following the bevelled incisions, horizontal incisions are made between each interdental space, with a No. 12 blade on a conventional scalpel handle, in order to separate the remaining interdental wedges of tissue.

Tissue removal If the incision has completely separated the pocket wall from the underlying tissue, the pocket wall can be removed easily with a large curette or scaler, e.g. the Cumene scaler (**Fig. 19.3B**). Remnants of fibrous connective tissue and granulation tissue are removed thoroughly with sharp curettes to reveal the root surface (**Fig. 19.3C**). Efficient suction is essential but once granulations have been removed bleeding reduces significantly.

Root scaling and planing The root surfaces should be inspected for evidence of residual calculus deposits and where necessary the root surfaces should be scaled and root planed.

If necessary, further trimming and reshaping of the gingivae can be carried out using scalpel, fine scissors or diathermy. Sterile swabs are placed over the wound to control bleeding so that the periodontal dressing can be applied to a relatively dry wound area.

The periodontal dressing A dressing to cover the wound serves a number of purposes:

1. To protect the wound from irritation
2. To keep the wound clean
3. To control bleeding
4. To control exuberant granulation tissue production.

The dressing thereby promotes healing and provides postoperative comfort.
The requirements of a satisfactory periodontal dressing are as follows:

1. It should be non-irritant and should not induce an allergic response
2. It should be adaptable to the teeth and tissues and flow between the teeth so that it is well retained. A slow setting-time allows manipulation
3. It should exclude food and saliva
4. It should have antibacterial properties to inhibit bacterial growth
5. It should set fairly hard so that it is not easily displaced
6. Its taste should be acceptable.

It is essential to apply the dressing carefully so that it covers the wound and fills the interdental spaces completely. It should be muscle trimmed by movement of the cheeks, lips and tongue, and all excess dressing on occlusal surfaces removed.

A number of dressings based on zinc-oxide-eugenol are available but many people find the taste of eugenol unacceptable and some reports of contact allergy to eugenol have been made. For these reasons eugenol-free dressings have been devised, e.g. Coe-Pack, Peripak, Septopak. These are easy to apply and well-tolerated by the patients.

Postoperative care

It is very important to provide the patient with comprehensive information about postoperative care. The following advice in writing should be given.

1. Avoid eating or drinking for 1 h
2. Avoid hot drinks and alcohol for 24 h. Do not rinse mouth for first day.

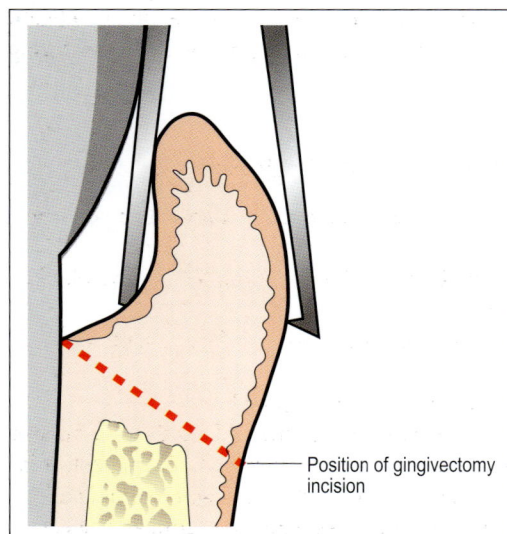

Position of gingivectomy incision

Fig. 19.2 Pocket marking forceps defining the approximate depth of the pocket. Note that the position of the gingivectomy incision is apical to the marking and that the angle of the incision is about 45°.

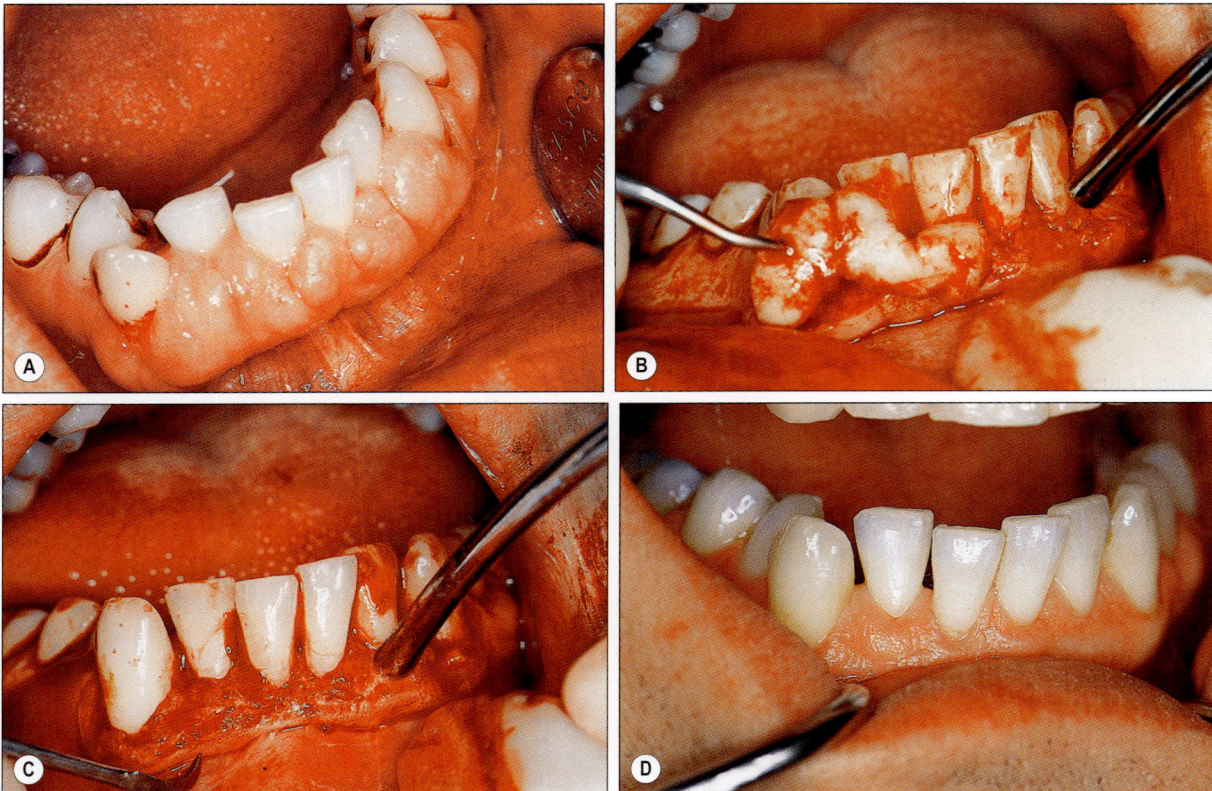

Fig. 19.3 Gingivectomy technique. (A) Hyperplastic gingivae with false pocketing before gingivectomy; (B) excised tissue being removed following gingivectomy incisions buccally and palatally; (C) tissue contour following tissue removal showing raw external wound; (D) healed, healthy gingivae with good contour, 2 weeks after the procedure.

3. Avoid eating hard, sharp or sticky foods and eat on the unoperated side
4. Take an analgesic if there is pain when the anaesthetic wears off. Aspirin is contraindicated for 24 h
5. Use warm saline mouthwashes after the first day. A 0.2% chlorhexidine mouthwash is used morning and night as mechanical plaque control is not possible. This can be used on the first day provided it is not swished around the mouth. Tea, coffee and smoking should be avoided when using a chlorhexidine mouthwash to reduce staining
6. If there is bleeding, exert pressure on the dressing for 15 min with a clean, boiled handkerchief; do not rinse; contact the surgery if the bleeding does not stop
7. Use the toothbrush only on unoperated parts of the mouth
8. If the immediate postoperative phase is uneventful but pain and swelling occur 2 or 3 days later, report immediately to the surgery.

A postoperative antibiotic is only prescribed in certain cases, e.g. a diabetic or any individual who may be debilitated. For routine purposes the dressing is usually removed after one week. All debris must be completely removed and the wound irrigated with warm water. If the wound is not sufficiently well epithelialized and is tender, a new dressing is applied for a further week.

After the dressing has been removed, further instruction in home care is needed. The chlorhexidine mouthwash can be used morning and night for a further week only, as prolonged use will cause staining which is very difficult to remove. The patient is encouraged to start gentle toothbrushing with a soft toothbrush in warm water that evening. Either a gentle roll or Charter's technique is used at this stage. The Bass technique and interdental cleaning are avoided for a week. The patient is advised to avoid cold and hard food.

After 2 weeks the wound is inspected and the teeth cleaned. The patient's oral hygiene must be reviewed until entirely satisfactory and the healing is complete, after which a 3–6 monthly recall regime, as appropriate, is established.

Healing after gingivectomy

The connective tissue wound is covered by a blood clot. The area beneath this undergoes a brief phase of acute inflammation, which is followed by demolition and organization. Epithelial cells migrate from the edge of the wound beneath the clot. They cover the wound in 7–14 days and keratinize in 2–3 weeks (**Fig. 19.3D**). The formation of a new epithelial attachment may take as long as 4 weeks. Good oral hygiene is essential during the healing period.

The limitations and drawbacks of gingivectomy

1. The gingivectomy procedure creates an open wound which heals by secondary intention
2. Tissue is wasted which could be used to close the wound and obtain healing by primary intention
3. Alveolar bone defects are not revealed and therefore cannot be treated adequately
4. The zone of attached gingiva may be eliminated
5. The clinical crown may be lengthened considerably and in the front of the mouth, this may be unsightly and unacceptable to the patient. It is important to explain before surgery that 'the teeth will look longer'
6. Exposed root may be sensitive. Some sensitivity to cold and sweet immediately after gingivectomy is extremely common but this symptom is usually transient. If it persists it will require the use of desensitizing agents.

Despite the above limitations, the gingivectomy technique has a place in periodontal treatment. It is extremely easy to carry out and gives an excellent result in the appropriate cases.

Flap techniques

The flap techniques have several obvious advantages over gingivectomy:

1. They allow access to the root and alveolar bone
2. Tissue is conserved which can be used to close the wound
3. The soft tissues can be manipulated if necessary to achieve an improved soft tissue morphology.

In raising a flap, certain basic requirements must be satisfied:

1. The flap must be big enough to expose any underlying bone defects
2. The base of the flap must be wide enough to maintain an adequate blood supply
3. The incisions must allow movement of the flap without tension
4. No important vessels or nerves should be damaged in raising the flap.

There are three basic flap shapes:

1. The full flap made by a gingival incision and two releasing incisions
2. The triangular flap with a gingival incision and one releasing incision
3. The modified flap with only a gingival incision and no releasing incisions.

Flaps have also been divided into two types:

1. A full-thickness flap, which consists of the complete mucoperiosteum and is raised by a periosteal elevator
2. The split-thickness flap, in which the gingiva is dissected from the underlying periosteum which is left on the bone. This type of flap is more difficult to raise and its use is restricted to special situations described below.

Flaps are further divided into those which are raised and replaced into their original position, and flaps which are moved into apical, coronal or lateral positions.

Flap procedures used to treat chronic periodontitis are described below.

THE REPLACED FLAP (MODIFIED WIDMAN TECHNIQUE)

The debate about 'open' and 'closed' approaches to subgingival scaling and root planing represents the most recent aspect of a historical conflict in periodontics between the conservative and radical approaches to treatment. In the early part of this century, as a reaction to gingivectomy, a mucoperiosteal flap approach to the periodontal lesion was described by Neuman (1912) and Widman (1918). This technique involved raising a full-thickness flap which, after scaling and root planing, was replaced in its original position to produce a closed wound which was more comfortable and healed more rapidly than the open wound produced by gingivectomy.

Morris (1965) introduced the internal bevel incision which separated the pocket wall from the rest of the mucoperiosteal flap and produced a healthy, thin and flexible margin to the flap. This was used by Ramfjord and Nissle (1974) in what they called the 'modified Widman flap' procedure, which allowed open access to the periodontal lesion and then much closer adaptation of the replaced flap to the tooth surface than had been possible with the unmodified full-thickness flap. The flap approach also allows access to alveolar bone defects (Ch. 20). A further advantage is that there is less postoperative root exposure than after gingivectomy, which is especially important in the front of the mouth.

When introduced it was thought that the technique would produce a physiological dentogingival junction, and therefore lead to permanent pocket elimination, but this is not possible (Caton & Nyman 1980; Caton et al 1980).

The long junctional epithelium produced by this procedure is inherently less stable than the physiological junctional epithelium and demands much higher standards of plaque control and higher frequencies of recall for maintenance than pocket elimination procedures.

However, it has been shown that this technique can successfully treat and stabilize cases with moderate and advanced chronic periodontitis. There have been many longitudinal studies, over periods ranging from 2 to 6 years, which have compared non-surgical and surgical treatment techniques including both replaced and pocket elimination flap techniques (Pihlstrom et al 1983; Ramfjord et al 1987). These all show that both non-surgical scaling/root planing and surgical replaced flap/pocket elimination techniques can effectively control moderate to advanced chronic periodontitis, preventing further attachment loss. However, all of these workers used regular and often long maintenance visits at intervals of 3 months or less throughout the period of study; this factor could have been at least as important as the technique itself in preventing relapse. The effect of maintenance in preventing deterioration following treatment has been clearly shown in a number of studies (Nyman et al 1975; Lindhe & Nyman 1984). These studies also showed that cases with deep pockets needed retreatment more often when treated with scaling alone. This is consistent with reports that residual deposits of subgingival calculus are commonly left in deep pockets following subgingival scaling and that this is significantly less common when surgical techniques are used (Ch. 15). Therefore this would seem to justify the use of periodontal flap techniques for open scaling and root planing which is the main purpose of the replaced flap technique.

A full course of basic periodontal therapy must be carried out before this procedure and surgery of this type should only be considered if there is persistent pocketing which makes effective subgingival scaling difficult and therefore prevents full resolution (**Fig. 19.5A**).

PROCEDURE

Incision An inverse bevel incision is made up to 1 mm from the gingival margin on both the facial and lingual sides of either the upper or lower arches. The aim of this incision, as with other flap techniques, is to separate the pocket epithelium and inflamed connective tissue (cervical wedge) from the flap (**Figs 19.4A, 19.5B, C**). No vertical relieving incisions are made unless necessary for reflection purposes. Two further incisions were described by Ramfjord and Nissle (1974). The first is an incision made from the base of the pocket to the bone crest. The second, which is made after flap reflection, is a horizontal incision made from the crest of the bone to the tooth surface. The purpose of these additional incisions is to allow the cervical wedge to be removed easily and to minimize damage to the underlying periodontal ligament. These incisions are not totally necessary and obviously serve no purpose if intrabony defects are present which have to be curetted.

Another suggested modification is to exaggerate the scalloping of the palatal inverse bevel incision in order to lengthen the interdental papillae so that they completely cover the interdental space on closure.

Reflection of flap A full-thickness mucoperiosteal flap is reflected with a periodontal elevator in order to expose the roots of the teeth and the bone margin (**Figs 19.4B, 19.5D–F**).

Curettage, scaling and root planning The cervical wedge is removed (**Fig. 19.5D**) and the root surfaces are scaled and root planed (**Fig. 19.5G, H**). Great care should be taken with this process as a totally clean and smooth

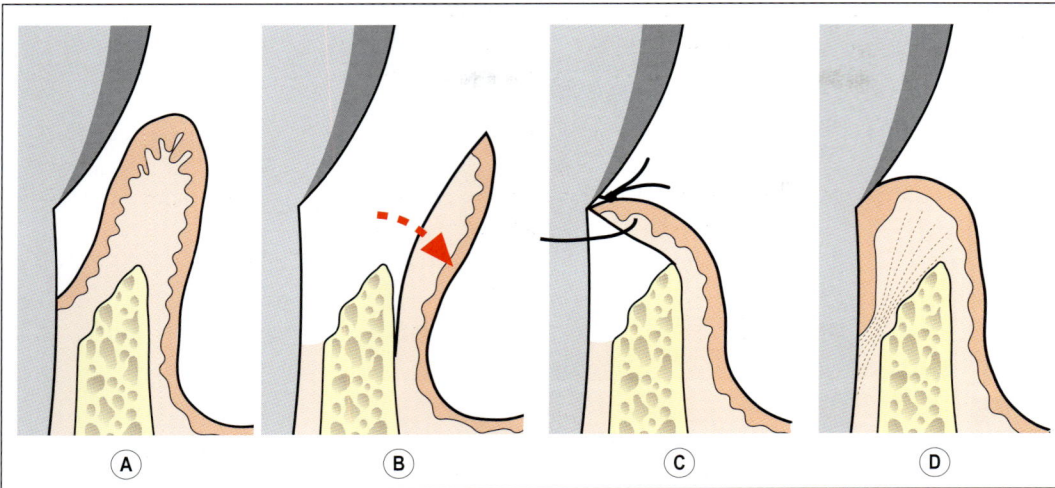

Fig. 19.4 Diagrams to show the replaced flap procedure. (A) inverse bevel incision; (B) the flap reflected to reveal alveolar margin; (C) following meticulous root surface debridement the flap is replaced and sutured in its original position; (D) long junctional epithelium following healing.

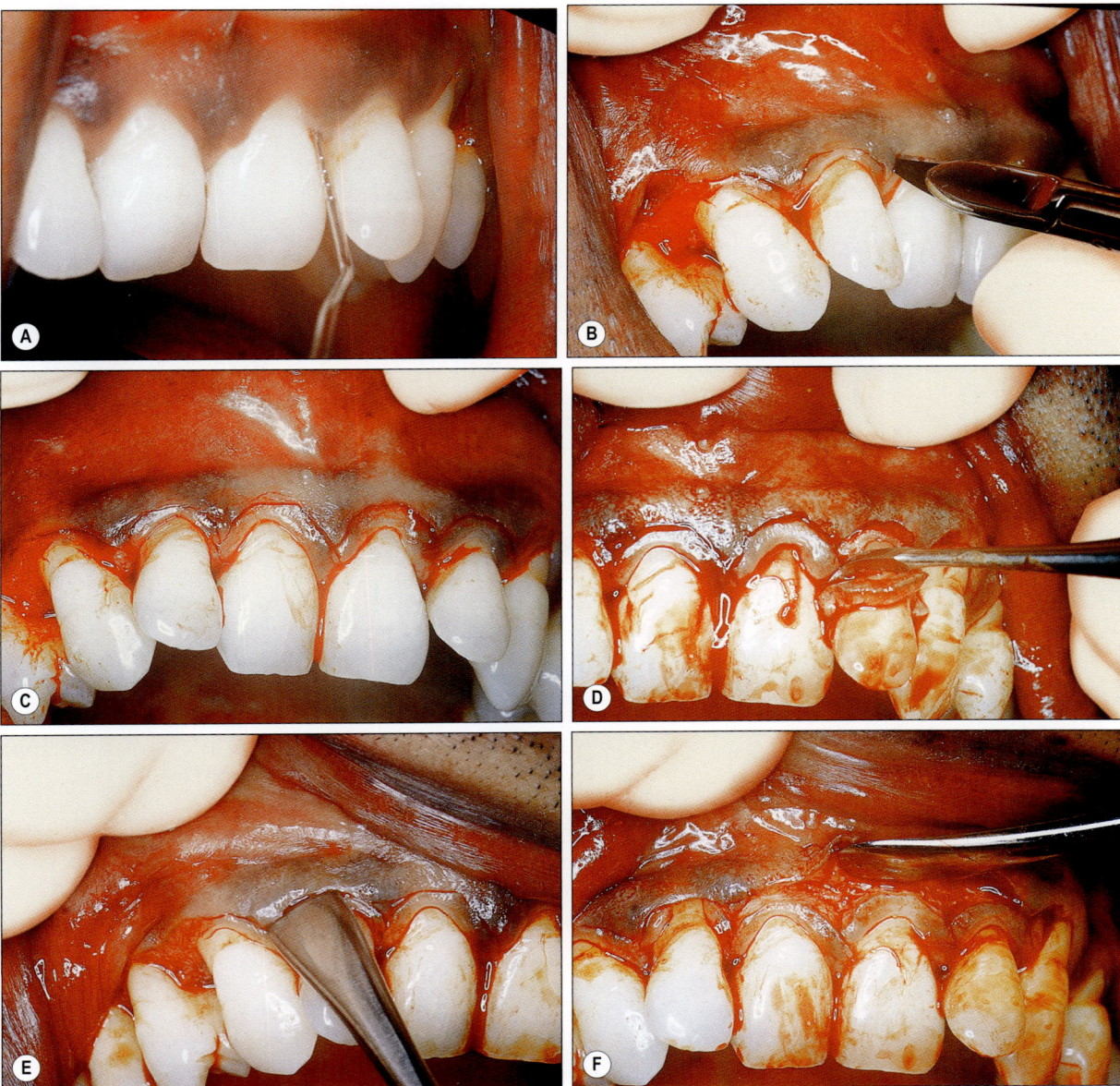

Fig. 19.5 Clinical pictures of the replaced flap procedure. (A) Preoperative appearance following basic periodontal treatment; (B) the inverse bevel incision being outlined; (C) the completed inverse bevel incision buccally (the same incision has also been carried out palatally, not shown); (D) following minimal raising of the flap the excised tissue is removed; (E) the flap is raised a little further to reveal the alveolar bone margin; (F) flap fully raised

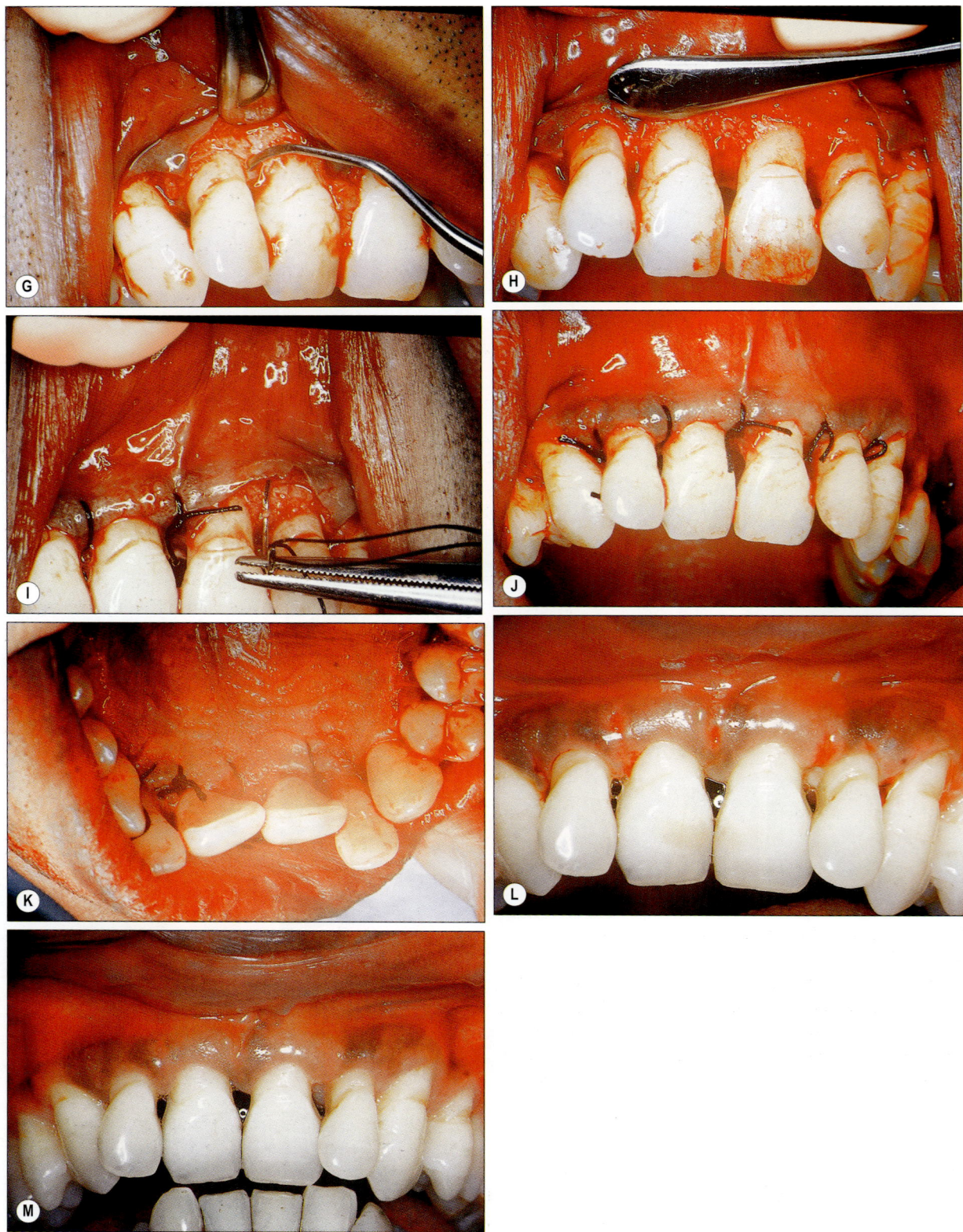

Fig. 19.5—Cont'd (G) the exposed root surfaces are carefully debrided of all deposits; (H) root debridement completed; (I) placement of interdental sutures to close buccal and palatal flaps in original position; (J) suturing completed, buccal view; (K) suturing completed, palatal view; (L) healing after 2–5 weeks; (M) 3 months after surgery showing complete healing and healthy tissues.

root surface is necessary to ensure that the long junctional epithelium, which will form following healing, will adhere to it. Failure of this adherence will lead to the reestablishment of pocketing. Any bony craters and deeper defects should be totally cleared of granulation tissue to create the best conditions for bone regeneration (Ch. 20).

Suturing The flaps are then replaced in their original position and secured by tight interdental suturing (**Figs 19.4C, 19.5I–K**). Every effort is made to ensure total interdental coverage and to avoid any root exposure. There is no need to place a periodontal dressing as it has no supporting function in this procedure. However, it can be placed if required for patient comfort and in this case it need cover only the gingival margin.

Postoperative management Postoperative instructions are the same as those for the gingivectomy. Postoperative swelling with this procedure is usually slight because of the smaller amount of flap retraction involved. Sutures are removed after a week and the chlorhexidine mouthwash is continued for a further week. Brushing is started with an extra soft brush. Flossing is usually started a week postoperatively, although some discretion needs to be exercised in this regard. It must be carried out with great care to avoid gingival trauma. The patient should be seen every 4 weeks until healing is complete and plaque control perfect. Maintenance visits will be necessary every 3 months thereafter as the long junctional epithelium is more liable to breakdown and a very careful check must be kept for pockets reforming. This procedure is likely to be more stable around single-rooted anterior teeth since they are more accessible for home care and for professional maintenance. Posterior teeth are likely to be complicated by furcation involvements which are extremely difficult to maintain if situated subgingivally.

Healing Following acute inflammation, healing will begin by the organization of the blood clot between the flap and the tooth into granulation tissue. This is then slowly replaced by collagenous connective tissue over the next 2–5 weeks (**Fig. 19.5L**). Epithelium proliferates over the connective-tissue wound to its preoperative position. If the root surface is free of irritant the long junctional epithelium can adhere to it. However, the longer the junctional epithelium, the more unstable this situation becomes and the greater the risk for the re-establishment of pocketing. A mature long epithelial attachment may take several weeks to form and care should be taken not to disrupt it by probing during this period (**Fig. 19.5M**). Quite frequently gingival recession will occur following replaced flaps and this has the effect of both producing some root exposure and reducing the length of the long junctional epithelium (**Fig. 19.4D**).

ROOT CONDITIONING WITH CITRIC ACID

Recently a fresh approach to obtaining new connective tissue attachment has been attempted using citric acid conditioning of the root surface (Polson & Proye 1982). Root cementum is first removed from the affected part of the root by planing with curettes. Citric acid at pH 1 is then applied to the dentine surface for 3 min. The superficial zone of the dentine becomes demineralized, leading to the exposure of collagen fibrils in the matrix. It has been claimed that a connective tissue attachment will reform by the interdigitation of new and existing collagen fibres on the root surface but if this occurs at all the amount is limited. The usual result is the development of a long junctional epithelium and this method does not therefore seem to offer any advantage over flap techniques alone (Moore et al 1987).

APICALLY REPOSITIONED FLAP

This procedure was first described by Friedman in 1962. It is indicated for the elimination of periodontal pocketing and increasing the zone of attached gingiva. Pocketing separates the attached gingiva from the tooth and deep pockets may extend below the mucogingival junction, i.e. through the whole width of the attached gingiva. In these circumstances gingivectomy techniques would leave either a narrow zone of attached gingiva or none at all and are contraindicated. Replaced flap techniques (see above) cannot increase the zone of attached gingiva and are thus not indicated for pockets extending to or beyond the mucogingival junction.

The apically repositioned flap achieves pocket elimination by moving the flap in an apical direction. Adequate mobility of the flap is necessary for this and is obtained by extending the releasing incisions to the base of the vestibule and further dissection of the flap from the underlying tissues. Apical repositioning will leave the flap just covering the alveolar crest, thus eliminating the pocketing. During healing the merging of the connective tissue on the inner surface of the flap with the bone will recreate a mucoperiosteal attached gingival zone.

A full course of basic periodontal treatment must be completed and repeated if necessary before surgery is considered for the treatment of persistent deep pocketing.

Procedure

Incisions Two vertical releasing incisions are made through to bone at either end of the operative area. They should be made mesial or distal to the last interdental periodontal pocket to be treated and must not be positioned interdentally. They should be parallel to each other and should extend into the alveolar mucosa at the base of the vestibule.

An inverse bevel incision is made along the gingival margin (**Figs 19.6A, 19.8A**). It should start up to 1 mm from the gingival margin and extend down to the crest of the alveolar bone (**Figs 19.6A, 19.8A**). It is

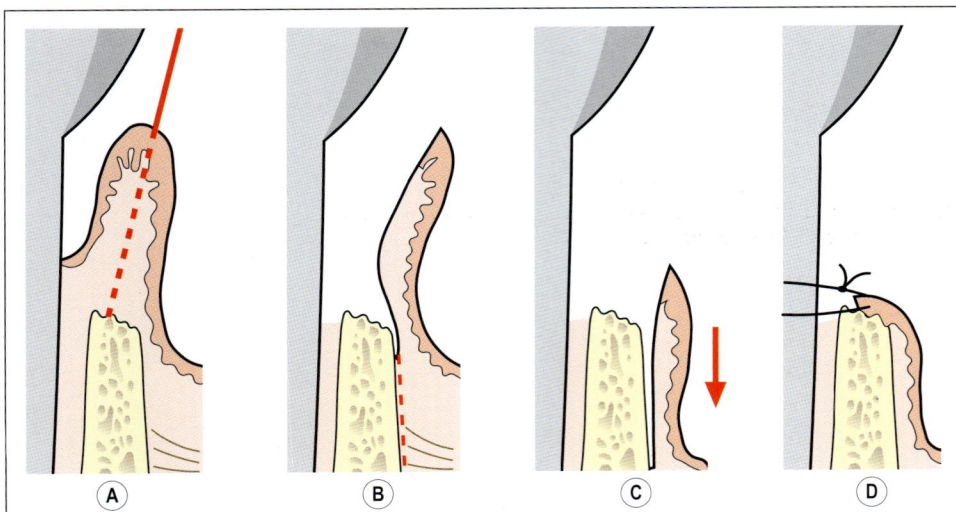

Fig. 19.6 The apically repositioned flap procedure. (A) Inverse bevel incision; (B) the flap is reflected and dissected from the alveolar process, so that (C) it can be moved in an apical direction; (D) the flap is sutured in an apical position, just covering the bone margin.

discontinuous and scalloped around the neck of each tooth and may be made in two stages, a superficial outlining incision and deepening incision. This allows the interdental papilla to be deflected outwards when making the deepening incision, which allows the blade to be angled more acutely. The aim of these incisions is to separate the pocket lining and inflamed connective tissue from the inner wall of the flap. This tissue is left on the surface of the tooth when the flap is raised and is referred to as the cervical wedge.

In the lower jaw, care should be taken lingually with the distal relieving incision to ensure that there is no risk to the lingual nerve. Care should also be taken not to damage or bruise the submandibular ducts in raising the flap. Palatal gingiva is treated by means of an inverse bevel gingivectomy incision, as obviously palatal tissue cannot be apically positioned (**Fig. 19.8B**). The angle of the incision can be varied according to the thickness of the tissue and may be used to fillet out hyperplastic tissue.

Raising the flap A periosteal elevator is used to separate attached gingiva from the alveolar process so that a full-thickness flap is lifted (**Figs 19.6B, 19.8C**). It should peel away easily from the tooth and bone and clearly separate from the cervical wedge. If it does not separate easily the marginal inverse bevel incision should be deepened.

The flap may be released in two stages, the first just to expose the bone to allow curettage and the second to detach the flap further, just before apical positioning. In this way bone exposure is reduced to the minimum.

In the case of upper teeth, the palatal tissue is raised to expose the margin of the bone and to give sufficient access for the removal of the large wedge of tissue produced by the inverse bevel gingivectomy incision.

Removing the cervical wedge and granulation tissue The separated cervical wedge is removed with curettes and scalers. All granulation tissue attached to the tooth surface, bone margin or within bone defects should be carefully and comprehensively curetted away to leave a clean tooth and bone surface. Efficient aspiration is necessary to ensure good visibility. Bleeding will reduce dramatically when this tissue has been removed. The treatment of intrabony pocketing and furcation involvement is discussed in Chapter 20.

Root scaling and planing The exposed roots must be scaled to remove any residual calculus and planed.

Apical repositioning The flap is reflected to the base of the vestibule. Once released the flap tends to contract and fold up so that apical positioning often takes place spontaneously. One should ensure that the flap is displaced apically so that its edge just covers the alveolar crest (**Fig. 19.6C**).

Suturing It is important to be sure that the flap is not pulled coronally when suturing. Sutures should be placed first at the mesial and distal vertical incisions. The suture should be placed near to the margin of the free flap and sufficiently apically on the attached gingiva of the fixed tissue to ensure the degree of apical positioning required.

The margin of the flap can be secured with either loose separate interdental sutures or by means of a continuous suspensory suture (**Figs 19.7, 19.8D**). Continuous suspensory suturing is useful in allowing manipulation of the flap margin where the bone margin is irregular and where the width of attached gingiva varies. Care should be taken not to pull the suture too tight as this will drag the flap coronally. The tension on the suture can be adjusted at each loop, rather like loosening or tightening the lace of a shoe. The tension should be adjusted so that the flap margin just covers the bone margin (**Figs 19.6D, 19.8D**). It must be remembered that the continuous suture does not hold the flap in an apical position but simply suspends it from the necks of the teeth. The degree of apical positioning will be maintained by the correct placement of the periodontal pack (**Fig. 19.8E**).

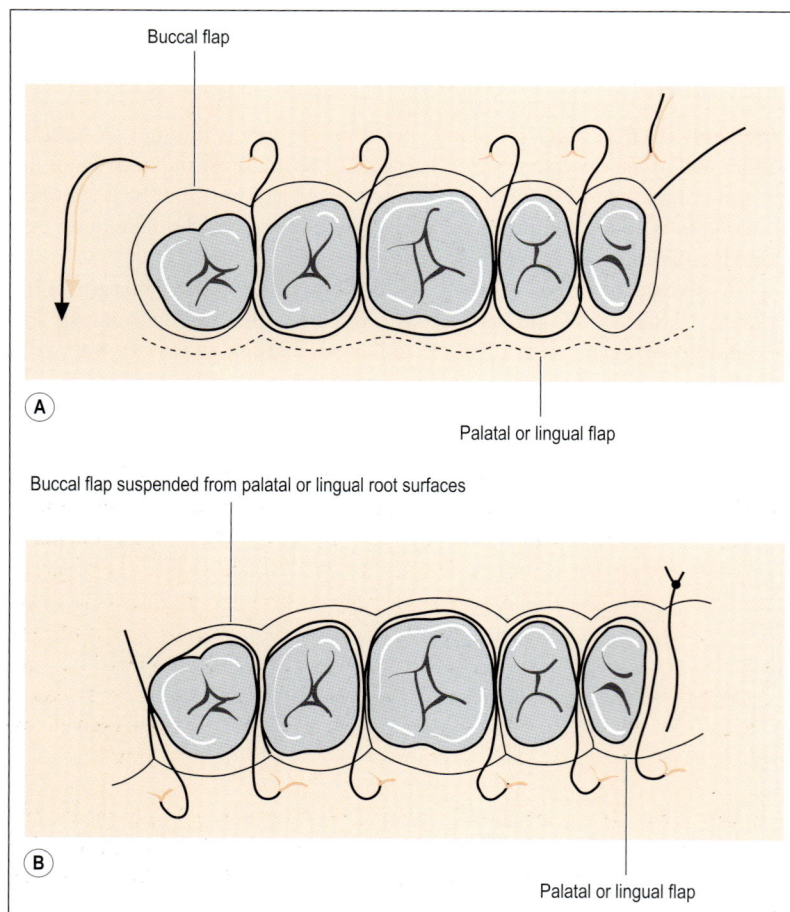

Buccal flap

(A)

Palatal or lingual flap

Buccal flap suspended from palatal or lingual root surfaces

(B)

Palatal or lingual flap

Fig. 19.7 The continuous suspensory suturing technique. (A) A single tie is made at the anterior papilla, buccally. The needle then passes interdentally to the palatal or lingual side, passes around the lingual surface of the tooth and then passes interdentally again at the next space to return to the buccal side. This process is repeated until the most distal interdental space is reached. The buccal flap is then suspended from the lingual root surfaces. (B) Following adjustment of the apical position of the suspended flap, the palatal or lingual flap is suspended in a similar fashion against the buccal root surfaces. When the positions of both flaps are ideal then the suture is tied off at the end which has been left at the single tie on the anterior papilla.

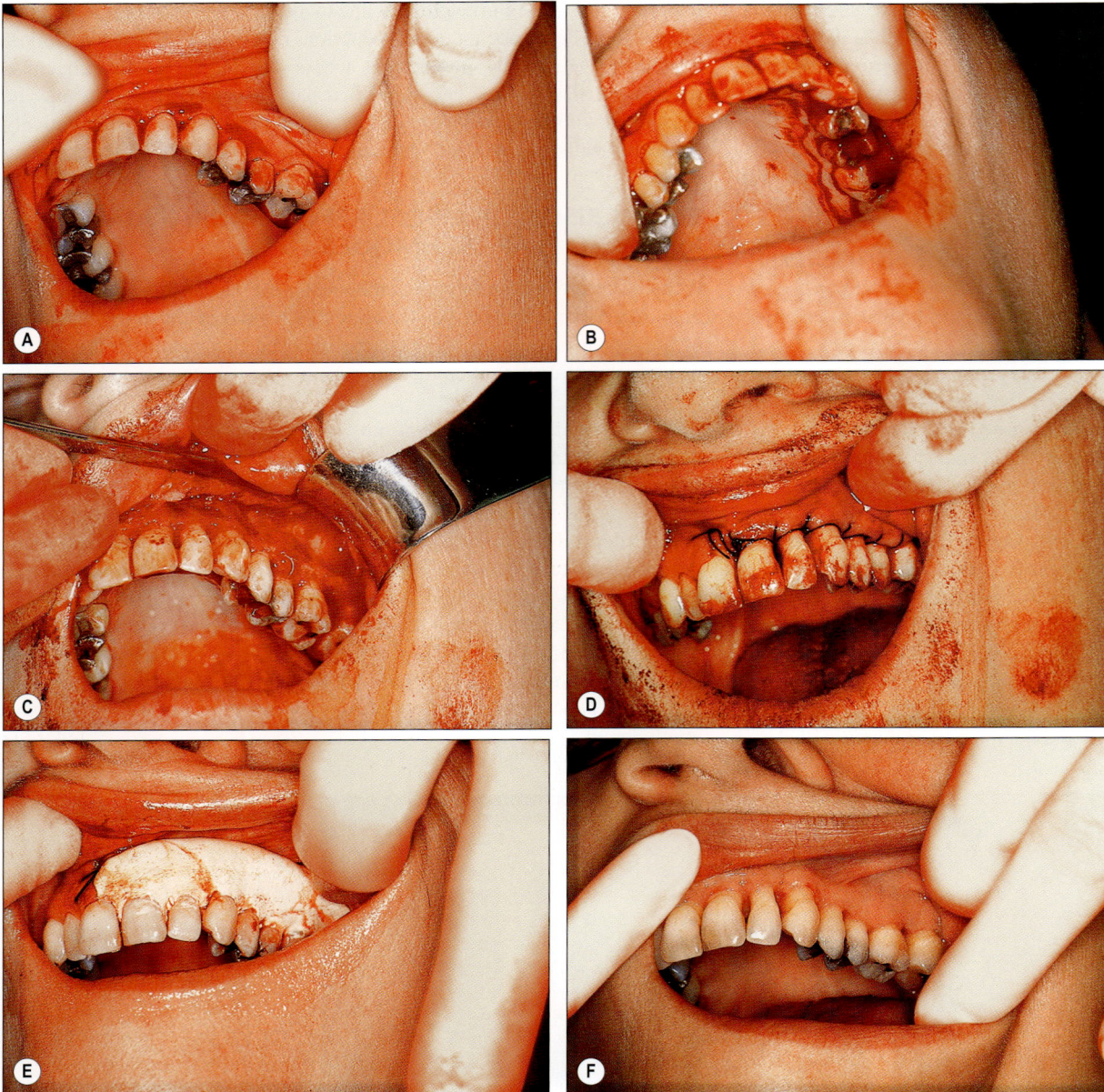

Fig. 19.8 Clinical pictures of apically repositioned flap procedure. (A) Inverse bevel incision buccally plus vertical relieving incisions mesially and distally to the flap to be raised (not visible distally); (B) inverse bevel gingivectomy incision palatally to excise pocket wall; (C) flap raised to allow root debridement and subsequently to below the mucogingival junction level to allow apical positioning to take place; (D) flap sutured in apical position by simple sutures at the mesial and distal margins and a continuous suspensory suture; (E) periodontal pack in position, buccally (shown) and palatally (not shown). This, in addition to protecting the area, maintains the apical positioning of the flaps; (F) 6 months after surgery showing healthy gingivae, exposure of root surfaces and elimination of pocketing.

Placing the periodontal dressing It is usual to use Coe-Pack. Close adaptation of the flap to the underlying bone can be assured by pressing damp swabs over the flap while the periodontal dressing is being mixed. The dressing must be placed when it is freely mouldable. It should occupy the area between the flap margin and the crowns of the teeth so that it prevents any coronal displacement of the flap (**Fig. 19.8E**). It should also extend down to the base of the vestibular to maintain the vestibular depth and should be carefully muscle trimmed (**Fig. 19.8E**).

Healing The inner surface of the flap in contact with the bone and tooth undergoes inflammation, demolition, organization and healing. The blood clot, which should be thin, is replaced by granulation tissue in about a week. This matures into collagenous connective tissue in 2–5 weeks. The inner surface of the flap will unite with the bone to produce a mucoperiosteum which increases the attached gingival zone. About 2 days after surgery the epithelium will begin to proliferate from the flap margin over the connective tissue wound. It will migrate apically at the rate of 0.5 mm/day to produce a new junctional epithelium. As the margin of the flap just covers the bone, this will be of physiological length. A mature epithelial attachment takes about 4 weeks to form. Some resorption of the alveolar bone margin will occur as the result of raising a flap but with careful management this will be in the order of 0.5 mm. Connective tissue attachment will reform between the marginal tissues and the root cementum from the bone margin to the base of the junctional epithelium. It will prevent further apical migration of the junctional epithelium.

Postoperative care The postoperative care is the same as for gingivectomy. The patient should however be additionally warned of facial swelling. This will develop over the first 3 postoperative days and then slowly reduce.

The dressing and sutures are removed after one week and the chlorhexidine mouthwash is usually discontinued a further week after this. The patient should be encouraged to return to normal brushing and flossing as soon as possible and certainly no longer than 7 days after suture removal. An extra soft toothbrush should be used for 2–3 weeks. Particular care is necessary with plaque control during the first few weeks after surgery since the tissues will be healing during this period and are particularly vulnerable to damage. Modification of these regimes must be made to take into account individual variation in healing.

Careful maintenance is necessary after this procedure (**Fig. 19.8F**). However, once immaculate plaque control is achieved recall periods can be extended to 6 months as all pockets have been eliminated and a physiological length of junctional epithelium results.

Because apical repositioned flaps are often carried out in cases where bone loss is quite advanced, it is inevitable that the clinical crown will be lengthened (**Fig. 19.8F**). Patients must be warned of this beforehand.

This procedure can give excellent long-term results providing that good oral hygiene is carried out by the patient and regular maintenance is carried out by the dentist and hygienist (**Fig. 19.9**).

Retzepi et al (2007) carried out a prospective randomized-controlled clinical trial which compared the gingival blood flow responses following simplified papilla preservation (test) versus modified Widman flap (control). Significant ischaemia was observed at all sites following anaesthesia and immediately post-operatively. At the mucosal flap basis, a peak hyperaemic response was observed on day 1, which tended to resolve by day 4 at the test sites, but persisted until day 7 at the control sites. The buccal and palatal papillae blood perfusion presented the maximum increase on day 7 in both groups and returned to baseline by day 15. Both surgical modalities yielded significant pocket depth reduction, recession increase and clinical attachment gain. Thus, periodontal access flaps represent an ischaemia-reperfusion flap model. The simplified papilla preservation flap may be associated with faster recovery of the gingival blood flow postoperatively compared with the modified Widman flap.

COMPARISON OF APICAL REPOSITIONING AND REPLACED FLAP TECHNIQUES

It can be seen from the foregoing that the apically repositioned flap results in pocket elimination and the formation of a normal or physiological length of junctional epithelium, whereas the replaced flap results in the formation of a long junctional epithelium which may adhere to the root surface (**Fig. 19.4D**).

A long junctional epithelium must be regarded as inherently unstable because it lacks the mechanical support of gingival fibres passing into it from the crest of the bone and adjacent cementum. The stability of the delicate biological seal between the junctional epithelium and the root would seem to depend on a very high standard of oral hygiene and frequent regular maintenance visits. If any plaque is allowed to mature at the margin there is the risk that subgingival plaque will become reestablished and will proliferate apically to detach the epithelium and reform the pocket.

The result of an apically repositioned flap is much more stable since pockets are eliminated (**Figs 19.8F, 19.9D**) and the dentogingival junction is normal. This is particularly important for posterior teeth with furcation involvement.

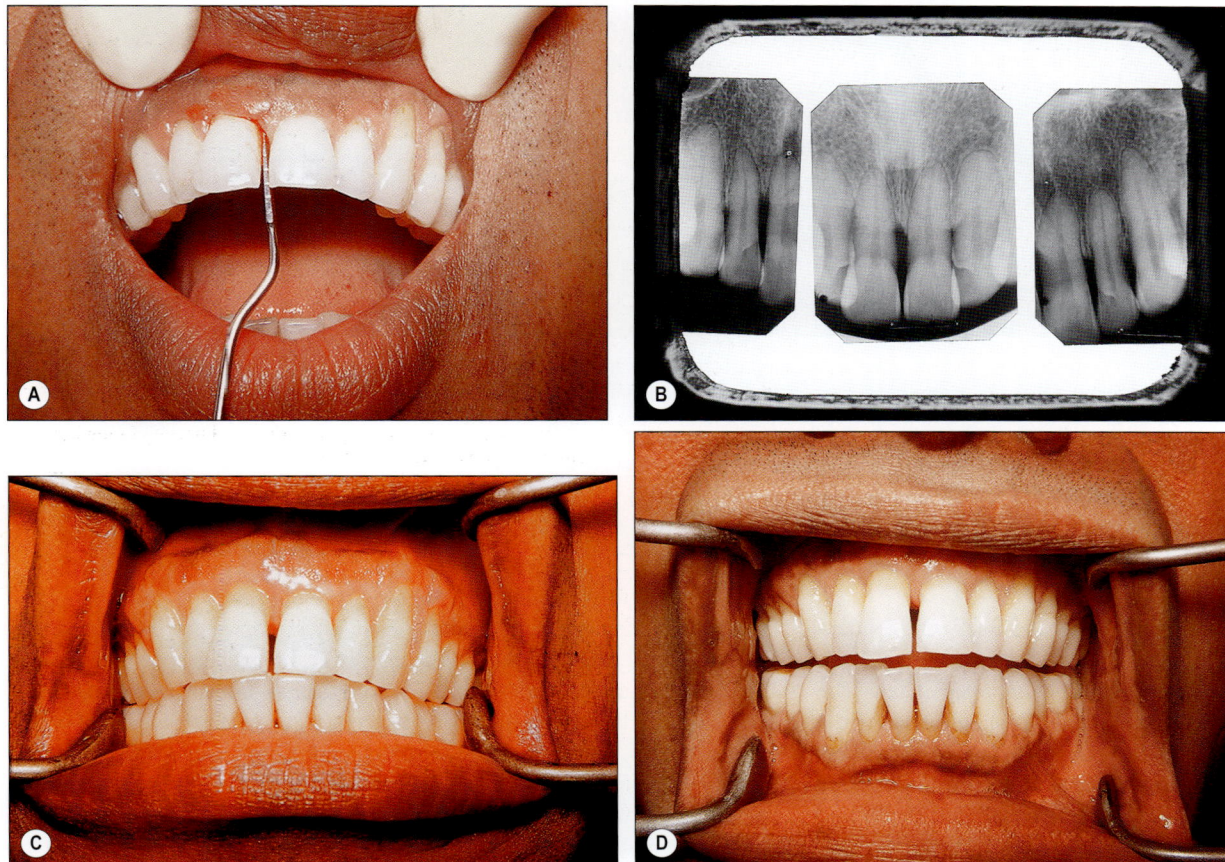

Fig. 19.9 Clinical pictures of the apically repositioned flap procedure showing long-term results after surgery and regular maintenance. (A) Patient aged 26 with rapidly progressive periodontitis is shown after basic periodontal treatment with a periodontal probe placed into a deep pocket mesial to the upper left central incisor; (B) radiographs of his upper anterior teeth showing 40–50% alveolar bone loss. There was at least this amount of bone loss throughout his mouth; (C) 2 weeks after apically reposition flap around his upper incisors and canines showing pocket reduction (similar surgery was carried out throughout his mouth by one of the authors (B.M.E.) in 1968); (D) appearance of the same area 27 years later showing healthy gingivae and no significant probing depths.

LOCAL AND SYSTEMIC CHANGES FOLLOWING PERIODONTAL SURGERY

Papapanou et al (2007) showed that surgical periodontal therapy may alter monocytic gene expression in a manner consistent with a systemic anti-inflammatory effect (see also Ch. 15).

TREATMENT OF TUBEROSITY INVOLVEMENT

The maxillary tuberosity may be large, flabby, unsupported by bone and related to a distal pocket on the last molar. It can be removed by making a radical gingivectomy incision but this creates a large open wound which bleeds readily, can be painful and heals slowly. The retromolar pad in the lower jaw can present similar problems. Both situations can be dealt with by using the 'distal wedge' technique (**Fig. 19.10**). Facial and lingual incisions are made through the tuberosity or retromolar pad to form a triangular wedge. The incisions must be deep enough to allow clean separation of the soft-tissue wedge from the underlying bone. When the wedge is removed, any loose tags of tissue are trimmed and the distal root surface of the adjacent tooth cleaned. The edges of the wound are then sutured and the wound closed as completely as possible.

This procedure works well where the tissue is firm and fibrous, as it usually is with the maxillary tuberosity. However, it may be difficult or impossible to produce the desired result in the lower retromolar area when the tissue is soft and flabby.

TREATMENT OF THE EDENTULOUS RIDGE

If teeth involved in surgery are adjacent to an edentulous ridge that is covered by fibrous or flabby tissue, this can be removed by gingivectomy but the situation is better managed using a flap technique. Inverse bevel incisions are continued from around the teeth along the facial and lingual aspects of the edentulous ridge to dissect out a wedge of tissue with its base on the bone. This wedge of tissue is removed with curettes from the surface of the ridge. Then the edges of the flaps are trimmed and sutured (**Fig. 19.11**). The apical movement of the flaps will remove soft-tissue pocketing mesial and distal to the two bordering teeth.

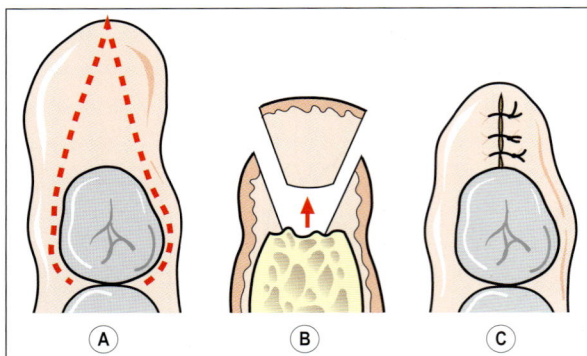

Fig. 19.10 Diagram to illustrate the distal wedge procedure to reduce a bulbous maxillary tuberosity and pocketing distal to the last standing molar. (A) Incision lines from occlusal surface viewpoint; (B) vertical section viewpoint to show the wedge of tissue; (C) suturing of the resulting wound.

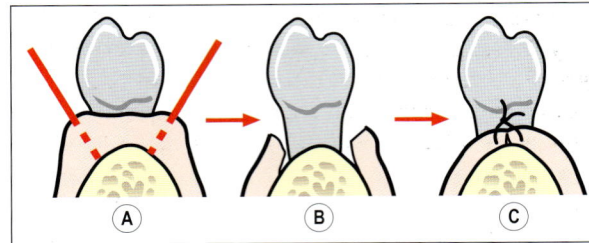

Fig. 19.11 Diagram to illustrate that the treatment of an edentulous space is similar to the distal wedge procedure. (A) Incisions mark out flabby ridge tissue, which is removed. (B) The wound is then sutured (C).

REFERENCES

Ah MKB, Johnson GK, Kaldahl WB, et al: The effect of smoking on the response to periodontal therapy, *J Clin Periodontol* 21:91–97, 1994.

Boström L, Linder LE, Bergström J: Influence of smoking on the outcome of periodontal surgery. A 5-year follow-up, *J Clin Periodontol* 25:194–201, 1998.

Brayer WK, Mellonig JT, Dunlap RM, et al: Scaling and root planing effectiveness: The effect of root surface access and operator experience, *J Periodontol* 60:67–72, 1989.

Caton J, Nyman S: Histometric evaluation of periodontal surgery. 1. The modified Widman flap procedure, *J Clin Periodontol* 7:212–223, 1980.

Caton J, Nyman S, Zander H: Histometric evaluation of periodontal surgery. II. Connective tissue attachment levels after four regenerative procedures, *J Clin Periodontol* 7:224–231, 1980.

Friedman N: Mucogingival surgery: the apically repositioned flap, *J Periodontol* 33:328–340, 1962.

Heitz-Mayfield LJA, Trombelli L, Heitz F, et al: A systematic review of the effect of surgical debridement vs. non-surgical debridement for the treatment of chronic periodontitis, *J Clin Periodontol* 29:S92–S102, 2002.

Hill RW, Ramfjord SP, Morrison EC, et al: Four types of periodontal treatment compared over two years, *J Periodontol* 52:655–662, 1981.

Kaldahl WB, Kalkwarf KL, Patil KD: A review of longitudinal studies that compared periodontal therapies, *J Periodontol* 64:243–253, 1993.

Lindhe J, Nyman S: Long-term maintenance of patients treated for advanced periodontal disease, *J Clin Periodontol* 11:504–514, 1984.

Moore JA, Ashley FP, Waterman CA: The effect on healing of the application of citric acid during replaced flap surgery, *J Clin Periodontol* 14:130–135, 1987.

Morris ML: The unrepositioned mucoperiosteal flap, *Periodontics* 3:141–151, 1965.

Neumann R: *Die Alveolar-Pyorrhea und ihre Behandlung*, Berlin, 1912, Meusser.

Nyman S, Rosling B, Lindhe J: Effect of professional tooth cleaning after periodontal surgery, *J Clin Periodontol* 2:80–86, 1975.

Papapanou PN, Sedaghatfar MH, Demmer RT, et al: Periodontal therapy alters gene expression of peripheral blood monocytes, *J Clin Periodontol* 34:736–747, 2007.

Pihlstrom BL, McHugh RB, Oliphant TH, et al: Comparison of surgical and non surgical treatment of periodontal disease. A review of current studies and additional results after 6.5 years, *J Clin Periodontol* 10:524–541, 1983.

Polson AM, Proye MP: Effect of root surface alterations on periodontal healing. II. Citric acid treatment of the denuded root, *J Clin Periodontol* 9:441–454, 1982.

Preber H, Bergstrom J: Effect of cigarette smoking on periodontal healing following surgical therapy, *J Clin Periodontol* 17:324–328, 1990.

Ramfjord SP, Nissle RR: The modified Widman flap, *J Periodontol* 45:601–607, 1974.

Ramfjord SP, Caffesse RG, Morrison EC, et al: 4 modalities of periodontal treatment compared over 5 years, *J Clin Periodontol* 14:445–452, 1987.

Retzepi M, Tonetti M, Donos N: Comparison of gingival blood flow during healing of simplified papilla preservation and modified Widman flap surgery: a clinical trial using laser Doppler flowmetry, *J Clin Periodontol* 34:903–911, 2007.

Scabbia A, Cho K-S, Sigurdsson TJ, et al: Cigarette smoking negatively affects healing response following flap debridement surgery, *J Periodontol* 72:43–49, 2001.

Serino G, Roslino B, Ramberg P, et al: Initial outcome and long-term effect of surgical and non-surgical treatment of advanced periodontal disease, *J Clin Periodontol* 28:910–916, 2001.

Widman L: The operative treatment of pyorrhoea alveolaris. A new surgical method, *Sven Tandlak Tidskr* (Dec. special issue), 1918.

Wylam JM, Mealey BL, Mills MP et al: The clinical effectiveness of open versus closed scaling and root planing on multi-rooted teeth, *J Periodontol* 64:1023–1028, 1993.

As the periodontal lesion advances the alveolar crest is resorbed and cancellous spaces are opened up. To compensate for resorption some deposition may take place at sites more distant from the inflammation. The result of this remodelling process is the formation of bone defects or 'intrabony' defects of an infinite number of shapes. In Chapter 8 these have been classified as marginal defects, intra-alveolar defects, furcation defects and perforations, and can be further subdivided according to the number of bone walls bounding the defect.

The objectives of treatment of these defects are:

1. To eliminate the periodontal lesion
2. To achieve a tissue shape which will allow the patient to carry out efficient plaque control
3. If possible, to obtain some bone formation, increase in tooth attachment and improved tooth support.

Careful radiographic examination is essential to diagnosis but even good radiographs may not reveal the presence of a bone defect or its precise morphology. This limitation can be overcome only by direct examination of the alveolar process and all bone lesions are approached by lifting full-thickness mucoperiosteal flaps. In all cases, granulations are curetted and root surfaces planed clean. When these procedures have been carried out, it should be possible to examine the alveolar crest, define the morphology of any bone defect and decide on the mode of treatment.

Three basic options are available:

1. To shape the bone so that after healing and remodelling the resultant alveolar architecture will allow effective oral hygiene measures to be carried out (**Fig. 20.1A**). This procedure, osteoplasty, must be undertaken with great care. Attempts to impose a stereotype of 'normal anatomy' are not justified. Cutting bone induces subsequent bone resorption so that the final result could be loss of tooth support. Therefore, osteoplasty should be resorted to only where gross bone deformity is present, e.g. buccal ledges often associated with craters which extend into furcation areas.
2. To attempt to obtain some fill-in of the bone defect. This may be achieved with or without a bone graft (**Fig. 20.1B**).
3. To attempt to obtain new connective attachment. To date, this has been obtained only by guided tissue regeneration techniques.

In practice, options 1 and 2 are frequently used together depending on the morphology of the bone defect. A three-walled intrabony defect offers a better chance of bony in-fill than a two-walled defect. A narrow, deep defect is more likely to be bridged by bone than a wide, shallow defect.

BONE RESHAPING

Osteoplasty is the term used for shaping bone that is not directly attached to the tooth. Ostectomy (osteo-ectomy) is the removal of bone that is directly involved in tooth support. Frequently these two procedures are carried out together. Bone may be removed by chisels or by rotating instruments, burs or diamond stones. If a rotating instrument is not adequately cooled, excessive bone loss may follow. If chisels are used to remove bone, the fragments may be used to fill in the bone defects. Small chisels, e.g. the Ochsenbein chisel, can be used with hand pressure. In attempting to obtain an acceptable bone shape, especially where there is a great deal of

bone loss, a compromise must often be made to effect a balance between adequate tooth support and a cleanable tissue shape. No attempt should be made to reproduce some ideal bone architecture as bone remodelling always follows surgery.

Bone reshaping is usefully applied to thickened and uneven alveolar margins, to marginal gutters providing they are not very deep, interdental craters and two-walled intrabony defects. When carrying out bone resection the removed fragments may be used as an autograft in an attempt to obtain some fill-in of the defect.

Bone 'swaging' is the name given to a technique whereby a piece of bone is incompletely detached from its base (by a chisel) and swung into a neighbouring bone defect with some of its blood supply maintained. There is some clinical evidence of success following this procedure.

PERIODONTAL TISSUE REGENERATION

The term 'reattachment' is used to describe the reunion of root and connective tissue separated by incision or injury and the term 'new attachment' to describe the union of connective tissue with a previously pathogenically altered root surface. The cells with regenerative potential in the periodontal wound are junctional epithelial cells, gingival connective tissue cells, bone

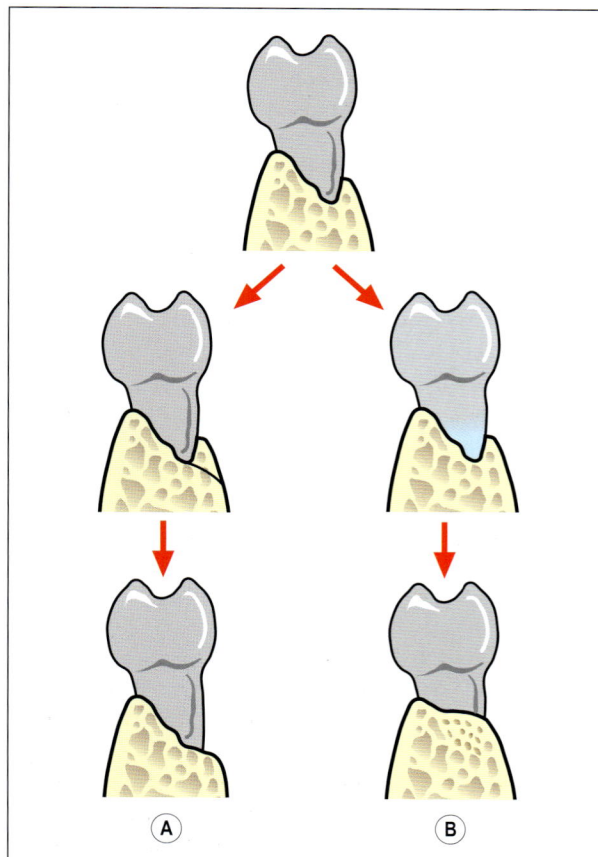

Fig. 20.1 A bone defect may be treated by (A) bone shaping to produce a cleanable overlying tissue contour, or (B) an attempt to obtain fill in (with or without a graft) and reattachment.

cells and periodontal ligament cells. The role of these tissues has been studied by clinical investigations and by the use of animal models, in particular the technique of producing experimental periodontitis in monkey teeth by placing orthodontic elastics into the gingival crevice (Caton & Zander 1975).

Clinical investigations have shown that:

1. Alveolar bone has good regenerative capacity within two- and three-walled intrabony defects following inverse bevel flap surgery and curettage to remove all granulation tissue. Claims of success in obtaining bony in-fill of such defects vary greatly from 15% to 70%. These assessments are based, however, upon measurements of clinical attachment levels, radiographic measurements and clinical observation following re-entry procedures, all of which are unreliable to varying degrees (Caton & Nyman 1980; Nyman et al 1990).

2. Bone regeneration may be encouraged or enhanced by the use of autograft cancellous bone or red bone marrow implants. With the latter material this may be complicated in some cases by root resorption and ankylosis unless it is frozen before use (Nyman et al 1990). Melcher (1976) postulated that the cells which populate the root surface after surgery determine the nature of the healing process. These tissues will now be considered separately below:

   ◆ *Junctional epithelium* – Junctional epithelium has a high regenerative capacity and will rapidly proliferate over the connective tissue wound surface. Using the monkey, Caton et al (1980) studied the effect of four surgical procedures on the healing of experimental periodontal lesions: (1) root planing and curettage; (2) replaced flap and curettage; (3) replaced flap followed by implantation of previously frozen autograft red marrow and (4) replaced flap followed by implantation of a bone substitute – beta tricalcium phosphate. They found that all four procedures resulted in the formation of a long junctional epithelium to the presurgical level and extending to the base of the intrabony defects. Where bone regeneration occurred in intrabony defects, which was a frequent occurrence with all the open techniques, the epithelium always interposed itself between the new bone and the root surface. No new connective tissue attachment occurred.

   ◆ *Gingival connective tissue and bone* – The effect of gingival connective tissue and bone on the healthy exposed root surface and the diseased root surface was studied in monkeys by Nyman et al (1990). Extracted, partially periodontally diseased roots were buried below the surface of the edentulous ridge with one surface in contact with gingival connective tissue and one with bone. Reattachment occurred around the healthy portion of the root but no reattachment occurred around the diseased portion. Both the bone and gingival connective tissue induced resorption of the diseased root surface. These experiments showed that granulation tissue derived from bone or gingival connective tissue does not have the capacity to form new connective tissue attachment to diseased root surfaces. It also shows that in the clinical situation the formation of a long junctional epithelium protects the root surface from resorption.

   ◆ *Periodontal ligament cells* – The fact that new cementum with connective tissue attachment may occasionally form at the most apical portion of the periodontal wound suggests that coronal migration of periodontal ligament cells may be responsible for this (Melcher 1976). This was confirmed by Nyman et al (1990) using a monkey model which prevented junctional epithelial cells and gingival connective tissue cells from populating the wound. A portion of the buccal root surface of the canine tooth was exposed between the apex and the margin, then root planed to remove the cementum. The preservation of the marginal tissues prevented interference from apical migration of junctional epithelium and

the placement of a plastic filter barrier over the bony fenestration prevented ingress of gingival connective tissue cells when the wound was closed. After 3 months new attachment had spread over the root surface from the margins of the fenestration and included new cementum, fibrous attachment and bone. This suggests that periodontal ligament cells have the capacity to develop new attachment if epithelium and gingival connective tissue are excluded from the wound during healing (Nyman et al 1990).

METHODS AIMED AT THE REGENERATION OF PERIODONTAL TISSUES

CURETTAGE FOR BONY IN-FILL

The complete removal of inflammatory tissue from bony defects and careful root planing will often result in some bone in-fill produced by the activity of osteoblasts from the surrounding marrow spaces. No new cementum will form on the root surface, which will be covered by the junctional epithelium, and this will interpose itself between the new bone and the root, preventing resorption. A number of factors can prevent this from happening:

1. Choosing the wrong type of defect, i.e. one that is too wide and shallow, with too few bone walls. The ideal is the deep three-walled defect
2. Failure to curette away all inflamed connective tissue and granulations
3. Failure to clean the root surface completely
4. Failure to close the flaps completely over the bone defect
5. Infection and disintegration of the blood clot
6. Excessive tooth mobility which can disturb the healing tissues. Temporary immobilization of a very mobile tooth may help to protect the lesion from mechanical stress.

The surgical procedure to gain access may be an apically repositioned or replaced flap procedure depending on the situation (Ch. 19). Particular attention is paid to closing the soft-tissue wound over the bone lesion.

Eliminating the bone defect by reshaping is a more predictable procedure than curettage; therefore in a situation where there is doubt about the treatment of the bone defect the position of the lesion may well provide an answer to the dilemma. However, it must be borne in mind that in many cases bone resection will further reduce tooth attachment and therefore be contraindicated. In the posterior segment it may be better to treat the bone defect definitively by bone reshaping, whereas in anterior segments one needs to conserve bone to preserve the appearance.

BONE GRAFTS

Attempting to obtain some fill-in of the bone defect and reattachment by simple curettage of the bone defect is an unpredictable procedure and a number of different types of graft material have been tried. Graft materials are of four general types:

1. *The autograft* which is bone from the same individual
2. *The allograft* which is from an individual of the same species
3. Xenografts which are bone from a different species, treated with ethylene diamine to remove the organic and antigenic fraction
4. Grafts of bone substitutes and synthetic materials. There are five types of alloplastic synthetic grafts which are available for clinical use. These are:
   a. Beta tricalcium phosphate
   b. Porous hydroxyapatite
   c. Non-porous hydroxyapatite
   d. HTR polymer (Mellonig 1990)
   e. Bio-active glasses and ceramics (Wilson & Low 1992).

One of these 'Periograft' or 'Durapatite', a non-porous hydroxyapatite is illustrated in **Figure 20.4**.

The essential requirements of a graft material are:

1. It should be immunologically acceptable
2. It should have osteogenic potential, i.e. it should contain viable bone cells which become active in the new site, or contain some chemical factor with osteogenic potential.

It would seem that graft materials which lack osteogenic potential act simply as a replacement for the blood clot which usually breaks down, or as an inert scaffold on which some bone formation takes place prior to the resorption of the graft. This is because cellular events of periodontal regeneration involve the controlled integration of a number of cell signalling systems for bone, cementum and periodontal ligament. Unless these are present in the graft material and/or the adjacent tissues in the right proportions, controlled regeneration cannot take place. However, regeneration of new cementum, periodontal ligament and alveolar bone can be achieved to some degree in intrabony defects with some grafting techniques including autograft bone and marrow (Hiatt & Schallhorn 1973; Rosenberg 1971), human freeze-dried, demineralized bone allograft (Mellonig et al 1976; Rummelhart et al 1989), with bone substitutes such as Bio-active glass (Wilson & Low 1992) and possibly HTR polymer (Stahl et al 1990) and with guided tissue regeneration, GTR (see below).

Bone autograft

Bone autografts using *iliac crest marrow* (Hiatt & Schallhorn 1973) or *cancellous bone from oral sites* (Rosenberg 1971) have been used with some success. Cancellous bone and marrow can be obtained from a number of sites in the mouth such as the tuberosity, extraction sockets or the edentulous ridge (**Fig. 20.2A–C**). The ideal autograft is obtained from the iliac crest but it is doubtful whether tapping this site is justifiable. Also, fresh marrow tissue often produces root resorption and ankylosis; it must be frozen before use to prevent this. Shavings of cortical bone obtained

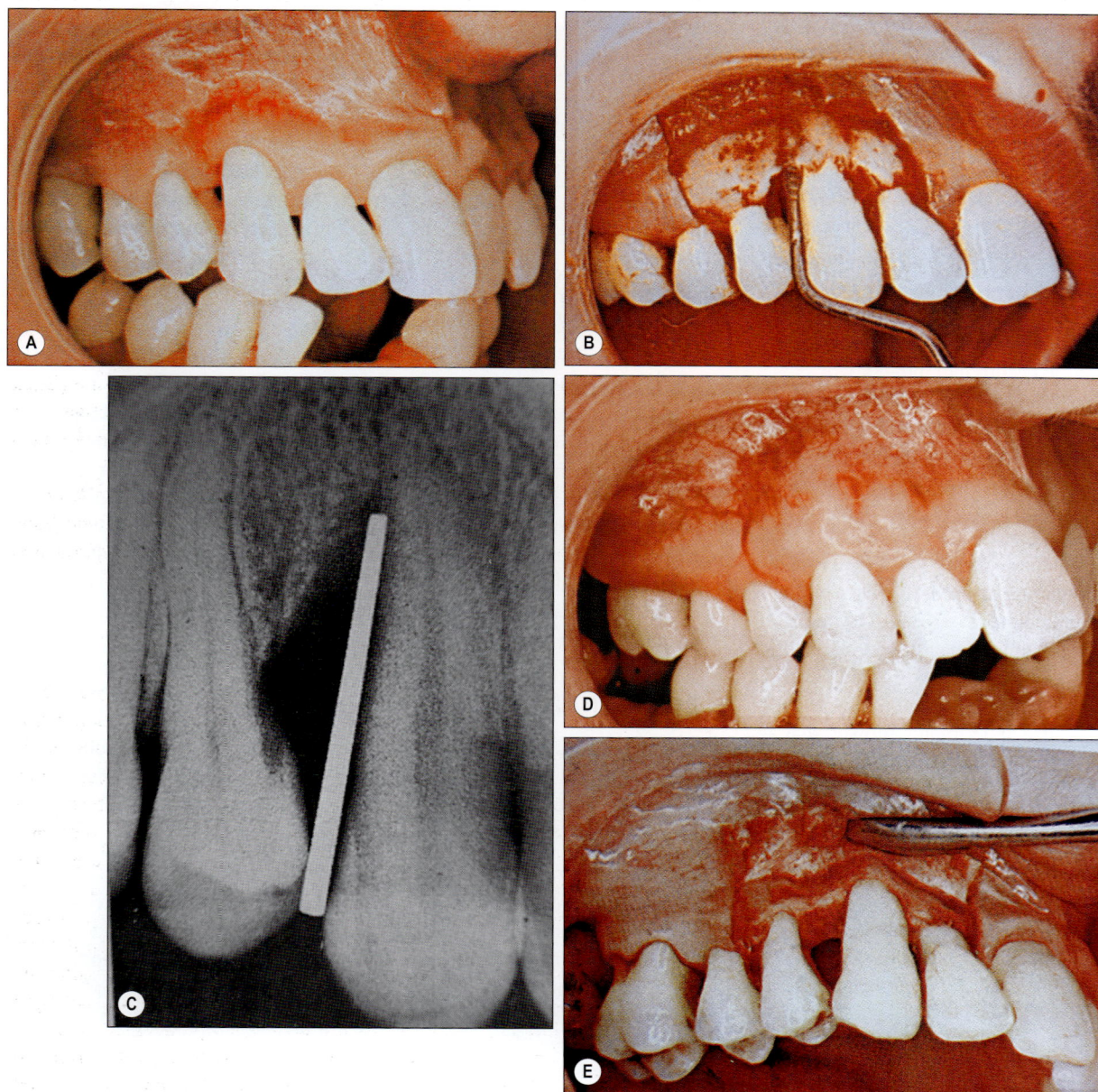

Fig. 20.2 A man of 35 years with a 2–3-walled intrabony defect distal to 3/ treated with a cancellous autograft bone from an adjacent edentulous site. (A) Preoperative clinical appearance; (B) operative appearance with flaps raised of bony defect; (C) radiograph with a radio-opaque marker with the pocket showing vertical bone resorption; (D) 6-months postoperative clinical appearance; (E) appearance of bony lesion after a 6-months re-entry procedure showing bony in-fill.

from the neighbourhood of the bone defect, although not as useful or as effective as cancellous bone, may also be used. Unless bone formation is very rapid, as with fresh bone marrow tissue, junctional epithelium will usually migrate apically over the connective tissue wound to cover the root surface and protect it from root resorption.

Good clinical results have been achieved with the use of cancellous autograft bone grafts from an adjacent edentulous site in 2- and 3-walled intrabony defects (**Figs 20.2, 20.3**). While these procedures may produce significant bony in-fill there is no evidence that they result in significant new attachment.

Bone allograft

More recently, *freeze-dried bone allograft* has been used to treat periodontal osseous defects. Two types of bone allograft are in clinical usage. These are *freeze-dried undemineralized bone allograft (FDBA)* and *freeze-dried demineralized bone allograft (FDDBA)*. Originally introduced as a periodontal material in 1976, it has been used successfully in clinical medicine for more than four decades (Mellonig 1990). The freeze drying permits storage within a vacuum for an indefinite shelf-life and also markedly reduces the antigenicity of the graft (Friedlaender 1987; Turner & Mellonig 1981; Quattlebaum et al 1988).

Clinical studies have shown that the use of the graft in intrabony defects following debridement produces more than 50% bony in-fill in 63% of the defects (Sanders et al 1983). Using a combination of FDBA and autograft bone to produce a composite graft produces this result in over 80% of defects (Sanders et al 1983). Although there is relatively little difference in the clinical results with FDBA and FDDBA, the latter has largely superseded the former as a periodontal grafting material (Rummelhart et al 1989). FDDBA appears to have superior bone induction properties and clinical studies indicate that sites grafted with this material produce >50% bony in-fill in 78% of sites comparing with only 38% of sites for debridement alone (Urist 1965; Urist & Strates 1971; Mellonig et al 1976, 1981; Quintero et al 1982). In addition, human histological studies (Bowers et al 1989a,b,c) have provided evidence for regeneration of new bone, ligament and cementum using this material (see below). Furthermore, it has been shown that bone matrix contains bone inductive proteins (Sampath & Reddi 1983) and several osteoinductive signal molecules have been purified from FDDBA powder. These include bone morphogenic proteins (BMP) 2 and 7 (Sampath et al 1990) and six other distinct bone derived growth factors (Hauschka et al 1986). It has also been suggested that the collagen matrix of the demineralized graft acts as a substrate for attachment, proliferation and differentiation of new osteoprogenitor cells (Sampath & Reddi 1983).

The fate of FDDBA grafts in human intrabony defects has been studied in 12 patients with 32 grafted sites (Reynolds & Bowers 1996). These lesions were removed *en bloc* after 6 months and were examined

histologically. This revealed that 72% of the grafted sites exhibited residual FDDBA particles and these appeared amalgamated with new viable bone. Defects harbouring residual graft material showed significantly greater amounts of new attachment formation including new bone, cementum and associated periodontal ligament than sites without evidence of residual graft material.

However, some difficulties have been encountered in the placement and retention of particulate FDDBA grafts especially in accessible and freely bleeding sites when the material may be flushed out. In an effort to overcome these difficulties and improve the biological and physical handling properties, these bone grafts have been combined with microfibrillar collagen (Blumenthal et al 1986). The combined graft helped to bind and retain the particles, created a space between the particles and acted as a scaffold for cell and blood vessel ingrowth. In addition, it was claimed that the collagen material became bound to the root surface and prevented epithelial downgrowth. The material consists of a combination of human freeze-dried bone powder with human tendon collagen. Following rehydration it can be layered into defect and expands to fill it. Clinical studies and experimental studies with dogs have been carried out with this material (Blumenthal et al 1986). Clinical re-entry was performed 5 months after the procedure and found a mean 61% bone in-fill. Histological studies showed evidence of bone formation, periodontal regeneration and prevention of epithelial migration. The material has also been used successfully in humans (Blumenthal 1994).

The possibility of disease transfer with bone allografts obtained from human cadaver material exists but is nonetheless very unlikely if the material is procured and processed using established tissue banking protocols which incorporate medical and social screening, antibody testing, direct antigen tests, serological tests, bacterial culturing and follow-up studies (Mellonig 1990; Friedlaender 1987; American Association of Tissue Banks 1984; Buck et al 1989, 1990; Martin et al 1985; Quinnan et al 1986; Resnick et al 1986). The risk of disease transmission with FDDBA is 1 chance in 8 million. The HIV virus has been cultured from bone (Buck et al 1990) but is likely to be detected by the above tests and inactivated in the event of being missed in the screening process by the sterilization procedures used in the preparation of these materials.

It seems likely that most grafts act both as a replacement for the blood clot which usually breaks down and as a scaffold on which some bone formation takes place. There then follows a progressive resorption and replacement of the graft by new bone.

Bone xenograft

In contrast to FDDBA, bone mineral for implantation has also been produced which is free of organic component. This product, a xenograft, is known as bovine anorganic cancellous bone (BACB) or commercially as Bio-Oss®, is produced from bovine bone by a special process which removes its organic components but retains its inorganic structure. This product contains biological apatite crystals and is either produced as cancellous blocks or granules. The same company also produces a porcine non-antigenic collagen (PNAC) known commercially as Bio-Oss® collagen. This is produced from healthy pigs and the collagen undergoes prolonged alkaline treatment which produces a bilayer structure and eliminates any risk of bacterial or viral contamination. During further processing the terminal peptides (telopeptides) (see Ch. 5) are split off from the collagen molecules and this process removes the areas most concerned with the antigenicity of the molecule. Also specific purification processes remove any residual fat or protein from the processed collagen. PNAC is produced as a block which can be cut or crushed to the desired size or consistency.

The antigenicity of grafts of BACB and composite BACB/PNAC have been compared with that of resorbable hydroxyapatite (see below) by implanting these materials subcutaneously into Wistar rats (Cohen

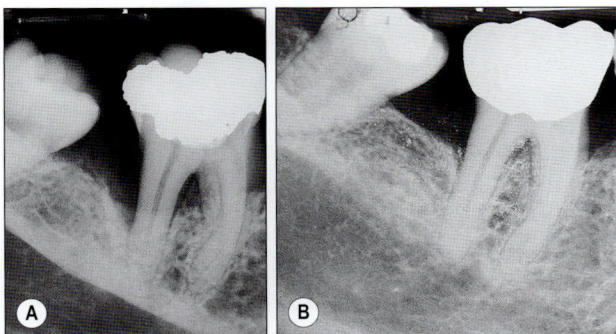

Fig. 20.3 Two radiographs of a 40-year-old woman before and after the placement of a cancellous autograft bone from an adjacent edentulous site. (A) Preoperative, (B) after 9-months, showing radiographical evidence of bony in-fill.

et al 1994). The nature of the cellular infiltration around these materials in biopsies taken at 3 days and 1, 2, 4, 6 and 8 weeks was examined using immunocytochemistry. Biopsies of sites with all of the materials showed a transient infiltration of macrophages which was maximal at 3 days but this had resolved to normal levels by 6–8 weeks. Lymphocytic infiltration was not seen and antibodies to bovine or porcine serum proteins or collagen were not detected. These data indicate that neither systemic nor local immune reactions developed in response to any of these materials.

The osteoconductive potential of BACB (Bio-Oss®), human FDDBA and resorbable hydroxyapatite (Osteogen®) have been compared in beagle dogs receiving dental implants (Wetzel et al 1995). Titanium dental implants (ITI®) (see Ch. 29) were placed into prepared edentulous sites which were extended into the maxillary sinus by elevating the sinus floor. The area below the raised sinus floor contained the protruding implant tip and was packed with one of these materials. The implanted material was placed so that it surrounded the implant tip and extended to the bone margin below. Sites implanted with human FDDBA showed no signs of new bone formation whereas those implanted with BACB (Bio-Oss®) or resorbable hydroxyapatite (Osteogen®) did show significant new bone formation in this area. The use of bone markers (tetracycline or calcein green) revealed rapid bone formation and remodelling, especially around the BACB particles. Thus, both BACB and resorbable hydroxyapatite were shown to be osteoconductive in this situation.

The regenerative potential of composite grafts of BACB (Bio-Oss®) and PNAC (Bio-Oss®collagen) were studied by placing them into intrabony periodontal defects prepared in 8 healthy beagle dogs (Clergeau et al 1996). The experimental lesions were either treated with a replaced flap plus curettage (control sites) or with additional composite BACB/PNAC grafts (test sites). After 6, 18 and 32 weeks postoperatively, non-decalcified block specimens were removed and examined by microscopy and contact microradiology. In the control sites, no significant bone regeneration was observed at any time period. In contrast, in the test sites bone trabeculae undergoing mineralization were seen at 6 weeks around the implanted particles above the reference notch. At 18 and 36 weeks, significant bone regeneration was seen. The periodontal ligament space adjacent to the new bone was always clear and the only signs of ankylosis were seen within the reference notch at 18 weeks in one animal of the test group and at 36 weeks in one animal of the control group. Therefore, this combined graft material appears to have osteogenic potential in periodontal intrabony defects. Similar favourable histological results using bovine bone mineral on a similar dog model over 2 years have also been reported (Artzi et al 2003a,b).

The main drawback with these materials is a very low risk of transmission of bovine or porcine viruses or other infective agents.

Synthetic bone substitutes

Synthetic bone substitutes are also available for clinical use. These materials avoid the problems of finding suitable autograft bone and the small infective risks inherent in the use of human cadaver materials or other animal tissue. Five types of synthetic bone substitute are available (see above) and all seem to produce better results than surgical debridement alone.

Porous and non-porous hydroxyapatite

Porous hydroxyapatite has a uniform pore size, which facilitates vascular ingrowth and subsequent new bone formation (Mellonig 1990). Controlled studies in humans show that it produces more bone in-fill in intrabony lesions than surgical debridement alone (Kenney et al 1985; Yukna et al 1986). Kenney et al (1986) also showed histological evidence of new bone formation on the surface of and within the pores of porous hydroxyapatite.

He placed this material into intrabony lesions of teeth with advanced periodontitis in human subjects and removed the teeth and surrounding tissues for light and scanning electron-microscopical examination. Spreading osteoblasts and new bone were seen in contact with the particles.

In a 5-year follow-up study (Yukna et al 1989) *non-porous hydroxyapatite* has also been shown to be superior to surgical debridement in producing bony in-fill. It also showed that the condition remained stable for long periods following this treatment. Porous and non-porous hydroxyapatite and surgical debridement have been compared in the treatment of intrabony defects (Krejci et al 1987) and this study showed that non-porous hydroxyapatite produced the most consistent results (**Fig. 20.4**). It is available commercially under the trade names of Periograf® and Alveolagraf®.

Tricalcium phosphate

Tricalcium phosphate has been shown to stimulate bone formation and is comparable or in most cases superior in this regard to the action of hydroxyapatite (Fetner et al 1994). It is also produced commercially under the trade names of Synthagraft® and Augmen®. Its use in periodontal intrabony defects has been compared with hydroxyapatite (see above) and bioactive glass, Bioglass®, (see below) in primates. It has been shown to stimulate bone formation to a greater extent than hydroxyapatite but to a much lesser extent than Bioglass® (Wilson & Low 1992; Fetner et al 1994). It, however, did not stimulate complete regeneration of the periodontium and did not retard epithelial downgrowth. In regard to these findings, it was similar to the effect of hydroxyapatite but unlike that of Bioglass® (see below).

HTR polymer

HTR polymer is a non-resorbable, microporous biocompatible composite of poly-methylmethacrylate (PMMA) and polyhydroxyethylmethacrylate (PHEMA). This material has been used in the fabrication of contact lenses, lens transplants and prosthetic heart valves over many years. The polymer does not produce an inflammatory or immune response in contact with bone or soft tissue (Yukna 1990). PMMA beads of 550–880 μm diameter with pores of 50–300 μm form the core of this material. These are coated with liquid PHEMA without the addition of any catalysts or inducers. The composite beads are then coated with calcium hydroxide/calcium carbonate. Thus, the actual surface interface with bone is the calcium surface layer and both fibrous tissue and bone can form on and attach to this layer. The composite is provided in a fine granular form for use in periodontal intrabony defects.

Stahl et al (1990) used this material in five volunteer patients with advanced periodontitis and they provided 11 intrabony defects. These were surgically debrided and implanted with HTR polymer and the lesions were

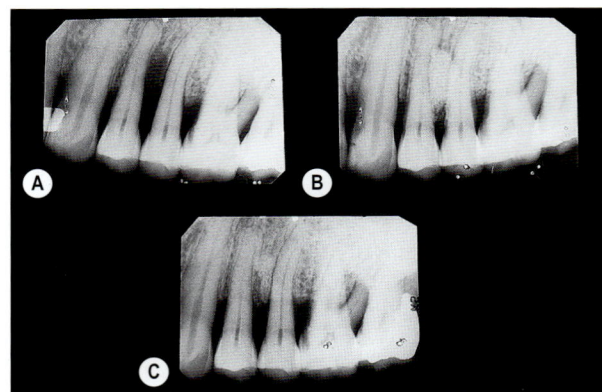

Fig. 20.4 Three radiographs showing a 50-year-old man. (A) Bone lesion between /45 caused by a lateral abscess; (B) postoperative radiograph after the placement of a hydroxyapatite graft (Periograft®); (C) 1 year postoperative radiograph showing graft partially resorbed.

followed for 4–26 weeks. After this time the teeth and blocks of tissue were removed for histological examination. The clinical observations showed a reduction in probing depth due both to gingival recession and a gain in clinical attachment level. The patients showed no untoward symptoms or signs during this period. Histological examination showed that the grafts became surrounded by connective tissue capsules and some limited bone deposition was present on the surface of some implanted particles. The 11 lesions showed varied responses and there were different responses both between patients and different sites in the same patient. In seven sites a long junctional epithelium was detected between the root surface and the graft, while in four sites there was limited evidence of new attachment.

Yukna (1990) investigated the effectiveness of HTR polymer in treating intrabony lesions in 21 adult patients with moderate to advanced chronic periodontitis. Some sites were treated by surgical debridement alone and some by debridement followed by implantation of HTR polymer. They were followed by clinical and radiographical measurements for 6 months after which surgical re-entry procedures were carried out. The re-entry procedures showed that the sites implanted with HTR polymer showed significantly better mean bony in-fill (60.8%) than those treated by debridement alone (32.2%). Clinical and radiological measurements also showed significantly better results for the polymer group. These studies show that HTR polymer synthetic alloplast does show some promise for repair of periodontal osseous defects.

Bio-active glasses and ceramics

Certain compositions of glasses, glass-ceramics and ceramics composed primarily of SiO_2-CaO-Na_2O-P_2O_5 have been widely used in conjunction with medical and dental implants because they develop a layer of hydroxy-carbonate-apatite on their surface following exposure to body fluids. When used on the surface of metal implants, this layer incorporates collagen fibrils and in this way produces a mechanically strong bond between the implant and the adjacent bone surface (Hench & Wilson 1984; Hench 1986, 1994; Hench & West 1996). Comparisons of SiO_2-CaO-Na_2O-P_2O_5 glasses with various other glass ceramics, SiO_2-CaO-P_2O_5 glasses, SiO_2 glasses, multi-component bio-active glasses and synthetic hydroxyapatites show that they all produce a strong interface bond with bone. However, most of these have a flexural strength, strain to fracture and fracture toughness less than bone. Also, the elastic modulus of the stronger and tougher bio-active glasses are greater than both cortical and cancellous bone. This would lead to excessive stress shielding of bone and could eventually produce fracture of bone distal and proximal to the implant. For these reasons their use with stress bearing implants is limited and their use is usually restricted to coating metal implants in non-load bearing areas or areas subject to compressive forces such as vertebrae.

They have also been used for the treatment of periodontal intrabony defects (Wilson & Low 1992), primarily because of their high bio-activity (see below).

Theory of bio-activity – The bio-activity of these materials is graded by their bio-active index which depends on the rate of bone stimulation by these materials. The index is defined as the inverse of the time required for 50% of the implant surface to be bonded to bone.

Larger differences in the rate of bone bonding to bio-active implants indicates that different biochemical factors may occur at the implant tissue interface with different materials. The highly bio-active glass particulates show both osteoproduction and osteoconduction whereas those with lower bio-activity show only osteoconduction (Hench 1994; Hench & Wilson 1995; Hench and West 1996). Osteoproduction has been defined as the process which the bio-active surface is colonized by osteogenic stem cells from the adjacent bone whereas osteoconduction relates to the properties of the bio-active interface surface which facilitates the migration of bone over it.

Wilson et al (1994) have compared the effectiveness of a highly bio-active glass, 45S5 Bioglass®, with autogenous bone in the augmentation of canine ribs. They have shown that the 45S5 Bioglass® produced more bone formation than autogenous bone. It also showed that equal mixtures of Bioglass® and autogenous bone was even more effective and resulted after 6 weeks in the formation of twice the amount of new bone compared with autogenous bone alone.

Oonishi et al (1994), using the rabbit tibial model, have shown that particulate 45S5 Bioglass® enhanced new bone formation many times faster than particulate hydroxyapatite.

The same research group (Oonishi et al 1997) compared particulate Bioglass® and hydroxyapatite as a bone graft substitute. 6 mm diameter holes were drilled bilaterally in the femoral condyles of mature rabbits and after haemostasis these were filled with either particulate Bioglass® or hydroxyapatite with one material on each side providing its own control. The animals were sacrificed after 1, 2, 3, 6, 12 weeks and the areas were examined histologically. By 1 week, new bone was present on the surface of the Bioglass® particles to the centre of the defect and by 2 weeks all the particles were covered and those at the periphery were joined by trabecular bone. By 3 weeks all the particles were connected by thick bony bridges and by 6 weeks they were all encased by new bone and by 12 weeks the calcium and phosphate rich area extended throughout the remaining parts of the particles. Bone formation was much slower with particulate hydroxyapatite and whereas full restoration of bone was complete in 2 weeks with Bioglass®, a comparable response took 12 weeks with hydroxyapatite. Particulate Bioglass® was used up in this process and therefore any problems associated with the production of a composite of bone and biological material are avoided in the fully restored bone.

In vivo studies have shown that there are probably 2 classes of bio-active materials known as classes A and B, Class A bioactivity leads to osteo-production and class B to osteoconduction. Osteoproduction is thought to occur (Hench 1994) when a material produces both intracellular and extracellular responses at its interface. Osteoconduction is thought to occur when a material only produces an extracellular response at its interface.

All class A bioactive materials release soluble silicon in the form of silicic acid due to surface ion exchange with H^+ and H_3O^+ on contact with body fluids and this reaction occurs immediately as contact occurs (Hench 1994). The concentration of silicon in the solution rises until the solubility limit is reached which is dependent on the pH and the relative concentrations of other chemical species which can lead to the formation of complex silicate phases. Class A compounds release silicon by ion exchange and network dissolution whereas class B materials have either low or zero ion exchange and release either very low or zero amounts of silicon.

It was first shown (Carlisle 1986; Schwartz & Milne 1972) that the released silicon is chemically combined with glycosaminoglycan-protein complexes which surround collagen and elastic fibrils and cover the surface of cells.

Studies by Keeting et al (1992) on human osteoblast-like cells have shown that soluble silicon is a potent mitogen for these cells. It was shown to increase by 3-fold the mitotic rate of these cells and enhanced the release of alkaline phosphatase and osteocalcin from these cells. They found that the induction of genetically controlled intracellular autocrine factors appeared to be responsible for this response and found that the levels of mRNA for transforming growth factor beta (TGF-β), which is a potent mitogen for osteoblasts, were increased. Soluble silicon increased the release of latent TGF-β into the medium within 6 h of stimulation.

Vrouwenvelder et al (1993) grew human osteoblast-like cells on the surface of 45S5 Bioglass® and class B (hydroxyapatite) materials. They found that by 6 days there was enhanced alkaline phosphatase release from the cells on 45S5 Bioglass® and by 8 days the amount released had doubled. The DNA content of the cells on this material was also increased. These changes were not seen with the cells grown on hydroxyapatite.

It has been proposed (Hench 1994; Hench & West 1996) that class A bio-active glasses provide both an intracellular effect by the release of silicon and an extracellular effect by the chemoabsorption of bone growth promoting factors such as TGF-β on to their surface. It has been shown that soluble silicon also accelerates the precipitation of an amorphous calcium phosphate phase from solution. This phase forms within the pores of the silica gel layer where the porosity and silanols provide a heterogeneous nucleation mechanism for hydroxy-carbonite-apatite crystallization. Thus, the crystalline hydroxy-carbonite-apatite layer develops within a few hours on class A materials whereas it may take many days or even weeks to develop on class B. The negatively charged silica gel and defect hydroxy-carbonite-apatite crystals provide sites for chemisorption of TGF-β and other growth factors released from proliferating osteoblasts. The absorbed growth factors are then thought to enhance differentiation and mitosis of stem cells which migrate into the area from the adjacent bone marrow spaces. This then may create an autocatalytic growth of bone and other tissues.

A study on the use of bioactive glasses in the treatment of periodontal intrabony defects – Wilson and Low (1992) compared the use of particulate 45S5 Bioglass® with commercially available hydroxyapatite (Periograf® and Alveolagraf®) and tricalcium phosphate (Synthagraft® and Augmen®) materials. Prepared periodontal intrabony defects were surgically created in the alveolar bone of six adult Patas monkeys. In order to resemble pathological periodontal lesions, the root surface of the adjacent tooth was root planed. Eighteen such sites were prepared and 12 were filled with Bioglass® particulate, two with hydroxyapatites, two with tricalcium phosphate materials and the remaining two were left unfilled. The animals were killed after 4 weeks (1), 4 months (2), 6 months (2) and 9 months (1). The alveolar bone and attached soft tissues were removed and examined microscopically with particular reference to the tooth/defect interface and the position and length of the junctional epithelium. It looked for particular histological evidence of regeneration of all the elements of the periodontium, i.e. bone, cementum and inserting periodontal ligament fibres.

Hydroxyapatite only resulted in partial restoration of bone by osteoconduction over the particles by 9 months. There was a long junctional epithelium and no new attachment was seen. Tricalcium phosphate was very reactive throughout the study period and there was significant bone production and in some sites root resorption and ankylosis. Cementoid lined the defect quite quickly but failed to allow the regeneration of normal periodontium and a long junctional epithelium formed. The use of particulate Bioglass® did however allow the regeneration of a normal periodontium. Immediately after implantation, fibroblasts laid down collagen above the level of the particulate material and this collagen appeared to attach to the superficial particles, immobilizing them in the soft tissue and restoring the transeptal connections of the periodontium. This appeared to prevent epithelial downgrowth which only occurs to the point at which it meets adherent collagen fibres overlying the restoring bone. Beneath this layer the particles induced a rapid production of bone and cementum and by 9 months the particles were seen within the repairing bone and cementum. A normal periodontal ligament was seen between these tissues.

Fetner et al (1994) compared the extent of periodontal regeneration in surgically created bony defects in six Patas monkeys of 45S5 Bioglass® (PerioGlas® and Fluoride PerioGlas®) and tricalcium phosphate (Synthagraft® or Augmen®) or hydroxyapatite (Alveolagraf®). Each animal had a total of 18 sites in which 4 mm osseous defects were prepared most of which were two walled interproximal defects but some were palatal and lingual three walled defects. Adjacent root surfaces were planed and existing periodontal ligament and cementum was removed. Twelve sites were filled with particulate Perioglas®, two each with hydroxyapatite and tricalcium phosphate and two remained as unfilled controls. Histological analyses were carried out at 1, 4 and 6 months. Histologically,

Perioglas® sites showed superior bone and cementum regeneration than the other materials with statistically higher percentage of both new cementum and bone. Perioglas® was also much more effective in retarding epithelial downgrowth than the other materials and this could be one reason for its superiority over the other materials.

The properties of the particulate Bioglass® which appeared to contribute to these favourable results seem to be first, the increased rate of reaction *in vivo* which it possess in comparison to the other materials as a result of its release of silicon (see above). Second, it appeared to bond with connective tissue collagen. Because of its high bioactivity the reaction layers appear to form within minutes of its implantation and the osteogenic cells freed by the surgery can rapidly colonize the particles. This process supplements the bone which grows by osteoconduction from the alveolus and these two processes combined have been termed osteoproduction (Wilson et al 1987). This results in more rapid filling of the defects than occurs with other less active materials such as hydroxyapatite. This may also result from a more rapid accumulation of bone morphogenic proteins and other growth factors on the surface of bioactive particles (Watanabe et al 1990). The prevention of epithelial downgrowth is probably the result of the rapid establishment of collagen over the coronal surface of the implanted particles and could be explained by a direct inhibitory effect on epithelium or to the rapid deployment and attachment of collagen fibres beneath the advancing epithelium.

Bioglass particulate has also been used to stimulate bone formation in extraction sockets and to thus maintain the alveolar ridge height (Hench et al 1991; Wilson et al 1993; Hench & Wilson 1995).

CEMENTUM FORMATION STIMULANTS

Enamel matrix derivative (Emdogain®)

The use of enamel matrix derivatives (EMD) for periodontal regeneration has been suggested because it is thought that this process might mimic the way these materials behave in normal tooth development. In this regard studies during the last 20 years have indicated that enamel-related proteins appear to be involved in the formation of cementum.

The initial formation of cementum and root formation are intimately related. It was previously thought that Hertwig's epithelial root sheath (HERS) induced mesenchyme cells of the dentine papilla to form mantle pre-dentine before it disintegrated to expose the mesenchymal cells of the dental follicle to the newly formed dentine. This event was then believed to induce cementogenesis (Bosshardt & Schroeder 1996). However, it has now been shown that exposure of follicular cells to slices of root dentine does not provide a sufficient stimulus for cementoblast differentiation (Thomas & Kollar 1989). The HERS is the apical extension of the dental organ and the inner layer of the sheath represents extension of the ameloblast layer in the dental organ and this has led to the proposal that enamel related proteins from the epithelial root sheath are involved in the formation of cellular cementum (Stavkin 1976).

Enamel matrix proteins were first demonstrated on the root-analogue surfaces of rabbit incisors (Schonfeld & Slavkin 1977) and its role was further supported by the finding that the HERS cells of the developing rat molars contained organelles suggestive of secretory activity (Owens 1978, 1979).

Further support was gained from scanning electron microscope and auto-radiographic studies on developing monkey incisors (Lindskog 1982a,b; Lindskog & Hammarström 1982). This demonstrated that the inner layer of the epithelial root sheath had a secretory stage and that an enamel-like material was formed in the root surface prior to cementum formation or as an initial step in this process. It was also shown that acellular cementum contains proteins that are immunologically related to proteins present in enamel matrix (Stavkin et al 1989a,b).

An association between enamel and cementum formation is also supported by the fact that coronal cementum is a normal structure on the enamel surface of a variety of rodents and Herbivora such as elephants, sheep, cows, rabbits and guinea-pigs (Ainamo 1970). Coronal cementogenesis seems to be initiated by the exposure of the cells of the dental follicle to the developing enamel.

The major proteins of the enamel matrix are known as amelogenins and they constitute about 90% of the matrix (Brookes et al 1995). The dormant protein known as amelogenin exists in several different sizes which together form aggregates. These are markedly hydrophobic and play a major role in crystal formation. Other enamel matrix proteins have been identified recently by cloning and DNA sequencing and these have been termed ameloblastin (Krebsbach et al 1996) and amelin (Cerny et al 1996).

Immunohistochemical (Thomas et al 1986) and *in situ* hybridization studies (Luo et al 1991) on developing rat molars have indicated that the enamel proteins expressed during root formation are not identical to amelogenin. It has also been shown by *in situ* hybridization that amelin is expressed by cells of HERs in rat molars during root formation (Fong et al 1996).

However, recently a number of further studies have been carried out on the role of enamel proteins in cementogenesis. The dominating constituent of enamel matrix, amelogenin, has been shown by immunohistochemistry to be expressed at the apical end of the forming root of human teeth and also to be present in the Tomes granular layer of such teeth (Hammarström 1997). This study, using a rat model, showed that when the mesenchymal cells of the dental follicle were exposed to enamel matrix a non-cellular hard tissue closely resembling cellular cementum was formed at the enamel surface. It was also shown that the application of porcine enamel matrix into prepared experimental cavities of the roots of monkey incisor teeth induced the formation of acellular cementum that was well attached to dentine. Control roots in these monkeys, that were sham operated and not treated with enamel matrix, formed a cellular, poorly attached hard tissue.

The ability of enamel matrix proteins to induce cementum formation and periodontal regeneration were first investigated in a buccal dehiscence monkey model (Hammarström et al 1997). Buccal mucoperiosteal flaps were raised from canine to first molar on each side of the maxilla and the buccal alveolar bone plate, the exposed periodontal ligament and cementum were removed. The exposed roots were then conditioned with citric acid and rinsed with saline. Then various preparations of porcine enamel matrix with or without vehicles were applied before the flaps were reapplied and sutured.

After 8 weeks, the healing was evaluated by light microscopy and morphometric measurements. It was found that the application of homogenized enamel matrix or acidic extract of the matrix containing the hydrophobic, low molecular weight proteins, amelogenins, resulted in almost complete regeneration of acellular cementum firmly attached to the dentine and with collagenous fibres extending over to newly formed alveolar bone, i.e. complete regeneration of periodontium. In contrast, application of fractions obtained by neutral EDTA extraction containing the acidic, high molecular weight proteins of enamel matrix produced very little new cementum and hardly any new bone. This lack of regeneration was also seen in control animals in which no test substance was applied before the repositioning of the flaps. Three vehicles for enamel matrix proteins, propylene glycol alginate (PGA), hydroxyethyl cellulose and dextran, were tried and it was shown that only PGA in combination with the amelogenin fraction resulted in significant regeneration of periodontium.

The regenerative effect of EMD on intrabony defects, experimentally produced in the mandibles of baboons, has been evaluated histologically (Cochran et al 2003). Defects of 1–6 mm were created around three mandibular teeth in each animal and pockets were produced with ligatures. The defects were treated either with EMD or placebo. EMD stimulated substantial periodontal regeneration. The height of new cementum was 45% and the height of new bone was 30% more at the EMD sites than the control ones. Furthermore, histological examination of the treated EMD sites showed new cementum and bone with inserting collagen fibres and a normal periodontal ligament space.

Viswanathan et al (2003) studied the effects of amelogenin on immortalized murine cementoblasts in culture. They found that low doses slightly enhanced and higher does dramatically reduced bone sialoprotein expression. This shows that an epithelial cell product can regulate mesenchymal cell activity and may act as a signalling molecule in periodontal regeneration.

Cementum and bone are very similar tissues so it is not surprising to find that EMD also affects bone cells. In this regard, EMDs have been shown (Yoneda et al 2003) to stimulate mouse osteoblastic cells (KUSA/A1 cells) to proliferate and to increase their alkaline phosphatase activity. It also stimulated the osteoblastic phenotype in these cells and their expression of type 1 collagen, osteopontin, osteocalcin and TGF-β1. These cells also secrete MMPs. In the same study EMDs were also found to stimulate new bone formation in a rat skull defect model. Suzuki et al (2005) have also shown that EMD-Gel contains both TGF-β- and BMP-like growth factors that contribute to the induction of biomineralization during periodontal regeneration.

A study of the action of EMD on osteoblast activity (Mizutani et al 2003) used RT-PCR and ELISA assays on samples from cultured human osteoblastic cells (SaM-1) in culture treated with EMD. EMD stimulated osteoblast proliferation and fibroblast growth factor-2 expression. It also increased cyclooxygenase (COX)-2 expression and decreased matrix metalloproteinase (MMP)-1 expression. The effects on FGF-2 and MMP-1 expression were nullified by an inhibitor of COX-2. The decreases in MMP-1 mRNA by EMD was prevented by treatment with an antisense oligonucleotide for FGF-2. This indicates that the activation of FGF-2 may underlie the actions of EMD on osteoblasts. In a further study Hägewald et al (2004) investigated the effects of enamel matrix derivative on proliferation, protein synthesis, and mineralization in primary mouse osteoblasts, from mouse calvaria. EMD treatments were found to increase the metabolic cell activity and 5-bromo-2′-deoxyuridine incorporation of osteoblasts. In the organoid cultures, alkaline phosphatase activity and calcium accumulation were enhanced by EMD treatment, but [3H]-proline incorporation was not. Morphologically, an increased deposition of mineralized nodules was found. Thus, EMD treatment enhanced the cellular activities of primary osteoblasts which might support its role in the regeneration of periodontal intrabony defects.

Another related study (Keila et al 2004) investigated the *in vitro* effects of EMD on rat bone marrow stromal cells and gingival fibroblasts. They found that EMD (25 μg/mL) increased the osteogenic capacity of the bone marrow, as evidenced by a 3-fold increase in bone marrow stromal cell numbers and a 2-fold increase in alkaline phosphatase activity and mineralized nodule formation. The presence of EMD in the initial stages (first 48 h) of the culture was crucial for these effects. In contrast, EMD did not induce osteoblastic development of gingival fibroblasts but did increase their number by up to 2-fold and the amount of intercellular matrix they produced. These results could explain the promotive effect of EMD on bone formation and connective tissue regeneration, respectively.

The action of EMD on osteoblasts is poorly understood but Carinci et al (2006) have attempted to address this question by using a microarray technique to identify genes that are differently regulated in osteoblasts exposed to enamel matrix proteins. They identified several upregulated and downregulated genes in the osteoblast-like cell line (MG-63) cultured with enamel matrix proteins. The differentially expressed genes covered a broad range of functional activities including signalling transduction, transcription, translation, cell cycle regulation, proliferation and apoptosis, activation of the immune system, vesicular transport and lysosome activity and cytoskeleton, cell adhesion and extracellular matrix production. This work could contribute to our understanding of the molecular mechanisms of bone regeneration and as a model for comparing other materials with similar clinical effects.

Palioto et al (2004) studied the effect of EMD, Insulin-like growth factor-I (IGF-I), and the combination of these two factors on the proliferation, adhesion, migration, and expression of type I collagen in PDL fibroblasts. IGF-I is a potent modulator of periodontal regeneration stimulating cell proliferation, differentiation, synthesis of type I collagen, and non-collagenous proteins. The fibroblast proliferation rate was measured by automated cell counting and immunohistochemical expression of proliferating cell nuclear antigen. The cell adhesion was analysed by a colorimetric assay and cell migration was measured in Boyden chambers. Type I collagen expression and production was determined by semi-quantitative reverse transcriptase-polymerase chain reaction and enzyme-linked immunosorbent assay, respectively. The proliferation of PDL fibroblasts was significantly stimulated by EMD and EMD plus IGF-I in a dose- and time-dependent manner. EMD, IGF-I, and the combination of both factors had no effects on cellular migration and adhesion or expression and production of type I collagen.

Rincon et al (2005) investigated, *in vitro*, the effect of EMD at three concentrations on proliferation, cell attachment and expression of mRNA for two mineralized tissue-related proteins (osteopontin and bone sialoprotein). Periodontal ligament fibroblasts, the epithelial cell rests of Malassez (ERM), alveolar bone cells and gingival fibroblasts were obtained from porcine periodontal ligament, alveolar bone and gingiva. As for other periodontal cells, the ERM proliferative response was enhanced by EMD. Attachment assays revealed a highly significant increase for ERM and gingival fibroblasts after EMD treatment at all concentrations. This study also showed that EMD stimulated expression of osteopontin mRNA by ERM and alveolar bone cells and provided evidence that EMD enhanced cellular events related with proliferation, attachment and osteopontin mRNA expression by porcine periodontal cells, in a manner consistent with its role in periodontal regenerative therapy.

Rodrigues et al (2007) evaluated the effects of enamel matrix derivative (EMD), transforming growth factor-β1 (TGF-β1), and a combination of both factors (EMD+TGF-β1) on periodontal ligament (PDL) fibroblasts. They found that treatment with EMD for 4, 7, and 10 days increased cell proliferation significantly compared with the negative control. At day 10, EMD and EMD+TGF-β1 showed a higher cell proliferation compared with TGF-β1. Cell adhesion was significantly upregulated by TGF-β1 compared with EMD and EMD+TGF-β1 ($p<0.01$). EMD enhanced *in vitro* wound healing of PDL cells compared with the other treatments. Total protein synthesis was significantly increased in PDL cells cultured with EMD compared with PDL cells treated with TGF-β1 or EMD+TGF-β1. EMD induced ALP activity in PDL fibroblasts, which was associated with an increase in bone-like nodules. Therefore these findings support the hypothesis that EMD and TGF-β1 may play an important role in periodontal regeneration. EMD induced PDL fibroblast proliferation and migration, total protein synthesis, ALP activity, and mineralization, while TGF-β1 increased cellular adhesion. However, the combination of both factors did not positively alter PDL fibroblast behaviour.

The effects of PGA formulations of enamel matrix proteins on cell kinetics and colonization were investigated using cell culture techniques and rat, pig and monkey models (Gestrelius et al 1997a). It was shown that enamel matrix derivatives (EMD) can be dissolved in PGA at an acid pH, resulting in a high viscous solution. At neutral pH and body temperature the viscosity decreases and EMD precipitates and it has been shown that it absorbs both to hydroxyapatite, collagen and denuded dental roots. By using radiolabelled preparations in rats and pigs it was shown that it forms insoluble spherical complexes on the tooth surface and remains in detectable amounts at the site of application for two weeks. Using a monkey

model they also showed by scanning electron microscopy that EMD in PGA promoted a repopulation of the root surface by fibroblast-like cells during the first weeks after application. This is supported by evidence that EMD can stimulate the proliferation and migration of periodontal ligament fibroblast *in vitro* in simulated wound production (Rincon et al 2003). This may also be one of the reasons that surgical wounds tend to heal more rapidly following the use of EMD. This is also supported by other evidence that EMD exhibits an angiogenic effect both *in vitro* and murine models of wound healing (Yuan et al 2003).

Further cell culture studies on periodontal ligament cells and EMD were carried out (Gestrelius et al 1997b). This investigated the effects of EMD on migration, attachment, proliferation, biosynthetic activity, mineral nodule formation of these cells and their ability to absorb a large range of polypeptide growth factors and cytokines. In culture EMD formed protein aggregates which appeared to provide ideal conditions for cell-matrix interactions. Under these conditions EMD enhanced the proliferation of periodontal ligament (PDL) cells but not epithelial cells, increased the protein and collagen production of PDL cells and promoted mineral nodule formation by these cells. However, it appeared to have no effect on the migration, attachment and spreading of these cells nor did they absorb any of the growth factors or cytokines that were tested.

The precise molecular events involved in EMD modulation of periodontal wound healing are not completely understood. In this regard one group (Parkar & Tonetti 2004) used cDNA micro array technology to examine EMD-mediated changes in gene expression in periodontal ligament (PDL) cells *in vitro*. They explored the selective effects of EMD on the activities of 268 cytokine, growth factor, and receptor genes in PDL. PDL cells were cultured in the absence and presence of EMD for 4 days. RNA was extracted and used to generate labelled cDNA probes. These were hybridized to cDNA arrays comprising 268 genes and exposed to X-ray films. Auto radiographs were digitized and analysed. 46% (125 of 268) of the tested genes were found to be expressed by the PDL cells. Of these 125 genes, 38 were differentially expressed by PDL cells which had been cultured in the presence of EMD. Among the 38, 12 were found to be downregulated, notably mostly inflammatory genes, whereas 26 genes demonstrated upregulation, many of these coding for growth factors and growth factor receptors. This study has shown that EMD downregulates the expression of genes involved in the early inflammatory phases of wound healing while simultaneously upregulating genes encoding growth and repair-promoting molecules and this may partly explain the apparent efficacy of EMD application in periodontal regeneration.

The ability of EMD to produce periodontal regeneration in the buccal dehiscence model was also tested in one human experimental defect (Heijl 1997). This defect was produced in a volunteer on a lower incisor which was to be removed for orthodontic treatment of incisor crowding. A defect was created on this tooth in a similar manner to that described in the monkey model above. The EMD was applied to the conditioned surface and the flaps were replaced and sutured. After 4 months, the experimental tooth together with the surrounding soft and hard tissues were removed surgically for histological evaluation. This revealed the formation of new acellular extrinsic fibre cementum, which was firmly attached to the underlying dentine. A new periodontal ligament with inserting and functionally orientated collagen fibres and associated alveolar bone was also present. The new cementum covered 73% of the original defect and the new bone covered 65% of the presurgical bone height.

The clinical safety of the commercially developed PGA-EMD product (Emdogain®) was tested in an open controlled study design in 10 Swedish specialist clinics and 107 patients were treated with the product (Zetterström et al 1997). Two surgical procedures were carried out on most patients at local intrabony sites. In addition a control group of 33 patients underwent flap surgery without the application of Emdogain® at one comparable site. Serum samples were taken from the test patients for the analysis of total and specific IgG and IgE antibody levels. None of the samples, even from allergy-prone patients, produced any deviations of antibody levels from baseline ranges and this indicates that the immunogenic potential of Emdogain® is extremely low when used in this way. Comparisons of test and control patients indicated the same frequency of post-surgical experiences. About half the patients were evaluated again after 3 years. There was a significant difference between the test and control results at 8 months post treatment and this difference increased further at the 3 year follow-up. There was a 2.5–3 mm gain of clinical attachment and bone levels, assessed clinically and radiographically, in the test subjects.

In a histometric animal study with 20 Wistar rats intrabony defects were created on the first molars (Nemcovsky et al 2006). In the test group EMD was applied, while the control group only received the vehicle. It showed that while EMD did not enhance bone formation it did enhance the formation of new cementum and did reduce gingival recession at the sites and reduced the downgrowth of junctional epithelium.

The ability of Emdogain® to effectively treat intrabony periodontal defects has also been studied in a placebo controlled, randomized multicentre trial involving 33 patients with 34 paired test and control sites (Heijl et al 1997). It was designed to compare the long-term effects of this material as an adjunct to modified Widman flap (MWF) surgery with the effect of MWF plus placebo treatment. The design required two comparable interproximal intrabony lesions appropriately separated in the same jaw with probing pocket depths greater than 6 mm and intrabony defects of at least 4 mm depth. Only predominantly 1- and 2-walled defects were included to allow radiographical assessment. Clinical and radiographic assessments were made at baseline, 8, 16 and 36 months post-treatment. Mean values for probing attachment level gain in test and control sites at 8 months were 2.1 mm and 1.5 mm respectively; at 16 months, 2–3 mm and 1–7 mm, respectively and at 36 months 2.2 mm and 1.7 mm, respectively. The radiographic bone level continued to increase over the 36 months at the test sites while it remained close to the baseline level at control sites. There was a statistically significant gain in radiographic bone level at 36 months of 2.6 mm at the test sites which corresponded to a 66% fill of the original bony defect. This study (Heijl et al 1997) has indicated that the topical application of Emdogain® to the conditioned root surface of diseased teeth with intrabony defects will promote a gain in clinical attachment and bone following MWF surgery compared with control (placebo application) in the same patient. Similar results have been shown in other multicentre studies (Bratthall et al 2001; Tonetti et al 2002).

Francetti et al (2004) compared the effects of a papilla preservation flap with or without the adjunctive use of Emdogain® in a 2-year clinical trial of 24 patients with intrabony defects. They showed that the adjunctive use of Emdogain® improved the clinical results particularly in respect to bony in-fill of the defects.

Cortellini and Tonetti (2007) carried out a minimally invasive surgical technique with an enamel matrix derivative in the regenerative treatment of intrabony defects in 13 patients. They found that it produced early wound healing, and primary wound closure was obtained and maintained in all sites with the exception of one site with a small wound dehiscence at week one. The 1-year clinical attachment level (CAL) gain was 4.8 ± 1.9 mm. The 1-year percentage resolution of the defect was 88.7 ± 20.7%, and reached 100% of the baseline intrabony component in seven sites. Residual probing depths (PPD) were 2.9 ± 0.8 mm. Differences between baseline and 1-year CAL and PPD were both clinically and statistically highly significant ($p<0.0001$). Thus it produced excellent clinical improvements while limiting patient morbidity.

Another prospective clinical study (Sculean et al 2001a) compared the effectiveness of the use of EMD and guided tissue regeneration (GTR), either separately or in combination and flap surgery alone (control) in 56 patients with a single intrabony defect. These defects were randomly

treated with one of these four modalities. They found both EMD and GTR produced a statistically greater gain in clinical attachment than the control but found no statistically significant differences between the results of EMD and GTR treatments either alone or in combination. They therefore found no advantage in combining EMD treatment with GTR. However, another study (Hoffmann et al 2006) showed better results from EMD than GTR for the treatment of class II furcation defects.

Another study by the same group (Sculean et al 2000) carried out a clinical and histological evaluation of two patients with localized deep intrabony defects adjacent to teeth scheduled for extraction. The defects were treated with EMD and allowed to heal for 6 months before extraction. Newly formed cementum with inserting collagen fibres were found on both specimens and in one this new attachment was accompanied by new bone formation.

Bosshardt et al (2005) investigated the tissues developing on the root surface following application of EMD. Twelve human periodontitis-affected teeth, scheduled for extraction, were treated with EMD. At 2–6 weeks later, the teeth were extracted, demineralized and processed for embedding in acrylic and epoxy resins. New tissue formation was analysed by light and transmission electron microscopy. They showed that treatment with EMD resulted in the development of a bone-like tissue resembling cellular intrinsic fibre cementum on the root surfaces rather than acellular cementum. This was the case on both scaled and unscaled root surfaces. They found that EMD may both induce de novo formation of a mineralized connective tissue on scaled root surfaces and stimulate matrix deposition on old native cementum.

The recent study of Lossdörfer et al (2007) suggested that EMD promoted periodontal ligament cell differentiation and osteoprotegerin production, potentially resulting in a micro environment supporting periodontal repair.

Taken together, all of these studies show that EMD will stimulate the regeneration of firmly attached acellular cementum in experimentally prepared root surfaces and will also produce complete regeneration of periodontium in the buccal dehiscence models. Furthermore, it has been shown to produce good clinical and radiographical indications of attachment and bone gain when used to treat naturally occurring, diseased intrabony defects. Furthermore, the role of EMD in promoting acellular cementum formation in these situations appears to mimic its role in the normal development of teeth.

Heden and Wennström, (2006) reported a prospective case series of the long-term (5 years) stability of clinical attachment level (CAL) gains following regenerative therapy with the use of enamel matrix proteins in intrabony defects. A total of 114 consecutively treated periodontal patients were initially included each with at least one deep proximal intrabony defect. A total of 82 patients (102 defects) were included in the analysis at one year and beyond. One year following the regenerative surgery, a mean CAL gain of 4.3 mm ($p<0.001$), a mean PPD reduction of 4.9 mm ($p<0.001$), and a mean increase in recession of 0.6 mm ($p<0.001$) were recorded. At the 5-year follow-up, a further mean PPD reduction of 0.3 mm ($p>0.05$), CAL gain of 1.1 mm ($p<0.01$), and reduction in recession of 0.8 mm ($p<0.01$) had taken place. Radiographs revealed that the bone defect had been reduced in depth with an average of 2.9 mm at 1 year ($p<0.001$). No statistically significant alteration in defect depth was observed between 1 and 5 years of follow-up. These results demonstrated long-term (5 years) stability of CAL gains following regenerative therapy with the use of enamel matrix proteins in intrabony defects.

There is no indication to give antibiotics after the use of EMD and in this regard a randomized, controlled, blinded study of 34 patients with intrabony defects treated with EMD (Sculean et al 2001c) has shown no statistical difference in the healing between one group not given post-operative antibiotics and one group given them (amoxicillin/metronidazole).

from the wound by the membrane to allow time for periodontal ligament cells to migrate coronally and to differentiate into functional cells for the three periodontal tissues–bone, cementum and periodontal ligament.

BARRIER MEMBRANES

There are five criteria which are considered to be important in the design of barrier membranes used for GTR (Greenstein & Caton 1993; Scantlebury 1993; Hardwick et al 1995). These are: (1) biocompatibility, (2) cell-occlusiveness, (3) spacemaking, (4) tissue integration and (5) clinical manageability. In order to achieve the mechanical tissue separation and support, various types of materials have been developed which can be grouped together as either non-resorbable or resorbable membranes.

Non-resorbable membranes

The first membranes used experimentally by Nyman's group in their initial work were constructed from Millipore (cellulose acetate) filters since these were easily available in the laboratory and were packed and stored in sterile conditions.

However, as the potential of this technique was realized commercial membranes were developed for clinical use. The first of these were made from Teflon (expanded polytetrafluoroethylene, ePTFE). This material was chosen because it had been found to be biocompatible in the human body and has been used for some time in reconstructive vascular surgery for replacement arteries.

This membrane consisted of two parts: (1) a collar portion, having open pores to allow ingrowth of connective tissue and to prevent epithelial migration and (2) an occlusive portion, preventing the flap tissues from coming into contact with the root surface (Scantlebury 1993). Because the space, which was defined and protected by the membrane, determined the volume of tissue that could be regenerated, the material was redesigned with a stiff central portion to treat osseous defects (Scantlebury 1993; Hardwick et al 1995) and reinforced with titanium for both osseous and periodontal defects (Hardwick et al 1995; Cortellini et al 1995; Sigurdsson et al 1995b).

Since these membranes are made of a non-resorbable material, a second surgical procedure is necessary to remove them. This procedure therefore has the disadvantage of the additional trauma to the patient as well as the healing periodontal tissues.

Clinical procedure

The area is first exposed by raising a flap developed with an intercrevicular incision to preserve keratinized gingiva. Pocket-lining epithelium is then removed from its inner aspect. All granulation tissue is removed and the roots are thoroughly planed (**Fig. 20.7A**). A flexible Teflon (ePTFE) membrane (Gore-Tex®) is carefully trimmed to cover the lesion (**Fig. 20.7B**). This consists of a narrow, open microstructure margin which is designed to allow connective tissue penetration to produce a seal at the coronal margin of the root, as well as an occlusive membrane (**Figs 20.6, 20.7B**). It is adapted to fit over the intrabony defect and the root of the tooth, extending from 2–3 mm below the bone margin to just below the CEJ on the root (**Figs 20.6, 20.7C, D**). This prevents the oral epithelium and gingival connective tissue contacting the root surface during healing. It is held in place by a Teflon sling suture which passes through both edges of the membrane upper margin and around the tooth (**Fig. 20.7B, C**). The flap is then sutured back with Teflon sutures to just cover the membrane. The membrane is left in place for 4–6 weeks and then removed. A further marginal incision exposes the membrane which is very carefully separated from the delicate healing tissue which appears like a gelatinous red jelly. The flap is then sutured back.

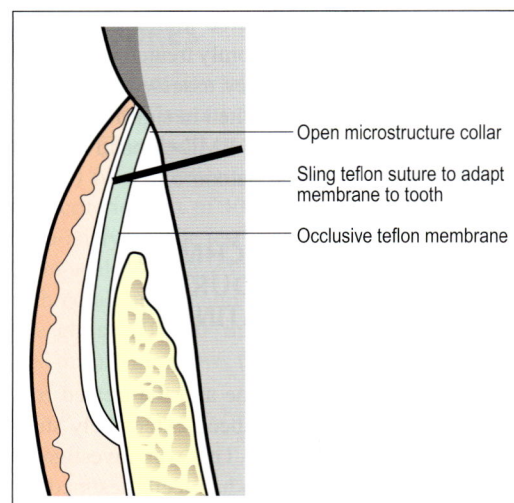

Fig. 20.6 Diagram to show the guided tissue regeneration technique described originally by Nyman et al (1983). After exposure of the area by raising a flap, all granulation tissue is removed and the root surface carefully root planed. A Teflon or bioabsorbable membrane is trimmed and adjusted to cover the root surface from just below the cemento-enamel junction to the apical extent of the bony lesion. It is interposed between these structures and the flap so that epithelium migrating apically over the exposed connective tissue surface is prevented from contacting the root. It also prevents gingival connective tissue from contacting the root.

It must be stressed that this technique is applicable only to the treatment of single teeth with two- or three-walled intrabony defects (**Fig. 20.7A**). This procedure underwent careful clinical assessments during the development stages. As explained in the following text GTR can be used to treat either intrabony or furcation defects.

Clinical trials of GTR using non-resorbable membranes

GTR techniques have been used for treatment of both the interproximal intraosseous defects and furcation defects in humans and there have been many short and long-term clinical studies of their use. Histological evaluation of the outcome of this therapy in humans has presented some difficulties due to ethical considerations. Clinical parameters are therefore used to assess the healing response in longitudinal investigations of patients undergoing this treatment. These parameters include clinical attachment level (CAL), probing pocket depth (PPD), gingival recession and bone fill as well as bone density and height using radiographs (Garrett 1996). The results are assessed by comparing pre- and post-treatment data over a reasonably long time scale. The response of the bone to GTR has also been assessed by quantitative digital subtraction radiology (see Ch.13 and Christgau et al 1996).

In human studies only clinical and radiographical measurements are possible and in this regard, Yun et al (2005) have shown, using beagle dogs, that measurements of the bone level with bone probing (sounding), radiographic measurement and histometric bone level, were closely comparable.

Human clinical studies using non-resorbable (ePTFE) membranes have demonstrated that GTR therapy significantly improves the clinical outcome compared to conventional flap surgery. Thus, several short-term clinical studies reported significant reductions in PPD (range 3.5–5.9 mm) and significant gains in CAL (range 3–6 mm) and bone levels (range 2.7–4.7 mm) following GTR treatment (Gottlow et al 1986; Schallhorn & McClain 1988; Becker et al 1988; Pontoriero et al 1988, 1989; Cortellini et al 1990; Caffesse et al 1990; Gottlow 1993; Tonetti et al 1993; Cortellini et al 1993a,b 1995b, 1996a; Kilic et al 1997; Eickholz et al 1998). All these studies have shown that a gain in clinical attachment level may occur on teeth with a variety of intrabony and furcation defects using this technique.

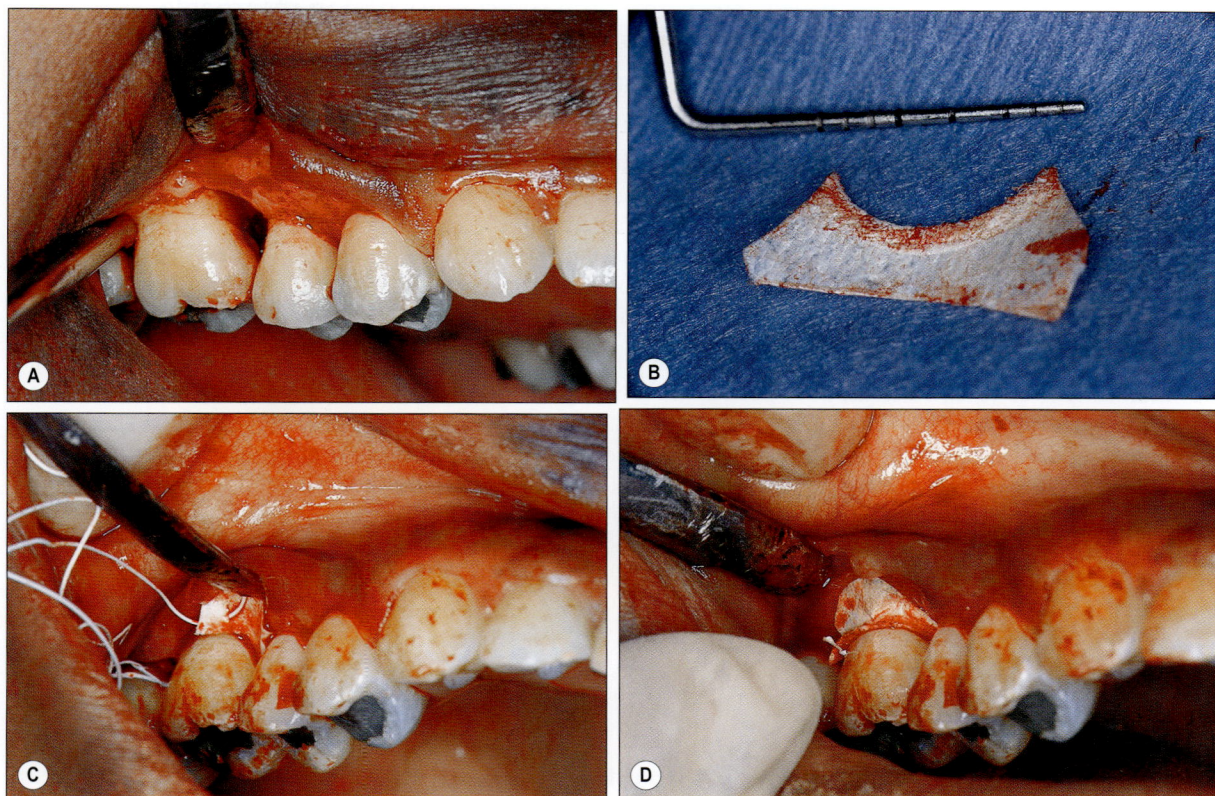

Fig. 20.7 Clinical views of the guided tissue regeneration technique using an ePTFE barrier membrane. (A) Operative view with the flaps raised of an intrabony defect mesial to upper right first molar; (B) trimmed ePTFE barrier membrane before placement; (C) membrane being secured with sling sutures; (D) barrier membrane in place covering the root surface and bony lesion and isolating these structures from the gingival connective tissue surface of the flap which will be closed over it.

Cortellini et al (1993a,b) treated interproximal intraosseous defects using ePTFE membranes and observed a significant gain in CAL, reduction in PPD and radiographic evidence of new formation of alveolar bone 1 year post-operatively, while Pontoriero et al (1988) demonstrated complete resolution of >90% furcation defects 6 months following GTR therapy.

Recently it has been also shown that these changes can be maintained over 1–5 years (Gottlow et al 1992; Weigel et al 1995; Machtei et al 1996; Cortellini et al 1996a). Gottlow et al (1992) found a continuous increase in bone density in both types of defect over the 13-month test period.

When the clinical efficacy of ePTFE membranes and titanium reinforced ePTFE membranes were compared, significant clinical improvements were obtained in both of the membrane groups, but the gain in CAL in the titanium-reinforced group was found to be greater than that in the ePTFE group (Cortellini et al 1995a).

Another recent study (Murphy 1996) investigated the effects of prolonged placement of ePTFE membranes on the amount of regeneration. A modified surgical technique was described which allowed substantial coverage of the barriers for a period of 4 months. Twelve intrabony defects were treated in this way and the amount of bone fill was assessed by a re-entry procedure after 1 year. The results showed a mean bony in-fill of 95% with three sites showing additional supracrestal bone growth. This suggests that the prolonged retention of a barrier membrane may increase the amount of regeneration. This relationship has also been found when membranes are used in connection with implants. In this situation the membrane can be completely buried and can be left *in situ* for 6 months (see Ch. 29).

The potential problem of prolonged retention with periodontal lesions is communication with the mouth via the gingival crevice which may result in progressive bacterial contamination (see below).

There are, however, some reports which show that the results of GTR are unpredictable and on many occasions show results that have no advantage over conventional surgery (Warren & Karring 1992; Proestakis et al 1992). In this regard, Pritlove-Carson et al (1993) reported on a series of matched intrabony lesions in patients. One lesion was treated with GTR and one with conventional surgery. They found no difference between the test and control sites in respect of probing depth, probing attachment level or recession.

With respect to the unpredictable nature of GTR treatment it has been shown that failures to achieve the formation of new attachment can be due to a number of clinical variables. Those reported are shortcomings in the surgical technique (Caffesse and Quiñones 1992; Becker & Becker 1990), restrictions in the size and configuration of the periodontal defect (Gottlow et al 1986) and limiting features of tooth anatomy (Lu 1992). These studies also show that the achievement of membrane stability and total coverage of the membrane are important in achieving success.

Experimental animal studies using non-resorbable membranes

Experimental studies using prepared defects in dogs and monkeys also showed histological evidence of regenerative new cementum with embedded collagen fibres at test sites in intrabony lesions and class II and III furcation defects (Nyman et al 1982b; Aukhil et al 1983, 1986; Gottlow et al 1984, 1990; Caffesse et al 1988, 1990; Pontoriero et al 1992). This did not occur at control sites. However, the results were variable at sites with Class III furcation involvement and extensive intrabony lesions. Thus, success was found to be partly dependent on the size, shape and apical extent of the lesion.

Bacterial contamination of membranes

The use of non-resorbable membranes has been associated with membrane contamination and/or infection when the membrane is exposed to the oral cavity (Selvig et al 1990; Tempro & Nalbandian 1993; Grevstad & Leknes 1993; Nowzari et al 1996; Nowzari & Slots 1994).

It has also been clearly shown that artificially buried defects in animals heal considerably better than exposed defects and this is also found in the clinical situation (Sander & Karring 1995a). One of the reasons for this is that exposed membranes become extensively contaminated and penetrated by bacteria from the oral and subgingival flora (Simion et al 1995) (see below) and this can significantly affect the outcome.

Several studies (Selvig et al 1992; Mombelli et al 1993; Nowzari & Slots 1994; Simion et al 1995; De Santos et al 1996a 1996b) have shown that the outcome of GTR procedures can be affected by bacterial contamination of the membrane. One of these studies (Nowzari & Slots 1994) compared the bacterial contamination of 11 barrier membranes used to treat intrabony defects or furcation involvement with 16 membranes used in conjunction with dental implants with associated bony defects. The nature of bacterial contamination was determined with non-selective and selective culture and by DNA probes. All the tooth-associated membranes yielded high levels of microorganisms. Four of the five teeth with membranes harbouring less than 10^8 microorganisms gained 3 mm or more in probing attachment level, whereas six teeth with membranes harbouring more than 10^8 microorganisms exhibited loss or only very small gains in attachment. In addition, three membranes with high levels of black pigmented anaerobes lost 1–2 mm of attachment. The membranes associated with dental implants were less commonly contaminated and when contaminated had considerably fewer bacteria present. There were 10 implant-associated membranes with no cultivatable microorganisms and these demonstrated a mean gain of 4.9 mm of supporting bone, while the six implants with infected membranes only gained an average of 2 mm. The lower rate of bacterial contamination of implant-associated membranes is undoubtedly because they are buried below the surface epithelium and were thus not in contact with the oral flora during the healing period. Also the lesser effects on the outcome seen with the implant cases probably relates to the lesser degree of contamination, which occurred during placement only, and the fact that periodontal pathogens are much less likely to contaminate these membranes.

These results seem to show a direct relationship between the amount of bacterial contamination of the membrane and the formation or lack of formation of new attachment. These findings apply equally to non-absorbable and bioabsorbable membranes (De Santos et al 1996a,b). Furthermore, these results would seem to indicate the importance in controlling or eliminating contamination of the membrane by periodontal pathogens by careful technique and possibly the use of antimicrobials.

In this last regard, it has been shown that the topical application of chlorhexidine (Simion et al 1995) or metronidazole gel (Sander et al 1994; Frandsen et al 1994) to GTR membranes during their application may reduce, but not completely prevent bacterial contamination of the membrane. In addition, this has been reported to result in improved clinical results (Sander et al 1994). Improved clinical results of GTR treatment for furcation defects have been also reported in patients given a systemic antibiotic (ornidazole) compared to patients given a placebo (Mombelli et al 1996). This is presumably because this reduced or delayed bacterial contamination of the membrane. However, using resorbable membranes (see below) Loos et al (2002) found no differences in the clinical result with or without systemic antibiotics. Therefore providing a careful technique avoids exposure of the membrane antibiotics should not be necessary.

Factors affecting the success of non-resorbable membranes

The main problems associated with the use of non-resorbable ePTFE barrier membranes which could affect the outcome can be summarized as:

- Shortcomings in the surgical technique
- The configuration of the periodontal defect
- Limiting features of tooth anatomy
- Membrane contamination and/or infection whenever the membrane is exposed to the oral environment
- The need for a second surgical procedure for membrane removal.

The success of GTR procedures and the stability of the result have also been found to be detrimentally affected by poor oral hygiene, poor compliance with maintenance programmes and smoking (Cortellini et al 1996a). Patients who are in any of these categories before this treatment is contemplated are best rejected as candidates for GTR.

In addition, the removal of the membrane is associated with increased morbidity for the patient, is time consuming for the surgeon, and can interfere with healing (Tonetti et al 1993, Cortellini et al 1995). Finally, the optimal timing of membrane removal has not been fully determined in humans (Caton et al 1992).

These factors have led to the development of bioresorbable membranes and these are discussed below:

Bioresorbable membranes

There are basically two types of biologically resorbable products – natural and synthetic membranes (Christgau et al 1995) and the various forms of these are listed below:

1. Synthetic polymers
   - Polyurethane
   - Polylactic acid
   - Lactide/glycolide copolymers e.g. polyglactin-910
   - Polylactic acid blended with citric acid ester.
2. Natural biomaterials
   - Collagen.

The commonest form of synthetic bioresorbable membrane commercially available is of the lactide/glycolide copolymer type developed by WL Gore and Associates under the trade name Resolute® and is supplied with a bioresorbable suture. It is a polylactate/polygalactate copolymer and has been used in many of the clinical trials reported below. Another commercially available synthetic bioresorbable membrane is composed of polylactic acid blended with citric acid ester and is made by Guidor AB, Huddinge, Sweden under the trade name Guidor®. This is also supplied with a bioresorbable suture incorporated into the top margin of the membrane. It has mainly been designed for use in GTR techniques to treat gingival recession (see Ch. 21) but can also be used for intrabony and molar furcation lesions. Also a new polylactate based membrane, which is fabricated from a kit at the chairside, has been developed by Atrix Laboratories Inc., Colorado, USA under the trade name of Atrisorb®.

Polylactide and polyglycoside membranes are broken down by the enzymes in the Krebs cycle with the formation of lactic and glycolic acids (**Fig. 20.8**). Whether this brings about any pH change in the tissues is uncertain but it is unlikely to be of any significance in healing since buffering would rapidly occur.

Polylactic acid (PLA) degradation (**Fig. 20.8**) appears to occur in two stages: first, a random non-enzymatic cleavage of the polymer and second, a loss of mechanical strength and weight (Pitt et al 1981). Degradation continues to free lactic acid, which is then further metabolized in the liver to carbon dioxide and water (Bergsma et al 1995). Several studies

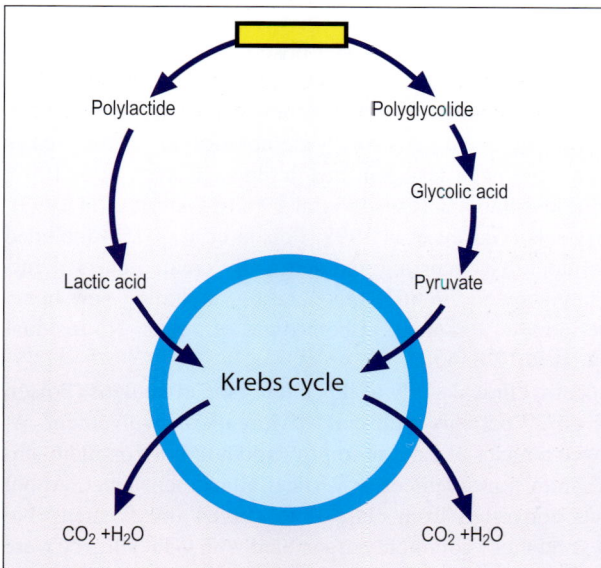

Fig. 20.8 A diagram of the polylactide and polyglycolide degradation pathways in relation to resorbable membranes of these materials.

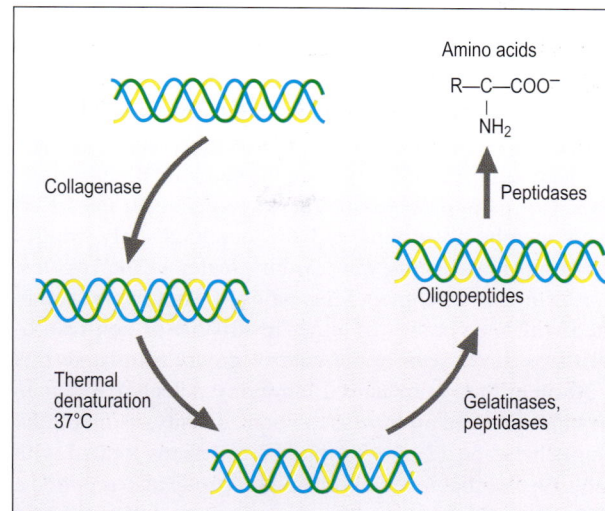

Fig. 20.9 The mechanism of collagen resorption in relation to resorbable membranes of this material.

have shown that PLA barrier membranes and sutures are safe and effective (Bergsma *et al* 1995; Cutright & Hunsuck 1971, 1972; Cutright et al 1971a,b).

The main difference with the Atrisorb® system is that it is fabricated from a kit at the chairside and can thus be customized for the use required. It is made by mixing polylactic acid with a solvent, *N*-methylpyrrolidone (NMP). This produces a flexible semi-solid film which can be cut to any size or shape required and each kit contains sufficient material for the fabrication of up to 10 membranes. Excess material cannot, however, be stored for future use and thus, this results in waste of this excess material. The resultant membranes can be moulded to the shape required and may be closely adapted to the shape of the defect. This obviates the need for sutures. This property is particularly useful for single surface defects on the buccal, lingual or palatal aspects of teeth such as class II furcation defects (see below). However, the semisolid, flexible nature of the membrane would make it impossible to pass it through an intact contact point. This makes this system much less useful for interproximal intrabony defects. If used for this situation two membranes usually have to be fabricated. The first passes under the contact to the other side to fit against the second membrane applied from this side. The two are then bonded together *in situ*. This may be difficult in a surgical field contaminated by blood and saliva. If there is sufficient space it may be possible to pass a single membrane under the contact point. The membranes solidify on contact with moisture in the mouth and thus retain their shape.

Many attempts to make resorbable collagen membranes have been attempted and recently a number of these membranes have been produced and tested (Wang et al 1994; Bluenthal 1993; Black et al 1994; Van Swol et al 1993). One such membrane has been produced and marketed by the German company, Geistlich Biomaterials under the trade name of Bio-Gide®. The collagen is prepared from pigs which have had veterinary examination to confirm their health. The manufacture of the collagen membrane involves several technological processing steps, one of which produces a collagen bilayer. An alkaline treatment is also carried out for several hours, according to EC-guidelines, to eliminate any possible viral or bacterial contamination of the material. Afterwards the structural quality of membrane is controlled by segment by segment analysis. Standardized processes under clean room condition guarantee a constituent, high quality biological product. It is composed of pure collagen fibres without any other organic residues or chemicals. Tests are finally carried out to confirm the biocompatibility and sterility of the end product.

It is important that a collagen membrane should be devoid of antigenicity. The locations of the collagen molecule concerned with antigenicity are the two terminal peptide regions and during the production of Bio-Gide®, the terminal peptides are split off. Also, specific purification processes remove any fat and protein residues. In this way the immunological properties of the resultant collagen are greatly reduced and appear not to be of clinical significance. Animal experiments (Möhler 1995) have confirmed that no inflammatory cells collect at the site of implantation of Bio-Gide®. Furthermore no antibodies against this material were found in the implanted animals.

The resorption of collagen membranes starts with the action of collagenase which splits the molecule at specific sites (see Ch. 1). The resultant large fragments become temperature sensitive and are denatured at 37°C to gelatin. Gelatinases and other proteinases then degrade gelatin down to oligopeptides and amino acids (**Fig. 20.9**).

Clinical trials and animal experiments with resorbable membranes

Some early trials with biodegradable membranes of polylactic acid or polyurethane failed to produce regeneration (Warren et al 1992). However, recently, several human and animal studies (Gottlow et al 1994; Caffesse et al 1994; Laurell et al 1994; Lindhe et al 1995; Sander & Karring 1995a,b; Christgau et al 1995, 1997; Becker et al 1996; Cortellini et al 1996b; Eickholz et al 1998) with improved resorbable membranes have shown that the placement of synthetic resorbable membranes in GTR procedures can result in the formation of similar amounts of new attachment to the placement of conventional e-PTFE membranes. This is the case both in the treatment of two- and three-walled intrabony defects and Class II and Class III furcation defects. The obvious advantage in using bioabsorbable membranes is the avoidance of a second surgical procedure.

Polson et al (1995b) demonstrated significant reduction in PPD and gain in vertical and horizontal attachment levels in furcation defects following the use of resorbable barrier membranes. However, Cortellini et al (1996b) obtained similar clinical outcomes in patients treated by GTR using either resorbable or non-resorbable membranes, whereas Hugoson et al (1995) found a significant improvement in gingival recession at the sites treated with resorbable membranes compared with non-resorbable membranes at 1 year postoperatively.

A recent controlled clinical trial (Cortellini et al 1996b) compared the periodontal regeneration produced in human intrabony defects using either synthetic bioresorbable membranes (Resolute®, polylactate/polygalactate copolymer), conventional ePTFE membranes or simple curettage of the defect.

A total of 36 patients were randomly assigned to one of these three groups and there were no significant differences in the baseline characteristics between the groups. The groups were carefully maintained for a year and clinical attachment levels were compared with those at baseline. Significant gains in clinical attachment levels were seen in all three groups. Although there were no significant differences in the clinical attachment levels between both the membrane groups there were significant differences between both membrane groups and the curettage only control group. In this regard the mean gains were 2 mm greater in the two test groups. Furthermore, clinical attachment level gains of 4 mm were seen in 83% of sites treated with membranes of either resorbable or non-resorbable type while this was never seen in the control group. Similar results were shown in a 30-month study of paired intrabony defects (Christgau et al 1997) and they also showed an increase in bone density, using digital subtraction radiology, between 12 and 30 months in lesions treated with either non-resorbable on resorbable membranes. This group also reported a virtually identically structured clinical study using two types of resorbable membrane, polylactic acid or polygalactin-910, at paired intrabony sites (Christgau et al 1998). The results were virtually the same as in their other studies and no significant differences were seen between them.

Another study assessed the degree of bony in-fill in intrabony lesions by reentry after 12 months in lesions treated by either non-resorbable (ePTFE) or resorbable (PLA) membranes (Weltman et al 1997). They found an average of 44% in-fill for the PLA and 58% for the ePTFE membranes with no significant difference between the two groups.

There is also a recent report of the success of GTR treatment of intrabony lesions using bioabsorbable membrane (Guidor®) carried out routinely in three specialist clinics (Falk et al 1997). They reported on the results of 203 consecutively treated intrabony defects using a bioabsorbable matrix barrier after 1 year using clinical and radiographical measurements. They found an average gain in probing attachment of 79% and that 78% of the sites treated gained 4 mm or more. They also found an average of 3 mm bone fill measured on serial radiographs. In addition, they found that sites with membrane exposure after 2 weeks gained less clinical attachment than fully covered sites as did sites in patients with poor plaque control. These changes in attachment were comparable to those found in clinical trials and this shows that GTR can be successful if carefully carried out in dental practice using resorbable membranes.

However, there is a study (Mayfield et al 1998) which shows that the use of bioresorbable (Guidor®) membranes did not result in any greater measurable gain in clinical attachment level than conventional flap surgery alone. A total of 40 patients with one suitable intrabony defect were divided into a control group receiving conventional flap surgery only and a test group treated with Guidor® membranes. They were assessed at baseline, 6 months and 12 months following surgery by pocket probing, bone sounding and radiography. Both groups of patients showed probing depth reductions and non-significant gains in bone sounding measurements. These results were confirmed by radiography. Thus, there were no significant differences between the procedures for the two groups. Another study (Loos et al 2002) also showed no difference between the use of a barrier membrane and conventional flap surgery alone. Both these studies highlight the unpredictability of GTR procedures.

The bioabsorption kinetics and safety of Atrisorb® membranes have been tested in the rabbit (Coonts et al 1996) and beagle dog (Garrett et al 1997) models. In the rabbit model test and placebo membranes were implanted subcutaneously for between 4 and 52 weeks. It showed that the Atrisorb® membranes degraded progressively with mass and molecular weight reductions and complete degradation occurred by 13–14 months. The histopathological results showed no differences between the test and control membranes and indicated that the Atrisorb® membranes were biocompatible and safe. The biocompatibility of N-methylpyrrolidone (NMP) has also been shown in other studies (Bartsch et al 1976; Becci et al 1983;

Ansell & Fowler 1988). The safety and biocompatibility of Atrisorb® membranes were confirmed by histological observations around retained barrier membranes used to treat naturally occurring furcation defects in beagle dogs (Garrett et al 1997).

The clinical effectiveness of Atrisorb® membranes in treating class II furcation lesions have been tested in beagle dogs (Garrett et al 1997; Polson et al 1995a) and humans (Polson et al 1995b; Garrett et al 1997). The beagle dog models (Garrett et al 1997; Polson et al 1995a) included treatment of both naturally occurring and surgically created class II furcation defects. They showed 70–80% regeneration, including new bone, cementum and periodontal ligament, in both types of defect. No residual barrier was seen after 9–12 months.

The first multicentre clinical study of this membrane in humans (Polson et al 1995b) was on 29 patients with class II furcation involvement. At 12 months it showed a mean of 2.5 mm improvement in horizontal attachment level and 1.7 mm improvement in vertical attachment level. About half of the defects converted from class II to class I involvement. No adverse effects beyond those commonly associated with GTR surgery were noted. The second multicentre clinical study (Garrett et al 1997) involved 162 patients with class II furcation involvement and compared the use of Atrisorb® resorbable membranes with conventional Gore-Tex® ePTFE membranes. A total of 82 patients were treated with resorbable membranes and 80 with ePTFE membranes. This study showed similar results for clinical improvement and tolerance between the two types of membrane with significant improvements in both vertical and horizontal attachment levels. A majority of lesions in both groups converted from class II to class I involvement.

Clinical testing of bioabsorbable collagen membranes has produced results which are closely similar to those achieved with synthetic bioresorbable and non-resorbable ePTFE membranes (Wang et al 1994; Bluenthal 1993; Black et al 1994; Van Swol et al 1993). The membrane function of Bio-Gide® has also been tested in various animal experiments. Standardized peri-implant defects in dogs were filled with a natural bone mineral (Bio-Oss®) (see below and above) and covered with Bio-Gide®. At re-entry after 4 months histological evaluation revealed the regeneration of organized cancellous and cortical bone (Hürzeler et al 1998). In addition, the repair of prepared circumferential intrabony defects in beagle dogs has been studied comparing the results of two different cross-linked bioabsorbable collagen membranes and a non-resorbable ePTFE (Crigger et al 1996). The animals were sacrificed after 6 months and the tissues were prepared for histological examination. The highly cross-linked, slowly resorbing collagen membranes did not integrate well with the tissues and produced membrane exposure and gingival recession. In contrast, the less cross-linked, rapidly resorbing collagen membranes and the ePTFE membranes produced good clinical results. Both these membranes also produced high levels of regeneration with connective tissue attachment to the root surface after 6 months. The collagen membrane produced 84% and the ePTFE 53% of connective tissue attachment but these differences were not statistically significant. Some areas of ankylosis were present with both membranes but these were more common with the collagen membrane. The areas of ankylosis seemed to originate from the furcation. The results indicated that both types of membrane produced good levels of periodontal regeneration in these defects.

These results seem to show that both clinically measurable gains in probing attachment level and histological verifiable periodontal regeneration can usually be obtained with GTR procedures using both bioresorbable or non-resorbable membranes. However, the lack of a second surgical procedure is a major advantage with bioresorbable membranes.

The fine details of the surgical techniques used in these procedures may also significantly affect the outcome of these procedures and it is particularly important to adapt the membrane carefully over the defect and fully close the flap over the membrane so that no part of it is exposed to the oral cavity. In this regard, Cortellini & Tonetti (2001) reported that careful microsurgical techniques using microsurgical instruments and an operating microscope with full wound closure and membrane coverage produced marked gains in clinical attachment and minimal recession. These gains appear to be greater than those produced with conventional surgical techniques but this is not yet proven since no direct comparisons of these two approaches have yet been made. This microsurgical technique has also been shown to enhance the regenerative effects of EMD in intrabony defects (Wachtel et al 2003).

The clinical procedure used with bioresorbable membranes is the same as that used with non-resorbable membranes except that they are secured with resorbable sutures. They, of course, do not need to be removed after the regenerative period.

Eickholz et al (2004) also showed attachment gain achieved after GTR therapy in intrabony defects using bioabsorbable barriers was stable after 5 years in 81% of defects. Similarly, Stavropoulos & Karring (2004) looked at the results of GTR treatment of intrabony defects with bioresorbable membranes after 6–7 years. They found that the clinical improvements could be maintained on a long-term basis with good maintenance.

Aimetti et al (2005) carried out a randomized controlled clinical trial of the treatment of wide, shallow, and predominantly one-wall intrabony defects with a bioabsorbable membrane in 18 paired defects in 18 non-smoking patients. They compared open flap debridement alone with the use of a bioabsorbable membrane.

They showed that the use of a bioabsorbable membrane produced significantly better results and found that it was also effective in the treatment of intrabony defects with unfavourable architecture without the use of filling materials.

GTR IN COMBINATION WITH BONE OR BONE SUBSTITUTE GRAFTS

In clinical studies using GTR, some of which were cited above, there were a number of variables in the GTR technique including the concurrent use of bone grafts, root surface conditioning and coronally positioned flaps (Gantes & Garrett 1991; Schallhorn & McClain 1988; Mellonig 1991).

Combinations of GTR with the use of bone grafts has been shown to have some advantages over either technique used alone (Schultz & Gager 1990). Schallhorn and McClain (1988) reported on a clinical study combining osseous composite grafting, root conditioning and GTR. They found a significantly greater gain of mean probing attachment with the combination compared to GTR alone.

Bowers et al (1989a,b,c) showed that periodontal regeneration could take place using human freeze-dried decalcified bone allograft (FDDBA) in intrabony defects (see previous section). They concluded that the combination of highly osteogenic material such as FDDBA with GTR might offer promise for increasing the predictability of periodontal regeneration procedures.

This combination approach was investigated by Anderegg et al (1991). They compared the use of FDDBA and GTR with GTR alone on human molar furcation defects. At the 6-month re-entry there was a distinct difference in the horizontal and vertical bone repair favouring the use of the graft. Stahl and Froume (1991) investigated the use of this combination on human intrabony defects and found gains in clinical attachment and histological evidence of new cementum, bone and periodontal ligament formation. However, the amount of new histological attachment varied from 0–1.7 mm in the four specimens studied.

This combination has been investigated by Guillemin et al (1993a,b) using two paired sites in each of 17 patients with advanced periodontitis, one of which was treated with FDDBA and GTR and the other with GTR alone. The results were compared for the extent of bony in-fill assessed at re-entry 6 months after the procedure and bone density was also assessed

by computerized densitometric analysis. No statistically significant differences were found for either comparison between the two groups. The average bony in-fill was 58% for the GTR alone sites and 70% for the combination sites. In addition the combination sites showed greater mean gingival recession (0.9 mm) than GTR alone sites (0.4 mm).

These studies would seem to indicate that both GTR and the use of FDDBA bone graft alone can produce some periodontal regeneration. Their combined use seems to produce good results, which may be slightly better than either used alone. However, the controlled studies do not show statistically significant differences between using GTR alone or with FDDBA.

GTR in combination with hydroxyapatite-collagen grafts have also been compared with GTR alone and surgical debridement (Kilic et al 1997). GTR alone and in combination with the graft produced significantly greater gains in attachment than debridement alone. The results of GTR with the graft were slightly better than GTR alone but these differences were not statistically significant.

The use of a combination of GTR with a resorbable collagen membrane (Bio-Gide®) and bovine anorganic cancellous bone (Bio-Oss®) in intrabony defects has been shown to result in significantly greater gains in clinical attachment level than surgical access and curettage (Sculean et al 2003; Vouros et al 2004). Mengel et al (2003) compared the use of bioabsorbable membranes with bioactive glass for the treatment of intrabony defects over 12-months using clinical and digital radiographical measurements. They showed that both agents produced good clinical gains in attachment and bony in-fill with no statistical differences between them.

In order to test the adjunctive effect of Bio-Oss® and bioactive glass (Biogran®) with GTR an experiment using rats was devised (Stavropoulos et al 2003, 2004a). The mandibular ramus was surgically exposed and a U-shaped Teflon membrane was placed on its outer surface either packed on its bone facing surface with Bio-Oss® or bioactive glass or nothing (control). After wound closure, the grafts were left in place for 1-year. The membranes were then removed at a re-entry procedure. Histological specimens of the grafted area were prepared and the volumes of new bone, graft particles and soft tissue in the space originally created by the membrane was estimated by a point counting technique averaged for 3–4 tissue sections. Newly formed bone was found to occupy only 23% of the total volume in the animals grafted by Bio-Oss® and 12.6% in those grafted with bioactive glass. The control animals (membrane alone) formed significantly greater volumes of new bone (88.2%, $p<0.01$). The major part of the space occupied in animals grafted with Bio-Oss® or bioactive glass consisted of the graft particles embedded in connective tissue. Thus in this experimental situation both Bio-Oss® and bioactive glass hindered rather than enhanced new bone material. This may call into question the clinical use of these materials with GTR particularly as the clinical situation is more unpredictable in terms of the formation of new periodontium.

In contrast, the results of a 124 patient, 10 centre, seven country, multicentre clinical trial (Tonetti et al 2004) indicated that regenerative periodontal surgery with a GTR and placement of bone replacement material produced additional benefits in terms of CAL gains, PPD reductions and predictability of outcomes compared with papilla preservation flaps alone. However, this was based on clinical criteria rather than the more reliable histological evidence of the experimental study above. This was supported by another study (Sculean et al 2005b). They compared clinically the treatment of deep intrabony defects with a combination of a composite bovine-derived xenograft (BDX Coll) and a bioresorbable collagen membrane for guided tissue regeneration (GTR) to access flap surgery only. A total of 32 patients, each of whom displayed one intrabony defect, were treated either with BDX Coll+GTR (test) or with access flap surgery (control). The results were evaluated at 1 year following therapy. It was found that the combination of BDX Coll+GTR resulted in significantly higher clinical attachment level gains than treatment with access flap surgery alone.

Pretzl et al (2008) published a short case series of GTR procedures after 10 years and showed that the gains in attachment were maintained over this period with both non-resorbable and resorbable membranes.

In spite of all this evidence, regenerative techniques remain unpredictable and the reasons for this may result from the complexity of the cellular events leading to the formation of these tissues. These are not as simple as originally conceived and some new views on connective tissue regeneration have a bearing on this.

GTR COMBINED WITH OTHER CLINICAL PROCEDURES

Although histological and clinical studies on the use of barrier membranes have provided extensive evidence that some periodontal regeneration is practically feasible, the clinical results remain variable and unpredictable. In addition, studies have shown that treatment of Class III furcation defects at mandibular molars using GTR results in partial healing and complete closure of the defect is obtained infrequently (Pontoriero et al 1989; Eickholz et al 1998). The biological principles of different regenerative procedures have therefore been combined in order to attempt to achieve a greater degree of clinical success.

GTR procedures have been used in combination with root conditioning and this has appeared to result in improved outcomes (McClain & Schallhorn 1993; Kilic et al 1997). Antimicrobial agents have either been applied topically before membrane placement (Sander et al 1994) or incorporated in the resorbable membranes (Dowell et al 1995), in order to reduce the possibility of bacterial contamination during healing. However, the addition of the antibiotic metronidazole did not appear to improve periodontal regeneration beyond that of the membrane alone (Sander et al 1994; Dowell et al 1995).

CLINICAL STUDIES COMPARING GTR WITH OTHER REGENERATIVE TECHNIQUES

Two clinical studies by the same research group have compared the use of GTR with a bioabsorbable membrane and Emdogain® (EMD) either separately or in combination. The first reported on 56 patients with paired intrabony defects over 1 year (Sculean et al 2001a) and the second on 12 patients with paired defects over 4 years (Sculean et al 2001b). All techniques produced significant gains in clinical attachment levels but with no statistical differences between them. Similar results were again reported by this group, this time for a five year time span (Sculean et al 2004).

The possible use of growth factors alone or in conjunction with other procedures including GTR is discussed in the sections below:

NEW VIEWS ON CONNECTIVE TISSUE REGENERATION

There have been very significant advances in this area recently (Hughes & McCulloch 1991; Hughes 1993, 1995). The cellular events of periodontal regeneration are not a simple race of cells but involve the controlled integration of a number of cell signalling systems. The following factors seem with our present knowledge to be the most important in determining the outcome of periodontal regenerative procedures:

■ Excluding epithelium and gingival connective tissue
■ Producing the conditions for the migration of stem and progenitor cells from the periodontal ligament and the bone marrow of the alveolar bone. This involves the integrated production of the appropriate signal molecules
■ Production of signal molecules for cementoblasts and cementum formation
■ Production of signal molecules for osteoblasts and bone formation
■ Production of signal molecules for synchronized periodontal ligament formation.

Substances that aid periodontal regeneration rely on accurate dissemination of active agents to their targets comprising connective tissue and bone. Healing is enhanced by incorporating a carrier agent and a time-release microshape containing the active agent for sustained release and improved uptake at the site of delivery. These concepts have been reviewed recently (Soory 2008). Chemotherapeutic agents range from antimicrobial, anti-inflammatory and tissue regenerative agents such as platelet rich plasma, enamel matrix proteins, bioactive glass, soy-bean based bone fillers, calcium phosphate and brushite cements. Cell recognition of tissue regenerative agents within a vehicular microcapsule for local delivery aid capture of relevant cells at the required site, enhancing its actions and sustenance. Gene-based therapies for tissue regeneration promote expression of specific proteins which lead to a steady supply of targeted stimulatory agents over stipulated periods. Techniques of tissue engineering and gene therapy are combined to enhance selective protein expression and expansion of specific cell populations on biodegradable scaffolds acting as carriers for dispensing the required agents. These concepts demonstrated the relevance of optimal targeting and host response which can enhance or detract from the outcome; these aspects have been reviewed recently by Soory (2008).

So far, we have only limited means of controlling these factors and the fine control of these systems in tissue healing almost certainly determines the type of tissue formed. Therefore, it is unlikely that periodontal regenerative procedures like GTR and bone grafting will be fully predictable until we have a better understanding of these processes and some practical means of controlling them. Some of the recent research in this area is discussed below.

CELLS AND EXTRACELLULAR MATRIX PROTEINS IN PERIODONTAL REGENERATION

The recognition that the cells involved in GTR are key factors which ultimately determine the success of periodontal regeneration has prompted a number of investigations aimed at understanding this process at the cellular and molecular levels. Morphological analysis of furcation defects treated by GTR in dogs showed that over the first 2 weeks the wound became occupied by granulation tissue containing numerous infiltrated inflammatory cells and blood vessels (Matsuura et al 1995). However, by 4 weeks the defect was nearly filled by new connective tissue containing many fibroblast-like cells. The cells colonizing the periodontal wound area at this stage were found to be derived from both the adjacent unwounded periodontal ligament (Gould et al 1980; Iglhaut et al 1988) and the marrow spaces of adjacent alveolar bone (Iglhaut et al 1988). By 8 weeks, some new periodontal ligament associated with newly-formed bone was present in the healing area (Matsuura et al 1995).

Nagatomo et al (2006) showed that periodontal ligament (PDL) cells possessed crucial stem cell properties, such as self-renewal and multipotency, and also expressed the mesenchymal stem cell markers CD105, CD166, and STRO-1 on their cell surface, although there were some variations. Thus, PDL cells may play a crucial role in periodontal regeneration.

A number of recent studies have investigated the cells and tissues adherent to ePTFE membranes and samples of regenerative tissue removed from periodontal surgical sites of patients (Pritlove-Carson et al 1992, 1994; Wakabayashi et al 1996, 1997; Grosso et al 1997; Kuru et al 1997a,b,c; 1998a; Kuru 1998). They showed that variable amounts of tissue was adherent to the membranes and that the coronal part of the membrane was colonized by oral bacteria. Immunohistochemical investigations showed that vimentin-positive mesenchymal cells and keratin-positive epithelial cells were present in these tissues (Pritlove-Carson et al 1992, 1994; Kuru 1998). Vimentin and keratin are markers of mesenchymal and epithelial cells respectively.

Recently, the cells harvested from removed ePTFE membranes and regenerated soft tissues taken from healing periodontal defects in GTR patients have been cultured and studied *in vitro* (Wakabayashi et al 1996, 1997;

Grosso et al 1997; Kuru et al 1997a,b,c 1998b; Kuru 1998). These cells appeared to be fibroblast-like in morphology and were shown to be vimentin-positive mesenchymal cells. Some of these cultured cells were also shown to express osteocalcin, osteonectin, bone sialoprotein (BSP) and high levels of alkaline phosphatase and to form mineralized nodules *in vitro* particularly when grown on media formulated for this purpose and stimulated by dexamethasone (Wakabayashi et al 1996, 1997; Grosso et al 1997; Kuru et al 1997b,c; Kuru 1998). Some of these cells thus appear to have osteoblast-like characteristics. Cultured cells were also found to produce extracellular matrix (ECM) proteins associated with both soft (Kuru et al 1997a) and hard connective tissues (Kuru et al 1997b), certain proteases (Wakabayashi et al 1996; Grosso et al 1997) and cytokines (Wakabayashi et al 1997). Furthermore, culture media in which these cells had been incubated *in vitro* was found to inhibit osteoclast differentiation (Rowe et al 1996).

The recruitment of the appropriate cells on to the root surface appears to be crucial for the formation of new periodontal attachment. A recent study (Zhao et al 2004) has investigated the ability of cementoblasts and dental follicle cells to promote periodontal regeneration in a rodent periodontal fenestration model. The buccal aspect of the distal of the first mandibular molar was denuded of its periodontal ligament (PDL), cementum and surface dentine through a bony window created bilaterally in 12 athymic rats. The treated defects were divided into three groups, carrier alone (biodegradable PLGA polymer sponges), carrier plus cultured murine primarily dental follicle cells and carrier plus immortalized cementoblasts. The mandibular molars were retrieved at 3 and 6 weeks post-surgery for histological evaluation. *In situ* hybridization for gene expression of bone sialoprotein (BSP) and osteocalcin (OCN) and histomorphometric analysis were also carried out on the 3-week specimens. Three weeks after surgery the defects treated with carrier alone showed some PLGA particles, fibrous tissue, and newly formed bone scattered within the defect area. Defects treated with carrier plus dental follicle cells had a similar appearance, but with less bone formation. In contrast, in the defects treated with carrier plus cementoblasts, mineralized tissues were found in the healing site with extension towards the root surface, PDL region, and laterally beyond the buccal plate envelope of bone. No PDL to bone attachment was noted at this stage in any of the groups. *In situ* hybridization showed that the mineralized tissue formed by the cementoblasts gave strong signals for BSP and OCN, confirming its nature as bone or cementum. At 6 weeks post-surgery, cementoblast-treated and carrier alone treated defects exhibited complete bone bridging and PDL formation, whereas follicle cell treated defects showed only minimal evidence of osteogenesis. No new cementum was formed on the root surface in the groups with carrier alone or carrier plus cultured dental follicle cell groups. Cementoblast-treated defects were filled with trabeculated bone which was more mature than at 3-weeks. Furthermore, the PDL region was maintained with well organized collagen fibres connecting the adjacent bone to a thin layer of cementum on the root surface. This study demonstrates that cementoblasts have a marked ability to produce periodontal regeneration while dental follicle cells seem to inhibit it. It also shows the selective behaviour of two different cell types in periodontal healing.

The identification and localization of ECM proteins, which are expressed during periodontal tissue regeneration, have been studied in animals and in a few human cases. Type I collagen, along with type III, was found to be sparsely distributed and not well organized (Matsuura et al 1995; Pritlove-Carson et al 1994). Collagen type IV was only found at basement membranes associated with blood vessels and epithelium (Pritlove-Carson et al 1994). Fibronectin was localized between the inflammatory cells in the newly-formed connective tissue and at the attachment sites of the periodontal ligament to the root surface (Matsuura et al 1995). The expression of bone-associated proteins, including osteocalcin, osteonectin and BSP, were observed in the newly-formed cementum and newly-formed bone as well as in the connective tissue in close proximity to the hard tissues (Amar et al 1995, 1997; Matsuura et al 1995; Ho et al 1995).

It has also been found that samples of regenerative tissue removed from GTR surgical sites of patients had upregulation of its platelet-derived growth factor (PDGF) and transforming growth factor beta (TGF-β) receptors in comparison to those found in gingival and periodontal ligament tissue (Kuru et al 1998b, Kuru 1998). Furthermore, PDGF and TGF-β have been detected in GCF from GTR patients and the levels of GCF TGF-β were found to be significantly higher than in GTR patients over GCF from conventional flap surgery patients (Kuru 1998).

A study by Nagatomo et al (2006) indicated that PDL cells possess crucial stem cell properties, such as self-renewal and multipotency, and express the mesenchymal stem cell markers CD105, CD166, and STRO-1 on their cell surface, although there were some variations.

In support of the view that all regenerative cells in the periodontium originate from stem cells it has been found that the culture of mesenchymal with periodontal ligament resulted in them expressing osteocalcin and osteopontin. They also showed a significant decrease in the expression of bone sialoprotein (Kramer et al 2004). This co-culture therefore seemed to induce them to differentiate into periodontal ligament cells.

Gonçalves et al (2008) studied surface cementum and found that it could alter osteopontin expression in the adjacent tissue (see also Ch. 5).

THE POSSIBLE USE OF GROWTH FACTORS AND CELL MEDIATORS TO PRODUCE PERIODONTAL REGENERATION

The new information described above has already begun to affect clinical methods to achieve periodontal regeneration. Melcher (1976) focused on the need to stimulate the regeneration of cementum and periodontal ligament as well as bone in periodontal regeneration. He postulated that if cells of the periodontal ligament and alveolar bone populated the healing tissue coronal to the residual alveolar bone, regeneration of new periodontium would occur.

Guided tissue regeneration seeks to produce these conditions by excluding epithelial downgrowth and thus proving an anatomical environment for the coronal migration of these cells. Bone grafts such as human freeze-dried, demineralized bone allograft (see bone graft section above) seek to provide a stimulus for bone regeneration. However, it would seem likely that predictable regeneration would not occur unless all cells capable of regenerating all the tissues of the periodontium, or their precursors, were stimulated by the necessary chemical messenger molecules. This would induce each cell line to differentiate and migrate into the healing area. It would also seem likely that cellular messenger molecules trigger all the stages of the complex events leading to periodontal regeneration. Recently some work has appeared in the literature which has experimentally tested some of these events.

The control of the stem and progenitor cell in the periodontal healing process is complex and is only just beginning to be unravelled. Various locally produced growth factors seem to play a role in recruiting cells into the healing area from the bone marrow spaces and periodontal ligament and their role has been studied in cell culture models.

Using cell culture techniques, platelet-derived growth factor (PDGF) has been found to be mitogenic and chemotactic for connective tissue cells (Ross et al 1986) and recently, the role of these factors has been studied on recruitment of osteogenic cells. This was investigated by recording the behaviour of cells which were enzymically released from rat fetal calvarium cultures. It was found that both PDGF and transforming growth factor alpha (TGF-α) were chemotactic for osteogenic cells (Hughes et al 1992) but the responses of different cell populations to these two factors were slightly different. The optimum concentration of PDGF was the same both for alkaline phosphate (AlkP) -positive and -negative cells while AlkP-positive cells showed two peaks of activity to different concentrations of TGF-α.

Sarment et al (2006) carried out a study using pyridinoline cross-linked carboxyterminal telopeptide of type I collagen (ICTP) release as a measure of active bone turnover following local delivery of PDGF-BB to periodontal osseous defects. The amount of ICTP released from the wound fluid of human subjects revealed an early increase for all treatment groups. Data from this study suggested that when PDGF-BB is delivered to promote periodontal tissue engineering of tooth-supporting osseous defects, there is a direct effect on ICTP released from the wound.

Teare et al (2008) investigated periodontal tissue regeneration enhanced by recombinant human transforming growth factor-β3 in *Papio ursinus*, a nonhuman primate. They found that when it was applied to the treated area in Matrigel® it significantly enhanced periodontal tissue regeneration.

Although the precise roles of different locally produced growth factors is unclear there is evidence for the involvement of epithelial growth factor (EGF), PDGF, fibroblast growth factor (FGF), insulin-like growth factor (IGF)-I and II and TGF-α in various stages of this process (Hughes 1995).

Sato et al (2004) investigated the effect of recombinant fibroblast growth factor on experimentally induced cementum defects of the root surface of beagle dogs. They showed that basic fibroblast growth factor in a collagen gel applied to the defective root surfaces induced new cementum and inserting collagen fibres linking it to the adjacent alveolar bone. This combination may then offer some promise in regenerative periodontal therapy but only if it works in a clinical situation.

In addition, the systemically produced steroid hormones, glucocorticoids, are known to modulate the effects of other hormones and local mediators of cell functions. In this regard they enhance the mitogenic activity of fibroblast growth factor (Hooley & Kieran 1974) and IGF-I (Conover et al 1986), but inhibit epidermal growth factor (Otto et al 1981). They could thus modulate the activities of growth factors in wound healing. In this regard a potent synthetic glucocorticoid, dexamethasone, has been shown to act synergistically with cartilage-derived growth factor to produce mitogenesis in cultured mouse cells while having no effect on PDGF produced mitogenesis (Levenson et al 1985). In contrast, it has been shown that dexamethasone acts synergistically with PDGF to induce proliferation of periodontal ligament and gingival tissue fibroblasts *in vitro* (Rutherford et al 1992b). Dexamethasone has also been shown selectively to stimulate the proliferation of osteoprogenitor cells (Bellows et al 1990) and to induce adult bone marrow cells to differentiate into osteoblasts (Kasuggai et al 1991). Glucocorticoids may therefore play a role in osteogenesis.

The behaviour of three groups of cells, cementoblasts, osteoblasts and periodontal ligament fibroblasts and their stem and progenitor cells is critical in the process of periodontal regeneration and the factors controlling these will be discussed in turn.

Cementoblasts associated with cellular cementum from fully formed teeth appear to share most of the phenotypical characteristics as osteoblasts. They would therefore be expected to respond to the same stimulating factors (Tenorio et al 1993, 1997; Tenorio & Hughes 1996). However, cementoblasts from acellular cementum do not appear to share these characteristics and may thus respond to different stimuli.

A primary requirement for periodontal regeneration is that the exposed root surface becomes populated by suitable cells from the periodontal ligament or bone marrow. Of particular importance are the cells which will develop into cementoblasts and form acellular cementum and those which will develop into periodontal ligament fibroblasts and form the inserting collagen fibrils.

The exposed root surface in periodontal disease is pathologically altered and this could deleteriously affect this process. In this regard it has been shown that periodontal ligament fibroblasts in culture failed to attach to or orientate to pathologically altered root surfaces (Tenorio et al 1997). It has been also shown (Hughes & Smales 1992) that their ability to attach to normal root surfaces can be reduced but not abolished by application of bacterial lipopolysaccharide (LPS). Furthermore, it has also been shown that acid conditioning of the root surface does not appear to alter this process (Tenorio et al 1997).

A number of locally produced factors have been shown to either stimulate or reduce the activity of osteogenic cells and these include interleukin (IL)-1, IL-6, IL-11, tumour necrosis factor alpha (TNF-α), interferon gamma (IFN-γ), bone morphogenic proteins (BMP) and the stimulation of nitrous oxide (NO) production by osteoblasts.

The role of bone morphogenic proteins (BMP) in periodontal healing seems to be considerable since they appear to be able to regulate all stages of this process from specifying cell commitment to regulating cell function (Hughes 1995; Hughes et al 1995). The effects of BMP-2, -4, -6 on the differentiation of osteoprogenitor cells in culture have been tested using a bone nodule formation assay system (Hughes et al 1995). All of these proteins produced differentiation of these cells right the way through to the formation of new bone although it was found that BMP-6 appeared to act on an earlier stage of the process than the others.

It has also been shown that the expression and production of nitrous oxide (NO) by osteoblasts, as the result of appropriate signals, has an important self regulatory role on these cells and the function of osteoclasts (Hukkanen et al 1995). Certain cytokines, IL-1β, TNF-α and IFN-γ, either alone or in synergistic combination stimulate the expression and production of NO by a variety of osteoblast cell lines *in vitro*. The secretion of NO by these cells significantly reduced osteoblast activity as evidenced by reduction in DNA synthesis, cell proliferation, alkaline phosphatase activity and osteocalcin production. In addition, IL-6 is a pluripotent cytokine which is synthesized by osteoblasts and this has also been shown to reduce osteoblast activity by inhibiting osteoblast differentiation (Hughes & Howells 1993a). Similar effects were produced by IL-11 but the effects were more potent than those produced by IL-6 (Hughes & Howells 1993b). Thus, there are now several known pathways which either stimulate or inhibit new bone formation.

In order for normal periodontal ligament attachment to form not only does new bone and acellular cementum need to form but also a normal periodontal ligament space between the two has to be maintained to accommodate the inserting fibres of the periodontal ligament. This process seems to be a function of the activity of specialized periodontal ligament fibroblasts and some knowledge of the mechanisms involved seems to be evolving. It has been shown that human periodontal ligament fibroblasts inhibit the formation of bone in rat marrow stromal cell cultures (Ogiso et al 1991). It has been further shown that these fibroblasts probably inhibit osteoblast differentiation and fulfil this function at least partially by the release of soluble factors including prostaglandins (PGs). The two most important PGs in this regard were found to be PGE_2 and PGF_2-α (Ogiso et al 1992).

The role of BMP-2 in promoting periodontal regeneration has been recently studied (King et al 1997). This was investigated using the rat buccal dehiscence model. The buccal aspect of the mandibular molars of Wistar rats was denuded of bone, periodontal ligament and some cementum and the exposed root surfaces were acid etched. The animals were then divided into test and control groups. Human recombinant BMP-2 in a collagen gel was applied to the exposed roots of the test animals while the control animals received the collagen gel alone. The flap was sutured back into their original position and the animals were then killed either after 10 or 38 days post-operation. The mandibular tissues were then examined histologically. In the test animals of the 10-day group there was more than twice the amount of new bone and cementum formation than was evident in the corresponding control animals. There was also no evidence of ankylosis. By 38 days there was complete periodontal regeneration of all tissues in both test and control animals with no differences between the groups.

Further studies by this group with this model have shown that recombinant human BMP-2 (rhBMP-2) increased cell recruitment in the healing area by increasing cell proliferation and migration from the unwounded periodontal ligament into the wounded area (King & Hughes 2001). These processes also led to a 3-fold increase in cementogenesis in the rhBMP-2 treated animals compared with controls. They also showed that the effects of rhBMP-2 on bone and cementum formation were affected by its rate of release from the gelatin carrier (Talwar et al 2001). In experiments using two carriers, one designed to release the protein slowly and the other rapidly, it was shown that slow release rhBMP-2 failed to stimulate bone formation while fast released rhBMP-2 did. However, slow release rhBMP-2 did significantly increase the rate of cementogenesis compared with both fast released rhBMP-2 and controls. These paradoxical results have relevance to the possible therapeutic use of rhBMP-2 in appropriately designed carrier systems. Thus, it appears that the local application of BMP-2 in a gelatin gel markedly increases the rate of periodontal regeneration in this model.

There are, however, important differences between this model and periodontal regeneration of periodontal defects since this model would have normal, healthy root surfaces, while the root surfaces of the periodontal defect would be pathologically altered by the disease process. This pathological alteration of the root surface is known to effect the colonization of the root surface by progenitor cells (Hughes & Smales 1992; Tenorio et al 1997).

It is generally not possible with GTR or grafting procedures or a combination of both to increase supra-alveolar bone height in periodontitis with horizontal bone loss. However, one study (Wikesjö et al 2003a) using dogs prepared supra-alveolar periodontal bone defects and treated them either with a combination of a polyglycolic acid trimethylene carbonate, space providing, macroporous, membrane and recombinant BMP-2 in a hyaluron bioabsorbable carrier or a placebo membrane and carrier without BMP-2. They showed that the membrane, BMP-2 combination significantly enhanced both supra-alveolar bone growth and healing compared with the placebo. They also showed that the membrane and carrier were completely bioabsorbed. This group also showed that this method using an e-PTFE membrane also enhanced bone formation in surgically produced intrabony defects in dogs compared with control dogs with membrane alone (Wikesjö et al 2003b).

Limitations of BMP administration to periodontal lesions include the need for a high dose bolus delivery, BMP transient biological activity and low bioavailability of growth factors at the wound site. These could be overcome by gene transfer and an experiment using this technique has been reported using a rat model with large surgically created mandibular alveolar bone defects (Jin et al 2003). Syngeneic dermal fibroblasts were transduced *ex vivo* with adenoviruses encoding either for green fluorescent protein (control virus) or BMP-7 (Ad-BMP-7), or an antagonist of BMP bioactivity, noggin (Ad-noggin). Transduced cells were seeded on to gelatin carriers and then transplanted into the mandibular alveolar bone defects in the rats. Ad-noggin inhibited osteogenesis as compared to control treated and Ad-BMP-7 treated specimens. The osseous lesions treated by Ad-BMP-7 gene delivery demonstrated rapid chondrogenesis with subsequent osteogenesis, cementogenesis and predictable bridging of the periodontal bone defects. This successful evidence of periodontal tissue engineering using *ex vivo* gene transfer of BMPs offers a possible new approach for repairing alveolar bone defects.

Several recent experimental studies in animals have used growth factors alone or in conjunction with either GTR or with GTR and root conditioning. The results have shown that growth factors had significantly increased potential for inducing regenerative healing of periodontal tissues (Sigurdsson et al 1995a,b; Cho et al 1995; Park et al 1995).

Platelet-derived growth factor (PDGF) in combination with insulin-like growth factor-1 (IGF-1) in a carboxymethylcellulose carrier has been tested in dogs with naturally-occurring periodontitis during treatment with periodontal surgery (Lynch et al 1991). In these experiments these factors appeared to produce regeneration of some new attachment with formation of some new cementum, bone and periodontal ligament. This same combination has also been tested on experimental periodontitis in monkeys (Rutherford et al 1992a, 1993) with similar results.

In these experiments, only the growth factors in the gel carrier separated the gingival tissue from the alveolar bone and root surface and no attempt was made to prevent the contact of gingival connective tissue with the root surface or the carrier as would be the case with GTR. In fact the amount and spatial distribution of the new periodontium formed suggested that cells present in the gingival connective tissue were induced by the growth factors and contributed cells to the healing process.

A combination of dexamethasone and PDGF in a collagen carrier matrix has also been tested on local experimental periodontitis lesions in monkeys. Paired lesions with horizontal and vertical bone loss and 3–5 mm of attachment loss were used. One site received an application of PDGF and dexamethasone in the collagen-carrier and the other the collagen-carrier only. A collagen matrix (CM) was used as the vehicle because it was thought that it might produce an environment which favoured connective tissue formation and also might act as a barrier to epithelial migration. The regeneration of some new periodontium, consisting of new cementum, bone and inserting periodontal ligament fibres coronal to the pre-treatment levels, was seen after 4 weeks in the PDGF/dexamethasone/CM sites but not in the control sites treated with CM alone. The application of PDGF/dexamethasone/CM produced 5-fold more new cementum and ligament and 7-fold more supracrestal bone than the control treatments over the full time period. This included the filling of intrabony defects and increased height of alveolar bone. In these experiments, it is possible that epithelial downgrowth was prevented both by the collagen matrix acting as a barrier and as a result of the inhibition of epithelial growth factor by PDGF (Otto et al 1981).

A combination of recombinant human transforming growth factor beta-1 (TGF-β1) and GTR with ePTFE membranes has been used on experimental periodontitis lesions in beagle dogs to evaluate bone and cementum regeneration (Wikesjö et al 1998). Supra-alveolar, critical size periodontal defects were surgically created around the 3rd and 4th mandibular molars on both sides of the jaw in five dogs. Alternative sides in consecutive animals received either a combination of TGF-β1 in a carrier and an ePTFE membrane (test) or an ePTFE membrane alone (control). The dogs were killed after 4 weeks and the histology of the healing lesions were assessed. Bone regeneration was seen in all animals but was limited to the very apical aspect of the lesion. Cementum was limited and no differences were seen between the test and control lesions. Statistical differences in favour of the test lesions were found for bone area growth and bone density. However, the amounts of bone and cementum formed were small and would have been clinically insignificant after this time period.

Periodontal therapies using the growth factors are considered to be in the experimental stage, and therefore no growth factor therapy has received approval by the USA Food and Drug Administration to treat periodontitis in humans (American Academy of Periodontology 1996). Nevertheless, Howell et al (1997) recently used recombinant human PDGF and insulin-like growth factor (IGF) to treat periodontal osseous defects in humans and reported that the application of these factors significantly increased the formation of alveolar bone compared with conventional flap surgery.

Thus, there is now good evidence that specific growth factors and cell mediators may interact with competent cells in the healing periodontal wound when applied locally in a suitable vehicle. The periodontal ligament cells would seem to react by differentiating and migrating into the wound area more rapidly than the rate of epithelial downgrowth to form the tissues of some new periodontium. These factors would seem to have great potential in promoting the formation of new attachment in human periodontitis lesions either alone in a suitable carrier or in combination with other methods such as GTR. However, with GTR it would probably be preferable to use a resorbable membrane, such as resorbable collagen, polygalactin, polylactide or polyurethane membranes, so that the healing process is not disturbed by membrane removal.

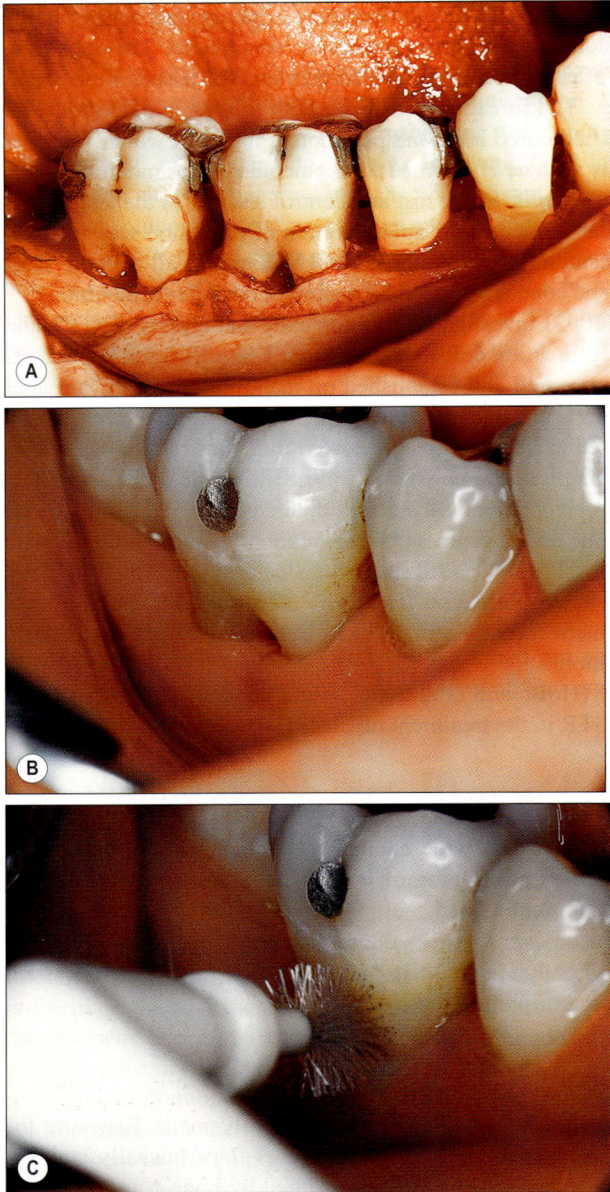

Fig. 20.10 The treatment of class III furcation involvement on the lower right first molar of a 40-year-old man. (A) The furcation is exposed by means of buccal and lingual inverse bevel flaps. The furcation space, the bone surface and the roots have been cleared of granulation tissue and deposits. The flaps were then repositioned apically to expose the furcation area. (B) The postoperative result (the picture was taken 6 months after surgery). (C) The use of a spiral brush to clean the exposed furcation area.

of individual roots after separation will exceed the mobility of the whole tooth. These techniques all require endodontic treatment prior to the surgery. In some cases lack of access to narrow, curved and partially obliterated canals will preclude this treatment. Very occasionally, in an emergency, e.g. when an unexpected problem is discovered during periodontal surgery, it may be necessary to amputate a root before endodontic treatment has been carried out. In this situation one must be sure that endodontic treatment is possible and that the tooth will be functional after the procedure. The exposed pulp at the amputation site should be dressed with calcium hydroxide and arrangements should be made for endodontic treatment soon after the surgery. In this situation it may be prudent to prescribe a course of antibiotics.

Presurgical endodontics should ensure that all of the roots to be retained are filled to the apex. A small cavity is made at the entrance of the canal of the root to be removed and packed with amalgam to produce a permanent seal at the point of amputation. The floor of the pulp chamber should also be packed with amalgam for a similar purpose. In the case of tooth division or hemisection the pulpal floor will be cut through and a permanent seal at this point is essential. The final restoration of these teeth will involve the provision of a crown(s) or a bridge.

Root amputation (Fig. 20.11A)

This is particularly applicable to three-rooted upper molar teeth when it will involve the removal of either the mesiobuccal or distobuccal root. This will allow access to the furcation area for cleaning between the remaining two roots from a buccal approach. Care should be taken to balance the occlusion on these teeth before this procedure.

Buccal and palatal inverse bevel flaps are raised to gain access. Palatal pocketing can be treated by an inverse bevel gingivectomy. Granulation tissue is curetted away to reveal the shape of the furcation and its relationship to the root to be amputated. Sectioning should start in the affected furcation and its path may be planned by passing a blunt probe through the space from buccal to palatal. The cut is made with a tapered diamond bur cooled by sterile water. A wide enough space should be made to elevate the root, taking care not to remove too much substance from the part of the tooth to be retained. The base of the crown should then be shaped so that it is cleanable from a buccal approach. The remaining roots are carefully scaled and planed and the buccal flap is placed apical to the furcation entrance between the two remaining roots. The position of the palatal gingival margin is determined by the position of the inverse bevel gingivectomy incision. A periodontal dressing is placed so that it passes between the margin of the flaps and the amputation site.

Tooth division (Fig. 20.11B)

This is carried out less frequently than the other techniques. It is indicated for extensive furcation involvement of lower molars where bone loss around both roots is similar. Buccal and lingual inverse bevel flaps are raised and the furcation revealed by curettage. The tooth is then completely divided by extending a cut from the roof of the furcation through the crown. Each half of the tooth is reshaped into a single-rooted tooth and will be subsequently prepared to receive a crown. In this way a two-rooted molar is converted into two single-rooted teeth.

Hemisection (Fig. 20.11C)

This is indicated for furcation involvement of lower molars where there is extensive bone resorption around one of the roots. It must be ensured that adequate restoration of the remaining half of the crown is possible before embarking on this procedure.

Buccal and lingual inverse bevel flaps are raised and the area is curetted. The sectioning process is begun at the roof of the furcation, extending upwards to divide the tooth. Tooth substance is preferentially removed from the half of the tooth to be sacrificed which is then removed with an elevator. The remaining root is scaled and planed. The remaining half of the crown is carefully contoured and smoothed and the flaps are repositioned to eliminate any pocketing. After healing the tooth will be crowned usually forming part of the bridge to replace the missing portion. Obviously a sufficient number of well-supported abutment teeth must be available.

Extraction

Advanced furcation involvement with extensive bone resorption around two or more roots will necessitate extraction. Teeth with uncertain prognosis may be retained on a temporary basis providing the patient is aware of

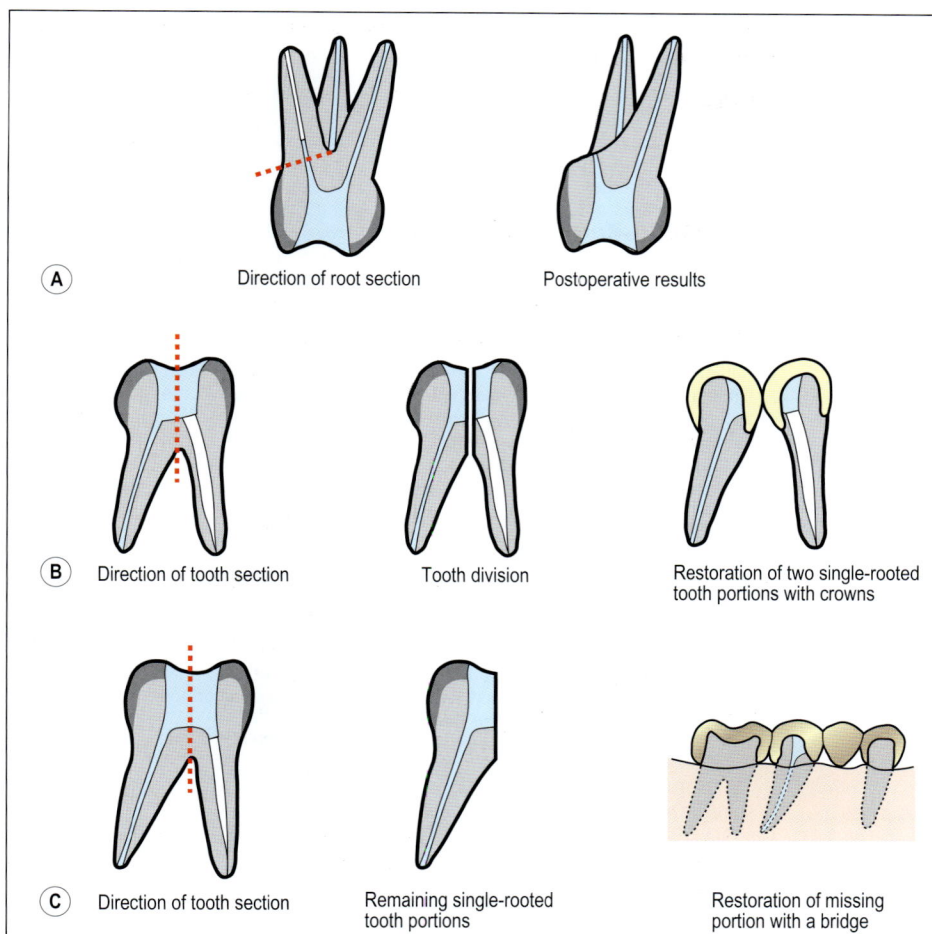

Fig. 20.11 Diagrams to show the procedures for treating more advanced Class III furcation involvement. (A) root amputation; (B) tooth division; (C) hemisection. In all cases, the tooth must be treated endodontically first.

(A) Direction of root section — Postoperative results

(B) Direction of tooth section — Tooth division — Restoration of two single-rooted tooth portions with crowns

(C) Direction of tooth section — Remaining single-rooted tooth portions — Restoration of missing portion with a bridge

the uncertainty, the teeth are symptomless and there are no signs of infection or increasing mobility. However, the effect of retaining these teeth on the prognosis of adjacent teeth should be carefully considered.

Maintenance

All teeth with furcation involvement require frequent and regular maintenance including careful subgingival scaling. The importance of careful oral hygiene measures using spiral-tufted interproximal brushes must be stressed and taught to the patients. Care must be taken to ensure effective plaque control while avoiding traumatic damage to the root surface. Successful long-term maintenance of teeth with furcation involvement can be achieved in many cases (Hirschfeld & Wasserman 1978; Knowles et al 1979).

REFERENCES

Aimetti M, Romano F, Pigella E, et al: Treatment of wide, shallow, and predominantly 1-wall intrabony defects with a bioabsorbable membrane: a randomized controlled clinical trial, *J Periodontol* 76:1354–1361, 2005.

Ainamo J: Morphogenic and functional characteristics of coronal cementum on bovine molars, *Scand J Dent Res* 78:378–386, 1970.

Amar S, Petrungaro P, Amar A, et al: Immunolocalization of bone matrix macromolecules in human tissues regenerated from periodontal defects treated with expanded polytetrafluoroethylene membranes, *Arch Oral Biol* 40:653–661, 1995.

Amar S, Chung KM, Nam SH, et al: Markers of bone and cementum formation accumulate in tissues regenerated in periodontal defects treated with expanded polytetrafluoroethylene membranes, *J Periodontal Res* 32:148–158, 1997.

American Academy of Periodontology: The potential role of growth and differentiation factors in periodontal regeneration (Position paper), *J Periodontol* 67:545–553, 1996.

American Association of Tissue Banks: Standards for tissue banking, Arlington VA, 1984, American Association of Tissue Banks.

Anderegg CR, Martin SJ, Gray JL, et al: Clinical evaluation of the use of decalcified freeze-dried bone allograft with guided tissue regeneration in the treatment of molar furcation invasions, *J Periodontol* 62:264–268, 1991.

Ansell JM, Fowler JA: The acute oral toxicity and primary ocular and dermal irritation of selected N-alkyl-2-pyrrolidones, *Food Chem Toxicol* 26:475–479, 1988.

Araújo MG, Lindhe J: GTR treatment of degree III furcation defects following the application of enamel matrix proteins. An experimental study in dogs, *J Clin Periodontol* 25:524–530, 1998.

Artzi Z, Givol N, Rohrer MD, et al: Qualitative and quantitative expression of bovine bone mineral in experimental bone defects. Part 1: description of a dog model and histological observations, *J Periodontol* 74:1143–1152, 2003a.

Artzi Z, Givol N, Rohrer MD, et al: Qualitative and quantitative expression of bovine bone mineral in experimental bone defects. Part 2: Morphometric analysis, *J Periodontol* 74:1153–1160, 2003b.

Aukhil I, Petterson E, Suggs G: Guided tissue regeneration. An experimental procedure in beagle dogs, *J Periodontol* 57:727–734, 1986.

Aukhil I, Simpson DM, Schaberg T: An experimental study of new attachment procedure in beagle dogs, *J Periodontal Res* 18:643–654, 1983.

Aukhil I, Pettersson E, Suggs C: Periodontal wound healing in the absence of periodontal ligament cells, *J Periodontol* 58:71–77, 1987.

Bartsch W, Spooner G, Dietmann K, et al: Acute toxicity to various solvents in the mouse and rat. Use of ethanol, dimethylacetamide, dimethylformide, dimethylsulfoxide, glycerine, N-methylpyrrolidone, polyethyleneglycol 400 and Tween 20, *Artzneimittelforschung* 26:1581–1583, 1976.

Becci PJ, Gephart LA, Koschier FJ, et al: Subchronic feeding study in beagle dogs of N-methylpyrrolidone, *J Appl Toxicol* 3:83–86, 1983.

Becker W, Becker B, Berg L, et al: New attachment after treatment with root isolation procedures. Report for treated class II and class III furcations and vertical osseous defects, *Int J Clin Periodontics Restorative Dent* 3:9–23, 1988.

Becker W, Becker BE: Guided tissue regeneration for implants placed into extraction sockets and for implant dehiscences: surgical techniques and case reports, *Int J Periodontics Restorative Dent* 10:377–391, 1990.

Becker W, Becker BE, Mellonig J, et al: A prospective multi-center study evaluating periodontal regeneration for Class II furcation invasions and intrabony defects after treatment with bioabsorbable barrier membrane: 1 year results, *J Periodontol* 67:641–649, 1996.

Bellows CG, Heersche JN, Aurin JE: Determination of the capacity for proliferation and differentiation of osteoprogenitor cells in the presence and absence of dexamethasone, *Dev Biol* 140:132–138, 1990.

Bergsma JE, Roseman FR, Boss RR, et al: Biocompatibility of as-polymerized poly (L-lactate) in rats using a cage implant system, *J Biomed Materials Res* 29:173–179, 1995.

Black BS, Gher ME, Sandifer JB, et al: Comparative study of collagen and expanded polytetrafluoroethylene membranes in the treatment of human class II furcation defects, *J Periodontol* 65:598–604, 1994.

Bluenthal NM: Comparison of collagen membranes with ePTFE membranes in the treatment of human class II defects, *J Periodontol* 64:925–933, 1993.

Blumenthal NM: Future directions in periodontal regeneration therapy – a combined human collagen-bone multifunction implant, *Ill Dent J* 34:35–38, 1994.

Blumenthal NM, Sabet T, Barrington E: Healing responses to grafting of combined collagen-decalcified bone in periodontal defects in dogs, *J Periodontol* 57:84–90, 1986.

Bogle G, Garrett S, Stoller NH, et al: Periodontal regeneration in naturally occurring class II furcation defects in beagle dogs after guided tissue regeneration with bioabsorbable barriers, *J Periodontol* 68:536–544, 1997.

Bosshardt DD, Schroeder HE: Cementogenesis reviewed. A comparison between human premolars and rodent molars, *Anat Rec* 245:267–292, 1996.

Bosshardt DD, Sculean A, Windisch P, et al: Effects of enamel matrix proteins on tissue formation along the roots of human teeth, *J Periodontal Res* 40:158–167, 2005.

Bouchard P, Giovannoli JL, Mattout C, et al: Clinical evaluation of a bioabsorbable regenerative material in mandibular class II furcation therapy, *J Clin Periodontol* 24:511–518, 1997.

Bowers GM, Chadroff B, Carnevale R, et al: Histologic evaluation of new attachment apparatus formation in humans. Part I, *J Periodontol* 60:664–674, 1989a.

Bowers GM, Chadroff B, Carnevale R, et al: Histologic evaluation of new attachment apparatus formation in humans. Part II, *J Periodontol* 60:675–682, 1989b.

Bowers GM, Chadroff B, Carnevale R, et al: Histologic evaluation of new attachment apparatus formation in humans. Part III, *J Periodontol* 60:683–693, 1989c.

Bratthall G, Lindberg P, Havemose-Poulsen A, et al: Comparison of ready-to-use EMDOGAIN® -gel and EMDOGAIN® in patients with chronic periodontitis. A multicenter clinical study, *J Clin Periodontol* 28:923–929, 2001.

Brookes SJ, Robinson C, Kirkham J, et al: Biochemistry and molecular biology of amelogenin proteins of developing enamel, *Arch Oral Biol* 40:1–14, 1995.

Buck B, Malinin T, Brown M: Bone transplantation and human immunodeficiency virus. An estimate risk of acquired immunodeficiency syndrome (AIDS), *Clin Orthop Relat Res* 240:129–136, 1989.

Buck B, Resnick L, Shah S, et al: Human immunodeficiency virus cultured from bone. Implications for transplantation, *Clin Orthop Relat Res* 251:249–253, 1990.

Caffesse RG, Dominguez LE, Nasjleti CE, et al: Furcation defects in dogs treated by guided tissue regeneration (GTR), *J Periodontol* 61:45–50, 1990.

Caffesse RG, Smith BA, Castelli WA, et al: New attachment achieved by guided tissue regeneration in beagle dogs, *J Periodontol* 59:589–594, 1988.

Caffesse RG, Quiñones CR: Guided tissue regeneration: biologic rationale, surgical technique, and clinical results, *Compend Contin Educ Dent* 13:166–178, 1992.

Caffesse RG, Nasjeti CE, Morrison EC, et al: Guided tissue regeneration: comparison of bioabsorbable and non-bioabsorbable membranes. Histologic and histometric study in dogs, *J Periodontol* 65:583–591, 1994.

Carinci F, Piattelli A, Guida L, et al: Effects of Emdogain on osteoblast gene expression, *Oral Dis* 12:329–342, 2006.

Carlisle E: *Silicon Biochemistry*, New York, 1986, Wiley, pp 123–136.

Caton J, Nyman S: Histometric evaluation of periodontal surgery. I. The modified Widman flap procedure, *J Clin Periodontol* 7:212–223, 1980.

Caton J, Nyman S, Zander H: Histometric evaluation of periodontal surgery. II. Connective tissue attachment levels after four regenerative procedures, *J Clin Periodontol* 7:224–231, 1980.

Caton J, Zander H: Primate model for testing periodontal treatment procedures. I, Histologic investigation of localised periodontal pockets produced by orthodontic elastics, *J Periodontol* 46:71–77, 1975.

Caton J, Wagener C, Polson A, et al: Guided tissue regeneration in interproximal defects in monkeys, *Int J Periodontics Restorative Dent* 12:267–277, 1992.

Caton J, Greenstein G, Zappa U: Synthetic bioabsorbable barrier for regeneration of human periodontal defects, *J Periodontol* 65:1037–1045, 1994.

Cerny R, Slaby I, Hammarström L, et al: A novel gene expressed in rat ameloblasts codes for proteins with cell binding domains, *J Bone Miner Res* 11:883–891, 1996.

Cho MI, Lin WL, Genco RJ: Platelet-derived growth factor modulated guided tissue regenerative therapy, *J Periodontol* 66:522–530, 1995.

Christgau M, Schmalz G, Reich E, et al: Clinical and radiographical split-mouth-study on resorbable versus non-resorbable GTR-membranes, *J Clin Periodontol* 22:306–315, 1995.

Christgau M, Wenzel A, Hiller KA, et al: Quantitative digital subtraction radiology for assessment of the bone density changes following periodontal guided tissue regeneration, *Dentomaxillofac Radiol* 25:25–33, 1996.

Christgau M, Schmatz G, Wenzel A, et al: Periodontal regeneration of intrabony defects with resorbable and non-resorbable membranes: 30 month results, *J Clin Periodontol* 24:17–27, 1997.

Christgau M, Bader N, Schmalz G, et al: GTR therapy of intrabony defects using 2 different bioresorbable membranes: 12 months results, *J Clin Periodontol* 25:499–509, 1998.

Clergeau LP, Danan M, Clergeau-Guérithault S, et al: Healing response to anorganic bone implantation in periodontal defects in dogs. Part I, bone regeneration. A microradiographic study, *J Periodontol* 67:140–149, 1996.

Cochran DL, King GN, Schoolfield J, et al: The effect of enamel matrix proteins on periodontal regeneration as determined by histological analyses, *J Periodontol* 74:1043–1055, 2003.

Cohen RE, Mullarky RH, Noble B, et al: Phenotypic characterization of mononuclear cells following anorganic bone implantation in rats, *J Periodontol* 65:1008–1015, 1994.

Conover CA, Rosenfeld RG, Hintz RL: Hormonal control of the replication of human fetal fibroblasts: the role of somatomedin C/insulin-like growth factor-1, *J Cell Physiol* 128:47–54, 1986.

Coonts BA, Whitman SL, Southard G, et al: Biodegradation and tissue response of a polymeric barrier membrane for guided tissue regeneration (GTR), *J Periodontol* 67:65, Abstract, 1996.

Cortellini P, Pini Prato G, Baldi C, et al: Guided tissue regeneration with different materials, *Int J Clin Periodontics Restorative Dent* 10:137–151, 1990.

Cortellini P, Pini Prato G, Tonetti MS: Periodontal regeneration of human infrabony defects. I. Clinical measures, *J Periodontol* 64:254–260, 1993a.

Cortellini P, Pini Prato G, Tonetti MS: Periodontal regeneration of human infrabony defects. II. Re-entry procedures and bone measures, *J Periodontology* 64:261–268, 1993b.

Cortellini P, Pini Prato G, Tonetti MS: Periodontal regeneration of human intrabony defects with titanium reinforced membranes. A controlled clinical trial, *J Periodontol* 66:797–803, 1995a.

Cortellini P, Prato GPP, Tonetti M: Interproximal free gingival grafts after membrane removal in guided tissue regeneration treatment of intrabony defects. A randomized controlled clinical trial, *J Periodontol* 66:488–493, 1995b.

Cortellini P, Prato GPP, Tonetti MS: Long term stability of clinical attachment following guided tissue regeneration and conventional treatment, *J Clin Periodontol* 23:106–111, 1996a.

Cortellini P, Prato GPP, Tonetti MS: Periodontal regeneration of human intrabony defects with bioresorbable membranes. A controlled clinical trial, *J Periodontol* 67:217–223, 1996b.

Cortellini P, Tonetti MS: Microsurgical approach to periodontal regeneration. Initial evaluation in a case cohort, *J Periodontol* 72:559–569, 2001.

Cortellini P, Tonetti MS: A minimally invasive surgical technique with an enamel matrix derivative in the regenerative treatment of intra-bony defects: a novel approach to limit morbidity, *J Clin Periodontol* 34:87–93, 2007.

Crigger M, Bogle GC, Garrett S, et al: Repair following treatment of circumferential periodontal defects in dogs with collagen and expanded polytetrafluoroethylene barrier membranes, *J Periodontol* 67:403–413, 1996.

Cury PR, Sallum EA, Nociti FH, et al: Long-term results of guided tissue regeneration therapy of class II furcation defects. A randomized clinical trial, *J Periodontol* 74:3–9, 2003.

Cutright DE, Hunsuck EE: Tissue reactions to the biodegradation of polylactic acid suture, *Oral Surg Oral Med Oral Pathol* 31:134–139, 1971.

Cutright DE, Hunsuck EE: The repair of fractures of the orbital floor using biodegradable polylactic acid, *Oral Surg Oral Med Oral Pathol* 33:28–34, 1972.

Cutright DE, Beasley JD, Perez B: Histological comparison of polylactic and poly glycolic sutures *Oral Surg Oral Med Oral Pathol* 32:165–173, 1971a.

Cutright DE, Hunsuck EE, Beasley JD: Fracture reduction using a biodegradable material, polylactic acid, *J Oral Surg* 29:393–397, 1971b.

Demolon IA, Persson GR, Ammons WF, et al: Effects of antibiotic treatment on clinical conditions with guided tissue regeneration: one year results, *J Periodontol* 65:713–717, 1994.

De Santos M, Zaccheli G, Clauser C: Bacterial contamination of barrier material and periodontal regeneration, *J Clin Periodontol* 23:1039–1046, 1996a.

De Santos M, Zaccheli G, Clauser C: Bacterial contamination of a bioabsorbable barrier material and periodontal regeneration, *J Periodontol* 67:1193–1200, 1996b.

Donos N, Sculean A, Reich E, et al: Wound healing of degree III furcation involvement following guided tissue regeneration and/or Emdogain®: a histologic study, *J Clin Periodontol* 30:1061–1068, 2003.

Dowell P, al-Arrayed F, Adam S, et al: A comparative clinical study: the use of human type I collagen with and without the addition of metronidazole in the GTR method of treatment of periodontal disease, *J Clin Periodontol* 22:543–549, 1995.

Eickholz P, Hausemann E: Evidence for healing of class II and III furcations after guided tissue regeneration therapy: digital subtraction and clinical results, *J Periodontol* 68:636–644, 1997.

Eickholz P, Kim TS, Holle R: Regenerative periodontal surgery with non-resorbable and biodegradable barriers: results after 24 months, *J Clin Periodontol* 25:666–676, 1998.

Eickholz P, Krigar D-M, Pretzl B, et al: Guided tissue regeneration with bioabsorbable barriers. II. long-term results in infrabony defects, *J Periodontol* 75:957–965, 2004.

Falk H, Laurell L, Ravald N, et al: Guided tissue regeneration procedures of 203 consecutively treated intrabony defects using a bioabsorbable matrix barrier. Clinical and radiographic findings, *J Periodontol* 68:571–581, 1997.

Fetner AE, Hartigan MS, Low SB: Periodontal repair using PerioGlas® in nonhuman primates: Clinical and histologic observations, *Compend Contin Educ Dent* 15:932–938, 1994.

Fong CD, Slaby I, Hammarström L: Amelin, an enamel related protein transcribed in the epithelial root sheath of rat teeth, *J Bone Miner Res* 11:892–898, 1996.

Francetti L, Del Fabbro M, Basso M, et al: Enamel matrix proteins in the treatment of intra-bony defects: a prospective 24-month clinical trial, *J Clin Periodontol* 31:52–59, 2004.

Frandsen EVG, Sander L, Arnbjerg D, et al: Effects of local metronidazole application on periodontal healing following guided tissue regeneration. Microbiological findings, *J Periodontol* 65:921–928, 1994.

Friedlaender G: Bone banking, *Clin Orthopaedics Rel Res* 255:17–21, 1987.

Gantes BG, Garrett S: Coronally displaced flaps in reconstructive periodontal therapy, *Dent Clin North Am* 35:495–504, 1991.

Garrett S: Periodontal regeneration around natural teeth, *Ann Periodontol* 1:621–666, 1996.

Garrett S, Polson AM, Stoller NH, et al: Comparison of a bioabsorbable GTR barrier to a non-absorbable barrier in treating human class II furcation defects. A multicenter. parallel design, randomized, single blind trial, *J Periodontol* 68:667–675, 1997.

Gestrelius S, Andersson C, Johansson A-C, et al: Formulation of enamel matrix derivative for surface coating. Kinetics and cell colonisation, *J Clin Periodontol* 24:678–684, 1997a.

Gestrelius S, Andersson C, Lidström D, et al: In vitro studies on periodontal ligament cells and enamel matrix derivative, *J Clin Periodontol* 24:685–692, 1997b.

Goncalves PF, Lima LL, Sallum EA, et al: Root cementum may modulate gene expression during periodontal regeneration: a preliminary study in humans, *J Periodontol* 79:323–333, 2008.

Gottlow J, Nyman S, Karring T, et al: New attachment formation as the result of controlled tissue regeneration, *J Clin Periodontol* 11:494–503, 1984.

Gottlow J, Karring T, Nyman S: Guided tissue regeneration following treatment of recession-like defects in the monkey, *J Periodontol* 61:680–685, 1990.

Gottlow J, Nyman S, Karring T: Maintenance of new attachment gained through guided tissue regeneration, *J Clin Periodontol* 19:315–317, 1992.

Gottlow J, Nyman S, Lindhe J, et al: New attachment formation in the human periodontium by guided tissue regeneration, *J Clin Periodontol* 13:604–616, 1986.

Gottlow J: Guided tissue regeneration using bioresorbable and nonresorbable devices: initial healing and long-term results, *J Periodontol* 64:1157–1165, 1993.

Gottlow J, Laurell L, Lundgen D, et al: Periodontal tissue response to a new bioresorbable guided tissue regeneration device. A longitudinal study in monkeys, *Int J Periodontics Restorative Dent* 14:437–449, 1994.

Gould TRL, Melcher AH, Brunette DM: Migration and division of progenitor cell populations in periodontal ligament after wounding, *J Periodontal Res* 15:20–42, 1980.

Greenstein G, Caton J: Biodegradable barriers and guided tissue regeneration, *Periodontol 2000* 1:36–45, 1993.

Grevstad HJ, Leknes KN: Ultrastructure of plaque associated with polytetrafluoroethylene (PTFE) membranes used for guided tissue regeneration, *J Clin Periodontol* 20: 193–198, 1993.

Grosso LT, Iha DK, Niu J, et al: Protease profiles of cells isolated from regenerative membranes are associated with clinical outcomes, *J Periodontol* 68:809–818, 1997.

Guillemin MR, Mellonig JT, Brusvold MA: Healing in periodontal defects treated by decalcified freeze-dried bone allografts in combination with ePTFE membranes. I. Clinical and scanning electron microscope analysis, *J Clin Periodontol* 20: 528–536, 1993a.

Guillemin MR, Mellonig JT, Brusvold MA, et al: Healing in periodontal defects treated by decalcified freeze-dried bone allografts in combination with ePTFE membranes. Assessment by computerised densitometric analysis, *J Clin Periodontol* 20: 520–521, 1993b.

Hägewald S, Pischon N, Jawor P, et al: Effects of enamel matrix derivative on proliferation and differentiation of primary osteoblasts, *Oral Surg Oral Med Oral Pathol Oral Radiol Endodontol* 98:243–249, 2004.

Hammarström L: Enamel matrix, cementum development and regeneration, *J Clin Periodontol* 24:658–668, 1997.

Hammarström L, Heijl L, Gestrelius S: Periodontal regeneration in a buccal dehiscence model in monkeys after application of enamel matrix proteins, *J Clin Periodontol* 24:669–677, 1997.

Hardwick R, Hayes BK, Flynn C: Devices for dentoalveolar regeneration: an up-to-date literature review, *J Periodontol* 66:495–505, 1995.

Hauschka P, Mavrakos A, Lafrati MD, et al: Growth factor in bone matrix. Isolation of multiple types by affinity chromatography on heparin Sepharose, *J Biol Chem* 261:12665–12674, 1986.

Heden G, Wennström JL: Five-year follow-up of regenerative periodontal therapy with enamel matrix derivative at sites with angular bone defects, *J Periodontol* 77:295–301, 2006.

Heijl L: Periodontal regeneration with enamel matrix derivative in one human experimental defect. A case report, *J Clin Periodontol* 24:693–696, 1997.

Heijl L, Heden G, Svärdström G, et al: Enamel matrix derivative (Emdogain®) in the treatment of intrabony periodontal defects, *J Clin Periodontol* 24:705–714, 1997.

Hench LL: Ceramic implants for humans, *Adv Ceramic Mater* 1:306–310, 324, 1986.

Hench LL: Bioceramics: theory and clinical applications. In Andersson H, Happonen R-P, Yli-Urpo A, editors: *Bioceramics 7*, 1994, Oxford, Butterworth-Heinemann, pp 3–14.

Hench LL, Wilson J: Surface-active biomaterials, *Science* 226:630–636, 1984.

Hench LL, Stanley HR, Clark AE, et al: Dental applications of Bioglass® implants. In Bonfield W, Hastings GW, Tanner KE, editors: *Bioceramics 4*, Oxford, 1991, Butterworth-Heinemann, pp 231–238.

Hench LL, Wilson J: Bioactive glasses and glass-ceramics: a 25 year retrospective, *Ceramic Transact* 48:11–21, 1995.

Hench LL, West JK: Biological applications of bioactive glasses, *Life Chem Rep* 13: 187–241, 1996.

Hiatt W, Schallhorn R: Intraoral transplants of cancellous bone and marrow in periodontal lesions, *J Periodontol* 44:194–208, 1973.

Hirschfeld L, Wasserman B: A long-term survey of tooth loss in 600 treated periodontal patients, *J Periodontol* 49:225–237, 1978.

Ho S, Ivanovski S, Bartold PM: An immunohistochemical study of the extracellular matrix associated with guided tissue regeneration, *Periodontol 2000* 16:61–66, 1995.

Hoffmann T, Richter S, Meyle J, et al: A randomized clinical multicentre trial comparing enamel matrix derivative and membrane treatment of buccal class II furcation involvement in mandibular molars. Part III: patient factors and treatment outcome, *J Clin Periodontol* 33:575–583, 2006.

Hooley RW, Kieran JA: Control of the initiation of DNA synthesis in 3T3 cells: serum factors, *Proc Natl Acad Sci USA* 71:2908–2911, 1974.

Howell TH, Fiorellini JP, Paquette DW, et al: A phase I/II clinical trial to evaluate a combination of recombinant human platelet-derived growth factor-BB and recombinant human insulin-like growth factor-1 in patients with periodontal disease, *J Periodontol* 68:1186–1193, 1997.

Hughes FJ: *Surgical intervention: repair, guided tissue regeneration (growth factors; bone morphogenic proteins)*, Oral presentation at British Society of Periodontology Scientific Meeting at the Royal College of Surgery, 1993, 5 June.

Hughes FJ: Cytokines and cell signalling in the periodontium, *Oral Dis* 1:259–265, 1995.

Hughes FJ, Howells GL: Interleukin-6 inhibits bone formation in vitro, *Bone Miner* 21:21–28, 1993a.

Hughes FJ, Howells GL: Interleukin-11 inhibits bone formation in vitro, *Calcif Tissue Int* 53:362–364, 1993b.

Hughes FJ, McCulloch CA: Stimulation of the differentiation of osteogenic rat bone marrow stromal cells by osteoblast cultures, *Lab Invest* 64:617–622, 1991.

Hughes FJ, Smales FC: Attachment and orientation of human periodontal ligament fibroblasts to lipopolysaccharide-coated and pathologically altered cementum in vitro, *Eur J Prosthodont restor Dent* 1:63–68, 1992.

Hughes FJ, Aubin JE, Heersche JN: Differential chemotactic responses of different populations of fetal rat calvaria cells to platelet-derived growth factor and transforming growth factor beta, *Bone Miner* 19:63–74, 1992.

Hughes FJ, Collyer J, Stanfield M, et al: The effects of bone morphogenic protein-2, -4, -6 on differentiation of rat osteoblast cells in vitro, *Endocrinol* 136:2671–2677, 1995.

Hugoson A, Ravald N, Fornell J, et al: Treatment of class II furcation involvements in humans with bioabsorbable and non-resorbable guided tissue regeneration barriers. A randomized multicenter study, *J Periodontol* 66:624–634, 1995.

Hukkanen M, Hughes FJ, Buttery LD, et al: Cytokine-stimulated expression of inducible nitric oxide synthase by mouse, rat and human osteoblast-like cells and its functional role in osteoblast metabolic activity, *Endocrinology* 136:5445–5453, 1995.

Hürzeler MB, Kohal R, Naghshbandi J, et al: Evaluation of a new bioabsorbable barrier to facilitate guided tissue regeneration around exposed implant threads. An experimental study in the monkey, *Int J Oral Maxillofac Surg* 27:315–320, 1998.

Iglhaut J, Aukhil I, Simpson DM, et al: Progenitor cell kinetics during guided tissue regeneration in experimental periodontal wounds, *J Periodontal Res* 23:107–117, 1988.

Jensen S, Eberhard J, Herrera D, et al: A systematic review of guided tissue regeneration for periodontal furcation defects. What is the effect of guided tissue regeneration compared with surgical debridement in the treatment of periodontal furcation defects? *J Clin Periodontol* 29(Suppl 3):103–116, 2002.

Jepsen S, Heinz B, Jepsen K, et al: A randomized clinical trial comparing enamel matrix derivative and membrane treatment of buccal class II furcation involvement in mandibular molars. Part I: Study design and results for primary outcomes, *J Periodontol* 75:1150–1160, 2004.

Jin Q-M, Anusaksathien O, Webb SA, et al: Gene therapy of bone morphogenetic protein for periodontal tissue engineering, *J Periodontol* 74:202–213, 2003.

Jones JK, Triplett RG: The relationship of cigarette smoking to intraoral wound healing: a review of evidence and implications for patient care, *J Maxillofac Surg* 50:237–239, 1992.

Kasuggai S, Todescan R, Nagata T, et al: Expression of bone matrix proteins associated with mineralised bone formation by adult marrow cells in vitro: inductive effects of dexamethasone on osteoblast phenotype, *J Cell Physiol* 147:111–120, 1991.

Keeting PE, Oursler MJ, Wiegand KE, et al: Zeolite A increases proliferation, differentiation, and transforming growth factor b production in normal adult human osteoblast-like cells in vitro, *J Bone Miner Res* 7:1281–1289, 1992.

Keila S, Nemcovsky CE, Moses O, et al: In vitro effects of enamel matrix proteins on rat bone marrow cells and gingival fibroblasts, *J Dent Res* 83:134–138, 2004.

Kenney EB, Lekovik V, Han T, et al: The use of porous hydroxyapatite implants in periodontal defects. I. Clinical results after 6 months, *J Periodontol* 56:82–88, 1985.

Kenney EB, Lekovik V, Sa Ferreira JC, et al: Bone formation within porous hydroxyapatite implants in human periodontal defects, *J Periodontol* 57:76–83, 1986.

Kilic AR, Efeoglu E, Yilmaz S: Guided tissue regeneration in conjunction with hydroxyapatite-collagen grafts for intrabony defects. A clinical and radiological evaluation, *J Clin Periodontol* 24:372–383, 1997.

King GN, King N, Cruchley AT, et al: Recombinant human bone morphogenic protein-2 promotes wound healing in rat periodontal fenestration defects, *J Dent Res* 76: 1460–1470, 1997.

King GN, Hughes JM: Bone morphogenic protein-2 stimulates cell recruitment and cementogenesis during early wound healing, *J Clin Periodontol* 28:465–475, 2001.

Knowles JW, Burgett FG, Nissle RR, et al: Results of periodontal treatment related to pocket depth and attachment level: 8 years, *J Periodontol* 50:225–233, 1979.

Kramer PR, Nares S, Kramer SF, et al: Mesenchymal stem cells acquire characteristics of cells in the periodontal ligament in vitro, *J Dent Res* 83:27–34, 2004.

Krebsbach PH, Lee SK, Matsuki Y, et al: Full length sequence, localization, and chromosome mapping of ameloblastin. A novel tooth-specific gene, *J Biol Chem* 271:4431–4435, 1996.

Krejci C, Bissada N, Farah C, et al: Clinical evaluation of porous and non-porous hydroxyapatites in the treatment of human periodontal defects, *J Periodontol* 58: 521–528, 1987.

Kuru L, Parkar MH, Griffiths GS, et al: Extracellular matrix production by cells associated with guided tissue regeneration, *J Dent Res* 76:444, Abstract 3447, 1997a.

Kuru L, Parkar MH, Griffiths GS, et al: Flow cytometry analysis of gingival and periodontal ligament fibroblasts, *J Dent Res* 76:1068, 1997b.

Kuru L, Griffiths GS, Parkar MH, et al: Osteoblast-like properties of regenerative periodontal cells, *J Dent Res* 76:1068, 1997c.

Kuru L, Parkar MH, Griffiths GS, et al: Flow cytometry analysis of gingival and periodontal ligament cells, *J Dent Res* 77:555–564, 1998a.

Kuru L, Griffiths GS, Parkar MH, et al: Expression of growth factor and their receptors by regenerated periodontal tissue, *J Dent Res* 77:999, 1998b.

Kuru L: *Cellular and molecular basis of periodontal regeneration*, PhD thesis, 1998, University of London.

Turner D, Mellonig J: Antigenicity of freeze-dried bone allograft in periodontal osseous defects, *J Periodontal Res* 16:89–99, 1981.

Urist MR: Bone formation by autoinduction, *Science* 150:893–899, 1965.

Urist MR, Strates B: Bone morphogenic protein, *J Dent Res* 60:1392–1406, 1971.

Van Swol RL, Ellinger R, Pfeifer J, et al: Collagen membrane barrier therapy to guide regeneration in class II furcations in humans, *J Periodontol* 64:622–629, 1993.

Viswanathan HL, Berry JN, Foster BL, et al: Amelogenin: a potential regulator of cementum-associated genes, *J Periodontol* 74:1423–1431, 2003.

Vouros I, Aristodimou E, Konstantinidis A: Guided tissue regeneration in intrabony periodontal defects following treatment with two bioabsorbable membranes in combination with bovine bone mineral graft. A clinical and radiographic study, *J Clin Periodontol* 31:908–917, 2004.

Vrouwenvelder WCA, Groot GP, de Groot K: Biochemical evaluation of osteoblasts cultured in bioactive glass, hydroxyapatite, titanium alloy and stainless steel, *J Biomed Mater Res* 27:465–475, 1993.

Wachtel H, Schenk G, Böhm S, et al: Microsurgical access flap and enamel matrix derivative for the treatment of periodontal intrabony defects: a controlled clinical study, *J Clin Periodontol* 30:496–504, 2003.

Wakabayashi RC, Wong F, Richards DW, et al: Protease repertoires of cells adherent to membranes recovered after guided tissue regeneration, *J Periodontal Res* 31:171–180, 1996.

Wakabayashi RC, Iha DK, Niu JJ, et al: Cytokine production by cells adherent to regenerative membranes, *J Periodontal Res* 32:215–224, 1997.

Wang HL, O'Neal RB, Thomas CL, et al: Evaluation of an absorbable collagen membrane in treating class II furcation defects, *J Periodontol* 65:1029–1036, 1994.

Warren K, Karring T: Guided tissue regeneration combined with osseous grafting in suprabony periodontal lesions. An experimental study in the dog, *J Clin Periodontol* 19:373–380, 1992.

Warren K, Karring T, Nyman S, et al: Guided tissue regeneration using biodegradable membranes of polygalactic acid or polyurethane, *J Clin Periodontol* 19:633–640, 1992.

Watanabe M: Implantation of hydroxyapatite granules mixed with atelocollagen and bone inductive protein in rat skull defects. In Yamamuro T, Hench LL, Wilson J, editors: *Handbook of Bioceramics*, Vol. II, Boca Raton, FL, 1990, CRC Press, pp 223–228.

Weigel C, Brägger U, Hämmerle CH, et al: Maintenance of new attachment 1 and 4 years following guided tissue regeneration (GTR), *J Clin Periodontol* 22:661–669, 1995.

Weltman R, Trojo PM, Morrison E, et al: Assessment of guided tissue regeneration procedures in intrabony defects with bioabsorbable and non-resorbable barriers, *J Periodontol* 68:582–591, 1997.

Wetzel AC, Stich H, Caffesse RG: Bone apposition onto oral implants in the sinus area filled with different grafting materials. A histological study in beagle dogs, *Clin Oral Implant Res* 6:155–163, 1995.

Wikesjö UME, Nilveus RE, Selvig KA: Significance of early healing events on periodontal repair: A review, *J Periodontol* 63:158–165, 1992.

Wikesjö UME, Razi SS, Sigurdsson TJ, et al: Periodontal repair in dogs: effect of recombinant human transforming growth factor-beta1 on guided tissue regeneration, *J Clin Periodontol* 25:475–481, 1998.

Wikesjö UME, Lee MB, Thomson RC, et al: Periodontal repair in dogs: evaluation of a bioabsorbable space providing macroporous membrane with recombinant human bone morphogenic protein-2, *J Periodontol* 74:635–647, 2003a.

Wikesjö UME, Xiropaidis AV, Thomson RC, et al: Periodontal repair in dogs: rhBMP-2 significantly enhances bone formation under the provisions for guided tissue regeneration, *J Clin Periodontol* 30:705–714, 2003b.

Wilson J, Low SB: Bioactive ceramics for periodontal treatment: comparative studies in the Patas monkey, *J Appl Biomater* 3:123–129, 1992.

Wilson J, Low S, Fetner A, et al: Bioactive materials for periodontal treatment: a comparative study. In Pizzoferrato A, Marchetti PG, Ravaglioli A, Lee AJC, editors: *Biomaterials and Clinical Applications*, Amsterdam, 1987, Elsevier Science B V, pp 223–228.

Wilson J, Clark AE, Hall M, et al: Tissue response to Bioglass® endosseous ridge maintenance implants, *J Implantol* 19:295–302, 1993.

Wilson J, Clark AE, Douek E, et al: Clinical applications of Bioglass® implants. In Andersson H, Happonen R-P, Yli-Urpo A, editors: *Bioceramics 7*, Oxford, 1994, Butterworth-Heinemann, pp 415–422.

Yoneda S, Itoh D, Kuroda S, et al: The effect of enamel matrix derivative (EMD) on osteoblastic cells in culture and bone regeneration in a rat skull defect, *J Periodontal Res* 38:333–342, 2003.

Yuan K, Chen C-L, Lin MT: Enamel matrix derivative exhibits an angiogenic effect in vitro and in a murine model, *J Clin Periodontol* 30:732–738, 2003.

Yukna RA: HTR-polymer grafts in human periodontal osseous defects. I, 6-months clinical results, *J Periodontol* 61:633–642, 1990.

Yukna RA: Clinical human comparison of expanded polytetrafluoroethylene barrier membrane and freeze-dried dura mater allografts for guided tissue regeneration of lost periodontal support. I. Mandibular molar class II furcations, *J Periodontol* 63:431–442, 1992.

Yukna RA, Cassingham R, Caudrill R, et al: Six months evaluation of Calcitite (hydroxyapatite ceramic) in periodontal osseous defects, *Int J Periodontics Restor Dent* 6:34–45, 1986.

Yukna RA, Mayer E, Amos S: 5-year evaluation of Durapatite ceramic alloplastic implants in periodontal osseous defects, *J Periodontol* 60:544–547, 1989.

Yun J-H, Hwang S-J, Kim C-S, et al: The correlation between the bone probing, radiographic and histometric measurements of bone level after regenerative surgery, *J Periodontal Res* 40:453–460, 2005.

Zetterström O, Andersson C, Eriksson L, et al: Clinical safety of enamel matrix derivative (EMDOGAIN®) in the treatment of periodontal defects, *J Clin Periodontol* 24:697–704, 1997.

Zhao M, Jin Q, Berry JE, et al: Cementoblast delivery for periodontal tissue engineering, *J Periodontol* 75:154–161, 2004.

As described in Chapter 1, the attached gingiva or 'functional mucosa' extends from the gingival groove to the mucogingival junction where it meets the alveolar mucosa. At the mucogingival junction the mucoperiosteum splits so that the alveolar mucosa is separated from the periosteum by a loose highly vascular connective tissue. The width of the attached gingiva can vary from zero (0) to about 9 mm, widest in the incisor regions and narrowest over canines and premolars. Its boundaries are defined on the buccal side by the insertion of the buccinator, the lip muscles and the frena, as well as by the morphology of the underlying bone. On the lingual side it is bounded by the insertion of the mylohyoid muscle, the insertions of lingual frena and the bone morphology.

Reduction in width of the attached gingiva is a consequence of gingival recession produced by atrophic changes, as described in Chapter 8, and/or as the result of progressive chronic periodontal disease.

In the past it had been assumed that some width of attached gingiva is necessary to maintain gingival health by separating the stable gingival margin from the mobile alveolar mucosa. It was also assumed that the depth of the vestibular sulcus was a significant factor in gingival health. As a result of this concept, a number of surgical 'vestibular extension' procedures were devised to achieve what were considered to be adequate anatomical dimensions. There was, however, no scientific evidence for these assumptions. Fortunately for the patient, notions of a normal vestibular depth were discarded, and ideas about the necessary width of attached gingiva questioned. Lang and Löe (1972) reported that a narrow band of 1–2 mm attached gingiva was necessary for gingival health, but other studies indicated that this is not the case. Miyasato et al (1977); Wennstrom et al (1982) and Salkin et al (1987) have shown that it is possible to maintain a healthy and stable gingival margin with little or no attached gingiva, providing the individual maintains a high standard of oral hygiene. Wennstrom (1987) confirmed these results in a 5-year study. Addy et al (1987) examined the relationship between frenal attachment, lip coverage and vestibular depth, and plaque and gingival bleeding scores in 1015 schoolchildren aged 11.5–12.5 years. They found that:

1. The position of the anterior maxillary frena appeared to affect plaque retention and gingival bleeding while the position of the mandibular labial frenum seemed to be unimportant
2. Plaque and bleeding scores in the anterior area of the mandible seemed to decrease with an increase in vestibular depth
3. Decreased upper lip coverage at rest (lack of lip-seal) was related to increased plaque and bleeding scores in both jaws.

These various findings point to the fact that variations in the width of attached gingiva are significant only when oral hygiene is poor, and even then, as Addy et al (1987) conclude, that significance is small, and alone does not justify surgical interference.

However, this study on children with gingival disease is not necessarily relevant to adults with various stages of periodontal disease. The precise form of treatment required depends on the anatomical and pathological variables involved in the lesion and in some cases the views of the patient.

Mucogingival problems can arise from the effects of:

- Chronic periodontitis
- Frenal pull
- Gingival recession.

THE EFFECTS OF CHRONIC PERIODONTITIS

1. Periodontal pocketing extending below the mucogingival junction where the apical limit of the pocket is:
   a. level with some point between the mucogingival junction and the vestibular fold (**Figs 21.1, 21.2**) so that after disease has been resolved there is enough healthy mucosa to cover the alveolar margin and produce a zone of attached mucosa and a vestibular sulcus. In this situation an apically repositioned flap may be indicated.

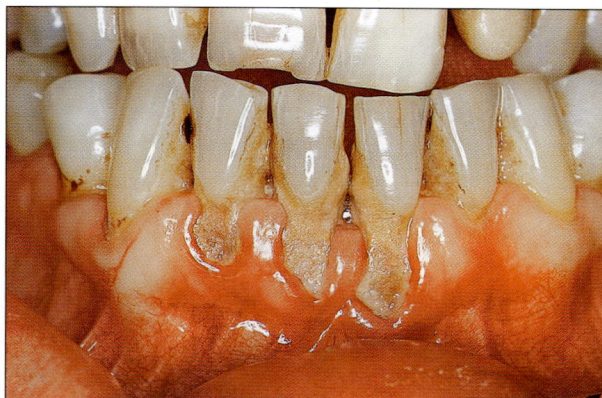

Fig. 21.1 A combination of gingival inflammation, periodontal pocketing and severe gingival recession as a result of progressive chronic periodontitis with marked attachment and bone loss. The recession and some of the pockets extend below the mucogingival junction and the gingival margin is subjected to pull from muscle and frenal attachments.

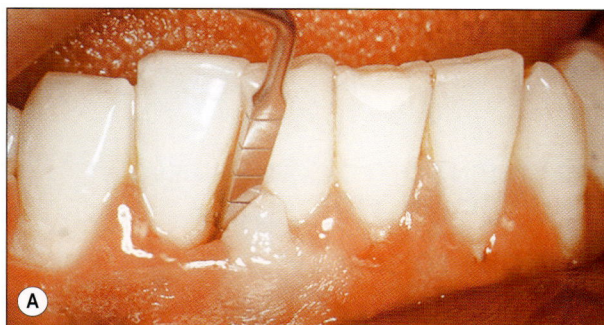

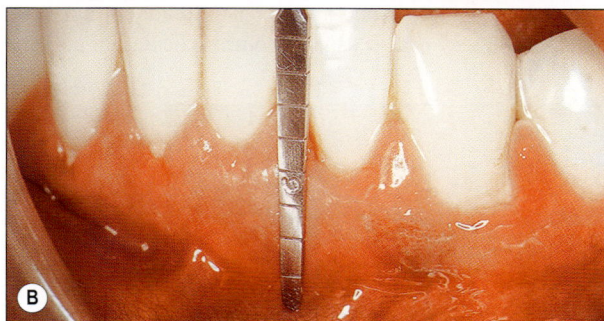

Fig. 21.2 A deep localized periodontal pocket extending below the mucogingival junction. (A) Clinical appearance with marked gingival inflammation and local inflammatory hyperplasia; (B) measuring probe indicating the depth of the pocket and its relationship to the mucogingival junction.

b. apical to the level of the vestibular sulcus so that any attempt at surgery to cover the alveolar margin would obliterate the gingival sulcus. In this case the apically displaced flap procedure could be used, plus a free gingival graft if tissue destruction is great.
2. Generalized gingival recession exposing root surfaces and reducing the zone of attached gingiva (**Fig. 21.1**). This can be treated conservatively or surgically. Several surgical procedures could be considered including the free gingival graft combined with the coronally repositioned flap or the free connective tissue graft.

THE EFFECTS OF FRENAL PULL

A frenum or muscle attachment which is inserted into an unhealthy gingival margin, which either:

1. interferes with effective plaque removal (**Fig. 21.3**) and/or
2. pulls on the wall of the pocket and thereby aggravates the lesion (**Fig. 21.2**). These lesions appear rather dramatic especially when related muscles are tensed by pulling (gently) on the lip or cheek.

Sometimes thorough scaling, root planing and efficient home care can keep the situation stable for several years. However, if gingival inflammation persists and/or there is evidence that the lesion is progressing surgical corrective treatment is indicated.

The first situation can be corrected by a simple *frenectomy*; the second may require a *free gingival graft*.

LOCALIZED GINGIVAL RECESSION

This may affect single or multiple teeth and may be caused by:

1. an underlying local bony dehiscence(s) with associated toothbrushing trauma (**Fig. 21.4**), or
2. direct gingival trauma from the occlusion such as from a deep overbite associated with an Angle's Class 2, division II occlusion (**Fig. 21.5**).

The first may be treated *conservatively* or *surgically*; surgical procedures include *pedicle grafts* and *free gingival grafts* and their variants (see below).

The second requires orthodontic treatment for the occlusal problem plus corrective surgery where this is possible. This is dependent on the precise nature of the defect.

SURGICAL TREATMENT OF POCKETING BELOW THE MUCOGINGIVAL JUNCTION

CONTRAINDICATIONS TO SURGERY

No surgical treatment should ever be contemplated unless the patient's plaque control is entirely satisfactory and all the basic treatment has been successfully completed. Surgery is also usually contraindicated in patients

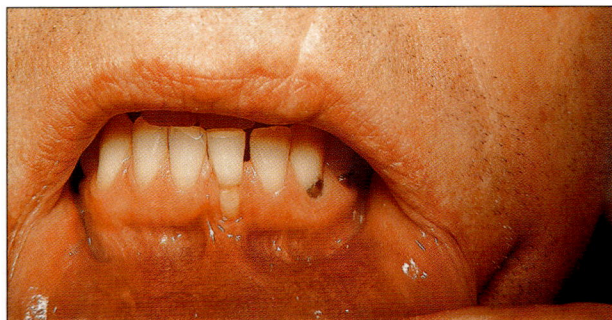

Fig. 21.3 Localized gingival recession on the lower right central incisor due primarily to a developmental bone dehiscence and secondarily affected by frenal pull.

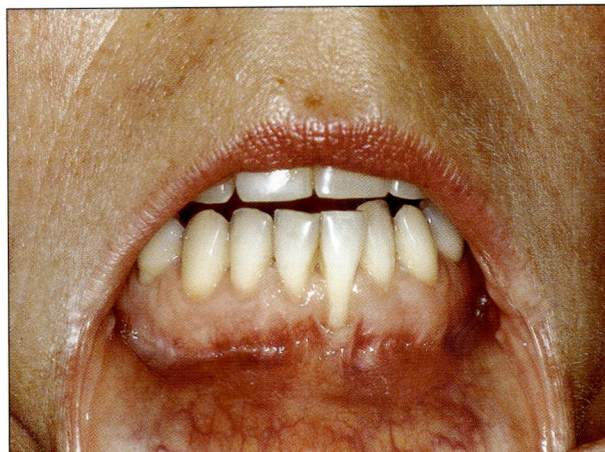

Fig. 21.4 Severe localized gingival recession on the lower left central incisor due primarily to a developmental bone dehiscence extending below the mucogingival junction.

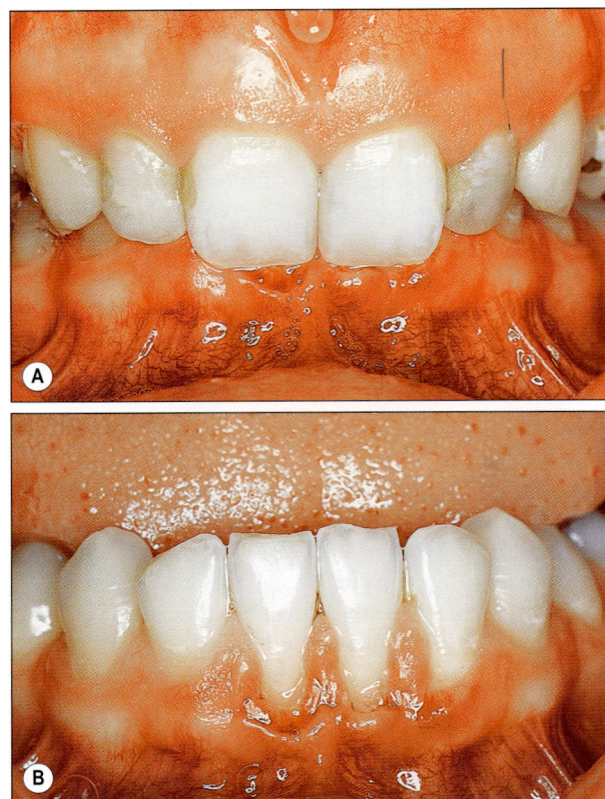

Fig. 21.5 Destruction of gingival tissue due to a combination of poor oral hygiene and direct physical gingival trauma from a Class 2, division 2 occlusion with a deep overbite, with the upper incisors impinging on the lower gingivae. (A) Jaws closed showing the contact of the upper incisors on the lower gingivae; (B) view of lower gingivae showing recession and trauma.

that smoke and refuse to give up since their response to surgical treatment is adversely affected (Preber & Bergström 1990; Ah et al 1994; Jones & Triplett 1992; Miller 1987).

SURGICAL PROCEDURES

A number of surgical procedures have been developed to correct mucogingival problems of this type. All have the common aims of:

1. the removal of disease
2. the production of a periodontal anatomy which allows effective plaque control, and therefore prevent disease recurrence.

Deep pocketing of this type may be treated by the *apically repositioned flap* or the *apically displaced flap* as appropriate. The former is described on Chapter 19.

THE APICALLY DISPLACED FLAP

The apically displaced flap technique can be used where the base of the pocket lies apical to the MGJ and a zone of keratinized gingiva is either absent or very narrow and the vestibular depth shallow (**Figs 21.6, 21.7**). For pocket elimination, the flap has to be moved apical by an amount equal to the depth of the pocket so that the flap margin coincides with the alveolar crest. However, where all or most of the attached gingiva has been destroyed, the flap has to be moved so that its margin is apical to the bone margin.

Procedure

If there is a usable zone of keratinized gingiva, then this is preserved by making an inverse bevel incision along the gingival margin (**Fig. 21.6A**). However, if very little keratinized gingiva remains and this is

grossly misshapen than it is best discarded. In this case there is little point in making a scalloped gingival incision. A straight incision can be made and the inflamed and frequently misshapen marginal tissue discarded. Vertical releasing incisions are made delineating the area of tissue to be moved apically and the flap is lifted by sharp dissection through the loose connective tissue of the alveolar mucosa plus any associated muscles (**Fig. 21.6B**), thus leaving the periosteum on the bone (**Fig. 21.7A**).

The flap is moved apical to the alveolar crest (**Fig. 21.6C**) into a position which will allow the production, by secondary intention healing, of a zone of attached gingiva free of frenal and muscle attachments. After curettage and root planing of the exposed root surfaces, the flap is fixed by sutures at the releasing incisions and, if necessary, by a suture in the midline fixing the flap to the underlying mentalis muscle. The exposed alveolar margin, which is covered by periosteum, will heal by secondary intention.

A periodontal dressing is essential (**Fig. 21.6D**). It is placed for 1 week and then removed; the wound is irrigated with a warm saline solution and the dressing is replaced for a further week. The surface of the wound

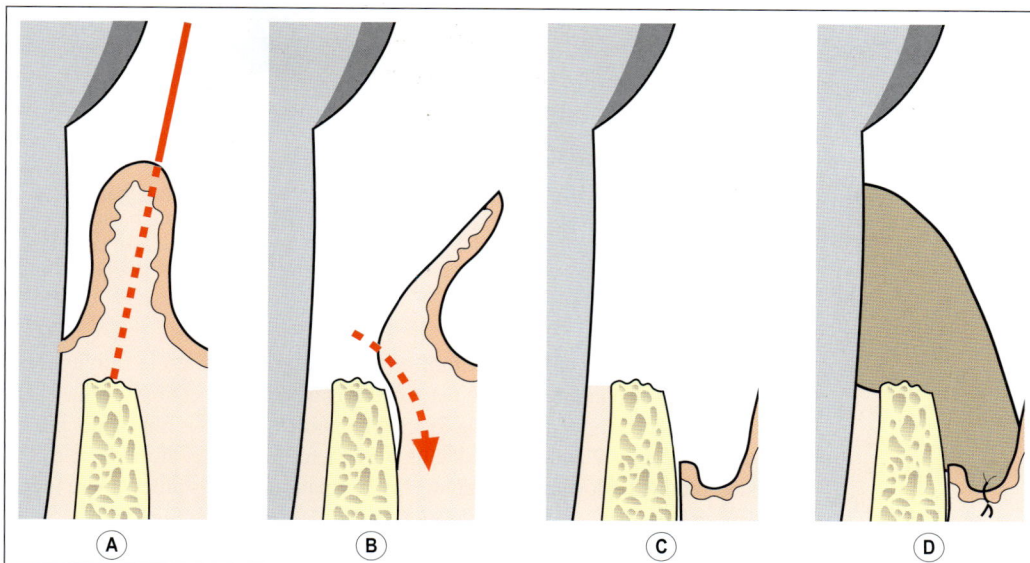

Fig. 21.6 The apically displaced flap technique. (A) An inverse bevelled incision is made (where there is considerable tissue destruction and distortion a horizontal incision may be made to excise the deformed tissue); (B) the flap is dissected from the underlying periosteum; (C) the tissue is displaced apical to the alveolar crest; (D) the displaced tissue is sutured to the underlying muscle with resorbable sutures and held in place by the periodontal pack. The healing of the exposed area takes place by secondary intention and is ultimately covered by keratinized epithelium (see Fig. 21.7B).

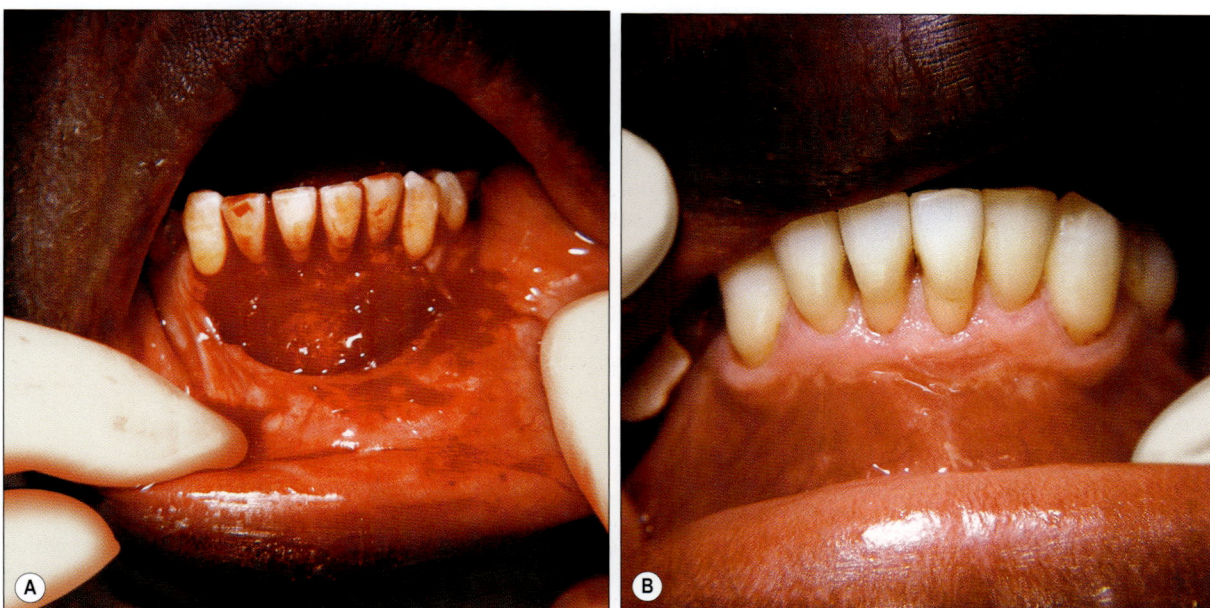

Fig. 21.7 Apically displaced flap. (A) A split-thickness has been dissected, leaving periosteum on bone surface; (B) final result shown 1 year after the procedure. There is pocket elimination with a functional zone of attached gingiva.

becomes covered by stratified squamous epithelium over this period but the healing period is much longer than that for flap procedures which cover the bone surface. The formation of mature connective tissue and well-keratinized attached gingiva can take up to 6 weeks. During this period, the patient needs to be kept on a chlorhexidine mouthwash and should receive professional cleaning every 2 weeks.

The final result of this procedure is good and should produce a functional zone of attached gingiva free from muscle and frenal pull and a good vestibular depth (**Fig. 21.7B**).

THE TREATMENT OF THE EFFECTS OF FRENAL PULL

This may be treated either by a frenectomy or a free gingival graft. The former is described below while the latter is included in the section on the treatment of gingival recession.

FRENECTOMY

A frenectomy is indicated where the attachment of a frenum or muscle attachment is so close to the gingival margin that it interferes with efficient plaque removal and contributes to persistent gingival inflammation. This problem is most frequently found on the labial surface between the upper central incisors, but can also occur in relation to the upper canines and premolars. In the lower jaw the frena are found labial to the lower incisors and rarely on the lingual aspect. Frenectomy may also be indicated prior to orthodontic treatment to close a midline diastema (**Fig. 21.8A**).

Procedure

1. After local anaesthesia, the lip is extended and the frenum is gripped with mosquito forceps. Incisions are made with a No. 15 Swann–Morton blade on either side of the forceps through the base of the frenum. The incisions should meet at the point of the instrument. The incision on the alveolar side is made close to the alveolar bone, leaving the periosteum in place.
2. The triangle of frenal tissue should come away easily if the incisions have been made correctly.
3. The edges of the lip wound are gently undermined so that they can be approximated without tension and sutured. It is not necessary to suture the alveolar wound (**Fig. 21.8B**).
4. Swabs are placed firmly over the wound to control bleeding and a periodontal dressing is applied. Retention of the dressing in this situation is often poor and the patient must be advised that if the dressing falls off it is not a calamity provided that the wound is kept clean with warm saline mouthwashes and a twice-daily rinse with 0.2% chlorhexidine solution.
5. After 1 week, the sutures and any dressing are removed. Usually healing is rapid and uneventful.

THE TREATMENT OF GINGIVAL RECESSION

LOCALIZED GINGIVAL RECESSION

Localized recession of the gingival margin with considerable exposure of the root is usually associated with the presence of an underlying bony dehiscence. It is most commonly seen on the buccal surface of teeth with buccally placed roots, associated with teeth with bulbous roots or in areas where the surface bone is naturally thin. Common teeth involved are lower incisors and upper canines, premolars or first molars. Recession progresses into the attached gingival zone, decreasing this as it deepens. If it progresses into the alveolar mucosa, below the mucogingival junction, the gingival margin is no longer protected from the pull of the muscles via frenal and mucosal attachments and

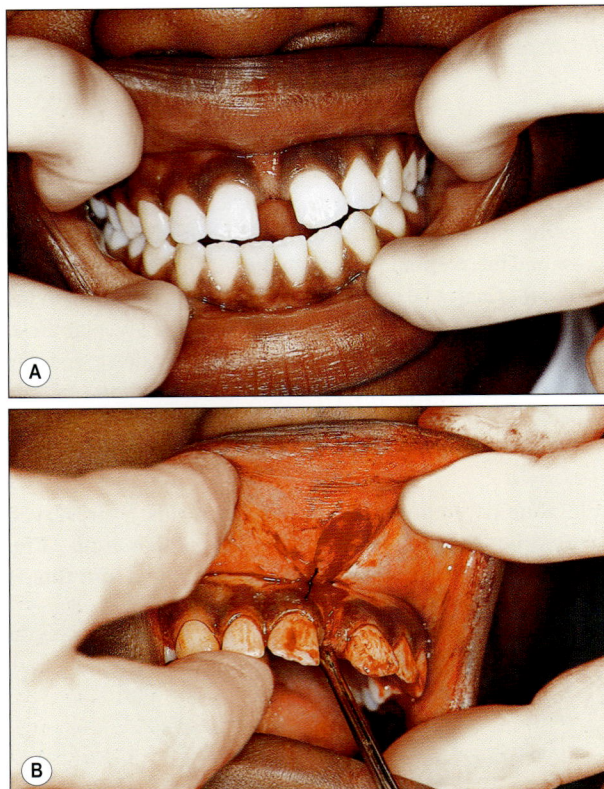

Fig. 21.8 Frenectomy. (A) Large frenum inserted close to the gingival margin and associated with a midline diastema in a 14-year-old girl. Gingivae are healthy and patient about to undergo orthodontic treatment which will seek to close diastema. (B) Frenectomy procedure after the removal of the frenum and after the first suture to close the mucosal wound.

it may be pulled away from the root surface during facial muscle activity. This relationship also interferes with plaque removal because the gingival margin at this point is no longer accessible for cleaning unless the lip is physically pulled back for access. Plaque and calculus may therefore collect at the base of the lesion producing localized gingivitis. Inflammation persists unless there is frequent professional cleaning. Lip movement also produces further tension on the gingival margin so that progressive destruction is almost inevitable.

Localized or generalized gingival recession may be managed conservatively or surgically and these are described below.

Conservative management of gingival recession

Gingival recession which is not accompanied by disease, i.e. inflammation or pocketing, does not require intervention other than good plaque control and scaling when necessary unless it presents a serious cosmetic problem. The patient must be reassured that recession, especially that produced by over enthusiastic toothbrushing, is of little significance, does not prejudice the life of the tooth and rarely justifies surgical intervention; it simply signals that a less harmful cleaning technique is needed. The main complications of gingival recession are:

- root dentine sensitivity
- abrasion/erosion
- root caries.

Root dentine sensitivity

The exposed root is potentially sensitive via exposed dentinal tubules which can transmit stimuli to the pain receptors in the pulp. When root is first exposed the small amount of cementum covering the dentine soon wears away to uncover the dentine. This usually has open tubules containing the odontoblastic processes passing from the surface to the odontoblast cell body on the pulpal surface. This recently exposed root dentine tends to be sensitive to cold, hot and sweet stimuli and also to drying with an air spray and the use of an ultrasonic scaler in the dental surgery. Repeated stimulation may lead to the formation of peritubular dentine which then reduces the sensitivity and therefore the sensitivity tends to reduce with time. The presence of fluoride ions on the surface of the root may encourage this process and therefore gentle brushing with a fluoride-containing toothpaste helps this process. The sensitivity can return if fresh open tubules are exposed again by abrasion from toothbrushing and/or acid erosion.

Root sensitivity to cold and sweet often deters the patient from brushing properly so that plaque accumulates on the root surface. This actually aggravates the root sensitivity and the patient needs to be reassured that proper cleaning is necessary. Initially it may be necessary to use warm water for brushing but in many cases adequate plaque control reduces the sensitivity. If sensitivity to cold and sweet persists, one of the toothpastes especially formulated to treat the problem (Sensodyne, Emoform, etc.) can be recommended. As stated earlier, sodium fluoride can be very effective as a desensitizing agent and it may be used as Lukomsky's paste (equal parts by weight of sodium fluoride, kaolin and glycerine) which is applied to the dried root on two or three occasions. An amine fluoride in a gel (Duraphat) applied to the dried root surface is also effective and convenient to use. Another useful medicament is 1% hydrocortisone solution applied several times to dried root. Topical guanethidine (1%) has also been recommended for rapid relief from dental hypersensitivity (Hannington-Kitt and Dunne 1993).

Generalized gingival recession resulting from periodontal disease tends to be less sensitive than single or multiple sites of localized recession from other causes. This is because the root dentine in the former situation has been irritated by the disease process over a considerable time leading to peritubular and secondary dentine formation.

One occasionally encounters intractable root sensitivity which does not respond to any topical applications. Usually, this points to pulp pathology, produced either by a large restoration or by a microscopic lateral pulp canal; in this situation endodontics is needed.

Abrasion/erosion

Toothbrushing using a hard brush, vigorous technique or an abrasive toothpaste can lead to surface wear which will progressively lead to the formation of abrasion cavities. Acid erosion from acid containing foods and drinks can lead to dissolution of the calcified content of the surface dentine. This can lead to loss of surface material *per se* or give rise to increased rates of abrasion of the softened surface. Eventually these lesions may become large enough to require restoration.

Root caries

Food stagnation as a result of avoidance of brushing due to sensitivity or within abrasion cavities can lead to conditions which favour the development of dental caries. Root caries demands caries removal and restoration of the resulting cavity. However, root caries may cover a wide area of the exposed root and also involve some surfaces with poor access. Therefore, these lesions may be difficult to restore. Combined abrasion and carious lesions are particularly difficult to restore because the cavities often lack mechanical retention. Furthermore, the only margin available for acid etching is the coronal enamel margin when this is present.

The most common restorative material for these lesions is glass ionomer cement and this produces a much better seal than composites in these situations. It also provides secondary caries protection by its ability to leach fluoride ions. However, it has low wear resistance and patients must be warned not to use hard toothbrushes or abrasive toothpastes.

Surgical treatment of gingival recession

Contraindications to surgery for gingival recession

This form of mucogingival surgery is contraindicated if the patient's oral hygiene is unsatisfactory, if there is any gingivitis and if there is any significant periodontal attachment loss due to chronic periodontitis. It is also contraindicated in smokers, since their response to this type of surgery is poor (Miller 1987).

Preoperative considerations

It must be stressed that surgical intervention is required in very few cases of recession. The chief criterion for such treatment is the presence of progressive disease which is definitely associated with the recession and which persists despite conservative measures.

Where there is inflammation and/or pocketing, i.e. the recession is involved in a progressive periodontal lesion, or where localized labial recession produces a significant cosmetic problem, intervention may be indicated.

If the recession is isolated and reflects an underlying dehiscence, a laterally repositioned graft can be an effective method of correction. If the recession is associated with a muscle attachment and a related inadequate zone of attached gingiva, a free gingival graft may be needed. These surgical techniques and other alternatives are described in the section below.

The type of surgical treatment possible depends on the nature of the lesion(s) and these are classified below:

CLASSIFICATION OF GINGIVAL RECESSION

The classification of gingival recession into type defects is based upon the relationships between the base of the defect, the mucogingival junction and the height of the interdental papillae (**Fig. 21.9**). This also gives a very reliable

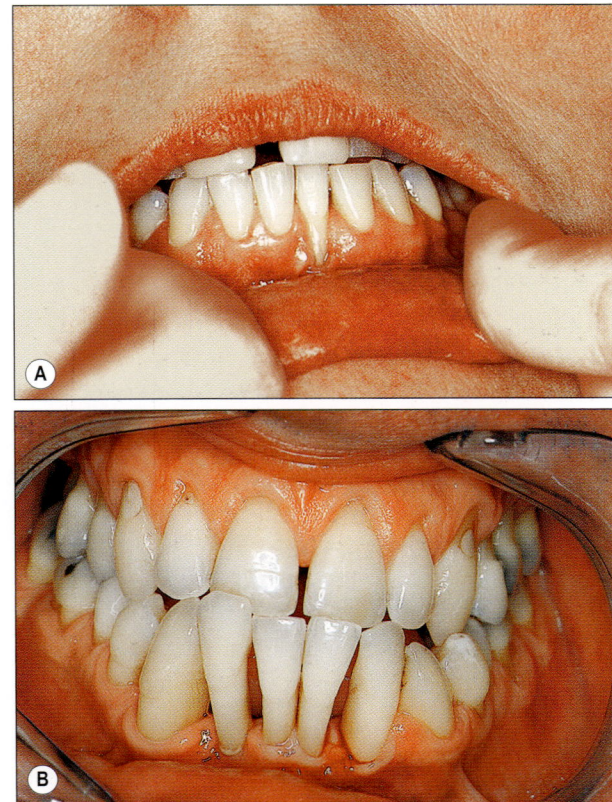

Fig. 21.9 Localized gingival recession. (A) Miller Class I, full height papillae, recession at/or below mucogingival junction, up to 100% coverage possible; (B) Miller Class IV, complete loss of papillary height, not possible to cover.

Table 21.1 *Defect classification, clinical criteria and degree of possible reconstruction*

Classification	Clinical criteria	Possible treatment result
Class I	Full height papillae	Recession within 100% coverage attached gingiva possible
Class II	Full height papillae	Recession at or beyond MGJ 100% coverage possible
Class III	Reduced papilla height	Recession at or beyond MGJ. Coverage only to level related to papilla height
Class IV	Gross flattening or loss of papillae	Not possible to cover

guide to the degree of reconstruction possible. These defects have been classified by Miller (1985a) and this is shown in Table 21.1, along with a summary of the clinical criteria for each group and the possible results of treatment.

As already stated above there are two approaches to the treatment of gingival recession:

1. *Accept and maintain* – If the degree of recession is acceptable to the patient then a decision can be taken to try to maintain the condition. (The appropriate treatment for this has been described above.) Study models should be taken and the condition should be reviewed at regular maintenance visits to determine whether it is stable. If the gingival recession is found to be progressing and the recession is still acceptable to the patient but is close to or beyond the mucogingival junction, then a free gingival graft can be carried out to increase the zone of attached gingiva and maintain the situation.

2. *Repair and eliminate recession* – If the recession is unacceptable to the patient and in one of the categories where successful repair is possible, then an appropriate surgical technique to repair the defect can be discussed with the patient, describing the probable outcome. The aim of these techniques is to cover the exposed root surface to the greatest degree possible and to increase and/or maintain a functional zone of attached gingiva. The possible techniques to consider are listed below:

PEDICLE GRAFTS

- coronally repositioned flap
- laterally repositioned flap
- double papillary flap.

FREE GRAFTS

- full thickness, thick epithelial
- connective tissue
- connective tissue with double papilla.

OTHER REGENERATIVE TECHNIQUES

- GTR with PTFE membranes
- GTR with resorbable membranes.

In reparative techniques, there is still debate about the need for root surface instrumentation or conditioning.

Root surface instrumentation

Miller (1992) states that root preparation will cause a reduction in inflammation which may result in a loss of papillary height by gingival shrinkage. This may affect the potential coverage of the exposed root surface.

The reduction in vascularity also may affect the nutrient supply to the graft. However, any plaque, calculus and stain must be removed from the root surface prior to surgery and patients undergoing these procedures must have immaculate oral hygiene.

Root surface preparation

There is still considerable debate about the need to prepare the surface, and also, if this is deemed necessary, about which method of preparation should be used. A number of clinical researchers have reported good results using citric acid at pH1 for between 2–3 min (Register & Burdick 1975, 1976; Crigger et al 1978; Garrett et al 1978; Nyman et al 1981; Miller 1982). This can be applied with a brush or a cotton bud, and may either be burnished into the root surface or left alone. Tetracycline has also been used as a solution in a similar manner to citric acid and beneficial results have been reported on its use (Wicksjö et al 1986; Demirel et al 1991; Terranova et al 1986). Terranova et al (1986) showed that biochemical manipulation of the dentine surface could affect the cells attaching to it and their growth. They found that treatment of the dentine surface with tetracycline increased the binding of fibronectin (Trombelli et al 1994, 1995) to its surface. They also found that the absorbed fibronectin stimulated the attachment of fibroblasts to its surface and stimulated their growth. Furthermore, they also showed that the absorbed fibronectin suppressed the attachment of epithelial cells to the dentine surface and their growth.

PEDICLE GRAFTS

LATERALLY REPOSITIONED FLAP

The laterally repositioned flap (LRF) is an effective procedure for treating an isolated area of gingival recession where a suitable donor site of keratinized tissue is present. The procedure was first introduced by Grupe and Warren (1956) and has been modified in small detail by several other clinicians. The exposed root is covered by mobilizing a pedicle graft from a suitable adjacent area which is then slid laterally to cover the defect. It is suitable to treat single tooth narrow areas of gingival recession with adequate interdental bone height and an adjacent donor area with an adequate zone of keratinized attached gingiva. This is a one-stage procedure, whereby a pedicle flap is elevated by split-thickness dissection from an adjacent area of keratinized tissue. The blood supply that nourishes the flap over the avascular root surface is supplied by the wide base of the pedicle flap and from the periosteum over the bone surrounding the denuded roots. The flap is secured into position over the denuded root with interrupted silk sutures. The colour blend and root coverage are excellent in well-chosen cases. However, it is generally not suitable for treating isolated wide areas of recession or multiple recessions.

Procedure

The area should receive preparatory periodontal treatment to remove all plaque and calculus from the root surface and resolve any gingival inflammation in the surrounding area and the rest of the mouth (**Fig. 21.10**).

Preparation of the recipient area

Incisions are made down the margins of the defect to remove epithelium from its edges (**Fig. 21.10A**). These incisions meet apically at the base of the defect where the incision is carried into the vestibule. More tissue should be removed from the margin of the defect which is to receive the leading edge of the sliding pedicle graft. This is to allow bone to be uncovered at this margin so that the sutured edge of the flap will lie over bone rather than root surface. This is very important to the success of this

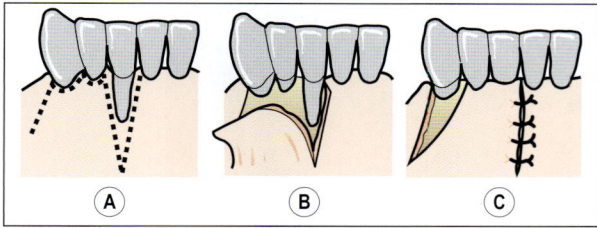

Fig. 21.10 Diagram to illustrate the laterally repositioned flap technique. (A) Incisions are made around the defect and along the gingival margin, then a releasing incision is made approximately two teeth away from the defect; (B) a part full-thickness and part split thickness flap is dissected away from the underlying bone and (C) moved laterally to cover the defect.

procedure and it dictates that the interproximal bone in this area must be at its normal height, i.e. there should be no interdental bone resorption. All the detached tissue should be carefully removed from around the exposed root surface and the root is carefully planed clean and smooth. Some clinicians have recommended root conditioning with citric acid for this procedure. Also if the recipient tooth has a bulky, outstanding root, this lessens the chances of success. Planing back of these prominent roots with a Kirkland No. 7 curette has also been advocated and this would normally be followed by root conditioning.

Preparation of the pedicle graft

A gingival crevicular incision is then made around the next two teeth and a releasing incision is made from the gingival incision into the vestibule (**Fig. 21.10A**). This should produce a flap which is twice as wide as the gingival defect. A part split thickness and part full thickness flap is then carefully developed. The full thickness mucoperiosteal flap is raised from the tooth which will provide the part of the flap covering the exposed root so that the root is directly covered by the periosteum. The part of the flap related to the adjacent tooth which, when raised, will expose the donor area bone, should be developed as a split-thickness flap. This allows the exposed donor area of bone to retain its periosteal covering for protection and additional blood supply. This part of the flap is dissected up to separate the gingival epithelium and connective tissue from the underlying periosteum over the bone (**Fig. 21.10B**). Great care should be taken with this stage of the procedure as perforation of the flap will mean inevitable failure. However, if this technique is attempted in an area potentially involving important nerves, such as in the lower premolar area then a total full thickness flap should be raised to avoid nerve damage. The dissection of the flap is carried into the alveolar mucosa so that the flap can be moved laterally without any tension.

Repositioning of pedicle graft

The flap is moved across the root surface so that its leading margin approximates the receiving edge of gingival tissue making sure that the resulting suture line will lie over bone (**Fig. 21.10C**). These margins are brought together and sutured using 4/0 or 5/0 silk sutures. Care must be taken that the flap fits tightly around the neck of the affected tooth. Three or four sutures may be needed to close the defect tightly and one of these is placed in the vestibule so that no residual eyelet defect is produced. An interdental suture is also placed in each interproximal space covered by the flap. A denuded area of periosteum-covered bone is left distal to the flap (or mesially to the flap if it was moved distally).

A moist sterile gauze is pressed firmly over the flap to fix it in position and minimize any underlying blood clot. A periodontal dressing such as Coe-Pack is placed over the wound area.

Postoperative care

The usual postoperative instructions are given with emphasis on the need to avoid vigorous lip movements. This procedure produces very little swelling or discomfort and healing is usually uneventful.

The dressing and sutures are removed after 1 week, by which time the suture line should be united and the denuded area covered by healing tissue.

Rarely does the wound need to be covered for more than 1 week. The patient is instructed to keep the area clean with a twice-daily chlorhexidine mouthwash and frequent warm saline washes. Irritation of the healing graft must be avoided. Careful toothbrushing with a soft brush can be started when the pack and sutures are removed but this should gently clean the tooth surface down to but not on to the gingiva.

Two weeks after surgery, the suture line should be fading and the denuded area should be covered with epithelium. One month after surgery, the wound is fully healed but it is still unwise to probe the gingival crevice over the defect. Probing is best left for about 6 months and should be carried out with great care.

Mode of healing

The exact form of healing that takes place after the laterally repositioned flap procedure is still debated. There are two possibilities:

1. Crevicular epithelium grows down the inner surface of the flap against the root surface to form a long epithelial attachment and the gingival fibre bundles keep the flap closely adapted to the root. It is also feasible that hemidesmosomes connect the epithelial downgrowth to the root surface so that a firm attachment is formed.
2. Epithelial downgrowth does not take place and a fibrous tissue connection forms between the flap and the root surface. This could imply the deposition of new cementum on to the root surface so that Sharpey's fibres can be formed. The differentiation of cementoblasts and formation of cementum seem unlikely without the concomitant formation of crestal bone and so far no evidence of such repair has been produced.

Whichever form of healing actually does take place, at a clinical level the graft can remain stable for many years providing that the gingival margin is free of plaque and therefore free of inflammation (**Fig. 21.11A, B**). Slight recession of the graft may take place but rarely recurrence of pocketing or of a new defect.

MODIFICATION OF LATERALLY REPOSITIONED FLAP

The standard laterally repositioned flap can sometimes result in some gingival recession in the donor area and a modification which spares the marginal gingiva at the donor site has been devised (Pennel et al 1965). This is only possible if a sufficiently wide zone of attached gingiva is present in the donor area to produce the desired zone of keratinized tissue at the recipient site. It has the advantage of leaving the interdental papillae *in situ* at the recipient site, which makes it easier to secure the pedicle graft at the required height. It also leaves a much smaller exposed area at the donor site than the conventional technique.

Procedure

Recipient site

Horizontal incisions are made across the base of the two interdental papillae of the recipient tooth so that these are retained in their original positions. These will form a butt joint against which the repositioned sliding flap will lie. Two vertical incisions are then made down to the vestibule on either side of the recession area to expose bone around its margin

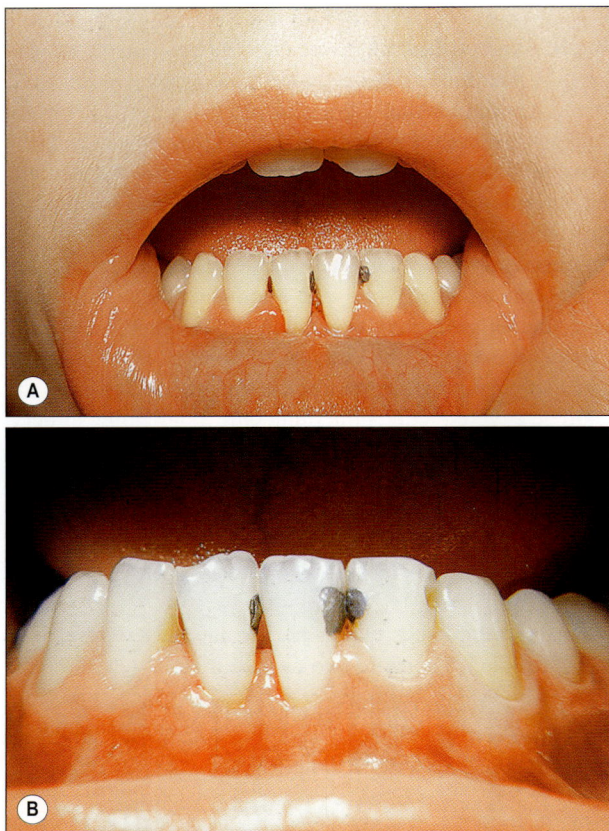

Fig. 21.11 Laterally repositioned flap. (A) Localized Miller Class II recession on both lower central incisors complicated by a gingival insertion of a lower labial frenum in a 14-year-old boy. The recession followed lower arch orthodontic treatment for crowding. (B) The clinical condition 12 months after a frenectomy followed (after healing) by a laterally repositioned flap. It shows good root surface coverage. The unsightly interproximal amalgams were replaced by composites after his high caries rate was brought under control by dietary changes.

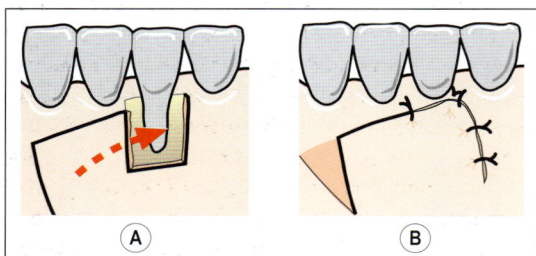

Fig. 21.12 Modified laterally repositioned flap. (A) Horizontal incisions below papillae of recipient tooth and below gingival margins of donor teeth. Bone is exposed around the root of the recipient tooth and a sloping vertical incision is made to delineate the flap; (B) flap slid over defect and sutured into place.

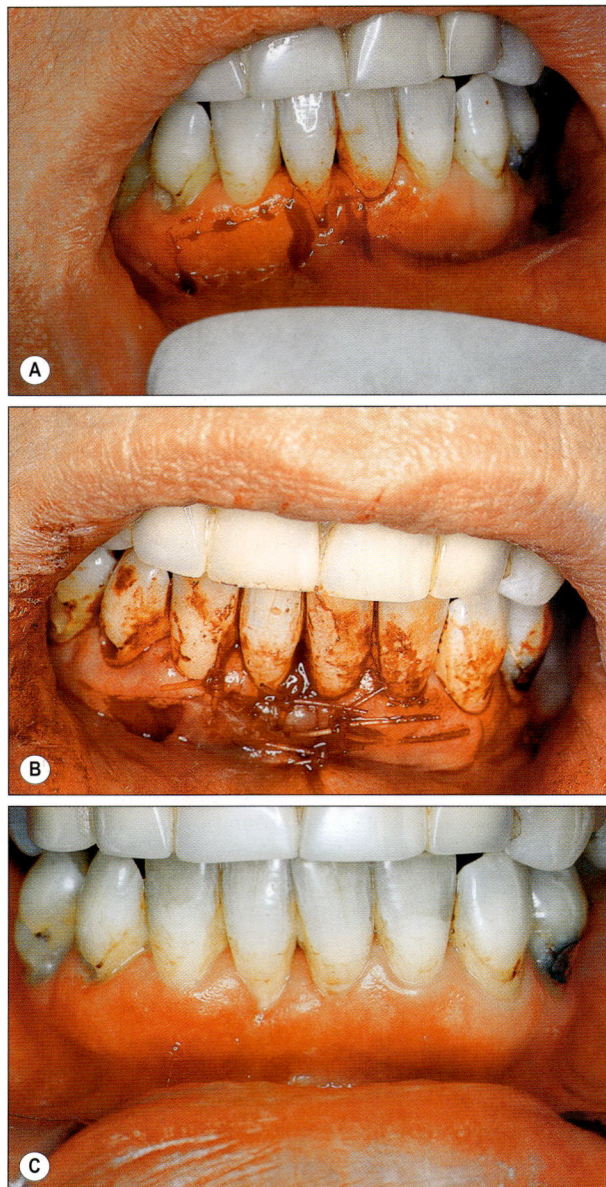

Fig. 21.13 Clinical pictures of the modified laterally repositioned flap in a 60-year-old woman. (A) Incisions; (B) sutured into new position; (C) 2 years after surgery showing improved coverage but some relapse. (Courtesy Dr C A Waterman).

(Figs 21.12A, 21.13A). This tissue is cut off by a further horizontal incision at its base and the tissue is removed. The root surface is carefully scaled and planed and may be conditioned if desired.

Donor site

A slightly sloping horizontal incision is then made from the tip of the distal vertical recipient site incision and is carried below the interdental papillae and marginal gingiva of the donor site teeth. A further slightly sloping vertical incision is then made distally down into the vestibule to delineate the donor flap (Figs 21.12A, 21.13A).

This flap is carefully dissected up as a split-thickness flap, leaving the periosteum in place. This flap is then fully mobilized and slid across to cover the defect where it fits into a butt joint with the recipient site papillae (Figs 21.12B, 21.13B). The flap is sutured into position with resorbable 5/0 gut sutures. Two sutures join it to the retained papillae at the recipient site and a further two or three join the vertical flap margin to the mesial edge of the recipient site. Only a small area of donor site periosteum is left uncovered with this procedure.

The area is covered with either a conventional pack such as Coe-Pack or a Surgicel/cyanoacrylate pack. With this latter method, Surgicel is placed over the area, and held in place using cyanoacrylate glue (Superglue). This can also be covered with Vaseline with tetracycline powder mixed into it if required (Miller 1982, 1985b, 1992). Coe-Pack is replaced after a week and replaced for a further week if necessary. The latter pack is left until it drops off, usually after 3 weeks.

Healing of both the donor and recipient sites is usually uneventful. Some relapse of root surface coverage occurs in a small proportion of these cases treated with either a conventional or modified laterally repositioned flap (Fig. 21.13C).

DOUBLE PAPILLARY FLAP

This technique was introduced by Cohen and Ross (1968) and is a variant of the laterally repositioned flap. The basic technique is similar except that the donor tissue is mobilized from the adjacent papillae rather than from an adjacent tooth. There is less exposure of donor site bone with this procedure and less tension is placed on the donor tissue. The interdental septum at the papillary area is of greater thickness than the facial or lingual alveolar plates and are less likely to be damaged when the overlying tissues are disturbed. A disadvantage of this technique is that the proximal papillae must be of sufficient bulk both mesio-distally and cervico-apically to cover the defect. Small papillae imply small interdental septa and under these conditions this procedure would both fail to cover the defect as well as possibly causing damage to the underlying bony septa.

Procedure

This procedure is suitable for a recession defect on a tooth with bulky mesial and distal papillae. The exposed root surface is scaled and root planed. A V-shaped incision is made around the margin of the recessed gingiva to expose connective tissue at its edge (**Fig. 21.14A**). The distal tissue is bevelled to expose a wider zone of connective tissue to accept the mesial portion of the graft. Mesial and distal vertical incisions are made and carried into the vestibule to mobilize the two papillae (**Fig. 21.14A**). The two papillary flaps are carefully raised and repositioned to cover the labial surface of the exposed root so that the join line coincides with the distal margin of the defect. The flaps are sutured together in this position with resorbable 5/0 medium gut sutures (**Fig. 21.14B**). This correct positioning is very important since placement of sutures at the midline of the exposed root will lead to inadequate coadaptation of tissue. This will result in the creation of a dehiscence at the suture line and failure of the procedure. The most apical suture is passed through the periosteum to stabilize the position of the graft. In addition, either mesial and distal sutures or a sling suture around the tooth can be placed to stabilize the graft further. A dressing such as Coe-Pack may be carefully placed over the area for a week.

CORONALLY REPOSITIONED FLAP

The coronally repositioned flap (CRF) (Harvey 1965; Bernimoulin et al 1975) can be used on its own or in combination with other procedures to treat multiple areas of recession. It can also be used in combination with other procedures to treat localized recession. On its own it cannot increase the amount of keratinized gingiva over that which is already present at the site. This however may be achievable if it is combined with other procedures which can fulfil this function. An example of this is its combination with the free gingival graft to treat the combined problem of gingival recession and lack of attached gingiva.

Leknes et al (2005) compared the treatment of gingival recession defects by coronally positioned flap procedures with or without biodegradable membranes (see below) in 22 patients over 6-year follow-up results for these two treatment approaches. They found similar favourable results with both procedures.

By contrast, Silva et al (2007) used a coronally positioned flap to treat a Miller Class I defect in a maxillary canine or premolar in 10 current smokers (≥10 cigarettes daily for ≥5 years) and 10 non-smokers (never smokers) and measured probing depth, clinical attachment level, recession depth, and width of keratinized tissue at baseline and 6, 12 and 24 months. They found that the long-term stability of CPF outcomes was less than desirable, particularly in smokers. Two years after a coronally positioned flap procedure, smokers had significantly greater residual recession compared to non-smokers both statistically and clinically.

Procedure

The free gingival graft is first carried out to increase the attached gingival zone (see full description in following section). After complete healing, a full-thickness mucoperiosteal flap is raised and extended to the base of the vestibule. It is then moved upwards in a coronal direction to cover the exposed roots of the teeth and maintained in this position by interdental suturing and the placement of a periodontal dressing. In the combined procedure the free gingival graft is used to provide new keratinized attached gingiva and the coronally repositioned flap to carry this up over the root surface.

FREE GRAFTS

FULL THICKNESS, THICK EPITHELIAL FLAP

The free gingival graft (FGG) was introduced by Nabors (1966). It is designed to increase the width of keratinized gingiva (Sullivan & Atkins 1968a) but can also be used to treat gingival recession (Sullivan & Atkins 1968b, 1969; Miller 1988). Unlike the pedicle graft, this procedure takes keratinized palatal epithelium and connective tissue from its original site and relocates it to a remote donor site. The graft is placed over a freshly prepared bed of connective tissue and sutured in place. The underlying connective tissue bed nourishes the graft until it builds its own blood supply. This forms as the result of blood vessels growing into it from the underlying connective tissue base (see below).

As this graft retains none of its own blood supply and is totally dependent on the bed of recipient vessels, it was originally developed to increase the zone of attached gingiva and not specifically to cover denuded root. New attached gingiva is produced by grafting keratinized palatal mucosa and its inductive connective tissue over a recipient bed previously covered by non-keratinized alveolar mucosa. However, several modifications have improved the root coverage capabilities of this procedure. Maynard (1977) developed two procedures: first, the placement of a free gingival graft to create a band of keratinized gingiva and second, a coronally repositioned flap (see above) to pull the tissue coronally over the exposed root(s). Holbrook and Ochsenbein (1983) used thick, stretched, free gingival grafts with intricate suturing to improve the graft's adaptation to the recipient bed

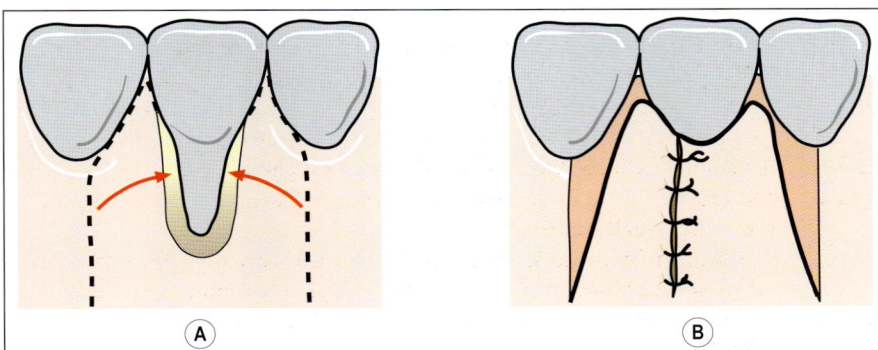

Fig. 21.14 Double papillary flap. (A) Incisions (i) around root to expose bone with wider zone distally to provide base for suture line; (ii) delineating flap margins. (B) Papillae transposed to cover defect and sutured over the bone exposed distal to defect.

and limit the amount of dead space, which could hinder vascularization. Miller (1982, 1985b) emphasized root planing and citric acid treatment of the exposed roots.

All of these modifications have improved the capability of free grafts to survive over avascular root surfaces. The coverage of wide or multiple areas of recession are best treated by the double procedure of Maynard (1977) (see below) while the free graft alone, using the modifications of Holbrook and Ochsenbein (1983) and Miller (1982, 1985b) can be used to cover single narrow root surface defects (**Fig. 21.16A**).

Procedures

The procedure differs in several details according to whether the aim is only to increase the zone of attached gingiva, leaving the existing gingiva undisturbed (Procedure 1) or whether the aim is additionally to cover area(s) of root exposed by gingival recession (Procedure 2).

Suitable donor and recipient sites are chosen and local analgesia given.

Preparation of recipient site

The following technique has been proposed by Miller (1982, 1985b).

For Procedure 1, an incision is made along the mucogingival junction (**Fig. 21.15A, C**). For Procedure 2 techniques, an incision made along the gingiva of the recipient site to allow butt joining of the graft to adjacent tissue

(**Fig. 21.15B, C**). The apical margin of the flap is raised and dissected through the connective tissue as a split thickness flap to delineate the connective tissue bed of the recipient site (**Fig. 21.15D**). This extends into the area previously covered by non-keratinized alveolar mucosa. Bulow Dry Foil is then placed over the bed to act as a template for the graft and trimmed to size.

Root preparation

This is only necessary for type 2 procedures and the method outlined is that proposed by Miller (1985b). If the exposed root surface is buccally prominent it is planed back to reduce the possibility of recurrence and to reduce localized pressures on the graft. This is done either using a Kirkland No. 12 curette or a Gracey curette. A butt joint is made at the cemento-enamel junction of the tooth. The root surface is then conditioned using pH1 citric acid using cotton buds or a burnishing technique. It is left until there is a frosted finish on the root surface after profuse rinsing.

Preparation of donor site

The template is placed on the palate and the graft outlined. It is delineated with a No. 15 Swann–Morton blade, making an incision about 3 mm deep so that the graft includes an adequate thickness of connective tissue. In fact it is this connective-tissue layer which is the functional part of the graft. A split-thickness graft is carefully dissected from the underlying deeper connective tissue with

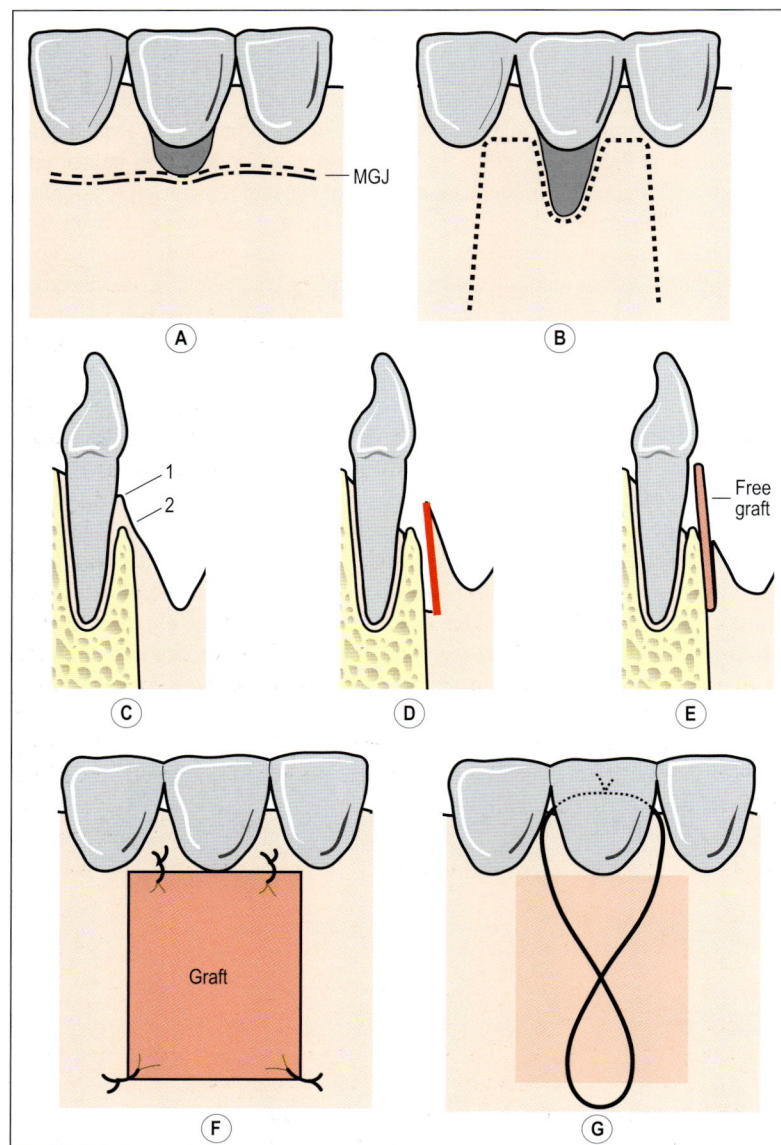

Fig. 21.15 Free gingival graft. (A) Incision for procedure 1 at mucogingival junction (MGJ). (B) Incisions for procedure 2 to cover exposed roots. Horizontal incision across base of papillae, which are left *in situ*. The incision continues around the recession area. Two vertical incisions delineate the flap. (C) Incision for procedure 1(1) and 2(2) in other plane. (D) Dissection of split-thickness flap to leave tissue over bone to nourish free graft. (E) Free graft in position. (F) Papillary and apical stretching sutures. (G) Vertical stabilizing suture.

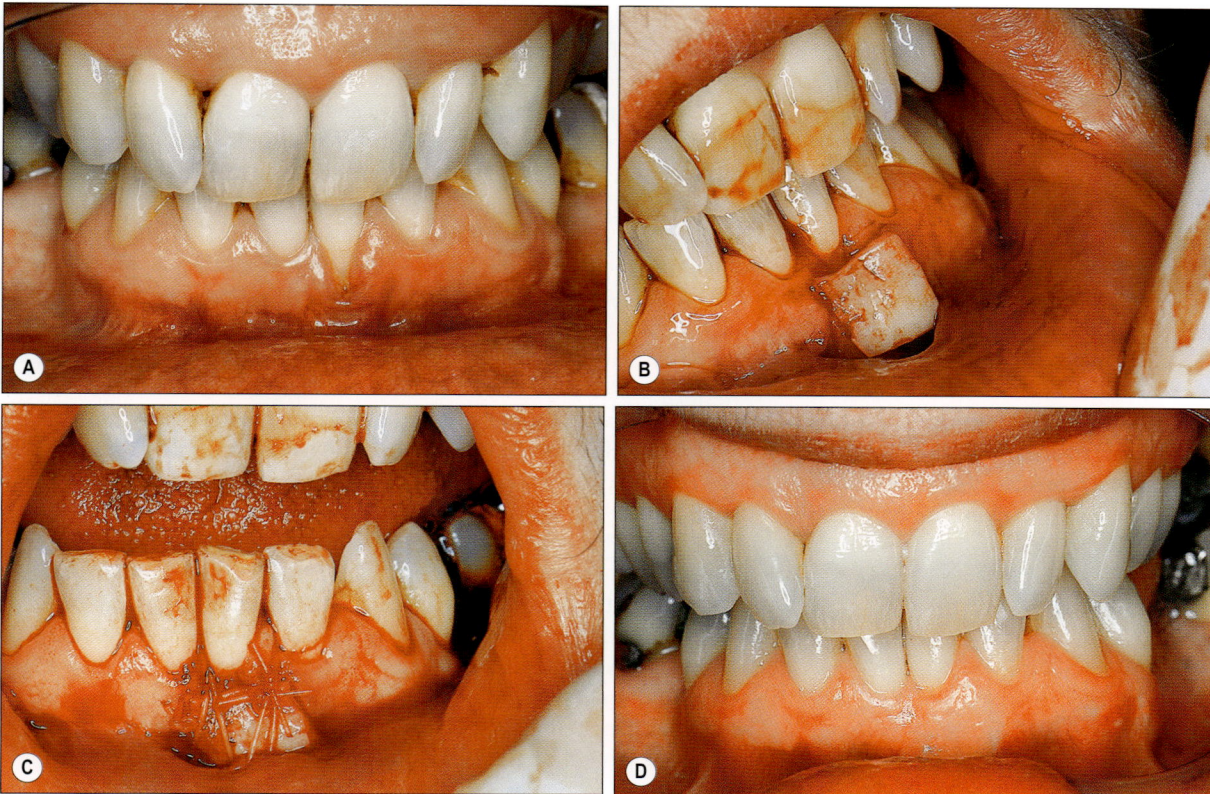

Fig. 21.16 Free gingival graft to treat localized recession in a 55-year-old woman. (A) Preoperative picture showing, recession on lower left central incisor extending to mucogingival junction; (B) free graft placed in position before suturing; (C) graft sutured in position; (D) postoperative result after five years. (Courtesy Dr C A Waterman).

the No. 15 blade. The graft should be at least 2–3 mm thick and any adipose tissue on the inner side can be left for root coverage. However, if root coverage is not being attempted then it should be 1–2 mm with no adipose tissue.

Placement of graft

The graft should be placed *in situ* (**Figs 21.15E, 21.16B**) and trimmed quickly, if necessary, to help to maintain its vitality. The flap raised at the recipient site can be cut off at this point as it is no longer needed, and the graft can be sutured in place.

Three types of suture have been described for use with this procedure (Miller 1982, 1985; Jahnke et al 1993). These are (**Fig. 21.15F, G**):

1. Papillary sutures positioned interdentally (**Fig. 21.15F**)
2. Apical stretching sutures (**Fig. 21.15F**)
3. Vertical stabilizing sutures (**Fig. 21.15G**).

The vertical stabilizing sutures (**Fig. 21.15G**) criss-cross over the graft without going through it. The suture passes from the palatal aspect of the tooth through the right interdental space. It then passes diagonally across the surface of the graft to its base at the opposite corner. It then penetrates through the periosteum at the base of the graft and crosses diagonally in the opposite direction to the left interdental space. It finally passes through this to meet the starting end to be tied off palatally.

These sutures allow the graft to be approximated closely to the root surface, while still allowing flow of nutrient. Resorbable catgut sutures are used to avoid trauma to the healing area. To protect the graft, Surgicel is placed over the area, and held in place using cyanoacrylate glue (Superglue). This is then covered with Vaseline into which tetracycline powder has been mixed (Miller 1982, 1985b, 1992). This is left until it drops off, usually

after 3 weeks and cleanliness is maintained using chlorhexidine mouthwashes. The patient may be placed on tetracycline for 2 weeks.

The palate can be similarly covered, or an acrylic stent may be used, although there is good healing after only 1 week.

The end-result can look extremely good (**Fig. 21.16A, C**), and this is a very predictable procedure with good long-term results (**Fig. 21.16D**). However, in some cases, it can look bulky or of a different colour.

Healing of the graft

Vascularization of the gingival graft takes place from the underlying connective-tissue bed. This can commence as early as the first 2–4 days, before which nutrients to the graft are supplied by tissue fluid. Capillary buds grow from the underlying connective tissue into the graft and these vessels anastomose and mature to form a new vasculature which is complete by about the 14th day. Because nutrition to the graft is minimal during the first 2–3 days the surface layers of the epithelium degenerate, necrose and are desquamated. A layer of new epithelium is present after 4–5 days, rete pegs are formed at 7–14 days and keratinization takes about 28 days. The maturation process takes place under the inductive influence of the palatal connective tissue.

Factors affecting success

1. Incorrect choice of site for procedure used, i.e. wrong class of gingival recession
2. The graft may be too thick. If such a graft becomes vascularized the tablet of tissue stands away from the rest of the tissue
3. If the graft is too thin it may perforate and necrose
4. If the underlying blood clot is too thick the graft may be discarded.

CONNECTIVE-TISSUE GRAFT (CTG)

This type of graft has a number of advantages over the free epithelial graft (Edel 1974; Langer & Langer 1985; Jahnke et al 1993). These are:

1. There is a closed palatal wound
2. The aesthetic result is claimed to be better
3. There is a better potential blood supply from the periosteum beneath and the split thickness flap above.

This procedure was introduced by Langer and Langer (1985) as a method of gaining root coverage in cases with severe recession involving either isolated or multiple teeth. The subepithelial connective tissue graft is a combination of a pedicle graft and a free autogenous connective-tissue graft performed simultaneously. In this procedure, the connective tissue receives a blood supply from the periosteum beneath and the split thickness flap above and this increases its chances of survival over the avascular root surface. The procedure also avoids an open palatal wound and produces a better aesthetic result because it avoids the problem of colour differentiation which occurs between a full thickness graft and the surrounding tissues (Schluger et al 1990).

Procedure

Preparation of recipient site

A horizontal incision is made around the teeth to be treated and the area is bounded by two vertical relieving incisions which extend well beyond the mucogingival junction to create a wide base for the flap. The horizontal incision passes along the base of each included interdental papilla and then into the gingival crevice buccally to each tooth (**Figs 21.17, 21.18A**). Great care must be taken not to lift the papillae. The incisions are carefully deepened and the flap is carefully dissected from the underlying periosteum and deep connective tissue as a split thickness flap. The edge of the flap is first raised and held under tension with fine tissue forceps to allow careful sharp dissection with a No. 15 blade. Great care must be taken not to perforate the flap as this will compromise its blood supply, which is an important source of nutrient to the connective-tissue graft (**Fig. 21.18E**). The flap is freed apically so that there will be very little tension when it is ultimately pulled coronally. The size of the connective-tissue graft is determined by the size of the recipient base and its height and length are measured. The graft must be large enough to cover the exposed roots and connective-tissue bed in all directions. The connective-tissue bed is the second important source of blood supply to the overlying graft.

Root preparation

Root planing of the exposed roots is carefully carried out. Additional preparation with citric acid or tetracycline may also be carried out as described in the last section. Opinion is divided as to whether this is necessary or beneficial.

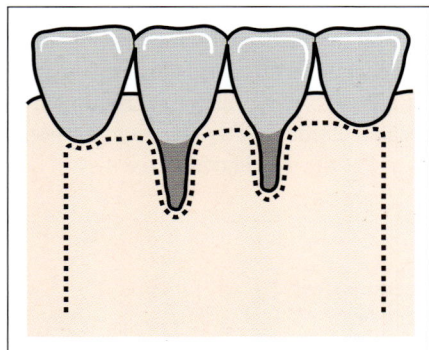

Fig. 21.17 Incisions for connective tissue graft at recipient site. The incision passes across the base of the papillae to leave these *in situ* for suturing.

Preparation of donor site

The donor site is prepared palatally by making two parallel horizontal bevelled incisions which are made 3 mm from the gingival margin using a No. 15 blade or a special two-blade scalpel (**Figs 21.18B, C, 21.19**). It is made from the canine to the first molar area since the connective tissue is thicker and better vascularized in this area and the rugae are of no concern because the graft is taken internally. A split thickness flap is raised with or without mesial and distal vertical relieving incisions. A wedge of connective tissue of about 1.5 mm thickness along with its thin border of epithelium is carefully dissected out (**Figs 21.18C, D, 21.19**). Care should be taken to avoid the palatine vessels but staying anterior to the first molar should avoid this problem. The length of the flap and the depth of the dissection depend on the size of the recipient area to be covered. This procedure leaves the outer epithelialized flap to be replaced for primary intention wound closure.

A special scalpel handle (**Fig. 21.18B, C**) has been devised to accept two blades 1.5 mm apart for use in obtaining a suitable connective-tissue graft. This was designed by Harris (1992) for use in the double papillary graft/connective-tissue graft (see below) but can be used in this procedure also if available.

It is advisable to suture the palatal flap back into position immediately after removing the donor tissue as this will reduce the size of the blood clot which will form. A method of suturing, which produces compression will also further this aim. Horizontal mattress sutures are used and they begin by passing through the mesial interproximal space on the buccal surface. They then penetrate the palatal mucosa apical and distal to the base of the graft and then exit the palate mesially. They finally cross to the distal interproximal space to be tied on the buccal surface. These sutures compress the palatal flap and approximate its edges. This should bring about rapid haemostasis. A dressing is optional and usually not necessary. The patient reports much less discomfort and bleeding problems than with the free gingival graft because of the full coverage.

Graft placement

The connective-tissue graft is carefully positioned over the denuded roots with its epithelialized border coronally (**Fig. 21.18F**). It is stretched slightly to extend mesially and distally to cover the full length of the prepared bed and should extend down apically over the full depth of the prepared bed. Some authorities advocate suturing the graft to the papillae separately using interrupted chrome gut interdental sutures and an atraumatic needle (**Fig. 21.18G**). Alternatively, the graft and the overlying flap may be secured into place together (see below). This second method does, however, depend on completely covering the connective-tissue graft right up to its thin epithelial border. This thin border of epithelium is left on the graft because it helps to colour blend it with the adjacent tissues. It must be placed coronally to the cement-enamel junction.

Replacement of the recipient overlying flap

The recipient flap is repositioned coronally to cover as much of the connective-tissue graft as possible (**Fig. 21.18H**). It is sutured in place using resorbable gut sutures either separately by interdental gut sutures or in combination with securing the graft. In this alternative form of suturing the gut sutures pass through the flap, the graft and finally the papilla. The graft is protected by using a surgical cyanoacrylate and Vaseline covering (see previous section). The patient is instructed to use chlorhexidine mouthwashes and may be put on tetracycline for 2 weeks. The area is left until the pack comes off naturally, usually after 2–3 weeks.

CONNECTIVE-TISSUE GRAFT WITH DOUBLE PAPILLARY FLAP

In both the above techniques when used separately, the graft over the root surface relies on the collateral circulation bringing nutrient from nearby areas. In this modification, proposed by Harris (1992), the graft is covered over the root

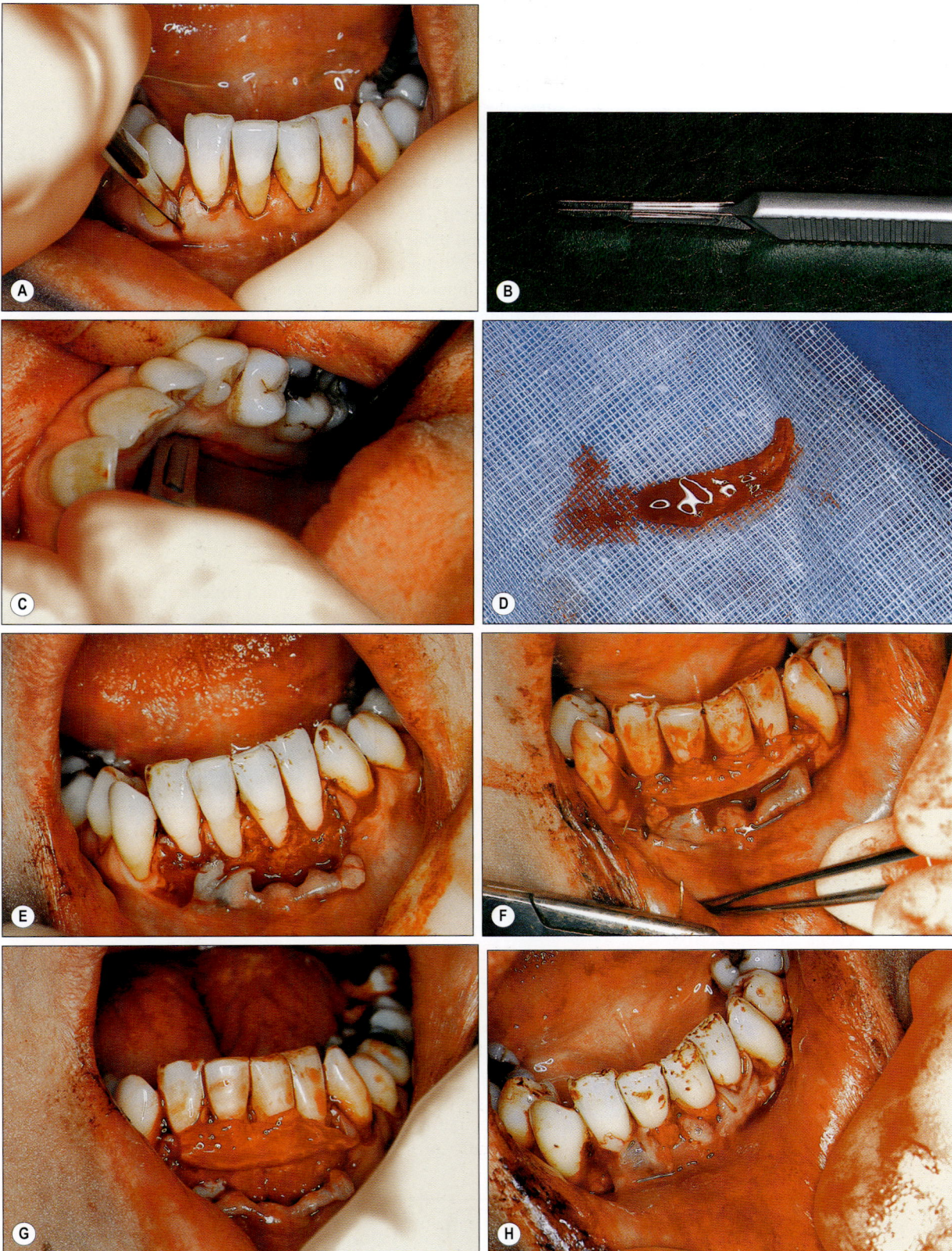

Fig. 21.18 Connective tissue graft in a 54-year-old woman. (A) Incisions: the papillae are left *in situ* for suturing. (B) A special scalpel handle with two blades 1.5 mm apart for taking optimum thickness connective tissue graft from the palate. (C) Incisions with special scalpel to obtain connective tissue graft from palate; (D) connective tissue graft so obtained. (E) Recipient site flap raised to expose bed for graft; (F) connective tissue graft in position over root surfaces and prepared bed; (G) connective tissue graft sutured in position. (H) The recipient site flap is then coronally advanced over graft and sutured. (Courtesy Dr C A Waterman).

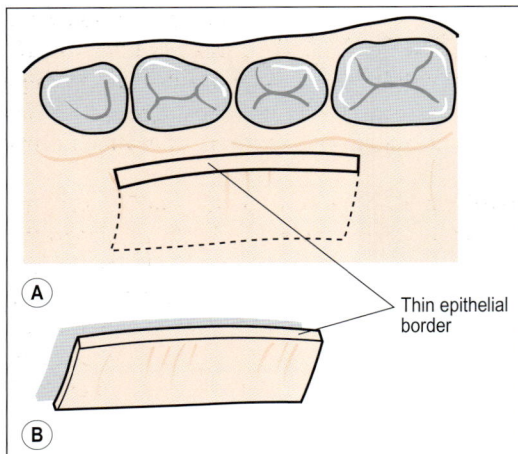

Fig. 21.19 (A) Incisions for connective tissue graft from palate. Two parallel incisions 1.5 mm apart are made from the canine to first molar. This can either be done with a conventional scalpel holder with a No.15 blade or more easily by a special two bladed scalpel (see Fig. 21.18B,C). The connective tissue graft is then dissected out. (B) The resultant graft with a thin epithelialized upper margin (see also Fig. 21.18D).

surface with tissue brought together by a double papillary type flap. The graft gets its blood supply both from the underlying periosteum, mesial, distal and apical to the exposed root, and from the covering double papillary pedicle flaps.

Procedure

Preparation of recipient site

The recipient site incisions are the same as those previously described for a double papillary graft coverage of a recession defect (see previous section). The tips of the papillae are left *in situ* (**Figs 21.20A, 21.21A**) to allow the graft to be sutured to them. For this combined procedure split thickness flaps are raised from both papillae (**Fig. 21.21A**).

Root preparation

The root surface is planed thoroughly to reduce any labial bulbosity of the affected tooth. It is then conditioned with tetracycline using a 250 mg tetracycline capsule dissolved in 2 mL saline.

Preparation of donor site

The procedure is the same as that described for the connective tissue graft (see previous section). A special scalpel handle (**Fig. 21.21B**) has been devised to obtain an optimum thickness connective tissue graft with this procedure (Harris 1992). It accepts two blades 1.5 mm apart which give an ideal incision in order to remove the graft (**Fig. 21.21C**).

Placement of the graft

The graft is tried in and its size slightly modified if necessary. It is sutured into position using 3/0 or 4/0 catgut in three parts.

1. Suture the connective-tissue graft to the remaining interdental papillae (**Figs 21.20B, 21.21D**)
2. To bring the flaps together as a double papilla (**Figs 21.20C, 21.21E**)
3. A sling suture to hold the flap over the graft (**Fig. 21.20D, 21.21F**).

The area is dressed using Surgicel and cyanoacrylate and this is covered with Vaseline and tetracycline. This last covering is made by mixing the contents of one 250 mg capsule of tetracycline into the Vaseline. Dietary restrictions are imposed and the patient is instructed to use a chlorhexidine mouthwash until normal oral hygiene can be carried out.

Resolution

The pack is left in position until it comes off naturally, usually after 2–3 weeks. Following this the resolution back to health and normal oral hygiene is usually quick and uneventful.

HISTOLOGICAL RESULT OF GRAFTING PROCEDURES OVER EXPOSED ROOT SURFACES

At best, all the grafting techniques which cover exposed root surfaces may result in a connective-tissue attachment to the root surface although this is extremely unlikely based on current knowledge of tissue relationships. Downgrowth of junctional epithelium occurs rapidly and may act to protect the root surface from the resorptive effects of gingival connective tissue (see Ch. 20). This results in the formation of a long junction epithelium which may be firmly adherent to the root surface. This relationship can be stable, but it is not as resistant to either inflammation or to trauma as would be the case if complete regeneration including bone had occurred. Regeneration in this context implies the restoration of the various components of the periodontium lost through disease or trauma in their appropriate locations, amounts and relationships to each other (Aukhil 1991).

Trombelli (1999) reviewed the various surgical techniques used to treat recession defects and their outcomes. It was concluded that pedicle and free gingival grafts heal for the most part by the downgrowth of long junctional epithelium with variable small amounts of new connective tissue attachment at the most apical margin of the lesion. Barrier membranes were shown in the reviewed studies to produce variable amounts of new connective tissue attachment and bone extending varying distances from the apical margin of the lesion.

The clinical success of root coverage with autogenous connective tissue (CT) or acellular dermal grafts (ADM) has been reported although limited histological results of these grafts have been reported (Cummings et al

Fig. 21.20 Connective tissue graft with double papillary flap. (A) Incisions: the tips of the papillae are left *in situ* for suturing of the graft. (B) Connective tissue graft sutured to papillae. (C) Double papillary flaps brought together and sutured over graft. (D) A sling suture tied lingually to hold the flap tightly over the graft.

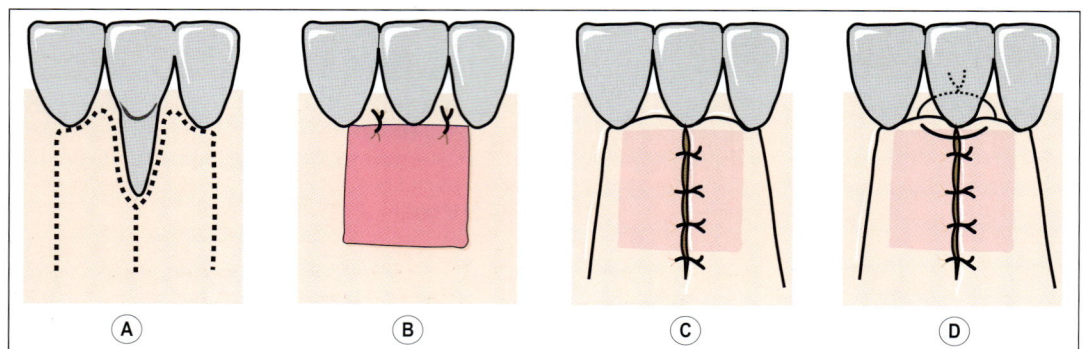

2005). These workers studied the histological results of CT grafts, ADM grafts, and coronally advanced flaps to cover denuded roots in humans. They obtained specimens from four patients previously treatment planned for extractions of three or more anterior teeth. Three teeth in each patient were selected and randomly designated to receive either a CT or ADM graft beneath a coronally advanced flap (tests) or coronally advanced flap alone (control). At 6 months postoperatively, block section extractions were performed and the teeth processed for histologic evaluation with hematoxylin–eosin (H&E) and Verhoeff's stains.

Histologically, both the CT and ADM were well incorporated within the recipient tissues. New fibroblasts, vascular elements, and collagen were present throughout the ADM, while retention of the transplanted elastic fibres was apparent. No effect on the keratinization or connective tissue organization of the overlying alveolar mucosa was evident with either graft. For both materials, areas of cemental deposition were present within the root notches, the alveolar bone was essentially unaffected, and the attachments to the root surfaces were similar. Although CT and ADM have a slightly different histological appearance, both can successfully be used to cover denuded roots with similar attachments and no adverse healing.

Hirsch et al (2005) carried out a 2-year clinical study in 101 patients treated for localized gingival recession by dermal matrix allografts. They showed that coverage of root by subpedicle acellular dermal matrix allografts or subepithelial connective tissue autografts is a very predictable procedure which is stable for 2 years postoperatively. They also showed that subepithelial connective tissue autografts resulted in significant increases in defect coverage, keratinized gingival gain and attachment gain.

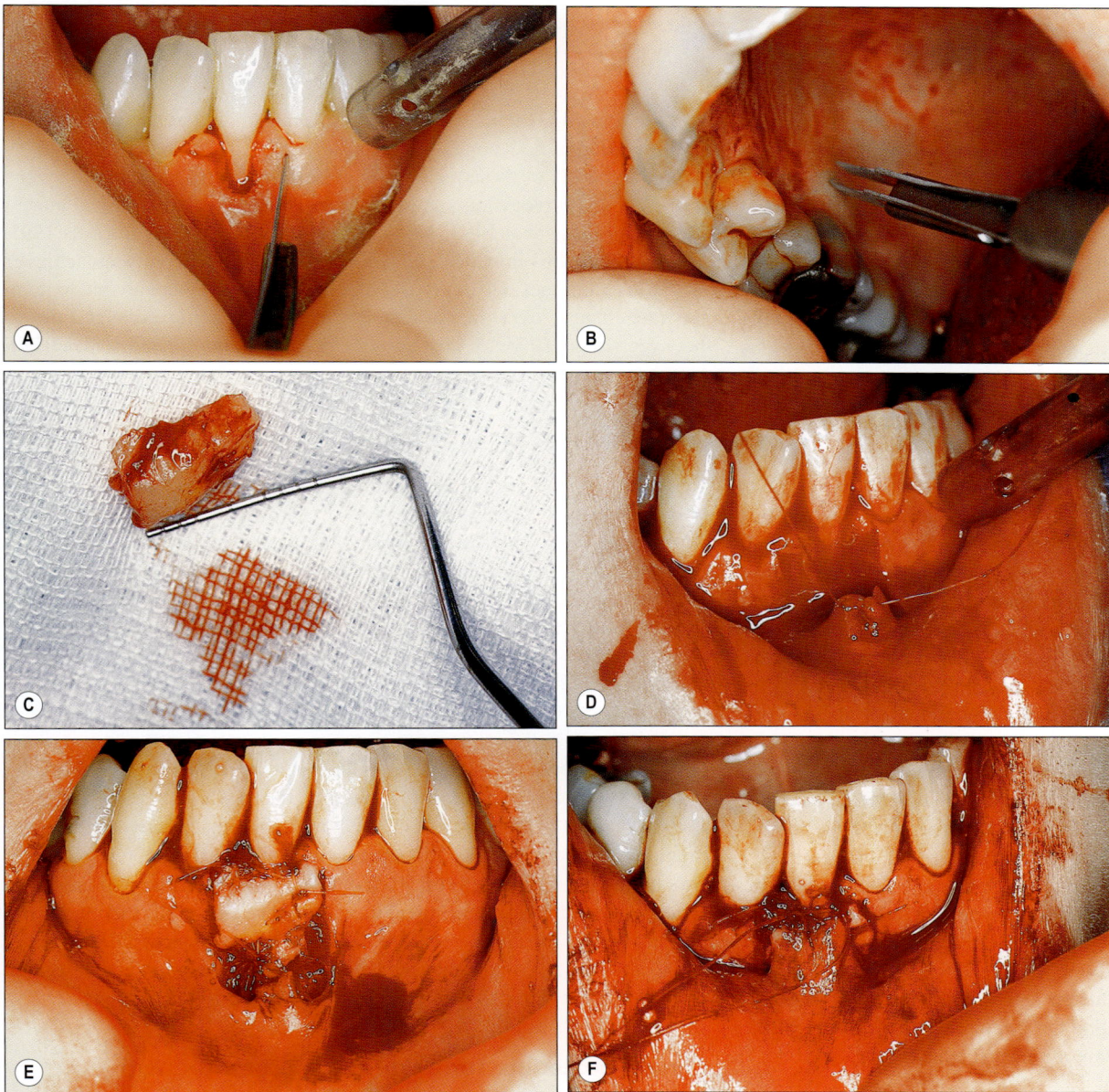

Fig. 21.21 Connective tissue graft with double papillary flap in a 29-year-old woman. (A) Incisions: the tips of the papilla are left *in situ* for suturing of the graft. (B) Harris knife used to obtain connective tissue graft from palate. (C) Connective tissue graft so obtained. (D) Graft placed and secured over root surface and recipient site. (E) Double papillary flaps sutured together over graft. (F) A sling suture tied lingually to hold the flap tightly over the graft. (Courtesy Dr C A Waterman).

GUIDED TISSUE REGENERATION

To have any chance of regenerating bone, cementum and periodontal attachment in these areas some form of guided tissue regenerative (GTR) technique needs to be performed. Standard GTR using Gore-Tex® membranes always require a secondary procedure to remove the PTFE membrane. This has the disadvantage of disturbing any newly formed osteoid material. Also flaps replaced over Gore-Tex® membranes may shrink and therefore coverage of any osteoid which might form may be difficult with this two-stage technique. However, the use of two-stage GTR techniques for buccal recession in monkeys has been shown to give rise to a reduction in gingival recession, a gain in connective tissue attachment and the formation of new bone (Gottlow et al 1990). They have been used successfully clinically to treat buccal gingival recession including defects in excess of 5 mm (Tinti & Vincenzi 1990a,b; Pini Prato et al 1992).

In addition, space maintenance is a problem with the use of PTFE membranes because they easily collapse and thus eradicate any space between the membrane and the root surface into which healing tissue from the periodontal ligament may grow (Nyman et al 1982). To avoid this disadvantage, techniques have evolved to help maintain this space with conventional PTFE membranes (Pini Prato et al 1992; Tinti et al 1992, 1993; Tinti & Vincenzi 1994). These include the use of a suture to tent the membrane inwards (Pini Prato et al 1992; Tinti & Vincenzi 1990a,b), the use of a cast gold framework (Tinti et al 1993) and the use of a titanium reinforced membrane which can be curved to produce the space.

If an area of localized recession is to be treated with GTR techniques it must have some remaining attached keratinized gingiva between the base of the defect and the mucogingival junction. This is because GTR procedures for gingival recession cannot increase the amount of keratinized gingiva already at the site and this must be provided over the grafted area by the coronal repositioning of the flap. Thus gingival recession defects must be treated at an earlier stage in their development than in the case of lesions treated with gingival grafting techniques.

Clinical procedure using two-stage GTR with PTFE membranes

A full thickness mucoperiosteal flap is developed from a crevicular horizontal incision, sparing the interdental papillae, and vertical relieving incisions. It is raised until freely mobile to allow subsequent coronal repositioning. A single tooth Gore-Tex® membrane is modified so that it can be tented out to give a space between the membrane and the root to allow tissue ingrowth. This is accomplished by either placing a suture to tent it inwards (**Fig. 21.22A**) or by tying it to a suitably bent gold bar or precast gold framework. Recently, Gore-Tex® membrane with an incorporated metal framework has been manufactured to allow the membrane to be tented to the correct shape (**Fig. 21.22B**). This membrane is then placed and secured by a sling suture to cover the exposed root surface, leaving a gap for tissue ingrowth (**Fig. 21.22C, D**). The flap is then coronally repositioned to cover the membrane and sutured into place with PTFE sutures.

After 4–8 weeks, a marginal flap is gently lifted to allow the membrane to be removed. This should leave a definite soft tissue attachment against the root of the tooth. The flap is sutured back after membrane removal and the sutures are removed one week later. The healing is usually uneventful thereafter. It is not yet known whether new hard tissues form after this procedure. In this connection it is also not known whether tenting of the membrane fully prevents downgrowth of gingival epithelium.

Clinical and laboratory trials of the two-stage technique

A clinical and histological investigation of the two-stage GTR techniques using ePTFE membranes for buccal recession has been carried out in monkeys (Gottlow et al 1990). It has shown that this technique can produce a

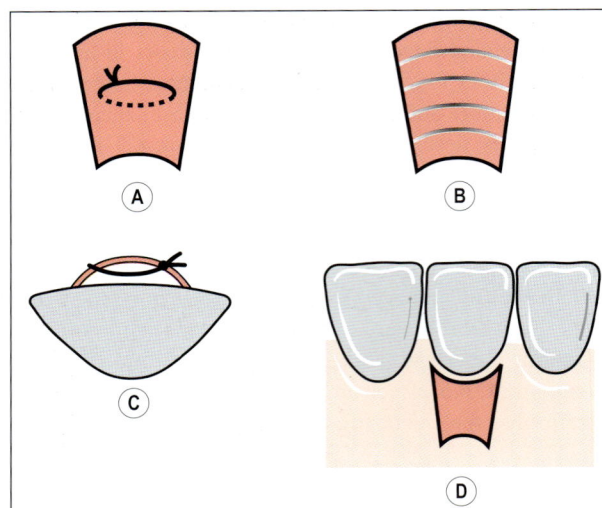

Fig. 21.22 Diagrams to show modifications of PTFE (Gore-Tex®) membrane for guided tissue regeneration for localized recession. (A) Membrane tented with a suture; (B) membrane with incorporated metal wires for tenting; (C) and (D) tented membranes in position over exposed root.

reduction in gingival recession, a gain in connective tissue attachment and the formation of new bone.

Clinical trials of these techniques in humans have shown that they can reduce gingival recession and produce an apparent gain in clinical attachment (Pini Prato et al 1992; Tinti et al 1992, 1993; Tinti & Vincenzi 1993, 1994). Reductions in soft tissue recession of 55–83% have been achieved by these techniques. However, Trombelli et al (2005) were unable to demonstrate changes over time in the clinical outcome achieved over a period between 4 and 10 years post-surgery in 20 patients treated with ePTFE membrane GTR.

RESORBABLE MEMBRANES

Resorbable membranes do not need to be removed as they are degraded by body tissues (see Ch. 20). They may also provide the suitable conditions for bone regrowth and the formation of new attachment (Brady et al 1973; Gottlow et al 1992; Laurell et al 1992). One advantage of these techniques is that they are one-stage procedures and are thus preferred by patients. Furthermore, because of the lack of a second surgical procedure to remove the membrane there is no interference with the healing tissue as could occur in the two-stage GTR procedure. The procedure is also considerably easier than other grafting procedures because it only involves a single surgical site and a full thickness mucoperiosteal flap is raised.

A multilayered resorbable membrane barrier membrane (Guidor® Guidor AB, Huddinge, Sweden) has been produced which is designed for use in the treatment of gingival recession by producing space between the membrane and the root surface. This membrane is unidirectional, having spacer bars on the inner surface to lift it away from the root surface and create the space required for new attachment formation. The use of this membrane has been shown to effectively prevent the downgrowth of junctional epithelium and to allow integration of the connective tissue flap with new attachment on the root surface (Lundgren et al 1994; Gottlow et al 1994a,b).

Clinical procedure for a one-stage procedure with a resorbable membrane

The procedure is similar to that described above for ePTFE membranes but differs in some minor details. It involves the raising of a full thickness mucogingival flap which will be subsequently coronally repositioned over the membrane. This flap must include some keratinized gingiva since this technique cannot increase this tissue (see above). It is thus suitable for Miller I and II categories of localized gingival recession (**Fig. 21.24A**). A flap is outlined (**Figs 21.23A, 21.24B**) with an inverse bevel incision which allows partial removal over papillae tips the remainder of which are left in situ to facilitate suturing. Vertical relieving incisions are made down to the vestibule to allow a full-thickness mucoperiosteal flap to be fully mobilized. The exposed root surface is cleaned and reduced in bulbosity using a Kirkland 13 and Gracey 11/12 and 13/14 curettes (**Fig. 21.24C**). The margin of a flap is slightly raised on the lingual side to accommodate the resorbable retaining suture tie submucosally. A bioresorbable membrane is placed

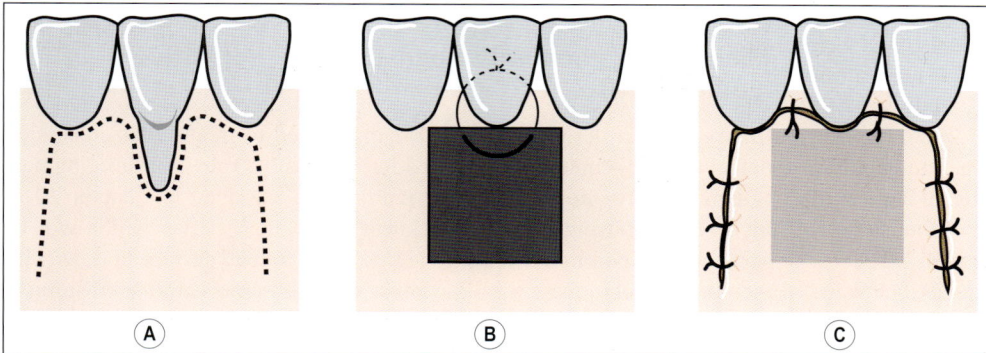

Fig. 21.23 Guided tissue regeneration for localized recession using resorbable membranes. (A) Incisions sparing tips of papillae; (B) membrane held in position with a sling suture; (C) flap coronally positioned over membrane. It is sutured to papillae and also vertically.

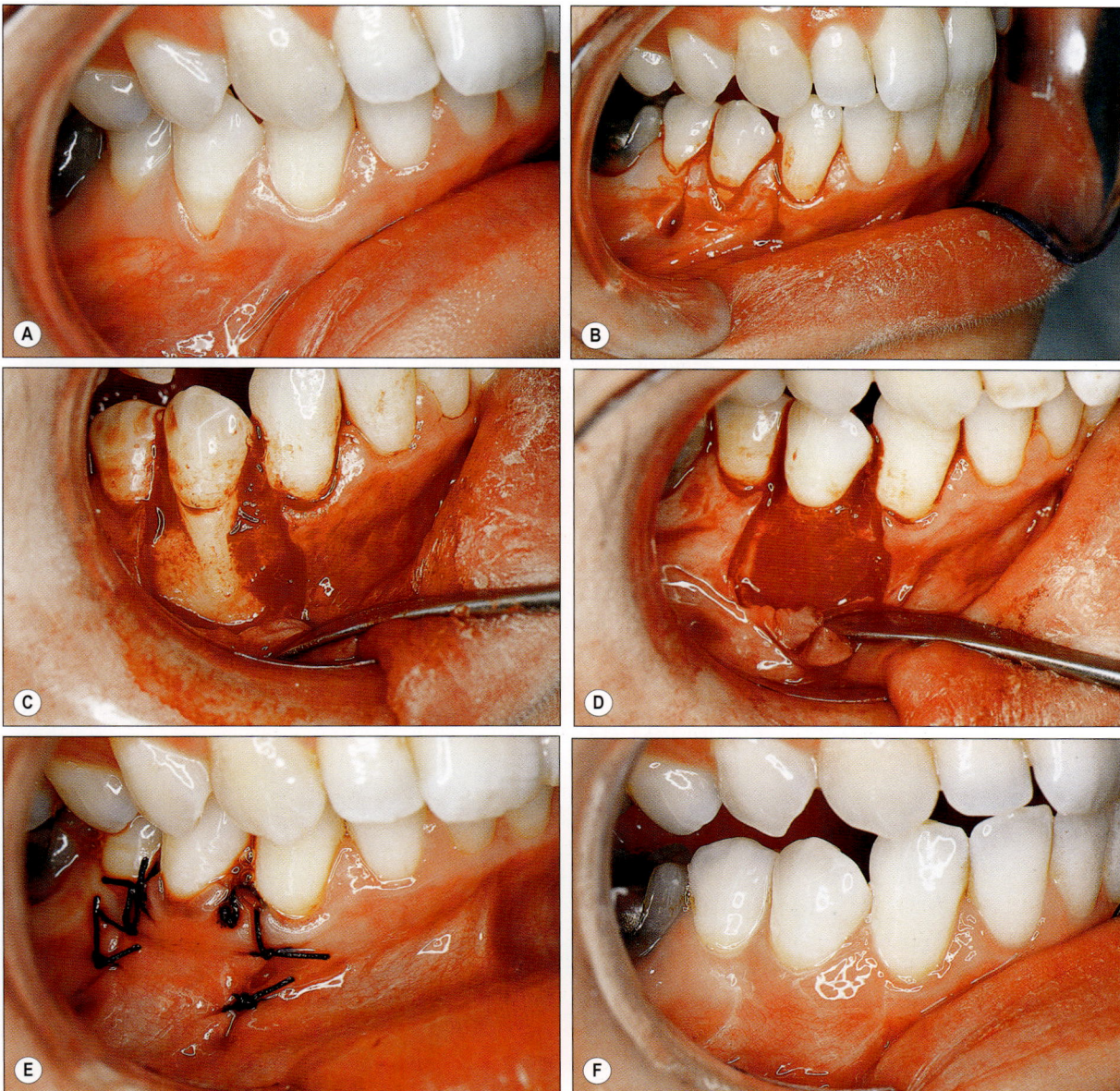

Fig. 21.24 Guided tissue regeneration using resorbable membrane to cover localized gingival recession in a 40-year-old woman. (A) Preoperative view of Miller Class I recession. (B) Incisions: sparing tips of papillae. Full thickness mucoperiosteal flap raised to expose root and bone. (C) Root surface prepared, conditioned and dried. (D) Guidor® resorbable membrane in position over root surface and surrounding bone. It adapts itself well to the shape of the root and adjacent bone. (E) Flap coronally repositioned and sutured over membrane. (F) Postoperative view 3 months after surgery. (Courtesy Dr C A Waterman)

and trimmed to cover the osseous recession defect and to cover the adjacent bone mesially, distally and apically by a few mm. A suitable membrane for this procedure is the Guidor® polylactate membrane (Guidor®, Guidor AB, Huddinge, Sweden) which has two layers with added spacers on the underside to lift it away from the root surface and so to aid the ingrowth of new cementum, bone and collagen fibre forming cells. It may be necessary to raise the apical edge of the retained interdental papilla in order to touch the edge of the membrane beneath. The membrane adapts itself well to the shape of the root and surrounding bone (**Fig. 21.24D**). It is then tied in place with resorbable sutures using a sling suture technique to suspend the membrane from the lingual surface of the tooth (**Fig. 21.23B**). It is tied off on the lingual aspect and the ends are tucked below a small lingual flap which is raised for this purpose taking care to avoid the lingual aspects of the papillae. The flap is sutured coronally using a minimum of four sutures, two through the papilla and two in the relieving incisions with black silk sutures (**Figs 21.23C, 21.24E**). No packing is applied or the space below the membrane would be eliminated, and there would be no ingrowth of healing tissue. The patients are instructed not to brush the operated area for 6 weeks and are told to rinse daily for 2 min with chlorhexidine mouthwashes. This is to minimize the risk of bacterial contamination of the membrane (Nowzari & Slots 1994). Two-weekly careful professional cleaning may also be undertaken during this period. As a further precaution against infection tetracycline may be prescribed for 2 weeks. The external sutures are removed after 4 weeks and at 6 weeks the patient is instructed to start cleaning this area with a careful non-traumatic brushing technique. The results of this procedure 3 months after normal cleaning resumed and healing was complete are shown in **Figure 21.24F**.

Unfortunately, the Guidor® membrane which was ideally manufactured for this procedure, with spacer bars on the inner surface to lift it away from the root surface and create the space required for new attachment formation, is no longer manufactured. Therefore the only resorbable membranes currently available for this procedure lack these spacer bars on their inner surface. There are other lactide/polyglycoside copolymer membranes such as: Resolute® and Atrisorb® and the resorbable collagen membranes such as Bio-Gide®. These produce good clinical results with regard to root surface coverage. They do not, however, produce the increases in bone level seen with the Guidor® membrane (Waterman, personal communication).

Yamada et al (2006) tried to avoid the possible risks of xenograft materials by fabricating a collagen membrane using tissue culture. They seeded gingival fibroblasts on to sponges of human recombinant type I or III collagen in medium. Fibroblast proliferation in these samples was compared using the cell-counting kit assay. Vascular endothelial growth factor (VEGF) and hepatocyte growth factor (HGF) released into the cultured media were examined by enzyme-linked immunosorbent assay.

The fibroblasts proliferated significantly in all six combinations of collagen and medium types. VEGF and HGF were released into the media. Thus, this new cultured gingival substitute containing no animal-derived materials produced good cell proliferation and VEGF release. The results suggested that the substitute may provide a new tool for the treatment of gingival recession.

Clinical procedure with enamel matrix derivative (Emdogain®)

Enamel matrix derivatives (EMD) can be used to treat certain recession defects and this method is justified by its possible role in promoting new cementum formation and new attachment as described in Chapter 20. It involves the raising of a full thickness mucogingival flap which will be subsequently coronally repositioned over the treated surface and, as with membrane techniques, this flap must include some keratinized gingiva since this technique cannot increase this tissue. The exposed root surface is carefully root planed, briefly conditioned, washed and dried before the placement of EMD. The coronally repositioned flap is then advanced and sutured over the treated root surface. Aftercare is as for membrane techniques. They produce excellent clinical results with regard to root surface coverage (**Fig. 21.25A, B**).

Cheng et al (2007) carried out a systematic review of coronally positioned flaps with or without EMD for the treatment of Miller Class I and II gingival recession. They found that the results of these procedures were unpredictable but became more predictable when the coronally positioned flap procedure was carried out with EMD.

Clinical trials of one-stage techniques

A clinical and histological investigation of the one-stage GTR technique using bioresorbable membranes for the treatment of buccal recession has been carried out on monkeys (Gottlow et al 1994a). It has shown that this technique can produce a reduction in gingival recession, a gain in connective tissue attachment and the formation of new bone. The amount of these tissues formed were of the same order as those seen for non-resorbable membranes (Gottlow et al 1990). In addition, clinical studies in humans have shown that bioresorbable membranes produce similar reductions in recession than those seen with non-resorbable membranes (Rachlin et al 1996; Roccuzzo et al 1996; Waterman 1997). Only these three studies of bioresorbable membranes have been reported to date but they show 60–83% reductions in gingival recession, which are similar or better than those seen with non-resorbable membranes. Only one clinical study of the use of Guidor® resorbable membranes for the treatment of buccal recession has used a re-entry technique 1 year after the placement of the membrane

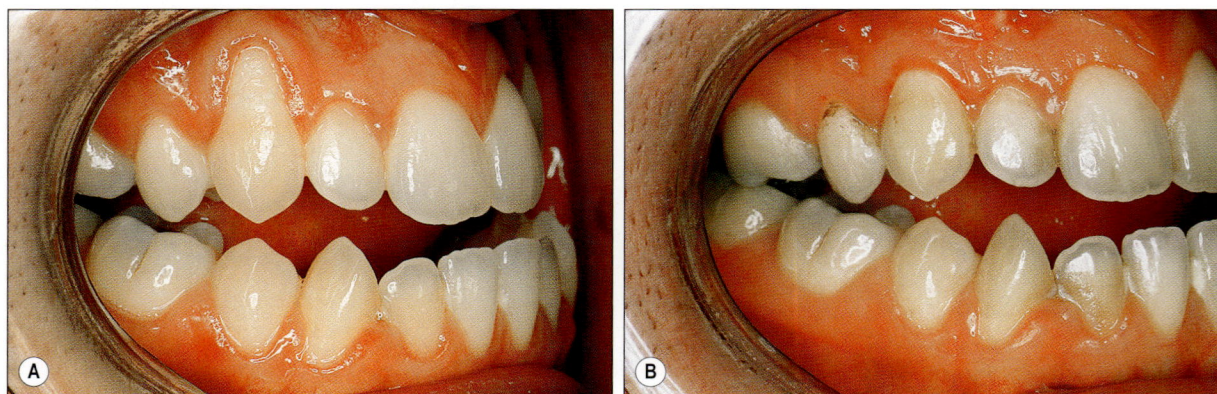

Fig. 21.25 Results of guided tissue regeneration using Enamel Matrix Derivative (Emdogain®). (A) Miller Class I recession on upper right canine of 26-year-old man. (B) 3 months after treatment. (Courtesy Dr C A Waterman).

to measure new bone growth in humans (Waterman 1997). It showed a mean increase in bone height of 1.95 ± 0.14 mm for all 17 sites, which included a variety of tooth sites, treated in 13 patients.

This technique therefore appears to have the potential to allow bone regeneration to occur in areas of buccal osseous defects such as those associated with localized gingival recession (Waterman 1997). The histology of the attachment of this bone to the root surface has not been studied in humans but results in monkeys (Gottlow et al 1994b) seem to indicate that new attachment is formed.

Clinical trials of the EMD technique

A blinded, split-mouth, placebo controlled study (Hagewald et al 2002) has compared the use of a coronally repositioned flap with either EMD application or placebo (propylene glycol alginate) to the root surface in 36 patients with paired buccal recession defects over 12 months. It found that both test and control sites had between 79–80% root coverage with no statistical difference between them. The EMD treated sites had a significantly greater gain of keratinized epithelium.

Castellanos et al (2006) carried out a clinical trial with 22 patients with Miller Class I or II gingival recessions of more than 2 mm. They showed that the coronally positioned flap alone or with EMD was an effective procedure to cover localized gingival recession. However, the addition of EMD significantly improved the amount of root coverage. Moses et al (2006) compared the effectiveness of root coverage between the use of a subpedicle connective tissue graft and the use of EMD and again found that the use of EMD produced significantly more coverage.

CLINICAL TRIALS COMPARING SURGICAL TECHNIQUES FOR TREATMENT OF RECESSION

Paolantonio (2002) compared a connective tissue graft with GTR using either a bioabsorbable membrane or a collagen membrane in 45 healthy adults with Miller Class I or II gingival recession defects at baseline and one year. Gingival coverage of the exposed root surface and probing attachment levels (PAL) were measured. All three techniques produced good root coverage of 90, 81 and 87%, respectively. There were no statistical differences between them in either coverage or PAL. The connective tissue graft produced a thicker gingival coverage than the GTR techniques.

Harris (2003) treated 50 patients with single molar root recession defects with connective tissue grafts. The study found that there was complete coverage in 585 of cases and overall there was a mean of 91% root coverage. This shows that this is a suitable technique for coverage of molar recession defects.

A systematic review of periodontal plastic surgical (PPS) procedures for localized gingival recession found 223 publications on these procedures of which only 20 were suitable for meta-analysis (Roccuzzo et al 2002). It found that all the PPS techniques (FGG, CTG, CRF, GTR) were effective in producing good root coverage with very slight differences between them. The only significant difference was that CTG produced statistically significantly more root coverage than GTR.

The treatment of labial recession on incisors and premolars by a coronally repositioned flap with either a connective tissue graft or EMD have been compared (McGuire & Nunn 2003a). They were found to produce similar favourable results although those treated with EMD healed quicker with fewer postoperative complaints. They also compared the histological results on one patient with two hopeless teeth with labial recession (McGuire & Nunn 2003b; Carvalho da Silva et al 2004). CTG was found to have adhered to the root surface by connective tissue and some root resorption while the use of EMD produced new cementum, organizing periodontal ligament fibres and islands of condensing bone at a constant distance from the root surface. Another study (Trabulsi et al 2004)

compared the adjunctive effect of EMD on GTR treatment of recession defects. They found that GTR root coverage utilizing a collagen membrane, with or without EMD could be successfully used in obtaining gingival recession coverage. All these studies show that EMD appears to simulate organized regeneration of periodontium.

Berlucchi et al (2005) evaluated the relationship of anatomical features such as tissue thickness, papillae height and width, recession depth, and vestibular bone height with the effectiveness of defect coverage of Miller Class I and II gingival recessions treated with a coronally advanced flap (CAF) in combination with enamel matrix derivative (EMD) in 30 non-smoking men. They found that their results suggested that baseline recession depth and flap thickness may influence the outcome of marginal tissue recession therapy with CAF plus EMD at 12 months. There was no clear correlation between root coverage and other anatomical features, such as papillary width, papilla height, and the amount of bone on the vestibular side.

COMBINED PROCEDURES

Some cases of localized gingival recession which are otherwise suitable for GTR or EMD regenerative procedures, lack the necessary keratinized gingiva to facilitate coverage by a coronally repositioned flap. In these cases an additional procedure, such as a free gingival graft may be first used to increase the amount of keratinized gingival tissue. When this has fully healed it may then be followed by a regenerative procedure. Good clinical results can be produced by these combined procedures. The results of combination treatments for multiple Miller Class II recession defects on lower incisors and canines with the use of free gingival graft to provide sufficient keratinized gingiva and subsequent Guidor® membrane regenerative procedures carried out in two stages are shown in **Figure 21.26A, B.** Also, the results of the use of free gingival graft to provide sufficient keratinized gingiva and the subsequent use of an Atrisorb resorbable membrane in a Miller Class I defect on lower right first premolar can be seen in **Figure 21.27A, B.**

It is also possible to treat two recession defects in the same mouth with different surgical procedures because of their nature and this is illustrated in **Figure 21.28A–E.** The buccal recession defect on the upper right canine was treated by GTR with a Guidor® membrane and a coronally repositioned flap (**Fig. 21.28A, B**). Three months later the buccal recession defect on the upper right lateral incisors was treated by an envelope flap and a connective tissue graft (**Fig. 21.28B–E**).

An envelope flap is a minimal, local access flap and is only suitable for Miller Class 1 buccal recession defects with full papillary height and a healthy gingival margin and crevice. The procedure is carried out as follows. A crevicular incision is made from the tip of the distal papilla to the tip of the mesial papilla (**Fig. 21.28C**). This should remove the crevicular epithelium which is gently curetted away after the flap has been gently raised to form a pocket. The exposed root surface is then scaled and possibly conditioned and a small connective tissue graft is removed from the palate using a Harris knife (see above). The connective tissue graft is then placed into the pocket and over the exposed root surface of the recession defect utilizing its epithelialized border for the defect coverage (**Fig. 21.28D**). Two interdental sutures at each end are placed to hold the flap down over the graft. These procedures heal over 6–8 weeks to produce full root surface coverage which is seen after 3 months in **Figure 21.28E.**

Tözüm et al (2005) compared the use of the subepithelial connective tissue graft with or without the use of an envelope tunnel technique on Miller Class I defects and found the latter slightly more effective although both techniques were found to be clinically satisfactory.

Spahr et al (2005) compared the root coverage of Miller Class I and II recession defects using enamel matrix proteins versus coronally advanced flap technique over 2 years and found the former to be more effective.

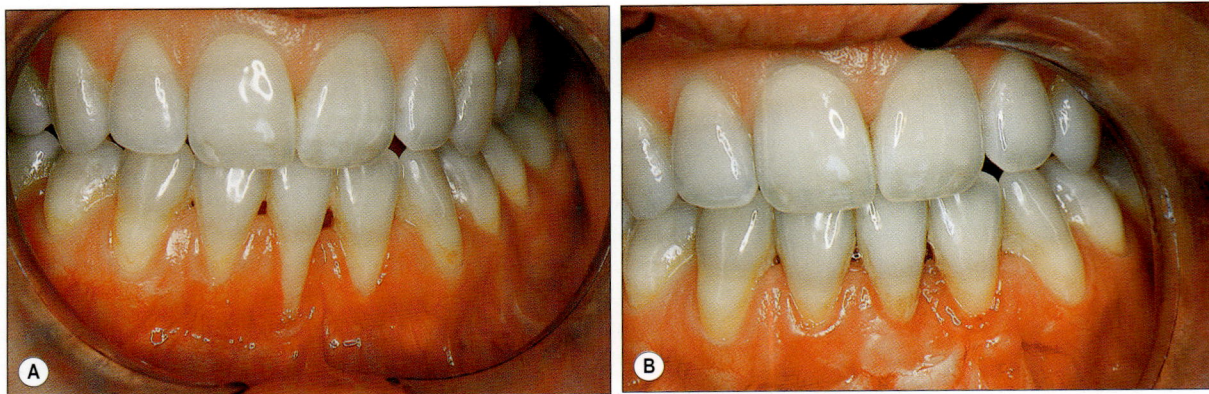

Fig. 21.26 Results of combination treatments in a 27-year-old woman: the use of a free gingival graft to provide sufficient keratinized gingiva and subsequently a Guidor® resorbable membrane. (A) Preoperative view showing multiple Miller Class II recession defects on lower incisors and canines (Guidor® treatment carried out in two stages). (B) Good root coverage 6-month after completion of treatment. (Courtesy Dr C A Waterman).

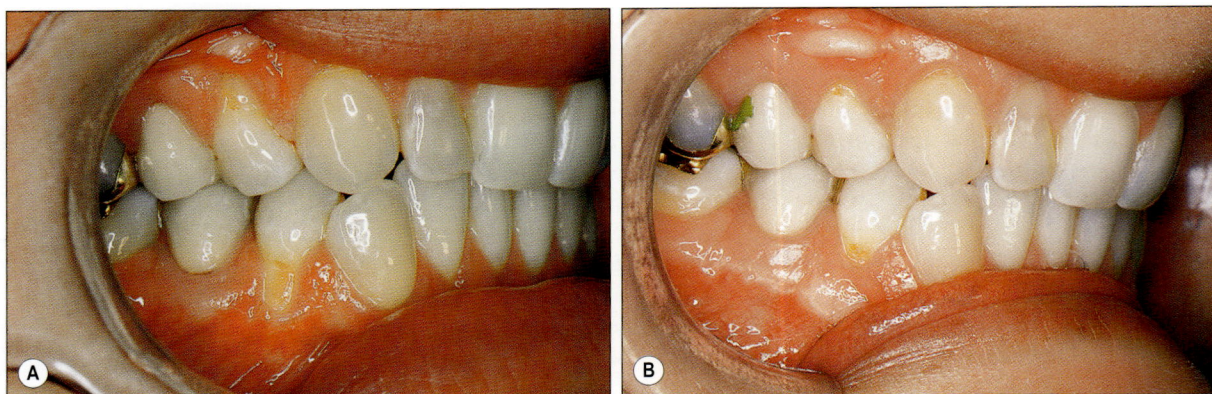

Fig. 21.27 Results of combination treatments in a 32-year-old woman: the use of a free gingival graft to provide sufficient keratinized gingiva and subsequently an Atrisorb resorbable membrane (A) Miller Class I defect on lower right first premolar; (B) good root coverage 6 months after treatment complete (Courtesy Dr C A Waterman).

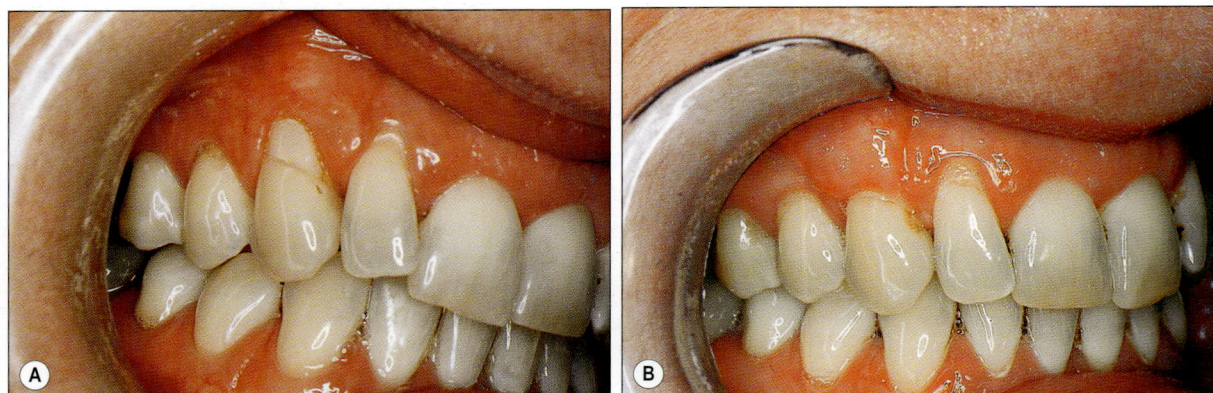

Fig. 21.28 Results of combination treatments in a 33-year-old woman: (A) Miller Class I recession defects before treatment on the upper right canine and lateral incisor. (B) 3 months after the treatment of the defect on the upper right canine with a Guidor® membrane and a coronally repositioned flap. It also shows the untreated defect on the upper right lateral incisor.

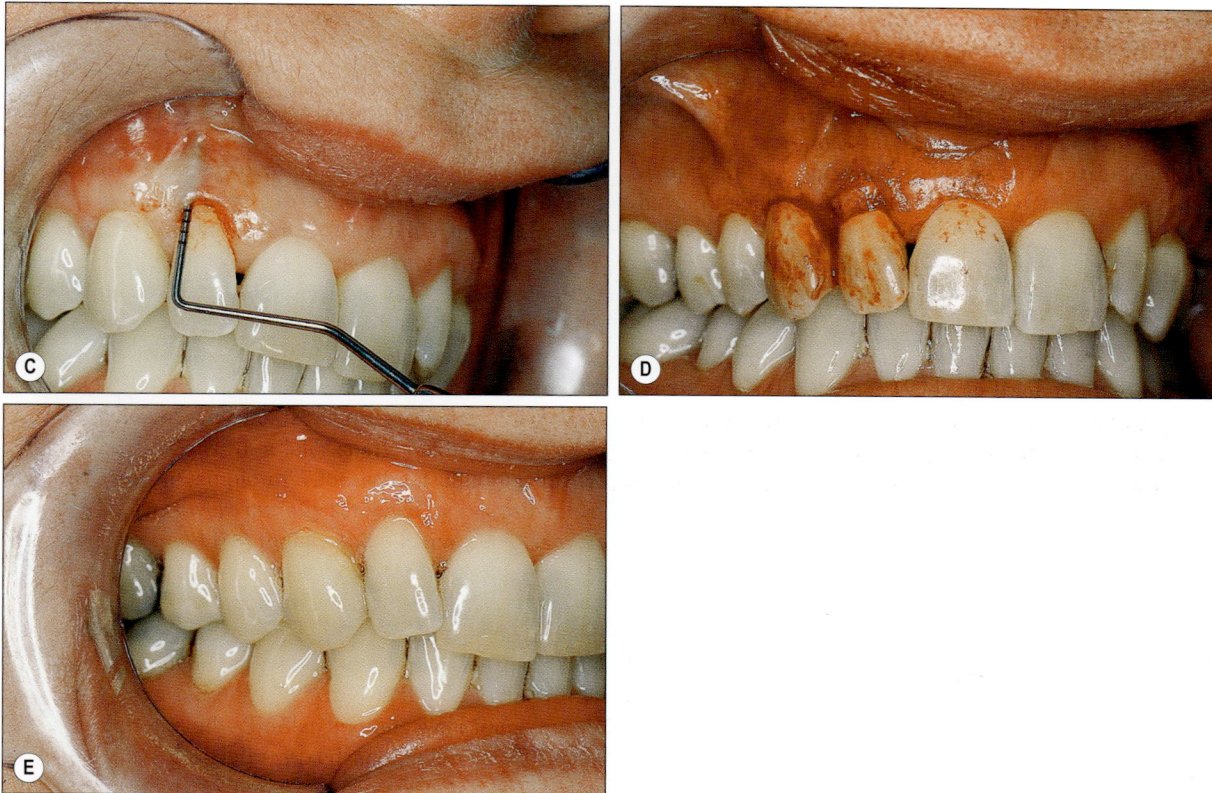

Fig 21.28—Cont'd (C) An envelope flap cut around the buccal defect on the upper right lateral incisor and deepened to form a pocket. (D) A connective tissue graft from the palate placed into the pocket and over the defect above the gingival margin using its epithelialized margin on its outer surface for this purpose. (E) The healed area after 3 months showing full root surface coverage over the defect on the upper right lateral incisor. (Courtesy Dr C A Waterman).

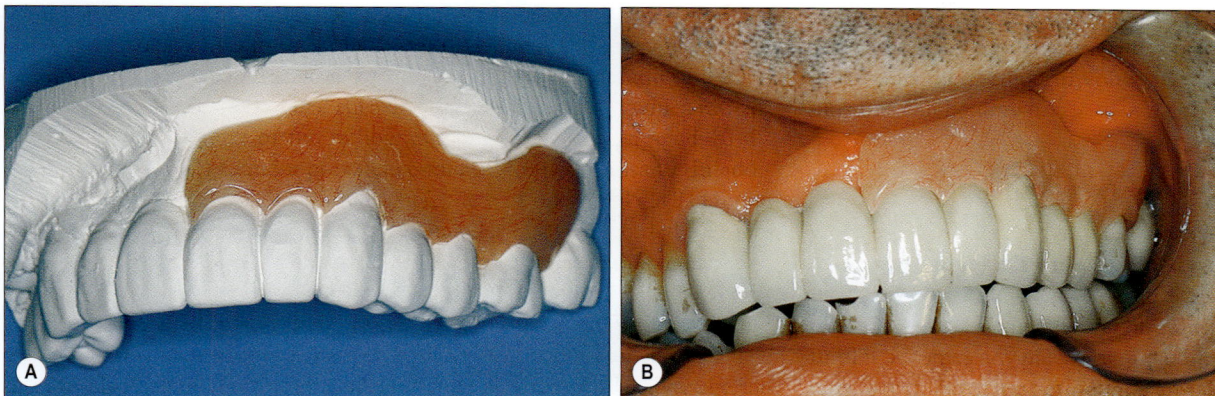

Fig. 21.29 A gingival veneer to mask uncorrectable generalized gingival recession which is otherwise unsightly and visible (A) on the model (B) in position in the mouth. (Courtesy Dr C A Waterman).

MASKING OF UNTREATABLE GENERALIZED GINGIVAL RECESSION

Uncorrectable generalized gingival recession when unsightly and visible may be masked by a gingival veneer made out of pink acrylic and made to resemble gingival tissue (**Fig. 21.29A, B**). It should not be worn at night and must be kept free of plaque to avoid it causing gingivitis in the underlying gingivae. Also, the underlying periodontal condition must be rendered stable before a gingival veneer is considered.

Smoking and treatment of mucogingival problems

A number of studies have shown that soft tissue grafting procedures (Miller 1987) and guided tissue regenerative procedures (Trombelli & Scabia 1997) used for the treatment of localized gingival recession are less likely to be successful in smokers than non-smokers. One should always take this into account in planning for these procedures. They should only be carried out in smokers if all other factors are favourable and the patient has been told of the relationship between smoking and poor healing and is aware that this may seriously affect the outcome.

REFERENCES

Addy M, Dummer PMH, Hunter ML, et al: A study of the association of frenal attachment, lip coverage and vestibular depth with plaque and gingivitis, *J Periodontol* 58:752–757, 1987.

Ah MKB, Johnson GK, Kaldahl WB, et al: The effect of smoking on the response to periodontal therapy, *J Clin Periodontol* 21:91–97, 1994.

Aukhil I: Biology of tooth-cell adhesion, *Dent Clin North Am* 35:359–468, 1991.

Berlucchi I, Francetti L, Del Fabbro M, et al: The influence of anatomical features on the outcome of gingival recessions treated with coronally advanced flap and enamel matrix derivative: a 1-year prospective study, *J Periodontol* 76:899–907, 2005.

Bernimoulin JP, Luscher B, Muhlemann HR: Coronally repositioned periodontal flap. Clinical evaluation after 1 year, *J Clin Periodontol* 2:1–13, 1975.

Brady JM, Cutright DE, Miller RA: Resorption rate, route of elimination and ultra structure of the implant site of polylactic acid in the abdominal wall of the rat, *J Biomed Mater Res* 7:155–166, 1973.

Carvalho da Silva R, Joly JC, Martorelli de Lima AF, et al: Root coverage using the coronally positioned flap with or without a subepithelial connective tissue graft, *J Periodontol* 75:413–419, 2004.

Castellanos AT, De la Rosa MR, De la Garza M, et al: Enamel matrix derivative and coronal flaps to cover marginal tissue recessions, *J Periodontol* 77:7–14, 2006.

Cheng YF, Chen, JW, Lin SJ, et al: Is coronally positioned flap procedure adjunct with enamel matrix derivative or root conditioning a relevant predictor for achieving root coverage? A systemic review, *J Periodontal Res* 42:474–485, 2007.

Cohen DW, Ross SE: The double papilla repositioned flap in periodontal therapy, *J Periodontol* 39:65–70, 1968.

Crigger M, Bogle G, Nilveus R, et al: The effect of topical citric acid application on the healing of experimental furcation defects in dogs, *J Periodontal Res* 13:538–549, 1978.

Cummings LC, Kaldahl WB, Allen EP: Histologic evaluation of autogenous connective tissue and acellular dermal matrix grafts in humans, *J Periodontol* 76:178–186, 2005.

Demirel K, Baer PN, McNamara TF: Topical application of doxycycline on periodontally involved root surfaces in vitro: comparative analysis of substantivity on cementum and dentin, *J Periodontol* 62:312–316, 1991.

Edel A: Clinical evaluation of free connective tissue grafts used to increase the width of keratinized gingiva, *J Clin Periodontol* 1:185–196, 1974.

Garrett JS, Crigger M, Egelberg J: The effects of citric acid on diseased root surfaces, *J Periodontal Res* 13:155–163, 1978.

Gottlow J, Karring T, Nyman S: Guided tissue regeneration following treatment of recession type defects in the monkey, *J Periodontol* 61:680–685, 1990.

Gottlow J, Lundgren D, Nyman S, et al: New attachment formation in the monkey using Guidor, a bioabsorbable GTR device, *J Dent Res* 71:1535, Abstract, 1992.

Gottlow J, Laurell L, Teiwik T, et al: Guided tissue regeneration using a bioresorbable matrix barrier, *Pract Periodontics Aesthet Dent* 6:71–81, 1994a.

Gottlow J, Laurell L, Lundgren D, et al: Periodontal response to a new bioresorbable guided tissue regeneration device: A longitudinal study in monkeys, *Int J Periodontics Restorative Dent* 14:437–449, 1994b.

Grupe HE, Warren RF: Repair of gingival defects by a sliding flap operation, *J Periodontol* 27:92–95, 1956.

Hagewald S, Spahr A, Rompola E, et al: Comparative study of Emdogain and coronally advanced flap technique in the treatment of human gingival recessions. A prospective controlled clinical study, *J Clin Periodontol* 29:35–41, 2002.

Hannington-Kitt JG, Dunne SM: Topical guanethidine relieves dental hypersensitivity and pain, *J R Soc Med* 86:514–515, 1993.

Harris RJ: The connective tissue and partial thickness double pedicle graft: A predictable method of obtaining root coverage, *J Periodontol* 63:477–486, 1992.

Harris RJ: Root coverage in molar recession: report of 50 consecutive cases treated with subepithelial connective tissue grafts, *J Periodontol* 74:703–708, 2003.

Harvey PM: Management of advanced periodontitis. I, Preliminary report of a method of surgical reconstruction, *N Z Dent J* 61:180–187, 1965.

Hirsch A, Goldstein M, Goultschin J, et al: A 2-year follow-up of root coverage using subpedicle acellular dermal matrix allografts and subepithelial connective tissue autografts, *J Periodontol* 76:1323–1328, 2005.

Holbrook T, Ochsenbein C: Complete coverage of denuded root surface with a one stage gingival graft, *Int J Periodontics Restorative Dent* 3:8–27, 1983.

Jahnke PV, Sandifer JB, Gher ME, et al: Thick free gingival and connective tissue autografts for root coverage *J Periodontol* 64:315–322, 1993.

Jones JK, Triplett RG: The relationship of cigarette smoking to intraoral wound healing: a review of evidence and implications for patient care, *J Maxillofac Surg* 50:237–239, 1992.

Lang NP, Löe H: The relationship between the width of keratinized gingiva and gingival health, *J Periodontol* 43:623–627, 1972.

Langer B, Langer L: Subepithelial connective tissue graft technique for root coverage, *J Periodontol* 60:715–720, 1985.

Laurell L, Gottlow J, Nyman S, et al: Gingival response to Guidor, a bioabsorbable device in GTR therapy, *J Dent Res* 71:1536, 1992.

Leknes, KN, Amarante ES, et al: Coronally positioned flap procedures with or without a biodegradable membrane in the treatment of human gingival recession. A 6-year follow-up study, *J Clin Periodontol* 32:518–529, 2005.

Lundgren D, Mathisen T, Gottlow J: The development of a barrier for guided tissue regeneration, *J Swed Dent Assoc* 86:741–756, 1994.

Maynard JG Jr: Coronal positioning of a previously placed autogenous gingival graft, *J Periodontol* 48:151–155, 1977.

McGuire MK, Nunn M: Evaluation of human recession defects treated with coronally repositioned flaps and either enamel matrix derivative or connective tissue. Part 1: Comparison of clinical parameters, *J Periodontol* 74:1110–1125, 2003a.

McGuire MK, Nunn M: Evaluation of human recession defects treated with coronally repositioned flaps and either enamel matrix derivative or connective tissue. Part 2: Histological evaluation, *J Periodontol* 74:1126–1135, 2003b.

Miller PD: Root coverage using a free soft tissue autograft following citric acid application. I Technique, *Int J Periodontics Restorative Dent* 2:65–70, 1982.

Miller PD: A classification of marginal tissue recession, *Int J Periodontics Restorative Dent* 5:9–13, 1985a.

Miller PD: Root coverage using the free soft tissue autograft following citric acid application. Part III. A successful and predictable procedure in areas of deep wide recession, *Int J Periodontics Restorative Dent* 5:15–37, 1985b.

Miller PD Jr: Root coverage with free gingival graft. Factors associated with incomplete coverage, *J Periodontol* 58:674–681, 1987.

Miller PD: Regenerative and reconstructive periodontal plastic surgery. Mucogingival surgery, *Dent Clin North Am* 32:287–306, 1988.

Miller PD: Personal communication, 1992.

Miyasato M, Crigger M, Egelberg J: Gingival condition in areas of minimal and appreciable width of keratinized gingiva, *J Clin Periodontol* 4:200–209, 1977.

Moses O, Artzi Z, Sculean A, et al: Comparative study of two root coverage procedures: a 24-month follow-up multicenter study, *J Periodontol* 77:195–202, 2006.

Nabors J: Free gingival grafts, *Periodontics* 4:243–245, 1966.

Nowzari H, Slots J: Microorganisms in polytetrafluoroethylene barrier membranes for guided tissue regeneration, *J Clin Periodontol* 21:203–210, 1994.

Nyman S, Lindhe J, Karring T: Healing following surgical treatment and root demineralization in monkeys with periodontal disease, *J Clin Periodontol* 8:249–258, 1981.

Nyman S, Gottlow J, Karring T, et al: The regenerative potential of the periodontal ligament, *J Clin Periodontol* 9:257–265, 1982.

Paolantonio M: Treatment of gingival recessions by combined periodontal regenerative technique, guided tissue regeneration and subpedicle connective tissue graft. A comparative clinical study, *J Periodontol* 73:53–62, 2002.

Pennel BM, Higgason JD, Towner JD, et al: Oblique rotated flap, *J Periodontol* 36:305–309, 1965.

Pini Prato G, Tinti C, Vincenzi G, et al: Guided tissue regeneration versus mucogingival surgery in the treatment of human buccal gingival recession, *J Periodontol* 63:919–928, 1992.

Preber H, Bergström J: Effect of cigarette smoking on periodontal healing following surgical therapy, *J Clin Periodontol* 17:324–328, 1990.

Rachlin G, Koubi G, Dejou J, et al: The use of resorbable membrane in mucogingival surgery. A case series, *J Periodontol* 67:621–626, 1996.

Register AA, Burdick FA: Accelerated reattachment with cementogenesis to dentin, demineralized in situ. I Optimum range, *J Periodontol* 46:646–655, 1975.

Register AA, Burdick FA: Accelerated reattachment with cementogenesis to dentin, demineralized in situ. II Defect repair, *J Periodontal Res* 47:263–267, 1976.

Roccuzzo M, Lungo M, Corrente G, et al: Comparative study of a bioresorbable and a non-resorbable membrane in the treatment of human buccal gingival recessions, *J Periodontol* 67:7–14, 1996.

Roccuzzo M, Bunino M, Needleman I, et al: Periodontal plastic surgery for the treatment of gingival recession: a systematic review, *J Clin Periodontol* 29:S178–S194, 2002.

Salkin LM, Freedman AL, Stein MD, et al: A longitudinal study of mucogingival defects, *J Periodontol* 58:164–166, 1987.

Schluger S, Youdelis R, Page RC, et al, editors: Mucosal reparative surgery. In *Periodontal Diseases*, Ch. 26. Philadelphia, Lea and Febiger, pp 560–578.

Silva CO, Martorelli de Lima AF, Sallum AW, et al: Coronally positioned flap for root coverage in smokers and non-smokers: stability of outcomes between 6 months and 2 years, *J Periodontol* 78:1702–1707, 2007.

Spahr A, Haegewald S, Tsoulfidou F, et al: Coverage of Miller Class I and II recession defects using enamel matrix proteins versus coronally advanced flap technique: a 2-year report, *J Periodontol* 76:1871–1880, 2005.

Sullivan HC, Atkins JH: Free autogenous gingival grafts. I. Principles of successful grafting, *Periodontics* 6:121–129, 1968a.

Sullivan HC, Atkins JH: Free autogenous gingival grafts. III. Utilization of grafts in the treatment of gingival recession, *Periodontics* 6:152–160, 1968b.

Sullivan HC, Atkins JH: The role of free gingival grafts in periodontal therapy, *Dent Clin North Am* 13:133–148, 1969.

Terranova VP, Franzetti LC, Hic S, et al: A biochemical approach to periodontal regeneration. Tetracycline treatment of dentin promotes fibroblast adhesion and growth, *J Periodontal Res* 21:330–337, 1986.

Tinti C, Vincenzi G: Guided tissue regeneration with Gore-Tex: new perspectives, *Quintessence Int* 6:45–49, 1990a.

Tinti C, Vincenzi G: Treatment of gingival recession with guided tissue regeneration with Gore-Tex membrane: clinical variations, *Quintessence Int* 6:465–468, 1990b.

Tinti C, Vincenzi G, Cortellini P, et al: Guided tissue regeneration in the treatment of human facial recession, *J Periodontol* 63:554–560, 1992.

Tinti C, Vincenzi G, Cocchetto R: Guided tissue regeneration in mucogingival surgery, *J Periodontol* 64:1184–1191, 1993.

Tinti C, Vincenzi G: Expanded polytetrafluoroethylene titanium-reinforced membranes for regeneration of mucogingival recession defects, A 12 case report, *J Periodontol* 65:1088–1191, 1994.

Tözüm TF, Keçeli GH, Güncü GN, et al: Treatment of gingival recession: comparison of two techniques of subepithelial connective tissue graft, *J Periodontol* 76:1842–1848, 2005.

Trabulsi M, Oh T-J, Eber R, et al: Effect of enamel matrix derivative on collagen guided tissue regeneration-based root coverage procedure, *J Periodontol* 75:1446–1457, 2004.

Trombelli L: Periodontal regeneration in gingival recession defects, *Periodontol 2000* 19:138–150, 1999.

Trombelli L, Schincaglia G, Checchi L, et al: Combined guided tissue regeneration, root conditioning, and fibrin-fibronectin system application in the treatment of gingival recession. A 15 case report, *J Periodontol* 65:796–803, 1994.

Trombelli L, Schincaglia G, Zangari F, et al: Effects of tetracycline HCl conditioning and fibrin-fibronectin system application in the treatment of gingival recession with guided tissue regeneration, *J Periodontol* 66:313–320, 1995.

Trombelli L, Scabia A: Healing response of gingival recession defects following guided tissue regeneration procedures in smokers and non-smokers, *J Clin Periodontol* 24:529–533, 1997.

Trombelli L, Minenna L, Farina R, et al: Guided tissue regeneration in human gingival recessions: A 10-year follow-up study, *J Clin Periodontol* 32:16–20, 2005.

Waterman C: A re-entry study to determine the hard and soft tissue changes following treatment of buccal defects using a bioabsorbable membrane, *J Periodontol* 68:982–989, 1997.

Wennstrom JL: Lack of association between the width of attached gingiva and the development of soft tissue recession. A 5 year longitudinal study, *J Clin Periodontol* 14:181–184, 1987.

Wennstrom J, Lindhe J, Nyman S: The role of keratinized gingiva in plaque associated gingivitis in dogs, *J Clin Periodontol* 9:75–85, 1982.

Wicksjö UME, Baker PJ, Christersson LA, et al: A biochemical approach to periodontal regeneration: tetracycline treatment conditions dentin surfaces, *J Periodontal Res* 21:322–369, 1986.

Yamada K, Yamaura J, Katoh M, et al: Fabrication of cultured oral gingiva by tissue engineering techniques without materials of animal origin, *J Periodontol* 77:672–677, 2006.

The periodontal abscess

THE PERIODONTAL OR LATERAL ABSCESS

A periodontal or lateral (as opposed to apical) abscess is a localized area of inflammation in which the formation of pus has taken place in the periodontal tissues. It is produced by endogenous pyogenic microorganisms, possibly toxic factors in the plaque and/or some reduction in host resistance caused by local or systemic factors. It most commonly complicates advanced periodontitis but can also more rarely occur when lesions of pulpal origin drain via the periodontal ligament and discharge from the gingival crevice. Thus the precise diagnosis must be established since in the latter situation rapid endodontic treatment needs to be carried out.

The factors that may provoke the formation of an abscess are listed below:

1. Obstruction of the opening to a deep pocket, frequently one which is tortuous, e.g. associated with a furcation defect
2. Gingival injury with a foreign body, e.g. toothbrush bristle or woodstick, etc. which carries bacteria into the tissues. Careless subgingival scaling may also carry microorganisms into damaged tissue, as can powerful irrigation of a pocket
3. Incomplete removal of plaque and subgingival calculus from the depths of a pocket. Frequently after scaling there is tightening of the gingival cuff which occludes a pocket containing bacteria
4. Infection of tissues damaged by excessive occlusal stress which may be produced by:
   a. A blow on a tooth
   b. Excessive orthodontic pressure
   c. Bruxism (see Ch. 27, p. 383).
5. As a consequence of pulp disease:
   a. Where a periapical lesion spreads up the lateral surface of a tooth
   b. Where lateral pulp canals link with the periodontal ligament. This is especially common in the furcation. Accessory pulp canals are extremely common and may not be evident on the radiograph. The furcation abscess produced by pulp pathology is frequently misdiagnosed as a primary periodontal lesion
   c. Perforation of the lateral wall of a tooth during endodontics
6. Altered host response as in diabetes. Diabetes has sometimes been diagnosed following the appearance of multiple periodontal abscesses.

The main direct cause of a lateral abscess is bacterial invasion of the soft tissue wall of the pocket and multiplication therein. This leads to an acute inflammatory response with the formation of pus. Bacterial invasion of the tissues in periodontitis has mainly been described in cases of advanced chronic periodontitis (Frank 1980; Saglie et al 1982a,b, 1985; Manor et al 1984) and an abscess is most common at this stage of the disease. Some studies have indicated that putative periodontal pathogens may penetrate epithelium, epithelial cells and connective tissue in this situation (Saglie et al 1986, 1988; Papapanou et al 1994; Sandros et al 1994) and if the defence mechanisms of the body do not control this situation quickly then it could easily lead to the formation of an abscess.

CLINICAL FEATURES

The onset of symptoms can be sudden with pain on biting and a deep throbbing pain. The involved tooth may feel high and mobile. The overlying gingiva becomes red, swollen and tender but at first there is no fluctuation or discharge of pus. There may be enlargement of the associated lymph glands.

The next stage is characterized by the presence of pus. This may discharge into a periodontal pocket when the symptoms reduce (**Fig. 22.1**), or the pus may track through the bone to form an abscess under the alveolar mucoperiosteum (**Fig. 22.2**). Once the pus enters the soft tissue the severe pain diminishes and the abscess appears as a red, shiny and very tender swelling over the alveolus. Sometimes a lateral abscess caused primarily by advanced periodontitis and deep pocketing may be precipitated by occlusal trauma such as secondary occlusal trauma or a tooth stressing habit (**Fig. 22.3**). The abscess usually points and discharges but if this does not happen the inflammation may spread into the surrounding connective tissue to produce a cellulitis. This occurs most commonly if the patient's resistance is low. If the abscess is in the upper jaw, depending upon the tooth involved, the lip, cheek, side of the nose or the infra-orbital area and lower eyelid may swell. Infection in the vicinity of the infra-orbital foramen is particularly dangerous. If the abscess is in the lower jaw, the lower

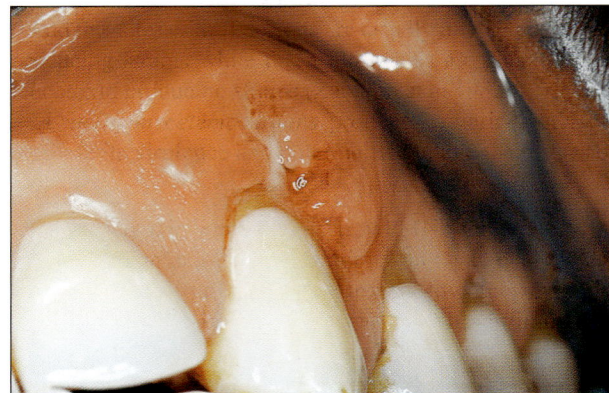

Fig. 22.1 A lateral periodontal abscess on the upper left canine of a 46-year-old man with advanced chronic periodontitis. It was associated with a 9 mm pocket buccal to this tooth and pus could be expressed from the gingival margin.

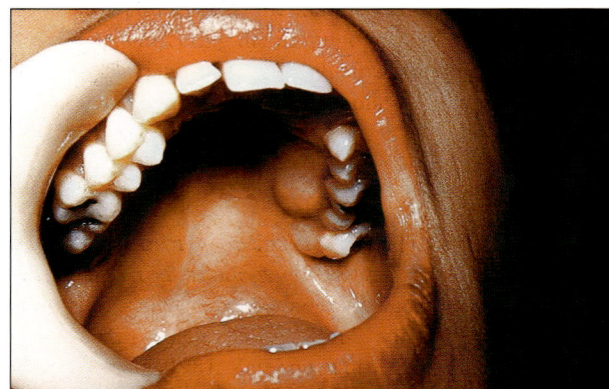

Fig. 22.2 A lateral periodontal abscess palatal to the upper left first molar in a 52-year-old woman with advanced chronic periodontitis. The abscess is associated with an 8 mm intrabony pocket palatal to this tooth. The pus has tracked through the bone to form an abscess under the alveolar mucoperiosteum with a fluctuant swelling palatal to this tooth which extends to the gingival margin. Pus could be expressed from the pocket.

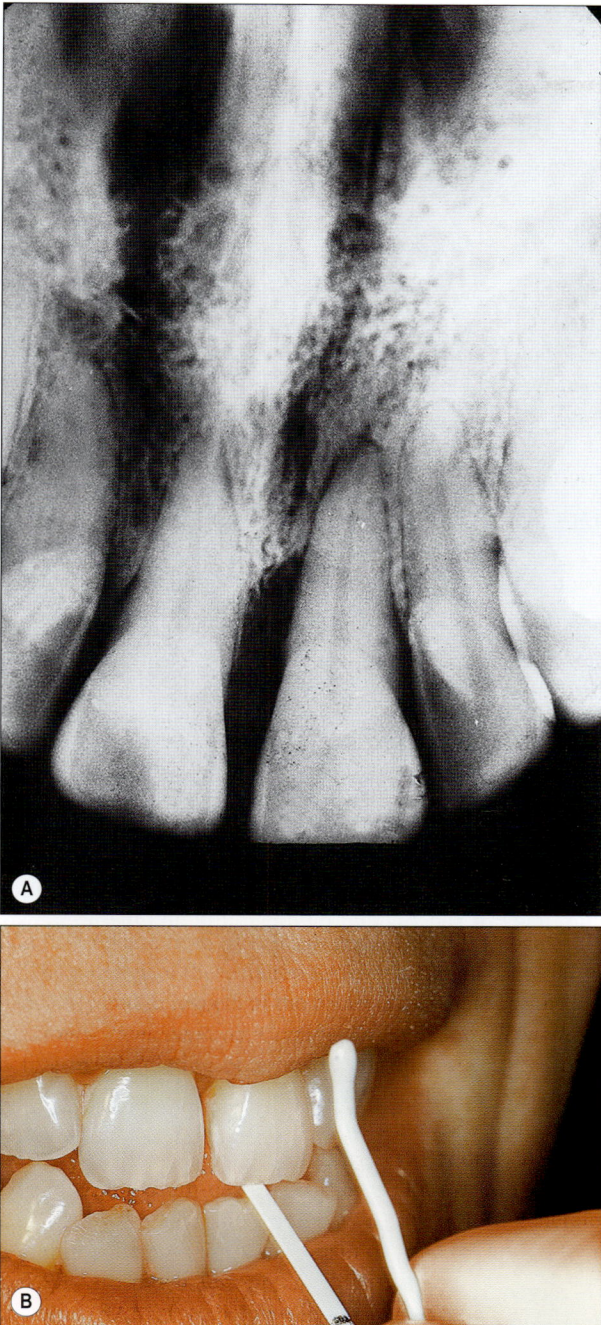

Fig. 22.3 (A) A radiograph of the upper anterior teeth of a 54-year-old woman with advanced chronic periodontitis showing a mixture of horizontal and vertical bone loss around the upper left central incisor. She presented with a lateral periodontal abscess distal to this tooth associated primarily with the 9 mm partly intrabony pocket on this tooth. The abscess appeared to be precipitated by occlusal trauma from her tooth stressing habit of holding her clips between her front teeth. (B) The same patient holding a clip between her front teeth in her accustomed manner.

lip, chin, cheek, angle of the mandible and neck may swell. If infection involves the lower third molar there may also be trismus and difficulty in swallowing. At this stage the patient is obviously unwell, in pain and distressed and his temperature may be elevated.

DIFFERENTIAL DIAGNOSIS

These clinical features can be produced by both periapical and periodontal abscesses and a differential diagnosis must be made because the treatment modalities for the two forms of abscess are different. Sometimes a differential diagnosis may not be easy. A number of features must be taken into account:

1. The position of the abscess swelling. If this is over the root apex it is more likely to be periapical.
2. The presence of periodontal disease with pocketing and bone destruction makes it more likely for the abscess to be of periodontal origin (**Fig. 22.4**), whereas if the periodontal condition is generally quite good and pocketing is absent or shallow this is unlikely.
3. If the involved tooth is heavily filled it is likely that pulp pathology is present, and a history of sensitivity to hot and cold tends to confirm this. If the tooth is non-vital the abscess could be either periapical or periodontal, or both as a combined abscess. Pulp vitality tests can be extremely misleading but if the tooth gives a normal reading this points to periodontal infection. If the tooth is caries free and unfilled the abscess is likely to be periodontal.
4. Radiographs taken in the earliest stages provide little useful information but once the lesion is established its position can be identified (**Fig. 22.3**). However, a periodontal abscess on the facial or lingual aspect of the tooth may not be clearly discernible on the radiograph. A radiograph taken with a gutta-percha point inserted gently into the suspected pocket can help to define the origin of the abscess.

BACTERIOLOGY OF LATERAL PERIODONTAL ABSCESS

The microflora of the lateral periodontal abscess resembles that of the periodontal pocket (Wade et al 1991; Leung et al 1993; Rajasuo et al 1996a,b; Herrera et al 2000a) (also see Ch. 2). It is a complex mixture of Gram-positive and Gram-negative cocci and rods, filaments, motile rods and spirochaetes which are either facultatively or totally anaerobic (Herrera et al 2000a,b). The predominating species found in these studies were *Porphyromonas gingivalis*, *P. melaninogenica*, *Prevotella intermedia*, *Tannerella forsythensis* (*Bacteroides forsythus*), *Fusobacterium nucleatum*, *Peptostreptococcus micros* and *Campylobacter rectus* (Herrera et al 2000b; Jaramillo et al 2005).

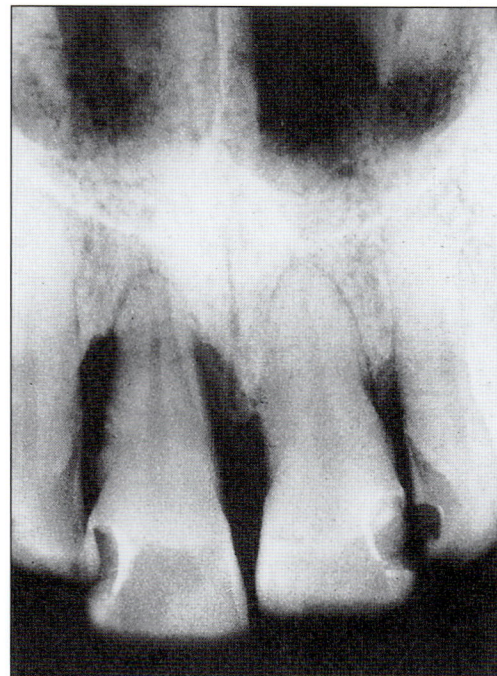

Fig. 22.4 The radiograph of the upper incisors of a 63-year-old man with a lateral periodontal abscess palatally. The radiograph shows vertical pattern bone loss mesially and distally in the upper right central incisor which had deep pocketing on all surfaces with the deepest palatally. The bone loss has reached to within 2 mm of the apex and could easily extend into the pulp via accessory canals and lead to a combined lesion.

Dahlén et al (2007) conducted a study to reveal phenotypic, serological subtypes and antibiotic susceptibility among fresh isolates of *Porphyromonas gingivalis* from a Swedish population with periodontitis and periodontal abscesses. They showed that the strains fell into two serotypes, of which serotype A predominated in the periodontitis cases and serotype B was over represented in periodontal abscesses. The same group (Yoshino et al (2007) also showed that the Swedish *P. gingivalis* isolates exhibited a wide variety of genotypes with only a weak clustering pattern. No predominant genotype at the whole chromosomal DNA level was present among Swedish *P. gingivalis* strains.

TREATMENT OF THE ABSCESS

Treatment depends upon the stage of abscess development, the amount of bone loss and whether pulp pathology is also involved. The initial aims of treatment are the relief of pain and control of infection by drainage. Once this has been achieved the residual lesion must be treated; otherwise recurrent abscess formation is inevitable. However, if the prognosis of the tooth is poor then it should be extracted and in this situation this is usually the only treatment needed. At the first episode of abscess formation the prognosis can be good but if recurrent abscesses have occurred then the prognosis is very poor.

DRAINAGE OF PUS

Drainage is essential and if the prognosis is hopeless then this will be achieved by extracting the tooth. If the tooth can remain functional and be retained then the abscess must be effectively drained under local anaesthesia. The injection must be made well away from the inflamed area. Regional anaesthesia or even general anaesthesia may be needed if the inflamed area is large.

When pus is discharging freely from the periodontal pocket then the pus may be drained from this site by easing it out and supplementing this by gentle irrigation of the pocket until all the pus is evacuated. If the abscess is fluctuant then it must be drained by incision. The drainage incision should be horizontal and made through the most fluctuant site. The margins of the wound may be spread to facilitate drainage. This is supplemented by regular hot salt water mouthwashes. If adequate drainage is established an antibiotic may not be needed. Relieving the occlusion by grinding the opposing tooth should allow the patient to eat on the other side of the mouth.

CONTROL OF THE ACUTE PHASE

Antibiotics are only needed if the tooth has a reasonable prognosis and is amenable to subsequent periodontal treatment. Furthermore, they are usually not necessary unless there are signs of spread of infection from the local site such as facial swelling, temperature rise or regional lymph node enlargement. As with other forms of infection, it is wise to obtain a pus sample by aspiration before starting antibiotic therapy in case empirical therapy proves ineffective (Lewis et al 1990).

Since the infection is varied and includes many anaerobes, it is best treated with amoxicillin or metronidazole, separately or in combination. In recent studies the predominating bacteria have been shown to be susceptible to these antibiotics (Herrera et al 2000a,c). The usual oral dosage is amoxicillin 250 mg/metronidazole 200 mg 8-hourly for 2–3 days (Gill & Scully 1991). Patients should be seen again after 2–3 days of antimicrobial therapy and if the temperature has returned to normal and clinical features resolved then therapy should be stopped (Martin et al 1997). In cases of penicillin allergy, the best alternatives are metronidazole alone or clindamycin 150 mg 6-hourly.

Metronidazole is contraindicated in patients who cannot be relied upon to refrain from alcohol and during pregnancy and in this situation the best alternative is oral clindamycin. It also helps to relieve the occlusion by grinding the opposing tooth.

Rarely if the infection has spread to produce a severe cellulitis or a tissue space infection an intramuscular or intravenous antibiotic may be indicated.

SUBSEQUENT TREATMENT

Once the acute condition is under control, treatment of the residual condition can be started. The periodontal condition of the whole mouth including the affected area must be treated by establishing good plaque control and carrying out subgingival scaling and root debridement. The affected tooth may need periodontal flap surgery to reduce periodontal pocketing and to treat any associated bone defect (see Chs 18 and 19). Frequently the abscess may perforate the facial or lingual plate of bone, leaving a bridge of marginal bone. If this bridge of bone is narrow it may have to be cut away. However, if the bridge is wide it may be conserved in the hope that the perforation will repair.

THE COMBINED PERIODONTAL–PERIAPICAL LESION

The combined lesion (**Figs 22.4, 22.5**) can develop in a number of ways:

1. Where an apical abscess has spread laterally to create a periodontal lesion or united with a pre-existing lateral lesion
2. Where pulp infection has spread via accessory canals into the periodontal tissues. This is most frequent in the furcation where accessory canals are common
3. Where a periodontal lesion extends close to the tooth apex and causes secondary pulpal infection.

At one time, the presence of a combined periapical–periodontal lesion justified extraction, especially occurring in a furcation. Today, endodontics has achieved a high level of success and predictability and the prognosis for a tooth involved in a combined lesion can be good.

TREATMENT

Once acute inflammation has been controlled and the occlusion adjusted, root-canal treatment should be initiated. A lateral compression technique is necessary to occlude accessory canals and when endodontics has been satisfactorily completed periodontal surgery can be carried out.

If a multirooted tooth is involved and (1) bone destruction around one root is much more advanced than that around the other root(s), or (2) the furcation defect is of such labyrinthine complexity that it cannot be kept clean, or (3) the divergent roots of neighbouring teeth, usually the buccal roots of upper molars, are very close together or actually touch, then root resection is indicated (see Ch. 20).

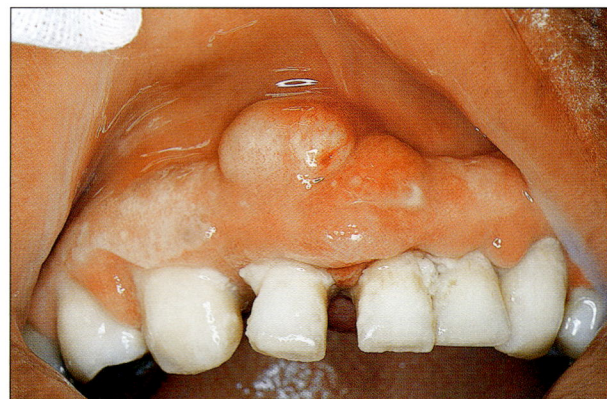

Fig. 22.5 A combined periodontal-pulpal-periapical abscess on the upper right central incisors of a man of 58 years. There is an apical fluctuant swelling and pus is also flowing from the gingival margin.

REFERENCES

Dahlén G, Gmür R, Yoshino T: Phenotypes, serotypes and antibiotic susceptibility of Swedish Porphyromonas gingivalis isolates from periodontitis and periodontal abscesses, *Oral Microbiol Immunol* 22:80–86, 2007.

Frank RM: Bacterial penetration in the apical pocket wall of advanced human periodontitis, *J Periodontal Res* 15:563–573, 1980.

Gill Y, Scully C: British oral and maxillofacial surgeons' views on the aetiology and management of acute pericoronitis, *Br J Oral Maxillofac Surg* 29:180–182, 1991.

Herrera D, Roldán S, Sanz M: The periodontal abscess: a review, *J Clin Periodontol* 27:377–386, 2000a.

Herrera D, Roldán S, González I, et al: The periodontal abscess (I). Clinical and microbiological findings, *J Clin Periodontol 2000;* 27:387–394, 2000b.

Herrera D, Roldán S, O'Connor A, et al: The periodontal abscess (II). Microbiological efficiency of 2 systemic antibiotic regimens, *J Clin Periodontol* 27:387–394, 2000c.

Jaramillo A, Arce RM, Herrera D, et al: Clinical and microbiological characterization of periodontal abscesses, *J Clin Periodontol* 32:1213–1218, 2005.

Leung WK, Theilade E, Comfort MB, et al: Microbiology of the pericoronal pouch in mandibular third molar pericoronitis, *Oral Microbiol Immunol* 8:306–312, 1993.

Lewis MA, MacFarlane TW, McGowan DA: A microbiological and clinical review of the acute dentoalveolar abscess, *Br J Oral Maxillofac Surg* 28:359–366, 1990.

Manor A, Lebendiger M, Shiffer A, et al: Bacterial invasion of the periodontal tissues in advanced periodontitis in humans, *J Periodontol* 55:567–573, 1984.

Martin MV, Longman LP, Hill JB, et al: Acute dentoalveolar infections: an investigation of the duration of antibiotic therapy, *Br Dent J* 183:135–137, 1997.

Papapanou PN, Sandros J, Lindberg K, et al: Porphyromonas gingivalis may multiply and advance within stratified human junctional epithelium, *J Periodontal Res* 29:374–375, 1994.

Rajasuo A, Leppanen J, Savolainen S, et al: Pericoronitis and tonsillitis: clinical and darkfield microscopy findings, *Oral Surg Oral Med Oral Pathol Oral Radiol Endod* 81:526–532, 1996a.

Rajasuo A, Jousimies-Somer H, Savolainen S, et al: Bacteriologic findings in tonsillitis and pericoronitis, *Clin Infect Dis* 23:51–60, 1996b.

Saglie FR, Carranza FA Jr, Newman MG, et al: Identification of tissue-invading bacteria in human periodontal diseases, *J Periodontal Res* 17:452–455, 1982a.

Saglie FR, Newman MJ, Carranza FA, et al: Bacterial invasion of gingiva in advanced periodontitis in humans, *J Periodontol* 53:217–222, 1982b.

Saglie FR, Carranza FA Jr, Newman MJ: The presence of bacteria within the oral epithelium of human periodontal disease. 1. A scanning and transmission electron microscopic study, *J Periodontol* 56:618–624, 1985.

Saglie FR, Rezende JH, Pertuiset J, et al: The presence of bacteria within the oral epithelium in periodontal disease II Immunochemical identification of bacteria, *J Periodontol* 57:492–500, 1986.

Saglie FR, Pertuiset J, Rezende JH, et al: In situ correlative immuno-identification of mononuclear infiltrates and invasive bacteria in diseased gingiva, *J Periodontol* 59:688–696, 1988.

Sandros J, Papapanou PN, Nannmark U, et al: Porphyromonas gingivalis invades the human pocket epithelium in vitro, *J Periodontal Res* 28:219–226, 1994.

Wade WG, Gray AR, Absi EG, et al: Predominant cultivable flora in pericoronitis, *Oral Microbiol Immunol* 6:310–312, 1991.

Yoshino T, Laine ML, van Winkelhoff AJ, et al: Genotypic characterization of Porphyromonas gingivalis isolated from Swedish patients with periodontitis and from periodontal abscesses, *Oral Microbiol Immunol* 22:195–200, 2007.

23 Early onset periodontitis (juvenile periodontitis/aggressive periodontitis)

A variety of names have been given to a form of periodontal disease characterized by deep pockets and advanced alveolar bone loss in the young, in children, adolescents and young adults, without any associated systemic disease. Gottlieb (1923, 1928) designated the condition(s) diffuse atrophy of alveolar bone, and subsequently other names were devised: deep cementopathia, paradontosis, periodontosis, juvenile periodontitis, prepubertal periodontitis, rapidly progressive periodontitis. Page and Baab (1985) suggested that all forms of the disease be designated early onset periodontitis (EOP). More recently the term localized aggressive periodontitis has been suggested (Armitage 1999).

At a population level there is direct correlation between oral hygiene status, the degree of gingival inflammation and the severity of periodontal destruction. However, at an individual level there is a great deal of variation in the way in which the tissues respond to plaque irritation. Some individuals with poor oral hygiene suffer little periodontal destruction while others with little plaque have advanced periodontal destruction. Two hypotheses have been proposed to account for this variation:

1. Certain plaque bacteria have a greater potential for tissue destruction than others and when they are present disease will occur
2. Host factors determine the tissue response to plaque.

Of course both of these factors could be important in both adult periodontitis and EOP.

Early onset periodontitis can be practically divided into three groups:

1. Prepubertal periodontitis – severe gingivitis and destructive periodontitis in primary dentition
2. Juvenile (aggressive) periodontitis:
   - Localized – severe localized attachment loss in permanent first molars and incisors
   - Generalized – involvement of these teeth and a few or many other teeth
3. Rapidly progressive periodontitis – generalized rapid attachment loss in the permanent dentition.

PREPUBERTAL PERIODONTITIS

This is an extremely rare form of periodontal disease characterized by rapid periodontal destruction of the primary dentition (Page et al 1983a). The gingivae are grossly inflamed and the patient commonly has other bacterial infections. In some cases the condition may affect the permanent dentition as well. In many instances there is a familial pattern to the disease and most if not all cases are probably genetically mediated. A number of inherited conditions described in Chapter 6 also produce these effects including hypophosphatasia, Papillon–Lefèvre syndrome, cyclic neutropenia, familial neutropenias, Chediak–Higashi syndrome.

Mutations in the cathepsin C gene (*CTSC*) have been identified as causal for the Papillon–Lefèvre syndrome (PLS), which includes prepubertal periodontitis (PP) (Loos et al 2005). Some *CTSC* mutations are causal for PP without PLS. No relationship has been demonstrated between *CTSC* mutations and other forms of periodontitis (see Ch. 6).

RAPIDLY PROGRESSIVE PERIODONTITIS

Rapidly progressive periodontitis (RPP) is characterized by severe generalized periodontal destruction and may affect any or all of the permanent dentition of patients between the ages of 20 and 35 (Page et al 1983b). The clinical features and subgingival flora resemble active chronic periodontitis with *Porphyromonas gingivalis*, *Prevotella intermedia*, *Eikenella corrodens* and *Aggregatibacter actinomycetemcomitans*, all being reported to be present. There is a lack of epidemiological evidence for this condition as a separate entity although there is evidence of some cases having a familial tendency. On present available evidence, it is difficult to justify the classification of this condition as a separate disease entity as it could well represent a rapidly progressive chronic periodontitis in a susceptible individual. In this regard, the IL-1A and B genetic pleomorphism that has been associated in some studies with susceptibility to periodontitis in the adult population (see Ch. 4) has not be found to be associated with RPP in young adult European Caucasians (Hodge et al 2001).

It is also important to distinguish this condition from post-juvenile periodontitis (see below) and to remember that some conditions such as Down's syndrome (see Ch. 6) have a high susceptibility to severe rapidly progressive periodontitis in the permanent dentition. It is also worth noting that this condition has also been referred to as generalized early onset periodontitis (Hart et al 1992).

JUVENILE (AGGRESSIVE) PERIODONTITIS

Usually multiple names for a disease entity indicate an ill-defined knowledge of the precise aetiology and pathogenesis; indeed it is possible for similar clinical manifestations to be produced by different causal factors and pathological processes. In this text, the term juvenile periodontitis (Butler 1969) is used because it refers to the general population affected and does not imply any particular cause or disease process. Baer (1971) described juvenile periodontitis as a well-defined clinical entity different from adult periodontitis in that it appears to start around puberty, is seen more commonly in girls, appears to occur in families, and is rapidly progressive.

Two forms of the disease were described, local and general. In the localized form the tissue destruction is restricted to the first molars and incisors, and is characterized by a symmetrical distribution; in the generalized form many or all the teeth are involved. Gradations between these two extremes are often seen. The variability of these forms was recently demonstrated by Yosof (1990) in a study of 47 Malaysian children (22 boys and 25 girls) with the condition. He divided the children into four groups according to the distribution of the bone loss:

Type 1: Bone destruction limited to first molars and incisors (14.9%)
Type 2: Bone destruction involving first molars and incisors and some other teeth (25.5%)
Type 3: Generalized destruction but worse around the first molars and incisors (14.9%)
Type 4: Generalized involvement of more than 14 teeth (44.7%).

Juvenile (aggressive) periodontitis (JP or AP) has distinctive clinical and bacteriological features which justify its classification as a separate disease entity.

The main epidemiological and clinical features of this disease are given below.

PREVALENCE

On the basis of the epidemiological studies detailed below, AP appears to occur in approximately 1 in 1000 adolescents and seems to have a racial predisposition, occurring most frequently in people of West African origin. Recent epidemiological studies using precise diagnostic criteria have reported an incidence of between 0.1 and 2.9% (Saxen 1980a,b; Saxby 1984, 1987; Kronauer et al 1986; Bial & Mellonig 1987; Melvin et al 1991; Hart et al 1991; Papapanau 1994). These studies all confirm that the prevalence varies amongst different ethnic groups and a study in Britain (Saxby 1984) showed an incidence of 0.02% for Caucasians, 0.8% for Afro-Caribbeans and 0.2% for Asians. In a later study, Saxby (1987) examined the prevalence of JP in a sample of 7266 school children in the West Midlands, UK. The subjects were initially screened by assessments of probing depths around incisors and first molars and positive subjects were then confirmed by full mouth clinical and radiological examination. An overall prevalence of 0.1% was found and subjects in both sexes were affected with equal frequency. However, highly significant differences were observed between different ethnic groups with a prevalence of 0.02% in Caucasians, 0.2% in Asians and 0.8% in Afro-Caribbeans which was virtually identical to the earlier study. Similar findings were found by Melvin et al (1991) who examined a racially mixed population in Florida, USA. A total of 3158 male and 1855 female armed service recruits were examined in a three-step procedure. First, panoramic radiographs of these subjects were screened and second, areas suggestive of bone loss were further examined with bite wing radiographs. Finally, the recruits with radiographic evidence of bone loss were subjected to careful clinical examination. A total of 38 cases of JP were identified with a female:male ratio of 1.1:1. There were significant ethnic differences with a prevalence of 2.9% in Blacks, 0.09% in Caucasians and 0.8% in those of Oriental and Hispanic origin. JP was more prevalent in Black males than females with a ratio of 0.52:1, while it was more prevalent in Caucasian females than males with a ratio of 4.3:1. In another study of the radiographs of 1038 children aged 10–12 years, Neely (1992) found a prevalence rate of 4.6 per thousand. In addition, an examination of 2500 children in Chile by Lopez et al (1991) found a JP prevalence of 0.32%, and in Iraq Albander (1993) recorded a prevalence of 1.8%. However, too many variables, e.g. oral hygiene, nutritional status and socioeconomic factors, enter into the picture to allow valid comparison, and in the Chilean study (Lopez et al 1991) the authors state that JP was found most commonly in people from low socioeconomic groups. The disease also seems more prevalent in Africa as exemplified by Nigerian studies (Hartley & Floyd 1988). This has been confirmed in a recent study (Albandar et al 2002) of 690 Ugandan students aged 12–25 years which showed a prevalence of 2.3% for generalized EOP and 4.2% for localized EOP and 22.3% of incidental EOP (involvement of only 1–3 teeth). It also found a slightly higher prevalence in boys than girls (33.8% vs 22.2%). These percentages are very much higher than in any other study including those from Africa and this may have been because the criteria used did not restrict the cases to localized JP and could have included some early onset chronic periodontitis cases in the older age groups. However, the percentages are still high if one restricts their data to the 12–16 age group where the percentages were 26.8% of the 77 subjects in that age group.

AGE OF PRESENTATION

The patient is usually an adolescent at the time of examination but may be much younger; the onset of the disease may be several years before the time of examination. Sjobin et al (1993) carried out a retrospective study of early radiographs of 118 young patients aged 13–19 with JP, taken when they were 5–12 years old, and compared these with early radiographs of 168 13–19-year-olds without JP. They found that some of the individuals with JP had bone loss around primary teeth.

A similar clinical picture to JP, but with obvious signs of gingival inflammation, has been found in individuals in their 20s and has been called post juvenile aggressive (A) periodontitis. It appears to result from the evolution of JP.

SEX RATIOS

Many of the earlier studies reported that the condition appeared more commonly in females than males, at a ratio of about 3:1 (Baer 1971; Manson & Lehner 1974). In Iraqi children Albander (1993) recorded a ratio of 3.5:1, and the ratio of girls to boys in the Lopez et al (1991) study was 7:1. However, there are certain qualifications that need to be applied to all epidemiological data before such assertions can be accepted. In this regard, it has been suggested that some of the findings reflect the way in which the data have been collected. In those studies based upon patients presenting at periodontal clinics, the adolescent girl who is usually more concerned about her appearance and wellbeing than the adolescent boy will figure more frequently. Also, the patient is more likely to be accompanied by the mother from whom the enquiries about the family are made. Fathers are often invisible, and prevalence in males may be underestimated simply because they are not examined.

When the data is obtained from balanced epidemiological surveys (Saxby 1987; Melvin et al 1991) an almost equal (1.1:1) sex prevalence is found. Furthermore, one of these studies (Melvin et al 1991) also showed very different sex ratios in Black and Caucasian subjects with a male to female ratio of 0.52:1 in Black subjects and 1:4.3 in Caucasians. It has also been pointed out that the apparent 2–10 times greater prevalence of JP in females in many studies may have been due to selection bias since more females than males seek treatment. They also found that there is no female preponderance of JP cases after correction has been made for selection bias. Thus the method of collecting data must be scrutinized before conclusions can be drawn.

CLINICAL MANIFESTATIONS

The gingivae usually show few if any signs of clinical inflammation and little or no supragingival plaque and calculus. Subgingival calculus deposits are usually absent from root surfaces and because of the absence of clinical inflammation and gingival bleeding the condition may escape detection until it becomes advanced when mobility and drifting of teeth, usually incisors, occur. An acute periodontal abscess may develop at this stage and the associated pain and swelling bring the patient to the dentist for examination. As stated, the condition is frequently localized to the incisors and first molars but may affect other teeth (Astemborski et al 1989).

In regularly attending patients, the disease should be diagnosed much earlier and at this stage treatment is more successful. The early clinical signs are periodontal pocketing and attachment loss, often on the mesial surface of the first molar (**Fig. 23.1**). Attachment loss may increase rapidly. Baer (1971) estimated that 50–75% of the attachment of affected teeth may be lost in 4–5 years.

BONE DESTRUCTION

The pattern of bone destruction and distribution of the lesions represent two of the intriguing aspects of the disease. In the classic case advanced bone destruction is localized to the incisors and first molars in a symmetrical or mirror-image distribution (**Fig. 23.2**). Deep angular or crescentic bone defects around these teeth, particularly the affected molars, are characteristic and the areas of bone resorption are sharply demarcated from the

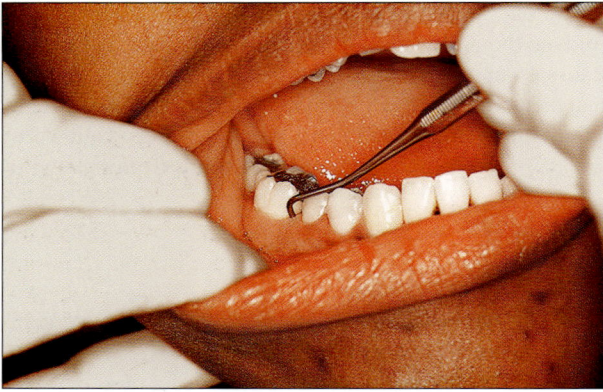

Fig. 23.1 Localized juvenile periodontitis. A periodontal probe measuring a 10 mm pocket mesial to the left lower first molar of an 18-year-old woman. Note the lack of clinical inflammation, plaque and calculus.

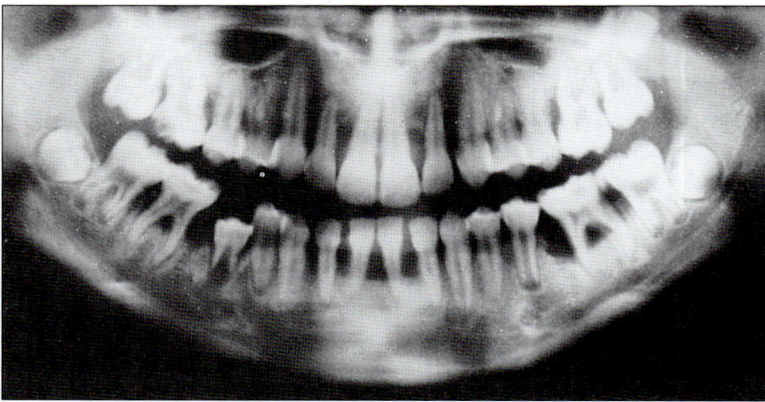

Fig. 23.2 Localized juvenile periodontitis. Classic first molar-incisor involvement in a 12-year-old boy. The orthopantogram shows advanced bone loss around upper and lower first molars and incisors.

neighbouring bone which on the radiograph appears completely healthy. Because the alveolar bone is thinner around incisors then these teeth often lose all the interdental bone and this appears on the radiographs as marked horizontal bone loss. Other teeth, in particular second premolars and second molars, may be involved.

With regular attenders, the first radiographical signs are likely to be seen on routine bite-wing radiographs usually on the mesial surface of the first molar. Any early signs of bone loss on these teeth should be taken seriously and should lead to a detailed examination of the patient. These radiographs should always be checked for any signs of bone loss since they clearly show the alveolar crest. They are probably the only means of early diagnosis of JP since children and adolescents are unlikely to have a detailed periodontal examination.

In a proportion of cases apparently random, asymmetrical involvement occurs. On rare occasions the condition may spread with time to other teeth so that the bone around almost every tooth is involved.

FAMILIAL TENDENCY

Many researchers have described a familial tendency in this disease. Benjamin and Baer (1967) described its occurrence in twins, siblings, cousins and other family connections. This has suggested a genetic transmission, and because of the apparently greater frequency in females an X-linked dominant inheritance has been suggested (Melnick et al 1976; Spektor et al 1985). However, reinterpretation of this evidence (Hart et al 1992) this supports the notion of autosomal transmission. In this connection some studies have suggested that it is an autosomal recessive condition

(Saxen 1980c; Long et al 1987) and still others that it is autosomal dominant (Roulston et al 1985; Boughman et al 1986). Boughman et al (1986) reported one child with JP and dentinogenesis imperfecta (a genetically transmitted autosomal dominant fault) which both showed genetic markers on chromosome 4, while the same group also discovered a family in which five generations displayed JP and dentinogenesis imperfecta always occurring together (Roulston et al 1985). In yet another study by one of these groups (Boughman et al 1988), genetic-model testing was used on 28 families with a history of JP. They showed that an autosomal recessive mode of inheritance was most applicable to the data.

The various genetic studies showed that if a patient has JP there is a 50% chance that the disease will develop in a brother or sister (Saxen 1980c; Spektor et al 1985; Van Dyke et al 1985).

It has also been shown that JP occurs frequently in blood group B (Kaslick et al 1971). Tissue typing has also been used to determine a possible predisposition to JP. The major histocompatibility complex, MHC (see Ch. 3) has at least six human leucocyte antigen (HLA) types and the composition of these is genetically determined and varies in different individuals. Available information indicates a great variation in HLA profiles amongst JP patients (Saxen 1980c; Saxen & Koskimies 1984), although there is an increased frequency of antigens A9, A28 and B15 in these patients (Reinholdt et al 1977). Thus although there is much evidence to support the genetic inheritance of JP, its mode of inheritance is still unclear. It is also not known how the genes are expressed.

Tai et al (2002) compared polymorphisms of the IL-1α, IL-1β and IL-1 receptor antagonist (IL-1ra) genes in 47 generalized early onset periodontitis (G-EOP) and 97 healthy Japanese subjects. They found no differences between the groups with regard to polymorphisms of IL-1α or IL-1β genes but did find a significant difference of polymorphisms of the IL-1ra gene. IL-1ra protein attaches to the IL-1 receptor to block IL-1 attachment and thus function. This therefore might be a mode of inheritance of some cases of generalized EOP.

GENERAL HEALTH

There seems to be no relationship with any systemic condition, although a somewhat similar dental picture is found in the rare Papillon–Lefèvre syndrome but with a generalized distribution and also involving the deciduous dentition.

The role of cementum

Gottlieb (1928) first suggested that the underlying cause of periodontosis was a defect in cementum formation. This concept has been reexamined more recently (Lindstog & Blomlöf 1983; Blomlöf et al 1986). They carried out a comparative histological study on teeth from patients with JP, adult chronic periodontitis and healthy controls. They found that the cementum on the teeth from JP subjects had extensive areas of hypoplasia in both the exposed and intra-alveolar root surfaces. This suggests that the defect is related to impaired cementum formation rather than the pathology of the pocket. This defect in cementum formation could be hereditary and could be an important aetiological factor.

BACTERIOLOGY

The subgingival microflora of JP is scanty when compared with that associated with adult periodontitis and its composition is very difficult. Examination with dark ground microscopy shows that it is dominated by coccoid and straight non-motile rods (Liljenberg & Lindhe 1980). The dominant cultivatable microflora consists of Gram-negative capnophilic and facultative rods and these make up about two-thirds of the isolates (Newman & Socransky 1977). The principal bacteria present are *A. actinomycetemcomitans*, *Capnocytophaga* spp. and *E. corrodens*. Some motile anaerobic rods, mainly *Campylobacter* (*Wolinella*) *recta*, may also be present in some cases (Slots 1976; Zambon et al 1983a). Using selective media for Peptostreptococcus *A. actinomycetemcomitans* can be isolated from nearly all JP patients (Slots et al 1980; Zambon et al 1983a). Mandell (1984) found 100-fold higher numbers of *A. actinomycetemcomitans* and 50-fold higher numbers of *E. corrodens* in active versus non-active sites.

Kamma et al (2004) characterized the bacterial profile of the periodontal pocket of early onset periodontitis/aggressive periodontitis patients using two different techniques, culture and immunofluorescence. The study group consisted of 66 systemically healthy individuals (41 females and 25 males, aged 23–35 years) with evidence of early onset periodontitis. Bacterial samples were collected from the deepest site in each quadrant, resulting in a total of 264 sites with a mean probing pocket depth of 6.6. Samples were cultured anaerobically and in 10% CO_2 using selective and nonselective media, and isolates were characterized to species level. Indirect immunofluorescence using monoclonal antibodies was applied to detect *A. actinomycetemcomitans*, *Porphyromonas gingivalis*, *Tannerella forsythia*, *Prevotella intermedia*, *P. nigrescens*, *C. rectus*, *Peptostreptococcus micros* and *Actinomyces israelii*.

Prevotella intermedia, *P. nigrescens*, *Porphyromonas gingivalis*, and *C. rectus* were detected in 77.3–85.9% of samples using culture methods and in 85.6–91.3% using immunofluorescence. *Peptostreptococcus micros* and *Aggregatibacter actinomycetemcomitans* were found respectively in 63.3% and 25.0% of all sites using culturing and in 58.7% and 27.7% sites using immunofluorescence. Significantly strong positive associations were observed between *T. forsythia* and *C. rectus* (odds ratio 109.46), and *T. forsythia* and *Porphyromonas gingivalis* (odds ratio 90.26), whereas a negative association was seen between *Prevotella intermedia*, *P. nigrescens* and *A. actinomycetemcomitans* (odds ratio 0.42). Coinfection by *Porphyromonas gingivalis*, *T. forsythia*, *Prevotella intermedia*, *P. nigrescens* and *C. rectus* was observed in 62.1% of the test sites, and in 89.4% of the studied subjects. The sensitivity of immunofluorescence for *T. forsythia*, *C. rectus*, *P. intermedia*, *P. nigrescens* and *Porphyromonas gingivalis* was found to be very high (0.99–0.94) using culture as the reference detection method. The agreement between culture and immunofluorescence in detecting the presence or absence of the investigated species was 85.2–88.1% for *P. gingivalis*, *Prevotella intermedia*, *P. nigrescens*, *C. rectus*, and *T. forsythia*, 75.9% for *A. actinomycetemcomitans* and 70.4% for *Peptostreptococcus micros*.

Thus, they found a complex microbial profile. However, the age range of the patients and the fact that a high proportion of the sites bled on probing suggests that none of these patients were LAP cases but rather post JP or RPP cases which would explain their findings.

The bacteria associated with JP may invade the periodontal connective tissue in this condition (Gillett & Johnson 1982; Carranza et al 1983; Christersson et al 1987) and *A. actinomycetemcomitans* is the principal invading species (Saglie et al 1982).

Several bacteria associated with JP produce substances capable of damaging the host defences and tissues and these will be described in association with each bacteria. By far the most important bacteria associated with this condition is *A. actinomycetemcomitans* and this has been the subject of most of the research on this subject. This is therefore the first bacteria described below.

Aggregatibacter actinomycetemcomitans

A. actinomycetemcomitans is a non-motile, capnophilic, Gram-negative coccobacillus that has been strongly implicated in aggressive periodontitis (Slots et al 1982; Zambon 1985). Numerous studies have shown the association between *A. actinomycetemcomitans* and JP and have suggested that it plays an important role in its pathogenesis (Haffajee et al 1984; Zambon

1985). *A. actinomycetemcomitans* is found in low numbers in the subgingival flora of healthy and adult chronic periodontitis sites whereas in JP it is found in 97% of affected sites and forms up to 70% of the total flora at these sites (Zambon 1985). Furthermore, resolution of JP coincides with a reduction or elimination of this bacteria from the subgingival flora and recurrence of disease is associated with a recolonization of the site with this bacteria (Slots & Rosling 1983).

However, there is now no doubt that a significant number of young healthy subjects also harbour *A. actinomycetemcomitans* in their oral flora. The global distribution of *A. actinomycetemcomitans* varies considerably and in normal periodontally healthy individuals its prevalence is about 13% in Finland (Alanuusua & Asikainen 1988), 20–25% in urban USA (Slots et al 1980) and 60% in Panama (Eisenmann et al 1983). Interestingly, this bacterial distribution seems to mirror the relative occurrence of JP in these three countries which was lowest in Finland, intermediate in the USA and highest in Panama (Lindhe & Slots 1989). Possibly if there is a higher infection rate with this bacteria in the population then there is a higher risk that susceptible individuals may acquire the bacteria and develop JP (Slots & Schonfeld 1991). This may to some extent explain the higher prevalence of JP in Black subjects in the USA and UK. It is possible that the high level of *A. actinomycetemcomitans* infection in these subjects represents a carriage of the bacteria from African populations with high prevalence of JP (Franklin 1978). Tracing *A. actinomycetemcomitans* transmission in racial and family groups is being aided by the development of sensitive microbial genetic methods to trace genotypes of this bacteria in various populations (Di Rienzo & Slots 1990; Zambon et al 1990).

Similarly, familial distribution of *A. actinomycetemcomitans* may be due to transmission of bacteria between family members and this could be particularly relevant in families with one or more members susceptible to JP. Convincing evidence of intra-familial transmission was produced by Zambon et al (1983a) who found that each infected subject in the family harboured the same biotype and serotype of the bacteria. This was also shown with genetic methods using restriction fragment length polymorphism (RFLP) typing of strains (Di Rienzo & Slots 1990). They showed at least one common RFLP type in each infected family member.

Transmission of putative periodontal pathogens between family members has been shown (van Winkelhoff & Boutaga 2005). Based on the current knowledge, screening for and prevention of transmission of specific virulent clones of *A. actinomycetemcomitans* may be feasible and effective in preventing some forms of early onset periodontal disease.

Dogan et al (2008) determined the periodontal status and occurrence of *A. actinomycetemcomitans* in family members of subjects with *A. actinomycetemcomitans*-positive aggressive periodontitis and evaluated the probability of its intrafamilial transmission. They found that in all families, the likelihood of intrafamilial transmission of *A. actinomycetemcomitans* was statistically significant. Members of most families also harboured additional clonal types of *A. actinomycetemcomitans*. Thus, parents and siblings of an individual with *A. actinomycetemcomitans*-positive AgP may have an increased susceptibility to periodontitis and may share other clonal types of oral *A. actinomycetemcomitans*.

Haubek et al (2005) showed in Moroccan adolescents that while sharing of toothbrushes did not seem to be associated with the presence of *A. actinomycetemcomitans*, eating and drinking habits conducive to exchange of saliva were positively associated with the presence of *A. actinomycetemcomitans*, and with a higher level of clinical attachment loss.

Various serotypes and genotypes of *A. actinomycetemcomitans* have been identified (Zambon et al 1990; Saarela et al 1992) and more than one serotype or genotype can colonize the oral cavity of an individual. Asikainen et al (1991) recovered two serotypes from 1 of 13 infected Finnish subjects and Chung et al (1989) found two serotypes in 3 of 12 infected Korean patients. In addition, Di Rienzo and Slots (1990) found two and three RFLP types in two Black families. Both the intra-familial

Extracellular outer membrane vesicles

A. actinomycetemcomitans produces numerous extracellular outer membrane vesicles which are shed from the surface of the bacteria (Holt et al 1980). These vesicles contain the leucotoxin (see above) and LPS (Lai et al 1981; Nowotney et al 1982; Tervahartiala et al 1989; Koga et al 1991). Their small size could easily permit them to cross epithelial barriers such as the pocket epithelium (Maryland & Grenier 1989).

Factors affecting the immune response

A. actinomycetemcomitans produces a potent polyclonal B-lymphocyte activating factor (Bick et al 1981) which may contribute to the pathogenesis of the condition by inducing B lymphocytes to produce antibodies with determinants unrelated to the bacterial antigens. This may in part be due to the LPS and SAM proteins present in outer membrane vesicles (see above).

IgG2 responses are gamma interferon (IFN-γ) dependent, and monocyte-derived dendritic cells (mDCs) promote IgG2 production (see Ch. 3). Dendritic cells spontaneously emerge from monocytes in cultures prepared from localized aggressive periodontitis (LAP) patients, and these patients have high levels of IgG2 that is reactive with *A. actinomycetemcomitans* (Kikuchi et al 2004). Furthermore, IFN-γ was found to promote both the immunopathologic and protective effects of IgG2. These researchers (Kikuchi et al 2004) investigated these relationships further and found that *A. actinomycetemcomitans* induced mDCs to produce IL-12, and the addition of *A. actinomycetemcomitans* and DCs to cultured peripheral blood lymphocytes elicited high levels of IFN-γ within 24h. In contrast, IL-4 was not detectable although DC-derived IL-10 production was apparent. *A. actinomycetemcomitans*-stimulated macrophages prepared from the same monocytes lacked the ability to induce IL-12 or IFN-γ responses. NK cells of the innate immune system were found to be the primary source of this early IFN-γ, although CD8 T cells also contributed some. The NK cell-derived IFN-γ was IL-12 dependent, and *A. actinomycetemcomitans*-DC interactions were Toll-like receptor 4 dependent. *A. actinomycetemcomitans* and *A. actinomycetemcomitans* lipopolysaccharide (LPS) were more potent than *Escherichia coli* and *E. coli* LPS in the ability to induce DC IL-12 and IFN-γ. The ability of *A. actinomycetemcomitans*-stimulated DCs to induce NK cells to rapidly produce IFN-γ in the absence of detectable IL-4 suggests their potential for skewing responses toward Th1 (see Ch. 3). This may also help explain the presence of Th1-associated cytokines in gingival crevicular fluid (GCF) from LAP patients and the high levels of IgG2 in their serum and GCF that is reactive with *A. actinomycetemcomitans*. It may also serve as an explanation of the lack of clinical gingival inflammation in early LAP cases.

Factors damaging host cells

A. actinomycetemcomitans produces an epitheliotoxin which can damage epithelial cells and could facilitate bacterial penetration of the junctional and pocket epithelium (Birkedal–Hansen et al 1992). It also produces a fibroblast-inhibiting factor which may impair tissue repair (Stevens & Hammond 1982).

The invasion of *A. actinomycetemcomitans* into epithelial cells may be aided by their release of an epitheliotoxin (Birkedal–Hansen et al 1992) and this may be a mechanism by which it might evade the host defences and may explain the episodic nature of this disease (Meyer et al 1991). In this regard these bacteria have been found in the connective tissue in contact with collagen and fibronectin and these proteins may be potential binding sites of *A. actinomycetemcomitans* (Mintz & Fives-Taylor 1999). Specific attachment of *A. actinomycetemcomitans* to host tissues is critical for infection and these bacteria adhere to and invade into epithelial cells (Fives-Taylor et al 1996).

Proteases that degrade immunoglobulins

A. actinomycetemcomitans produces proteolytic enzymes which degrade immunoglobulins (Killian 1981). This could reduce the local effectiveness of antibodies produced against this bacteria.

Collagenase

A. actinomycetemcomitans produces a collagenolytic proteinase which can attack collagen (Robertson et al 1982). This could contribute to degradation of collagen and connective tissue breakdown in the periodontal tissues. In this regard an arginine- and lysin-specific protease of approximately 50kDa in molecular weight has been purified from the culture supernatant of *A. actinomycetemcomitans* and this enzyme showed collagen degrading activity (Wang et al 1999).

This purified protease (Wang et al 1999) has also been shown to reduce the cell growth rate, DNA synthesis rate and fibronectin level of human gingival epithelial cells in a dose dependent way *in vitro* (Wang et al 2001). Thus, this protease may inhibit the proliferation of these cells.

Factors released by the other Gram-negative, capnophilic bacteria associated with aggressive periodontitis could also contribute to the pathology of this disease. The most important of these are *E. corrodens* and *Capnocytophaga* species.

Eikenella corrodens

Both the SAM and LPS from *E. corrodens* stimulate bone resorption *in vitro*. The SAM appears to do this by first releasing IL-1 and TNF from its target cells which then stimulates the release of PGE$_2$ and collagenase (Holt & Ebersole 1991; Henderson & Blake 1992). It has been shown that the inhibition of bone DNA and collagen production by osteoblasts in murine calvaria produced by low titres of this SAM may be due to this mechanism because it is blocked by indomethacin, an inhibitor of prostaglandins (Meghji et al 1992a). This SAM also produces polyclonal B-lymphocyte activation (Bick et al 1981).

E. corrodens also produces factors which inhibit PMN chemotaxis (Van Dyke et al 1982).

Capnocytophaga species

The LPS of *Capnocytophaga* species produces weak bone resorption *in vitro* by the same mechanism as *E. corrodens*.

These bacteria also produce proteases which can degrade types I and IV collagens, immunoglobulins and the glycosaminoglycan components of proteoglycans (Killian et al 1983; Seddon & Shah 1989; Söderling et al 1991).

Finally, they produce factors which inhibit PMN chemotaxis (Van Dyke et al 1982).

THE HOST RESPONSE IN AGGRESSIVE PERIODONTITIS

Local

The primary defence of the periodontal pocket is provided by PMNs and reduction in their function gives rise to severe disease. It has been shown that PMNs from the periodontal pockets of JP cases have reduced chemotactic activity and phagocytic function which could in part be related to the secretion of leucotoxin by *A. actinomycetemcomitans* (Murray & Patters 1980).

The local lesion of JP in the connective tissue adjacent to the pocket and junctional epithelium is mainly populated by plasma cells and blast cells (Liljenberg & Lindhe 1980). Gingival explant cultures have been shown to produce immunoglobulins against the associated bacteria and this shows that plasma cells in the local tissues are capable of local production of these immunoglobulins (Hall et al 1990).

Patients with localized aggressive periodontitis have type-1 cytokines in gingival crevicular fluid and high titres of IFN-dependent IgG2 reactive with *Porphyromonas gingivalis* in gingival crevicular fluid and serum. Localized aggressive periodontitis monocytes spontaneously differentiate into dendritic cells that can stimulate IFN-production by NK cells (Kikuchi et al 2005). These workers have shown that *P. gingivalis*-dendritic cell–NK cell interactions apparently result in reciprocal stimulation and increased type-1 cytokine production by both dendritic cells and NK cells, and increased *P. gingivalis*-specific IgG2. This may enhance protection against this bacterium in this condition and reduce its numbers in the subgingival flora.

General

Leucocyte function

The majority of patients with JP have peripheral blood PMNs with an impaired ability to react to chemotactic stimuli (Clark et al 1977; Van Dyke et al 1980). This appears to be caused by a cell-associated defect.

In the normal chemotactic response, receptor stimulation triggers a rise of intracellular calcium level in two separate stages. In this regard, another study (Daniel et al 1993) has measured the level of intracellular calcium in the neutrophils of six JP patients following chemotactic stimulation and have reported a decreased cytosolic calcium response. The initial phase was not affected but the second stage was reduced. They suggested that the second phase of reduced calcium response, possibly caused by defective calcium channels, was the cause of the reduced chemotaxis. This could thus be an important factor in the aetiology of JP.

Another study (Hurttia et al 1998) has measured the adhesion of neutrophils from patients with JP and compared them with those from healthy controls. They found that the neutrophils from patients with JP had significantly increased adherence. They suggested that this hyper-adherence could inhibit the migration of neutrophils from the circulation to the infection site.

Some retrospective and cross-sectional studies also suggest that all forms of early onset periodontitis may be associated with genetic deficiencies in phagocytic leucocyte function such as chemotaxis, degranulation or adhesion (Schenkein & Van Dyke 1994; Novak & Novak 1996; Hart & Kornman 1997; Kornman et al 1997). The latter mechanism may be mediated by leucocyte adhesion deficiencies (LAD) which occur in humans as the result of genetic faults (Springer 1994; Frenette & Wagner 1996a,b; Malech & Nauseef 1997).

Leucocytes use the selectin glycoprotein and integrin-Iγ-superfamily interactions to migrate from blood vessels to sites of infection (Springer 1994; Frenette & Wagner 1996a,b). In particular, selectin-glycoprotein interactions are responsible for the initial rolling adhesion between leucocytes and vascular endothelium and involve three selectin family members, P (platelet), E (endothelium) and L (leucocyte). Selectins bind to glycoprotein ligands expressed on the surface of both leucocytes and vascular endothelial cells.

Fucosylation of these glycoproteins is deficient in human leucocyte adhesion deficiency II (LAD-II) (Von Andrian et al 1993). These patients are highly susceptible to infections and have leucocytosis but much reduced pus formation. They also present with early onset prepubertal periodontitis (Etzioni et al 1992). Similarly, patients with a L-selectin deficiency exhibit rapidly progressive periodontitis (Macey et al 1998; Gainet et al 1998, 1999).

Mice can be genetically engineered to be P and E selectin deficient and these animals resemble in many ways human LAD-II (Wilson et al 1993b; Bullard et al 1995, 1996; Ley et al 1995; Frenette et al 1996; Mizgerd et al 1996, 1999; Munoz et al 1997). These mice exhibit leucocytosis and their leucocytes have a much reduced ability to emigrate to sites of infection (Socransky et al 1984; Trudel et al 1986). These mice have also recently been studied in relationship to their susceptibility to periodontal bone loss (Niederman et al 2001).

It has been shown (Niederman et al 2001) that P/E-selectin-deficient mice exhibit spontaneous rapidly progressive early onset periodontal disease which does not occur in the wild type mice. Significant alveolar bone loss was seen from 6 weeks of age and then progressively increased with time. The affected mice also had a 10-fold increase in the numbers of bacteria in the oral cavity in comparison to the control mice.

The oral flora of mice is different from that of primates and in this study a total of nine species were detected in the wild type in comparison to 5 with the P/E-selectin-deficient mice. Three of these species, *Enterococcus gallinarum*, *Proteus mirabilis*, *Staphylococcus aureus*, were not seen in the wild-type mice. Also the severe alveolar bone loss in the P/E-selectin-deficient mice was prevented by the prophylactic administration of antibiotics showing that the bacteria were necessary for the disease to occur. The affected mice also showed a leucocytosis.

The P/E-selectin-deficient mice had elevated gingival tissue levels of the bone resorptive cytokine IL-Iα in comparison to control mice. They also had significantly lower levels of the anti-inflammatory cytokines IL-4 and IL-10 and the anti-bone resorptive cytokine IFN-γ. The age of onset and kinetics of this early onset periodontitis in P/E-selectin-deficient mice is different to that seen in previous mice models (Baer & Bernick 1957; Baer & Lieberman 1959, 1960; Sheppe 1965; Gilbert & Sofaer 1988, 1989: Baker et al 1994).

The ability of the oral microbiota to produce disease in P/E-selectin-deficient mice suggests that their susceptibility is due to decreased leucocyte emigration into the gingival tissue and gingival crevice. This in turn probably allows unchecked growth of the plaque in the crevice and would also not prevent bacteria from invading the gingival tissues thus producing early-onset progressive periodontal disease. The cytokine changes described above are consistent with similar findings in humans with active periodontitis (Stashenko et al 1991; Wilton et al 1992; Lee et al 1995; Tsai et al 1995). They also support the observation in monkeys that the specific inhibition of IL-1 blocked periodontal bone loss (Assuma et al 1998).

This appears at the present time to be the only animal model of spontaneous, rapid onset periodontal disease and is one in which the host responses can be genetically manipulated. Although it is very different in terms of the oral flora to human and other primate disease it may none the less provide important insights into key factors in the host responses.

Recently, it has been found that the PMNs associated with LAP are not hypofunctional or deficient but rather hyperfunctional (Kantarci et al 2003) and their amplified activity may be responsible for the tissue destruction. Several signal transduction abnormalities are associated with the elevated PMN function in LAP. There is strong correlation between defective chemotaxis and decreased intracellular Ca^{2+} levels. Furthermore, the total calcium-dependent protein kinase C activity of PMNs in LAP is significantly lower than healthy subjects. There is also a marked increase in diacylglycerol (DAG) levels which is accompanied by a marked decrease in DAG kinase activity. In addition, GCF from LAP subjects was found to contain PGE_2, leukotriene B_4 (LTB_4) and lipoxin A_4 (LXA_4). Peripheral blood PMNs of LAP patients, but not PMNs from blood from healthy volunteers, also generated LXA_4, suggesting that this immunoregulatory molecule could play a role in LAP with its relationship to PGE_2, and LTB_4. Thus it appears that the hyper-responsiveness of PMNs in LAP enhances tissue damage and may be due either to cell priming or genetic predisposition.

Diacylglycerol kinase (DGK) metabolizes diacylglycerol (DAG), an endogenous activator of protein kinase C, to phosphatidic acid (Oyaizu et al 2003). This group has also reported that there were increased levels of DAG in neutrophils from patients with localized juvenile (aggressive) periodontitis (LAP), which was associated with reduced DGK activity (see above). This reduced activity could have been due to a mutation, post-translational modification, differential expression, or lack of expression of a particular isoform(s). They have also investigated the mRNAs for DAG isoforms in normal and LAP neutrophils (Oyaizu et al 2003). The three main isoforms of

Thus, providing there is sufficient support remaining on the affected teeth then the aim of the primary treatment is elimination of *A. actinomycetemcomitans* from the pockets by a combination of a course of antibiotics followed by oral hygiene instruction and scaling and root planing. This should be followed by regular 3-monthly maintenance scaling to prevent recolonization.

If *A. actinomycetemcomitans* reinfects a site(s), then the patient may be retreated with the appropriate antibiotic(s) based on the results of microbiological sensitivity tests. Regular microbiological monitoring of *A. actinomycetemcomitans* in the subgingival flora should be carried out if such facilities are available. Practitioners should refer patients to a dental hospital if oral microbiological facilities are not available to them locally.

Where appropriate, periodontal surgery may be considered for the treatment of residual deep pockets. Where there is insufficient support remaining extractions and prosthetic replacement need to be considered. A plan for such treatment is set out below:

1. Samples of subgingival flora of affected sites should be taken for microbiological investigation and in particular to monitor *A. actinomycetemcomitans* and its antibiotic sensitivity. A suitable collection and transport system using an appropriate medium must be worked out with the microbiology laboratory.

2. Oral hygiene instruction and counselling of the patient with emphasis laid on the special nature of the condition and therefore the special responsibility of the patient in maintaining a high level of home care.

3. Administration of antibiotics: either metronidazole 200 mg and amoxicillin 250 mg 3 times daily for 7 days or metronidazole 200 mg 3 times daily for 10 days or tetracycline 250 mg four times daily for 14 days.

4. Scaling and root planing of affected sites. Subgingival calculus deposits are usually absent. However, debridement and root planing help to create conditions unfavourable to the microflora.

5. Extraction when necessary, with immediate replacement of anterior teeth, of teeth with a hopeless prognosis due to excessive bone loss and drifting.

6. Periodontal surgery: Localized inverse bevel periodontal surgery should only be carried out if the patient's cooperation is good and is best done with preoperative and postoperative antibiotic administration. Any suprabony pockets in posterior teeth can be eliminated by apical positioning but, with anterior teeth, replaced flaps are necessary because of aesthetic considerations. A majority of teeth with this condition will have deep intrabony pocketing with associated angular bony defects. These lesions should be curetted with the aim of producing bony in-fill with or without the placement of a bone or bone substitute graft. Certain isolated intrabony lesions with suitable morphology can be treated with guided tissue regenerating and/or bone grafting techniques (see Ch. 20). The tissues heal rapidly after surgery and often show evidence of in-fill of bone defects. In some cases, advanced bone loss around one of the roots of a first molar may be treated by root amputation or hemisection.

7. Occlusal adjustment: Migration of incisors is a late characteristic of AP but orthodontic treatment of these cases is usually contraindicated. If teeth which are to remain have drifted into premature contact, these should be treated by selective grinding. In a few cases after successful periodontal treatment and after the condition has become fully stable, gentle orthodontic retraction of labially drifted upper incisors might be considered if they can be stabilized behind the lower lip or splinted in a stable position.

8. Prosthetics: Any necessary partial dentures must be carefully designed so that gingival irritation is avoided and abutment teeth loaded as near axially as possible. Chrome cobalt skeleton dentures are usually indicated and acrylic dentures should only be used in the immediate replacement phase.

9. Maintenance: The observation by Waerhaug (1977) that successfully treated cases can subsequently show signs of relapse indicates that long-term maintenance is essential. These patients should be recalled every 3 months for oral hygiene reinforcement and scaling. The affected sites should be monitored and if any deterioration occurs, samples of subgingival flora be taken for microbiological investigation in order to monitor possible recurrence of *A. actinomycetemcomitans*. If this bacteria is found by the microbiologists, its antibiotic sensitivity should be determined. Appropriate antibiotic treatment can then be given to eliminate this bacteria from the flora. For these reasons it is usually appropriate to refer these cases to a dental hospital where microbiological facilities are available.

EVALUATION OF TREATMENT PROCEDURES FOR AP

Antibiotics and scaling and root planing

It has been shown by Christersson et al (1985) that scaling and root planing alone may improve the clinical condition somewhat but fails to reduce significantly the number of *A. actinomycetemcomitans* in the subgingival flora. However, a number of studies have shown that a 2-week course of tetracycline or related drugs both brought about clinical improvement and significantly reduced the numbers of *A. actinomycetemcomitans* (Slots & Rosling 1983; Christersson et al 1985; Novak et al 1991). However, tetracycline often fails to eliminate *A. actinomycetemcomitans* from the subgingival flora (Mandell et al 1986). Penicillin and metronidazole used separately have been reported to be ineffective in treating AP (Mitchell 1984; Kunihira et al 1985) but in contrast metronidazole and amoxicillin used in combination have been found to be very effective (van Winkelhoff et al 1989, 1992). In a 2-year follow-up study (Pavicic et al 1994) this combination of drugs with scaling and root planing (see above) has been shown to eliminate totally *A. actinomycetemcomitans* from the subgingival flora for 2 years. Recently, however, the administration of metronidazole alone has been shown to be effective in eliminating *A. actinomycetemcomitans* from the flora (Saxen & Asikainen 1993).

Antibiotics and surgery

A combination of antibiotics and surgery seems to be very effective in controlling AP. A 2-week course of tetracycline plus replaced flap surgery (Lindhe & Liljenberg 1984) controlled the progress of the disease in 16 study patients, although 2 patients had recurrence and needed retreatment. After 5 years of follow-up there was improvement in all clinical measurements and evidence of bony in-fill of bone defects. Bacterial monitoring of this combination of treatment (Kornman & Robertson 1985) showed that sites with high levels of *A. actinomycetemcomitans* showed a better response to surgery plus tetracycline than scaling plus tetracycline. It has also been shown that surgery plus tetracycline can completely eliminate *A. actinomycetemcomitans* from the subgingival flora for up to 12 months (Mandell & Socransky 1988). However, it has now been shown (Pavicic et al 1994) that this can be achieved for 2 years with metronidazole and amoxicillin plus scaling and root planing (see above). There are as yet no reported studies of these antibiotics in combination with surgery.

REFERENCES

Alanuusua S, Asikainen S: Detection and distribution of Actinobacillus actinomycetemcomitans in the primary dentition, *J Periodontol* 59:504–507, 1988.

Albander JM: Juvenile periodontitis – pattern of progression in relationship to clinical periodontal parameters, *Community Dent Oral Epidemiol* 21:185–189, 1993.

Albandar JM, Muranga MB, Rams TE: Prevalence of aggressive periodontitis in school attendees in Uganda, *J Clin Periodontol* 29:823–831, 2002.

Armitage GC: Development of a classification system of periodontal diseases and conditions, *Ann Periodontol* 4:1–6, 1999.

Asikainen S, Lai C-H, Alanuusua S, et al: Distribution of Actinobacillus actinomycetemcomitans serotypes in periodontal health and disease, *Oral Microbiol Immunol* 6:115–118, 1991.

Assuma R, Oates T, Cochran D, Amar S, Graves DT: IL-I and TNF antagonists inhibit the inflammatory response and bone loss in experimental periodontitis, *J Immunol* 160:403–409, 1998.

Astemborski JA, Boughman JA, Myrick PO, et al: Clinical and laboratory characteristics of early onset periodontitis, *J Periodontol* 60:557–563, 1989.

Baehni PC, Tsai C-C, McArthur WP, et al: Interactions of inflammatory cells and oral microorganisms. VII. Detection of leukotoxic activity of a plaque-derived Gram negative microorganism, *Infect Immun* 24:233–243, 1979.

Baer PN: The case for periodontitis as a clinical entity, *J Periodontol* 42:516–519, 1971.

Baer RN, Bernick S: Age changes in the periodontium of the mouse, *Oral Surgery* 10:430–436, 1957.

Baer RN, Lieberman JE: Observations on some genetic characteristics of the periodontium in three strains of inbred mice, *Oral Surgery* 12:820–829, 1959.

Baer RN, Lieberman JE: Periodontal disease in 6 strains of inbred mice, *J Dent Res* 39:215–225, 1960.

Baker RJ, Evans RT, Roopenian DC: Oral infection with Porphyromonas gingivalis and induced alveolar bone loss in immunocompetent and severe combined immunodeficient mice, *Arch Oral Biol* 39:1035–1040, 1994.

Balashova NV, Crosby JA, Ghofaily LA, et al: Leukotoxin confers beta-hemolytic activity to Actinobacillus actinomycetemcomitans, *Infect Immun* 74:2015–2021, 2006.

Benjamin SD, Baer PN: Familial patterns of advanced alveolar bone loss in adolescence (periodontosis), *Periodontics* 5:82–88, 1967.

Bial JJ, Mellonig JT: Radiographical evidence of juvenile periodontitis (periodontosis), *J Periodontol* 58:321–326, 1987.

Bick PH, Betts-Carpenter A, Holdman LV, et al: Polyclonal B-cell activation induced by extracts of gram negative bacteria isolated from periodontally diseases sites, *Infect Immun* 34:43–49, 1981.

Birkedal-Hansen H, Caulfield PW, Wannameumier Y, et al: A sensitive screening assay for epitheliotoxins produced by oral organisms, *J Dent Res* 61:192, 1992.

Blomlöf L, Hammerström L, Linskog S: Occurrence and appearance of cementum hypoplasias in localized and generalized juvenile periodontitis, *Acta Odontol Scand* 44:313–320, 1986.

Boughman JA, Beaty TH, Yang P, et al: Problem of genetic model testing in early onset periodontitis, *J Periodontol* 59:332–337, 1988.

Boughman JA, Halloran SL, Roulston D: An autosomal dominant form of juvenile periodontitis (JP): its localization to chromosome No. 4 and linking to dentinogenesis imperfecta, *J Craniofac Genet Dev Biol* 6:341–350, 1986.

Buduneli N, Biçakçi N, Keskinoglu A: Flow-cytometric analysis of lymphocyte subgroups and mcd14 in patients with various periodontitis categories, *J Clin Periodontol* 28:419–424, 2001.

Bullard DC, Qin L, Lorenzo I, et al: P-selectin/Icam-I double mutant mice: acute emigration of neutrophils into the peritoneum is completely absent but is normal into pulmonary alveoli, *J Clin Invest* 95:1782–1788, 1995.

Bullard DC, Kunkel EJ, Kubo H, et al: Infectious susceptibility and severe deficiency of leukocyte rolling and recruitment in E-selectin and P-selectin double mutant mice, *J Exp Med* 183:2329–2336, 1996.

Butler JH: A familial pattern of juvenile periodontitis (periodontosis), *J Periodontol* 40:115–118, 1969.

Califano JV, Pace BE, Gunsolly JC, et al: Antibody reactive with Actinobacillus actinomycetemcomitans leukotoxin in early onset periodontitis, *Oral Microbiol Immunol* 12:20–26, 1997a.

Carranza FA, Saglie FR, Newman MG, et al: Scanning and transmission electron microscopic study of tissue-invading microorganisms in localized juvenile periodontitis, *J Periodontol* 54:598–617, 1983.

Christersson L, Slots J, Rosling B, et al: Microbiological and clinical effects of surgery treatment of localised juvenile periodontitis, *J Clin Periodontol* 12:465–476, 1985.

Christersson LA, Wikesjö UMA, Albini B, et al: Tissue localization of Actinobacillus actinomycetemcomitans in human periodontitis. 1. Light, immunofluorescent and electron microscopic studies, *J Periodontol* 58:529–539, 1987.

Chung H-J, Chung C-P, Son S-H, et al: Actinobacillus actinomycetemcomitans serotypes and leukotoxicity in Korean localized juvenile periodontitis, *J Periodontol* 60:509–511, 1989.

Clark RA, Page RC, Wilde G: Defective neutrophil chemotaxis in juvenile periodontitis, *Infect Immun* 18:694–700, 1977.

Daniel MA, McDonald G, Offenbacher S, et al: Defective chemotaxis and calcium response in localized juvenile periodontitis, *J Periodontol* 64:617–621, 1993.

Di Rienzo JM, Slots J: Genetic approach to the study of epidemiology and pathogenesis of Actinobacillus actinomycetemcomitans in localized juvenile periodontitis, *Arch Oral Biol* 35:79S–84S, 1990.

Dogan B, Kipalev AS, Ökte E, et al: Consistent intrafamilial transmission of Actinobacillus actinomycetemcomitans despite clonal diversity, *J Periodontol* 79:307–315, 2008.

Ebersole JL, Taubman MA, Smith DC, et al: Humoral immune responses and the diagnosis of human periodontal disease, *J Periodontal Res* 17:478–480, 1982.

Ebersole JL, Taubman MA, Smith DJ, et al: Human immune responses to oral microorganisms. II. Serum antibody responses to antigens from Actinobacillus actinomycetemcomitans and correlation with localized juvenile periodontitis, *J Clin Immunol* 3:321–331, 1983.

Eisenmann AAC, Eisenmann R, Sousa O, et al: Microbiological study of localized juvenile periodontitis in Panama, *J Periodontol* 54:712–713, 1983.

Etzioni A, Frydman M, Pollack S, et al: Severe recurrent infections due to a novel adhesion molecule defect, *N Engl J Med* 327:1789–1792, 1992.

Farida R, Wilson M, Ivanyi L: Serum IgG antibodies to lipopolysaccharide on various forms of periodontal disease in Man, *Arch Oral Biol* 31:711–715, 1986.

Fives-Taylor PM, Mintz KP: Virulence factors of the periodontopathogen Actinobacillus actinomycetemcomitans, *J Periodontol* 67:291–297, 1996.

Franklin ER: Periodontal diseases, a socioeconomic problem in Black Africa, *Odonto-Stomatolo Trop* 6:16–28, 1978.

Frenette PS, Wagner DD: Adhesion molecules. Part I, *N Engl J Med* 334:1526–1529, 1996a.

Frenette PS, Wagner DD: Adhesion molecules. Part II, *N Engl J Med* 335:43–45, 1996b.

Frenette PS, Mayadas TN, Rayburn H, et al: Susceptibility to infection and altered hematopoesis in mice deficient in both P- and E-selectins, *Cell* 84:563–574, 1996.

Fujita T, Kantarci A, Warbington ML, et al: CD38 expression in neutrophils from patients with localized aggressive periodontitis, *J Periodontol* 76:1960–1965, 2005.

Gainet J, Chollet-Martin S, Brion M, et al: Interleukin-8 production by polymorphonuclear neutrophils in patients with rapidly progressive periodontitis: an amplifying loop of polymorphonuclear neutrophil activation, *Lab Invest* 78:755–762, 1998.

Gainet J, Dang RM, Chollet-Martin S, et al: Neutrophil dysfunctions, IL-8, and soluble L-selectin plasma levels in rapidly progressive versus adult and localized juvenile periodontitis: variations according to disease severity and microbial flora, *J Immunol* 162:5013–5019, 1999.

Garrison SW, Holt SC, Nichols FC: Lipopolysaccharide-stimulated PGE2 release from human monocytes. Comparison of lipopolysaccharide prepared from suspected periodontal pathogens, *J Periodontol* 59:684–687, 1988.

Gilbert AD, Sofaer JA: Host genotype, pathogenic challenge and periodontal bone loss in the mouse, *Arch Oral Biol* 33:855–861, 1988.

Gilbert AD, Sofaer JA: Neutrophil function, genotype and periodontal bone loss in the mouse, *J Periodontal Res* 24:412–414, 1989.

Gillett R, Johnson NW: Bacterial invasion of the periodontium in a case of juvenile periodontitis, *J Clin Periodontol* 9:93–100, 1982.

Gottlieb B: Die diffuse Atrophie des Alveolarknochens Weitere Beitrage zur Kenntnis des Alveolarschwandes und dwssen Wiedergutmachung durch Zementwachstum, *Zeitschrift für Stomatologie* 21:195–262, 1923.

Gottlieb B: The formation of the pocket: diffuse atrophy of alveolar bone, *J Am Dent Assoc* 15:462–476, 1928.

Gu K, Bainbridge B, Daveau RP, et al: Antigenic components of Actinobacillus actinomycetemcomitans lipopolysaccharide recognized by sera from patients with localized juvenile periodontitis, *Oral Microbiol Immunol* 13:150–157, 1998.

Haffajee AD, Socransky SS, Ebersole JL, et al: Clinical, microbiological and immunological features associated with treatment of active periodontal lesions, *J Clin Periodontol* 11:600–618, 1984.

Hagewald S, Bernimoulin JP, Kottgen E, et al: Total IgA and Porphyromonas gingivalis – reactive IgA in the saliva of patients with generalized early onset periodontitis, *Eur J Oral Sci* 108:147–173, 2000.

Hall EP, Falkler WA, Suzuki JB: Production of immunoglobulins in gingival tissue explant cultures from juvenile periodontitis patients, *J Periodontol* 61:603–608, 1990.

Hart TC, Marazita ML, Schenkein HA, et al: No female preponderance for juvenile periodontitis after correction for ascertainment bias, *J Periodontol* 62:745–749, 1991.

Hart TC, Marazita ML, Schenkein HA, et al: Reinterpretation of the evidence for X-linked dominant inheritance of juvenile periodontitis, *J Periodontol* 63:169–173, 1992.

Hart TC, Kornman KS: Genetic factors in the pathogenesis of periodontitis, *Periodontol 2000* 14:202–215, 1997.

Hartley AF, Floyd PD: Prevalence of juvenile periodontitis in school children in Lagos, Nigeria, *Community Dent Oral Epidemiol* 16:299–301, 1988.

Harvey W, Kamin S, Meghji S, et al: Interleukin 1-like activity in capsular material from Haemophilus actinomycetemcomitans, *Immunology* 60:415–418, 1987.

Haubek D, Ennibi O-K, Abdellaoul L, et al: Attachment loss in Moroccan early onset periodontitis patients and infection with the JP2-type Actinobacillus actinomycetemcomitans, *J Clin Periodontol* 29:657–660, 2002.

Haubek D, Ennibi O-K, Poulsen K, et al: The highly leukotoxic JP2 clone of Actinobacillus actinomycetemcomitans and progression of periodontal attachment loss, *J Dent Res* 83:767–770, 2004.

Haubek D, Ismaili Z, Poulsen S, et al: Association between sharing of toothbrushes, eating and drinking habits and the presence of Actinobacillus actinomycetemcomitans in Moroccan adolescents, *Oral Microbiol Immunol* 20:195–198, 2005.

Henderson B, Blake S: Therapeutic potential of cytokine manipulation, *Trends Pharmacol Sci* 13:145–152, 1992.

Henderson D, Poole S, Wilson M: Bacterial modulins: a novel class of virulence factors which cause host tissue pathology by inducing cytokine synthesis, *Microbiol Rev* 60:316–341, 1996.

Hodge PJ, Riggio MP, Kinane DF: Failure to detect an association with IL-1 genotypes in European Caucasians with generalized early onset periodontitis, *J Clin Periodontol* 28:430–436, 2001.

Holt SC, Ebersole JL: The surface of selected periodontopathic bacteria: possible role in virulence. In Hamada S, Holt SC, McGhee JR, editors: *Periodontal Disease Pathogens and Host Immune Response*, Tokyo, 1991, Quintessence, pp 79–96.

Holt SC, Tanner ACR, Socransky SS: Morphology and ultrastructure of oral strains of Actinobacillus actinomycetemcomitans and Haemophilus aphrophilus, *Infect Immun* 30:588–600, 1980.

Hopps RM, Sisney-Durrant HJ: Mechanisms of alveolar bone loss in periodontal disease. In Hamada S, Holt SC, McGhee JR, editors: *Periodontal Disease Pathogens and Host Immune Response*, Tokyo, 1991, Quintessence, pp 307–320.

Hurttia H, Saarinen K, Leino L: Increased adhesion of peripheral blood neutrophils from patients with localised juvenile periodontitis, *J Periodontal Res* 33:292–297, 1998.

Iino Y, Hopps RM: The bone resorbing activities of lipopolysaccharides from the bacteria Actinobacillus actinomycetemcomitans, Bacteroides gingivalis and Capnocytophaga ochracia isolated from human mouths, *Arch Oral Biol* 29:59–63, 1984.

Iwase M, Lalley ET, Berthold P, et al: Effects of cations and osmotic protectants on cytolytic activity of Actinobacillus actinomycetemcomitans leukotoxin, *Infect Immun* 58:1783–1788, 1990.

Johnstone AM, Koh A, Goldberg MB, et al: A hyperactive neutrophil phenotype in patients with refractory periodontitis, *J Periodontol* 78:1788–1794, 2007.

Kamin S, Harvey W, Wilson M, et al: Inhibition of fibroblast proliferation and collagen synthesis by capsular material from Actinobacillus actinomycetemcomitans, *J Med Microbiol* 22:245–249, 1986.

Kamma JJ, Nakou M, Gmür R, et al: Microbiological profile of early onset/aggressive periodontitis patients, *Oral Microbiol Immunol* 19:314–321, 2004.

Kantarci A, Oyaizu K, Van Dyke TE: Neutrophil-mediated tissue injury in periodontal disease pathogenesis: findings from localized aggressive periodontitis, *J Periodontol* 74:66–75, 2003.

Kaslick RS, Chasens AI, Tuckman MA, et al: Investigation of periodontosis with periodontitis: literature survey and findings based on ABO blood groups, *J Periodontol* 42:420–427, 1971.

Kikuchi T, Hahn CL, Tanaka S, et al: Dendritic cells stimulated with Actinobacillus actinomycetemcomitans elicit rapid gamma interferon responses by natural killer cells, *Infect Immun* 72:5089–5096, 2004.

Kikuchi T, Willis DL, Liu M, et al: Dendritic-NK cell interactions in P. gingivalis-specific responses, *J Dent Res* 84:858–862, 2005.

Kiley P, Holt SC: Characterization of the lipopolysaccharide from Actinobacillus actinomycetemcomitans T Y4 and N27, *Infect Immun* 30:862–873, 1980.

Killian M: Degradation of immunoglobulins A1, A2, and G by suspected principal periodontal pathogens, *Infect Immun* 34:757–765, 1981.

Killian M, Thompson B, Petersen PE, et al: Occurrence and nature of bacterial IgA proteases, *Ann N Y Acad Sci* 409:612–624, 1983.

Kinane DF, Mooney J, MacFarlane TW, et al: Local and systemic antibody response to putative periodontal pathogens in patients with chronic periodontitis. Correlation with clinical indices, *Oral Microbiol Immunol* 8:65–68, 1993.

Kirby AC, Meghji S, Nair SP, et al: The potent bone-resorbing mediator of Actinobacillus actinomycetemcomitans is homologous to the molecular chaperone groel, *J Clin Invest* 96:1185–1194, 1995.

Koga T, Nishihara T, Amano K, et al: Chemical and biochemical properties of cell-surface components of Actinobacillus actinomycetemcomitans. In Hamada S, Holt SC, McGhee JR, editors: *Periodontal Disease Pathogens and Host Immune Response*, Tokyo, 1991, Quintessence, pp 117–127.

Kolodrubetz D, Dailey T, Ebersole J, et al: Cloning and expression of leukotoxin gene from Actinobacillus actinomycetemcomitans, *Infect Immun* 57:1465–1469, 1989.

Kornman KS, Robertson PB: Clinical and microbiological evaluation of juvenile periodontitis, *J Periodontol* 56:443–446, 1985.

Kornman KS, Page RC, Tonetti MS: The host response to the microbial challenge in periodontitis: assembling the players, *Periodontol 2000* 14:33–53, 1997.

Kronauer E, Borsa G, Lang NP: Prevalence of incipient juvenile periodontitis at age 16 in Switzerland, *J Clin Periodontol* 13:103–108, 1986.

Kunihira D, Caine F, Palicanis K: A clinical trial of phenoxymethyl penicillin for adjunctive treatment of juvenile periodontitis, *J Periodontol* 56:352–360, 1985.

Lai C-H, Listgarten MA, Hammond BF: Comparative ultrastructure of leukotoxic and non-leukotoxic strain of Actinobacillus actinomycetemcomitans, *J Periodontal Res* 16:379–389, 1981.

Lee HJ, Kang IK, Chung CR, et al: The subgingival microflora and gingival crevicular fluid cytokines in refractory periodontitis, *J Clin Periodontol* 22:885–890, 1995.

Lehner T, Wilton JMA, Ivanyi L, et al: Immunological aspects of juvenile periodontitis (periodontosis), *J Periodontal Res* 9:261–272, 1974.

Leung WK, Ngai VKS, Yau JYY, et al: Characterization of Actinobacillus actinomycetemcomitans isolated from young Chinese aggressive periodontitis patients, *J Periodontal Res* 40:258–268, 2005.

Ley K, Bullard DC, Arbones ML, et al: Sequential contribution of L- and P- selectin to leukocyte rolling in vivo, *J Exp Med* 181:669–675, 1995.

Liljenberg B, Lindhe J: Juvenile periodontitis. Some microbiological, histopathological and clinical characteristics of juvenile periodontitis, *J Clin Periodontol* 7:48–61, 1980.

Lindhe J, Liljenberg B: Treatment of localized juvenile periodontitis results after 5 years, *J Clin Periodontol* 11:399–410, 1984.

Lindhe J, Slots J: Periodontal disease in children and young adults. In Lindhe J, editor: *Textbook of Clinical Periodontology*, Copenhagen, 1989, Munksgaard, pp 193–220.

Lindstog S, Blomlöf L: Cementum hypoplasia in teeth affected by juvenile periodontitis, *J Clin Periodontol* 10:443–451, 1983.

Long JC, Nance WE, Waring P: Early onset periodontitis: a comparison and evaluation of two proposed modes of inheritance, *Genet Epidemiol* 4:13–24, 1987.

Loos BG, John RP, Laine ML: Identification of genetic risk factors for periodontitis and possible mechanisms of action, *J Clin Periodontol* 32:159–179, 2005.

Lopez NJ, Rios V, Pareja MA, et al: Prevalence of juvenile periodontitis in Chile, *J Clin Periodontol* 18:529–533, 1991.

Löwick CW, van der Pluijm G, Bloys H, et al: Parathyroid hormone (PTH) and PTH-like protein (PLP) stimulate interleukin-6 production by osteogenic cells: a possible role of interleukin-6 in osteoclastogenesis, *Biochem Biophys Res Commun* 162:1546–1552, 1989.

Macey MG, McCarthy DA, Howells GL, et al: Multiparameter flow cytometric analysis of polymorphonuclear leucocytes in whole blood from patients with adult rapidly progressive periodontitis reveals low expression of the adhesion molecule L-selectin (Cd62L), *Cytometry* 34:152–158, 1998.

Malech HL, Nauseef WM: Primary inherited defects in neutrophil function: etiology and treatment, *Semin Hematol* 34:279–290, 1997.

Mandell RL: A longitudinal microbiological investigation of Actinobacillus actinomycetemcomitans and Eikenella corrodens in juvenile periodontitis, *Infect Immun* 45:778–780, 1984.

Mandell RL, Socransky SS: Microbiological and clinical effects surgery plus doxycycline on juvenile periodontitis, *J Periodontol* 59:373–379, 1988.

Mandell RL, Tripodi LS, Savitt E, et al: The effect of treatment on Actinobacillus actinomycetemcomitans in localized juvenile periodontitis, *J Periodontol* 57:94–99, 1986.

Manson JD, Lehner T: Clinical features of juvenile periodontitis (periodontosis), *J Periodontol* 45:636–640, 1974.

Maryland D, Grenier D: Biological activities of outer membrane vesicles, *Can J Microbiol* 35:607–613, 1989.

McArthur WP, Tsai C-C, Baehni PC, et al: Leucotoxic effects of Actinobacillus actinomycetemcomitans, *J Periodontal Res* 16:159–170, 1981.

Meghji S, Henderson B, Nair S, et al: Inhibition of bone DNA and collagen production by surface-associated material from bacteria implicated in the pathology of periodontal disease, *J Periodontol* 63:736–742, 1992a.

Meghji S, Wilson M, Henderson B, et al: Antiproliferative and cytotoxic activity of surface associated material from periodontopathic bacteria, *Arch Oral Biol* 37:637–644, 1992b.

Meghji S, Barber P, Wilson M, et al: Bone resorbing activity of surface-associated material from Actinobacillus actinomycetemcomitans and Eikenella corrodens, *J Med Microbiol* 41:197–203, 1994.

Melnick M, Shields ED, Bixler D: Periodontitis: a phenotypic and genetic analysis, *Oral Surg Oral Med Oral Pathol* 42:32–41, 1976.

Melvin WL, Sandifer JB, Grey JL: The prevalence and sex ratio of juvenile periodontitis in a young racially mixed population, *J Periodontol* 62:330–334, 1991.

Meyer DH, Sreenivasan PK, Fives-Taylor PM: Evidence for invasion of human cell line by Actinobacillus actinomycetemcomitans, *Infect Immun* 59:2719–2726, 1991.

Mintz KP, Fives-Taylor PM: Binding of the periodontopathogen Actinobacillus actinomycetemcomitans to extracellular matrix proteins, *Oral Microbiol Immunol* 14:109–116, 1999.

Mitchell D: Metronidazole: its use in clinical dentistry, *J Clin Periodontol* 11:145–158, 1984.

Mizgerd JR, Meek BB, Kutkoski GJ, et al: Selectins and neutrophil traffic: margination and Streptococcus pneumoniae-induced emigration in murine lungs, *J Exp Med* 184:639–645, 1996.

Mizgerd JR, Bullard DC, Hicks MJ, et al: Chronic inflammatory disease alters adhesion molecule requirements for acute neutrophil emigration in mouse skin, *Journal of Immunology* 162:5444–5448, 1999.

Munoz FM, Hawkins ER, Bullard DC, et al: Host defense against systemic infection with Streptococcus pneumoniae is impaired in E-, P-, and E-/P-selectin-deficient mice, *J Clin Invest* 100:2099–2106, 1997.

Murray P, Patters M: Gingival crevice neutrophil function in periodontal lesions, *J Periodontal Res* 15:463–469, 1980.

Nair SP, Meghji S, Wilson M, et al: Bacterially induced bone destruction: mechanisms and misconceptions, *Infect Immun* 64:2371–2380, 1996.

Nakagawa T, Yamada S, Oosuka Y, et al: Clinical and microbiological study of local minocycline delivery (Peri cline) following scaling and root planing in recurrent periodontal pockets, *Bull Tokyo Dent Coll* 32:63–70, 1991.

Nakashima K, Usui C, Koseki T, et al: Two different types of humoral immune response to Actinobacillus actinomycetemcomitans in higher responding periodontal patients, *J Med Microbiol* 47:509–575, 1998.

Neely AL: Prevalence of juvenile periodontitis in a circumpubertal population, *J Clin Periodontol* 19:367–372, 1992.

Newman MG, Socransky SS: Predominant cultivatable microbiota in periodontitis, *J Periodontal Res* 12:120–128, 1977.

Nibali L, Griffiths GS, Donos N, et al: Association between interleukin-6 promoter haplotypes and aggressive periodontitis, *J Clin Periodontol* 35:193–198, 2008.

Niederman R, Westernoff T, Lee C, et al: Infection-mediated early-onset periodontal disease in P/E-selectin-deficient mice, *J Clin Periodontol* 28:569–575, 2001.

Nishihara T, Koga T, Hamada S: Extracellular proteinous substances from Haemophilus actinomycetemcomitans induce mitogenic responses in murine lymphocytes, *Oral Microbiol Immunol* 2:48–52, 1987.

Nishihara T, Koga T, Hamada S: Suppression of murine macrophage interleukin-1 release by the polysaccharide portion of the lipopolysaccharide of Haemophilus actinomycetemcomitans, *Infect Immun* 56:619–625, 1988.

Novak MJ, Stamatelakys C, Adair SM: Resolution of early lesions of juvenile periodontitis with tetracycline therapy alone: long term observations in 4 cases, *J Periodontol* 62:628–633, 1991.

Novak MJ, Novak KE: Early onset periodontitis, *Curr Opin Periodontol* 3:45–58, 1996.

Nowotney A, Behling UH, Hammond B, et al: The release of toxic microvesicles by Actinobacillus actinomycetemcomitans, *Infect Immun* 37:151–154, 1982.

Ohta H, Kato K: Leucotoxic activity of Actinobacillus actinomycetemcomitans. In Hamada S, Holt SC, McGhee JR, editors: *Periodontal Disease Pathogens and Host Immune Response*, Tokyo, 1991, Quintessence, pp 143–154.

Oyaizu K, Kantarci AZ, Maeda H, et al: Identification of mRNA for the various diacylglycerol kinase isoforms in neutrophils from patients with localized aggressive periodontitis, *J Periodontal Res* 38:488–459, 2003.

Page RC, Bowen T, Altman L, et al: Prepubertal periodontitis. 1. Definition of a clinical disease entity, *J Periodontol* 54:257–271, 1983a.

Page RC, Altman LC, Ebersole JL, et al: Rapidly progressive periodontitis, a distinct clinical condition, *J Periodontol* 54:197–200, 1983b.

Page RC, Baab DA: A new look at the etiology and pathogenesis of early onset periodontitis, *J Periodontol* 56:748–751, 1985.

Page RC, Sims TJ, Engle LD, et al: The immunodominate outer membrane antigen of Actinobacillus actinomycetemcomitans is localized in the serotype-specific high-mass carbohydrate moiety of liposaccharide, *Infect Immun* 59:3451–3462, 1991.

Papapanau PN: Epidemiology and natural history of periodontal disease. In Lang NP, Karring T, editors: *Proceedings of the 1st European Workshop on Periodontology*, London, 1994, Quintessence Publishing Co. Ltd, pp 23–41.

Pavicic MJ, van Winkelhoff AJ, de Graaff J: Synergistic effects between amoxicillin, metronidazole and its hydroxy-metabolite against Actinobacillus actinomycetemcomitans, *Antimicrob Agents Chemother* 35:961–966, 1991.

Pavicic MJ, van Winkelhoff AJ, de Graaff J: Susceptibilities of Actinobacillus actinomycetemcomitans to a number of antimicrobial combinations, *Antimicrob Agents Chemother* 36:2634–2638, 1992.

Pavicic MJ, van Winkelhoff AJ, Douqué NH, et al: Microbiological and clinical effects of metronidazole and amoxicillin in Actinobacillus actinomycetemcomitans associated periodontitis: a 2 year evaluation, *J Clin Periodontol* 21:107–112, 1994.

Preus HR, Olsen I, Namork E: The presence of phage-infected Actinobacillus actinomycetemcomitans in localized juvenile periodontitis, *J Clin Periodontol* 14:605–609, 1987.

Ranney RR, Yanni NR, Burmeister JA, et al: Relationship between attachment loss and precipitating antibody to Actinobacillus actinomycetemcomitans in adolescents and young adults having severe periodontal destruction, *J Periodontol* 53:1–7, 1982.

Reddi K, Poole S, Nair S, et al: Comparison of the IL-6 inducing activity of periodontopathic bacterial surface-associated proteins, *J Dent Res* 73:81, 1994.

Reddi K, Henderson B, Meghji S, et al: Interleukin-6 production by lipopolysaccharide-stimulated fibroblasts is potentially inhibited by naphthoquinone (vitamin K) components, *Cytokine* 7:287–290, 1995a.

Reddi K, Meghji S, Wilson M, et al: Comparison of the osteolytic activity of surface-associated proteins of bacteria implicated in periodontal disease, *Oral Dis* 1:26–31, 1995b.

Reddi K, Wilson M, Poole S, et al: Relative cytokine stimulating activities of surface components of the oral periodontopathic bacterium, Actinobacillus actinomycetemcomitans, *Cytokine* 7:534–541, 1995c.

Reddi K, Wilson M, Nair S, et al: Comparison of the pro-inflammatory cytokine-stimulating activity of surface-associated proteins of periodontopathic bacteria, *J Periodontal Res* 31:120–130, 1996a.

Reddi K, Nair S, White PA, et al: Surface-associated material from the bacterium, Actinobacillus actinomycetemcomitans, contains a peptide which in contrast to lipopolysaccharide, directly stimulates interleukin-6 gene transcription, *Eur J Biochem* 236:871–876, 1996b.

Reddi K, Nair S, White PA, et al: Surface-associated material from the bacterium Actinobacillus actinomycetemcomitans contains a peptide which, in contrast to lipopolysaccharide, directly stimulates fibroblasts IL-6 gene transcription, *Eur J Biochem* 236:871–876, 1996c.

Reinholdt J, Bay I, Svjgaard A: Association between HLA antigens and periodontal disease, *J Dent Res* 56:1261–1263, 1977.

Robertson PB, Lantz M, Marucha PT, et al: Collagenolytic activity associated with Bacteroides species and Actinobacillus actinomycetemcomitans, *J Periodontal Res* 17:275–283, 1982.

Roodman GD: Interleukin-6: An osteotropic factor? *J Bone Miner Res* 7:475–478, 1992.

Roulston D, Schwartz S, Cogan MM, et al: Linkage analysis of dentinogenesis imperfecta and juvenile periodontitis: creating a 5 point map of 4q, *Am J Hum Genet* 37:A206, 1985.

Saarela M, Asikainen S, Alaluusua S, et al: Frequency and stability of mono- or poly-infection by Actinobacillus actinomycetemcomitans: serotypes a,b,c,d or e, *Oral Microbiol Immunol* 7:277–279, 1992.

Saglie FR, Carranza Jr FA, Newman MG, et al: Identification of tissue-invading bacteria in human periodontal disease, *J Periodontal Res* 17:452–455, 1982.

Sakellari D, Socransky SS, Dibart S, et al: Estimation of serum antibody to subgingival species using checkerboard immunoblotting, *Oral Microbiol Immunol* 12:303–310, 1997.

Sakurada S: Leucotoxic mechanism of Actinobacillus (Haemophilus) actinomycetemcomitans leukotoxin on human neutrophils, *Japanese Journal of Oral Biology* 32:103–114, 1990.

Sandholm L, Gronblad E: Salivary immunoglobulins in patients with juvenile periodontitis and their healthy siblings, *J Periodontol* 55:9–11431–9–11438, 1984.

Sandholm L, Tolo K, Olsen I: Salivary IgG, a parameter of periodontal disease activity? High responder to Actinobacillus actinomycetemcomitans Y4 in juvenile and adult periodontitis, *J Clin Periodontol* 14:289–294, 1987.

Saxby M: Prevalence of juvenile periodontitis in a British school population, *Community Dent Oral Epidemiol* 12:185–187, 1984.

Saxby M: Juvenile periodontitis. An epidemiological study in the West Midlands of the United Kingdom. *J Clin Periodontol* 14:594–598, 1987.

Saxen L: Prevalence of juvenile periodontitis in Finland, *J Clin Periodontol* 7:177–186, 1980a.

Saxen L: Juvenile periodontitis, *J Clin Periodontol* 7:1–19, 1980b.

Saxen L: Heredity of juvenile periodontitis, *J Clin Periodontol* 7:276–288, 1980c.

Saxen L, Koskimies S: Juvenile periodontitis – no linkage with HLA-antigens, *J Periodontal Res* 19:441–444, 1984.

Saxen L, Asikainen S: Metronidazole in the treatment of juvenile periodontitis, *J Clin Periodontol* 20:166–171, 1993.

Schenkein HA, Van Dyke TE: Early onset periodontitis: systemic aspects of etiology and pathogenesis, *Periodontol 2000* 6:7–25, 1994.

Seddon SV, Shah HN: The distribution of hydrolytic enzymes among Gram-negative bacteria associated with periodontitis, *Microbial Ecology in Health and Disease* 2:181–190, 1989.

Sheneker BJ, McArther WP, Tsai C-C: Immune suppression induced by Actinobacillus actinomycetemcomitans. I, Effects on human peripheral blood lymphocyte responses to mitogens and antigens, *J Immunol* 128:148–154, 1982a.

Sheneker BJ, Kushner ME, Tsai C-C: Inhibition of fibroblast proliferation by Actinobacillus actinomycetemcomitans, *Infect Immun* 38:986–992, 1982b.

Sheppe W: Periodontal disease in the deer mouse, Peromyscus, *J Dent Res* 44:506–508, 1965.

Sigusch BW, Wutzler A, Nietzsch T, et al: Evidence for a specific crevicular lymphocyte profile in aggressive periodontitis, *J Periodontal Res* 41:391–396, 2006.

Sjobin B, Mattson L, Unell L, et al: Marginal bone loss in the primary dentition of patients with juvenile periodontitis, *J Clin Periodontol* 20:32–36, 1993.

Slots J: The predominant cultivatable organisms in juvenile periodontitis, *Scand J Dent Res* 49:248–255, 1976.

Slots J: Salient biochemical characters of Actinobacillus actinomycetemcomitans, *Arch Microbiol* 131:60–67, 1982.

Slots J, Reynolds HS, Genco RJ: Actinobacillus actinomycetemcomitans in human periodontal disease: a cross-sectional microbiological investigation, *Infect Immun* 29:1031–1020, 1980.

Slots J, Zambon JJ, Rosling B, et al: Actinobacillus actinomycetemcomitans in human periodontal disease: association, serology, leukotoxicity and treatment, *J Periodontal Res* 17:447–448, 1982.

Slots J, Rosling B: Suppression of periodontopathic microflora in localized juvenile periodontitis by systemic tetracycline, *J Clin Periodontol* 10:465–486, 1983.

Slots J, Schonfeld SE: Actinobacillus actinomycetemcomitans in localized juvenile periodontitis. In Hamada S, Holt SC, McGhee JR, editors: *Periodontal Disease Pathogens and Host Immune Response*, Tokyo, 1991, Quintessence, pp 53–64.

Socransky SS, Haffajee AD, Goodson JM, et al: New concepts of destructive periodontal disease, *J Clin Periodontol* 11:21–32, 1984.

Söderling E, Mäkinen PL, Syed SA, et al: Biochemical comparison of proteolytic enzymes present in rough- and smooth-surfaced Capnocytophaga isolated from the subgingival plaque of periodontitis patients, *J Periodontal Res* 26:17–23, 1991.

Spektor MD, Vandersteen GE, Page RC: Clinical studies of one family manifesting rapidly progressing juvenile periodontitis and prepubertal periodontosis, *J Periodontol* 56:93–101, 1985.

Springer TA: Traffic signals for lymphocyte recirculation and leukocyte emigration: the multistep paradigm, *Cell* 76:301–314, 1994.

Stashenko R, Fujiyoshi P, Obernesser MS, et al: Levels of interleukin Ib in tissue from sites of active periodontal disease, *J Clin Periodontol* 18:548–554, 1991.

Stevens RH, Hammond BF: Inhibition of fibroblast proliferation by extracts of Capnocytophaga spp. and Actinobacillus actinomycetemcomitans, *J Dent Res* 61:347, 1982.

Tai H, Endo M, Shimada Y, et al: Association of interleukin-1 receptor antagonist gene polymorphisms with early onset periodontitis in Japanese, *J Clin Periodontol* 29:882–888, 2002.

Taichmann NS, Dean RT, Sanderson CJ: Biochemical and morphological characterization of the killing of human monocytes by leukotoxin derived from Actinobacillus actinomycetemcomitans, *Infect Immun* 28:258–268, 1980.

Tanaka S, Barbour SE, Best AM, et al: Prostaglandin E2 mediated regulation of immunoglobulin G2 via Interferon gamma, *J Periodontol* 74:771–779, 2003.

Tervahartiala B, Uitto V-J, Kari K, et al: Outer membrane vesicles and leukotoxic activity of Actinobacillus actinomycetemcomitans from subjects with different periodontal status, *Scand J Dent Res* 97:33–42, 1989.

Trudel L, Amand St L, Bareil M, et al: Bacteriology of the oral cavity of BALB/c mice, *Can J Microbiol* 32:673–678, 1986.

Tsai C-C, McArthur WP, Bachni PC, et al: Serum neutralizing activity against Actinobacillus actinomycetemcomitans leukotoxin in juvenile periodontitis, *J Clin Periodontol* 8:338–348, 1981.

Tsai C-C, Sheneker BK, Di JM, et al: Extraction and isolation of a leukotoxin from Actinobacillus actinomycetemcomitans with polymyxin B, *Infect Immun* 43:700–705, 1984.

Tsai C-C, Taichmann NS: Dynamics of infection by leukotoxic strain of Actinobacillus actinomycetemcomitans in juvenile periodontitis, *J Clin Periodontol* 13:330–331, 1986.

Tsai CC, Ho YR, Chen CC: Levels of interleukin-l beta and interleukin-8 in gingival crevicular fluids in adult periodontitis, *J Periodontol* 66:852–859, 1995.

Van Dyke TE, Bartholomew E, Genco RJ, et al: Inhibition of neutrophil chemotaxis by soluble bacterial products, *J Periodontol* 53:502–508, 1982.

Van Dyke TE, Horoszewicz HO, Cianciola LJ, et al: Neutrophil chemotactic dysfunction in human periodontitis, *Infect Immun* 27:124–132, 1980.

Van Dyke TE, Schweinebraten M, Cianciola LJ, et al: Neutrophil chemotaxis in families with juvenile periodontitis, *J Periodontal Res* 20:503–514, 1985.

Van Winkelhoff AJ, Rodenberg AJ, Goené RJ, et al: Metronidazole plus amoxicillin in the treatment of Actinobacillus actinomycetemcomitans associated periodontitis, *J Clin Periodontol* 16:128–131, 1989.

Van Winkelhoff AJ, Tijhof CJ, De Graaff J: Microbiological and clinical results of metronidazole plus amoxicillin therapy in Actinobacillus actinomycetemcomitans – associated periodontitis, *J Periodontol* 63:52–57, 1992.

Van Winkelhoff AJ, Boutaga K: Transmission of periodontal bacteria and models of infection, *J Clin Periodontol* 32:16–27, 2005.

Von Andrian UH, Berger EM, Ramezani L, et al: In vivo behavior of neutrophils from two patients with distinct inherited leukocyte adhesion deficiency syndromes, *J Clin Invest* 91:2893–2897, 1993.

Waerhaug J: Plaque control in the treatment of juvenile periodontitis, *J Clin Periodontol* 4:29–40, 1977.

Wang P-L, Shirasu S, Daito M, et al: Purification and characterization of a trypsin-like protease from the culture supernatant of Actinobacillus actinomycetemcomitans Y4, *Eur J Oral Sci* 106:1–7, 1999.

Wang P-L, Azuma Y, Shinohara M, et al: Effect of Actinobacillus actinomycetemcomitans protease on the proliferation of gingival epithelial cells, *Oral Dis* 7:233–237, 2001.

White PA, Wilson M, Nair SP, et al: Characterization of an anti-proliferative surface-associated protein from Actinobacillus actinomycetemcomitans which can be neutralized by sera from a portion of patients with localized juvenile periodontitis, *Infect Immun* 63:2612–2618, 1995.

Wilson M: Bacterial activities of lipopolysaccharides from oral bacteria and their relevance to the pathogenesis of chronic periodontitis, *Scientific Progress* 78:19–34, 1995.

Wilson M, Kamin S, Harvey W: Bone resorbing activity from purified capsular material from Actinobacillus actinomycetemcomitans, *J Periodontal Res* 20:484–491, 1985.

Wilson M, Meghji S, Harvey W: Effect of capsular material from Haemophilus actinomycetemcomitans on bone collagen synthesis in vitro, *Microbios* 54:181–185, 1988.

Wilson M, Meghji S, Barber P, et al: Biological activities of surface associated material from Porphyromonas gingivalis, *FEMS Immunol Med Microbiol* 6:147–155, 1993a.

Wilson M, Henderson B: Virulence factors of Actinobacillus actinomycetemcomitans relevant to the pathogenesis of inflammatory periodontal diseases, *FEMS Microbiological Reviews* 17:365–379, 1995.

Wilson M, Reddi K, Henderson D: Cytokine-inducing components of periodontopathic bacteria, *J Periodontal Res* 31:393–407, 1996.

Wilson RW, Ballantyne CM, Smith CW, et al: Gene targeting yields a CD I 8-mutant mouse for study of inflammation, *J Immunol* 151:1571–1578, 1993b.

Wilton JM, Bampton JL, Griffiths GS, et al: Interleukin-l beta levels in gingival crevicular fluid from adults with previous evidence of destructive periodontitis, *J Clin Periodontol* 19:53–57, 1992.

Yang H-W, Asikainen S, Dogan B, et al: Relationship of Actinobacillus actinomycetemcomitans serotype b to aggressive periodontitis: frequency in pure cultured isolates, *J Periodontol* 75:592–599, 2004.

Yosof ZA: Early-onset periodontitis: radiographic patterns of alveolar bone loss in 55 cases from a selected Malaysian population, *J Periodontol* 61:751–754, 1990.

Zambon JJ: Actinobacillus actinomycetemcomitans in human periodontal disease, *J Clin Periodontol* 12:1–20, 1985.

Zambon JJ, Christersson LA, Slots J: Actinobacillus actinomycetemcomitans in human periodontal disease. Prevalence in patient groups and distribution of biotypes and serotypes within families, *J Periodontol* 54:707–711, 1983a.

Zambon JJ, de Louca C, Slots J, et al: Studies of leukotoxin from Actinobacillus actinomycetemcomitans using the promyelocytic HL-60 cell line, *Infect Immun* 40:205–212, 1983b.

Zambon JJ, Slots J, Genco RC: Serology of oral Actinobacillus actinomycetemcomitans and serotype distribution in human periodontal disease, *Infect Immun* 41:19–27, 1983c.

Zambon JJ, Gregory GJ, Smutko JS: Molecular genetic analysis of Actinobacillus actinomycetemcomitans epidemiology, *J Periodontol* 61:75–80, 1990.

INTRODUCTION

Acute lesions are by definition of sudden onset, limited duration and with well-defined clinical features; by contrast with chronic gingivitis which is frequently not obvious, acute gingival lesions are usually easier to diagnose.

There are some pathological conditions that can affect other parts of the oral mucosa, as well as the gingivae, which are impossible to classify because their aetiology is uncertain, e.g. erythema multiforme, or because they may be chronic with acute episodes, e.g. the fungal disease candidiasis. Syphilis, tuberculosis and other bacterial and viral infections may occasionally involve the gingiva but the lesions are widespread, involving many parts of the mouth as well as other parts of the body.

The gingival lesions to be described are:

- Traumatic lesions, both physical and chemical
- Viral infections
  - Acute herpetic gingivostomatitis
  - Herpangina
  - Hand, foot and mouth disease
  - Measles
  - Herpes varicella/zoster virus infections
  - Glandular fever
  - HIV infection and AIDS (see Ch. 7)
- Bacterial infections
  - Acute ulcerative necrotizing gingivitis (see Ch. 25)
  - Tuberculosis
  - Syphilis
- Fungal infections
  - Candidiasis
- Gingival abscess
- Aphthous ulceration
- Erythema multiforme
- Drug allergy and contact hypersensitivity.

TRAUMATIC LESIONS

Physical injury can be mechanical or thermal. A carelessly wielded toothbrush or woodstick, a sharp piece of food such as a fish-bone, hot food and drink are the most common causes of injury. Occasionally, the cause is rather more bizarre, a cigarette burn, a pencil pushed into the mouth, a hair-grip, a musical instrument – the range of human oral activity is extensive. Self-inflicted injury to the lips, particularly the lower lip is common due to lip biting (**Fig. 24.1**) and more severe accidental trauma to the lips and mucosa can occur with loss of sensation following local anaesthesia (**Fig. 24.2**).

Chemical causes of damage include aspirin placed against the gum to alleviate toothache, escharotics such as silver nitrate, even hydrogen peroxide solution used too strong and too frequently. Careless use of a caustic by the dentist, e.g. phenol, trichloroacetic acid, can cause considerable tissue damage.

Usually there is little doubt about the diagnosis. The patient is aware of the accident and may suffer immediate and fairly severe pain. The acute symptoms may last for a day or so and be followed by several days of soreness and sensitivity to further irritation. A localized area of inflammation and ulceration

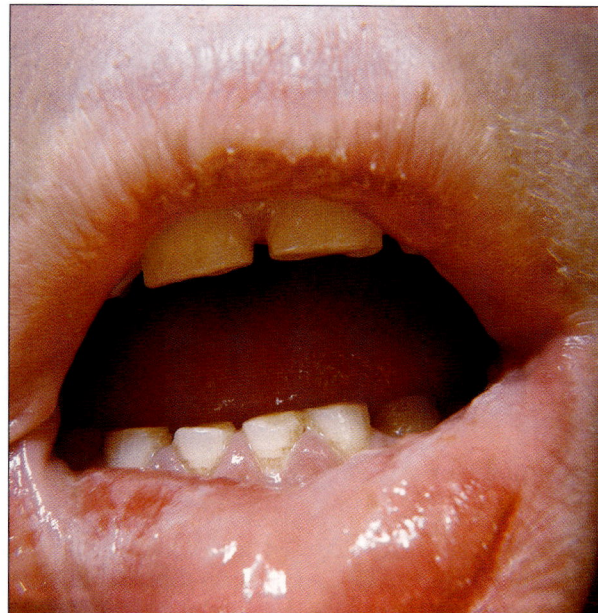

Fig. 24.1 Self-inflicted trauma to the lower lip mucosa producing ulceration in a 19-year-old woman.

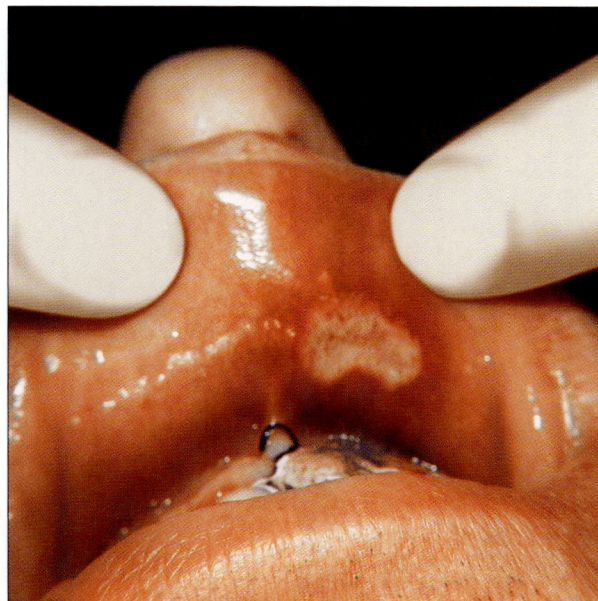

Fig. 24.2 Large ulcer of upper lip mucosa due to accidental trauma to the upper lip mucosa of a 38-year-old man following loss of sensation following local anaesthesia for periodontal surgery. Trauma from the edge of the periodontal pack may have also contributed to the lesion.

may form. In the case of a burn there may be vesicle formation followed by ulceration. The wound is seen as a bright red area denuded of epithelium and with a ragged edge of necrotic tissue which can be felt by the tongue. The healing wound is quickly covered by epithelium unless secondary infection takes place as it might do in the debilitated individual. In this case pain persists, the wound may suppurate and this may be accompanied by lymph gland enlargement and malaise. Abscess formation may follow damage by a piece of woodstick or bone if the foreign object is not removed.

Treatment

Frequently, the wound heals without any active intervention. The patient should and probably will avoid irritant foods or hot drinks. Rinsing with cold water or a very dilute saline solution might soothe. Strong antiseptics should be avoided. Troches containing a topical anaesthetic, e.g. benzocaine lozenge, can be recommended and some analgesic such as aspirin or paracetamol prescribed. If the cause of the injury is still there, e.g. a fishbone, it should be removed as gently as possible.

If there is secondary infection an antibiotic may need to be prescribed.

It can be helpful to protect the wound with a bland dressing such as carboxymethylcellulose gelatin paste (Orabase), which is spread gently over the wound several times a day.

INFECTIONS

VIRAL INFECTIONS

Acute herpetic gingivostomatitis

Primary infection by the herpes simplex virus (HSV) type I usually occurs in children (1–10 years) but may affect older children or adults. The virus is transmitted by infected saliva or skin lesion contact. Infection in neonates can produce encephalitis or meningitis but in children or adults it produces either a febrile illness or subclinical infection. The incubation period is about 5 days. Symptoms appear abruptly with mild to severe fever. Temperature may be raised as high as 39.4°C. There is lymph gland enlargement and malaise, and the mouth and throat may be very painful.

In young children there is irritability, profuse salivation and refusal to eat, even before the oral lesions become apparent. Small vesicles form on the gingivae, the tongue, buccal mucosa and lips, in fact anywhere in the mouth (**Fig. 24.3A, B**). Usually the vesicles burst before they are seen and the resultant round or irregular ulcers form a grey membrane surrounded by bright red mucosa. There is an acute gingivitis with redness, swelling and bleeding (**Fig. 24.3C**). This tends to be more severe in older patients with this condition (**Fig. 24.3D**). Symptoms subside in 10–21 days as the titre of protective antibodies rises.

A large proportion (30%) of patients who have had a primary herpetic infection early in life develop recurrent infection years later. The commonest recurrent lesion is on the lip (herpes labialis or cold sore). The lesion develops at the mucocutaneous junction of the upper lip (**Fig. 24.4**) and on the skin up to the nostril (**Fig. 24.5**), although it can occur on the lower lip (**Figs. 24.5, 24.6**), and rarely on the gingiva or palate. An itching or burning sensation precedes the appearance of the lesion and a blister or cluster of blisters form which burst, crust and heal after about 10 days. The blisters occur as a result of reactivation of latent virus in the trigeminal ganglion. This can occur as a result of any infection which lowers the resistance or dries the skin, or as a result of excessive exposure to sunlight.

Laboratory diagnosis may be made by direct smear to show characteristic giant cells or by staining with specific fluorescent antisera to HSV. The virus can be isolated in tissue culture. A considerably raised antibody titre indicates recent infection.

Treatment

Treatment of the oral infection is largely symptomatic and supportive, i.e. bed-rest, cool, soft food and plenty of fluid. In the infant, milk of magnesia or 55% Dequadin paint may be gently applied on cotton wool to the lesions. Benzocaine lozenges are useful in the older child or adult.

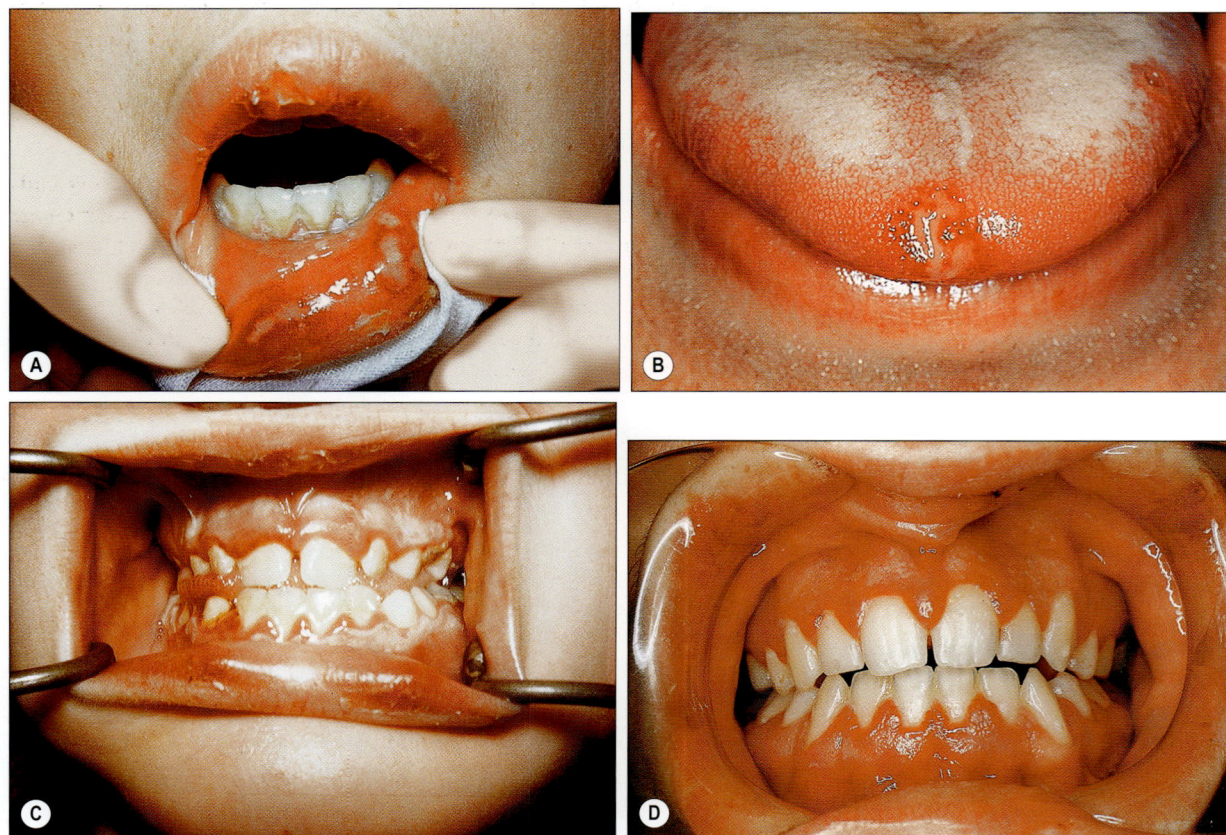

Fig. 24.3 Acute herpetic gingivostomatitis. (A) Herpetic vesicles and ulcers on the lower lip of an 8-year-old boy with primary acute herpetic gingivostomatitis. He has a high temperature and malaise. (B) Herpetic vesicles and ulcers on the tongue of the same boy. (C) Acute gingivitis and ulceration of the mucosa in a febrile 5-year-old boy. (D) more severe acute gingivitis in a 20-year-old febrile woman with primary acute herpetic gingivostomatitis.

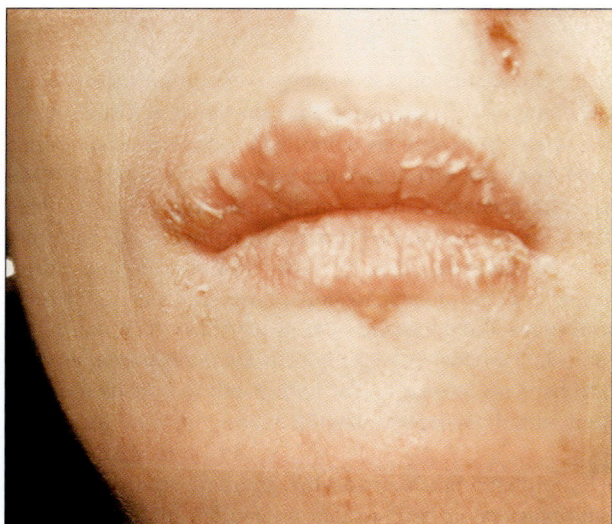

Fig. 24.4 Secondary herpes simplex: 'cold sore' consisting of herpetic vesicles and ulcers on the upper and lower lip in a 27-year-old woman.

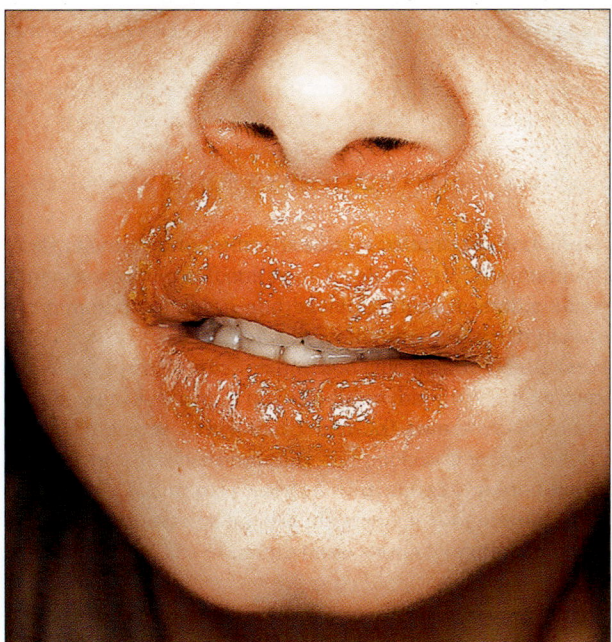

Fig. 24.5 Secondary herpes simplex: recurrent severe and widespread secondary herpetic vesicles and ulcers on both the mucosa of both lips and the skin under the nose of a 20-year-old man.

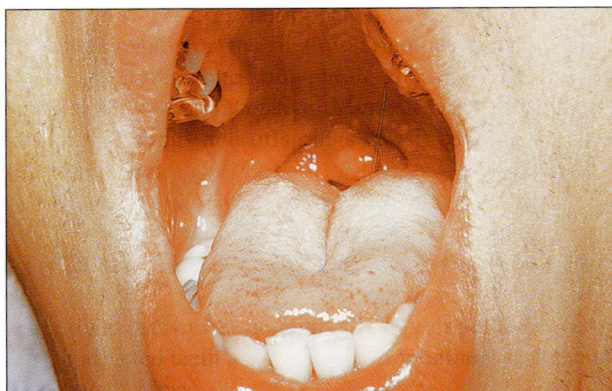

Fig. 24.6 Herpangina: Ulcers on the anterior faucial walls, uvula, soft palate, posterior pharyngeal wall and tongue of a 12-year-old febrile boy with herpangina.

Aspirin or paracetamol will help to reduce pain and temperature. Phenergan is a useful sedative in the child.

In severe cases, acyclovir (Zovirax) tablets (200 mg 5 times daily for 5 days) or suspension (5 mL of suspension 5 times daily for 5 days) may be prescribed. Acyclovir cream (apply 5 times daily for 5 days) may also be used as a preventive measure for herpes labialis.

Herpangina

This is an acute febrile illness caused by infection with Coxsackie A types 1–6, 8, 10, 16 or 22. It occurs in sporadic outbreaks mainly in children. The patient complains of a sore throat due partly to oral ulceration. Small ulcers appear mainly on the anterior faucial walls but also on the hard and soft palate, posterior pharyngeal wall, buccal mucosa and tongue (**Fig. 24.7**). They heal in a few days and recovery is uneventful in 7–10 days.

Hand, foot and mouth disease

This is an acute febrile illness caused by infection with Coxsackie A type 16 or occasionally 5 or 6. It occurs in sporadic outbreaks affecting mainly young children. Maculopapular and vesicular lesions appear on the skin and oral mucosa. The skin lesions mainly affect the hands, arms and feet. The oral vesicles break down into small ulcers. Recovery is uneventful in 10–14 days.

Measles

Measles is a severe febrile illness affecting mainly children and protective vaccination against it is available. There is fever, malaise, cough, conjunctivitis, photophobia and lacrimation; and a typical blotchy macular rash. Oral lesions known as Koplik's spots precede the skin lesions by a number of days. These are bluish-white specks surrounded by a bright red margin and they occur mainly on the buccal mucosa.

Recovery takes place in 2–3 weeks in otherwise healthy, fit and well-fed children but the infection can be serious in previously unexposed populations particularly when poor and malnourished. Vaccination against measles is available for all children as part of their vaccination programme.

Herpes varicella/zoster virus infections

Varicella or chickenpox is an acute febrile illness mainly affecting children. It produces a widespread maculopapular or vesicular eruption on the skin. Small vesicles also form on the oral mucosa including the tongue and gingiva. Recovery is uneventful in 2–3 weeks.

Herpes zoster or shingles is caused by reactivation of latent varicella virus or reinfection of a person who has previously had chickenpox. It is commonest in middle-aged to older adults and affects sensory nerves

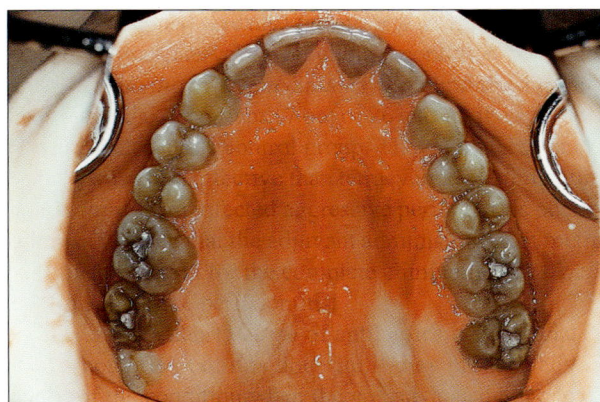

Fig. 24.7 Chronic atrophic candidiasis (denture sore mouth): bright red and spongy candidal infection of the palate under a removable orthodontic appliance in a 16-year-old man.

producing a severe neuralgia. A vesicular eruption occurs on the skin or mucosa innervated by the affected sensory nerve. If the trigeminal nerve or sensory portion of the facial nerve is affected the vesicles can affect the skin of the face and oral mucosa.

Glandular fever

Glandular fever is caused by infection with the Epstein–Barr virus (EBV) which is a herpes-like virus. It is thought to spread via infected saliva and is most common in children, adolescents and young adults. The infection may be prolonged and this occurs particularly in adults. It is characterized by fever, malaise, sore throat, headache, chills, cough and widespread lymphadenopathy. The liver and spleen may also be enlarged. There is oral involvement with a pharyngitis and oral lesions which take the form of palatal petechiae. There is also an acute gingivitis and stomatitis.

Good oral hygiene and regular professional cleaning are important to treat the gingivitis. Sometimes acute necrotizing ulcerative gingivitis (ANUG) may occur and require treatment.

HIV infection and AIDS

The oral features and other aspects of this infection are fully discussed in Chapter 7.

Antiviral agents

These generally function by interfering with nucleotide synthesis (Neu 1991). Some agents interfere with purine and pyrimidine synthesis or the interconversion or utilization of nucleotides. Others act as nucleotide analogues that are incorporated into polynucleotides resulting in nonsense sequences.

Adenosine arabinoside is phosphorylated in virus-infected cells and acts as a competitive analogue of dATP, inhibiting the incorporation of dATP into DNA.

Acyclovir is a nucleotide analogue which is first converted in the virus-infected cell into a triphosphate. It then inhibits the thymidine kinase and DNA polymerase of Herpes viruses. Zidovudine (AZT) inhibits human immunodeficiency virus (HIV) replication by interfering with viral RNA-dependent DNA polymerase (reverse transcriptase).

If antiviral agents are used it should be remembered that resistance can develop against these agents.

Resistance to antiviral agents

Resistance has evolved and is still evolving in response to the 20 or more antiviral drugs available to treat a number of serious viral infections (Drew & Bubbles 1997). It results from viral mutation and selection of resistant forms by the widespread use of the drug in question. Resistance has emerged to acyclovir used to treat Herpes simplex and zoster infections (Reyes et al 1998; Pottage & Kessler 1995; Safrin et al 1991a,b), also to ganciclovir for *Cytomegalovirus* infections (Standing Medical Advisory Committee 1999; Drew & Bubbles 1997; Dienstay et al 1995; Slavin et al 1993), lamivudine and famciclovir for Hepatitis B infections (Dienstay et al 1995; Bartholmeusz & Locarnini 1997; Kellam et al 1992; Main et al 1996), zidovudine and lamivudine for human immunodeficiency virus infections (Kellam et al 1992; Larder et al 1995; Japour et al 1995) and amantadine and its analogue rimantadine for influenza (Drew & Bubbles 1997; Standing Medical Advisory Committee 1999).

BACTERIAL INFECTIONS

The commonest acute gingival bacterial infection, ANUG, is described separately in Chapter 25. Other bacterial infections affecting the oral mucosa are described below.

Tuberculosis

Oral lesions are rare and are usually secondary to sputum infection from open pulmonary tuberculosis. Deep ulcers may occur on any part of the oral mucosa and a tuberculous gingivitis has been reported (Shafer et al 1983). Tuberculosis is once again on the increase in immigrant, immuno-suppressed and poor groups.

Syphilis

Secondary syphilis occurs about 6 weeks after primary infection and it produces a widespread skin rash and oral eruption. In the mouth ulcers known as mucous patches form and also irregular long winding ulcers known as snail track ulcers. These lesions are teeming with spirochaetes and are highly infectious.

FUNGAL INFECTIONS

These include *Candida* infections and other opportunistic fungal infections such as aspergillosis of the lung and *Cryptococcus* infections seen in immunocompromised patients.

Treatment of fungal infections

Fungal infections may need treatment with antifungal agents. These include agents that are active against true filamentous fungi, such as *Aspergillus* spp and yeasts, such as *Candida albicans*. The three principal groups in this regard are the polyene, imidazole and triazole antimicrobials (Green & Harris 1993).

Most *Candidal* infections in healthy individuals respond to topical agents but more serious candidal and other opportunistic fungal infections such as aspergillosis of the lung and *Cryptococcus* infections seen in immunocompromised patients require systemic therapy.

The two best examples of *polyene antimicrobials* are *nystatin* and *amphotericin*. Neither are absorbed orally and may be administered as lozenges, gels, creams or mouthwashes for treating oropharyngeal candidiasis (Green & Harris 1993). Amphotericin may be administered parenterally for serious systemic fungal or yeast infections but it is toxic and may cause severe renal damage even at low dosages. In this situation it may also be used in combination with flucytosine an antimetabolite of cytosine.

The first *imidazoles clotrimazole, econazole* and *miconazole* are used topically and miconazole gel is a useful alternative for the treatment of oropharyngeal candidiasis (Green & Harris 1993). Parenteral miconazole is less toxic than amphotericin but is usually less effective.

The newer related agents are classified as *triazole antifungal agents* (Green & Harris 1993). They are well absorbed and the first orally active agent was ketoconazole. However, when given in high doses or long courses this produced severe hepatotoxicity. The newer agents, *fluconazole* and *itraconazole*, with this property are less toxic and useful for the treatment of resistant candidiasis.

These agents either function by interfering with fungal membranes or by interfering with nucleotide synthesis (Neu 1991). Unlike bacterial membranes, fungal membranes contain sterol. The polyene antibiotics appear to act by binding to membrane sterols. The polyene antibiotics contain a rigid hydrophobic centre and a flexible hydrophilic section. They are composed of tightly packed rods held in rigid extension by the polyene portion. They interact with the fungal surface membrane to produce a membrane-polyene complex that alters the membrane permeability and results in acidification of the fungus and eventual leakage of cell protein. Prokaryotic cells neither bind nor are inhibited by the polyenes.

The imidazoles, miconazole, ketoconazole, clotrimazole and fluconazole also interfere with fungal membrane synthesis (Neu 1991). They inhibit the incorporation of subunits into ergosterol and may also directly damage the membrane. It should be noted that miconazole can interact with a number of other drugs such as warfarin and antidepressants (Pemberton et al 2004) and can affect their actions.

Flucytosine is an antifungal agent that interferes with nucleotide synthesis (Neu 1991). It is converted in the fungal cell to 5-fluorouracil, which inhibits thymidylate synthetase resulting in a deficit of thymine nucleotides and impaired DNA synthesis.

Candidiasis

The fungus *Candida albicans* is normally found in the mouth as a saprophyte until some changes in the balance of the oral flora or alteration in the local and systemic defence mechanisms occur, producing lowered resistance. Then the fungus proliferates and infects the tissues. It is the most common fungal infection of the mouth. Factors which predispose to infection are prolonged use of antibiotics, steroids, and immunosuppressive drugs. It is also associated with diabetes, leukaemia and conditions of the gastrointestinal tract which promote malabsorption and malnutrition. *Vaginal candidiasis* is common in pregnancy and the newborn infant may be infected from the vagina. It is also a very common feature of HIV infection and its presence in a severe form should alert one to the possibility of this infection.

C. albicans has been found in the oral cavities of a high proportion of adults (Arendorf & Walker 1979; Odds 1988) and has been found to colonize the tongue, palate and buccal mucosa (Arendorf & Walker 1980). It may also occur in the subgingival plaque of adults with severe periodontitis (Slots et al 1988). Yeasts, especially *C. albicans* have been recovered from the periodontal pockets of 7–19% of chronic periodontitis patients (Dahlén & Wikström 1995; Rams et al 1997; Reynaud et al 2001, Slots et al 1988; Järvensivu et al 2004). Using electron microscopy, yeasts were also found in the gingival connective tissues in 26 out of 60 samples from juvenile periodontitis subjects (González et al 1987). Using specific monoclonal and polyclonal antibodies for immunochemistry *C. albicans* hyphae have been found in the gingival connective tissues of 4 out of 25 (16%) tissue samples from chronic periodontitis patients (Järvensivu et al 2004). Interestingly, *C. albicans* hyphae were not found in the pocket epithelium but in the adherent subgingival plaque and in the connective tissue below the epithelium. It therefore seems unable to invade intact pocket epithelium. However, in chronic periodontitis the pocket epithelium is ulcerated allowing *C. albicans* easy access to the underlying connective tissue. Like bacterial penetration into the gingival tissue in periodontitis, candidal penetration into the gingival connective tissue is likely to be transient in subjects with an intact immune system.

Increased induction of interleukin 8 (IL-8) and intercellular adhesion molecule 1 (ICAM-1) by oral epithelial cells may play a role in the host defense mechanism in oropharyngeal candidiasis. in this regard, Egusa et al (2005) investigated the expression of these molecules on human gingival epithelial cells (HGECs) during *C. albicans* infection. They showed that neutralization with antibody against ICAM-1 inhibited both the adherence of *C. albicans* to HGECs and the *Candida*-induced production of IL-8. This suggested a role for ICAM-1 in recognition and signalling of HGECs to express IL-8 upon infection with *C. albicans.*

Candidiasis occurs in many forms. Four forms tend to be confined to the mouth and the first three of these are usually transient and tend to respond to treatment. However, the last form described, oropharyngeal candidiasis, seen in immunocompromised patients, is often persistent and difficult to treat.

Acute pseudomembranous candidiasis (thrush)

Thrush is found in infants, debilitated older adults and patients with HIV infection. Lesions occur in the gingivae, tongue, cheeks and throat. They are creamy white, elevated patches which can be wiped away to leave a raw red base. The patient complains of a sore dry mouth or throat. Diagnosis can be made by demonstrating the yeasts in scrapings from the lesion.

In infants, a suspension of nystatin (100 000 IU/mL) can be painted on the lesions two or three times a day. In adults amphotericin B lozenges BP (10 mg) or nystatin pastilles DPF (100 000 IU) are sucked 3–4 times a day. In severe cases miconazole oral gel DPF can be used.

Acute atrophic candidiasis

This form is usually associated with an upset in balance between tissues and oral flora which follows the prolonged use of steroids or antibiotics. The mucosa is thin, fiery red and painful. Nystatin or amphotericin B reduces the symptoms.

Chronic atrophic candidiasis (denture sore mouth)

This condition is produced by *Candida* infection of tissue which is being irritated by a denture, often one which is worn day and night. The most usual site is the palate where the tissue is bright red and spongy (**Fig. 24.8**).

The condition is often accompanied by an angular cheilitis which is produced by overclosure following alveolar resorption under the denture. The corners of the mouth become folded and wet and subsequently infected by *C. albicans*.

Treatment consists of: (1) leaving the denture out as much as possible; (2) coating the lesions and the denture when worn with nystatin or amphotericin B; (3) remodelling the dentures and remaking them when the infection is controlled.

Oropharyngeal candidiasis

More serious oropharyngeal candidiasis are usually seen in immunocompromised patients including HIV-infected patients and these are often treated by their physicians with systemic triazole antifungal agents.

In treating candida infections with antifungal agents it should be remembered that resistance can develop to these agents particularly to prolonged use.

Resistance to antifungal agents

The unwelcome rise in the number of serious fungal infections has resulted in a marked increase in the use of antifungal agents. This has contributed to the emergence of resistance to a number of important compounds, although the clinical impact of this problem has differed from one group of patients to another. However, drug resistance has been identified as a major cause of treatment failure among patients treated with flucytosine

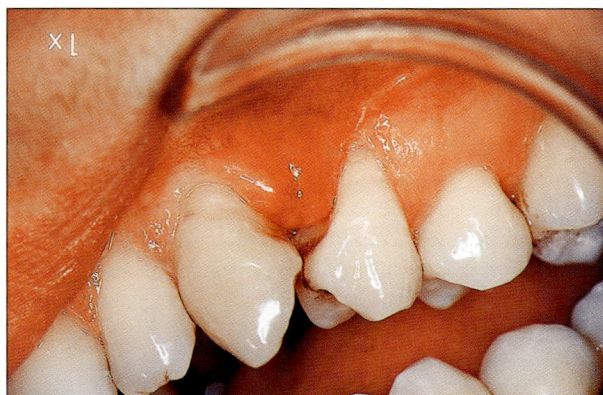

Fig. 24.8 Gingival abscess: caused by with physical damage to the gingival margin by a woodstick with subsequent infection of the wound in a 29-year-old man.

(Voss et al 1996). Fortunately, use of this compound has been declining. Until the 1990s, acquisition of resistance to azole antifungal agents (which are the most important group of ergosterol biosynthesis inhibitors) was low (Vanden et al 1994). In recent years, however, resistance to these agents has become a significant problem in several groups of patients, notably those with AIDS (Denning et al 1997).

Oral candidosis is usually the earliest infectious complication encountered in HIV-infected individuals (Schulten et al 1989), and occurs in up to 90% of patients with AIDS. Furthermore, it becomes more prevalent and less responsive to treatment as the immunological defence mechanisms of the patient become more impaired. These infections are mostly caused by *C. albicans*.

Fluconazole, introduced in the late 1980s, proved an excellent agent for the treatment of mucosal candidosis (Standing Medical Advisory Committee 1999). It is well-tolerated and safe and these factors led to a rapid expansion in its use to prevent relapse in patients with HIV-related mucosal candidosis. These prophylactic regimes often used low dosages for long periods, a situation which favours the development of resistance.

In 1992, the first reports appeared, from Madrid and Paris, of failures of fluconazole treatment in significant numbers of AIDS patients with oral or oesophageal candidosis. Since then, strains of *C. albicans* resistant to this agent have been reported worldwide (Schulten et al 1989). The recent introduction of the antiretroviral protease inhibitors has led to a reduction in the number of new cases of azole drug resistance in fungi from AIDS patients, but it remains to be seen whether this improvement can be sustained.

The impact of fluconazole on the management of other groups of immunocompromised and debilitated patients has also been considerable (Standing Medical Advisory Committee 1999). In addition to treatment of intensive care and surgical patients, this agent has been used on a large scale for prophylaxis in neutropenic cancer patients and following bone marrow transplantation (BMT). Over the period of such use, it has been possible to document a shift from azole susceptible organisms, such as *C. albicans*, to intrinsically fluconazole-resistant species such as *C.glabrata* and *C. krusei* as the infective agents in these subjects. This shift has been best reported in data from BMT recipients exposed to fluconazole prophylaxis (Wingard et al 1991). However, it has also occurred in other hospital populations. In one report from the USA, the proportion of blood culture isolates identified as *C. albicans* fell from 89% to 30%, in the period between 1987 and 1992, while the proportion of isolates identified as *C. glabrata*, *C. parapsilosis* or *C. tropicalis* increased consecutively (Price et al 1994). This shift in species distribution is not solely related to increased fluconazole use, but it may be an important factor in this process. Up to 50%, of *C. tropicalis* isolates are resistant to fluconazole (Law et al 1996) and many are cross-resistant to other azoles (Johnson et al 1995).

Koray et al (2005) compared the influence of fluconazole capsules and/or hexetidine mouthrinses for the management of oral candidiasis associated with denture stomatitis in 61 patients. Patients in group 1 ($n=21$) were given only fluconazole capsules (Zolax 50 mg once a day), those in group 2 ($n=18$) were given only hexetidine mouthrinses (Heksoral 0.1%, twice daily), whereas those in group 3 ($n=22$) were given both fluconazole capsules and hexetidine mouthrinses for 14 days. The yeast colonies of the saliva samples were counted and calculated as the number of colony forming units per millilitre. The presence of yeasts in the lesion and denture samples were evaluated as present or absent according to their growth on cultures. *C. albicans* was identified by means of germ tube analysis. Patients in groups 1, 2 and 3 had a statistically significant decrease in the amount of *C. albicans* in saliva, lesions and dentures after treatment, when compared with pretreatment results ($p<0.05$). *C. albicans* counts in saliva, lesion and denture after treatment detected no statistically significant difference when the three groups were compared.

Of the three study groups, group 2, where hexetidine was the only medication prescribed, was found to be superior on account of fewer potential complications. They concluded that dentists should employ a more conservative intervention with oral mouthrinses rather than risk adverse effects and complications of systemic drugs for the management of oral candidiasis.

Manfredi et al (2006) assessed the antifungal susceptibility of *Candida* isolates to six antifungal agents using a commercially available kit. The isolates were collected from patients affected by diabetes mellitus from two different geographic localities (London, UK and Parma, Italy) and from a group of healthy non-diabetic subjects. No differences in antifungal susceptibility to the six agents tested were observed between *Candida* isolates from diabetic and non-diabetic subjects. However, differences were observed between the two geographically different diabetes mellitus populations. Oral yeast isolates from diabetes mellitus patients in the UK more often displayed resistance or intermediate resistance to fluconazole ($p=0.02$), miconazole ($p<0.0001$), and ketoconazole ($p=0.01$) than did isolates from diabetes mellitus patients in Italy. In addition, more *C. albicans* isolates were found in diabetic and non-diabetic subjects that were susceptible to fluconazole than non-*albicans* isolates. The difference in the antifungal resistance of isolates from the two populations of diabetes mellitus patients may have been related to differences in the therapeutic management of candidal infections between the two centres.

Vaginal candidosis is one of the commonest infections seen in general practice in the UK. Up to 75% of all women will suffer at least one episode of this condition, and many have recurrent disease. *C. albicans* accounts for 80–95% of these infections, but 5–10%, of cases are due to *C. glabrata*. Unfortunately in marked contrast to *C. albicans*, isolates of *C. glabrata* become resistant to azole antifungal agents after short periods of exposure (Hitchcock et al 1993). Once azole treatment has failed to control vaginal infection with *C. glabrata*, management of the condition becomes much more difficult and chronic or recurrent disease is common (White et al 1993).

GINGIVAL ABSCESS

The term 'gingival abscess' should be used for abscesses confined to the gingivae. It is often associated with physical damage to the gingival margin by a woodstick, fish-bone, etc. with subsequent infection of the wound but it can also arise within the wall of a gingival pocket where drainage has been impeded.

The abscess appears as a localized, shiny red swelling, which is painful (**Fig. 24.9**); associated teeth are sensitive to percussion. The abscess may discharge spontaneously or spread into the underlying tissue to form a periodontal abscess.

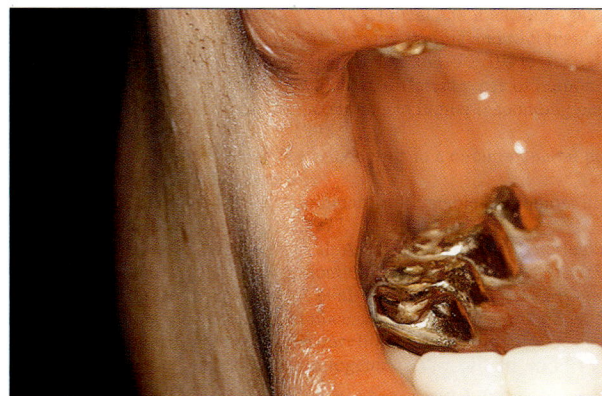

Fig. 24.9 Minor aphthous ulcers on the buccal mucosa of a 24-year-old man.

Treatment

If the cause of the abscess is still present it should be removed carefully. Drainage can be established by hot salt water mouthwashes used every 2 h. If the lesion persists it can be curetted under local anaesthesia or incised if it is pointing. If persistent and severe a systemic antibiotic may be needed. Any residual pocketing can be removed by thorough subgingival curettage or localized gingivectomy.

APHTHOUS ULCERATION

Recurrent mouth ulcers are the most common lesions of the oral mucosa (Scully & Felix 2005a). There are three types of ulcer: minor aphthous ulcers, major aphthous ulcers and herpetiform ulcers. Their common characteristics are that they are painful lesions which appear without any reason, last for several days or weeks, heal and then after a variable interval recur. The cause is as yet unknown but it is thought that the ulcers may be a manifestation of auto immunity to a component of the oral mucosa. Several related factors have been suggested, such as emotional stress and hormonal change. In a number of patients the ulcers appear to be related to the menstrual cycle, the peak incidence being found in the post-ovulation period. There may be a relationship between ulceration and iron-deficiency anaemia, deficiency of folic acid and vitamin B12.

Guimarães et al (2007) investigated the possible association of functional gene polymorphisms IL-1α, IL-6, IL-10 and TNF-α in individuals with recurrent aphthous stomatitis. Their findings demonstrated that polymorphisms of IL-1α and TNF-α were associated with an increased risk of RAS development and their findings also gave additional support to a genetic basis for RAS pathogenesis.

MINOR APHTHOUS ULCERS (*MIKULICZ'S APHTHAE*)

These are the most common type. One or several small ulcers occur on non-keratinized oral mucosa, especially the lips, cheeks, vestibule and margins of the tongue (**Fig. 24.10**). They are shallow ulcers less than 10 mm in length with a surrounding zone of inflammation and slight swelling. They may be very painful or scarcely noticed by the patient unless traumatized. Sometimes tissue breakdown is heralded by localized paraesthesia. The ulcer(s) may last 4–14 days, heal without scarring and recur after weeks or months. They are found in the age group 10–40 years, slightly more frequently in females than males.

MAJOR APHTHOUS ULCERS (*PERIADENITIS MUCOSA NECROTICA RECURRENS*)

These are much less common than the minor variety. They are larger (up to 30 mm), last as long as 40 days and are much more painful (**Fig. 24.11**). Sometimes they recur so rapidly that involvement seems continuous. They

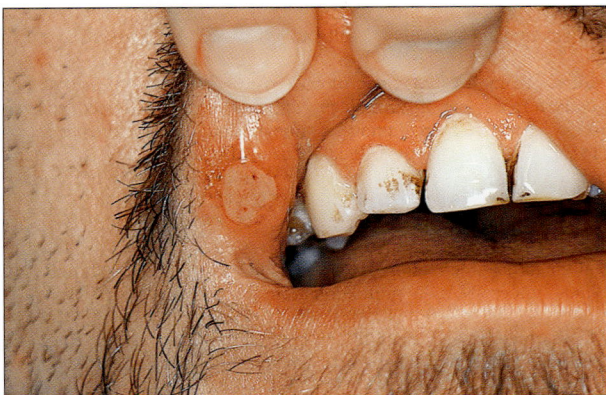

Fig. 24.11 Herpetiform aphthous ulcers on the palatal mucosa of a 24-year-old woman. The original small ulcers have coalesced to form larger ulcers.

can be found anywhere on the oral mucosa. They start as a submucosal nodule which breaks down to form a deep crater-like ulcer with considerable tissue destruction which heals with a scar.

HERPETIFORM ULCERS

Despite their name, they are not related to herpes. They are most frequent in females and occur as a group of pin-head ulcers which may coalesce to form larger painful ulcers (**Fig. 24.12**). They can occur on any part of the oral mucosa, including the tongue, palate and oropharynx in which case they cause dysphagia (discomfort or pain on swallowing).

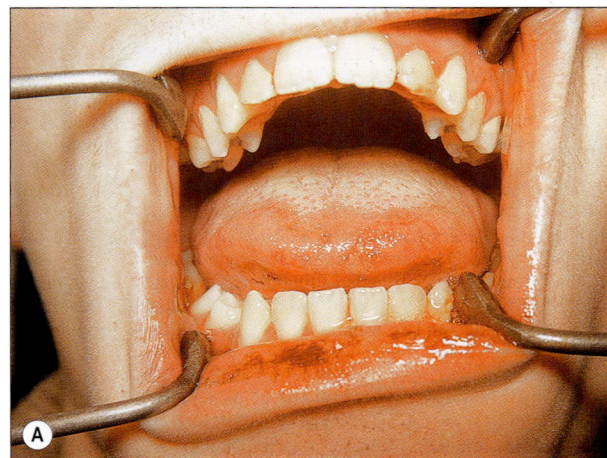

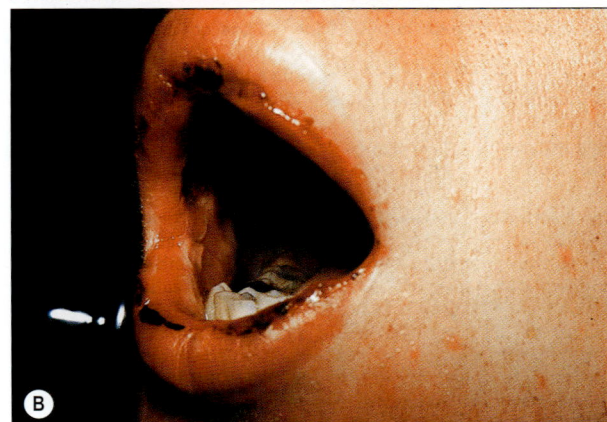

Fig. 24.12 Erythema multiforme. (A) Diffuse inflammation of the oral mucosa and some crusting vesicles on the lips of a 40-year-old man with this condition. (B) More severe condition with widespread crusting lesions on the oral mucosa particularly of the lips in a 22-year-old man with this condition.

Fig. 24.10 Major aphthous ulcer on the inner upper lip mucosa of a 31-year-old man.

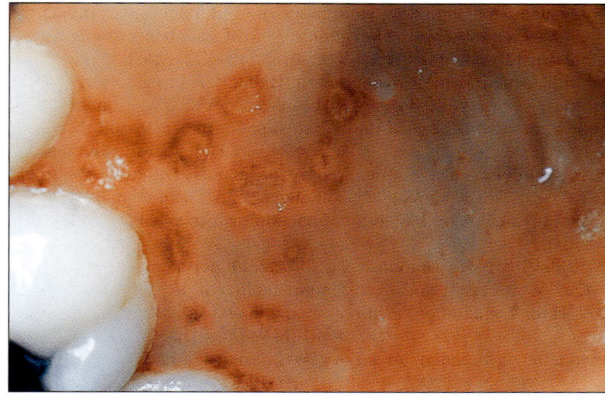

Treatment

Treatment for all aphthous ulceration is symptomatic and depends on the frequency and severity of the ulceration. The patient needs to be reassured that the ulcer is not malignant. In the case of minor ulcers treatment may be unnecessary but if they are painful topical anaesthetics or applications of Bonjela can be useful. Where the ulcer is more painful and persistent the application of topical corticosteroid preparations, such as 0.1% triamcinolone (Adcortyl A in Orabase), may be beneficial. Tablets of hydrocortisone hemisuccinate (2.5 mg, Corlan) can be used four times a day, allowing the tablet to dissolve next to the ulcer.

Tetracycline mixture BP as a mouthwash is useful for herpetiform ulcers in adults.

Very rarely, systemic corticosteroids may be needed in severe cases but in these patients it is essential to have comprehensive blood tests and assessment of iron, folic acid and vitamin B_{12} levels.

If the patient has a problem keeping the mouth clean a 0.2% chlorhexidine mouthwash is useful and can speed-up the rate of healing.

ERYTHEMA MULTIFORME

This is a syndrome of multiple aetiology, with a wide spectrum of clinical features. The oral and cutaneous lesions may occur separately or together. In about one-third of cases the condition is recurrent (Scully & Felix 2005b).

The aetiology of the syndrome may involve several underlying mechanisms. Drug allergy can cause the condition, especially to long-acting sulphonamides, penicillin and barbiturates. Several cases have also been associated with *Mycoplasma pneumoniae* infection which causes primary atypical pneumonia. In many cases no cause can be found.

The major form of the disease produces systemic involvement whilst the minor form produces local manifestations only. The patient is usually a child or young adult. In the major form there is a skin eruption with conjunctivitis and lesions of the mouth and upper respiratory tract. The patient becomes progressively ill over 7–14 days with fever and malaise.

In the mouth there is diffuse inflammation of the oral mucosa and gingivae. There are widespread erosions on the mucosa and these have a red, velvety base and bleed freely. Some vesicles also form. The lips are severely involved with extensive crusting and they may crust together at night. Eating, talking and oral examination are painful.

On the skin there is an extensive erythematous and macular rash. Iris target lesions with a central bulla which breaks down to crust may be seen. The hands, feet and flexural surfaces are most involved.

There is a diffuse conjunctivitis which can become secondarily infected to produce corneal ulceration. The upper respiratory tract is often involved with epistaxis, dysphagia and tracheitis. Pneumonia, urinogenital involvement, nephritis and myocarditis can occur in severe cases.

In the minor form there are only local manifestations in the mouth or the skin or both and no fever or prostration.

The patient should be referred to a physician. In the minor form topical corticosteroids may be used in the mouth. In the major form systemic steroids and supportive treatment are necessary. If *Mycoplasma pneumoniae* infection is present a course of tetracycline is given.

DRUG ALLERGY AND CONTACT HYPERSENSITIVITY

As the number and variety of drugs and chemicals used as food additives increase, oral manifestations of hypersensitivity become more common.

Adverse reactions are basically of two types:

1. Those following systemic administration of a drug or chemical
2. Those following direct contact with the oral mucosa.

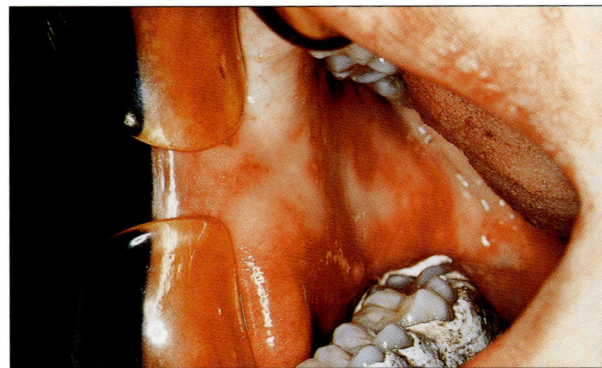

Fig. 24.13 Contact hypersensitivity: type IV hypersensitivity reaction on the buccal mucosa of a 40-year-old man to a component of Coe Pack®. The reaction followed the placement of Coe Pack® following periodontal surgery and resolved shortly after removing the pack.

DRUG ALLERGY

These reactions can be provoked by penicillin, diazepam, local anaesthetics, codeine, tetracycline, barbiturates and many other drugs in common use.

Manifestations depend on the type of allergic response provoked, ranging from simple drying of the mouth to the most severe response, anaphylactic shock, which is potentially fatal. A severe reaction is angioneurotic oedema in which there is swelling of the face, eyelids, lips, tongue and even pharynx. A fairly common response, especially to penicillin, is urticaria, skin rash, pains in the joints and fever. In the mouth, patches of inflammation, vesicles and ulcers may appear.

CONTACT HYPERSENSITIVITY

Reactions of the oral mucosa have been reported to chewing gum, mouthwashes, toothpaste, sweets, cosmetics, topical antibiotics, periodontal dressings, etc. Often flavouring agents, such as peppermint, menthol, cinnamon, eugenol, are implicated.

Symptoms start with a burning sensation of the oral mucosa and swelling and redness of the tongue, lips and gingivae (**Fig. 24.13**). The epithelium may peel off to leave very sore ulcerated areas. The gingivae are characteristically bright red and sensitive and because the patient cannot clean the mouth it can become very dirty.

Management

The drug or chemical suspected must be immediately withdrawn. Antihistamines, such as Piriton, are useful where symptoms are mild but more severe reactions, e.g. angioneurotic oedema, may require injection of hydrocortisone hemisuccinate.

In anaphylactic shock, intramuscular injection of 0.5 mL of 1:1000 adrenaline (epinephrine) is necessary.

The mouth can be kept clean by frequent warm water or weak saline mouthwashes.

REFERENCES

Arendorf TM, Walker DM: Oral Candidal populations in health and disease, *Br Dent J* 147:267–272, 1979.

Arendorf TM, Walker DM: The prevalence and intraoral distribution of Candida albicans in man, *Arch Oral Biol* 2S:1–10, 1980.

Bartholmeusz A, Locarnini S: Mutations in the hepatitis B virus polymerase that are associated with resistance to famciclovir and lamivudine, *International Antiviral News* 5:123–124, 1997.

Dahlén G, Wikström M: Occurrence of enteric rods, staphylococci and Candida in subgingival samples, *Oral Microbiol Immunol* 10:42–46, 1995.

Denning DW, Baily GG, Hood SV: Azole resistance in Candida, *Eur J Clin Microbiol Infect Dis* 16:261–280, 1997.

Dienstay JL, Perillo RP, Schiff ER, et al: A preliminary trial of lamivudine for chronic hepatitis B infection, *Lancet* 333:1657–1661, 1995.

Drew W, Bubbles W: Antiviral drug resistance. In Richman D, editor: *Drug Resistance*, London, 1997, Wiley.

Egusa H, Nikawa H, Makihira S, et al: Intercellular adhesion molecule 1-dependent activation of interleukin 8 expression in Candida albicans-infected human gingival epithelial cells, *Infect Immun* 73:622–626, 2005.

González S, Lobos I, Guajardo A, et al: Yeasts in juvenile periodontitis, *J Periodontol* 58:119–124, 1987.

Green RJ, Harris ND: Infections and antimicrobial therapy. In *Pathology and Therapeutics for Pharmacists. A Basis for Clinical Pharmacy Practice*, Ch. 12. London, 1993, Chapman and Hall, pp 548–558.

Guimarães AL, Correia-Silva J de F, Sá AR, et al: Investigation of functional gene polymorphisms IL-1a, IL-6, IL-10 and TNF-a in individuals with recurrent aphthous stomatitis, *Arch Oral Biol* 52:268–272, 2007.

Hitchcock CA, Pye GW, Troke PF, et al: Fluconazole resistance in Candida glabrata, *Antimicrob Agents Chemother* 37:1962–1965, 1993.

Japour A, Welles S, D'Aquila R: Mutations in human immunodeficiency virus isolated from patients following long-term zidovudine treatment, *J Infect Dis* 171:1172–1179, 1995.

Järvensivu A, Heitanen J, Rautemaa R, et al: Candida yeasts in adult periodontitis tissues and subgingival microbial biofilms in vivo, *Oral Dis* 10:106–112, 2004.

Johnson EM, Davey KG, Szekely A, et al: Itraconazole susceptibilities of fluconazole susceptible and resistant isolates of five Candida species, *J Antimicrob Chemother* 36:787–793, 1995.

Kellam P, Boucher CA, Larder BA: Fifth mutation in human immunodeficiency virus type 1 reverse transcriptase contributes to the development of high-level resistance to zidovudine, *Proc Natl Acad Sci USA* 89:1934–1938, 1992.

Koray M, Ak G, Kurklu E, et al: Fluconazole and/or hexetidine for management of oral candidiasis associated with denture-induced stomatitis, *Oral Dis* 11:309–313, 2005.

Larder BA, Kemp SD, Harrigan PR: Potential mechanism for sustained antiretroviral efficacy of AZT-3TC combination therapy, *Science* 269:696–699, 1995.

Law D, Moore C, Joseph L: High incidence of antifungal drug resistance in Candida tropicalis, *Int J Antimicrob Agents* 7:241–245, 1996.

Main L, Bown JL, Howells C, et al: A double blind, placebo controlled study to assess the effect of famciclovir on virus replication in patients with chronic hepatitis B virus infection, *J Viral Hepat* 3:211–215, 1996.

Manfredi M, McCullough MJ, Polonelli L, et al: In vitro antifungal susceptibility to six antifungal agents of 229 Candida isolates from patients with diabetes mellitus, *Oral Microbiol Immunol* 21:177–182, 2006.

Neu HC: Antimicrobial chemotherapy. In Baron S, Jennings PM, editors: *Medical Microbiology*, ed 3, New York, 1991, Churchill Livingstone, Ch. 11, pp 179–201.

Odds FC: *Candida and Candidosis*, London, 1988, Baillière Tindall.

Pemberton MN, Oliver RJ, Theaker ED: Miconazole oral gel and drug interaction, *Br Dent J* 196:529–531, 2004.

Pottage JC Jr, Kessler HA: Herpes simplex virus resistance to acyclovir: clinical relevance, *Infect Agents Dis* 4:115–124, 1995.

Price MF, LaRocco MT, Gentry LO: Fluconazole susceptibilities of Candida species and distribution of species recovered from blood cultures over a 5-year period, *Antimicrob Agents Chemother* 38:1422–1427, 1994.

Rams TE, Flynn MJ, Slots J: Subgingival microbial associations in severe human periodontitis, *Clin Infect Dis* 25:S224–S226, 1997.

Reyes M, Grabber JM, Weatherall N, et al: Acyclovir-resistant herpes simplex virus; preliminary results from a national surveillance system, *Antiviral Res* 37:44, 1998.

Reynaud AH, Nygaard-Østby B, Bøygard G-K, et al: Yeasts in periodontal pockets, *J Clin Periodontol* 28:860–864, 2001.

Safrin S, Berger TG, Gilson I: Foscarnet therapy in five patients with AIDS and acyclovir-resistant varicella zoster infection, *Ann Intern Med* 115:19–21, 1991a.

Safrin S, Crumpacker C, Chatis P, et al: A controlled trial comparing foscarnet with vidarabine for acyclovir-resistant mucocutaneous herpes simplex in the acquired immunodeficiency syndrome. The AIDS Clinical Trials Group, *N Engl J Med* 325:551–555, 1991b.

Schulten EA, ten Kate RW, van der Waal I: Oral manifestations of HIV infection in 75 Dutch patients, *J Oral Pathol Med* 18:42–46, 1989.

Scully C, Felix DH: Oral medicine – update for the dental practitioner. Aphthous and other common ulcers, *Br Dent J* 199:259–264, 2005a.

Scully C, Felix DH: Oral medicine -update for the dental practitioner. Mouth ulcers of more serious connotation, *Br Dent J* 199:339–343, 2005b.

Shafer WG, Hine MK, Levy BM: *A Textbook of Oral Pathology*, ed 4, Philadelphia, 1983, Saunders.

Slavin MA, Bindra RR, Gleaves CA, et al: Ganciclovir sensitivity of cytomegalovirus at diagnosis and during treatment of cytomegalovirus pneumonia in marrow transplant recipients, *Antimicrob Agents Chemother* 37:1360–1363, 1993.

Slots J, Rams TE, Listgarten MA: Yeasts, enteric rods and pseudomonads in the subgingival flora of severe adult periodontitis, *Oral Microbiol Immunol* 3:47–52, 1988.

Standing Medical Advisory Committee, Subgroup on Antimicrobial Resistance Current resistance problems in the UK and worldwide. In DoH, *The Path of Least Resistance*, Ch. 10, London, 1999, Department of Health, pp 33–54.

Vanden Bossche H, Warnock DW, Dupont B, et al: Mechanisms and clinical impact of antifungal drug resistance, *J Med Vet Mycol* 32:S189–S202, 1994.

Voss A, Kluytmans JA, Koeleman JG, et al: Occurrence of yeast bloodstream infections between 1987 and 1995 in five Dutch university hospitals, *Eur J Clin Microbiol Infect Dis* 15:909–912, 1996.

White DJ, Johnson EM, Warnock DW: Management of persistent vulvo vaginal candidosis due to azole-resistant Candida glabrata, *Genitourin Med* 69:112–114, 1993.

Wingard JR, Merz WG, Rinaldi MG, et al: Increase in Candida krusei infection among patients with bone marrow transplantation and neutropenia treated prophylactically with fluconazole, *N Engl J Med* 325:1274–1277, 1991.

This condition has many synonyms including acute ulcerative gingivitis (AUG), acute necrotizing gingivitis (ANG), Vincent's disease, trench mouth and fusospirochaetal gingivitis. Acute necrotizing ulcerative gingivitis (ANUG) is an acute necrotizing inflammatory disease produced by endogenous infection where systemic changes, as yet not precisely defined, predispose the gingiva to invasion by some bacteria in the oral flora, in particular spirochaetes and fusiform bacteria.

In Western countries, ANUG is usually seen in the 16–30 age group. Epidemiological studies from 1950–1960 reported a 5% incidence of this condition in young adults particularly in large groups living in cramped conditions such as military recruits and college students. However, the prevalence of the disease has reduced markedly over the past 20 years and this may reflect improved general health and nutrition and better standards of plaque control. More recently, the disease has been seen in patients with HIV infection and AIDS (see Ch. 7) and this now needs to be considered in the diagnosis of this condition.

In some developing countries, such as those in Africa, ANUG is often seen in children and is often associated with malnutrition and infectious disease such as measles and herpes simplex infections (Osuji 1990). Environmental factors are entirely responsible for this situation because it occurs in the poor malnourished children and not in those children from rich families who are of the same race and tribe. In a few of these affected children with severe malnutrition and recent infections the infection may spread from the gingiva to involve the oral and facial tissues producing a condition known as cancrum oris or noma. This may result in massive orofacial necrosis and is life-threatening. If the child recovers from the infection gross facial deformity results.

A study of 58 Nigerian children with ANUG, Osuji (1990) found five cases of cancrum oris. All these children had a recent history of febrile illness. Predisposing factors for cancrum oris are severe malnutrition, infectious childhood diseases, HIV infection and any disease in which the immune system is compromised, as well as poor oral hygiene.

CLINICAL FEATURES OF ANUG

In developed countries, the condition is a disease of young adults and occurs equally in both sexes. It appears to be seasonal, occurring most frequently in autumn and winter months. The condition rarely occurs in a clean mouth and then only if there is a major predisposing factor.

The condition is very painful and plaque accumulates around the affected areas. Patients complain of gingival soreness, which is sometimes severe, and eating becomes difficult. There may be spontaneous gingival bleeding, an objectionable taste and a powerful halitosis.

ANUG is characterized by necrotic ulceration of the affected gingival margins (**Fig. 25.1**). In the early stages of the disease the gingival papillae become red and swollen and the tips of the papillae become ulcerated. Necrotic ulceration of the papillae increases and the ulcers may spread laterally along the gingival margins. The ulcers are painful to touch and are covered by a yellowish-grey slough. They have a characteristic 'punched out' appearance and if the 'false membrane' of sloughing tissue is removed a raw and bleeding surface is exposed.

The ulceration may be localized to one area or involve the whole mouth (**Figs 25.1, 25.2**). Localized infections are most often seen around the lower anterior teeth. They may also be related to sites of bacterial stagnation such as a partially erupted lower third molar.

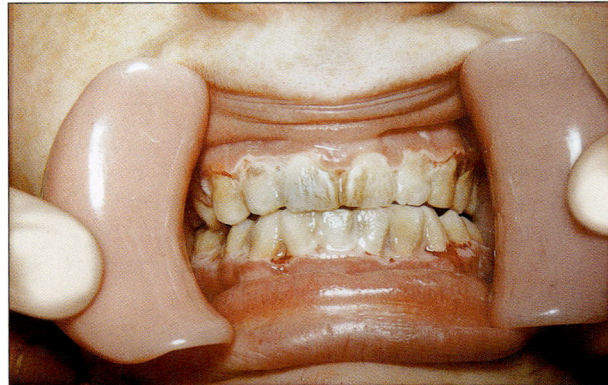

Fig. 25.1 Generalized severe ANUG in a 25-year-old man who was a heavy smoker, poorly nourished and stressed by loss of employment. It is characterized by necrotic ulceration of the interdental papillae and gingival margins. The ulcers are painful to touch and are covered by a yellowish-grey slough.

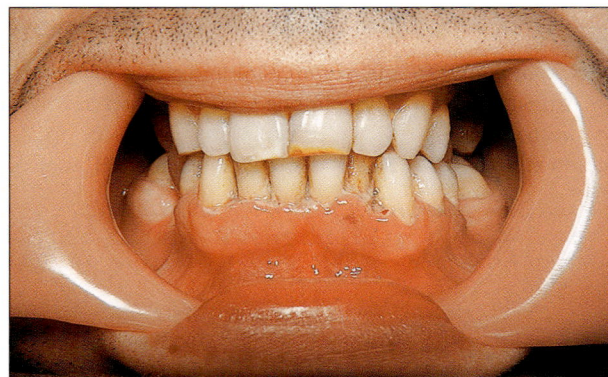

Fig. 25.2 Localized ANUG affecting the lower anterior teeth of a 30-year-old man who was a heavy smoker and night worker with an additional day job and was deprived of sufficient sleep. There is necrotic ulceration of the interdental papillae and gingival margins.

There are frequently no systemic symptoms, although cervical or submandibular lymphadenopathy is commonly present. In some severe cases, there may be mild to moderate fever and malaise and more marked lymphadenopathy. In a study of 35 ANUG patients presenting at an urban USA dental school, Falker et al (1987) found lymphadenopathy in 61% and fever in 39% of their cases.

Ulceration can also rarely occur on the contacting surface of the tongue or cheek, the palate and the fauces (Vincent's angina) but only when there is very severe debilitation. When ANUG occurs in association with HIV infection the lesion may spread more deeply and lead to exposure and infection of the underlying bone (Ch. 7).

Even without active intervention the acute symptoms will subside and the ulcers heal in 10–14 days. However, the normal gingival form does not return and the gingival margin becomes thickened by fibrous repair tissue and the papillae retain the concave shape of the healed ulcer. This saucer-shaped deformity of the gingiva is so characteristic of ANUG that an episode of previous infection can be diagnosed years later.

Once an episode of ANUG has occurred there is a tendency for recurrence (**Figs 25.3, 25.5**) and in a susceptible individual this can occur more

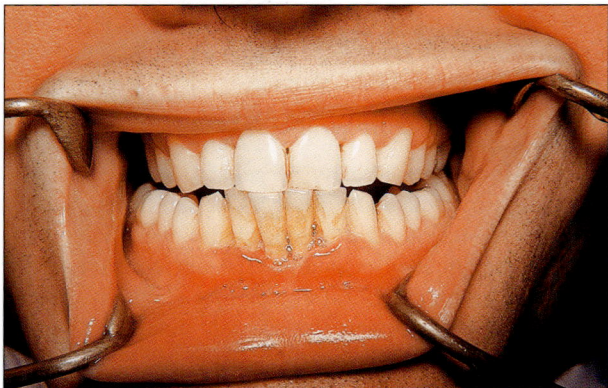

Fig. 25.3 Recurrent ANUG in a heavy smoking 29-year-old woman with a large young family. She has had recurrent attacks over the last 5 years affecting the lower incisors. Combined with periodontal disease this has resulted in loss of gingival tissue and deformity of the gingival contour. Some necrotic ulceration of the interdental papillae and gingival margins can be seen.

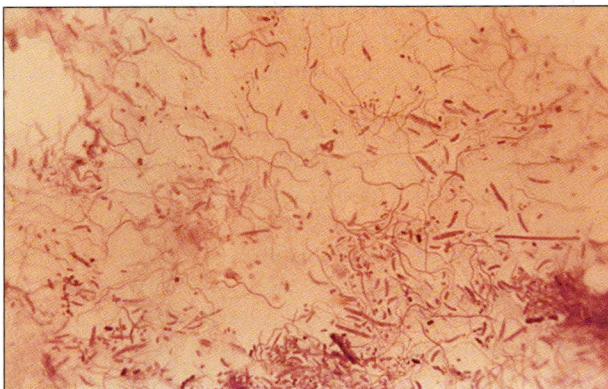

Fig. 25.4 A Gram-stained smear taken from an active lesion of ANUG. It shows a Gram-negative, fusospirochaetal flora characteristic of this condition.

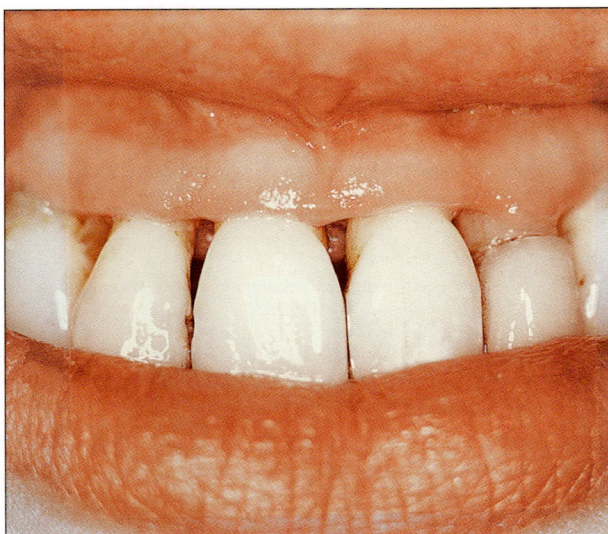

Fig. 25.5 Complete loss of interdental papillae and gingival deformity due to recurrent ANUG in a 32-year-old woman who smoked heavily.

than once a year. This can result in progressive destruction of the periodontal tissues with typical loss of the interdental papillae and the formation of characteristic gingival craters. The additional stagnation produced by this tissue deformity also encourages the progression of any underlying chronic periodontitis.

PREDISPOSING FACTORS

The main predisposing factors in most cases are poor oral hygiene, smoking and emotional stress. However, it can be precipitated by malnutrition, blood dyscrasias such as acute leukaemia, infections such as AIDS and glandular fever, malignant neoplasms and chemotherapy. Probably any condition in which the immune and defence systems are compromised would act in the same way.

The reduction in this condition in recent times probably reflects better standards of oral hygiene and improved health and nutrition. The name trench mouth derives from the high prevalence of ANUG in soldiers suffering the appalling conditions of trench warfare in the First World War. The disease occurred in groups living together in these grossly unhygienic conditions and under immense stress.

MICROBIOLOGY

ANUG is a mixed bacterial infection caused by a group of anaerobes consisting of spirochaetes and fusiform bacteria, which is often termed a fusospirochaetal complex (**Fig. 25.4**). These bacteria include *Treponema vincentii*, *T. denticola*, *T. macrodentium*, *Fusobacterium nucleatum*, *Prevotella intermedia* and *Porphyromonas gingivalis* (Loesche et al 1982). These bacteria are all found in large numbers in the slough and necrotic tissue at the surface of the ulcer and also invade a small distance into the underlying intact tissue at the base of the ulcer (Courtois et al 1983). Spirochaetes can be seen under electron microscopy to invade the greatest distance into the tissue. The aetiological role of these bacteria is suggested by the fact that ANUG resolves rapidly following short-term treatment with metronidazole.

Other bacterial species commonly found in the subgingival flora are also present on the surface of the lesion in lesser numbers.

There are many reports of ANUG in closely confined groups of young adults (see above). However, there is no evidence that the condition is transmissible. This view is supported by experiments in which the inoculation of microorganisms from affected to healthy animals did not result in development of ANUG except when the recipients were severely immunosuppressed. It is therefore thought that the reported group outbreaks of ANUG were due to common exposure to stressful conditions and poor oral hygiene rather than direct transmission of an infecting agent. This view is also supported by the fact that all of the bacteria infecting the tissues in ANUG are bacteria found in the subgingival flora of patients with chronic gingivitis and periodontitis who do not develop ANUG.

SMOKING

A clear association between smoking and the prevalence of ANUG was demonstrated over 40 years ago (Stammers 1944; Pindborg 1947, 1949). A number of more recent studies (Macgregor 1992) have also indicated that smoking is an important predisposing factor in ANUG (see also Ch. 4). Stammers (1944) examined over 1000 cases of ANUG and found that nearly all of them were smokers. More recently, in a study in Edinburgh, Kowolik and Nisbet (1983) found that 98 out of 100 cases of ANUG were smokers. Similarly, Falker et al (1987), in a study of 35 ANUG patients in an urban dental school, found that 83% of them were smokers.

Smokers tend to have poorer levels of oral hygiene and greater deposits of calculus than non-smokers but this is not sufficient to explain the association. Smoking may cause vasoconstriction of gingival blood vessels (Bergström & Floderus-Myrhed 1983) and might in this way favour the colonization of an anaerobic bacterial flora. Of more possible relevance would seem to be the effects of smoking on serum IgG antibodies to subgingival bacteria (Haber 1994), on the numbers of T-helper lymphocytes (Ginns et al 1982; Costabel et al 1986) and neutrophil function (Eichel & Shahrik 1969; Armitage et al 1975; Bridges et al 1977; Kenny et al 1977; Codd et al 1987; Nowak et al 1990; Kalra et al 1991; Lannan et al 1992; Selby et al 1992; MacFarlane et al 1992; Totti et al 1994; Ryder et al 1994) (see Ch. 4).

HOST RESPONSES

The exact way in which the predisposing factors trigger the infection is not clear. However, the fact that ANUG occurs in AIDS and in severely immunosuppressed animals suggests that immunosuppression might be an important factor.

ANUG usually develops when there is poor oral hygiene and pre-existing gingivitis. It will, however, rarely occur in a clean mouth when a severe debilitating factor is present, e.g. acute leukaemia.

Emotional stress as a predisposing factor in ANUG has been long recognized by clinicians. However, there are only a few well-controlled studies which demonstrate the association between ANUG and stress. Stress may alter behaviour such as decreasing oral hygiene, reducing salivary flow and local blood flow and probably affects immune function. In spite of these effects it is not entirely clear how these effects operate as predisposing factors for this condition.

There is a clear relationship between nutritional deficiency and ANUG in developing countries. This may operate by compromising the defence mechanisms to such a degree that the disease spreads more easily.

HISTOPATHOLOGY

The histopathological changes of ANUG are largely non-specific. The surface epithelium and adjacent connective tissue on the surface of the lesion is necrotic. There is a dense acute inflammatory infiltration of the underlying tissues with large numbers of polymorphonuclear neutrophil leucocytes (PMNs) in the tissues. Bacteria can be seen invading this area, with the spirochaetes spreading deepest. Below this area is viable tissue infiltrated with plasma cells, lymphocytes and some macrophages.

DIAGNOSIS

The diagnosis is easily made on clinical grounds without the need to take a bacterial smear to show the fusospirochaetal flora. Nevertheless, it is important to take a very careful history to determine the underlying predisposing factors in each individual case.

TREATMENT

Treatment is divided into two stages:

1. Control of the acute phase
2. Management of the residual condition.

CONTROL OF THE ACUTE PHASE

This is achieved by cleaning the wound and using an antibacterial agent. The lesion is irrigated with warm water or 5-vol hydrogen peroxide solution, gently cleaned and the teeth lightly scaled. The patient is prescribed an oxygen-releasing mouthwash, such as hydrogen peroxide DPF or sodium perborate (Bocasan) DPF, to be used three times daily. The scaling of the affected teeth is completed over the next few days. This may suffice in very mild cases but most cases require an antibiotic in addition. ANUG is an anaerobic infection, thus oral metronidazole (200 mg three times daily for 3–5 days) is the first choice (Shinn 1962; Shinn et al 1965). It gives rapid relief of symptoms and is not likely to produce hypersensitivity reactions. Side-effects may include nausea, headaches, a metallic taste and tachycardia. It should not be prescribed in early pregnancy, if there is blood dyscrasia or in patients drinking alcohol heavily. Alcohol must be totally avoided when taking metronidazole since it precipitates nausea and vomiting. In these cases, phenoxymethyl penicillin (250 mg four times daily for 5 days) is an effective alternative. Erythromycin or clindamycin may be used if both metronidazole and penicillin are contraindicated. A 2% chlorhexidine mouthwash might also be helpful in some cases but should only be used during the short period in which mechanical oral hygiene is compromised.

It is also vital to determine the predisposing factors in each individual case and to counsel the patient on controlling these when appropriate.

MANAGEMENT OF THE RESIDUAL CONDITION

This is essential if recurrence is to be avoided. Meticulous supra- and subgingival scaling is carried out together with the removal of all predisposing local factors, such as overhanging filling margins, partially erupted teeth and food impaction.

Residual gingival deformity (**Figs 25.3, 25.5**) needs to be corrected by gingivoplasty in early cases and by inverse bevel flap procedures in all other cases. Any underlying chronic periodontitis lesion, e.g. pocketing, can be dealt with at the same time.

The maintenance of a high standard of oral hygiene is essential, therefore regular inspection and scaling should be organized.

Patients suffering unexplained recurrence should undergo medical examination and blood screening for major predisposing factors.

REFERENCES

Armitage AK, Dollery CT, George CF, et al: Absorption and metabolism of nicotine from cigarettes, *Br Med J* 4:313–316, 1975.

Bergström J, Floderus-Myrhed B: Co-twin study of the relationship between smoking and some periodontal disease factors, *Community Dent Oral Epidemiol* 11:113–116, 1983.

Bridges RB, Kraal JH, Huang LJT, et al: The effects of tobacco smoke on chemotaxis and glucose metabolism of polymorphonuclear leucocytes, *Infection and Immunology* 15:115–123, 1977.

Codd EE, Swim AT, Bridges RB: Tobacco smokers neutrophils are desensitized to chemotactic peptide-stimulated oxygen uptake, *J Lab Clin Med* 110:648–652, 1987.

Costabel U, Bross KJ, Reuter C, et al: Alterations in immunoregulatory T-cell subsets in cigarette smokers. A phenotypic analysis of bronchoalveolar and blood lymphocytes, *Chest* 90:39–44, 1986.

Courtois G, Cobb C, Killoy W: Acute necrotizing ulcerative gingivitis. A transmission electron microscope study, *J Periodontol* 54:671–679, 1983.

Eichel G, Shahrik HA: Tobacco smoke toxicity: loss of human oral leucocyte function and fluid cell metabolism, *Science* 166:1424–1428, 1969.

Falker WA Jr, Martin SA, Vincent JW, et al: A clinical and demographic and microbiologic study of ANUG patients in an urban dental school, *J Clin Periodontol* 14:307–314, 1987.

Ginns LC, Goldenheim PD, Miller LG: T-lymphocyte subsets in smoking and lung cancer. Analysis of monoclonal antibodies and flow cytometry, *Am Rev Respir Dis* 126:265–269, 1982.

Haber J: Cigarette smoking: a major risk factor for periodontitis, *Compend Contin Educ Dent* 15:1002–1014, 1994.

Kalra J, Chandhary AK, Prasad K: Increased production of oxygen free radicals in cigarette smokers, *Int J Exp Pathol* 72:1–7, 1991.

Kenny EB, Kraal JH, Saxe SR, et al: The effects of cigarette smoke on human polymorphonuclear leukocytes, *J Periodontal Res* 12:227–234, 1977.

Kowolik MJ, Nisbet T: Smoking and acute ulcerative gingivitis, *Br Dent J* 154:241–242, 1983.

Lannan S, McLean A, Drost E, et al: Changes in neutrophil morphology and morphometry following exposure to cigarette smoke, *Int J Exp Pathol* 73:183–191, 1992.

Loesche WJ, Syed SA, Laughton BE, et al: The bacteriology of acute necrotizing ulcerative gingivitis, *J Periodontol* 53:223–230, 1982.

MacFarlane GD, Herzberg MC, Wolff LF, et al: Refractory periodontitis associated with abnormal polymorphonuclear leucocyte phagocytosis and cigarette smoking, *J Periodontol* 63:908–913, 1992.

Macgregor IDM: Smoking and periodontal disease. In Seymour RA, Heasman PA, editors: *Drugs, Diseases and the Periodontium*, Oxford, 1992, Oxford University Press, pp 118–119.

Nowak D, Ruta U, Piasecka G: Nicotine increases human polymorphonuclear leukocytes' chemotactic response – possible additional mechanism of lung injury in cigarette smokers, *Exp Pathol* 39:37–43, 1990.

Osuji OO: Necrotising ulcerative gingivitis and cancrum oris in Ibadan, Nigeria, *J Periodontol* 61:769–772, 1990.

Pindborg JJ: Tobacco and gingivitis. I. Statistical examination of the significance of tobacco in the development of acute ulceromembranous gingivitis and in the formation of calculus, *J Dent Res* 26:261–264, 1947.

Pindborg JJ: Tobacco and gingivitis. II. Correlation between consumption of tobacco, acute ulceromembranous gingivitis and calculus, *J Dent Res* 28:460–463, 1949.

Ryder MI: Nicotine effects on neutrophil F-actin formation and calcium release: implications for tobacco use and respiratory disease, *Exp Lung Res* 20:283–296, 1994.

Selby C, Drost E, Brown D, et al: Inhibition of neutrophil adherence and movement by acute cigarette smoke exposure, *Exp Lung Res* 18:813–827, 1992.

Shinn DL: Metronidazole in acute ulcerative gingivitis, *Lancet* 1:1191, 1962.

Shinn DL, Squires S, McFadzean JA: The treatment of Vincent's disease with metronidazole, *Dental Practitioner* 15:275–280, 1965.

Stammers A: Vincent's infection: observations and conclusions regarding the aetiology and treatment of 1,017 civilian cases, *Br Dent J* 76:147–155, 1944.

Totti N, McCuster KT, Campbell EJ, et al: Nicotine is chemotactic for neutrophils and enhances neutrophil responsiveness to chemotactic peptides, *Science* 227:169–171, 1994.

26 Epulides and tumours of the gingivae and oral mucosa

EPULIDES

The term 'epulis' means a 'lump on the gum' and these lesions are the commonest localized enlargements of the gingiva. They are best described as chronic inflammatory hyperplasias. These can be fibrous epulides, pyogenic granulomata or giant-cell granulomata, the first two being much more common than the third.

FIBROUS EPULIS (FIBROEPITHELIAL POLYP)

This usually arises from an interdental papilla and is a firm, pink nodule of varying shape (Fig. 26.1). They usually associate with a source of chronic irritation such as calculus or the rough edge of a restoration. Similar lesions can occur on the cheek as the result of cheek biting or related to the margin of an ill-fitting denture (denture granuloma).

Histologically the lesion consists of hyperplastic connective tissue covered by stratified squamous epithelium. These lesions should be treated by excision with care to remove any irritating factor. The whole lesion should be placed in formal saline fixative and sent for histological confirmation of the diagnosis.

PYOGENIC GRANULOMA

The pyogenic granuloma usually arises from the interdental papilla. It appears as an elevated, pedunculated or sessile mass with a smooth or lobulated surface (Fig. 26.2). It is deep red or reddish-purple in colour and the surface may be ulcerated. It also has a tendency to bleed either spontaneously or on provocation with slight trauma. It may develop rapidly to a variable size and then remain stable for an indefinite period.

The lesion appears to result from local irritation but in some cases there may be a hormonal conditioning factor such as in the lesions occurring in pregnancy (pyogenic granulomata of pregnancy) and at puberty (Ch. 6).

Histologically, the overlying stratified squamous epithelium is usually thin and atrophic but may show signs of hyperplasia in some parts of the lesion. The connective tissue contains vast numbers of endothelium-lined vascular spaces and proliferation of endothelial cells and fibroblasts. There is a moderately intense infiltration of polymorphonuclear neutrophil leucocytes (PMNs), lymphocytes and plasma cells with high numbers of PMNs at the surface of the lesion particularly when ulceration is present.

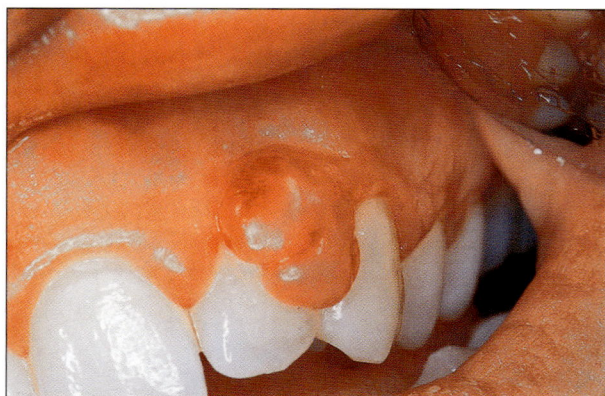

Fig. 26.2 A pyogenic granuloma arising from the interdental papilla between the lower left first and second premolar in a 15-year-old boy.

The lesion should be carefully excised with care to remove all affected tissue and any local irritating factor. Lack of care in these respects can lead to recurrence of the lesion. The whole lesion should be placed in formal saline fixative and sent for histological confirmation of the diagnosis.

GIANT-CELL EPULIS

The giant-cell epulis or granuloma is usually found growing from the gingival margin between teeth anterior to the permanent molars and its development may be related to the resorption of the deciduous molars (Fig. 26.3). The lesion is rounded, soft and purplish-red in colour. It may grow rapidly in its early stages and tends to bleed easily.

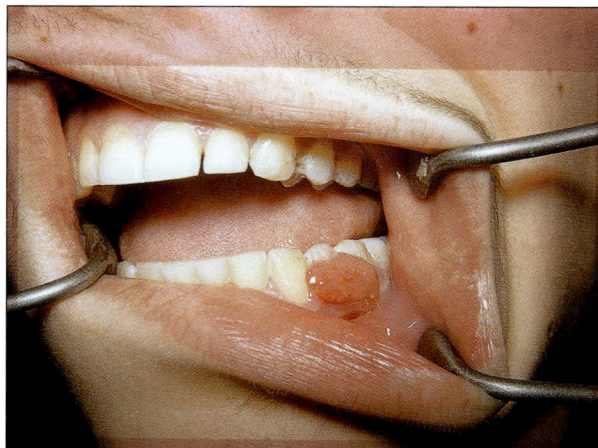

Fig. 26.1 A fibrous epulis arising from the interdental papilla between the upper right second incisor and canine teeth in a 17-year-old woman.

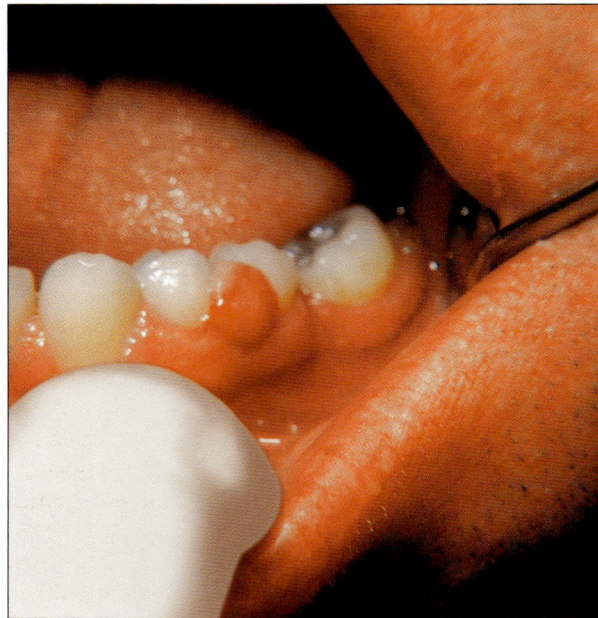

Fig. 26.3 A giant-cell epulis arising from the interdental and buccal tissues between the lower left first and second premolar in a 15-year-old boy.

Histologically, the connective tissue consists of numerous multinucleated giant-cells (macrophage polykaryons) and plump spindle-shaped cells in a loose fibrous stroma. It is covered by stratified squamous epithelium.

A giant-cell granuloma of the jaw may erode through the outer alveolar plate and appear as a gingival swelling. This should be distinguished from the epulis by radiological investigation.

The treatment is total excision of the lesion along with the basal tissue from which it arose. The alveolar bone at the base of the lesion should also be curetted thoroughly. Histological confirmation of the diagnosis is essential and the lesion must be immediately placed in formal saline fixative for this purpose.

NEOPLASMS OF THE GINGIVA

True benign or occasionally malignant neoplasms may arise from the gingival or periodontal tissue and may sometimes resemble an epulis.

EPITHELIAL NEOPLASMS

Squamous-cell papilloma

The squamous-cell papilloma usually appears as a warty nodule with a white surface if keratinized and a pink one if not (**Fig. 26.4**). It may be related to the common wart of the skin and be due to infection with human papilloma virus (HPV).

The whole lesion should be excised and submitted for histological examination to confirm the diagnosis.

Squamous-cell carcinoma

These tumours may occasionally occur on the gingiva but are more common on other parts of the oral mucosa such as the tongue (**Fig. 26.5**), lips, buccal mucosa, floor of the mouth or alveolar mucosa. Carcinoma of the gingiva usually presents as an ulcerated lesion with rolled edges but it may sometimes have an exophytic or verrucous type of growth (Sully & Felix 2005). Any fast growing lesion or ulcer which fails to heal should be regarded with suspicion; 95% of oral cancer occurs after the age of 40 and it becomes more common with increasing age. Gingival carcinomas are closely related to the underlying bone and rapidly invade the periosteum

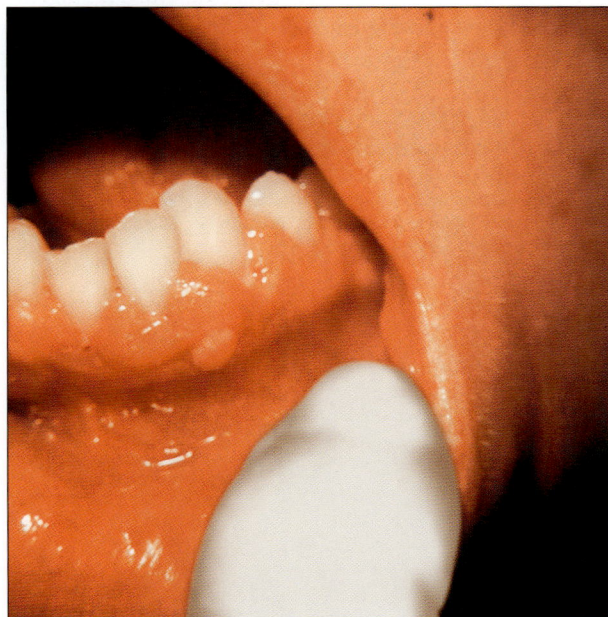

Fig. 26.5 A squamous cell carcinoma of the tongue in a 61-year-old, heavy smoking and drinking man. Note the ulceration and rolled margins. There is also evidence of smoker's keratosis of the other parts of the tongue.

and bone. Metastasis is common and early diagnosis is essential if treatment is to have any chance of success. Suspicious lesions should be quickly referred to a specialist oral surgeon and oral pathologist to confirm the diagnosis by biopsy and treatment instituted.

The incidence of oral cancer amongst young adults is increasing in many European and other countries with a previously high incidence. Most oral cancer has been linked to the use of tobacco and alcohol but more recently there has been evidence produced for the presence of viral nucleic acids in oral squamous cell carcinoma (OSCC) (Sully 2005). This suggests that there may be viral involvement in a least some OSCCs. Subsequently, human papillomaviruses (HPV) have been implicated in OSCC (Sully 2005). Antibody responses have been seen and HPV-DNA detected in some tumours and that found is usually HPV-16 which has also been implicated in ano-genital cancer. More recently, HPV has been found in oropharyngeal cancer and some tonsillar carcinomas and may represent an alternative pathway in carcinogenesis to the established factors of tobacco and alcohol. It has also been suggested that some OSCCs with a viral association may be sexually transmitted.

CONNECTIVE-TISSUE NEOPLASMS

Benign and occasionally malignant neoplasms arising in the connective tissue can sometimes involve the gingival tissues. They may present as firm masses which stretch the overlying mucosa and may displace adjacent teeth. They may also sometimes resemble epulides. Suspicious lesions should be referred to a specialist oral surgeon and oral pathologist for definitive diagnosis.

These neoplasms may include benign fibromas (**Fig. 26.6**) and myxomas and their equivalent malignant sarcomas. It should also been borne in mind that benign and malignant bone tumours and bony malformations may also resemble gingival swelling (**Fig. 26.7**). Tumours may also arise from salivary gland tissue including minor salivary glands beneath the oral mucosa (**Fig. 26.8**).

LYMPHOID NEOPLASMS

Lymphomas such as Hodgkin's and non-Hodgkin's lymphoma may produce deposits beneath the oral mucosa including the gingiva. In addition deposits from a leukaemia may seed in the gingiva and multiply (see Ch. 6). All such cases should be quickly referred to specialists for these conditions.

DENTAL TISSUE NEOPLASMS

Tumours of odontogenic origin may be found in the jaws and occasionally arise from dental epithelial remnants in the periodontium, such as the epithelial rests of Malassez, and occur in the periodontium or gingiva.

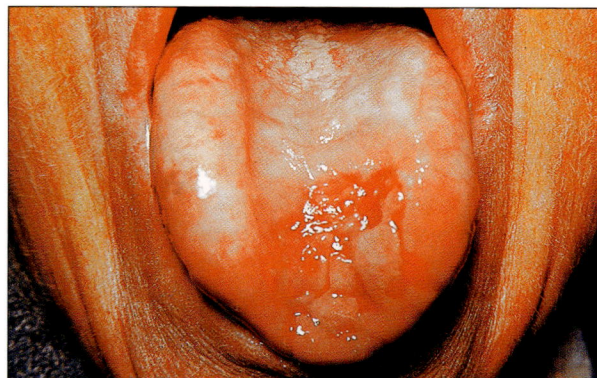

Fig. 26.4 A squamous cell papilloma on the gingiva between the lower left second incisor and canine teeth in a 40-year-old woman.

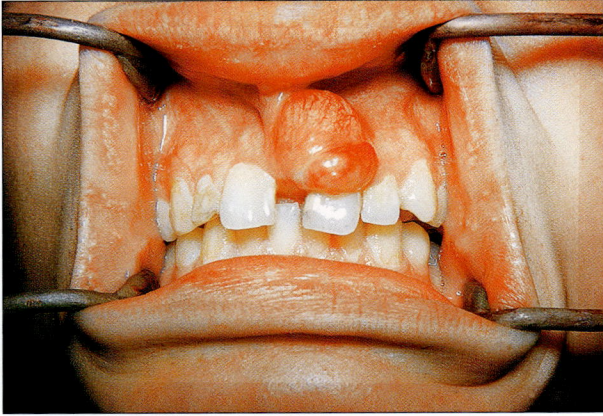

Fig. 26.6 A benign true fibroma arising from fibrous tissue beneath the gingival and alveolar mucosa related to the upper left central incisor in a 25-year-old woman. The tumour has caused displacement of the involved incisor tooth.

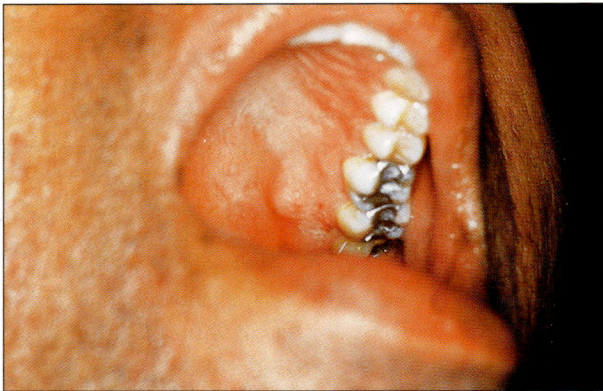

Fig. 26.7 A bony exostosis causing stretching of the overlying mucosa palatal to the upper first molar of a 50-year-old man. Palpation of the enlarged tissue will reveal its bony origin.

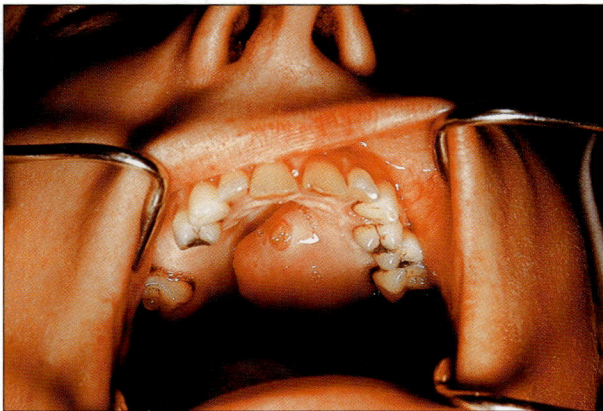

Fig. 26.8 A pleomorphic adenoma arising from minor salivary gland tissue beneath the palatal mucosa in a 45-year-old woman.

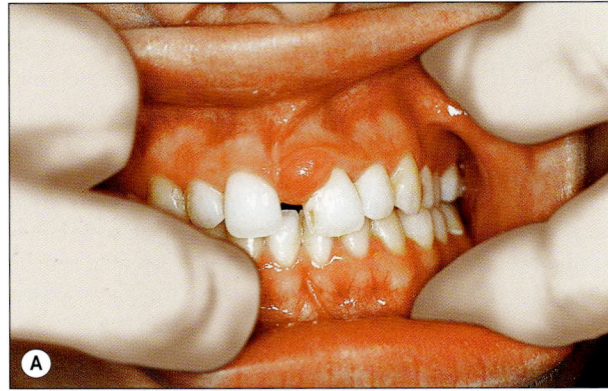

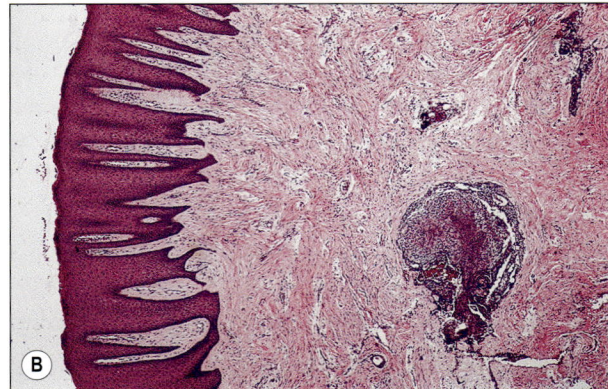

Fig. 26.9 (A) A tumour of dental tissue origin, resembling an epulis, arising from epithelial cell rests of Malassez within the periodontal ligament of the upper left central incisor of a 16-year-old girl. (B) Photomicrograph of a low-power view of a histological section of the above lesion. It shows the features of an adenomatoid odontogenic tumour.

Those in the gingiva may resemble epulides and those within the bone may expand the alveolar plate and produce a gingival swelling. They include adenomatoid odontogenic tumours, squamous odontogenic tumours and calcifying epithelial odontogenic tumours. Careful radiographic examination is necessary in these cases and they should be referred to a specialist oral surgeon and oral pathologist for definitive diagnosis and treatment. The clinical appearance and histology of an adenomatoid odontogenic tumour of the gingiva are shown in **Figure 26.9**.

REFERENCES

Sully C: Oral cancer; the evidence for sexual transmission, *Br Dent J* 199:203–207, 2005.
Sully C, Felix DH: Oral medicine – update for the dental practitioner. Mouth ulcers of more serious connotation, *Br Dent J* 199:339–343, 2005.

The term 'occlusion' applies to any contact between the mandibular and maxillary teeth in any position of the mandible. The occlusion is therefore of importance to restorative and prosthetic dentistry as well as to orthodontics and periodontics. Unfortunately, each of these specialties has been concerned with a particular aspect of occlusion and has developed its own beliefs and vocabulary, leading to confusion. Many of the concepts valuable to prosthetics or orthodontics may be irrelevant or even contrary to an understanding of the role of occlusal relationships and occlusal stresses in periodontics. The concept of 'balanced occlusion' in which bilateral cuspal contacts are made in lateral excursions may well be important in prosthetics but under certain circumstances can be contrary to periodontal health. Health of the tooth-supporting tissues does not depend primarily on the conformity of the occlusion to any particular anatomical stereotype. However, occlusal stresses can play a role in periodontal pathology (Ch. 8). These concepts have been reviewed recently (Harrel et al 2006).

Three important aspects of masticatory function need to be considered:

1. During normal mastication teeth are separated by the food bolus and make contact at the end of the chewing cycle and during swallowing. It has been estimated that the total duration of tooth contact in a 24 h period is 17.5 min made up of 9 min chewing contact and 8.5 min swallowing contact. Therefore normal functional tooth-to-tooth contact is occasional and transient and by itself unlikely to cause damage.
2. The activity of the masticatory system is largely under the control of the trigeminal nerve nucleus which, subject to the control of the higher centres, operates various forms of reflex activity. These constitute a feedback mechanism which protects the various tissues of the masticatory system, including the periodontium. For example, the presence of a hard object such as a piece of bone or nut in the bolus of soft food stimulates proprioceptors in the periodontal ligament which by reflex activity causes the jaw to open. In this way stress on the teeth and supporting tissues is controlled, unless the higher centres dictate that a conscious effort be made to crack the nut.
3. All the tissues of the masticatory system except the teeth have considerable powers of adaptation and bone, connective tissue and epithelium are in a state of constant activity and renewal. The masticatory system is not a rigid system; like other vital tissues it is immensely flexible and allows a range of environmental changes to be absorbed without damage.

EXCESSIVE OCCLUSAL STRESS

Attempts to define the word 'excessive' in most situations tend to beg the question. Excessive occlusal stresses are those which exceed the limits of tissue adaptation and therefore cause occlusal trauma. Supra-physiological forces would be excessive for a well supported dentition while physiological loading may be excessive in a compromised dentition. Forces generated during mastication depend largely on the consistency of the food. Peak pressures on an adult molar have been estimated at 0.4–1.8 kg, but because of the powers of adaptation of the periodontal tissues it is impossible to define excessive occlusal stress in precise numerical terms.

Excessive stresses appear to be engendered by:

1. Abnormal or parafunctional activity
2. Dental treatment
3. Occlusal disharmony
4. Destruction of the periodontal tissues by disease, i.e. chronic periodontitis.

These factors are frequently interrelated.

PARAFUNCTION

Parafunctional activity is outside the range of functional activity. It is usually habitual and the patient is often unaware of such habits during which contact may be made between the upper and lower teeth as in clenching and grinding, between the teeth and the soft tissues, cheeks, lips and tongue or between the teeth and some foreign body, e.g. pencil, pipe, etc. These habits may be associated with psychological factors, e.g. anxiety, anger, frustration, or with occupational or recreational activity.

BRUXISM

The most common tooth-to-tooth habits are clenching and grinding, i.e. bruxism. A large proportion of patients with periodontal disease indulge in this habit. Many patients are aware of clenching their teeth when under stress during the day but few people are aware of a night grinding habit unless complained of by someone else. It has been estimated that during clenching or grinding the individual might impose a load of over 20 kg on a tooth over periods of 2.5 s at a time. This is far in excess of normal functional stresses and causes 'flow' within the viscoelastic periodontal ligament and distortion of the alveolar bone, from which the tissues are slow to recover. Furthermore, the excessive load tends to affect the proprioceptive nerve endings which are either overridden or set at a higher tolerance level, thereby impairing the protective reflex mechanism. Muscle activity becomes abnormal and the habit is perpetuated. Such disturbed muscle activity may also interfere with temporomandibular joint function. Bruxism is the most usual cause of advanced attrition in the Western world.

In the absence of gingival inflammation or periodontal destruction the supporting tissues may adapt to the load of primary occlusal trauma. Where there is pre-existing inflammatory periodontal disease the tissues usually similarly adapt. In early to moderate periodontitis the adaptive response is the same but in advanced periodontitis the rate of disease progression may be accelerated by the fusion of the marginal inflammatory and the intra-alveolar 'trauma' lesions (Ch. 8).

There are two causes of bruxism: nervous tension and occlusal interference. These two factors often act together so that an occlusal interference in an anxious person may provoke bruxism, whereas in a relaxed individual interference may be adapted to.

Diagnosis of bruxism

There may be a definite history of bruxism but as stated many patients are unaware of parafunction. A number of signs help in its detection:

1. Advanced attrition is the most obvious clue, also wear facets which could be produced only in extreme positions of mandibular movements
2. Increased tooth mobility patterns which are not commensurate with the amount of attachment loss or degree of gingival inflammation
3. The presence of widened periodontal ligament spaces seen in radiographs
4. Hypertonicity of the muscles of mastication
5. Temporomandibular joint discomfort.

DENTAL TREATMENT

One of the most common causes of excessive occlusal stress in the partially dentate patient is the badly designed partial denture. Many abutment teeth suffer abnormal loading because the stress is either greater than normal or applied in an abnormal direction. The tooth used as an abutment for a free-end saddle denture is particularly vulnerable, especially when clasps without occlusal rests are used. As the denture sinks into the soft tissues, lateral and distal forces are imposed on the abutment teeth. In most cases oral hygiene is poor and the combined effect of gingival inflammation under the denture and excessive occlusal loads make loss of abutment teeth more than likely. In denture design axial loading of abutment teeth is imperative and where soft-tissue support is necessary this should be spread over as large an area as possible.

Orthodontic treatment can cause excessive occlusal stress in two ways. Large forces can cause rapid tooth movement and damage to the supporting tissues. If the alveolar plates of bone are thin they may be perforated; thus, tipping a lower incisor forward against a thin labial plate may produce a dehiscence. Slow orthodontic movement allows tissue adaptation and less likelihood of trauma. Tooth movement can also produce occlusal disharmonies with harmful results.

Failure to contour the cusps of restorations or to check the occlusion in both intercuspal and functional positions can produce cuspal interference. Unfortunately, modern dental amalgams set rapidly and leave little time for careful occlusal adjustment which is very important if the restoration is to have correct occlusion relationships.

Failure to replace a lost tooth can result in drifting of other teeth with resultant disharmonies.

OCCLUSAL DISHARMONY

Functional harmony is a very important attribute of the healthy masticatory system, with all parts of the unit – muscles, ligaments, temporomandibular joints – working smoothly together. Occlusal disharmonies are tooth contacts which interfere with smooth closing movement along any pathway into intercuspal position. A common mistake is to assume that malocclusions are always associated with occlusal disharmonies. So flexible is the tooth eruption mechanism that even gross tooth malalignment does not necessarily produce cuspal interference; rather it is external interference with the fully erupted dentition which produces disharmony. Badly executed dentistry can create interferences but the most common cause is tooth loss. After tooth extraction, neighbouring teeth may tip and drift and opposing teeth overerupt until a new position of stability is reached. Thus after extraction of the lower first molar the second and third molars tip mesially and lingually and the distal cusps of these teeth come into interfering contact with upper molar cusps. Moreover, because of the tilt, plaque may be allowed to collect on the mesial and lingual aspects of these teeth producing gingival inflammation and pocketing.

EFFECTS OF OCCLUSAL INTERFERENCE

1. The path of closure of the mandible may alter to avoid the interference. This may put an excessive load on other teeth, e.g. occlusal interference between molar cusps may produce a path of closure forward of the normal pathway and forward posturing of the mandible so that the upper incisors become overloaded (**Fig. 27.1B**). This may result in drifting of the incisors which is more likely when there is already loss of tooth support caused by periodontal disease.
2. If there is no adaptation to the interference, the involved teeth make contact in what is called an initial or premature contact from which a slide carries the mandible into the position of maximum intercuspation (**Fig. 27.1A**). This may produce excessive stress on those teeth involved directly as well as on those teeth indirectly stressed at the end of the slide. Drifting and occlusal trauma may result.
3. The interference may also initiate parafunctional habits. Parafunctional habits are more likely to induce occlusal trauma due to sustained contact between teeth; in comparison with relatively minimal contact of 17–20 min encountered in a 24 h physiological cycle associated with mastication and swallowing.

THE DIAGNOSIS OF OCCLUSAL TRAUMA

A number of clinical features point to the presence of occlusal trauma. A diagnosis should be based not on the presence of only one but several features together.

1. Tooth mobility is affected by the load on the tooth and its duration, by the proportion of tooth invested in supporting tissue and by the morphology of the root(s). It is also affected by inflammation of the attachment apparatus. Increased tooth mobility may be a sign of occlusal trauma or of hyperfunction, i.e. increased loading of the tooth without evidence of tissue breakdown. Assessment of mobility (outside the laboratory) is entirely subjective, teeth being given a score from 0 to 3 (Ch. 12). It can be detected by having the patient grind the teeth from side to side while the operator rests his fingers on the facial surfaces of the teeth. It is more usually tested for by pressing the blunt end of an instrument against one side of the tooth while a finger rests on the tooth under examination and a neighbouring tooth which acts as a fixed point.
2. Tooth wear which appears to be greater than one might expect in a patient of that age and which cannot be attributed to any special diet or deficiency in tooth mineralization.
3. The migration of one or more teeth: this is usually seen in the anterior segment often related to (a) loss of posterior support and/or (b) an abnormal path of closure due to tooth interference between posterior teeth (**Fig. 27.1**). Where bone loss due to periodontal

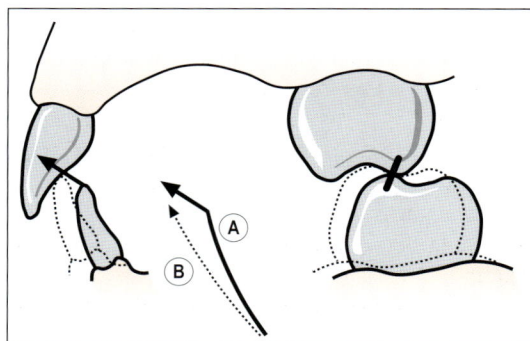

Fig. 27.1 An interference between the posterior teeth may produce: (A) a slide from the initial contact into the intercuspal position, or (B) forward posturing of the mandible to avoid the contact resulting in it closing through a forward path.

disease has taken place tooth migration can be rapid and a common cause of patient alarm. Food impaction may occur following tooth drifting and breaking of interproximal contacts.

4. Operators with a sensitive ear may be able to detect that the percussion note of an affected tooth is dull rather than resonant.

5. There may be hypertrophy and hypertonicity of the muscles of mastication, most obviously of the masseters. This is detected by palpation but sometimes can actually be seen, especially in the bruxist patient.

6. Signs of temporomandibular pain dysfunction syndrome with jaw deviation, joint clicking, discomfort and even pain due to muscle spasm.

7. Radiographic evidence together with mobility offers evidence of occlusal trauma. The signs are:

   a. Widening of the periodontal space

   b. Funnel-like or crescentic resorption of the alveolar crest around a tooth

   c. Loss of definition of the lamina dura; this is an unreliable sign as other factors including root morphology affect the radiographic appearance of the socket wall.

8. Tooth sensitivity may be associated with both occlusal trauma and pulp pathology brought about by excessive loading. Sometimes patients have an awareness of a discrepancy in their occlusion, a positive occlusal sense, and a patient may be able to point to the tooth involved.

ANIMAL RESEARCH

There were two predominant research groups in the 1970s who carried out animal studies on occlusal trauma from the Eastman Dental Center, Rochester NY and the University of Gothenburg in Sweden. These American (1) and Scandinavian (2) studies utilized: (1) repeated application of simulated orthodontic forces on squirrel monkeys and (2) cap splints with intermaxillary elastics on beagle dogs respectively in order to induce occlusal traumatic forces in the presence or absence of plaque induced inflammation.

Despite differences in the animal models used, results showed that when tissues were maintained free of inflammation, occlusal trauma resulted in increased mobility and loss of bone density with no loss of attachment, with reversal on removal of traumatic forces (primary occlusal trauma with mobility and widening of the ligament space).

There was evidence of attachment loss only when inflammation was superimposed on compromised bone levels of beagle dogs (secondary occlusal trauma with mobility and crestal bone loss).

Osteoclast differentiation and activation play an important role in inflammatory bone resorption. RANKL (receptor activator of nuclear factor kappa B ligand) stimulates osteoclast differentiation. A recent study on rats has demonstrated that inflammation and traumatic occlusion enhance the expression of RANKL on endothelial, inflammatory and periodontal ligament cells (Yoshinaga et al 2007), using *Escherichia coli* LPS as the stimulant and gold inlays to raise the bite and induce occlusal trauma. Other workers confirm the role of LPS in causing apoptosis of osteoblasts by inducing release of TNF-α from macrophages (Thammasitboon et al 2006). Regulation of osteoclastogenesis is determined by the balance between RANKL and osteoprotegerin. Reduced expression of osteoprotegerin has been demonstrated in periodontal ligament cells *in vivo* in response to a combination of LPS and mechanical stress (Tsuji et al 2004). Collectively, expression of RANKL appears to be enhanced in response to traumatic occlusion during inflammatory bone resorption (Yoshinaga et al 2007) and could be a more definitive marker than the surrogate clinical parameters of occlusal trauma.

OCCLUSAL ANALYSIS

This is an analysis of static jaw relationships as well as of the relationships of the teeth during mandibular movements. A large number of articulators have been designed to replicate jaw movement but each of them has its limitations and the almost inevitable errors in bite registration and model mounting frequently nullify the accuracy of the articulator. A more fundamental criticism of mechanical aids is that they simply cannot reproduce the flexibility of vital tissues. However, fully adjustable articulators are necessary in carrying out complex restorative procedures. In a periodontal analysis study models are useful but careful oral examination is essential.

The examination of static jaw relations should include a record of the teeth in the arch, tooth alignment and such tooth deviations as tilting, over-eruption and plunger cusps. Inter-arch examination records the Angle's classification, overbite, overjet, gross malocclusions such as crossbite and any details of cusp to fossa relationships which appear abnormal.

The examination of functional relationships is a great deal more difficult and can be carried out properly only with experience and great attention to detail. The starting point for this examination has been the subject of much debate. The intercuspal position (ICP) as the end point of functional movement would appear to be the natural starting point for analysis but it is not a fixed position and may well be the end point of a habitual mandibular closing path which compensates for and therefore masks the disharmonies we are trying to detect. The only fixed and reproducible position is the retruded contact position (RCP) where the jaw rotates around its hinge axis. Although some people swallow in RCP, it is an abnormal and strained position in most people. However, it is useful because of its reproducibility.

The essential requirement for recording RCP is to have the patient sitting in a relaxed position. Some operators even go as far as to hypnotize the patient. With the dental chair slightly reclined and the patient sitting comfortably the operator puts one hand on the patient's chin with the thumb resting on the incisal edge of the lower incisors. The patient is instructed to relax the jaw and allow the operator to move it freely up and down. When the muscles relax the mandible can be rotated around its hinge axis without discomfort and when the thumb is removed the jaw can come together in RCP. Once the patient has learned the feel of this position he or she can reproduce it at will and allow the operator to register a number of contact relations with coloured bite papers or soft occlusal indicator wax a number of contact relations. Sometimes muscle tension is so great that closing pathways cannot be altered in this way and a bite-guard may be needed as an aid to overcome abnormal patterns of muscle activity.

An initial cuspal contact in centric relation can be detected by placing coloured paper or indicator wax over the upper posterior teeth, guiding the patient into tooth contact in RCP and then sliding from there into complete closure (ICP). The direction of the slide can be observed and the point of initial contact will be marked on the teeth or seen by perforations in the indicator wax. Similarly, tooth contacts in working and non-working sides during lateral excursions, and tooth contacts in protrusive movement can be defined. These techniques can be learned only by practical experience.

It should be possible to link signs of occlusal disharmony such as drifting, mobility and faceting with the site of an occlusal disharmony and an associated slide. Thus a premature contact in RCP between the distal slope of an upper molar cusp will produce a forward slide so that the lower incisors come forward against the upper incisors.

OCCLUSAL ADJUSTMENT

In a clinical trial of 89 patients with periodontitis, Harrel and Nunn (2001) showed a slight but significant improvement in periodontal outcome following correction of occlusal discrepancies associated with premature contacts and balancing contacts in lateral excursion. However one would not carry out routine occlusal equilibration in periodontally compromised patients unless specific signs and symptoms justify such intervention. In certain cases, traumatic occlusion can exacerbate progressive periodontal destruction (Harrel et al 2003).

Adjustment can be carried out by:

1. Selective grinding
2. Restorative dentistry
3. Orthodontics.

Whatever technique is used the objectives remain the same:

1. To direct occlusal forces along the long axis of the tooth and as far as possible reduce lateral components of force
2. To distribute forces over as many teeth as possible in maximum intercuspation and to establish 'group function' during lateral and protrusive movements by creating simultaneous gliding contacts between working teeth
3. To establish bilateral contact between posterior teeth in RCP and a sagittal movement of no more than 1 mm between RCP and ICP
4. And thereby eliminating the signs and symptoms of occlusal disharmony.

Selective grinding

The greatest danger of selective grinding is that it can be indiscriminate. One is faced with a bewildering array of coloured dots and smudges and multiple perforations in the occlusal wax. Before any tooth grinding is carried out the consequences of any adjustment must be determined. Central to this analysis is the location of cuspal inclines which act as centric stops or supporting cusps in maximum interdigitation and thus maintain the vertical dimension of the face (**Fig. 27.2**). Selective grinding is carried out with a handpiece and diamond stones and should proceed in a methodical manner.

1. Elimination of gross occlusal disharmonies which are obvious to the eye, such as plunger cusps, malposed and extruded teeth, discrepancies in marginal ridge height. Where there is a widened buccolingual diameter caused by attrition the diameter can be reduced. Keeping the positions of supporting cusps in mind these obvious sources of occlusal disharmony can be corrected to a considerable degree as a first step.
2. Correction of prematurities in RCP. These may be divided into two groups, with or without prematurities in lateral excursions. These situations and their corrections are shown in **Figure 27.3**.
3. Correction of protrusive disharmonies. The contact between incisors and canines should be a smooth glide into the edge-to-edge position with as many anterior teeth as possible in contact. In adjustment of

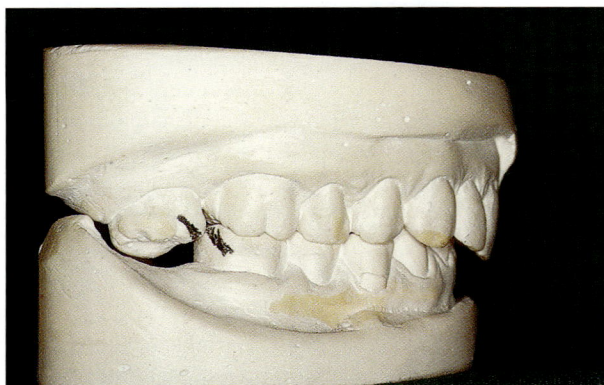

Fig. 27.2 Articulated study models showing the position of a cuspal interference between right upper and lower first molars.

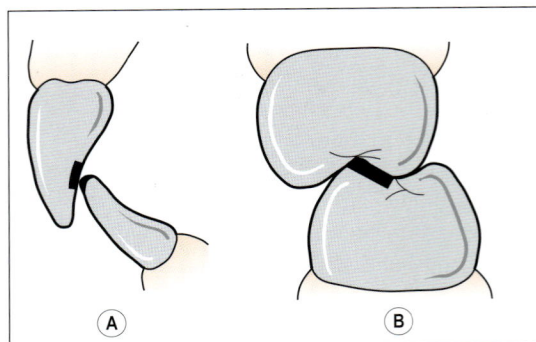

Fig. 27.3 Centric stops (A) on incisors and (B) on posterior teeth.

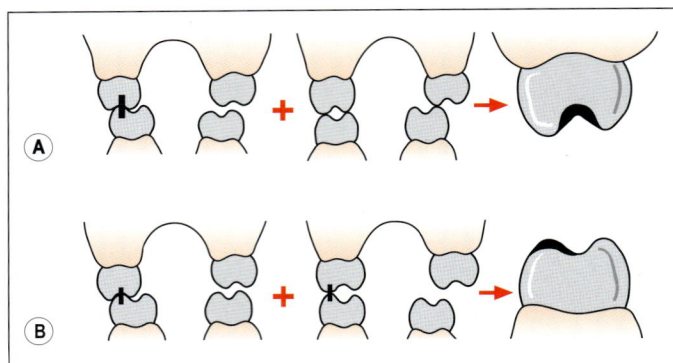

Fig. 27.4 Correction of interferences between posterior teeth in RCP. If there is no interference in lateral excursions, the fossa is ground as in (A). If there is interference in lateral excursions, the cusp is ground as in (B).

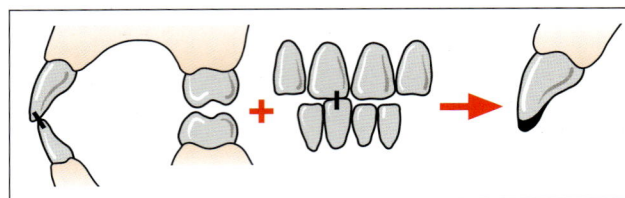

Fig. 27.5 Correction of interference between incisors in protrusive movements. The adjustment should not disturb the centric stop.

protrusive contact it is essential to remember that the incisal edge (or close to it) of the lower incisors is a centric stop (**Fig. 27.4**). One of the most common mistakes is the reduction of an incisal edge obviously above the line of the rest of the incisors in order to achieve an improved appearance. The almost inevitable result is overeruption of the reduced tooth with recreation of the interference and consequent aggravation of the problem.

4. Correction of disharmonies in lateral excursions (**Figs 27.5, 27.6**). The objective of this adjustment is group function on the working side and disarticulation of the non-working side. Non-working side contacts (in prosthetics called balancing contacts) are frequently associated with advanced periodontal destruction and TMJ dysfunction. A premature contact between/buccal cusps in working movement and position is corrected by grinding the buccal cusp of the upper tooth, while a lingual cusp contact is corrected by grinding the lingual cusp of the lower tooth. This is the so-called BULL rule (**Fig. 27.6**).

Correcting a non-working side contact can be a problem as the contact is frequently between the buccal incline of the palatal cusp of the upper tooth and the lingual incline of the lower buccal cusp, i.e. supporting cusps. It is almost impossible to avoid cutting these surfaces and the adjustment will depend upon the form of contact made by these surfaces in other positions

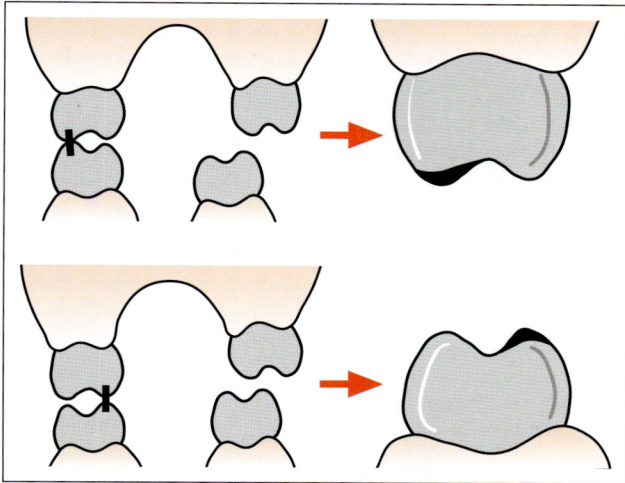

Fig. 27.6 Correction of working side interference according to the BULL rule.

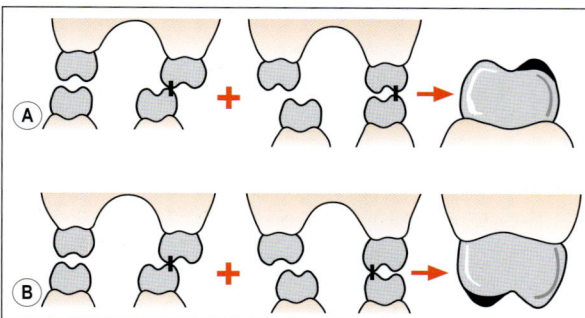

Fig. 27.7 The correction of lateral movement on the non-working side depends on the relationships of the interfering cuspal inclines in other excursions. In (A) the buccal cusp of the lower tooth is in an interfering contact in two positions, while in (B) the palatal cusp of the upper tooth is an interfering contact in two positions and is therefore the one to be corrected.

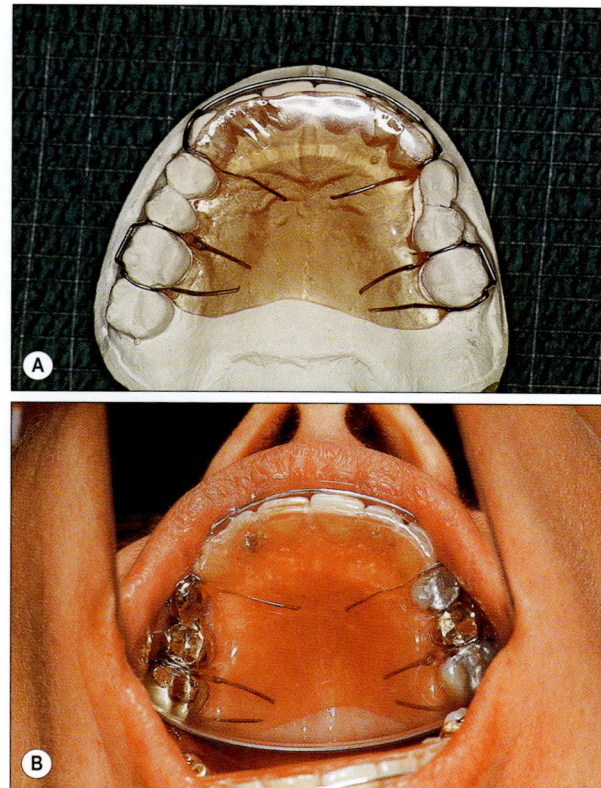

Fig. 27.8 Upper bite-guard with anterior bite plane (A) on model and, (B) in place in the patient's mouth.

(**Fig. 27.7**). If a cuspal incline is in premature contact in both working and non-working positions, this can be adjusted. On other occasions very precise adjustment of the cuspal incline is needed so that the cusp tip, as the centric stop, is retained, thus avoiding overeruption. If grinding a centric stop is unavoidable the occlusion will need to be supervised in case there is resultant tipping of involved teeth which would create a further interference.

Finally, the adjusted surfaces are polished smooth. Not infrequently the patient remarks on an improvement in the feel of the occlusion. After some weeks mobility and other features of occlusal disharmony should reduce if the adjustment has been carried out correctly.

Treatment of bruxism

The first step in the control of any parafunctional habit must be discussion with the patient. Frequently once the individual becomes aware of a habit and the damage that it can do, he or she can bring it under some degree of daytime control.

If occlusal disharmonies play a role in provoking or aggravating a clenching or grinding habit, selective grinding should help to relieve the parafunction. However, the psychological substrate of stress will remain and apart from reassuring the patient that the dental problems can be controlled, attempts to alleviate psychological problems have no place in dental treatment. Further dental treatment involves the use of bite-guards aimed at limiting the effects of excessive occlusal stress.

There are basically two forms of bite-guard, both of which are made in acrylic:

1. The occlusal shield which fits over the occlusal surfaces, incisal edges and facial and lingual tooth convexities
2. The anterior bite plate (**Fig. 27.8**).

Where attrition is severe or where there has been collapse of the posterior segments so that the free-way space is increased, the occlusal shield can be useful, especially in cases where there has been considerable periodontal destruction. Usually it is fitted over the teeth of the jaw in which there is most periodontal destruction. The occlusal surface must be flat and highly polished so that the teeth in the opposing jaw can skid across the surface without impediment. The thickness of the bite-guard must be adjusted so that the freeway space is not encroached upon, otherwise muscle tension will be intensified rather than diminished. 'Opening the bite' can be a dangerous procedure which may accelerate periodontal destruction.

Where there is an obvious bruxing habit with symptoms of muscle spasm a maxillary bite-guard with occlusal coverage or the anterior bite plate are useful. They disengage cuspal contact thus eliminating any cuspal interference and interrupting the reflex activity which causes muscle spasm. The anterior bite plate is also useful where the freeway space is small. Depending on the habit pattern the bite-guard is worn at night or during the day, and any necessary adjustments are made until the minimal thickness compatible with comfort and efficiency is obtained. Relief from symptoms in response to using a bite guard is usually diagnostic of the existence of an occlusal problem; it is best used in the short-term until definitive treatment is carried out.

Patients with bite-guards must adhere to a strict oral hygiene regime and avoid sugar between meals.

REFERENCES

Harrel SK: Occlusal forces as a risk factor for periodontal disease, *Periodontol 2000* 32:111–117, 2003.

Harrel S, Nunn M: The effect of occlusal discrepancies on periodontitis. Part II: relationship of occlusal treatment to the progression of periodontal disease, *J Periodontol* 72:495–505, 2001.

Harrel SK, Nunn ME, Hallmon W, et al: Is there an association between occlusion and periodontal destruction? *J Am Dent Assoc* 137:1380–1392, 2006.

Thammasitboon K, Goldring SR, Boch JA: Role of macrophages in LPS-induced osteoblast and PDL cell apoptosis, *Bone* 38:845–852, 2006.

Tsuji K, Uno K, Zhang GX, et al: Periodontal ligament cells under intermittent tensile stress regulate mRNA expression of osteoprotegerin and tissue inhibitor of matrix metalloprotease-1 and -2, *J Bone Miner Metab* 22:94–103, 2004.

Yoshinaga Y, Ukai T, Abe Y, et al: Expression of receptor activator of nuclear factor kappa B ligand relates to inflammatory bone resorption, with or without occlusal trauma, in rats, *J Periodontal Res* 42:402–409, 2007.

When the periodontal tissues are no longer capable of withstanding the stresses of function, teeth become mobile. This mobility can interfere with function. In many cases, treatment of the periodontal lesion and occlusal adjustment, if necessary, is all that is required to strengthen the supporting tissues, reduce mobility and re-establish function. When such local treatment fails to achieve these ends and chewing is uncomfortable, and/or where periodontal support is so reduced that increased mobility is inevitable, further tooth support is needed. Nyman and Lang (1994) have distinguished between increased tooth mobility due to compromised bone levels which may be stable following treatment and increasing tooth mobility indicative of an unstable periodontium requiring periodontal management to control inflammation.

There is growing acceptance of the fact that residual mobility of severely compromised teeth following treatment does not preclude them as stable long term components of the dentition. They need to be correctly managed in order to provide optimal function as a group rather than as individual teeth; this can be achieved with suitably designed splints (Ruhling 2004).

Splinting periodontally compromised teeth that have been treated and are stable with residual mobility, could aid their retention and function in the arch by distributing occlusal loading more evenly and preventing individual tooth loss (Mosedale 2007). Labial drifting and spacing are typical examples of compromised teeth being overloaded by physiological forces resulting in orthodontic effects.

Any splint is likely to compromise plaque control and patients must be instructed on suitable measures for gaining access to splinted teeth for optimal plaque control.

A splint is a device for supporting weakened tissues. It serves two purposes:

1. It facilitates treatment of mobile teeth and provides rest where wound healing is in progress
2. It permits function where the tooth/teeth and its/their periodontium alone cannot perform adequately.

There has been a great deal of debate about the role of splinting in periodontal treatment, largely because the role of the splint has been misunderstood. A splint does not make loose teeth tight. A splint controls mobility when the splint is in place and when the splint is removed, tooth mobility is manifested again. Only the removal of disease and subsequent healing can achieve a real reduction in tooth mobility.

The aim of splinting teeth is:

1. To protect the tooth-supporting tissues during the healing period after an accident or following surgery
2. To bring into function teeth which cannot be used to eat efficiently or in comfort without artificial support.

If splinting is carried out incorrectly it may make firm teeth loose, as for example when a loose first premolar is linked to a stable second premolar, overloading the latter tooth and producing two loose teeth.

There are many types of splint, temporary and permanent, fixed and removable, but every splint should meet certain requirements:

1. It should incorporate as many firm teeth as is necessary to reduce the extra load on individual teeth to a minimum
2. It should hold the teeth rigid and not impose torsional stresses on any incorporated teeth

3. It should extend around the arch, so that anteroposterior forces and faciolingual forces are counteracted
4. It should not interfere with the occlusion. If possible, gross tooth disharmonies should be eliminated before the application of the splint
5. It should not irritate the pulp
6. It should not irritate the soft tissues, gingivae, cheeks, lips or tongue
7. It should be designed so that it can be kept clean. Interdental embrasure spaces should not be blocked by the splint.

TEMPORARY AND PROVISIONAL SPLINTS

Temporary splints are used to assist healing after injury or after surgical treatment. They should be reasonably easy to apply to mobile teeth and also easy to remove after healing has taken place. They should not be left in place for longer than 2 months. If adequate stabilization has not taken place in that time a more permanent form of splinting is necessary. Most temporary splints do not involve destroying tooth tissue.

Composite filling materials can be acid-etched to the surface of mobile teeth and linked together. This is the simplest form of temporary splinting and one which is especially useful in emergencies (**Fig. 28.1**).

The wire and acrylic splint (**Fig. 28.2**) is also fairly easy to apply and is frequently used for the stabilization of incisors. It is stronger and more

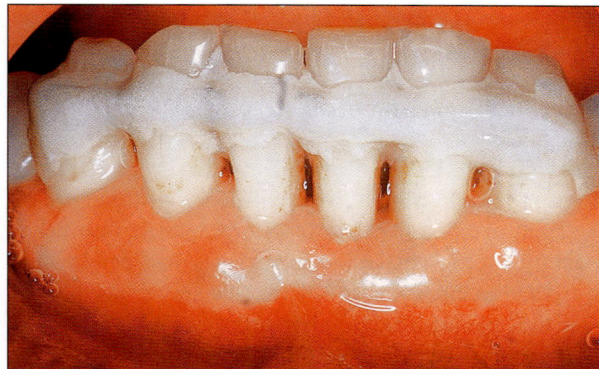

Fig. 28.1 Emergency splint made with composite filling material.

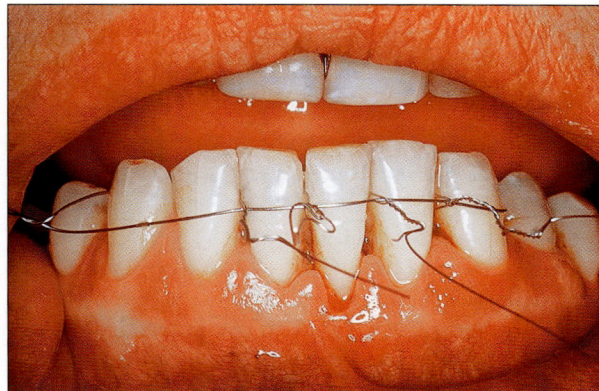

Fig. 28.2 Temporary splint made of wire which is passed around the teeth to be splinted, pulled tight and then pulled to a close fit to each tooth by wire ties at each interdental space. It will then be covered with acrylic resin. It is only suitable for anterior teeth.

reliable than the composite filling splint. Usually the teeth from canine to canine, or first premolar to first premolar, are included in the splint. A length of 0.05 mm (0.002 inch) stainless-steel wire is looped around the teeth with the lingual arch wire just incisal to the cingula. The ends of the wire are twisted together distal to the last tooth included. The interdental wires are looped around both lingual and facial arch wires and twisted tight so that the arch wire is pulled tight around the teeth just apical to the contact point. After any necessary adjustment in the correct position, the arch wire and interdental wires are finally tightened, their ends trimmed and tucked out of the way into embrasure spaces. A thin mix of quick-set acrylic is run over the wire, care being taken to avoid blocking out embrasure spaces. When set the acrylic is trimmed smooth and polished so that it is comfortable to the soft tissues. This method may be used with or without tooth preparation as a permanent or temporary measure, respectively.

Etch-retained composite splints may be constructed with fibre glass cord, metal mesh or stainless steel wire. When pre-impregnated glass fibre reinforcement material is used, additional use of wire may not be necessary. The permanent reinforced composite splint is an inexpensive method, but technically exacting at placement (Samama et al 2004). It usually allows simple root resection if required at a later stage. Rehabilitation of the dentition of a young patient presenting with severely advanced aggressive periodontal disease, using a glass fibre-reinforced composite has been reported (Sewon et al 2000). Following periodontal stabilization with root surface debridement and surgical intervention, a cavity retained internal fibre-reinforced composite splint was applied. A 12-month follow-up showed a good functional and aesthetic result with a healthy periodontium. Obtaining an aesthetic result with the fibre-reinforced composite splint is a challenge due to limited space in the connector region in order to create the appearance of individual teeth (Strassler & Serio 2007).

Orthodontic bands may also be used, especially in posterior segments where they are not obvious; 0.13 mm (0.005 inch) stainless-steel bands are fitted to the teeth to be splinted and welded together. Alternatively, the splint can be fabricated on a model and cemented into position. The edges of the bands must be contoured and polished to reduce plaque retention and avoid soft-tissue irritation.

Acrylic bite-guards already described for the treatment of bruxism may also be used as splints. The splint should cover the occlusal surface of the teeth and extend 1–2 mm over the facial surfaces of the teeth. In order to obtain adequate stability and rigidity in the upper jaw considerable palatal coverage is needed and in the lower jaw the lingual acrylic needs to be brought well down in the lingual vestibule without impeding muscle activity. The occlusal surface must be designed to allow free excursion of the mandible with no greater than 1 mm increase in vertical dimension in the molar regions. Very careful adjustment of the occlusion in the mouth is essential otherwise opposing teeth will be subject to excessive stress.

The intracoronal splint can be regarded as a semi-permanent rather than temporary splint and many consist of either a continuous intracoronal bar, or sections of wire in the so-called A-splint.

1. The continuous intracoronal bar. A transverse groove, 2–3 mm wide, is cut in the lingual surface of anterior teeth coronal to the cingulum, or in the occlusal surface of posterior teeth. The groove is made about 1.5 mm deep and slightly undercut. A stainless-steel wire is bent to fit the groove which is filled with self-curing acrylic and the wire quickly pressed home. After the acrylic has set it is shaped and polished. Alternatively, a gold bar may be cast to fit the preparation and cemented in place. As occlusal pressures may push anterior teeth away from the bar, it is advisable to improve retention by making pin-hole preparations in the base of the groove, but even with this added retention it is not advisable to splint upper anterior teeth in this way. The horizontal-pin splint represents a variation of

the continuous intracoronal bar. It is strong and well retained but can be used only where some pulp recession has taken place. A form of continuous intracoronal bar which is used to stabilize a posterior segment consists of MOD amalgam fillings placed in the teeth to be stabilized and then subsequently linked by a bar cemented with acrylic into a channel cut through the amalgams.

2. The Rochette splint: Acid-etch composite materials provide an opportunity for splinting without radical tooth preparation. An impression of the teeth to be splinted is taken and a chrome-cobalt splint, fitting the lingual surface of these teeth, is constructed. The lingual tooth surfaces are dried and etched and the splint is glued into position with the composite material. If carefully prepared and in good occlusal balance, this form of splinting provides excellent stability and may be regarded as a semi-permanent splint.

PERMANENT SPLINTS

Permanent splints may be fixed or removable.

FIXED SPLINTS

Fixed splints provide the most reliable form of immobilization but do require considerable tooth preparation, skill and time (**Fig. 28.3**). They consist of linked inlays or crowns.

Linked inlays are self-descriptive. Inlays which fit into dovetail preparations in the lingual surfaces of anterior teeth may be displaced if an excessive anterior force is exerted on any individual tooth. In the posterior region a series of linked MOD inlays with occlusal coverage can make a satisfactory and permanent splint.

Linked crowns provide the most reliable form of immobilization and support (Mosedale 2007). The splint is extremely strong, holds the teeth rigidly and is the most aesthetically satisfying and unobtrusive type of splint. If teeth are missing, the multiple abutment fixed bridge may be used to replace these teeth and to stabilize a segment or a complete arch. This type of splint allows one to modify the form of the teeth and in fact provides one of the most satisfactory methods of occlusal rehabilitation. This splint is difficult to make and requires a great deal of chairside time and skill. Considerable tooth preparation is necessary and there is often the possibility of pulpal involvement. Alternatively, telescope crowns soldered together may be used. These are fitted over gold copings which are cemented on to the teeth. The telescope superstructure may be fixed with temporary cement so that it may be removed periodically for inspection and cleaning.

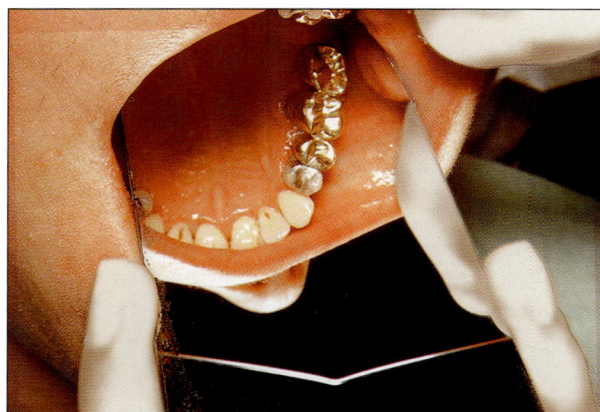

Fig. 28.3 A small fixed splint stabilizing class II mobility of the upper first molar to the upper second molar and second premolar. All three teeth have full crowns which are linked. Periodontal health and stability were first achieved by periodontal treatment.

One modification of the linked crown splint is the multiple pinlay splint which reduces tooth-tissue loss to a minimum. Three parallel pin-holes are made in each tooth to be splinted. Usually six teeth are incorporated into the splint and paralleling 18 pin-holes presents some difficulty. Pin retention is not as good as that provided by inlays or crowns, therefore this appliance can only be used with success where functional forces are not acting to separate the appliance from the tooth, as they may be where upper incisors are under some occlusal stress. This factor restricts the application of the pinlay splint to the lower incisors.

REMOVABLE SPLINTS

The removable splint does not involve cutting tooth tissue, it is easier to construct than a fixed splint and can be altered or discarded at will. Like all removable appliances the splint may act as a plaque-retention factor and source of gingival irritation unless oral hygiene is good.

The most common type of splint is the lingual coverage splint which is essentially a partial denture in chrome-cobalt with extensions covering the lingual surfaces of the teeth to be protected. The continuous clasp splint (**Fig. 28.4**) is a variation in which support is reinforced by a labial arch bar. However, removable splints have been largely superceded by fixed acid-etched splints.

Designing splints provides the opportunity for considerable ingenuity but the choice of splint should reflect patient need rather than the artistic aspirations of the operator. Many forms of splint are complex, difficult to execute and costly and are justified only when a good prognosis is likely. Where the prognosis is doubtful, a simple form of splint is indicated. If the prognosis is poor the removable chrome-cobalt lingual coverage splint allows for the addition of weak teeth as they are lost. The long-term retention of periodontally compromised teeth and their effective function can be aided by well planned and executed splints.

Patient motivation and compliance with plaque control measures are an essential component of maintenance. A 6-week follow up of 82 cases of post-traumatic splinting demonstrated that professionally maintained cases showed significantly lower plaque scores than those that did not have this schedule (Pasini et al 2006), reinforcing the importance of a good maintenance programme following splinting. Patients also need to be made aware of the consequences of tooth loss in the long-term and consented for replacement options which may be necessary in the future.

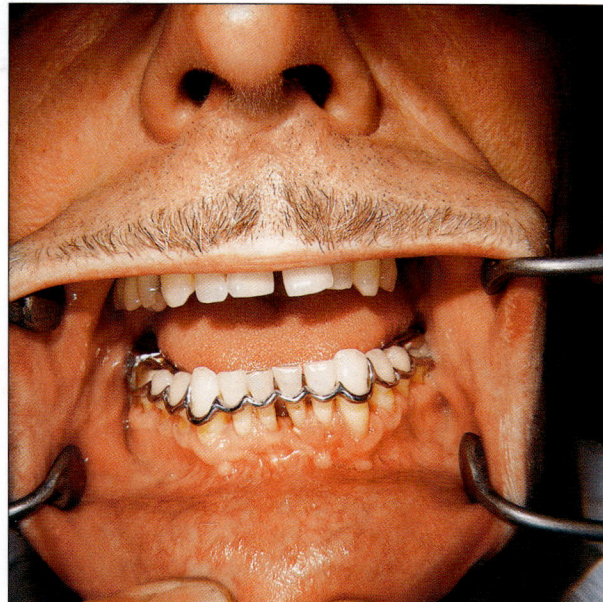

Fig. 28.4 A chrome cobalt removable splint utilizing a continuous clasp for stabilizing loose teeth. Periodontal health and stability were first achieved by periodontal treatment.

REFERENCES

Mosedale R: Current indications and methods of periodontal splinting, *Dent Update* 34:168–180, 2007.

Nyman S, Lang N: Tooth mobility and biological rationale for splinting, *Periodontol 2000* 4:15–22, 1994.

Pasini S, Bardellini E, Casula I, et al: Effectiveness of oral hygiene protocol in patients with post-traumatic splinting, *Eur J Paediatr Dent* 7:35–38, 2006.

Ruhling A: Strategies in the case of advanced attachment loss. Part 2, *Periodontal Practice Today* 1:213–224, 2004.

Samama Y, Lboukili L, Purer R: Predictability of resin bonded splints in the treatment of patients with periodontitis: a retrospective study, *Periodontal Practice Today* 1:227–235, 2004.

Sewon LA, Ampula L, Vallittu PK: Rehabilitation of a periodontal patient with rapidly progressing marginal alveolar bone loss: 1-year follow-up, *J Clin Periodontol* 27:615–619, 2000.

Strassler HE, Serio CL: Aesthetic considerations when splinting with fibre-reinforced composites, *Dent Clin North Am* 51:507–524, 2007.

29

Dental implants and peri-implantology

This account is merely meant to be an introduction to this subject from the periodontal standpoint, and not to be a comprehensive account which can be obtained from a specialist text devoted to this subject.

DEVELOPMENT OF OSSEOINTEGRATED DENTAL IMPLANTS

The successful development of titanium endosseous implants over the last two decades has made it possible to place these with a degree of predictability not previously attainable. It was first shown that titanium implants could achieve a bone-to-implant contact (Brånemark et al 1969) and this was demonstrated in undecalcified ground sections by Schroeder et al (1976). They referred to this contact as functional ankylosis but Brånemark et al (1977) later created the term 'osseointegration' which they referred to as a direct structural and functional connection between the bone and the surface of a load bearing implant.

Titanium is a highly reactive metal which spontaneously forms an oxide layer in contact with air and this layer is almost resistant to further corrosion. This protects it against chemical attacks in biological tissues and gives it excellent biocompatible properties. Also functional loading of implants transfers masticatory forces to the jawbone and for this reason the stiffness of the implant should be similar to that of bone. Titanium approaches this more closely than other materials (Brånemark et al 1969). The implant requires retention to achieve ankylotic anchorage and this is usually in the form of screw threads (Brånemark et al 1985), perforations and also micro-retentions in the form of plasma coatings (Schroeder et al 1976). This provides resistance to shearing forces essential to successful osseointegration.

CLINICAL FACTORS RELATED TO OSSEOINTEGRATION

Successful osseointegration occurs at 3–6 months after placement of the implant. Osseointegration has been shown to be achievable with either two-stage or one-stage techniques. In the two-stage technique (Brånemark et al 1977) the implant fixtures are submerged under the mucosal tissues at the time of the installation and this has been claimed to be necessary for success by the advocates of this technique. Over the decades, implant therapy has become a reliable approach for replacing missing teeth. The concept of immediate implant loading has recently become popular due to decreased trauma, reduction in overall treatment time, anxiety and discomfort of patients resulting in increased acceptance by patients, with better function and aesthetics (Avila et al 2007). However there are contradictory reports in this area. Results from the literature reviewed indicate that immediate loading achieved similar success rates to those with a delayed protocol. This was dependent on careful case selection, good treatment planning, meticulous surgery and suitable design of prostheses when this method was adopted (Avila et al 2007). Suitable preparation of the implant bed would be critical. Drilling in bone generates considerable heat which can result in bone necrosis. Therefore it is essential to use low drilling speeds (i.e. under 800 r.p.m.) and abundant irrigation with chilled sterile saline to minimize injury. The sequential use of drills of increasing diameter also helps to minimize thermal trauma. There must be a minimal gap between the prepared site and the implant which is achieved by the careful use of matched precision drills in the chosen implant system.

Piezoelectric surgery developed by Vercellotti (2003) uses ultrasound at ideal frequencies for bone surgery in orthopaedics, maxillofacial, periodontal and endodontic surgical procedures; it helps to overcome some of the limitations of drilling in bone by being precise, protective of delicate anatomical structures and maintaining a clear surgical field with less bleeding. A biomolecular and histological comparative analysis of osseointegration around porous implants has been reported recently for traditional implant placement using drills versus a piezoelectric bone surgical technique (Preti et al 2007). A total of 16 porous titanium implants were inserted in minipig tibias, using either a drilling technique following the Brånemark protocol or the piezoelectric surgical method using specific steel inserts of 2 and 3 mm diameter and a frequency of 27 000 to 30 000 kHz. Histological examination showed that there were more inflammatory cells isolated from drilled sites. Implant sites that underwent piezoelectric bone surgery demonstrated a consistently greater degree of osteoneogenesis, with an earlier increase in the key regulators BPP-4 and TGF-β2 and reduced levels of pro-inflammatory cytokines. Piezoelectric surgery appeared to be effective in the first phase of bone healing with evidence of bone remodelling at 56 days post-treatment.

A recent study evaluated a software system for virtual planning of implant placement and its reliability in directly transferring this data to a surgical template used as a drill guide (Nickenig & Eitner 2007). Virtual planning of implant position was carried out using cone-beam CT data for pre-operative assessment of implant size, position and anatomical complications, with applications for installation of implants without flaps. The postoperative panoramic radiographic control showed that it was possible to avoid anatomical structures such as the maxillary sinus, mental foramen, mandibular canal and adjacent teeth with this method.

If stability is achieved new bone will grow and replace damaged bone resulting in an intimate bone-to-implant contact with a gap of about 20 µm or less. If an implant lacks primary stability healing will occur by fibrous replacement of the damaged bone preventing osseointegration.

THE HISTOLOGY OF THE PERI-IMPLANT TISSUES

The head of the implant fixture penetrates through the crest of the alveolar bone and relates to the gingival or alveolar mucosa. Once the implant head penetrates the mucosa, at the second operation in the two-stage technique or at the first operation in the one-stage technique, a tight soft tissue collar will form around it. This consists of fibrous tissue with fibres running parallel to the long axis of the implant and an epithelial cuff. The junctional epithelium attaches to the implant surface by hemidesmosomes and a basal lamina similar to that seen with natural teeth.

In a series of experimental studies on the beagle dog model, aspects of the histology and pathology of the gingival and periodontal tissues around normal teeth and the peri-implant mucosa around osseointegrated implants were studied, using light and electron-microscopical techniques which enabled examination of tissues adjacent to the implant. It was shown that the gingival and peri-implant mucosal tissues had several features in common. In this regard, both tissues exhibited a junctional epithelium adjacent to their respective surfaces of about 2 mm in length. Apical to the junctional epithelium there was a zone of connective tissue forming a barrier between the epithelium and the bone. However, the gingiva and peri-implant mucosa also differed in several important respects. The implant surface, as expected, was devoid of cementum and this prevented the collagen fibres in this area from inserting into its surface.

A recent experimental study investigated the histopathology of the mucosal attachment to titanium implants placed in the mandibles of 20 Labrador dogs (Berglundh et al 2007). All mandibular premolars were extracted and after a 3-month healing period four implants (ITI Dental Implant System) were placed on each side of the mandible. A non-submerged method was used to place the implants. This method has been described previously (Berglundh et al 2003). A plaque control regime was instituted postoperatively. Healing was uneventful following implant placement at all 160 sites and the animals were sacrificed periodically in order to elicit data on sequential healing. The implants used were solid screw implants with a diameter of 4.1 and length of 10 mm; their configuration was either a turned or sandblasted and acid-etched surface topography with a polished transmucosal surface of 2.8 mm, also used in previous studies (Abrahamsson et al 2004).

In the present study (Berglundh et al 2007), there was some inflammation around the implants in the first 2 weeks of healing, with improved stability of the mucosa at 4 weeks. At 4 days, there was a heavy infiltrate of PMNs and a mucosal seal consisting of a clustering of leucocytes in a dense fibrin network. This was present at 1 week, with a smaller zone and the more apical area was dominated by collagen and fibroblasts.

At 2 weeks after surgery, the peri-implant mucosa adhered to the implant surface by connective tissue rich in cells and blood vessels. There was marginal epithelial proliferation indicative of the formation of a junctional epithelium (JE) as a barrier. There was intensive bone modelling at this stage and the level of bone to implant contact was at a more apical position than at 1 week of healing.

At 4 weeks following implant placement, the formed barrier epithelium (JE) comprised about 40% of the mucosal interface to titanium. The connective tissue was well organized and contained large amounts of collagen and fibroblasts. Bone remodelling resulted in distinct crestal bone situated 3.2 mm apical to the soft tissue.

At 6–12 weeks of healing, tissue maturation and collagen fibre organization was evident with complete maturation of the JE at 6–8 weeks. There was a dense layer of elongated fibroblasts forming the connective tissue interface to titanium. There were a few vascular structures lateral to this zone interposed with fibroblasts between collagen fibres which were mainly parallel to the implant surface.

The overall height of the mucosa assessed from the margin of the soft tissue to the most coronal point of bone to implant contact (BIC) increased gradually and ranged from 3.1–3.5 mm at 2–12 weeks of healing. The apical position of the JE from the mucosal margin extended from 0.5 mm at 2 weeks, 1.42 mm at 6 weeks and 1.7–2.1 mm between 6 and 12 weeks. These findings indicate that it takes about 6 weeks for a robust soft tissue barrier to form, comprising a stable JE and mature connective tissue.

The connective tissue interface with titanium implants was analysed in dogs using light and electron microscopy (Abrahamsson et al 2002). Fibroblasts were found to be orientated both parallel and perpendicular to the long axis of the implant surface and it was suggested that this fibroblast rich barrier played an important role in maintaining soft tissue apposition.

The blood supply of the peri-implant mucosa has also been studied by several workers using a Beagle dog model for comparison with that in the gingiva adjacent to natural teeth. The blood supply of the peri-implant mucosa differs from that of the gingiva in important respects. The gingiva receives a copious blood supply (see Ch. 1) from two major sources, namely the supra-periosteal vessels lateral to the alveolar process and the vessels of the periodontal ligament which anastomose freely with the alveolar bone supply. In contrast the blood vessels of the peri-implant mucosa were found to be terminal branches of the larger vessels of the periosteum of the bone. In addition, the blood vessels lateral to the junctional

epithelium in both the peri-implant mucosa and gingiva formed a characteristic crevicular plexus. However, while the supra-alveolar mucosa of the gingiva is richly vascularized, the corresponding area of the peri-implant mucosa has a limited blood supply.

CLINICAL INDICATIONS FOR DENTAL IMPLANTS

Only a few total edentulous and partially edentulous patients will benefit from dental implants and these must be carefully selected both on clinical grounds and the patient's wishes after they have been fully informed about everything necessary to make an informed judgement. Successful implants may need a team approach with co-operation between oral surgeons, periodontologists, restorative and prosthetic dentists. Any dentist or dental specialist carrying out any part of this work needs to have undergone a lengthy course of postgraduate academic and practical training in the subject. Oral surgeons or periodontologists will easily be able to acquire the necessary surgical skills but will need to acquire considerable restorative and prosthetic knowledge, skills and experience if they wish to carry out the full treatment.

Implants can be considered for stabilizing a full lower or upper denture. The use of anterior mandibular implants is probably the commonest use. They can also be used in the partially edentulous mouth to act as abutments for bridgework (**Fig. 29.1**) or as single tooth replacements (**Fig. 29.2**). A very careful clinical assessment has to be made to plan any of these procedures.

CLINICAL CONSIDERATIONS

A careful evaluation of the prognosis of the existing dentition must precede any decisions on partial cases. If implants are clinically indicated, regardless of the implant system used, success mainly depends on the patients' health and cooperation, the design of the prosthesis and the amount and quality of the bone at the implant site. All of these factors need very careful assessment and this involves comprehensive clinical and radiographical examinations of the soft tissue and bony anatomy. Relationships of the proposed implants with vital structures such as the inferior dental canal, maxillary sinus and floor of the nose must be carefully assessed. Adequate radiographs are necessary to assess these relations as well as to assess the amount and quality of the supporting bone. These may include panoral, lateral and occlusal views. Manual examination also is necessary in conjunction with this to assess the width of the available bone and the presence of undercuts and exostoses.

Since the long-term future of remaining natural teeth must be assured, there should not be any caries or periodontal activity on any of the remaining teeth and the patient must be willing to carry out all the necessary preventive

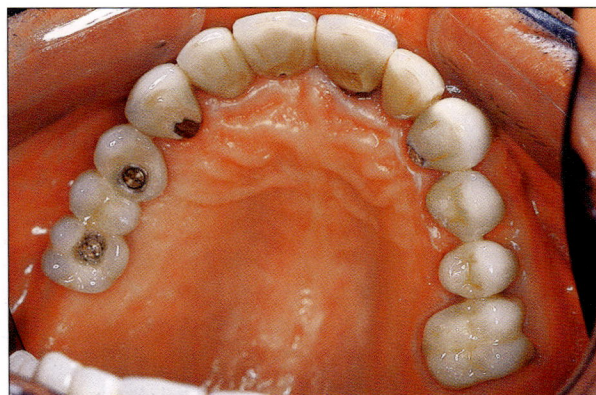

Fig. 29.1 Two Brånemark osseointegrated implants in the position of the upper right 6 and 4 acting as two of the abutments of a full arch bridge (Courtesy Dr C. Waterman).

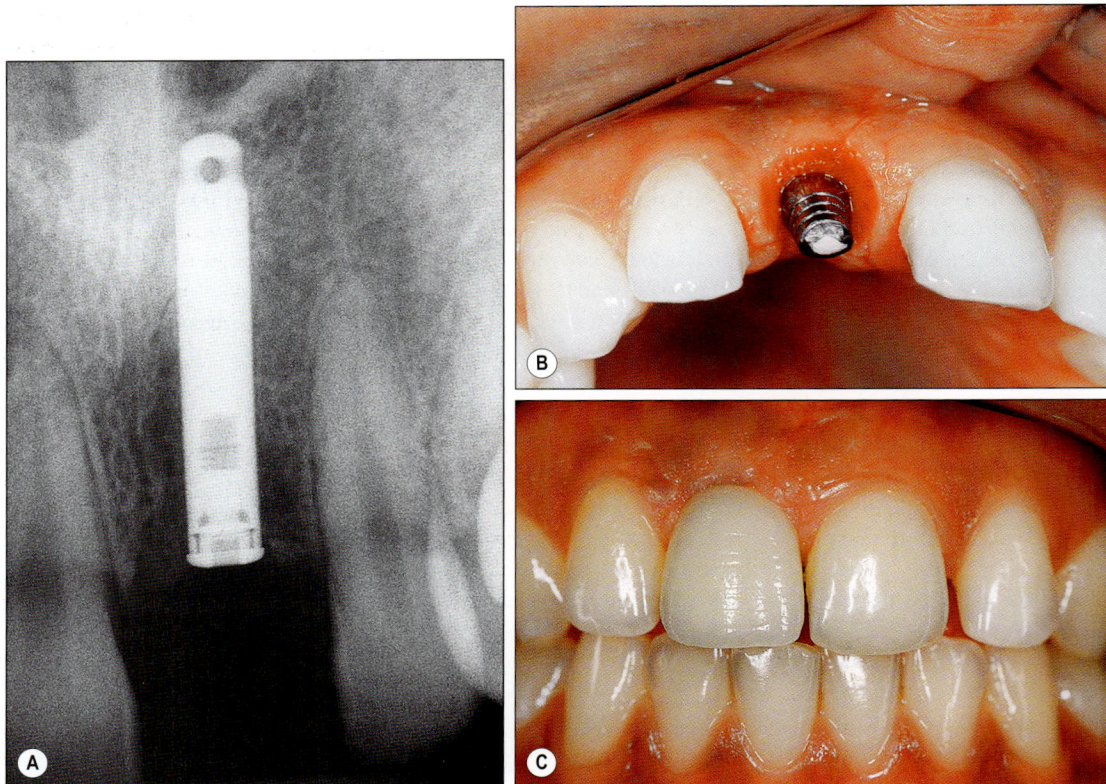

Fig. 29.2 A Calcitek® hydroxyapatite coated titanium osseointegrated dental implant used as the support to replace the missing upper right central incisor. (A) A radiograph of the implant in position in the alveolar bone following stage 1. The upper right central incisor was lost due to trauma. Root resorption can be seen on the upper right lateral incisor. (B) The superstructure in position (stage 2). (C) Jacket crown tried in prior to glazing and cementation. (Courtesy Professor R. Watson).

measures to avoid this in the future. All necessary periodontal and restorative treatment must have been successfully completed on the remaining natural teeth. Periodontal stability is of critical importance because the bacterial flora associated with active periodontal disease can spread from adjacent natural teeth to the implant resulting in peri-implant infections (see below).

It is extremely important to relate the final position of the artificial teeth of a full denture in edentulous cases or the abutment teeth of a bridge in a partially edentulous case to the position of the implant fixtures before these are decided upon. The final occlusion is of critical importance and this is best determined by making up a planning appliance which acts as a stent for determining the eventual positions of the implant fixtures. The occlusion of the natural teeth must be in balance in all functional positions before any implant work is planned and any necessary occlusal equilibration must be undertaken prior to implant planning.

No details will be given here of the basic techniques since these are best obtained from books solely devoted to this subject or books where specialist authors write separate chapters on this subject. A good detailed account from a periodontal standpoint can be found in the implant section of Belser et al (2003).

USE OF GUIDED BONE REGENERATION (GBR)

The biological principles of GTR (see Ch. 17) have been applied to the treatment of osseous defects in the alveolar ridge and around endosseous dental implants when it is termed GBR. The barrier membrane is adapted over the bony defect to allow cells of osseous origin to populate the area to form new bone. This procedure has been shown to be capable of forming new bone to increase the alveolar bone height or to increase bone support around the implant at the time of installation. Either non-resorbable ePTFE or bioresorbable membranes can be used for this purpose (see Ch. 19).

The membrane function of a resorbable collagen membrane (Bio-Gide®) has also been tested in animal experiments. Peri-implant defects in dogs were filled with a bovine bone mineral (Bio-Oss®) (see Ch. 19) and covered with Bio-Gide®. Histological evaluation after 4 months showed the regeneration of organized cancellous and cortical bone.

It is also very important to avoid bacterial contamination of the membrane since this can seriously affect the success of the procedure (see Ch. 19). In this regard one study has investigated the effect of bacterial contamination of 16 membranes used in conjunction with dental implants with associated bony defects. The nature of bacterial contamination was determined with non-selective and selective culture and by DNA probes. The 10 implant-associated membranes with no cultivatable microorganisms demonstrated a mean gain of 4.9 mm of supporting bone while the six implants with infected membranes only gained an average of 2 mm. This seems to show a direct relationship between bacterial contamination of the membrane and the extent of new bone formation. Furthermore, these results would seem to indicate the importance in controlling or eliminating contamination of the membrane by periodontal pathogens in some cases by the use of antibiotics.

These results seems to show that clinically significant gains in bone formation on the alveolar ridge and around implants can be obtained with GTR procedures using both bioresorbable or non-resorbable membranes. The lack of a second surgical procedure is a major advantage with bioresorbable membranes.

USE OF BONE OR BONE SUBSTITUTE GRAFTS

Allograft and xenograft bone and synthetic bone substitutes such as hydroxyapatite and bioceramics and bioglass have all been used to enhance the bone support around implants either alone or in conjunction with barrier membranes (see Ch. 20). This can be in the form of ridge augmentation via advanced flaps with autogenous and alloplastic grafting material or the placement of grafting materials into extraction sockets to preserve ridge height or to build support for a subsequent implant.

The osteoconductive potential of bovine anorganic cancellous bone (BACB) (Bio-Oss®), human freeze-dried demineralized bone allograft (FDDBA) and resorbable hydroxyapatite (Osteogen®) have been compared in beagle dogs receiving dental implants. Titanium dental implants (ITI®) (see below) were placed into prepared edentulous sites which were extended into the maxillary sinus by elevating the sinus floor. The area below the raised sinus floor contained the protruding implant tip and was packed with one of these materials. The implanted material was placed so that it surrounded the implant tip and extended to the bone margin below. Sites implanted with human FDDBA showed no signs of new bone formation whereas those implanted with BACB (Bio-Oss®) or resorbable hydroxyapatite (Osteogen®) did show significant new bone formation in this area. The use of bone markers (tetracycline or calcein green) revealed rapid bone formation and remodelling, especially around the BACB particles. Thus, both BACB and resorbable hydroxyapatite were shown to be osteoconductive in this situation.

Bioglass particulate (Bioglass®) has also been used to stimulate bone formation in extraction sockets and to thus maintain the alveolar ridge height.

Implants placed with the aid of GBR and/or bone or bone substitute grafts share the same success rates as those placed conventionally (Berglundh et al 2002; Hämmerle et al 2002).

At 9–14 years following implant placement, survival rates of dental implants are high (95.7%), related to patient factors and the presence or absence of radiographic evidence of periodontitis at remaining teeth prior to implant placement (Roos-Jansaker 2007). A history of smoking and periodontitis were often patient factors associated with peri-implantitis. Animal research has shown that re-osseointegration can occur, while human studies have been case reports: bone fill has been shown to occur in peri-implant defects using submerged healing and bone transplants, bone substitutes with or without resorbable regenerative membranes with defect fill of ≥2 threads in 81% of the implants, associated with reduction in pockets and attachment gain (Roos-Jansaker 2007).

IMPLANT SYSTEMS

Numerous implant systems are available but most clinicians in this field limit themselves to one or two systems. They include the Brånemark (Nobel Pharma), Astra (Astratec), IMZ (General Medica) and Maestro (Biohorizons Implant Systems, Inc.) systems which are all two-stage and Bonefit and ITI (Straumann Institute) which are one-stage.

THE EFFECT OF SMOKING ON THE SUCCESS OF DENTAL IMPLANTS AND ITS RELATION TO PERI-IMPLANT INFECTIONS

In view of documented evidence that smoking imposes increased risk of impaired bone healing and implant failure, a 5-year retrospective analysis aimed to evaluate the implant survival rates among non-smokers (NS) and smokers categorized as light (LS), moderate (MS) or heavy (HS) using clinical and radiographic data (Sánchez-Pérez et al 2007). Records of 66 consecutive patients who had received a total of 165 dental implants were examined. A total of 16 implants (9.7%) failed and had to be removed. Smokers showed 15 failures and a success rate of 84.2%. Group NS had only one failure, giving a success rate of 98.6%. The risk of implant failure was approximately 31% among HS who smoked more than 20 cigarettes per day. There were significant differences between HS and NS or LS but

not MS. Within the limits of this study, it was concluded that the use of tobacco involves a 15.8% risk of implant failure, with a 13.1 odds ratio, showing a 10.1% relative risk of implant loss for LS or MS and a 30.8% risk for HS consuming >20 cigarettes per day.

A meta-analysis and systematic literature review were performed to compare the prognosis of implants in smokers and non-smokers with and without accompanying augmentation procedures (Strietzel et al 2007). Meta-analysis revealed a significantly enhanced risk for implant failure among smokers compared with non-smokers and the implant related odds ratio (OR) was 2.25, CI 95% 1.96–2.59; patient-related OR was 2.64; CI 95% 1.70–4.09 and for smokers receiving implants with accompanying augmentation procedures the implant related OR was 3.61; CI (95%) 2.26–5.77. The systematic review indicated significantly enhanced risk of biological complications among smokers. Five studies revealed no significant impact of smoking on prognosis of implants with particle-blasted, acid-etched or anodic oxidized implant surfaces. It was concluded that smoking is a significant risk factor for dental implant therapy and augmentation procedures accompanying implant placement.

For these reasons, smoking is usually a strong contraindication to the placement of dental implants and they should only be carried out in smokers if all other factors are favourable and the patient has been informed of the possible effects of smoking on the outcome.

THE RESPONSE OF THE PERI-IMPLANT MUCOSAL TISSUES TO PLAQUE

The relationship between periodontal pathogens, pro-inflammatory cytokines and bone pathophysiology is an important emerging area of osteoimmunology (Nowzari et al 2008). Levels of selected pro-inflammatory cytokines: interleukin (IL)-8, IL-1β, IL-6, IL-10, tumour necrosis factor (TNF)-α, and IL-12p70 were examined from clinically healthy peri-implant and periodontal sites in relation to subgingival microbial and viral (human cytomegalovirus HCMV) pathogens. The percentage frequency and levels of periodontopathic bacteria were higher around teeth than implants. Cytokine levels were significantly greater, almost 2-fold in some cases around implants than natural teeth. However when periodontal pathogens were present cytokine levels were high, both around implants and natural teeth. The high levels of cytokines around implants in the absence of periodontal pathogens could be related to the buffering capacity of the periodontium compared with implants during functional loading.

The response of the gingiva adjacent to normal teeth and peri-implant mucosa adjacent to the suprabony surface of the implant have been compared in the Beagle dog model. Both tissues responded to *de novo* plaque formation with an increased migration of leucocytes through the junctional epithelium and the establishment of an inflammatory cell infiltrate in the adjacent connective tissue. The location and composition of these lesions were similar in both situations but the lesions in the peri-implant mucosa tended to be larger.

The response of these tissues to long standing plaque irritation has been studied. In this situation the peri-implant mucosa was much less effective than the gingiva in preventing apical proliferation of the bacterial plaque. As a consequence, with increasing exposure times, the lesion in the peri-implant mucosa became larger and extended apically to become closer to the bone margin than in the corresponding gingiva. This much poorer response to plaque on the part of the peri-implant mucosa may be partly explained by the structural differences between peri-implant mucosa and gingiva (see above). It indicates a susceptibility of the peri-implant tissues to plaque-mediated damage and if allowed to proceed unchecked can result in peri-implant infections.

PERI-IMPLANT INFECTIONS

Since the superstructure of dental implants share the same environment as the teeth and are surrounded like them by a gingival cuff, it is to be expected that bacterial plaque will form on their surfaces. In edentulous mouths the flora associated with the natural teeth is absent and therefore they appear to accumulate plaque less readily than implants in dentate mouths. This suggests that the presence of natural teeth may influence the composition of the subgingival flora around implants. It seems likely that the early colonization of implants by putative periodontal pathogens could be more frequent in patients with poorly controlled periodontal disease on adjacent teeth. These teeth may therefore serve as a reservoir for potentially pathogenic bacteria to colonize adjacent implant surfaces.

Further studies over 5 years (Mombelli & Mericske-Sterne 1990) in 18 edentulous implant patients have shown that a predominantly Gram-positive coccal flora persisted around healthy implant sites over this period. Gram-negative rods such as *Fusobacterium nucleatum* and *Prevotella intermedia* were found in 9% of the samples but *Porphyromonas gingivalis* and spirochaetes were never seen at the healthy sites. Most other studies of successful implants over recent years have shown a similar pattern. Failing implants which had probing depths exceeding 5 mm, suppuration and radiological loss of alveolar bone demonstrated the presence of *P. gingivalis, Prevotella intermedia, F. nucleatum* and other putative periodontal pathogens; spirochaetes, fusiform bacteria, motile and curved rods were commonly seen by dark field microscopy in samples from failing sites. In contrast, the healthy sites maintained a predominantly Gram-positive coccal flora. There was also a 20-fold lower bacterial count in the healthy as compared with the failing sites.

A recent study assessed the microbiology of implants diagnosed with peri-implantitis and implant mucositis versus clinically healthy implants (Renvert et al 2007). A total of 40 species were identified by the checkerboard DNA–DNA hybridization method on 976 functional implants after 10.8 years in 213 subjects of mean age 65.7 (± 14) years. There was periodontitis in 44.9% of subjects, implant mucositis in 59% and peri-implantitis in 14.9% of all cases. The submucosal implant microbiota were dominated by *Neisseria mucosa, F. nucleatum sp. nucleatum, F. nucleatum sp. polymorphum* and *Capnocytophaga sputigena*. Implant sites with the deepest probing depths were associated with *Eikenella corrodens, F. nucleatum sp. vincentii, Porphyromonas gingivalis* and *Micromonas micros*. Tooth loss due to periodontitis in these subjects was associated with increased amounts of *F. nucleatum sp. vincentii* and *N. mucosa*. Subjects with teeth had significantly higher levels of *P. gingivalis* and *Leptotrichia buccalis*, independent of implant status. Implant and dentate status did not affect the microbiota isolated at the implant sites investigated.

In animals ligature-induced disease has been produced around dental implants and has been shown to be clinically, radiologically and microbiologically similar to ligature induced periodontitis. All of these studies would seem to indicate that implant failures after osseointegration have taken place (i.e. after 4–6 months) are most likely due to bacterial infection rather than an effect of occlusal overload.

A systematic review was carried out to assess the effect of anti-infective therapy in the treatment of peri-implantitis (Klinge et al 2002). No randomized, controlled clinical trials (RCTs) were found and of 145 retrieved publications on this subject only 21 (6 human and 15 animal studies) passed the inclusion criteria. The antibiotic regimes varied between the studies and no standardized medication protocol was used in any of them. The type of antibiotic, its dosage, duration and initiation time varied in all the studies. In many cases much of this information was not given. A non-medicated control was only included in one animal study. The reported clinical outcomes were extremely variable and the evidence for a clinically relevant advantage for using antibiotics was lacking. Therefore, there is no data to support a specific treatment protocol and there is a need for well designed RCTs for the treatment of peri-implantitis to resolve this issue.

It has also been shown that after infection has been controlled regenerative procedures can result in the formation of some new bone in intrabony peri-implant defects that may form following peri-implantitis (Roos-Jansaker et al 2003).

MONITORING OF IMPLANT SITES AND DIAGNOSIS OF POSSIBLE IMPLANT FAILURE

Dental implants should be regularly monitored by careful clinical and radiological measurements for signs of possible implant failure. Probing depths are best measured from a fixed reference point such as the occlusal surface or incisal edge of implant retained crowns or the occlusal edge of the implant head in implants retaining dentures. They may be more accurately measured with constant pressure, electronic probes such as the Florida disk probe (see Ch. 13). However, this must be carried out very gently to avoid damage to the delicate junctional epithelium. Certainly. any pain elicited during probing is indicative of tissue damage and should warn the operator to stop. Thus, there is some evidence to indicate that probing should not be used around healthy implants. If this advice is adhered to then implant failure can only be detected by radiographical evidence of bone loss, clinical signs of soft tissue inflammation or infection or a novel method based on examination of a peri-implant sulcus fluid component (see below).

Radiographs should be very carefully localized so that a constant bite block, film position and tube angulation are achieved (see Ch. 13). Only in this way can serial radiographs be compared and measured (Hollender & Rockler 1980). Comparability of serial radiographs can also be checked by measuring the distance between the implant screw threads on each radiograph. Careful measurements can then be made of the distance from an identifiable and reproducible point on the neck of the implant to the crest of the alveolar bone. Any change in attachment level in sequential clinical measurements should be verified and if confirmed should be regarded as possible evidence of loss of implant support. Any measurable change in the position of the alveolar bone level in respect to the implant on radiographs should be regarded as stronger evidence of loss of implant support. Gingival inflammation, bleeding on gentle probing and the presence of calculus should also be noted.

In addition, paper point samples of the bacterial flora in the peri-implant sulcus may be taken and placed into anaerobic transport medium for anaerobic bacterial culture. Samples could also be taken for darkground microscopy (see Ch. 14). The presence of or an increase in the numbers of black-pigmented anaerobes or spirochaetes could be taken as a possible indication of impending peri-implant infection (Mombelli et al 1990).

Finally, in the future the measurement of proteolytic enzymes in peri-implant sulcus fluid (PISF) may be of possible diagnostic value in the future. In this regard, the total enzyme activity and enzyme concentration of several host derived proteinases, cathepsin B, elastase and dipeptidyl peptidase (DPP) IV and a bacterial protease, trypsin-like protease, in 30 s paper strip PISF samples have been shown to significantly correlate with increased attachment and bone loss around osseointegrated dental implants (Eley et al 1991).

Kivela-Rajamaki et al (2003) investigated the levels and molecular forms of MMP-7 (matrilysin-1) and MMP-8 (collagenase-2) in PISF from healthy and diseased implant sites in 72 dental implant patients. The effects of synthetic inhibitors on MMP-7 were also assessed. They found that the levels of the active forms of MMP-8 and MMP-7 were significantly elevated in fluid from diseased as compared with healthy implant sites. The synthetic inhibitors failed to inhibit the activity of MMP-7 which was only affected by its specific human inhibitor. Thus the levels of these MMPs appear to be related to the presence of disease at implant sites.

PISF samples are very easy to obtain and if these relationships were shown to be predictive in a longitudinal study of dental implants then one or more of these proteases could be used as a diagnostic test of possible impending implant failure as described in Chapter 14. This would, of course need confirmation from the other clinical and radiological measurements described above.

TREATMENT OF IMPLANT SITES

In many ways, the treatment of dental implant sites is similar to that of natural teeth since the aim is to prevent the development of a pathogenic bacterial flora which would lead to resorption of supporting bone. Careful oral hygiene with soft toothbrushes and dental floss should be carefully taught. Specially designed interproximal brushes that can penetrate into the peri-implant crevice can also be used.

Metallic scalers cannot be used with dental implants because they would damage the titanium surfaces of the implant and for this reason good plaque control is also necessary to prevent calculus formation. Specially designed plastic scalers can be used to remove soft deposits but these are ineffective for calculus removal. Recently plastic tips have also been produced for ultrasonic scalers for use with implants. However, if calculus does form it is usually impossible to remove with these instruments. In this case the calculus should be chipped away very carefully with curettes, taking extreme care not to damage the surface. During maintenance visits the implants can be polished with a rubber cup and non-abrasive polishing paste. Regular applications of antiseptic agents such as 0.2% aqueous chlorhexidine have also been shown to be beneficial in addition to mechanical oral hygiene in some cases.

A recent study on the treatment of peri-implantitis monitored the clinical and radiographic responses to adjunctive local delivery of minocycline microspheres (Salvi et al 2007). Thirty one implants diagnosed with peri-implantitis were treated in 25 partially edentulous subjects. Three weeks after completion of patient motivation, thorough debridement and cleaning with 0.2% chlorhexidine gel minocycline microspheres (Arestin) were delivered locally to sites with bone loss and probing depths ≥5 mm, and followed up at 10 days, 1, 2, 3, 6, 9 and 12 months for measurement of probing pocket depths (PPD), clinical attachment level (CAL), bleeding on probing (BOP) and plaque index. There was significant reduction in PPD of 1.6 mm ($p<0.001$) and BOP up to 12 months, proving to be an effective therapy for peri-implantitis. Systemic antimicrobials such as metronidazole with or without adjuvant amoxicillin have also been effective in most cases with the additional benefit of eradicating black-pigmented Gram-negative anaerobic rods and spirochaetes from subgingival implant sites.

Takasaki et al (2007) evaluated the effects of Er:YAG laser therapy on implant surface debridement in experimentally induced peri-implantitis in dogs. Treatment was carried out using an Er:YAG laser or a plastic curette. The animals were sacrificed at 24 weeks and undecalcified histological sections were examined. The Er:YAG laser provided effective and safe treatment for implant surface debridement and degranulation; laser treated implant surfaces showed favourable new bone formation with better defined bone to implant contact than the curette group. The results of this study indicate that Er:YAG therapy shows potential for effective management of peri-implantitis.

THE FAILURE RATE OF OSSEOINTEGRATED ORAL IMPLANTS

The variables associated with primary implant stability were analysed in a retrospective study of 1084 Brånemark implants placed in 316 patients, by multivariate analysis (Mesa et al 2008). The site of implant placement showed the greatest correlation with implant failure. Implants in the anterior mandible showed 6.4-fold lower risk of stability failure. Those in the maxilla had a 2.7-fold greater risk of failing than those in the mandible and females showed a 1.5-fold greater risk of implant stability failure than males, while implants less than 15 mm in length had a 1.5-fold higher risk of failing than longer implants. These factors are of relevance when considering immediate or early loading of implants.

This analysis of Medline data between 1980 and 2004 was done to consider the benefits of bone augmentation surgery compared with using short implants (das Neves et al 2006). The study examined 7, 8.5 and 10 mm implants which were analysed according to the period of failure and risk factors implicated in the failure. 16 344 implants were analysed; there were 786 failures (4.8%). Implants of 3.75 mm diameter and 7 mm length failed at a rate of 9.7% compared with 6.3% for 3.75×10 mm implants. It was found that 54.9% of failures occurred before the prosthesis connection. A total of 66.7% of all failed implants occurred due to poor bone quality, 45.4% due to location (maxilla or mandible), 27.2% in response to occlusal overload, 24.2% based on location within the arch and 15.1% due to infection. Clearly multiple risk factors are associated with the failure of implants. Among the risk factors analysed, poor bone quality associated with short implants were significantly associated with failure. Increasing implant width to 4 mm reduced failure rates in these cases. This may provide a useful alternative to bone augmentation procedures which could elevate cost, result in extended recovery periods and increase morbidity.

A recent study evaluated survival of implants following immediate versus delayed loading and identified risk factors (Susarla et al 2008). Those who had at least one Bicon implant (Bicon, Boston, MA) placed over 13 years were included in the study. The primary variable was immediate loading (on insertion) versus delayed (3–6 months after placement) and other variables included demographic, anatomic, abutment and reconstructive, on 855 study patients. In this study implants loaded immediately were 2.7 times more likely to fail at the end of the first year than those subjected to delayed loading. Other factors associated with failure were current tobacco use, maxillary implants and shorter implants.

It is relevant that when the success rate and marginal bone loss associated with loading at 8 weeks for the maxilla and 6 weeks for the mandible were evaluated, the fixation success rate was 98.1% with mean bone loss of 0.58 mm after 1 year of loading (Boronat et al 2008). This is similar to the values reported in the literature. Early loading as described seems to be safe and predictable and reduces treatment time. Immediate loading may have different implications, based on primary implant stability as mentioned above.

A recent study carried out a retrospective evaluation of marginal bone loss (MBL) around rough-surface dental implants, placed in a private clinic, and constructed a multivariate model based on patient-based prognostic variables (Tandlich et al 2007). MBL was calculated using current annual dental records and radiographs of patients treated previously. A total of 82 patients and 265 implants were evaluated with a follow-up period of up to 30 months. The overall survival rate was 95.8% (2.6% early loss and 1.5% late loss). The single implant was the unit of data analysis and MBL was correlated with time. Higher MBL values were found in smokers and around implants supporting removable prostheses with odds ratios of 1.95 and 2.57 respectively. There was no correlation with time or other anticipated variables. These results confirm the view that smoking correlates with higher MBL and indicate that implants supporting removable prostheses tend to display more bone loss, as substantiated by others (Berglundh et al 2002).

A systematic review of the incidence of biological and technical complications in implant dentistry over 5 years has been reported (Berglundh et al 2002). Out of 1310 retrieved publications only 51 passed the inclusion criteria and allowed meta-analysis. It found a failure rate of 2.5% before functional loading. Implant loss during function was found to occur in 2–3% of implants supporting fixed constructions and >5% of implants supporting over dentures. 1–2% of implant patients reported sensory disturbances for more than 1 year. Implant fracture was rare and occurred in <1% of cases. Information on the loss of bony support and peri-implantitis was lacking in the included studies.

A new implant two stage design (Maestro System®, Biohorizons Implant Systems, Inc) has been the subject of a 5-year, independently monitored, multicentre clinical trial (Kline et al 2002). The implants were designed to limit the sheer forces on the bone at placement and functional loading by using square rather than V-shaped threads. Four types of these implants progressing to a finer pitch and varied in surface roughness, were plasma sprayed or coated with hydroxyapatite. A total of 151 cases with 495 implants were included in the study. Radiographs were taken at stage I and stage 2, the time of prosthetic loading, 6 months after loading and then annually. The radiographs were digitized and computer analysed for bone changes. This system produced a 99.5% success rate and showed a mean bone loss of 0.06 mm at 1 year and a mean bone gain of 0.04 mm 2 years after loading. There were no statistical differences in the results between centres or between implant type, D1–4, bone density at placement, area of the mouth placed or prosthetic type. These results compared favourably with those of other systems and were better than the Albrektsson et al (1986) success criteria of 1 mm of bone loss during the first year of functional loading and 0.2 mm additional loss annually.

A retrospective study was done to assess the influence of systemic factors, local bone and intra-oral factors on the occurrence of early implant failures, prior to connection of abutments (Alsaadi et al 2007). Surgical records of 2004 consecutive patients from the total patient population who had been treated in the period 1982–2003 (with a total of 6946 Brånemark system implants) at the Department of Periodontology of the Catholic University, Leuven were evaluated. For each patient, the medical history was carefully checked. Data collection and analysis mainly focused on endogenous factors such as hypertension, coagulation problems, osteoporosis, hypo/hyperthyroidism chemotherapy, diabetes type I or II, Crohn's disease, some local factors (e.g. bone quality and quantity, implant length, diameter, location, type of edentulism, Periotest value at implant insertion), radiotherapy, smoking habits and breach of sterility during surgery. A total failure rate of 3.6% was recorded. Osteoporosis, Crohn's disease, smoking habits, implant length, diameter, location and proximity to the natural dentition were all significantly associated with early implant failure ($p<0.05$). It was concluded that the indications for the use of oral implants should sometimes be reconsidered when alternative prosthetic treatments are available in the presence of possible interfering local or systemic factors.

REFERENCES

Abrahamsson I, Berglundh T, Linder E, et al: Early bone formation adjacent to rough and turned endosseous implant surfaces. An experimental study in the dog, *Clin Oral Implants Res* 15:381–392, 2004.
Abrahamsson I, Zitzmann NU, Berglundh T, et al: The mucosal attachment to titanium implants with different surface characteristics: an experimental study in dogs, *J Clin Periodontol* 29:448–455, 2002.
Albrektsson T, Zarb G, Worthington P, Eriksson AR: The long-term efficacy of currently used dental implants: A review and proposed criteria of success, *Int J Oral Maxillofac Implants* 1:11–25, 1986.
Alsaadi G, Quirynen M, Komárek A, et al: Impact of local and systemic factors on the incidence of oral implant failures, up to abutment connection, *J Clin Periodontol* 34:610–617, 2007.
Avila G, Galindo P, Rios H, et al: Immediate implant loading: current status from available literature, *Implant Dent* 16:235–245, 2007.
Belser U, Bernard J-P, Buser D: Implant placement in the aesthetic zone. In Lindhe J, editor: *Clinical Periodontology and Implant Dentistry*, ed 4, Ch. 40, 2003, Blackwell, Munksgaard, pp 915–944.
Berglundh T, Abrahamsson I, Lang NP, et al: De novo alveolar bone formation adjacent to endosseous implants, *Clin Oral Implants Res* 14:251–262, 2003.
Berglundh T, Abrahamsson I, Welander M, et al: Morphogenesis of the peri-implant mucosa: an experimental study in dogs, *Clin Oral Implants Res* 18:1–8, 2007.
Berglundh T, Persson L, Klinge B: A systematic review of the incidence of biological and technical complications in implant dentistry reported in prospective longitudinal studies of at least 5 years, *J Clin Periodontol* 29:S197–S212, 2002.
Boronat A, Peñarrocha M, Carrillo C, et al: Marginal bone loss in dental implants subjected to early loading (6 to 8 weeks post-placement) with a retrospective short-term follow-up, *J Oral Maxillofac Surg* 66:246–250, 2008.
Brånemark T-I, Breine U, Adell R, et al: Intraosseous anchorage of dental prostheses. Experimental studies, *Scand J Plast Reconstr Surg* 3:81–100, 1969.
Brånemark T I, Breine U, Adell R, et al: Osseointegrated implants in the treatment of the edentulous jaw. Experience from a 10 year period, *Scand J Plast Reconstr Surg* 11:S1–S132, 1977.
Brånemark PI, Zarb GA, Albrektsson T: *Tissue-integrated prostheses: Osseointegration in Clinical Dentistry*, Chicago, 1985, Quintessence.
das Neves FD, Fones D, Bernardes SR, et al: Short implants – an analysis of longitudinal studies, *Int J Oral Maxillofac Implants* 21:86–93, 2006.
Eley BM, Cox SW, Watson RM: Protease activities in peri-implant sulcus fluid from patients with permucosal osseointegrated dental implants. Correlation with clinical parameters, *Clin Oral Implant Res* 2:62–70, 1991.
Hämmerle CHF, Jung RE, Feloutzis A: A systematic review of the survival of implants in bone augmented by barrier membranes (guided bone regeneration) in partially edentulous patients, *J Clin Periodontol* 29:S226–S231, 2002.
Hollender L, Rockler B: Radiographic evaluation of osseointegrated implants of the jaws, *Dentomaxillofac Radiol* 9:91–95, 1980.
Kivela-Rajamaki M, Maisi P, Srinivas R, et al: Levels and molecular forms of MMP-7 (matrilysin-1) and MMP-8 (collagenase-2) in diseased human peri-implant sulcus fluid, *J Periodontal Res* 38:583–580, 2003.
Kline R, Hoar JE, Beck GH, et al: A prospective multicenter clinical investigation of a bone quality-based dental implant system, *Implant Dent* 11:224–234, 2002.
Klinge B, Gustafsson A, Berglundh T: A systematic review of the effect of anti-infective therapy in the treatment of peri-implantitis, *J Clin Periodontol* 29:S213–S225, 2002.
Mesa F, Muñoz R, Noguerol B, et al: Multivariate study of factors influencing primary dental implant stability, *Clin Oral Implants Res* 19:196–200, 2008.
Mombelli A, Mericske-Sterne R: Microbiological features of stable osseointegrated implants used as abutments for overdentures, *Clin Oral Implant Res* 1:1–7, 1990.
Nickenig H-J, Eitner S: Reliability of implant placement after virtual planning of implant position using cone beam CT data and surgical (guide) templates, *J Cranio-Maxillofac Surg* 35:207–211, 2007.
Nowzari H, Botero JE, DeGiacomo M, et al: Microbiology and cytokine levels around healthy dental implants and teeth, *Clin Implant Dent Relat Res* 10:166–173, 2008.
Preti G, Martinasso G, Peirone B, et al: Cytokines and growth factors involved in the osseointegration of oral titanium implants positioned using piezoelectric bone surgery versus a drill technique: A pilot study in minipigs, *J Periodontol* 78:716–722, 2007.
Renvert S, Roos-Jansaker AM, Lindahl C, et al: Infection at titanium implants with or without a clinical diagnosis of inflammation, *Clin Oral Implants Res* 18:509–516, 2007.
Roos-Jansaker AM: Long time follow up of implant therapy and treatment of peri-implantitis, *Swed Dent J Suppl* 188:7–66, 2007.
Roos-Jansaker AM, Renvert S, Egelberg J: Treatment of peri-implant infections: a literature review, *J Clin Periodontol* 30:467–485, 2003.
Salvi GE, Persson GR, Heitz-Mayfield LJ, et al: Adjunctive local antibiotic therapy in the treatment of peri-implantitis II: clinical and radiographic outcomes, *Clin Oral Implants Res* 18:281–285, 2007.
Sánchez-Pérez A, Moya-Villaescusa MJ, Caffesse RG: Tobacco as a risk factor for survival of dental implants, *J Periodontol* 78:351–359, 2007.
Schroeder A, Pohler O, Sutter F: Gewebsreaktion auf ein Titan-Hohlzylinderimplantat mit Titan-Spritzschichtoberfläche, *Schweiz Monatsschr Zahnheilkd* 86:713–727, 1976.
Strietzel FP, Reichart PA, Kale A, et al: Smoking interferes with the prognosis of dental implant treatment: a systematic review and meta-analysis, *J Clin Periodontol* 34:523–544, 2007.
Susarla SM, Chuang SK, Dodson TB: Delayed versus immediate loading of implants: survival analysis and risk factors for dental implant failure, *J Oral and Maxillofac Surg* 66:251–255, 2008.
Takasaki AA, Aoki A, Mizutani K, et al: Er:YAG laser therapy for peri-implant infection: a histological study, *Lasers Med Sci* 22:143–157, 2007.
Tandlich M, Ekstein J, Reisman P, et al: Removable prostheses may enhance marginal bone loss around dental implants: a long-term retrospective analysis. *J Periodontol* 78:2253–2259, 2007.
Vercellotti T: The bone piezoelectric surgery, *Dentista Moderno* 5:21–55, 2003.

The relationship between periodontal and restorative treatment

30

Dental restorations should be designed both to minimize plaque accumulation at the gingival margin and to avoid physical injury to the periodontal tissues. The main areas where restorative dentistry and periodontics interrelate are as follows:

- The relationship between dental restorations and gingival margins
- The occlusal relations of dental restorations
- The support from the periodontium for partial dentures or fixed bridgework
- The consequences of gingival recession
- Crown lengthening for cast restorations
- Periodontal/pulpal infections
- Dental implants.

THE RELATIONSHIP BETWEEN DENTAL RESTORATIONS AND GINGIVAL MARGINS

Dental caries usually attack smooth enamel surface, interproximally and buccal or lingual surfaces cervically, immediately coronally to the gingival margin. The enamel carious lesion tapers towards the amelodentinal junction and then spreads laterally along the junction. In this way, it involves a greater area of dentine and may result in it progressing subgingivally towards the alveolar crest (**Fig. 30.1**). Breakdown of the unsupported enamel may then result in damage to the attached junctional epithelium.

When the tooth is restored the margin of the restoration often has to extend slightly subgingivally in order to eliminate the caries and unsupported enamel (**Fig. 30.1**). Whatever restorative material is used, amalgam, composite, glass ionomer, gold or porcelain, the junctional epithelium fails to adhere to its surface and a pocket results. A further important factor in this process is the restorative margin itself, since even apparently perfect margins accumulate plaque at this site. The lack of protective seal from the junctional epithelium results in the pocket becoming colonized by the bacteria found in subgingival plaque. Thus all subgingival restorations, even those judged clinically sound, will cause gingivitis of some degree extending at least to the margin of the restoration (**Fig. 30.2**). This situation could eventually promote the development of chronic periodontitis. However, if a restoration such as an anterior crown is very carefully prepared so that the resulting margins can be cleaned by the patient then the surrounding gingival margin will remain healthy (**Fig. 30.3**).

Obviously if the restorative margin is poor then much more damage may result. Deficient or overhanging margins become completely covered with plaque over their whole complex surface and are impossible to clean (**Fig. 30.4**). Therefore, they are a potent source of gingival irritation and result in severe gingivitis which frequently progresses to periodontitis (see Ch. 4).

CLINICAL CONSIDERATIONS

In view of these problems a cavity margin should not extend subgingivally except when absolutely necessary for caries removal (Reeves 1991). Major precautions should also be taken to avoid deficient or overhanging cervical margins. Furthermore, all restorations with deficient or overhanging cervical margins should be removed and replaced by satisfactory ones.

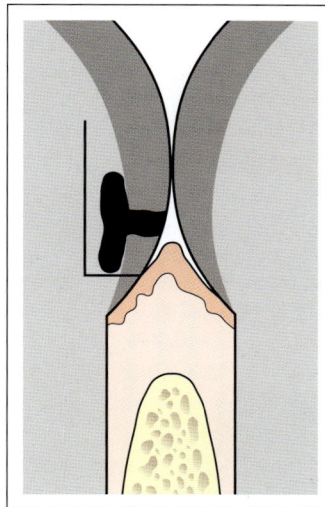

Fig. 30.1 Diagram showing the restoration of interproximal caries. Caries as it progresses spreads below the contact area by extending into dentine and spreading along the amelodentinal junction. The resultant restoration, in order to remove all caries, will invariably, in this situation, extend into the gingival crevice and thus result in a gingival pocket.

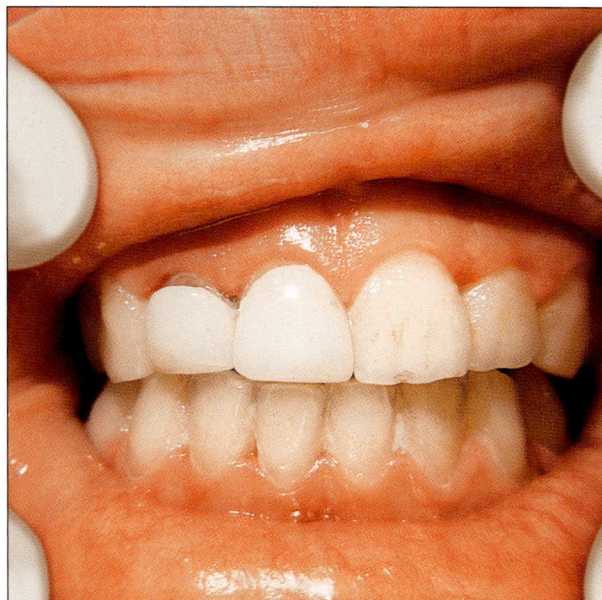

Fig. 30.2 Porcelain jacket crowns on the upper right central and lateral incisors with poorly fitting and subgingival margins which are impossible to clean effectively. Severe localized gingivitis is present associated with these restorations.

AMALGAM RESTORATIONS

Careful cavity preparation should avoid any unnecessary cervical extension. Class II preparations should be fitted with a tightly fitting and appropriately adapted matrix band and this should be firmly wedged cervically. If the cervical floor of the restoration is at or below the cement-enamel junction the proximal surface will be concave. In this situation a conventionally shaped wedge will fail to adapt the matrix to the cervical floor (**Fig. 30.5**). A carefully contoured wedge should be used to adapt the

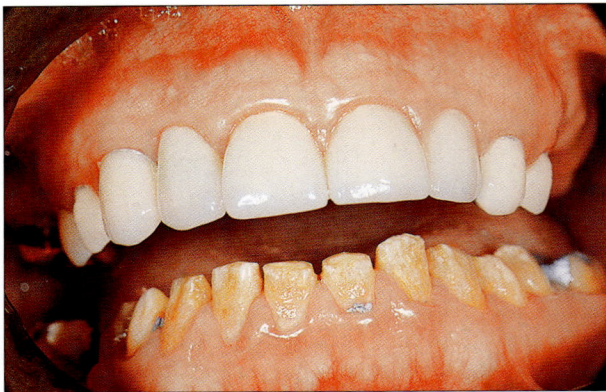

Fig. 30.3 Carefully prepared metal bonded porcelain crowns on upper left and right central and lateral incisors and upper right canine with buccal margins coincident with the gingival margin and the non-visible interproximal and palatal margins placed supragingivally. The gingivae are totally healthy since the patient had good oral hygiene and was able to keep the margins of the crowns free from plaque.

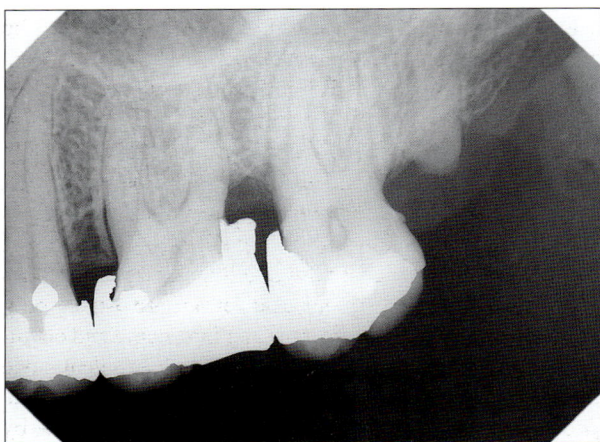

Fig. 30.4 A paralleling technique intra-oral radiograph showing grossly overhanging amalgam restorations associated with severe gingivitis and moderate periodontitis. There is horizontal bone loss between the upper right first and second molars. A retained root of the third molar can also be seen.

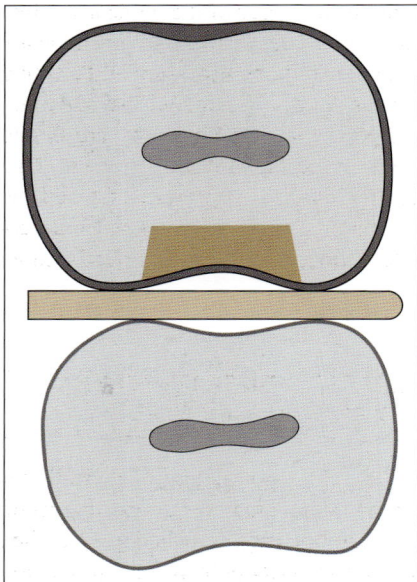

Fig. 30.5 Diagram showing a section through a class II cavity at the level of the cervical floor. It shows how a conventional wedge may fail to adapt the matrix to a proximal furrow on the tooth.

matrix (Eli et al 1991). The cervical margin should be carefully checked with a fine explorer immediately the matrix is removed so that any small excesses can be trimmed with a fine instrument.

COMPOSITE AND GLASS IONOMER RESTORATIONS

A wide range of composite filling and veneering materials are now available for anterior and posterior teeth. In posterior teeth they should only be used for small restorations. Glass ionomers are used to restore buccal and lingual cervical cavities and as a secondary base material for composite restorations. Both types of restoration should ideally be placed using a rubber dam since they are very moisture sensitive.

Careful cavity preparation should avoid any unnecessary cervical extension. Matrices should be very carefully adapted, placed and wedged to avoid cervical excess. Any thin excess should be carefully fractured away after the material has fully set to leave a good tooth-restoration junction. When necessary, composites can be carefully contoured and trimmed with fine diamond stones and abrasive discs specially made for this purpose. The cervical margin should be carefully assessed with a probe and dental floss before accepting the restoration as satisfactory. Excesses with this material will not adhere to the tooth and plaque will rapidly form between its inner surface and the tooth. This actively promotes the development of secondary caries, gingivitis and periodontitis.

Very great care indeed should be taken with the use of composite as a veneer material on anterior teeth for aesthetic purposes. Its use must be fully justified since the potential for gingival damage is great. If it is considered appropriate to use this technique then sufficient tooth substance must be removed labially to accommodate the veneer without over contouring. The use of a rubber dam is mandatory. The cervical margin should be placed level with the gingival margin and the material must be very carefully contoured to avoid it acting as a plaque trap. It must be possible to clean the margin effectively with a toothbrush.

GOLD AND PORCELAIN RESTORATIONS

Careful cavity preparation should avoid any unnecessary cervical extension. The margins must be very precise and a very accurate full arch master impression should be taken along with a full arch impression of the opposing arch and appropriate bite registration. Supragingival placement of margins makes it much easier to take an accurate impression. The restoration must precisely fit the margins without any deficiency or excess. This depends both on the skills of the dentist and the dental technician.

PERIODONTAL CARE OF TEETH WITH SUBGINGIVAL RESTORATIONS

There will be a tendency for buccal or lingual subgingival restorations to stimulate gingival recession which may expose their cervical margin. Perhaps in this instance the gingiva knows what is good for it! The effects on the gingiva can be reduced interproximally by the regular use of floss, taking it down to just below the margin of the restoration. Obviously, any excess material at the margin will prevent this procedure. Buccally and lingually, the use of Bass technique brushing will be effective only providing the bristles of the brush can reach the cervical margin of the restoration. Regular subgingival scaling should also be carried out. These areas should be regularly checked by periodontal probing and when appropriate, radiographs to watch for any loss of attachment.

Ideally, surgical pocket elimination should be carried out to expose the margin and produce a physiological sulcus. However, this is only possible if a sufficiently deep periodontal pocket is present with the alveolar bone margin 4 mm apical to the restorative margin. If this is

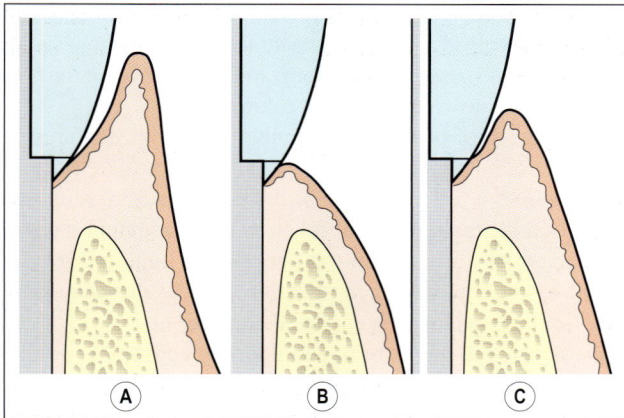

Fig. 30.6 Diagram showing an apically repositioned flap used to expose the margin of a subgingival restoration with a restoration-to-bone distance less than 4 mm: (A) before surgery; (B) healing after surgery; (C) months later when gingival regeneration is complete. The gingival margin has migrated coronally to cover the restoration margin again.

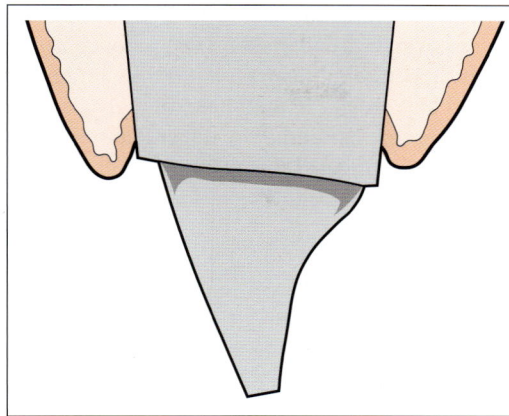

Fig. 30.7 Diagram showing a section through an anterior crown preparation for a bonded porcelain–metal crown. The palatal finishing line is located supragingivally. The buccal finishing line is located just (<1 mm) within the gingival crevice for aesthetic reasons. This margin must be carefully cleaned by the Bass technique of toothbrushing. The interdental finishing line joins these two points.

attempted for situations with a lesser distance the procedure is only temporarily successful in exposing the margin (Van der Velden 1982). This is because during repair, following the surgery, the gingiva will gradually reform its physiological form and relationships and will extend coronally so that its margin is 4 mm above the bone margin (**Fig. 30.6**). If a deeper pocket is present then pocket elimination surgery using as appropriate gingivectomy or an apically repositioned flap will be successful in exposing the margin.

However, Santos et al (2007) carried out a 6-month study which evaluated the effects of resin-modified glass-ionomer cement and microfilled composite subgingival restorations on periodontal tissues and subgingival biofilm. It showed that well-finished resin-modified glass-ionomer cement or microfilled composite subgingival restorations did not negatively affect periodontal health.

CROWN MARGINS

There is a strong case for supragingival margins on crowns (**Figs 30.2, 30.3**), provided the crown length is sufficient for retention. If not, a crown lengthening procedure should be considered (see below). Supragingival margins greatly simplify impression taking, provision of temporary crowns, the inspection of the final restoration and its cementation. Most importantly, the crown margins are accessible for cleaning.

The only possible exception to this rule is the buccal aspects of visible anterior teeth for aesthetic purposes. In this situation, the labial margin only of the crown is extended to a maximum of 0.5 mm (i.e. just) into the gingival crevice (**Fig. 30.7**). Obviously, there must be complete gingival health before the provision of any crown is considered. Provided the labial surface consists of highly glazed porcelain, has a precise fit and is reachable by Bass technique toothbrushing then little harm should result. Good plaque control is essential to maintain this situation and it should be remembered that gingivitis in this area is very unsightly.

THE OCCLUSAL RELATIONS OF DENTAL RESTORATIONS

All dental restorations should be in a balanced occlusion in the functional intercuspal, protrusive, retruded and lateral positions. If this is not achieved then occlusal trauma lesions may result (Ch. 27). In addition, the contact areas should be correctly restored to avoid food impaction and drifting of adjacent teeth.

With plastic restorations such as amalgam these relationships must be checked and corrected by carving before the material reaches its final set. Composites in posterior teeth are more difficult to deal with and this is one of their disadvantages. The intercuspal occlusion can be roughly produced by placing a cling-film membrane over the occlusal surface so that the patient can bite on this. Since this impedes light curing, the patient can only close on this material and grind immediately after placement of the composite and then open again to allow curing. This is also difficult with a rubber dam in position, which is essential to avoid moisture contamination. Therefore, composites involving the occlusal surface are usually only roughly shaped before curing and then need grinding into shape and occlusion using occlusal registering paper or wax. This is far from ideal since it destroys the original surface of the composite and makes it impossible to achieve good occlusal contouring. These problems can be overcome by using composite inlays, which are fabricated on models outside the mouth. Their initial fit and occlusion depend on the accuracy of the impressions and bites but their marginal seal is no better than that of conventional composites because they are luted in with composite acid etched to the enamel surface. Their life is therefore similar to conventional composites.

With caste gold or fused porcelain or bonded metal–porcelain restorations the correct occlusion depends on the accuracy of the models and bite registration and the skill of the dental technician. If all these functions are carried out correctly then no adjustments should be necessary at the fitting stage and the restoration(s) should be in balance in the intercuspal and functional lateral, protrusive and retruded positions (Ch. 27). Great care should also be taken to restore the correct contact area(s) with adjacent teeth. This requires accurate impressions of the arch with the restoration(s) and the opposing arch and accurate bite registration using a face bow when necessary and functional wax bites in order to place the models correctly on an articulator.

THE SUPPORT FROM THE PERIODONTIUM FOR PARTIAL DENTURES OR FIXED BRIDGEWORK

When teeth are lost and replaced by dentures or bridges, the occlusal forces applied to the prosthesis are transmitted to the remaining supporting teeth. Obviously, the greater number of teeth lost, the larger are the forces applied to the remaining teeth. In addition, chronic periodontitis can significantly reduce the support of teeth which are therefore less able to resist occlusal forces placed upon them and more particularly additional forces placed upon them by prostheses.

It is essential that all periodontal disease is successfully treated before any prosthetic work, fixed or removable, is undertaken. If periodontal health cannot be achieved and advanced periodontitis persists then the prognosis for the remaining dentition and any prosthesis will be extremely poor. In some situations with advanced chronic periodontitis, transitional dentures may have to be provided as part of a planned transition to a full denture. However, these dentures are never stable and always to some extent reduce the life of the remaining dentition.

The aim of any prosthesis is to spread the occlusal load of missing teeth to as many remaining teeth as possible and to avoid overloading any supporting teeth. In periodontally controlled mouths, the choice usually lies between a tooth supported, skeleton, chrome cobalt partial denture and a fixed bridge. The tendency is to restrict the use of bridgework to short edentulous spans, where the abutment teeth have good periodontal support and health and to use dentures for patients with greater numbers of missing teeth and consequently fewer abutment teeth. The design of a chrome cobalt denture aims to distribute the occlusal load to as many supporting teeth as possible using occlusal rests. It also aims to minimize the stress on abutment teeth by reciprocating the forces placed upon them by retention clasps. In addition, it aims by its skeleton design, where possible, to leave the gingival margins of supporting teeth uncovered and thus to reduce its plaque retentiveness and to avoid gingival trauma. However, chrome cobalt dentures can still overstress abutment teeth if the edentulous span is long and particularly where there is a free end saddle. In these situations, tilting and rocking of abutment teeth can occur and this can reduce their functional life. In addition, the movements of a free end saddle may cause gingival and mucosal trauma. These tendencies can be minimized with a wide distribution of occlusal loads and careful reciprocation of clasps.

These forces are much more damaging with poorly designed acrylic partial dentures. Teeth with reduced periodontal support may be rocked by ill-fitting clasps and denture components and considerable gingival trauma may be caused by tissue coverage and denture movement. These dentures are also plaque retentive and will cause gingival irritation if not kept scrupulously clean.

A period of periodontal adaptation will follow the placement of a new partial denture and the result will greatly depend on its design.

The problems described above may be overcome by the provision of bridgework. This is, however, extremely expensive and very demanding on clinical and technical expertise.

A 15-year longitudinal study of 108 bridges made in 102 patients made by senior students in a Norwegian dental school was carried out by Valderhaug et al (1993). They found that the amount of plaque was similar on crowned and control teeth but marked gingivitis was seen more frequently in crowned teeth with subgingival margins. A slight increase in mean pocket depth was seen with crowned teeth but not in control teeth although no differences could be detected in bone levels. There was also a steady increase in secondary caries around the abutment teeth from 3.3% at the 5th year to 12% at the 15th year. These findings make it clear that abutment crowns should have supragingival margins wherever possible; oral hygiene and diet should be continually monitored as should periodontal and caries status.

The amount of support provided by abutment teeth is crucial in the success of a bridge. This is usually based on Ante's law which proposes that in a fixed bridge the attached root surface area of the abutment teeth should be equal to or greater than the equivalent root surface area of the teeth to be replaced. The blanket application of this 'law' places great restraint on the use of bridges in subjects with reduced periodontal support. However, provided that periodontally healthy conditions are first produced and then maintained, it has been shown that satisfactory function can be achieved with bridges of a cross-arch design supported by teeth with markedly reduced periodontal support (Nyman & Lindhe 1979; Nyman & Ericsson 1982). In many of these cases, successful bridges were produced with the support of as little as 16% of the presumed root area of the teeth replaced. However, these bridges involved the whole arch and took maximum advantage of cross arch support.

Such bridges can also take advantage of the increased clinical crown length of treated periodontally involved teeth with attachment loss. This allows the preparation of abutments with good retention form and also allows for the provision of supragingival margins when aesthetics allows.

These types of bridges are probably preferable to partial dentures in cases with reduced periodontal attachment especially where there is tooth mobility. This is because the full arch fixed bridge has greater rigidity and provides a more favourable distribution of function to the remaining teeth. Moreover, the mechanoreceptors within the periodontal ligament restrict the force generated by the muscles of mastication by a feedback mechanism, and thereby limit the occlusal forces on the bridge.

However, as already stated, there are three important constraints on this type of work. First, it is extremely expensive which puts it out of reach of most patients in this category. Second, and most importantly, it will only be successful if existing periodontal disease is first effectively treated and then maintained both by immaculate oral hygiene and regular 3-monthly subgingival scaling. Third, this work is extremely demanding on the clinical expertise of the dentist and the technical expertise of the dental technician. This is because all of the abutment crowns must fit perfectly with superb leak-free margins which are easy to clean and the whole occlusion must be in balance in the functional intercuspal, retrusive, lateral and protrusive positions.

PONTIC DESIGN

Pontics should be designed so that the interproximal cleaning of the abutment teeth can be effectively carried out. This means that it must be possible to thread dental floss through the interproximal space between the abutments and the pontic(s). It should also be possible to pass floss under the inner surface of the pontic to clean the surface adjacent to the bridge mucosa. If such a design is provided, then floss can be threaded through using a floss threader or by using superfloss with its stiffened end. It can then reach the proximal surfaces of both abutments and the undersurface of the pontic.

The ideal design for a posterior pontic is the so-called bullet-shaped pontic (Fig. 30.8A). This has a point contact with the ridge mucosa and is shaped to produce wide interproximal spaces to allow floss access.

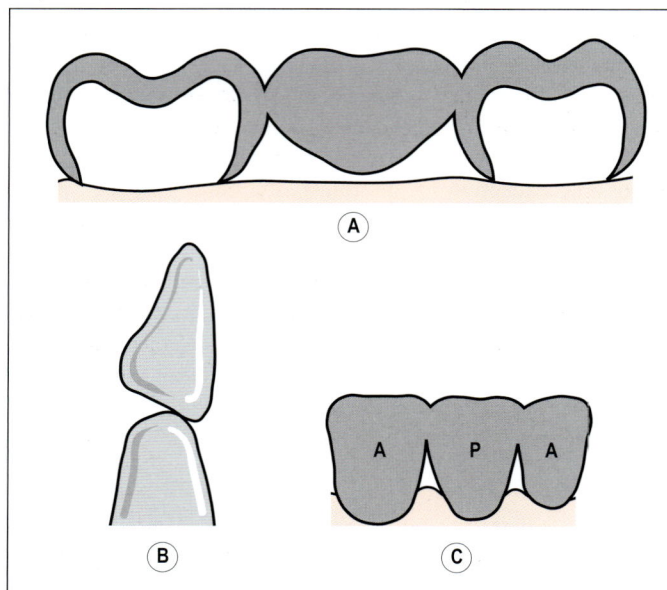

Fig. 30.8 Diagram showing bridge design to allow cleaning. (A) A 'bullet-shaped' posterior pontic. This has wide interproximal spaces to allow the easy passage of floss and a point contact with the ridge. (B) An anterior single ridge lap pontic (buccolingual view). It laps the labial ridge but remains clear palatally. (C) Labial view of a diagram of anterior supporting crowns and pontic. The pontic (P) has wide interproximal spaces to allow the easy passage of floss to clean the proximal surfaces of the abutments (A) and the undersurface of the pontic.

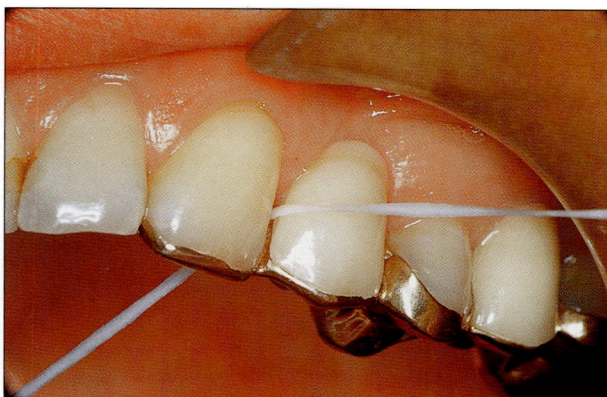

Fig. 30.9 Floss being used to clean between an abutment and a pontic of a fixed bridge. It was introduced using a floss threader but superfloss could also have been used.

Its occlusal surface is also somewhat narrowed in comparison to a corresponding natural tooth in order to reduce the occlusal loads placed upon it. This design is not possible for anterior pontics because of aesthetic considerations. These usually have a single ridge-lap design, slightly lapping over the labial aspect of the ridge (**Fig. 30.8B**). However, the undersurface should slope upwards from the labial edge so that it passes clear of the ridge surface palatally. The undersurface should be smooth and slightly convex for easy cleaning. The anterior-posterior dimensions of the labial aspect should resemble the tooth it is replacing but should also have wide enough interproximal spaces to allow good floss access (**Fig. 30.8C**). It is essential that all the interproximal surfaces of crowns and bridges can be reached by floss (**Fig. 30.9**).

THE CONSEQUENCES OF GINGIVAL RECESSION

Gingival recession results either from developmental bony dehiscences, periodontal disease, orthodontic movement or periodontal surgery (see Chs 8, 19 and 21). Trauma from toothbrushing can result in abrasion and acids from foods and drinks cause erosion. These processes may quickly remove the surface cementum and progressively the root dentine to produce abrasion/erosion cavities. These can occur on buccal and lingual surfaces but are much more common buccally.

These cavities are often periodically sensitive to hot and cold stimuli and become retentive of food debris. These cavities or unaffected exposed root surfaces may also become carious if conditions for this are present and this will necessitate restorative treatment. Abrasion cavities also need restoring if progressive loss of dentine is taking place or if there is persistent sensitivity.

These cavities are usually restored with glass ionomer materials using the newer dentine bonding agents. These materials are moisture sensitive and the work is best carried out using a rubber dam. These restorations need to be very carefully placed if a good marginal seal and smooth edge-free margins are to be achieved. Failure to do this will lead to restoration failure and gingival irritation. Obviously, further trauma and erosion need to be avoided by correct oral hygiene training and dietary advice.

CROWN LENGTHENING FOR CAST RESTORATIONS

Since the subgingival placement of restorative margins is undesirable, crown lengthening will have to be considered if the clinical crown is too short to achieve a retentive preparation (Allen 1993). This is usually a problem with full crown preparations on molar teeth but can also affect other teeth. Crown lengthening would usually need to be carried out with an apically repositioned flap as it is extremely important to preserve the full amount of keratinized attached gingiva. The only possible exception to this would be where the problem is caused by gingival hyperplasia when a gingivectomy could be considered. Soft tissue surgery alone will not achieve the objective unless there is sufficient periodontal pocketing and/or gingival hyperplasia to expose the desired amount of clinical crown. Furthermore, tooth exposure will only be permanent if the bone–gingival margin distance is kept to approximately 4 mm. Therefore, in all other cases marginal bone will also have to be reduced, usually by 1–2 mm, to achieve the desired length of clinical crown.

Where these procedures are carried out, crown preparation should be delayed for at least 20 weeks until the position of the gingival margin is stable (Wise 1985). This is particularly important with anterior crowns when aesthetics are important.

PERIODONTAL/PULPAL INFECTIONS

There may be communication between the pulp and periodontal ligament (**Fig. 30.10**) via:

- Dentinal tubules
- Lateral and accessory root canals
- The apical foramen
- Cracks and fracture lines
- Iatrogenic perforations.

These may sometimes give rise to:

- Pulpal disease with secondary periodontal involvement
- Periodontal disease with secondary pulpal involvement
- Combined lesions where coincidental periodontal and pulpal origin lesions have merged.

PULPAL DISEASE WITH SECONDARY PERIODONTAL INVOLVEMENT

Infection from the pulp may pass into the periodontal ligament space through the apical foramen or through lateral canals (Hiatt 1977). Lateral canals are most common in the apical third of the root but may also occur less commonly in the middle and coronal thirds. In addition, lateral canals are relatively common in the furcation areas of multirooted teeth (**Figs 30.10, 30.11**).

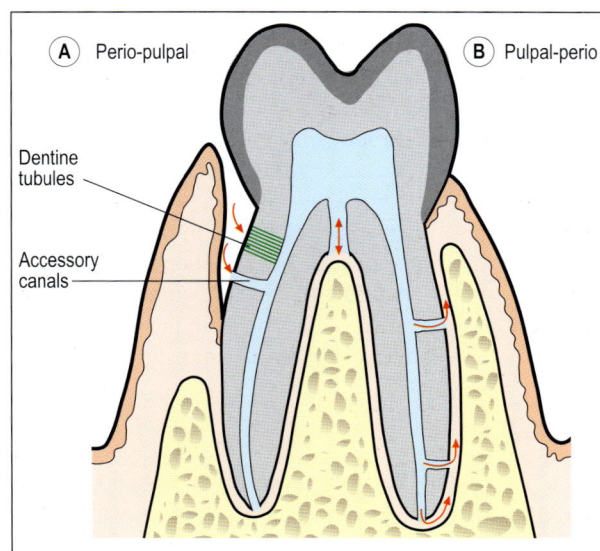

Fig. 30.10 Pathways between the pulp and the periodontium: (A) Perio-pulpal via dentinal tubules and accessory canals. (B) Pulpal-perio via accessory canals and the apical foramen.

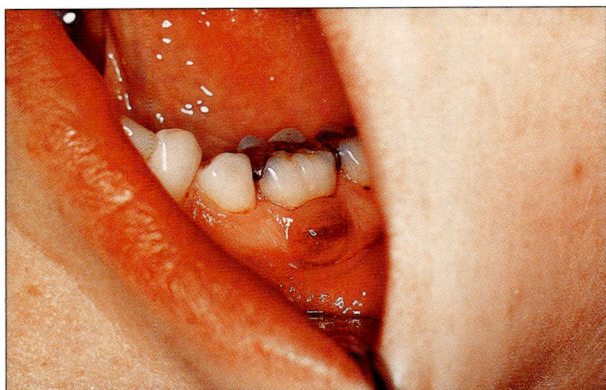

Fig. 30.11 An abscess in the furcation area of the lower first molar with pus discharging from the gingival margin in a 19-year-old woman. The condition was associated with a primary pulpal infection and drained into the periodontium via accessory furcation canals. The condition resolved following successful endodontic treatment started immediately after the diagnosis.

Infection passing from the pulp into the apical periodontium via the apical foramen or lateral canals in the apical third usually produces an apical granuloma or abscess. Infection usually tracks through the bone to form a subperiosteal abscess which drains into the vestibule. A very small percentage of apical abscesses, less than 1%, drain via the periodontal ligament to discharge from the gingival margin. This route is, however, more likely if infection passes via a lateral canal in the coronal or middle third of the root. This is also very likely if the infection passes via a lateral canal in the furcation area of a molar tooth (**Figs 30.10, 30.11**) and in this situation it may simulate periodontal furcation infection (**Fig. 30.11**). Fortunately, this is most likely to occur in a young patient with no signs of periodontal disease elsewhere in the mouth and is therefore less likely to deceive.

Infection may also pass from the pulp to the periodontal ligament space via fracture line due to trauma or iatrogenic perforations which may occur during endodontic treatment or post-preparation (Tidmarsh 1979). This also may lead to discharge of pus from the gingival margin and could lead to misdiagnosis of a lesion of periodontal origin.

PERIODONTAL DISEASE WITH SECONDARY PULPAL INVOLVEMENT

Gingival recession may expose dentinal tubules to irritation from the oral involvement and lead to hypersensitivity. It can also lead to abrasion and erosion. However, secondary and peritubular dentine formation in these instances usually minimizes pulpal irritation.

Within periodontal pockets the root surface is exposed to bacteria and their products. Scaling and root planing will remove diseased cementum and expose the dentine tubules, which may transmit irritants (**Fig. 30.10**). However, secondary dentine formation usually protects the pulp from irreversible damage.

Periodontal pockets may also involve lateral canals in the coronal and middle thirds of the root and the furcation area and infection could pass via these communications into the pulp (**Fig. 30.10**). Finally, teeth with advanced chronic periodontitis could pass secondary infection from the pocket to the pulp via lateral canals in the apical third or the apical foramen.

COMBINED LESIONS

In these cases there is no clear indication from the history or examination of a primary causal link with chronic periodontitis or pulpal disease. A true combined lesion is the result of the fusion of two separate lesions, one marginal periodontal and the other pulpal. The pulpal lesion spreads to the periodontium via apical foramen or lateral canals and both lesions enlarge and merge together.

Diagnosis

The correct diagnosis of these conditions involves a careful history of the onset and development of the symptoms and signs followed by a careful clinical examination. This should be backed up by the appropriate radiographs and vitality tests. It is much more difficult to get a clear history from a chronic periodontal-pulpal lesion than immediately after an acute episode.

Clinical examination

One should be alerted to the possibility of a periodontal-pulpal lesion by discoloured clinical crowns, pus discharge from the gingival margin buccally or palatally or from the furcation area between the molar roots and by deep localized pocketing uncharacteristic of the mouth as a whole.

When a primary pulpal lesion spreads to the periodontal ligament and thence to the previously healthy marginal periodontium, it usually spreads along a narrow pathway. When this area is carefully probed it reveals a localized narrow pocket in an otherwise healthy mouth. The pocket contains pus but no plaque or calculus. The age of the patient may also give a clue to its origin since pulpal disease is more common in the young than periodontitis. In particular, the discharge of pus from the furcation area of a single molar in a young patient with an otherwise healthy mouth is very suggestive of a primary pulpal lesion (**Fig. 30.11**).

Vitality testing

The response of the pulp to vitality testing depends on an intact nerve supply, whereas pulpal vitality may be maintained with an intact blood supply alone. Testing may be carried out electrically, thermally or by using a bur in a cavity within a non-anaesthetized tooth. None of these tests are infallible and both false positives and negatives may occur. They are particularly likely in heavily filled, multirooted molar teeth.

Radiography

Careful long-cone paralleling radiographs should be taken of the suspected tooth. Where appropriate, radiographs of the rest of the mouth may also be needed. The radiographs of the suspected tooth should show an undistorted view of both the apical and marginal periodontium. The radiographs should be checked for widening of the apical periodontal space, apical or lateral areas of radiolucency, furcation radiolucency and the presence, extent and pattern of marginal bone loss. It should be remembered that the furcation radiolucency can be either pulpal or periodontal in origin.

Treatment

Pulpal disease with secondary periodontal involvement

The pulpal disease will have progressed to partial or total necrosis and endodontic treatment should be commenced immediately. If drainage of pus from the gingival margin is not rapidly controlled by mechanical cleaning of the pulp chamber and root canals then a course of an appropriate antibiotic should be given. This is best based on a sample of pus which is sent to a microbiology laboratory for antibiotic sensitivity testing. However, as speed is the essence in these cases, treatment can usually be started with amoxicillin provided that the patient is not hypersensitive to penicillin. If the infection is rapidly controlled by these measures then the involved marginal periodontium may regenerate and successful endodontic treatment will lead to a return to full periodontal health. However, if the infection is allowed to become chronic the healing is much less predictable. This is because the chronic infection can cause pathological changes to occur on

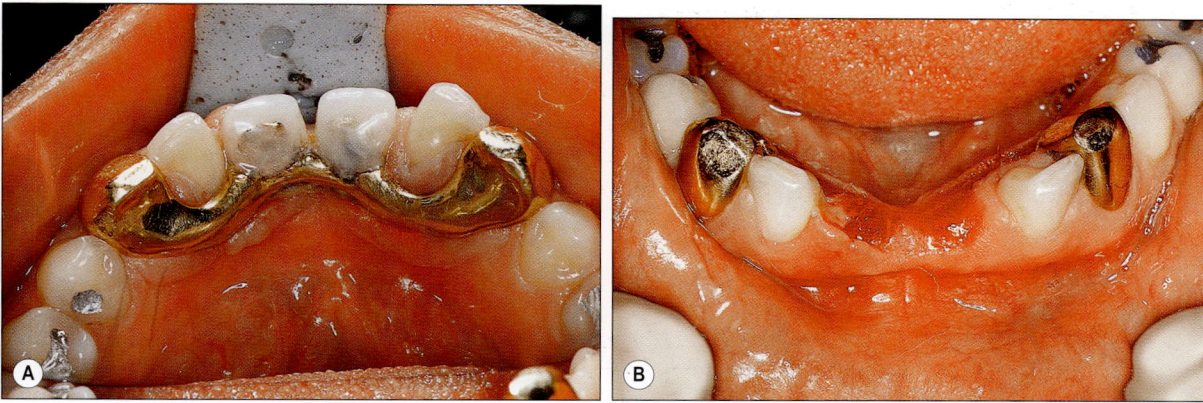

Fig. 30.12 An inappropriately designed gold and acrylic partial denture which is causing both gingival and mucosal damage and inflammation by both direct trauma and plaque retention. (A) Denture in the mouth. (B) Denture removed showing damage to the ridge mucosa and gingivae.

the root surface with the cementum becoming infected and necrotic. This leads to a downgrowth of junctional epithelium along the changed root surface which leads to the establishment of a deep chronic periodontal pocket. For this reason, rapid diagnosis and treatment of the primary pulpal disease in these cases are essential for a successful outcome. Chronic lesions will need both endodontic and periodontal treatment including periodontal surgery. The outcome of the periodontal treatment of such lesions is doubtful.

Periodontal disease with secondary pulpal involvement

An assessment of the prognosis of the tooth in terms of its remaining alveolar bone support should be made before further treatment is planned and instituted.

Lesions of periodontal origin are invariably chronic. An assessment should first be made of the state of the pulp and it should be ascertained whether the pulpal disease is reversible or irreversible, i.e. whether the pulp is hyperaemic or necrotic. If the pulp is necrotic then endodontic treatment should be carried out first. If, on the other hand, the pulp appears to be still vital but hypersensitive then periodontal treatment should be carried out first to see whether the reduction in the source of irritation will lead to pulpal recovery.

The periodontal lesion should be first treated by careful, meticulous subgingival scaling and root planing. The condition of the rest of the mouth should be taken into account in the overall treatment plan. Meticulous oral hygiene must be established. The periodontal lesion will invariably require periodontal surgery and the precise technique employed will depend upon the depth of the pocket and pattern of bone resorption (Chs 19 and 20).

The outcome can be difficult to determine in cases associated with advanced periodontitis and all cases should receive regular maintenance treatment.

Combined lesions

If the prognosis is reasonable both periodontal and endodontic treatment is carried out as outlined above. The endodontic treatment should be carried out first. The periodontal treatment invariably includes periodontal surgery in these cases. The outcome of treatment is uncertain in cases associated with advanced periodontitis.

PARTIAL DENTURES

As well as a possible cause of occlusal trauma (see above), partial dentures can also cause gingival damage either by direct trauma, if they both cover the gingival margins and move inappropriately, or by encouraging plaque

retention (**Fig. 30.12**). This can be avoided, providing there is sufficient tooth support available, by carefully designed cobalt-chrome skeleton dentures. These can be kept away from gingival margins and the occlusal loads can be distributed by the correct placement of occlusal rests. They can also be prevented from moving by the correct placement of clasps. Finally, it is essential that patients keep dentures free of bacterial plaque by careful cleaning.

DENTAL IMPLANTS

Osseointegrated dental implants and their clinical implications have been discussed in Chapter 29. They require very careful design and great clinical and technical expertise. They also require careful maintenance to prevent peri-implant disease.

REFERENCES

Allen EP: Surgical crown lengthening for function and aesthetics, *Dent Clin North Am* 37:163–180, 1993.

Eli I, Weiss E, Kozlovsky A, et al: Wedges in restorative dentistry: principles and applications, *J Oral Rehabil* 18:257–264, 1991.

Hiatt WH: Pulpal periodontal disease, *J Periodontol* 48:598–609, 1977.

Nyman S, Ericsson I: The capacity of reduced periodontal tissues to support fixed bridgework, *J Clin Periodontol* 9:409–414, 1982.

Nyman S, Lindhe J: A longitudinal study of combined periodontal and prosthetic treatment for patients with advanced periodontitis, *J Periodontol* 50:163–169, 1979.

Reeves WG: Restorative margin placement and periodontal health, *J Prosthet Dent* 66:733–736, 1991.

Santos VR, Lucchesi JA, Cortelli SC, et al: Effects of glass ionomer and microfilled composite subgingival restorations on periodontal tissue and subgingival biofilm: A 6-month evaluation, *J Periodontol* 78:1522–1528, 2007.

Tidmarsh BG: Accidental perforation of the roots of teeth, *J Oral Rehabil* 6:235–240, 1979.

Valderhaug J, Ellingsen JE, Jokstad A: Oral hygiene, periodontal condition and carious lesions in patients treated with dental bridges. A 15-year clinical and radiographic follow-up study, *J Clin Periodontol* 20:482–489, 1993.

Van der Velden U: Regeneration of the interdental soft tissue following denudation procedures, *J Clin Periodontol* 9:455–459, 1982.

Wise WD: Stability of the gingival crest after surgery and before anterior crown placement, *J Prosthet Dent* 53:20–23, 1985.

FURTHER READING

Nevins M: Periodontal considerations in prosthodontic treatment. In Yukna RA, Newman MG, Williams RC, editors: *Current Opinion in Periodontology*, Philadelphia, 1993, Current Science, pp 151–156.

Wilson RD: Restorative dentistry. In Wilson T, Kornman K, Newman M, editors: *Advances in Periodontics*, Chicago, 1992, Quintessence, pp 226–244.

Index